GNRS

Geriatric Nursing Review Syllabus

A Core Curriculum in Advanced Practice
Geriatric Nursing

2nd edition

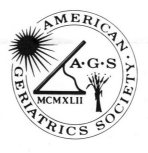

A Collaboration with
The John A. Hartford Foundation Institute for Geriatric Nursing
• New York University • Steinhardt School of Education • Division of Nursing

The editors were Carolyn Auerhahn, EdD, APRN, Elizabeth Capezuti, PhD, RN, APRN, Ellen Flaherty, PhD, APRN, and Barbara Resnick, PhD, CRNP.

Many thanks to Fry Communications for assistance in organizing the *GNRS* material onto an editorial content management website and for all production work, including typesetting, graphic design, and printing. With more than 60 years in the information industry, Fry offers printing and ancillary services to publishers and other content providers.

Citation: Auerhahn C, Capezuti E, Flaherty E, and Resnick B, eds. *Geriatric Nursing Review Syllabus: A Core Curriculum in Advanced Practice Geriatric Nursing*, 2nd edition. New York: American Geriatrics Society; 2007.

Geriatric Nursing Review Syllabus: A Core Curriculum in Advanced Practice Geriatric Nursing, 2nd edition. Cataloging in publication data are available from the Library of Congress.

Library of Congress Control Number: 2007925464

ISBN 978-1-0886775-2-0

Printed in the United States of America

10   9   8   7   6   5   4   3   2   1

TABLE OF CONTENTS

DISEASES AND DISORDERS

GNRS2 EDITORIAL BOARD

The *Geriatric Nursing Review Syllabus: A Core Curriculum in Advanced Practice Geriatric Nursing*, 2nd edition *(GNRS2)* is a collaborative effort between the American Geriatrics Society (AGS) and The John A. Hartford Foundation Institute for Geriatric Nursing. Nursing faculty modified the AGS's *Geriatrics Review Syllabus: A Core Curriculum in Geriatric Medicine*, 6th edition *(GRS6)* to be used primarily by advanced practice geriatric nurses.

EDITORS

Carolyn Auerhahn, EdD, APRN, BC, NP-C, FAANP
Clinical Associate Professor
Coordinator, Geriatric and Adult/Geriatric Nurse
 Practitioner Programs
New York University College of Nursing
New York, New York

Ellen Flaherty, PhD, APRN, BC
Vice President for Quality Improvement
Village Care of New York
New York, New York

Elizabeth Capezuti, PhD, RN, APRN, BC, FAAN
Associate Professor and Co-Director,
The John A. Hartford Foundation Institute for
 Geriatric Nursing
New York University College of Nursing
New York, New York

Barbara Resnick, PhD, CRNP, FAAN, FAANP
Professor
University of Maryland School of Nursing
Baltimore, Maryland

CONSULTING EDITOR

Judith L. Beizer, PharmD, CGP, FASCP
Clinical Professor
Department of Clinical Pharmacy Practice
College of Pharmacy and Allied Health Professions
St. John's University
Jamaica, New York

GNRS2 EDITORIAL STAFF

Managing Editor
Andrea N. Sherman, MS

Medical Editor
Susan E. Aiello, DVM, ELS

American Geriatric Society Staff
Linda Hiddemen Barondess,
 Executive Vice President
Nancy E. Lundebjerg, MPA,
 Deputy Executive Vice President of Education,
  Communications and Special Projects
Elvy Ickowicz, MPH,
 Assistant Vice President, Education,
  Communications and Special Projects

Indexer
L. Pilar Wyman, Wyman Indexing

Fry Communications, Inc.
Melissa Durborow,
 Information Services Manager
Terry Plyler,
 Content Management Architect
Jason Hughes,
 Technical Services Manager
Julie Stevens,
 Project Manager
Gwen Eckenrode,
 Compositor

ORIGINAL *GRS6* PROGRAM EDITORIAL BOARD AND AUTHORS

This *Geriatric Nursing Review Syllabus*, 2nd edition is based upon the *Geriatrics Review Syllabus*, 6th edition, which was developed by the following Editorial Board and chapter authors. For a complete listing of the *GRS6* Editors, Chapter Authors, and Question Writers and their professional affiliations, please see p. 597.

Chief Editor, Syllabus
Peter Pompei, MD

Chief Editor, Questions
John B. Murphy, MD

Syllabus Editors
Colleen Christmas, MD
Steven R. Counsell, MD
G. Paul Eleazer, MD
Anne R. Fabiny, MD
Susan K. Schultz, MD

Question Editors
William J. Burke, MD
Alison A. Moore, MD, MPH
Gail M. Sullivan, MD, MPH

Special Advisors
James T. Pacala, MD, MS
Stephanie Studenski, MD, MPH

Consulting Question Reviewers
Itamar B. Abrass, MD
Jane F. Potter, MD

Consulting Editor on Ethnogeriatrics
Carmel Bitondo Dyer, MD

Consulting Editor on Pharmacotherapy
Todd P. Semla, PharmD, MS

AUTHORS OF ORIGINAL *GRS6* CHAPTERS

Current Issues in Aging
Demography — Lynda C. Burton, ScD, Judith D. Kasper, PhD
Biology — Bruce R. Troen, MD, Donald A. Jurivich, DO
Psychosocial Issues — Kenneth W. Hepburn, PhD
Legal and Ethical Issues — Margaret A. Drickamer, MD
Financing, Coverage, & Costs of Health Care — Chad Boult, MD, MPH, MBA

Approach to Patient
Assessment — Thomas M. Gill, MD
Cultural Aspects of Care — Reva N. Adler, MD, MPH
Physical Activity — David M. Buchner, MD, MPH
Prevention — Harrison G. Bloom, MD
Pharmacotherapy — Todd P. Semla, PharmD, MS, Paula A. Rochon, MD, MPH
Complementary and Alternative Medicine — Barbara E. Moquin, PhD(c), MSN, APRN, Marc R. Blackman, MD
Elder Mistreatment — Terry T. Fulmer, PhD, RN
Hospital Care — William L. Lyons, MD, C. Seth Landefeld, MD
Perioperative Care — Colleen Christmas, MD, Peter Pompei, MD
Rehabilitation — Stephanie A. Studenski, MD, MPH, Cynthia J. Brown, MD, Pamela W. Duncan, PhD
Nursing-Home Care — Paul R. Katz, MD, Jurgis Karuza, PhD
Community-Based Care — G. Paul Eleazer, MD, Robert McCann, MD

Contributing Question and Critique Authors

Reva N. Adler, MD, MPH
Kathryn A. Atchison, DDS, MPH
Sidney T. Bogardus, Jr., MD
Kenneth Brummel-Smith, MD
Susan Charette, MD
Pejman Cohan, MD
Leo M. Cooney, Jr., MD
Robert S. Crausman, MD, MMS
James Cummins, MD
Margaret A. Drickamer, MD
Edmund H. Duthie, Jr, MD
Carmel Bitondo Dyer, MD
Michelle S. Eslami, MD
Mark H. Fleisher, MD
Alastair J. Flint, MB
David G. Folks, MD
Christine Himes Fordyce, MD
Andrea R. Fox, MD, MPH
Angela Gentili, MD
Mary Kane Goldstein, MD, MS
Shelly L. Gray, PharmD, MS, BCPS
Nathan Herrmann, MD
Kevin Paul High, MD, MSc
Michele Iannuzzi-Sucich, MD
Gail Ishiyama, MD
Thomas Vincent Jones, MD, MPH
Fran E. Kaiser, MD
Anne Kenny, MD
Mary B. King, MD
George A. Kuchel, MD
Robert K. Lee, DPM
Michael C. Lindberg, MD

Shari M. Ling, MD
Constantine G. Lyketsos, MD, MHS
Mathew S. Maurer, MD
Ellen McMahon, MD
Lynn McNicoll, MD
Daniel Ari Mendelson, MS, MD
Laura Mosqueda, MD
Benoit H. Mulsant, MD
Arash Naeim, MD, PhD
Joseph G. Ouslander, MD
Ronald Frederick Pfeiffer, MD
James T. Pacala, MD, MS
Joe W. Ramsdell, MD
Anthony E. Ranno, PharmD
Michael W. Rich, MD
Debra Saliba, MD, MPH
Gary Schiller, MD
Nancy Shafer Clark, MD
Alan M. Singer, DPM
Upinder Singh, MD
Monica Stallworth Kolimas, MD
David H. Stern, MD
Gwen K. Sterns, MD
Dennis H. Sullivan, MD
Mark Supiano, MD
Robert A. Sweet, MD
David C. Thomas, MD, MS
Corina M. Velehorschi, MD
Katherine Ward, MD
Michael R. Wasserman, MD
Barbara E. Weinstein, PhD
Steven P. Wengel, MD

PROGRAM INFORMATION

CONGRUITY OF CONTENT BETWEEN SYLLABUS AND QUESTIONS

Since the *Syllabus* chapters and the questions with critiques were written by different authors, questions may not always correlate directly with the *Syllabus*. In the event that a question's content is not addressed in the correlating chapter, its answer is fully supported in the critique.

In an effort to provide greater consistency of content between chapters and questions, editors asked the chapter authors and question writers to address topics from similar outlines of their area. However, regardless of whether the question material is covered adequately in the corresponding chapter text, the questions rely on the accompanying critiques to provide supportive information for the question content.

The *GNRS2* review questions are provided as learning aides but not as practice items for the Geriatric Nurse Practitioner Examination for the American Nurses Credentialing Center or the American Academy of Nurse Practitioners.

SELF-ASSESSMENT PROGRAM

For self-assessment testing, answer sheets are available for download at: http://www.americangeriatrics.org/products/gnrs_2.shtml.

AGS GERIATRICS RECOGNITION AWARD

The Geriatrics Recognition Award (GRA) recognizes nurses who are committed to advancing their continuing education in geriatrics/gerontological nursing. The GRA was developed by the American Geriatrics Society to encourage nurses to acquire special knowledge and keep abreast of the latest advances in geriatrics/gerontological nursing through continuing education programs.

Although CEU hours are not offered for this activity, the AGS has evaluated the number of hours it would take an individual to complete the *GNRS2* syllabus and self-assessment questions and determined that individuals can submit for up to 50 hours toward the GRA.

To receive more information and an application for the AGS GRA, please see http://www.americangeriatrics.org/products/gnrs_2.shtml.

USER EVALUATION

The AGS would appreciate participants' comments about the *GNRS2* program through the User Survey located at: http://www.americangeriatrics.org/products/gnrs_2.shtml. Comments and suggestions will be taken into consideration by those planning the next edition.

UPDATES AND ERRATA

Important updates, such as medication alerts, will be posted as necessary on the AGS Web site: http://www.americangeriatrics.org/products/gnrs_2.shtml.

Please report any errata to: info.amger@american geriatrics.org, Attention: *GNRS* Manager. Identified errata will be posted on the AGS Web site: http://www.americangeriatrics.org/products/gnrs_2.shtml.

LEARNING OBJECTIVES

At the conclusion of this program, participants will be better able to:

- Describe the general principles of aging and the biomedical and psychosocial issues of aging;

- Discuss legal and ethical issues related to geriatric medicine;

- Evaluate the financing of health care for older persons;

- Identify the basic principles of geriatric medicine, including assessment, pharmacology, prevention, exercise, palliative care, rehabilitation, and sensory deficits;

- Diagnose and manage geriatric syndromes, including dementia, delirium, urinary incontinence, malnutrition, osteoporosis, falls, pressure ulcers, sleep disorders, pain, dysphagia, and dizziness;

- Use state-of-the-art approaches to geriatric care while providing care in hospital, office-practice, nursing-home, and home-care settings;

- Adjust patient care in the light of evidence-based data regarding the particular risks and needs of ethnic, racial, and sexual patient groups; and

- Employ evidence-based data to increase the effectiveness of teaching geriatrics to all health professionals.

INTRODUCTION

The core mission of the American Geriatrics Society (AGS) is to promote the optimal health, function, and well-being of older persons. In order to accomplish this goal, AGS members must possess a current fund of knowledge that is evidence based and incorporates the most recent advances in health care. In 1989 the AGS published its first *Geriatrics Review Syllabus (GRS)*. This publication was enormously successful and has become the standard resource in the field of geriatric medicine to assist clinicians in staying current and providing the best possible care to their patients. Recognizing the need for a text specifically tailored for the advanced practice nurse, the AGS, in collaboration with The John A. Hartford Foundation Institute of Geriatric Nursing at New York University, has created the *Geriatric Nursing Review Syllabus*, 2nd edition *(GNRS2)*, which is based on the *Geriatrics Review Syllabus, 6th edition* and adapted for advanced practice geriatric nurses. It is with a great sense of accomplishment that the AGS publishes this second edition of the *GNRS*, authored largely by AGS members and leaders in the field of geriatrics.

The *Syllabus* text is divided into five sections: Current Issues in Aging; Approach to the Patient; Syndromes; Psychiatry; and Diseases and Disorders.

The *GNRS2* consists of 59 chapters, each of which provides a synopsis of the current thinking about a particular topic or field. It must be recognized, however, that the *GNRS* is not intended to be a comprehensive textbook of geriatrics. Accordingly, discussion of certain subjects must be brief, and the reader is referred to more in-depth discussions in a bibliography. In addition, references specific to advanced practice nursing can be found at the end of the chapters. In compiling the bibliography, the interdisciplinary Editorial Board has made every attempt to restrict the references to journals listed in *Index Medicus*. Finally, the *GNRS2* devotes little attention to topics that are core components of medicine and nursing and not unique to the care of older persons; this information can be found in standard medical texts.

The Question Review Committee, using questions drafted by a team of question writers, has developed 100 case-oriented, multiple-choice self-study questions. These questions are designed to complement material in the chapters, and they draw on the entire knowledge base of geriatrics, rather than limiting themselves to the *GNRS2* text. We recommend that participants prepare for answering these questions by first carefully reading through the *Syllabus* chapters. Any material addressed in the questions that is not discussed in the chapters is amply discussed in the critiques. The *GNRS2* review

questions are provided as learning aides but not as practice items for the Geriatric Nurse Practitioner Examination for the American Nurses Credentialing Center or the American Academy of Nurse Practitioners. They are not, and will not be, part of any certifying examination.

The authors were encouraged to include information on health disparities among racial and ethnic minorities in those areas where accurate data exist. Although there has been an increase in the understanding of the health outcomes and diseases among older minorities, these populations remain insufficiently studied. Readers of the *GNRS2* must recognize the differences between various ethnic groups and are encouraged to be sensitive to cultural issues in the care of older persons.

Topics for inclusion have been carefully selected by the editorial team. Authors were selected on the basis of their in-depth knowledge of a particular area and their ability to condense large amounts of information into clinically applicable, succinct essays. Editors and authors are experienced in caring for geriatric patients and emphasize the geriatric perspective in the preparation of *GNRS* content.

With each new edition, the *Syllabus* has included increasing amounts of information about drugs commonly used in treating older adults, though no effort is made to provide comprehensive coverage of available drugs for each disease or disorder. (See the AGS *Geriatrics At Your Fingertips*, published annually, for details about individual agents.) When *Syllabus* authors have chosen to discuss specific drugs, we have made certain that the information provided was up to date at the time of publication and that any mentions of uses not specifically approved by the U.S. Food and Drug Administration (so called "off-label" uses) are so tagged.

Chapters new to *GNRS2* include those on perioperative care, cultural aspects of care, persistent pain, and diabetes mellitus. Also new to the *GNRS2* are key points provided at the beginning of each chapter. The Appendix offers material that clinicians find useful in clinical practice.

We hope the *GNRS* will meet our goal of improving participants' knowledge base in geriatrics and thus enhancing the practice patterns of clinicians who care for older persons by providing a self-study tool that is current, concise, scholarly, and clinically relevant. We encourage your comments and suggestions, as the AGS continually strives to better serve its members, other health professionals, and the older persons they treat.

CURRENT ISSUES IN AGING

CHAPTER 1—DEMOGRAPHY

KEY POINTS

- The aging of baby boomers, ethnic differentials in aging, and particularly increases in the old-old age group will significantly shift the composition of older adult population in the United States.

- The older segment of the U.S. population is changing: (a) becoming better educated; (b) becoming better off financially (though ethnic minorities lag behind white Americans); and (c) altering living arrangements, especially with the growth of assisted living.

- Population heterogeneity continues to increase, with wider variations in ethnicity, functional ability, and chronic conditions.

- Among older adults, heart disease, cancer, and stroke remain the leading causes of death, and age-specific conditions such as Alzheimer's disease are becoming more common; other diseases (influenza, pneumonia) become more lethal than among younger adults.

DEMOGRAPHIC TRENDS

In 2000 about one in eight Americans living in the United States was aged 65 or older, but by 2030 that rate is expected to be one out of every five. This major demographic shift has prompted numerous concerns regarding U.S. social and health policy in recent years. Not only will the sheer number of older adults increase dramatically, but the composition and characteristics of the older population will also change. Although clinicians are primarily concerned with the needs of individual patients, some of the attributes that an older patient brings to the patient-clinician relationship are a function of the cohort to which he or she belongs. Aging baby boomers (the generation born between 1940 and 1960) are expected to have a major impact on the health and social service systems of the United States, although the exact nature of this impact remains unclear.

During the 20th century the U.S. population under age 65 tripled, while the age group 65 years and older increased by a factor of more than 11, growing from 3.1 million in 1900 to 35.6 million in 2002. This group will more than double by the middle of the next century, to 82 million people, with most of this growth occurring between 2010 and 2030. The United States

is not unique in its growing share of older people. At present it is surpassed by many other developed countries, including Italy, Japan, Germany, Sweden, and the United Kingdom, where the proportion of people aged 60 and older is already at 20% or above.

The older population of the United States is not evenly distributed geographically. Half of persons aged 65 or older live in nine states, led by California, Florida, New York, and Texas. The midwestern states, however, have the highest percentages of older persons living alone (30% or greater). The older U.S. population is predominantly white, but the proportion of older persons of other races is expected to grow from about one in 10 currently, to two in 10 in the next 50 years. The number of older black Americans is expected to triple in this period, whereas the size of the older Hispanic American population, which is growing much faster, may exceed that of the older black population within 30 years.

LIFE EXPECTANCY

In the United States the average life expectancy is currently highest for white women, followed by that for black women and white men, who have nearly identical in life expectancies, and black men (Table 1.1). Women who survive to age 65 can, on average, expect to live to age 84, and those surviving to age 85 can expect to live to age 92. Up to age 85, the life expectancy of white American men and women exceeds that of their black counterparts. At age 85, these racial differences in life expectancy largely disappear. There is disagreement about whether these findings reflect errors in documenting age (for older black Americans) or a true cross-over in mortality rates.

The exact number of centenarians in the United States is difficult to gauge, but their numbers are growing and are expected to be over 800,000 by 2050. For persons born in 1899, the odds against living to 100 were 400 to 1; for persons born in 1980, the odds are estimated at 87 to 1.

SOCIOECONOMIC STATUS

Improvements in the Social Security system and the adoption of Medicare have had an important impact on the economic well-being of older persons in the United States. In the early 1960s, 35% of people aged 65 or older had incomes below the federal poverty

Table 1.1—Years of Life Expectancy at Birth and Ages 65, 75, 85, by Gender and Race, 2000

	All Races			White			Black		
	Both sexes	Male	Female	Both sexes	Male	Female	Both sexes	Male	Female
At birth	76.9	74.1	79.5	77.4	74.8	80.0	71.7	68.2	74.9
Age 65	17.9	16.3	19.2	17.9	16.3	19.2	16.2	14.5	17.4
Age 75	11.3	10.1	12.1	11.3	10.1	12.1	10.5	9.4	11.2
Age 85	6.3	5.6	6.7	6.2	5.5	6.6	6.3	5.7	6.5

SOURCE: Data from *National Vital Statistics Report.* 2002; 51(3):2. Available at http//www.cdc.gov/nchs/ (accessed July 2005).

level, and only 70% received Social Security pensions. By the early 1970s, over 90% of older people received Social Security retirement benefits (accounting for at least 50% of income for 63% of beneficiaries, and 90% or more of income for 26%), and 97% were covered by Medicare. The percentage of older people with incomes below the poverty line today is about 10%. Another 6.5% are classified as "near poor," that is, with an income between the poverty level and 125% of this level. For impoverished seniors (generally having an income well below the poverty line), Medicaid plays a key role in filling in the gaps in Medicare by covering prescription drugs, nursing-home and other long-term care services, and health care services not covered by Medicare, as well as paying for Medicare premiums and cost sharing. Currently there are approximately 4.5 million seniors enrolled in both Medicare and Medicaid (ie, "dual eligibles").

Although the overall economic position of older people in the United States has improved significantly over the past three decades, these gains have not been shared by all. Poverty rates among older people are higher among black Americans (22%), Hispanic Americans (22%), persons aged 85 and older (12%), those who never finished high school (21%), those living in rural areas (13%) and central cities (14%), and those living alone (21%). Rates in some groups of older persons are much higher—half of older black American women living alone are poor, for example.

Older workers have declined as a share of the U.S. work force, and this trend is expected to continue. In 1950, 60% of men aged 65 to 69 were still in the work force, whereas in 1990, 28% of the same age group were working. Overall, in the early 1990s, 16% of older men and 8% of older women were working. Today, more than half of those who continue to work do so part time and largely by choice, rather than because of restricted opportunities for full-time work.

Compared with their parents at the same age, baby boomers typically have higher income, are preparing for retirement at largely the same pace, and have accumulated more private wealth. On the whole, boomers are on track to have higher incomes in

retirement than their parents and appear much less likely to live in poverty after they retire.

One of the most dramatic changes in the older U.S. population of the future will be in levels of educational attainment. Between 1970 and 2001, the percentage of those aged 65 or older who completed high school increased from 28% to 70%. By 2030, 83% of older people will have completed high school. The percentage with a bachelor's degree or more will have increased to 24% from the current level of 15%. Education is closely related to lifetime economic status, and, as many studies have shown, those with more education generally are in better health and at lower risk of disability than those with low levels of educational attainment. There is also speculation that the better-educated older baby boomers will be both more activist health care consumers and more demanding of the health care system. Today, approximately 50% of U.S. households have personal computers, but Internet use is much more common among persons under the age of 55. Despite concerns about the accuracy of much of the health and medical information available on various Internet Web sites, the use of these alternative information sources is likely to grow. In addition, pharmaceutical companies are increasingly marketing directly to consumers as a means of developing demand.

LIVING ARRANGEMENTS AND MARITAL STATUS

Among Americans living in the United States who are aged 65 to 74 years, two thirds are married and living with their spouse; in contrast, only about one fifth of those aged 85 and older are living with their spouse (Table 1.2). Not surprisingly, given older women's greater life expectancy, older men are far more likely to be married than are older women. Conversely, widowhood is much more common among older women; 56% of women aged 75 to 84 and 82% of women aged 85 and older are widows.

Older men and women who live alone, often having lost a partner, usually prefer to remain independent and continue living alone as long as their health

Table 1.2—Marital Status and Living Arrangement of Medicare Beneficiaries, by Age, 2000 (beneficiaries as a percentage of total in each age group)

	All (%)			Male (%)			Female (%)		
	65–74	75–84	85+	65–74	75–84	85+	65–74	75–84	85+
Marital status									
Married	64.1	49.1	21.9	79.0	70.5	50.9	51.7	34.2	9.8
Widowed	21.0	41.4	70.4	7.2	19.9	41.8	32.5	56.2	82.3
Other	14.9	9.5	7.7	13.8	9.6	7.3	15.8	9.6	7.9
Living arrangement									
Lives alone	24.5	33.6	38.8	14.9	20.1	28.9	32.6	43.0	42.9
With spouse	62.6	46.8	18.4	76.8	67.5	43.5	50.7	32.4	8.0
With children	6.8	9.6	14.9	2.5	4.9	9.4	10.4	12.9	17.2
With others	4.7	4.7	5.1	4.3	3.7	4.2	5.1	5.4	5.5
In nursing home	1.4	5.3	22.8	1.5	3.8	14.0	1.2	6.3	26.4

SOURCE: Data from *Medicare Current Beneficiary Survey*, 2000; Table 1.2. Available at http://www.cms.hhs.gov/mcbs/PubCNP00.asp (accessed October 2005).

and economic means allow them to do so. Many of those who live alone have families or friends nearby, and about three in five have lived in the same place for 10 years or more. These persons may also be vulnerable, however. They are more likely than older people who live with others to use community services and to report greater levels of loneliness and social isolation.

THE OLDER FOREIGN-BORN POPULATION

In 2000, there were 3.1 million foreign-born persons aged 65 or older in the United States. More than one third (39%) of this older foreign-born group are from Europe, and another 31% are from Latin America; 22% are from Asia, and 8% are from other parts of the world. In the future, the older foreign-born resident is more likely to be from Latin America or Asia. Almost two thirds of the older foreign-born group have lived in the United States for more than 30 years. About one third of them live in the western states.

Older foreign-born persons are more likely than their native counterparts to live in family households. Eight of 10 older foreign-born men are married; nearly half of older foreign-born women are widowed. Older foreign-born women are much more likely than older foreign-born men to live alone. The poverty rate is higher for the older foreign-born population than for the older native population. Households with older foreign-born householders participate in means-tested programs at higher rates than households with older native householders.

ASSISTED-LIVING FACILITIES

Assisted living represents one of the fastest-growing trends in residential settings for older people in the United States. This type of facility seeks to fill the need for greater supervision and assistance than may be possible in a private home. Approximately 800,000 people were estimated to be living in 33,000 assisted-living facilities in the United States in 2002. A typical assisted-living resident is a woman between 75 and 85 years of age who is mobile but needs assistance with about two activities of daily living (ADLs). Residents move to assisted-living residences from a variety of settings. Just under half (46%) come from their home, 20% come from another assisted-living residence, 14% come from a hospital, and 10%, from a nursing home. The average length of residency is 2 years. (See also the section on assisted living in "Community-Based Care," p 124, and the AGS statement on assisted living in the Appendixes, p 456.)

TRENDS IN NURSING-HOME USE

The 1999 National Nursing Home Survey showed 1.6 million residents in 18,000 homes and an 87% occupancy rate. The rate per thousand population for those aged 65 and over was 429.2: 108 per 1000 for those aged 65 to 74, 429.7 for those 75 to 84, and 182.5 for those 85 years and over. Nationally, the percentage of older people residing in nursing homes has remained fairly constant, at about 5% overall, rising to 20% of persons aged 85 and older. The lifetime chance of ever being in a nursing home is much higher, however, at nearly 1 in 2. In part, this is due to increased use of nursing homes for short stays for recovery and rehabilitation following hospital discharge, stays that are paid for by Medicare if preceded by a 3-day hospital stay. The resident population is older and more disabled today. Over the past decade, the proportion of residents aged 85 and older has risen from 49% to 56% for women, and 29% to 33% for men; the proportion needing help with three or more ADLs rose from 72% to 83%.

TRENDS IN HEALTH AND FUNCTIONING

The burden of disease and disability is greater for older people than for those under age 65. In the United States in 2000, 84% of persons aged 65 or older had one or more chronic conditions. Hypertension is the most common chronic condition reported, followed by arthritic symptoms, heart disease, chronic obstructive pulmonary disease, and cancer (Figure 1.1). Although 80% of very old persons (aged 85 and older) report two or more chronic conditions, only 36% report being in fair or poor health (Figure 1.2). There is great heterogeneity in health status among older people (Table 1.3). Data on self-assessed health, which has been shown in several studies to correlate highly with mortality and risk of functional decline, illustrate this. Among white non-Hispanic Americans aged 65 to 74, 18% regarded their health as excellent and another 31% as very good; 13% indicated only fair health and 5%, poor health (Table 1.3). As might be expected, the percentages who viewed their health as only fair or poor increases with age. Also, self-reports of only fair or poor health were higher for older black and Hispanic Americans than for older white Americans.

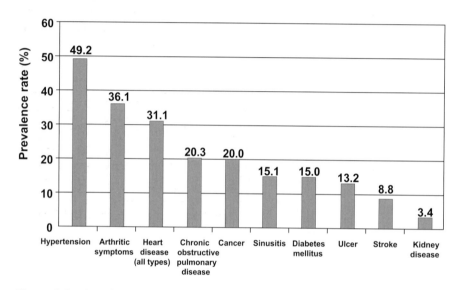

Figure 1.1—Prevalence of selected chronic conditions among persons aged 65 and over, all races.

SOURCE: Data from Data Warehouse on Trends in Health and Aging: Health Status and Chronic Conditions, 1997–2001, from the National Health Interview Survey. Estimates for 2000–2001. See http://www.cdc.gov/nchs/agingact.htm (accessed October 2005).

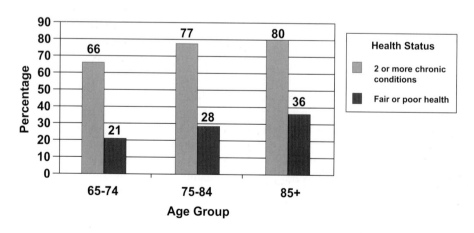

Figure 1.2—Percentage of all Medicare beneficiaries with two or more chronic conditions and self-reporting fair or poor health, by age group, 2000.

SOURCE: Data from Medicare Beneficiary Survey, 2000. See http://www.cms.hhs.gov/mcbs/ (accessed October 2005).

Functional disability also increases with age and is closely associated with chronic disease. In the United States, the majority of people under the age of 85 report no difficulty in ADLs or instrumental activities of daily living (IADLs); much lower proportions of those aged 85 and older report little or no difficulty (Figure 1.3). Older women exhibit a higher percentage of limitations at all ages than older men do. Differences between racial and ethnic groups exist as well. Among those aged 70 and older, black Americans are 1.5 times as likely as white Americans to be unable to perform one or more ADLs.

In the United States older persons who need assistance with functioning in routine ADLs rely first and foremost on family. In 1995, of those providing assistance to community-dwelling persons aged 70 or older, 73% were unpaid or informal helpers. Nine out of 10 informal or unpaid caregivers were family members, one fourth were spouses, and about half were children. Half of these informal caregivers resided with the person receiving help. Estimates of the use of paid helpers vary across studies, but use is consistently found to be higher among persons living alone and to rise with increasing age.

Deaths of older persons make up nearly 75% of all deaths in the United States. About one fifth of all deaths occur at age 85 or older, but this proportion is expected to grow. For many decades, heart disease, cancer, and stroke have been the leading causes of death among people 65 or older, accounting for six out of 10 deaths (Table 1.4). Causes of death vary by race, ethnicity, and gender, however. Diabetes mellitus

Table 1.3—Perceived Health of Medicare Beneficiaries, by Age and Race or Ethnicity, 2000

	White, non-Hispanic (%)			Black, non-Hispanic (%)			Hispanic (%)		
	65–74	75–84	85+	65–74	75–84	85+	65–74	75–84	85+
Excellent	18.23	13.79	11.19	10.93	7.42	8.31	13.17	12.86	8.19
Very good	31.06	26.97	22.98	22.58	18.73	17.13	21.61	17.48	20.56
Good	31.87	32.96	31.30	35.05	34.84	30.70	30.06	32.11	28.46
Fair	13.40	18.78	25.82	24.31	29.85	30.90	25.26	29.08	32.48
Poor	5.44	7.50	8.70	7.13	9.56	12.97	9.91	8.47	10.32

SOURCE: Data from *Medicare Current Beneficiary Survey*, 2000; Table 2.3. Available at http://www.cms.hhs.gov/mcbs/PubCNP00.asp (accessed October 2005).

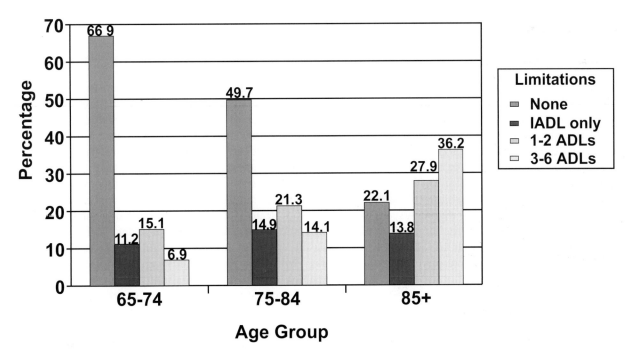

Figure 1.3—Self-reported functional limitations of Medicare beneficiaries, by age group, 2000. Key: ADLs = activities of daily living; IADL = instrumental activity of daily living.

SOURCE: Data from Medicare Beneficiary Survey, 2000; Table 2.1. See http://www.cms.hhs.gov/mcbs/ (accessed October 2005).

Table 1.4—Leading Causes of Death and Numbers of Deaths, for Persons Aged 65 and Over, 1999

Rank	Cause of Death	Number of Deaths	% of Deaths
	All Causes	1797,331	100.0
1	Diseases of heart	607,265	33.8
2	Malignant neoplasms	390,122	21.7
3	Cerebrovascular diseases	148,599	8.3
4	Chronic lower respiratory disease	108,112	6.0
5	Influenza and pneumonia	57,282	3.2
6	Diabetes mellitus	51,843	2.9
7	Alzheimer's disease	44,020	2.4
8	Unintentional injuries	32,219	1.8
9	Nephritis, nephrotic syndrome, and nephrosis	29,938	1.7
10	Septicemia	24,626	1.4

SOURCE: *Health, United States, 2002 With Chartbook on Trends in the Health of Americans.* Hyattsville, MD: National Center for Health Statistics; 2002:132 (Table 33).

was the fourth leading cause of death among older Hispanic and black Americans, while ranking sixth for older white Americans. Alzheimer's disease ranked seventh among all causes of death.

Some causes of death usually associated with younger people also are of concern in the older population. In the United States, older men have motor vehicle accident death rates two to three times those of older women, overall and within racial and ethnic groups. The highest suicide rates among older people are for white men (43.7 per 100,000, compared with 6.5 per 100,000 for older white women), who are more likely to commit suicide than die in a motor vehicle crash.

TRENDS IN DISABILITY

There are conflicting opinions about whether rates of disability in the United States are declining among people aged 65 and over. Some studies suggest a decline in the past decade in the proportion unable to do some activities (one or more ADLs or IADLs), but there is also evidence for an increase in the proportion unable to perform one or more ADLs. Differences in study populations and measures contribute to conflicting findings. The measurement of disabilities varies across studies, and assessments of the presence and severity of disability can differ when histories are taken from an older person, the family caregiver, or the clinician.

Trends in disability are of special interest because increases in life expectancy overall and for people aged 65 and older have led to debate over whether these additional years will be free of disability. Studies of active life expectancy, which use mortality and disability estimates to project disability-free years, suggest an advantage for persons with more education. Because of

their greater total life expectancy, older women also experience both greater active life expectancy and more years of disability than do older men. It has also been suggested that if there is a limit to increases in life expectancy, increases in disability-free years could produce a *compression of morbidity*, with the period of disability prior to death gradually compressed as active life expectancy (or disability-free years) increases. Increases in active life expectancy must occur if compression of morbidity is to be achieved, but debate continues regarding whether there is a maximum human life span, and whether compression of morbidity is possible if total life expectancy continues to increase.

As more longitudinal studies are conducted and other evidence is brought to bear, the trend in active life expectancy among older people may become clearer. Regardless of its true direction, however, preventing and reducing disability among older people remains a major objective of much geriatrics research.

The assumption has been that disability is irreversible, but studies show that up to one third of persons who experience disability in a basic ADL recover. Age less than 85 years, good nutritional status, and greater mobility are all associated with increased likelihood of recovery from basic ADL disability.

TRENDS IN HEALTH CARE

On average, older people in the United States have more contacts with health care professionals than do younger adults, from a mean of 10 per year among those aged 65 to 74, to nearly 15 per year among those aged 85 and older. Those who assess their health as fair or poor have twice as many contacts per year as do persons in excellent or good health. Older adults accounted for 20% of the hospital discharges and used a third of the days of care in 1970; in the year 2000 they made up close to 40% of discharges and used almost one-half of the hospital days. Variations in length of stay can be considerable, however.

Diseases of the heart were the leading discharge diagnosis in the United States for older people, with heart disease and stroke together accounting for more than one fourth of all hospital discharges among older men and women aged 85 and older. Malignant neoplasms were the next most common discharge diagnosis, followed by pneumonia and bronchitis. Fracture-related hospitalizations were more common among women than men and accounted for nearly 10% of discharges for those aged 85 and older.

Home-health care, including medical treatment, physical therapy, and homemaker services, is an alternative to institutional care for older people. Nursing care is the most commonly used service (85% of older home-health patients received nursing care in 1996), and 29% of patients use homemaker services. Medicare has been a major payer for home-health care (nearly half of expenses in 1996), and changes in payment methods have resulted in a dramatic drop in use of these services (both in the numbers of persons served and visits per user).

Prescription drugs have become a major component of medical treatment. Eighty percent of older people in the United States are using one or more prescribed medicines; among those with three to five ADL limitations, 93% use at least one.

OTHER ISSUES

The older U.S. population is among the most heterogeneous subgroups, encompassing the entire spectrum of health and functioning, from the bedridden Alzheimer's patient to the marathon runner. One of the important unresolved questions is whether gains in longevity after age 65 are accompanied by gains or declines in years of disability-free life. It is unlikely that one answer will fit this large and diverse group. There are many questions in other areas as well. While levels of education continue to rise, so do rates of early retirement. Will the increasing numbers of better-educated, longer-lived persons contribute to the larger society, and in what ways? Will the sheer numbers of older people strain to the breaking point the medical care system and public programs that finance health care and retirement, as some analysts fear? Or will improvements in health behavior, medical breakthroughs, and financial prosperity diminish these threats?

Under any scenario, chronic illness will remain a constant in the lives of many older people. Clinicians treating this population face the challenge not only of treating chronically ill persons but of assisting all older people in preventing or at least delaying the onset of chronic disease.

REFERENCES

■ Administration on Aging, U.S. Department of Health and Human Services. *A Profile of Older Americans: 2002.* Available at http://www.aoa.gov/prof/statistics/profile/2002profile.pdf (accessed July 2005).

■ American Association of Retired People (AARP). Public Policy Institute Releases—Topics in Health and Wellness: Disabilities; Spring 2005.

■ Federal Interagency Forum on Aging-Related Statistics. *Older Americans 2000: Key Indicators of Well-Being.* Washington, DC: U.S. Government Printing Office; August 2000. Available at http://www.agingstats.gov/chartbook2000/default.htm (accessed October 2005).

■ Hall MJ, Owings MF. 2000 National Hospital Discharge Survey. *Advance Data from Vital and Health Statistics,* No. 329, June 19, 2002. Available at http://www.cdc.gov/nchs/data/ad/ad329.pdf (accessed July 2005).

■ Stone R. *Long-Term Care for the Disabled Elderly: Current Policy, Emerging Trends and Implications for the 21st Century.* New York: Milbank Memorial Fund; 2000.

CHAPTER 2—BIOLOGY

KEY POINTS

■ Aging changes are caused by multiple factors, including genetics, wear and tear, oxidative and glycative damage, and environmental factors.

■ Animal models have shown that maximum life span can be extended by caloric restriction, genetic mutations, and genetic manipulation.

■ Human studies indicate that hereditary factors account for approximately 10% to 58% of longevity.

■ Genetic factors may regulate aging or life span through a variety of mechanisms, including insulin signaling, control of oxidative damage, predisposition to (or suppression of) age-associated diseases (including cancer), DNA maintenance, and altered gene expression at the level of transcription or translation, or both. There may be no "master control" or single pathway that controls senescence.

Knowledge about age-dependent changes in cellular and organ function is important in the care of older persons. The rate of physiologic aging varies from person to person, with large interindividual variations. At the cellular and molecular levels, provocative scientific findings have begun to unravel the question of why we age. Some determinants of longevity now can be understood in terms of gene expression. Importantly, temporal expression of aging resembles a rheostatic switch with small incremental changes. Attempts to answer questions about what controls the rheostatic switch and the rate of senescence have resulted in several theories on aging (Table 2.1).

CHARACTERISTICS OF AGING

Common traits of aging processes include the following:

- Mortality increases with age after maturation, and the increases become exponential with increasing age.
- The biochemical composition of tissue changes with age; examples are lipofuscin and extracellular matrix cross-linking, protein oxidation, and altered rates of gene transcription.
- Physiologic capacity decreases.
- The ability to maintain homeostasis diminishes, especially with regard to adaptive processes under physiologic stress.
- The susceptibility and vulnerability to disease increase.

Loss of physiologic reserve and decreased homeostatic control may be a consequence of changes in allostasis and development of homeostenosis. *Allostasis*, "maintaining stability through change," refers to the normal response to stress, that is, the activation of the neuroendocrine, immune, and autonomic systems with a stressor, such as a surgical operation. The responses to the stress include changes in cortisol, epinephrine, and cytokines that are adaptive in the short run but that may be harmful if prolonged. *Allostatic load* refers to the effects of prolonged or overactive allostatic response. A possible example of allostatic load is the relationship between the subtle increase in cortisol levels seen in many older people, possibly leading to hippocampal damage and memory loss. Conversely, it has been hypothesized that brief or recurrent exposures to stress such that specific signaling pathways and expression of genes are stimulated or suppressed, or both, may be beneficial and ultimately promote longevity of an organism. This phenomenon is known as *hormesis* and is likely to be found occurring alongside examples of allostatic load. Hormesis has been observed in a variety of organisms (yeast, flies, worms, rodents) and in human cells in vitro.

Homeostenosis is the altered response to physiologic stresses often seen in older people. Examples include decreased ability to manage fluid and electrolyte derangements, including diminished thirst perception, decreased glomerular filtration, and changes in the renin-aldosterone system, urinary concentrating, and dilutional capacity.

One axiom of aging had been the irreversibility of changes that occur over time, and although this is

Table 2.1—Representative Theories of Aging

Theory	Synopsis	Support
Oxidative stress	The result of homothermia and metabolism is the accumulation of protein, lipid, and DNA damage mediated through highly reactive, oxygen-derived substances (free radicals).	Mutations in oxidative stress pathway can extend life span. Mutations of genes in other pathways (including in mammals) that increase longevity also exhibit enhanced resistance to stress and oxidative damage.
Chromosomal alterations	Deletions, mutations, translocations, and polyploidy have been suggested as age-acquired chromosomal instabilities that contribute to gene silencing or expression of disease-related genes, such as those seen in cancer.	Mitochondrial DNA mutations of genes in the oxidative stress pathway may contribute to reduced resistance to oxidative stress. However, the practical impact in normal nondiseased aging may be minimal.
Immunologic	Time-acquired deficits, primarily in T-cell function, predispose elderly persons to infections and cancer.	Impact upon diseases associated with aging, but not apparently directly related to a healthy organismic aging
Neuroendocrinologic	The cortisol surge leading to death in spawning salmon has served as a model for explaining the decline of humans after their maximal reproductive years.	No direct support in humans
Developmental-genetic	Because the maximum life span appears fixed, a genetically programmed induction of senescence is thought to occur, resulting in the activation or suppression of specific "aging" genes.	Longevity in humans appears heritable. However, evolution selects for reproductive fitness to maintain the species, not for postreproductive senescence.
Metabolic and insulin signaling, caloric restriction	Alterations in body size and composition, and in insulin-signaling pathways act independently and in concert to extend life span.	Caloric restriction and mutations in insulin-signaling pathways in a wide variety of species (yeast, worms, flies, rodents) enhance resistance to oxidative stress and extend life span.

generally true, the rate of aging can be influenced by environmental and genetic factors. Thus, the prevention of deleterious changes with age and the reversal of certain aspects of senescence are promising possibilities.

THEORIES OF AGING

The oxidative stress theory is one widely accepted explanation of the aging process. This theory posits that oxygen converted during metabolism into superoxide anions, hydrogen peroxide, and hydroxyl radicals causes damage over time. Untoward events are indiscriminate and cumulative. Key observations include the following:

- Free-radical damage to lipids, protein, and DNA have been found in aging heart, liver, and kidney tissue.
- Short-lived species accumulate this damage quickly.
- Transgenic animal models that concurrently overexpress copper and zinc superoxide dismutase and catalase have extended life spans.
- Antioxidant compounds such as vitamin E can enhance the average life span in animal models. Interestingly, the expression of human SOD (super oxide dismutase) gene in *Drosophila* neurons has been found to increase life span by 40%, which suggests that the central nervous system plays a key role in longevity.
- Caloric restriction, which extends life span, and single gene mutations that increase longevity enhance resistance to oxidative stress in yeast, worms, flies, and rodents.

Skeptics of the oxidative stress theory point out that knockout of the SOD gene does not accelerate aging. This observation attests to redundant systems that counter damage. On a pragmatic level, no evidence exists that antioxidants delay human senescence or disease. In fact, sufficient levels of these compounds may not reach critical areas such as the brain to prevent age-associated oxidant injury.

Mitochondria play a key role in biologic aging. Damage induced by free radicals results in mitochondrial-DNA (mtDNA) mutations in muscle and brain. These lead to defective mitochondrial respiration and further oxidant injury, which creates a cycle of damage and continued loss of mitochondrial function. Mitochondrial mutations and defective respiration have been linked to neurodegeneration in conditions such as Alzheimer's disease and Parkinson's disease. Given maternal inheritance of mtDNA, human longevity potentially is linked to the maternal genome.

Longevity is greater in family members of extremely old humans. Epidemiologic studies of twins suggest that heritability of life span is between 22% and 33%. Similar studies in families yield a wider range of estimates, between 10% and 58%. If this is true, the question is "Which genes are responsible for longevity?" It has been proposed that genes regulate the rate of aging (longevity assurance) and disease acquisition (disease-resistance genes). Genes also exist for damage repair. Thus, the human life span may depend upon multiple components that counter deleterious changes. The question remains whether a "master switch" is turned on over time so as to down-regulate repair mechanisms or perhaps exude a systemic factor for aging.

Differences in life spans observed among various mammalian species suggest a developmental-genetic theory of aging. Some aspects of aging resemble developmentally regulated programs; however, it is difficult to understand why evolutionary pressures would preferentially select senescence, unless a genetically controlled program for aging might be a mechanism to assure gene-pool turnover. On the other hand, genetically regulated programs that delay the onset of aging might be selected in human evolution if this enhanced the reproductive years. There is a growing literature documenting the association of single nucleotide polymorphisms with longevity in humans. Some of these gene alleles are actually associated with increased prevalence of disease at younger ages, suggesting that they may be examples of antagonistic pleiotropy (exerting deleterious effects early in life, but beneficial effects at later ages). Irrespective of potential selective evolutionary pressures, comparable longevity between monozygotic and not dizygotic twins hints that normal aging is influenced by a genetic program. Genetic disorders leading to accelerated aging, such as that seen in Hutchinson-Gilford progeria syndrome (HGPS) and Werner's syndrome, provide insight into the genetic components of processes associated with aging, such as alopecia, arteriosclerosis, osteoporosis, and skin atrophy. One of the progeria conditions, Werner's syndrome, is due to a perturbation on chromosome 8 and is linked to a gene that codes for a helicase. This enzyme is responsible for unwinding DNA during replication and repair. Chromosomal instability appears to mediate cumulative cellular pathology that contributes to death in the middle-aged adult. It has been discovered that mutations in the lamin A gene on chromosome 1 result in HGPS. Lamins are a family of nuclear intermediate filament proteins that establish and maintain the shape and strength of the interphase nucleus. HGPS fibroblasts exhibit abnormalities of the nuclear membrane. Lamin A mutations also cause at least six other genetic disorders, including forms of muscular dystrophy and cardiomyopathy. Clearly, both HGPS and Werner's syndrome, as well as accelerated aging observed in trisomy 21 syndrome (Down syndrome), indicate that the phenotype of human senescence has several genetic loci that can mediate the pace of aging.

Although indirect evidence supports a genetic link to the rate of aging, little direct evidence exists for a genetic program that actively triggers the aging processes. Indeed, animal models show that environmental manipulations, such as caloric restriction, can significantly extend life span. Thus, the relationship between environmental factors and gene expression appears to drive the aging process.

CELLULAR CHANGES WITH AGE

Senescence induces functional changes in cells. Perturbations are observed in cells with full replicative potential, as well as in those in a postmitotic state. Cells with proliferative capacity, such as lymphocytes and fibroblasts, typically demonstrate diminished proliferative potential over time. For instance, cultured lymphocytes from human blood start to divide after being provided a growth stimulus (plant lectin, phytohemagglutinin, and interleukin-2). The onset of proliferation is slower in old than in young donor lymphocytes, and the peak number of dividing cells is lower in elderly donor lymphocytes. The main reason for loss of lymphocyte proliferation with age is decreased secretion of interleukin-2 and expression of T-cell populations that have an altered affinity for this cytokine. Mixed populations of T cells from old donors express a high percentage of memory cells that exhibit different proliferative characteristics than naive T cells, which are more plentiful in young donor samples.

To circumvent concerns about mixed subpopulation dynamics characteristic of polyclonal T-cell cultures, researchers have stimulated single T-cell clones from young and elderly donor cells. In these instances, the cloning efficiency of T cells from old donors is reduced, with many fewer of them reaching benchmarks of 20, 30, and 40 population doublings than young donor cells that have identical cell surface markers. Thus, it appears that age alters both the population dynamics of T-cell growth and individual cellular capacity to sustain clonal expansion. The net result is diminished T-cell responses with age, which could account for the increasing infection and cancer rates observed over the human life span.

The loss of proliferation in cultured cells is broadly known as *clonal senescence*. Other cell types, such as endothelial and fibroblast cells, also exhibit loss of proliferative potential over time during in vitro tissue culture. A well-established model for replicative senescence entails serial passage of fetal or primary fibroblasts in well-defined cell culture media. At a certain

point, these cells enlarge and no longer divide. A number of studies have suggested that donor fibroblasts from old individuals undergo fewer population doublings than do donor cells from young individuals. However, an important consideration is that the loss of replicative potential varies among aged individuals. Thus, a wide range exists whereby some young donor cells divide only a few times and old donor cells replicate comparably to many young donor cells. Furthermore, other studies fail to reveal a reproducible age-related alteration in donor cell proliferative capacity and demonstrate no change in replicative capacity when cells from the same individuals are examined at older ages. Skin biopsy experiments suggest an age-dependent accumulation of senescent fibroblasts as indicated by staining for β-galactosidase; however, the percentage of these cells in old donor skin is surprisingly small. Furthermore, this putative marker of senescence may be indicative of quiescent or damaged cells rather than the age of the cell. The body of evidence implies that changes in function other than loss of proliferation contribute to cellular aging.

It is possible that cellular senescence evolved as a mechanism of tumor suppression and that aging is an antagonistically pleiotropic manifestation of evolutionary pressures to prevent malignant transformation. Consequently, cellular senescence is good for the organism, and aging may be the price we pay to avoid, for the most part, cancer. However, even this concept has been qualified by the demonstration that senescent cells can foster the growth of premalignant and malignant epithelial cells in culture and the tumorigenesis of these cells in mice. Although these findings seem to be at odds with the beneficial effects of cellular senescence, they are themselves another example of antagonistic pleiotropy, wherein a process that has evolved to protect us against cancer in fact may predispose us to cancer later in life.

DNA AND GENE EXPRESSION DURING SENESCENCE

DNA Mutations or Deletions

The concept that age alters the integrity of DNA, primarily through mutations, originally led to the somatic mutation theory of aging. That aging results in DNA template errors, thus leading to errors in or loss of gene expression, has not held up experimentally. However, certain "hot spots" of DNA change have been observed in human and animal aging. These hypermutable DNA foci are thought to accumulate changes that produce functional cellular problems over time. Structural changes in DNA range from deletions to aberrant expansions. These changes occur in both somatic and germ cells. Importantly, several hypermutable areas are juxtaposed with key regulatory elements, such as the insulin gene and oncogene *ras1* locus. Changes over vast distances of DNA sequences can affect downstream gene activity, which suggests that age-related changes observed in nonfunctioning DNA areas can potentially exert untoward effects on critical regulatory genes.

A similar concern exists with age-dependent changes in mtDNA. The circular mtDNA is reported to undergo a mutation rate that is 10,000-fold greater in elderly than in younger adult tissue. A nearly exponential increase in mtDNA mutations occurs over time, with up to 10% of extremely old donor tissue exhibiting deletions. Because mitochondria and mtDNA are amply redundant, subtle, if any, age-dependent changes in respiratory chain activities are noticed, and it is most likely that aging results in a reduced functional reserve of energy production.

Telomeres

Perhaps the most provocative data concerning DNA changes with age relates to chromosomal end points. These chromosomal tips contain redundant DNA sequences or tandem repeats that cannot be replicated by DNA polymerase. To solve this problem, a ribonucleoprotein called *telomerase* deals with end chromosomal replication.

A fundamental problem observed in aged donor cells with replicative potential is that their telomeres shorten. Telomere shortening and loss of telomerase activity has been observed during clonal senescence of fibroblasts and T cells. Telomeric DNA loss is also a function of donor age. The consequence of this diminished activity is thought to be alterations in the immune system and deficient wound healing.

Conversely, telomerase hyperactivity is linked to cellular transformation and cancer. Given the relationship of telomeres to aging and cancer, some have proposed measurement of telomere length and telomerase activity as potential clinical markers of human aging and oncogenesis. Thus, targeted disruption of telomerase activity would be important as cancer therapy, whereas reactivation of this enzyme might reverse age-dependent changes in replicative potential. Such an approach may have to be tumor specific, since some cancerous cells do not have telomerase.

Gene Expression

Age affects gene expression at several levels. Age-related changes depend upon the cellular state, such as quiescence, proliferation, or physiologic stress.

When side-by-side comparisons of gene expression from mature adult and aged donors are conducted, the rates of gene expression either decrease, stay the same, or increase in elderly donors. An important and, as yet, unresolved consideration is whether differences in gene expression with age are functionally significant. The inability of cells to withstand physiologic stress with age is the strongest evidence that changes in stress-related gene expression contribute to poor functional outcomes.

A variety of mechanisms can influence gene expression with aging. For instance, mutations in DNA sequences in or around certain genes can influence their expression. Similar effects can be expected from latent viral infections (eg, herpes viruses), as well as from accumulation of environmentally induced cell damage. Targets for altered gene expression and aging would be reduced activity of transactivators, enhanced activity of DNA silencers or repressors, and intrinsic changes in RNA polymerase activity.

Because the overall total messenger ribonucleic acid (mRNA) content does not appear to change with age, aging has been characterized as a state with a decline in mRNA turnover and transcriptional rate. RNA polymerase per se does not appear to change with age, so most of the change in mRNA expression appears to be due to changes in the gene-promoter regions. Gene promoters are areas of DNA upstream of the target gene that have constitutively and inducibly bound DNA-binding proteins. Through proper assemblage of these DNA-binding proteins, DNA conformational changes that enhance RNA polymerase recruitment and efficiency are affected. Expected age-dependent changes would include alterations in DNA-protein interactions (transcription factors), accumulation of proteins interfering with DNA binding proteins, and unfavorable conformations of DNA during transcriptional activation. Importantly, there is no evidence that age leads to an increased error rate during transcription and translation.

In sum, the primary changes in gene expression with age are as follows:

- decreased transcription rates for key genes;
- decreased mRNA turnover;
- decreased inducibility of genes, such as immediate early genes, acute phase reactants, and stress genes.

Constitutive levels of gene expression remain intact.

Typically, aging alters the morphology of the nucleus, including multilobulation and irregular membranes. Micronucleation is commonly noted in old donor cells, and more cells from elderly donors than from young donors manifest abnormal chromosomal DNA content.

Of 6000 known human genes analyzed, only 61 or 1% showed changes in expression between young and middle-aged donors. Most of these changes were reduced gene expression involving cell cycle progression and maintenance or repair of the extracellular matrix. The functional consequence of declining gene expression related to cell cycle is possibly to predispose elderly individuals to increased DNA strand breaks and other chromosomal instabilities.

When gene expression in fibroblasts from progeria donors and elderly donors are compared, some interesting linkages between normal and premature aging are manifest. For example, down-regulation of bone- and joint-associated genes is found in normal aged and progeric individuals. Cathepsin C, a lysosomal protease, is similarly down-regulated sixfold in aged donors and likely contributes to dermal changes with senescence. A tumor-suppressor gene, BARD1, is down-regulated 4.5-fold with age and may account for age-related increases in breast cancer. Because the most extensive gene-expression data are derived from human fibroblasts, information about changes in gene expression with age that are specific to other tissues may reveal additional underlying mechanisms of senescence and increased susceptibility to disease.

Not all genes examined during senescence are found to be attenuated in their expression. Curiously, basal expression of genes related to the stress response is up-regulated in aged donor cells. One of these genes, alpha-B-crystallin, is associated with the maintenance of the cellular cytoskeleton. The consequence of up-regulation of gene expression in human aging remains to be determined. Possibly these changes are simply adaptations to accumulated ravages of environmental or metabolic (oxidative) stress.

Some of the most definitive age-dependent changes in gene expression are observed when aged donor cells are analyzed during different forms of physiologic stress. This observation is perhaps not surprising, given clinical observations that elderly persons often respond less well than young adults to physiologic stress, such as infections, environmental extremes, and hypoxic events.

CELLULAR DEFENSE MECHANISMS

Age results in altered responses to physiologic stress. Cells have specific reactions to thwart injury and death. Damage may result from ultraviolet light, heat, lack of oxygen, absent nutrients, and metabolic oxidants. Cells have multiple strategies to cope with various forms of stress by means of stress-inducible transcription factors. For instance, ultraviolet radiation affects the transcription factor NF-κB, whereas thermal stress causes the transcription factor heat-shock factor (HSF1) to be activated. The thermal stress response can also be evoked by hypoxia, heavy metals, and other types of injury. Damaged intracellular proteins trigger the cytoplasm-located transcription factor to translocate to the nucleus and bind to a gene promoter region containing consensus nucleotide sequences GAA. HSF1 binding to the heat-shock element increases RNA polymerase activity, leading to elevated expression of mRNAs for various heat-shock proteins.

Heat-shock proteins have multiple functions. They primarily function as chaperones to allow protein trafficking and organelle transmembrane transport. Other functions include refolding damaged proteins and newly synthesized polypeptides. Heat-shock proteins interact with transcription factors, such as the steroid receptor, and serve as a type of molecular brake or attenuator of the transcription factor when conditions do not require its activation. During stress, increased need of heat-shock proteins causes the protein synthetic machinery to exclusively translate mRNA for heat-shock proteins. These proteins protect enzymatic function under stress. In short, heat-shock proteins assure proper protein levels and function so that cells may survive. Once overexpressed, their efficacy is sustainable, as witnessed by the increased ability of cells to withstand subsequent lethal stress.

The study of the human heat-shock response is an excellent paradigm for understanding how aging affects basic responses to cellular injury. One reason is that all species studied thus far have consistently revealed age-related decrements in various components of the heat-shock response. This fact illustrates how inducible responses, rather than constitutive responses, go awry with age.

The primary age-dependent defect of the heat-shock response occurs in the transcriptional trigger. Age causes approximately a 50% reduction in observable DNA binding after stress of old donor cells. Loss of HSF1–DNA binding with age appears to be multifactorial. This age-dependent change in stress-inducible HSF1 binding results in marked reduction in the rate of mRNA production for all the heat-shock proteins. No one knows exactly what levels are necessary for full protection from cell death; however, levels are likely proportional to the degree and duration of cell stress. In other words, higher levels of heat-shock proteins are needed if the cellular stress is severe, whereas lower levels are capable of handling mild to moderate stress. Most importantly, increased susceptibility to cell death results from altered heat-shock gene expression. For example, heat-shocked human lymphocytes from elderly donors aged 75 years and older result in earlier cell death and involve more cells than young donor lymphocytes. Despite this observation, controversy exists whether age represents a defect in apoptosis or programmed cell death. When fibroblasts are serially passaged, the cells passaged very late minimally produce heat-shock genes when thermally stressed, yet these cells are resistant to another form of death, namely, serum deprivation. These seemingly paradoxical observations are reconcilable when one considers that apoptosis can occur through several pathways, not all of which are equally affected by age.

Observations regarding senescence and cell stress demonstrate an emerging principle, that inducible responses requiring enhanced gene expression are attenuated by aging. The attenuation of inducible stress responses may be due to the accumulation or overexpression of heat-shock proteins in the nonstress state, which raises a provocative question, whether senescent cells are in a state of low-grade stress.

One concern is whether age results from elevated expression of certain genes, perhaps triggered by some internal chronometer. So far, no clear evidence exists for genes that evoke the senescence phenotype. However, experiments with nematode aging show that manipulation of *daf-2*, a mutation that confers longevity, may result in secretion of a factor that regulates the pace of aging. Similarly, in *Drosophila* studies, manipulation of the methuselah gene, which is homologous with G-regulatory proteins, can extend life span. By comparison, the decline in estrogen levels in aging women has been cited as a waning systemic factor that prevents bone, brain, and vascular deterioration. However, there is no hormonal factor known to extend human life span, and it is not clear whether changes in the hormonal axis with aging influence the rate of aging or merely represent an adaptive response to intrinsic tissue changes.

CELL DEATH

Experimental investigations have assessed the impact of aging on cell death. Cell death may occur by necrosis or apoptosis. In the former case, massive cell injury results in chromatin clumping and disorderly breakdown of cellular components. On the other hand, apoptosis is an active suicidal mechanism in response to external or internal stimuli. Apoptosis is essential to tissue maintenance, and it is especially important in down-regulating immune responses, such as clonally expanded lymphocytes, when infections resolve. Age-dependent problems with apoptosis could result in leukemias, lymphomas, and abnormal tissue repair.

Apoptosis is recognized by compaction and segregation of chromatin adjacent to the nuclear membrane, condensation of the cytoplasm, and nuclear fragmentation. DNA "ladders," detected in acrylamide gels, represent the orderly enzymatic degradation of DNA. Membrane-bound apoptotic bodies are phagocytized. Gene products activate and block apoptosis. For instance, cysteine proteases (ICE, CPP32, and ICH-1)

initiate apoptosis, whereas *bcl-2* and HIAP (human inhibitor of apoptosis protein) block or prevent apoptosis.

It has been suggested that apoptosis plays a role in neurodegenerative diseases associated with aging. The neuronal loss observed in Alzheimer's disease is possibly due to cytotoxicity of aggregated β-amyloid, which can induce apoptosis in cultured cells. Putative toxins such as free radicals created during neuronal transmission have also been implicated in neuronal cell death seen in Parkinson's disease; however, the exact role of apoptosis in aging and diseases of aging remains an area of ongoing research.

CALORIC RESTRICTION AND METABOLIC AND INSULIN SIGNALING

Dietary restriction without malnutrition can increase both the average and maximum life spans in a wide variety of species, including yeast, worms, flies, spiders, fish, hamsters, rats, and mice. Although calories are severely restricted (up to 40%), essential nutrients such as vitamins and minerals are maintained at levels equivalent to those found in ad libitum diets. The diet-restricted animals exhibit a delay in the onset of physiologic and pathologic changes with aging. These include hormone and lipid levels, female reproduction, immune function, nephropathy, cardiomyopathy, osteodystrophy, and malignancies. Size, weight, fat percentage, and some organ weights are markedly less in calorically restricted animals. Leanness per se is not necessarily an important feature in life span extension (see below). However, small body weight early in life is a predictor of longevity in genetically heterogeneous mice. Caloric restriction in rhesus monkeys leads to reductions in body temperature and energy expenditure, consistent with changes seen in rodent studies in which aging is retarded by dietary restriction. Calorie restriction also increased high-density lipoprotein and retards the postmaturational decline in serum dehydroepiandrosterone sulfate in the rhesus monkeys. However, it is too soon to assess whether life span is affected in these primates, given that they can live 50 years or more. Caloric restriction in mice retards the age-associated accumulation of mtDNA mutations. Perhaps very importantly, caloric restriction reduces oxidative damage in flies, rodents, and primates.

In yeast, the benefits of caloric restriction are mediated by the enzyme Sir2. Overexpression of Sir2 in both yeast and worms enhances longevity. Sir2 belongs to the sirtuin family of proteins, which are present in other animals and humans. Screening of sirtuin-activating compounds (STACs) has revealed that resveratrol, a plant polyphenol that is commonly found in red wine, potently activates Sir2 and thereby prolongs life span in yeast. Furthermore, resveratrol also enhances life span in fruit flies and worms, and does so without impairing reproduction. Resveratrol has also been found to exert anti-inflammatory, antioxidant, anticancer, and vasoactive effects upon human cells. These studies hold out the possibility that STACs may act to enhance life span in humans. They may also explain some of the potential benefits of red wine consumption and lay the foundation for the development of calorie restriction mimetics to be used in humans.

There are multiple single gene mutations that extend life span in yeast, worms, flies, and rodents. Many of the products of these genes appear to play roles in metabolic and insulin-signaling pathways and also enhance the organism's resistance to oxidative stress. Animals lacking expression of the growth hormone–releasing hormone are long lived, but are small and exhibit delayed puberty. Similarly, knockout of the growth-hormone receptor results in small subfertile animals that are long lived. Growth hormone acts via the insulin or insulin-like growth factor 1 (IGF-1) pathway. In worms, flies, and mice, mutations in insulin receptor substrate (IRS) genes, the insulin receptor, and the IGF-1 receptor enhance longevity. A study in transgenic rats suggests that caloric restriction may also act, in part, independently of the GH-IGF-1 axis. The first single gene mutation that was described in worms to extend life span is in the AGE-1 gene, which appears to code for the homologue of the human phosphoinositol-3-kinase gene, which in turn is a downstream effector of IGF-1. In worms, a neuron-specific mutation in the insulin-signaling system extends life span. In addition, reducing the activity of heat-shock factor 1 (HSF-1) shortens life span, whereas overexpression of heat-shock protein 70F

increases life span in worms. Interestingly, HSF-1 is required for insulin–IGF-1 signaling. Mice with a knockout of the insulin receptor specifically in adipose tissue are longer lived. Furthermore, mice heterozygous for a knockout of the IGF-1 receptor (homozygous knockouts are lethal) are longer lived, while exhibiting normal fertility and essentially normal size. These mice display increased resistance to oxidative stress, as do many of the long-lived mutants noted above. Polymorphisms in the IGF-1 receptor gene and the phosphoinositol-3-kinase gene result in lower plasma IGF-1 levels in humans and are more represented in long-lived individuals. Therefore, there appears to be an evolutionarily conserved endocrine regulation of aging by insulin-like signals. Though more research is needed, these pathways represent potential targets for drug development that may delay or even prevent physiologic and pathologic concomitants of aging.

REFERENCES

- Barzilai N, Rossetti L, Lipton RB. Einstein's Institute for Aging Research: collaborative and programmatic approaches in the search for successful aging. *Exp Gerontol.* 2004;39(2):151–157.

- Finkel T. Ageing: a toast to long life. *Nature.* 2003;425(6954):132–133.

- Kim S. Molecular biology of aging. *Arch Surg.* 2003; 138(10):1051–1054.

- Longo VD, Finch CE. Evolutionary medicine: from dwarf model systems to healthy centenarians? *Science.* 2003;299(5611):1342–1346.

- Troen BR. The biology of aging. *Mt Sinai J Med.* 2003;70(1):3–22.

CHAPTER 3—PSYCHOSOCIAL ISSUES

KEY POINTS

- The older adult faces many psychosocial issues. Stressors can be modified or mediated by factors both internal and external to the individual. Positive modification of the stressors can improve outcomes.

- Stressors such as caregiving, loss and grief, and changes in social status and social roles are more common in the lives of older adults; successful adaptation to stressors can improve

health outcomes; unsuccessful adaptation can lead to health declines.

- Implementing healthy behaviors can be beneficial, regardless of age.

- Social networks and positive interpersonal relationships can significantly moderate age-related stressors and lead to improved health.

Appreciating the role and scope of psychosocial aspects of aging improves clinicians' ability to address and treat factors that have important bearing on the overall well-being of older persons. Health events have broad ramifications. When they are viewed within a framework that includes both the stressors and the means to ameliorate the impact of stress, other factors besides the treatment of the disease itself can be seen to need clinical attention.

Stressors are any demands that call forth a physiologic, behavioral, or emotional response; often, such demands are perceived as threats. Unchecked stressors can lead to negative outcomes directly related to the situation as well as to more indirect negative outcomes across the whole spectrum of physical and mental health, economic welfare, and family life. Given the range of demands posed by the stressors, it is evident that they can greatly affect a person's physical and mental health, including every aspect of his or her well-being. The person's ability to function in the world may be reduced; the enthusiasm the person brings to and the pleasure he or she takes from social interaction may also be reduced. The use the person makes of financial, health, and social service resources may also be strongly affected.

Figure 3.1 offers a framework for considering the complex interaction of physical and psychosocial factors shaping the outcomes of stressors confronting older persons; the figure also structures the material presented in this chapter. The chapter briefly discusses common psychosocial threats faced by older persons, but it is principally focused on immutable and mutable factors that bear on the direct and indirect outcomes of stress situations, all with an eye to offering the clinician important tools for treatment as well as targets for therapeutic intervention. The chapter highlights findings from social science research that indicate ways in which unchangeable facts about a person's life (eg, gender) contribute to the outcome of stress situations—and to a person's ability to respond to them. In particular, the chapter discusses mediators and moderators, factors that can serve to filter, though not entirely protect against, the impact of stress through different mechanisms. Mediators involve the older person's perceptions of and responses to the stress situation. Moderators—which may be constituents of an older person's environment or behaviors in which the person engages—can be thought of as acting on the stressor itself to lessen its intensity or buffer its effect; they also affect a person's ability to respond to the stressor. Assisting older persons to see and work toward health outcomes that impact the quality of their life is an appropriate and effective clinical strategy for helping them to confront declines in physical health and the issues of mortality.

STRESSORS

The older person faces a great number and variety of stressors that are produced by a broad range of events and conditions. The stressors may be chronic, or they may have sudden, dramatic onset. They may be based in diseases or they may be of a more social nature. A chronic stressor may be health related (eg, the pain and mobility limitation of arthritis) or it may be psychologic (eg, the prolonged worry over a chronically ill spouse). An acute stressor might also be physical or psychologic (eg, learning of a newly diagnosed medical condition or experiencing the unex-

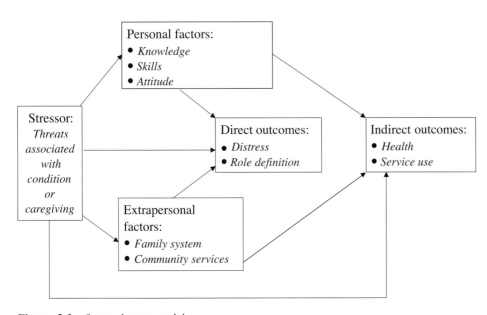

Figure 3.1—Stress theory model

pected death of a close friend). Other stress demands include changes in social identity due to role loss in retirement or the function-driven need to move to a more supportive living arrangement. Losses in physical capacity and reserve may place demands on the person, not only because he or she perceives them as threats or increased physical demands, but also because of their accompanying psychologic component, the perception that he or she may have diminished capacity to respond to other demands. Always in the background for older persons are the various risk factors for incident or recurrent morbidity and mortality.

Some risk factors—particularly those involving behaviors over which the person (with some encouragement, teaching, and counseling) might exert control—may be modifiable. Other risk factors, such as gender and race, are not modifiable and produce accumulated assaults that may amplify other stressors. The increasing incidence of diseases with age means that the number and frequency of stressors are likely to increase as a person ages.

Caregiving

Caregiving is nearly endemic; more than 44 million Americans care for family members of all ages. Gender is an important factor; more than 70% of all caregivers are women. Many older persons are caregivers for a family member. Chronic diseases affect a large proportion of elderly persons, and much of the care they receive is provided by family members, especially spouses. The burden of caregiving for dementing disorders like Alzheimer's disease is typical. Dementia caregivers spend many hours each day in caregiving activities, and they do so for many years (20% are caregivers for more than 5 years). Such caregiving exacts a heavy toll. Caregivers are at twice the risk as their noncaregiving peers for adverse physical and mental health outcomes and more than twice as likely to be taking psychotropic medications. Social isolation, family disharmony, and economic hardships are common sequelae of caregiving.

Caregivers need training, information, and support, and they should be regularly observed for signs of the known effects of caregiving. Attention to family dynamics may also be useful in identifying issues contributing to stressors that are modifiable. A number of intervention programs (eg, those providing education, counseling, and cognitive-behavioral therapy) have proven effective in ameliorating the stress associated with caregiving. Disease-specific support activities offer only modest relief but may be the conduit for more focused help.

Loss and Grief

Being widowed, especially for women, is a common occurrence in old age; so, too, are deaths in one's extended family and larger social network. More than 1 million spouses will be widowed in the United States in 2003; by 2030, more than 1.5 million spouses will be widowed annually. In 2000, 8.3% of those between 65 and 74 years of age were widowed; 22.7% of those older than 75 were widowed. Other losses, such as sensory and functional losses imposed by the onset of chronic or acute illnesses, also produce grief. Such losses are generally understood to be among the major negative life events, and they place a substantial demand on a person. For most, the intense experience of grief lasts 6 to 12 months, generally a time of withdrawal and depression. After about a year, a more accepting period ensues, during which a re-emergence into a social milieu occurs or a less affecting form of more permanent memorialization of the lost person is established. Acknowledgment and monitoring of the grieving process and active treatment for the depression associated with loss can help in avoiding prolongation of this process. (See also "Depression and Other Mood Disorders," p 247.)

Role Loss and Acquisition

People typically encounter a large number of role shifts in aging. They leave work and social roles that may have provided economic rewards as well as status. For example, the Social Security administration made 1.8 million new awards in 2001, a year in which 2 million Americans turned 65. The average age of retirement has been in steady decline, dropping to slightly under 62 years of age in 1995–2000 (down more than 5 years since 1950–1955). Within relationships, roles may change, and wage-earning spouses, after retirement, may find themselves in significantly greater contact with each other. Grandparenthood and great-grandparenthood provide both new demands and opportunities. Functional losses may place older persons in help-seeking rather than help-providing roles, or, as noted above, another's losses may place one in a caregiving role. These role changes can be stressful and can negatively affect mental or physical health. Retirement planning can help make these positive experiences. The clinician's assessment of an older person's role loss and acquisition may suggest the need for interventions.

Social Status

Three factors are consistently associated in the United States with a broad range of negative psychosocial and physical outcomes: being nonwhite, being a woman, and being poor or poorly educated (usually a surrogate for being poor). They should serve as warnings for clinicians, as the presence of one or more of these factors may add to the person's stress load. They may also affect the kinds of coping mechanisms the person has available. Lack of disposable income, for example, may exclude the use of some formal services or involvement in community activities that come with a fee. Cultural status may present other challenges; women from some cultures, for example, may face special barriers to exercising in public.

Race has a direct bearing on health stresses and longevity in old age. A 65-year-old black American man can expect to live nearly 2 years less than a 65-year-old white American man (a pattern mirrored among black American and white American women). A person's ethnic or cultural background and community context may substantially affect the outlook she or he brings to bear on a situation, the kinds of moderating activities she or he deems acceptable, and the importance she or he places on various outcomes. Older persons may understand disease through frameworks specific to other cultures, and treatment may need to include or rely principally on culturally centered options. A concept like autonomy that has become so central in issues of patient choice and advance directives has a different weight and value in cultures where choice belongs more to the community as a whole (as with some American Indian groups) or to a community or family leader (eg, in Hmong societies). Choices like hospice care may be viewed in some cultures as tantamount to wishing for and bringing about the death of the person. A procedure like autopsy may strongly violate cultural or religious beliefs. The clinician is advised to proceed attentively in cross-cultural situations. (See also "Cultural Aspects of Care," p 46.)

MEDIATORS

Mediators shape a person's responses to stress. They are the internal and external resources the person can bring to bear to assess and interpret the stress, to assess his or her own capacities for addressing it, and to formulate a coping response to it. Many key mediators are modifiable through psychosocial intervention. Instruction and information can affect the person's understanding of a situation. Various forms of psycho-education have been shown to be effective in enhancing an older person's sense of mastery within a stress situation and in increasing his or her awareness and use of formal services. Family counseling and therapy can strengthen older person's involvement with his or her social network.

Self-efficacy Beliefs

A number of constructs have been studied that relate to a person's sense of his or her own ability to manage situations. The concept of self-efficacy is comparable to concepts such as mastery, internal locus of control, resilience, and competence, and although it is singled out here, it resembles these in representing a key personal quality to be considered when dealing with an older person facing any stress situation. Self-efficacy is an important consideration for the mental and physical health of older persons for two reasons.

First, there is a relationship between strong or positive self-efficacy and a number of important health and mental health outcomes (Table 3.1). A large number of longitudinal studies—most notably the MacArthur study of "successful" or healthy aging—have produced a coherent set of conclusions about self-efficacy. The way a person approaches a situation—whether it be a specific threat, like the onset of an acute condition, or a more pervasive one, like change of life roles or decline in physical performance—affects the eventual outcome. Of particular note in Table 3.1 is the broad range of effects of strong self-efficacy beliefs, which influence physical and mental health as well as overall function. In addition, self-efficacy seems to contribute to a person's ability to be actively engaged in life, an important moderating factor.

The second reason self-efficacy is important is that it is modifiable. It can be weakened by repeated assaults and poor outcome, but it can also be strengthened. Among the strategies effective for strengthening self-efficacy are the following:

- performance accomplishment (seeing oneself succeed in a series of increasingly difficult tasks);
- vicarious learning and social modeling (seeing others like oneself succeed in a targeted area);

Table 3.1—Physical and Mental Health Impacts of Self-Efficacy Beliefs

Strong self-efficacy beliefs

- Buffer the effects of stress exposure on physical and mental health
- Contribute to overall physical performance, independently of ability
- Help maintain good function
- Slow functional decline among those with poor physical performance
- Contribute to good choice making, good performance, and persistence of effort (especially in women)
- Contribute to increased productivity

Weak self-efficacy beliefs

- Are associated with declines in functional status, especially in those with decreased physical performance

- encouragement (being persuaded to undertake a targeted activity); and
- reinforcement (experiencing pleasure from success).

A number of training programs aimed at improving specific performance (eg, reducing the fear of falling or increasing adherence to an exercise regimen following a heart attack) have succeeded by working to strengthen participants' self-efficacy beliefs in the targeted area. Strong self-efficacy beliefs appear to be better predictors of performance than are measures of physical ability. In falls prevention studies, for example, those with strong self-efficacy beliefs related to falling were found to show reduced fear of falling, despite low objective measures for risk of falling. Self-efficacy appears to play an important role in coping and overall well-being in older persons. Clinicians should assess the older person's sense of his or her own competence and intervene, where possible, to strengthen it.

Coping Strategies

A number of theorists have studied the manner in which older persons meet and address the accumulated challenges of aging. Cultivating an emotional response to a stressor can mediate its effect and produce a better outcome. Thus, invoking confidence and optimism in the face of bad news helps a person to meet the challenge and strengthens the likelihood of a positive outcome. One strategy older people may use consists of selection, optimization, and compensation. In this strategy, as people age, they begin to hone down the number and kinds of things in which they engage on the basis of what they believe they do well, selecting activities in which they are more likely to succeed. They also reframe the way they judge their own performance, looking, for example, at people their own age or older for a source of comparison. They do the selected things more, and they derive optimal credit for doing them. As losses continue and performance diminishes, people employ compensatory strategies that allow them to put their remaining performance capacities in the best light possible. A person known for preparing elaborate dinners might, for example, choose a simpler main course (selection) that she does well and has prepared many times (optimization) and surround it with numerous but very simple courses and side dishes as a way of favorably setting it off (compensation). Other coping strategies (eg, assimilation, accommodation, immunization, or resilience) also build essentially on the notion of reframing the self or one's performance in order to provide positive reinforcement and to reinforce self-esteem. Clinicians should attempt to learn how their patients typically form successful responses to challenges and help them to address new challenges in these same terms.

Social Involvement

Like people at all ages, older persons are faced with developmental tasks and challenges. In Erikson's theory of staged development, the task of old age is integration—putting the pieces together in a way that both celebrates and continues to act on the learning and accomplishments of life. In this conception, and consistent with many other findings, involvement (sometimes termed *productivity*) plays an important role. Becoming more involved, actively seeking out ways to contribute to and participate in the broader world, even engaging in paid work are all mediators that can lead to better outcomes. Taking part, making a contribution—through volunteering, productive (sometimes paid) labor, active family roles (especially child care), and participation in group activities—are all associated with older persons' continued well-being.

In terms of the framework of factors affecting health outcomes, social involvement can be understood as a positive, problem-focused coping response, a way of filtering the effects of a stressor by strengthening the connection of the person to the community (affirming the person's value in the community). Older theories of normal aging saw disengagement—the systematic withdrawal of ties to the social world—as normative. In current thinking, however, such disengagement is not encouraged and might even be considered an abnormal behavior. At the very least, there is an association between lack of social involvement and affective disorders such as depression.

MODERATORS

Moderators are components of a person's life or behaviors in which the person engages that act to affect the demands of the various stressors he or she faces. Moderators may be in place before the onset of a stressor or they might be developed in response to it. A person who has a long history of exercise already has a good base of conditioning to deal with an emergent condition affecting mobility (eg, arthritis). Alternately, making a decision to begin to exercise, to control diet or alcohol consumption, or to cease smoking is a possible—and healthy—response to stressors ranging from the onset of illness to a realization that one has slowed down. These healthy behaviors directly moderate the effect of the threat or demand and contribute to better physical and mental health outcomes. Having a strong social network and calling on it in a time of crisis (rather than withdrawing) may help moderate age-related demands (for example the loss of a loved one).

The literature points to three major activities that moderate stress or demand and that appear to contribute to healthy aging: social involvement, spiritual or religious activity, and engaging in healthy behaviors. Older persons' activities in these areas should be assessed regularly and encouraged, as appropriate.

Social Networks

The older person's social network is a critical resource for overall well-being, and social isolation is a powerful risk factor for broad declines and mortality. The effect of their social networks on older persons' overall well-being has been extensively studied, and the results of these studies are conclusive (Table 3.2). The literature points to the importance of quality over quantity but does not discount the latter. The closeness of social relationships is most important; thus, a well-functioning marital or familial relationship—a relationship that provides a person with a confidante—will offer the kinds of support and protection suggested in Table 3.2. Dysfunctional close relationships—those characterized by negative and conflict-filled interactions—appear to work in the contrary direction. The size of an older person's social network appears to work in both directions. On the one hand, having a larger social network offers the opportunity for greater involvement and contribution; on the other hand, it presents the likelihood of experiencing a greater number of losses within the network (because of death or increased disability).

A robust social network both mediates and moderates age-related stresses. Social networks provide emotional and instrumental help in times of crisis. Families help older persons, for example, weather the death of a spouse or close friend, but they also provide direct and indirect help when more functional losses occur. The social network can provide a person under stress with a context within which to envision and frame responses to various demands. Social networks seem to exert a positive effect on older persons by strengthening their self-efficacy beliefs (the person feels valued within the social network, and this contributes to a sense of self-value). It also provides opportunities for taking action to address demands (eg, calling on family for specific functional assistance, spending more time with children following the death of a spouse, increasing time spent with friends following retirement).

The literature is clear that the provision of such help is positive and contributes to recovery, unless it sends the wrong message. Too much instrumental assistance provided to older people (particularly men) by the social network may contribute to continued disability. Rather than being encouraged to work toward restored function, a person may receive too much help or not be encouraged to self-care and may,

Table 3.2—Physical and Mental Health Impacts of Robust Social Networks

- Reduced mortality risks
- Better physical health outcomes
- Better mental health outcomes
- Reduced risk of ADL disability or decline
- Increased likelihood of ADL recovery
- Buffered impact of major negative life events
- Promotion of strong self-efficacy beliefs
- Assistance that does not preclude self-care but that may increase risk of new or recurrent ADL disability (especially in men)

NOTE: ADL = activities of daily living.

therefore, accept a modifiable condition as permanent. Thus, although assistance from the social network should be encouraged, it should be done with attention to promoting maximum function by the person receiving the help.

Spiritual or Religious Involvement

Studies have consistently demonstrated two important facts about religion and older people. First, religion plays a more important part in the lives of older persons; older persons are more actively involved than younger persons in attending religious services and in carrying out regular private religious practices. More than 50% of older persons report frequent attendance at religious events (with little variation by gender or race). Second, there are consistent positive relationships between religious involvement and indicators of good health. Whether religious activity contributes to social integration, promotes involvement, or assists in the developmental tasks of aging, it seems clear that it is a positive force—at least for those already inclined to it.

Healthy Behaviors

Implementing positive behaviors (eg, exercise; controlling intake of food, tobacco, and alcohol; and active relaxation or stress-reduction techniques) have all been shown to have positive effects on overall well-being, no matter at what age they are begun. Although these are physical behaviors, they often rely on and benefit from strong psychosocial mediators, particularly self-efficacy and social networks. Clinicians should use these mediators when proposing older persons begin or strengthen healthy behaviors. It can help to invoke a person's understanding of benefits and appreciation of his or her own proven ability to make change while at the same time offering suggestions about how the targeted behavior might contribute to a strong social network (eg, "you could walk every day with your daughter," "you and your husband could take the healthy cooking class together").

REFERENCES

- Blazer DG. Self-efficacy and depression in late life: a primary prevention proposal. *Aging Ment Health.* 2002;6(4):315–324.

- Fry PS, Debats DL. Self-efficacy beliefs as predictors of loneliness and psychological distress in older adults. *Int J Aging Human Dev.* 2002;55(3):233–269.

- Krause N. Exploring age differences in the stress-buffering function of social support. *Psychol Aging.* 2005;20(4):714–717.

- Krause N. Exploring the stress-buffering effects of church-based and secular social supporton self-rated health in late life. *J Gerontol B Psychol Sci Soc Sci.* 2006;61(1):S35–S43.

- Pinquart M, Sorensen S. Associations of stressors and uplifts of caregiving with caregiver burden and depressive mood: a meta-analysis. *J Gerontol B Psychol Sci Soc Sci.* 2003;58(2):P112–P128.

- Rowe JW, Kahn RL. *Successful Aging.* New York: Pantheon Press; 1998.

- Smith J, Maas I, Mayer KU, et al. Two-wave longitudinal findings from the Berlin aging study: introduction to a collection of articles. *J Gerontol B Psychol Sci Soc Sci.* 2002;57(6):P471–P500.

CHAPTER 4—LEGAL AND ETHICAL ISSUES

KEY POINTS

- Four guiding ethical principles of American medical practice are beneficence, nonmaleficence, justice, and the respect for autonomy.

- A clinician may evaluate a patient's *capacity* to make decisions; *competence* is a legal term implying that a court has taken action.

- Substituted judgment is the process of constructing what a person would have wanted.

- Living wills are advance directives that describe the decisions a person would make under specified circumstances.

Normative ethics is the inquiry into the standards of what we see as right or wrong action. It focuses on the question "What *ought* I do?" Medical ethics is based on a utilitarian ethical structure; that is to say, it is not based on deontological overarching moral imperatives (as a religious ethic would be), but rather seeks the answer to the *ought* question through the principles that are applied in the context of the clinical situation with the goal of providing the greatest beneficence (ie, maximizing good consequences and minimizing bad consequences). These principles are tethered to values and perspectives that are unique to each culture and that may differ, depending on whether one is talking about a specific case (situational ethics) or about public policy.

The four guiding principles for American health care practice most often cited are the following: respect for autonomy, nonmaleficence, beneficence, and justice. How each of these principles guides the practice of medicine today is different from even 50 years ago. These principles and their application also differ widely within various subcultures within the American culture.

The primacy of individual autonomy is a foundation of American culture, from the early pioneers to modern health care practice. Respect for individuals' autonomy should include respect for their right to subjugate their individualism to family, culture, or religion. In many cultures, family structure dictates who will be the decision maker for individuals within that family, and that person is deferred to even when the individual involved retains the ability to make his or her own decisions. However, even when such dictates are absent, clinicians all too often consult with and defer decisions to the adult child of an elderly patient who is capable of making decisions for him- or herself.

Nonmaleficence is, in essence, the Hippocratic "do no harm." What a culture or an individual may view as harm differs widely. The most frequently cited conflict between mainstream and subculture perspectives is that concerning blood transfusions for a Jehovah's Witness. For a Jehovah's Witness, blood transfusion causes more harm than the alternative, even if that alternative is death. But views of harm will also vary from individual to individual. Understanding the values of subcultures within our society may help to give us clues as to the spectrum of the values that underlie that individual's perspective on harm. Similarly, what constitutes beneficence, doing more good than harm, is very culture bound as well as specific to the individual. (See "Cultural Aspects of Care," p 46.)

Finally, the concept of justice and health care in our society is still very ambiguous. There is not a recognized right to health care in the United States. The distribution of health care benefits and the use of health care technologies continue to be very uneven and reflect biases regarding gender, age, race, and ethnic origin. Researchers have typically not included older adults in their study populations, and the lack of knowledge on the relative effectiveness of interventions when they are used for older patients may lead to the under- or overutilization of interventions in this age group. Furthermore, assumptions that equate age with chronic illness and comorbidity may deny beneficial treatment to healthy elderly patients. Patients from groups that have long been denied many of the benefits of our society, especially our health care dollars, may be more reluctant than more historically privileged patients to step back from aggressive treatments because of a perception of continued prejudice.

It is important to keep these differences in mind when considering the following discussions of ethical decision making and its application to the individual patient. These are, in a true utilitarian sense, guiding principles, not moral imperatives. Just as the "laws" of medical science differ from case to case, these principles need to be used as they apply to each individual situation.

DECISIONAL CAPACITY

Because of the nature of the diseases affecting older persons, clinicians are often called on to assess a person's decision-making capacity and to use other, appropriate sources of decisional authority when that capacity is impaired. Although the focus of much of the literature has been on clinicians' assessments of patients' capacity to make medical decisions, clinicians are also asked to render opinions on patients' ability to make decisions about other matters, such as managing money, writing a will, continuing to drive, or possessing firearms. It is important to use the correct terminology in discussing the clinician's responsibility. A clinician may evaluate a patient's capacity to make decisions, but *competence* and *incompetence* are legal terms, and they imply that a court has taken a specific action.

Assessment of Patients' Decisional Capacity

Assessing the patient's ability to understand the consequences of a decision is the overarching principle used in making a judgment of decisional capacity. To make a medical decision, the patient must be able to understand the basic information about his or her condition and the probable outcomes of the disease and of various potential interventions. This requires the ability to understand the disease process; the proposed therapy and alternative therapies; the advantages, adverse effects, and complications of each therapy; and the possible course of the disease without intervention. The patient needs to be able to understand the broad consequences of accepting, deferring, or rejecting a proposed intervention. Admittedly, even clinicians cannot predict the full implications of complex medical decisions, since they can rarely know all the consequences of an intervention or the precise natural history of an illness. Nonetheless, the patient should be able to make decisions that are based on his or her beliefs and values. Therefore, it is often most helpful for the clinician to explore a patient's hopes and fears and to help the patient clarify his or her goals so that the treatment options that are offered are based on these goals. Cultural differences of the members of ethnic minority groups can make assessing decision-making capacity a more difficult task than it already is. Capacity assessment involves abstract concepts not easily communicated in another language. It also involves interpreting value judgments on the basis of what is considered reasonable; this may differ according to culture. Clinicians must avoid assuming on the sole basis of ethnic background that a patient holds certain beliefs and evaluate each patient by considering his or her own biopsychosocial circumstances.

The capacity to make a living will is similar to that of being able to make treatment decisions, although it is somewhat more complicated, since the patient is being asked to think in the abstract, with a "what if?" frame of reference. The ability to choose a health care proxy (see below) is much less complex, and even fairly impaired patients are often able to choose someone to make decisions for them.

The requirements are even less stringent for *testamentary competence* (the ability to make a last will and testament). In general, a person's ability to decide how he or she wishes to dispose of belongings after death is felt to be preserved even when the person is very cognitively incapacitated in other ways. As long as the person can identify the individuals involved, is not delusional or in other ways psychiatrically ill such that judgment is impaired (eg, paranoia), and is capable of understanding the consequence of signing the will, he or she is considered to have testamentary competence.

Table 4.1 summarizes the elements of decisional capacity in each of these four areas.

Table 4.1—Decisional Capacity

Medical decisions
- Ability to understand relevant information
- Ability to understand the consequences of the decision
- Ability to communicate a decision

Decisions of self-care
- Ability to care for oneself *or*
- Ability to accept the needed help to keep oneself safe

Finances
- Ability to manage bill payment
- Ability to appropriately calculate and monitor funds

Last will and testament
- Ability to remember estate plans
- Ability to express logic behind choices

Standardized Tests of Decisional Capacity

Traditional tests of cognitive function have some, but limited, utility in determining decisional capacity. An overall score on the Folstein Mini–Mental State Examination (MMSE) of 10 or less indicates such diminished cognitive ability that it is unlikely that the person retains decisional capacity. Some deficits uncovered by the use of the MMSE may be relevant (eg, immediate memory, attention, word finding, understanding simple verbal or written instructions, and ability to express simple ideas in writing). Others are not (eg, calculation and visual-spatial relationships). As we come to appreciate the influence of frontal lobe dysfunction on a patient's capacity to function, especially to perform complex activities of independent living, we are also coming to appreciate the influence that the cognitive domains tested with executive function have on decisional capacity. Executive functions include problem solving, planning (including appreciating consequences of an action), initiation, capacity to monitor one's own behavior, and inhibition of inappropriate behaviors. The Executive Interview 25-item examination (EXIT 25) of executive function has been shown to correlate well with subjective measures of decisional capacity. Observation of the patient while completing tasks on the examination may reveal poor insight, impulsivity, intrusion of irrelevant material, poor self-monitoring, and impaired ability to form and follow through on a plan. Clinicians may make similar observations by observing a patient draw a clock.

Specific tests of decisional capacity have been developed. The Capacity to Consent to Treatment Instrument asks the person to read two vignettes and then decide between two treatment options. The Competency Assessment Test helps judge the person's ability to understand advance directives. Both instruments deal with hypotheticals, thereby adding more abstraction than is necessary for deciding real-time issues. The MacArthur Competency Assessment Tool—Treatment tests the person's ability to make a specific decision and has the advantage of dealing with real-time decisions. Assessment of decisional capacity is a functional assessment; therefore, there is no substitute for critical observation of the process itself.

Principles Governing Decision Making for Patients Who Lack Decisional Capacity

The hierarchy of decision-making strategies for those making the decisions for incapacitated patients is as follows: 1) respect their last competent indication of their wishes, 2) use substituted judgment, and 3) determine their best interests (ie, an analysis of benefits versus burden). Table 4.2 summarizes the hierarchy.

The last competent indication of wishes is most relevant in cases when patients are able to foresee that they will become incapacitated and can foresee what decisions will need to be made. Patients entering the terminal phase of an illness who know that at some point they will become confused or unconscious can give very clear advance directives (also called *advance care plans* in some contexts) stating their preferences for care. As long as the circumstances remain substantially as predicted, other persons should not be allowed to reverse these decisions.

Substituted judgment is the process of constructing what the person would have wanted if he or she had been able to foresee the circumstances and give directions for care. In theory, those who know the person best and understand what his or her fears, pleasures, and goals were (ie, what the patient's rationale for a decision would have been) can provide substituted judgment. This is usually, but not always, the next of kin. A patient can appoint someone to hold durable power of attorney for health affairs (designating that person as what is also referred to as a *health care agent* or *proxy*). The patient chooses the person who can best represent him or her. Any such surrogate makes decisions only if the patient has become incapable of making decisions. The person granted durable power of attorney takes precedence over the next of kin.

The best-interest standard or the principle of beneficence guides clinicians in making a medical decision for an incapacitated patient on the basis of the benefits and burdens an intervention poses for that person. When there is no expressed wish by the patient and no one to offer substituted judgment, then the surrogate decision maker must weigh the benefits and the burdens of treatment for that person in order to make a decision. Such analysis is best done by someone

Table 4.2—Hierarchy of Decision Making

Patient's current wishes

- If the patient has decisional capacity, this ALWAYS takes precedence

Substituted judgment

- Done by the surrogate decision maker only when the patient is not fully capable of making the decision
- Based on the patient's prior values and wishes
- Advance directive is used as guide
- Patient input is used when possible even if the patient is not fully capable of making the decision

Beneficence

- Done by the surrogate decision maker when the patient lacks decisional capacity and evidence does not exist for substituted judgment
- Weighing of benefits and burdens as based on the patient's present indications of pleasures and burdens
- Input from caregivers is very important

who is very aware of what gives that patient pleasure, what causes agitation, fear, pain, or discomfort, and how the patient reacts to a change in setting, use of restraints, and similar matters.

Conservatorships and Living Wills

In the absence of next of kin or durable power of attorney for a patient lacking decisional capacity, the court may appoint a conservator (called a *guardian* in some states). There are usually two types of conservatorship: conservator of finance and conservator of person. Incompetence in matters of finance is usually determined either by the demonstrated incapacity of the patient to manage financial matters (eg, unpaid bills, uncashed checks) or through specific testing by either an occupational therapist or a neuropsychologist. A conservator of person is required when the patient has demonstrated that he or she can no longer make personal decisions (such as medical decisions) or care for him- or herself to the point that the patient endangers him- or herself and cannot understand and accept the need for help (eg, neglecting oneself or risking injury)

Living wills are advance directives that attempt to demonstrate what decisions a person would make under certain circumstances. Most living wills address a couple of hypothetical clinical situations (eg, vegetative state, terminal illness) and four possible treatment options (cardiopulmonary resuscitation, respirator therapy, artificial feeding and hydration, and dialysis). A living will has limited utility because of its vagueness and lack of generalizability to the decisions that most commonly need to be made. Some living wills offer a detailed set of hypothetical case scenarios and treatment decisions, but these can be difficult for patients

to understand and may not add information about the person's rationale for decisions. An individual's reaction to a hypothetical event may differ from how he or she will deal with reality. Nonetheless, a living will can be used as evidence of preferences when one is trying to construct how a patient who lacks decisional capacity might have felt about an intervention.

The Role of the Incapacitated Patient in Decision Making

Even when patients may not be fully capable of making decisions, often they can still participate in decision making at many levels. A task assessment of decision-making ability around a specific issue is always appropriate. A patient with even very little cognitive ability can give some indication when something causes discomfort or displeasure or when something brings pleasure. The surrogate decision maker must consider these indications when analyzing the benefits and burdens of an intervention. Case law supports the idea that the patient's indications of preference should be given consideration.

The perceived relative burden of an intervention may vary from one person to the next because of differences in mental status and ability to cope with change or disability. A demented patient who is accustomed to one environment will have a much harder time adjusting to hospitalization and may need restraints in order to undergo even something as simple as intravenous antibiotic therapy. The relative benefit of this therapy should be weighed against the burden of hospitalization for such a patient.

It is nearly impossible to perform some interventions without the cooperation of the patient. If the conservator recommended a cataract operation but the patient refuses to cooperate, for instance, it is doubtful that the procedure could be performed. In other situations it may be hard to justify doing a major invasive procedure against the will of an alert and mildly to moderately impaired person, even though it could be done. An example is a patient with frontal lobe dementia who adamantly refuses cardiac surgery. A surrogate decision maker must consider the present status of the patient and the patient's wishes, concerns, pleasures, and pains. Even though a person may not be intellectually capable of consenting to (or refusing) a treatment, on some level his or her assent may be needed to administer that treatment.

Temporary Loss of Decisional Capacity

Patients may temporarily lose the ability to make decisions during acute confusional states, acute psychotic episodes, periods of unconsciousness from anesthesia or illness, or during an acute central nervous system event. Although in these cases, the patients can be expected to regain this ability over time, the rules described above still apply. Decisions that the patient has made before becoming temporarily incapacitated should be respected. A patient may reverse his or her do-not-resuscitate status while undergoing anesthesia with the understanding that it can be reinstated postoperatively. However, a patient who has stated that he would never agree to resuscitation should not have this reversed by a family member during a temporary confusional state due to an intercurrent illness.

When using either substituted judgment or best-interest standards in surrogate decision making for a patient with a transient loss of decisional capacity, the decision maker should err on the side of more aggressive intervention if there are situations in which the patient's wishes are not known or the circumstances are substantively different from what the patient had anticipated.

Informed Consent for Research

The new emphasis on the quality of consent obtained for participants in research must extend to the vulnerable populations of elderly persons. Still, it is imperative that researchers study dementia and related problems so that the care of these patients may improve. The two most vulnerable populations are those with cognitive impairment, by virtue of their inability to understand the study or their role in it, and institutionalized patients, who may feel coerced to consent. Research involving vulnerable populations needs to be particularly well designed and focused on issues of importance to that population because of their lack of free will in having others agree to their participation.

Guidelines developed by the American Geriatrics Society for informed consent for research on cognitively impaired persons are shown in Table 4.3.

DECISIONS NEAR THE END OF LIFE

Although the issues discussed in this section focus on the period near the end of life, the decision-making process and ethical principles described are the same for all medical decisions. All patients make decisions, consciously or subconsciously, concerning treatment of minor conditions, adherence with medical regimens, and related issues by weighing competing values and needs. When a person is faced with a terminal illness or a chronic, disabling, or progressive disease, decision making becomes more acute and focused. Patients, families, and clinicians must attempt to balance benefits

Table 4.3—AGS Guidelines for Research Using Cognitively Impaired Persons as Subjects

- The research must be justified on scientific, clinical, and ethical grounds but can be focused on conditions other than dementia itself.

- The capacity to give consent should be assessed for each individual for each research protocol since decision-making capacity is task specific and some cognitively impaired individuals will be able to give consent.

- Advance consent to participate in research given prior to the loss of decisional capacity should, in general, be respected.

- The traditional surrogates for decision making can be used to obtain consent.

- Research protocols that involve more than minimal risk or do not have a likelihood of direct benefit for the subjects should be offered only to persons who are able to consent or who have an advance directive consenting to participate in research. Exceptions might be made for exceptionally promising treatments, but this should be reviewed at a national level.

- Surrogates can refuse participation or withdraw the person from participation if the surrogate determines that the research protocol is not what the person intended to consent to or is not in the person's best interest, even if there is advance consent.

- Only in very unusual circumstances would the refusal to participate of even an incapacitated patient be overridden.

NOTE: AGS = American Geriatrics Society.
SOURCE: Data from AGS Ethics Committee. Informed consent for research on human subjects with dementia. *J Am Geriatr Soc.* 1998;46(10):1308–1310.

and burdens when making many health care decisions. This difficult task is further complicated by the fact that only probabilities of the benefits and burdens can be known, not certainties.

See also the section on end-of-life decision making in "Cultural Aspects of Care" (p 50).

Forgoing and Discontinuing Interventions

A patient's right to refuse unwanted treatment was confirmed by the Supreme Court of the United States in the 1991 case of *Cruzan* v. *Director, Department of Health of Missouri*. This refusal can occur before the intervention has been instituted or after it is in place. There is no ethical or legal distinction made between these two situations, often referred to in the more dramatic terms of *withholding* or *withdrawing* therapies. For example, in the case of uremia, a patient with kidney failure may decline to begin dialysis, thus increasing the risk of death from uremia. Alternatively, a patient may try dialysis for a period of time, even years, and then choose to stop this treatment and die from uremia. The same principle holds for discontinuing ventilatory support for a patient. The patient will die from his or her underlying respiratory disease whether ventilatory support is never started or if it is discontinued. The act of extubating a patient with the expectation that he or she will die is difficult for many clinicians because of the proximity of the act performed by the clinician and the death of the patient, but the decision is informed by the same ethical principles as is the decision to discontinue dialysis or to decline other medical interventions.

Clinicians and families often feel uncomfortable when a patient declines tube feeding and intravenous fluids. Case law, as well as the *Cruzan* case, characterizes these methods of delivering food and fluid as medical interventions; therefore, they are subject to the same ethical right of refusal that applies to any other medical intervention. Many people worry that the terminally ill patient will suffer without these interventions, but accumulated experience in hospice care has shown that it is usually easier to make someone comfortable without them: intravenous and gastric administration of food and fluid can cause discomfort through decreased gastric emptying and gastric distention, the need to replace intravenous lines or nasogastric tubes, and fluid overload as membranes become more permeable. These interventions may dampen or eliminate some of the natural comfort measures that occur, such as the release of endorphins.

Interventions That May Hasten Death

Palliative care, defined here as interventions that are given in order to relieve discomfort or suffering, may at times have the unintended effect of hastening death. We have come to accept that there may be two effects of a treatment, one (intended) effect of palliation, and the other possible (unintended) effect of hastening death. This is sometimes referred to as *the rule of double effect*. The intention of the application of the medical intervention is not to hasten death, but to palliate symptoms. Aggressive pain management, when respiratory depression is foreseeable but not intended, is generally seen as an ethical practice. Further, most evidence shows that gradually increasing narcotic dosage does not hasten death. The rule of double effect has been extended by some to cover the use of terminal sedation (without hydration) in cases in which any level of consciousness will constitute continued suffering, as is frequently the case in death from head and neck cancer, for example.

Physician-assisted suicide and euthanasia occur when an intervention is made with the clear intention of ending the patient's life. The underlying motivation of patients who wish to hasten death varies. In population-based surveys, people commonly cite fear of pain and of other suffering (such as shortness of breath, anorexia, nausea, constipation, insomnia, and anxiety) as the reason for considering physician-assisted suicide. Fear of being dependent or a burden to others is mentioned at least as often.

In the United States, unlike in some other countries that have addressed this issue, only physician-assisted suicide (and not euthanasia) is being considered for legalization. Because suicide is an act committed by the person who will suffer the consequences, it is felt that such a death is more clearly voluntary than a death that results from another person's administration of a lethal intervention. Although the Supreme Court has ruled that there is not a constitutional right to physician-assisted suicide, it did not rule that it is unconstitutional, either. Each state has been left to make its own laws in this regard. Some states have yet to act; many have made physician-assisted suicide explicitly illegal. Oregon has had legalized physician-assisted suicide since 1997. Experience there has shown that relatively few terminally ill patients request physician assistance with suicide. In the first 3 years after legalization, 91 patients out of 90,000 who died in Oregon availed themselves of physician-assisted suicide, yielding a rate of 1 per 1000 deaths. Prominent motivating factors were loss of autonomy and determination to control the way in which one dies.

Ability to Predict Time of Death

Despite increasingly sophisticated prediction models, especially for patients who are critically ill, patients still rely on their clinician's judgment for most assessments of prognosis. Instruments such as the APACHE III (the third version of the acute physiology and chronic health evaluation scoring system), which uses a combination of age, diagnosis, cause of acute illness, and a scale of physiologic parameters to predict mortality risk in acute illness, are unable to address issues of the burden of treatment or the patient's quality of life. Long-range predictions for patients with slowly deteriorating conditions are even more difficult. Physicians must certify that a patient has 6 months or less to live in order for that patient to qualify for the Medicare hospice benefit. Similarly, the Oregon Death with Dignity Act asks physicians to predict, using reasonable judgment, whether a terminal illness will result in death within 6 months. Patients often seek a precise prognosis from their clinicians as they weigh the benefits and burdens of interventions and consider quality-of-life issues as well as survival. Unfortunately, neither clinician judgment nor prediction rules have proven accurate in predicting prognosis under these circumstances.

The Continuum of End-of-Life Decisions Based on Goals

Decisions near the end of life are not all-or-nothing choices. The absence or presence of do-not-resuscitate orders (more accurately referred to as do-not-attempt-resuscitation orders) is often misinterpreted as instruction to the clinician either to do everything or to do nothing. This dichotomy is false.

Other medical interventions for seriously ill patients with similar prognoses may have very different outcomes. For example, a patient with New York Heart Association Class 4 heart failure from a cardiomyopathy may ask not to receive cardiopulmonary resuscitation but might choose to accept placement of an automatic implantable cardiovascular defibrillator or be given a "dobutamine holiday." A patient who is dying from lung cancer might weigh the relative burdens and benefits of antibiotic treatment for pneumonia before deciding whether to treat the infection. The benefits and burdens of enteral feeding are highly influenced by the condition being treated. Most studies that have been done on the utility of enteral feeding for patients who aspirate have grouped all patients with feeding tubes together, which may not be appropriate. These scenarios illustrate some of the variables:

- Patient 1 has had surgery for a localized pharyngeal cancer followed by radiation. The procedure has left the patient freely aspirating, making it difficult for him to take sufficient calories by mouth. The patient's overall prognosis is still uncertain.
- Patient 2 has Parkinson's disease and still functions well. His pharyngeal muscle coordination is slow, and he recurrently chokes on his food, especially thin liquids.
- Patient 3 has end-stage Alzheimer's disease. Although she has evidence of aspiration on a swallowing examination and has had two documented pneumonias that are probably related to aspiration, she seems comfortable when she eats. One of her few remaining discernible pleasures is eating.

The balance between benefits and burdens is very different for each of these patients. Enteral feeding may or may not prolong their lives, and restrictions on eating could have a different meaning for each. The recommendations by clinicians to each patient or patient's surrogate might include everything from feeding-tube placement and avoidance of taking food or drink by mouth to oral intake, as tolerated, for pleasure and the use of antipyretic medications for fevers. Before a choice is made, the patient or family must first clarify their priorities. The clinician can then decide how different approaches can best meet these goals.

SPECIAL ETHICAL ISSUES IN DEMENTIA

Although most of the topics discussed above intimately involve the ethics of caring for cognitively impaired persons, some areas of particular concern for patients with dementia merit further discussion.

Truth Telling

The ethics of truth telling has evolved considerably through the last half of the 20th century in mainstream American culture, breaking with the longstanding tradition of paternalism in medicine that advocated withholding bad news from patients in order to do no harm. In many other cultures, telling the truth is still not felt to be appropriate. In the United States, however, telling a patient that he or she has a dementing illness may be the last area of controversy about truth telling. Increasingly, both professional and lay people agree that patients with dementia should be given a chance to understand what is happening to them. The opportunity for the older person with early dementia to prepare legal documents (powers of attorney, a will, advance directives), to address personal issues, and to make plans is important. As therapies become available and research advances, it is imperative that persons with dementia be informed of their options and given the opportunity to voice their preferences, even though they may no longer be capable of giving fully informed consent.

Autonomy

Ensuring personal safety and avoiding harm to others are important concerns in caring for patients with dementia. Because of the very nature of the disease process and its effect on recent memory, patients may not perceive how they have changed; they may not be able to recognize when their problem interferes with their ability to make decisions. Some patients with dementia may not understand the consequences of their actions and may have difficulty planning because of frontal lobe dysfunction. This puts them at risk for behaviors that may endanger themselves or others, including unsafe driving, the continued possession of firearms, wandering, and socially inappropriate behaviors. Their care needs may exceed what their caregivers can provide, and they may be unable to understand the rationale for seeking help at home or for a sitter, day care, or nursing-home care. The clinician plays a crucial role in being able to objectively recognize when this has happened and to help the family or others to take the necessary steps to protect the patient and others.

Definition of Personhood and Advance Directives

Adults with intact decisional capacity not only have the right to make their own decisions but also always have the right to change their minds. Even when they become unconscious, their last competent statement was usually made close to the event, often with full knowledge of the decisions that will need to be made; the likelihood is low that their rationale for the decision or that their goals, fears, and pleasures had changed significantly. If life experiences do mold their thinking, or if new interventions or approaches to problems occur, they can alter their directive to fit with these changes. A person with a progressive cognitive disorder can change substantially over time. What brings pleasure and what causes fear or pain can change substantially from year to year; almost certainly a patient's perceptions change greatly as the disease progresses. The demented person is unable to comprehend the future and slowly becomes more and more disconnected from the past. In some ways, the person with advancing dementia becomes suspended in time: the person loses his or her connection to previous and future selves, the essence of what many define as personhood. A demented person is tied to the decisions and perceptions of a previous self whom he or she may not even remember. The decisions made by this prior "self" may inform current decision making, even though that person did not know what he or she would need or want at this time. Therefore, conflict can arise between the previous directives made by that patient and what is best for the demented patient in the here-and-now (ie, what gives the patient pleasure and what may disturb him or her).

Genetic Testing and Alzheimer's Disease

Relatives of persons with Alzheimer's disease are increasingly interested in knowing their risk of having the disease. For relatives of those who have a clear autosomal dominant, known single-gene mutation, as is the case with Huntington's chorea, genetic testing has proven useful when accompanied by safeguards of counseling and follow-up. In familial, early-onset Alzheimer's disease, several gene mutations have been found that cause clusters of Alzheimer's disease in families. For those clusters in which the mutation is known, mapping and phenotyping may be helpful in conjunction with counseling. For most familial clusters, however, the genes responsible have not been identified, and testing is not useful.

The value of testing is less certain in the case of apolipoprotein E alleles, which may influence a person's susceptibility or probability of having Alzheimer's disease sometime in the future. Many people with the high-risk alleles do not get the disease, and many without it do. As long as there is no intervention that has been shown to significantly alter the course of the

dementing process, it does not seem advisable to create anxiety when the predictive value of the test is so low.

See also "Dementia" (p 204).

ETHICS IN THE NURSING HOME

Although the ethics that apply to the treatment of patients in other settings apply to patients in the nursing home, some issues are brought more acutely into focus because of the setting and the concentration of patients with chronic and end-stage disease.

Treatment Decisions

Until policymakers and clinicians paid attention to the resuscitation status of patients in nursing homes, residents were assumed not to be candidates for attempted resuscitation. It was rarely, if ever, attempted. Studies that have looked at the outcomes of attempted resuscitation of patients in long-term-care facilities show that it is used infrequently and is associated with low long-term survival. However, the number of patients in long-term-care settings for short-term recuperation and rehabilitation has grown, which may change the statistics concerning the utility of attempted resuscitation of nursing-home patients.

Staff perceptions of the utility of resuscitation efforts differ by profession. Nursing staff strongly prefer to limit interventions in this setting, especially for older patients and those with cognitive impairments. On the other hand, clinicians tend to overestimate the benefit of interventions for these patients and sometimes hesitate to honor a do-not-resuscitate request for those who are not clearly terminally ill. Patient participation in the process is variable. Federal legislation requires the systematic inquiry into advance directives for all patients in institutions receiving federal funds. With the advent of this more systematic approach to discussions about treatment status, nursing homes have transferred fewer patients to acute-care settings, and yet patient and family satisfaction have not declined.

Regulatory agencies have encouraged enteral feeding of patients in nursing homes to prevent nutritional deficits in patients who may not be able to get enough nourishment by eating. Although the motives for enacting these regulations were compassionate, the usefulness of enteral feeding, especially for patients with advanced dementia, is questionable. Also, it is not ethical to use enteral feedings for a patient capable of taking oral sustenance but who may not be getting enough nutrition because a facility fails to provide patients with the help they need in eating. (See "Malnutrition," p 161.)

Restraints

The use of restraints in the long-term-care setting has become closely regulated and monitored. Studies have shown that using physical restraints has little, if any, value in preventing injuries from falls. Less restrictive alternatives are usually available. Clinicians and patients' surrogates must consider several factors in deciding whether to use restraints. If the patient is engaging in activities that might harm other residents or staff, and when intervention is ineffective or the patient's surrogate refuses it, then the institution's responsibility to protect others may require that it send the patient elsewhere.

Conflicts of Interest

The allocation of resources in nursing homes is closely linked to the ability of nursing-home care to prevent complications of chronic illness. When staffing falls below a critical level, pressure ulcers, functional decline, depression, agitation, and the need for restraints may increase. Appropriate activities to meet the patient's physical, cognitive, and emotional needs, although sometimes referred to as the "hotel" functions or "recreation," are also part of the good medical care of these patients. The role of the nursing-home medical staff in monitoring and participating in this process needs further clarification.

MISCELLANEOUS ISSUES

Driving

Older persons with physical and cognitive impairments have as high a risk of motor vehicle collisions per mile driven as do teenage drivers. Health care providers face complex ethical problems when caring for older patients who endanger themselves and others by driving. The conflicting values are powerful: respect for the patient's autonomy, duty to protect the patient from harm, duty to protect others from predictable danger, and respect for patient-doctor confidentiality. Educating the patient and family members is often the key to developing a practical solution. Legal requirements regarding reporting of unsafe older drivers by physicians, nurse practitioners, or other health care providers vary from state to state. In some states, physicians are required to report patients who may be unsafe; in other states they are permitted to do so; and in a few states, reporting may be considered a violation of patient-doctor confidentiality. (See also the section on the older driver in "Assessment," p 45.)

Ethics and Health Care Financing

The ethical issues regarding the financing of health care have become much more salient in an era of rapidly rising costs and managed care. Health care professionals need to be aware of the forces, both positive and negative, exerted by payment structures on the nature of the care delivered. Ideally, providers, aware of these forces, will take maximal advantage of the positive forces and work to guard against the negative forces when caring for patients. The two major care payment structures to health care providers, fee-for-service and capitation, influence care differently.

Fee-for-Service Structures

Fee-for-service (FFS) care means that the provider receives payment for each service rendered. The built-in advantage of an FFS method is that providers have an incentive to be thorough in the diagnosing and treating of patients; the more services a provider performs (and documents), the more he or she is paid. Patients receiving FFS care may be more reassured that the provider is doing everything possible to care for them. The potential disadvantage of FFS care is overtreatment of patients, resulting in unnecessary iatrogenic morbidity and mortality as well as increased costs.

About 85% of older adults receive care from "traditional" Medicare, a system that compensates providers under an FFS arrangement (see "Financing, Coverage, and Costs of Health Care," p 29). Medicare FFS providers have relative incentives to provide covered benefits and disincentives to perform noncovered services. The primary method of controlling overall costs in an FFS system is to carefully delineate which services are covered and to discount payments for those services. The catalogue of Medicare-covered services is published as the *Current Procedural Terminology* coding system. One of the most common areas in which providers may feel pressured to stretch the truth, or to lie outright, is in the coding of conditions and procedures in order to make sure that patients will not be left liable for bills.

Capitation Structures

Capitation means prepayment for the care of a patient population on the basis of the number of patients, regardless of the amount of care the provider performs. Under the Medicare Advantage option (formerly the Medicare Plus Choice option), which is selected by about 15% of Medicare beneficiaries, health plans (not individual providers) receive capitation from the Centers for Medicare and Medicaid Services based on the number of enrollees (see "Financing, Coverage, and

Costs of Health Care," below). Capitation arrangements provide incentives for the prevention of serious (and costly) conditions, commonly through the use of disease management programs, health promotion efforts, and care management. Analysts describe capitated care as proactive and FFS as reactive. The chief concern regarding capitation is an inherent underservice bias; the less that is spent on the patient, the more the provider or plan may profit. Providers receiving capitation, or any other incentive to restrict costs, have an ethical obligation not to undertreat their patients.

REFERENCES

- AGS Ethics Committee. Informed consent for research on human subjects with dementia. *J Am Geriatr Soc.* 1998; 46(10):1308–1310.

- Marson DC. Loss of competency in Alzheimer's disease: conceptual and psychometric approaches. *Int J Law Psychiatry.* 2001; 24(2–3):267–283.

- Post SG, Whitehouse PJ. Fairhill guidelines on ethics of the care of people with Alzheimer's disease: a clinical summary. Center of Biomedical Ethics, Case Western Reserve University, and the Alzheimer's Association. *J Am Geriatr Soc.* 1995; 43(12):1423–1429.

- Quill TE, Lee BC, Nunn S. Palliative treatments of the last resort: choosing the least harmful alternative. *Ann Intern Med.* 2000;132(6):488–493.

- Sullivan AD, Hedberg K, Fleming DW. Legalized physician-assisted suicide in Oregon—the second year. *N Engl J Med.* 2000;342(8):598–604.

- The Hastings Center. *Guidelines for the Termination of Life-Sustaining Treatment and the Care of the Dying.* Bloomington, IN: Indiana University Press; 1987.

CHAPTER 5—FINANCING, COVERAGE, AND COSTS OF HEALTH CARE

KEY POINTS

- Medicare Part A covers hospital, skilled nursing home, and home-health and hospice services; Medicare Part B covers physicians, nurse practitioners, social workers, psychologists, therapists, laboratory tests, and durable medical equipment. Medicare Part D (optional) covers some of the cost of prescription medications.

- Medigap supplemental insurance plans are available that cover Medicare Part A and Part B deductibles and co-insurance costs, as well as preventive care and other health-related goods and services.

- The Medicare Personal Plan Finder (http://www.medicare.gov/MPPF/home.asp) can assist patients in selecting a Medigap plan or Medicare HMO and in comparing nursing facilities and home-health-care agencies.

- Medicaid is a joint federal and state program that provides supplemental health insurance (including long-term custodial care in nursing homes) to people of all ages who have low incomes and limited savings.

In 1965, the U.S. government passed legislation designed to improve access to acute health care for people who are old, disabled, or poor. During the decades that followed, the resulting Medicare and Medicaid programs expanded, evolved, and spawned thousands of supplemental commercial insurance plans. Today, a complex and often confusing array of personal payments, public programs, and private insurance plans (see Figure 5.1) pays for and thereby determines much of the health care that older Americans receive.

This chapter describes, through the eyes of patients and providers, how these programs influence the day-to-day care of older people. It illustrates their effects during a year in the life of Mrs. Rose Murat, an imaginary 79-year-old retired schoolteacher who lives with her 83-year-old husband in a small older home. Mrs. Murat has hypertension, coronary artery disease, and mild heart failure, for which she takes hydrochlorothiazide, metoprolol, lisinopril, and nitroglycerin. Her total out-of-pocket payments for these medications are $104.67 per month.

OUTPATIENT CARE

At the end of her quarterly office visit, Mrs. Murat asks for advice on joining a health maintenance organization (HMO) that has been marketing a Medicare health plan in her county. She is impressed by the HMO's offer of free eyeglasses, hearing aids, and

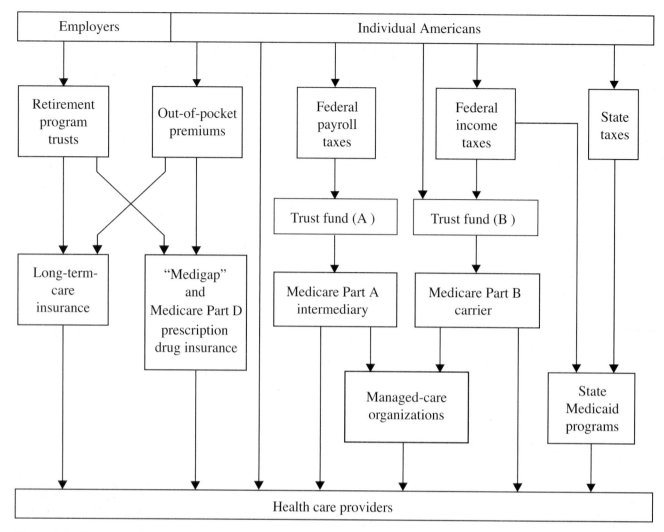

Figure 5.1—The flow of funds for the health care for older Americans.

preventive check-ups, all of which she has purchased out-of-pocket in the past. Her options, summarized in Table 5.1, are as follows: staying with traditional fee-for-service (FFS) Medicare as her only coverage; keeping FFS Medicare and applying for either Medicaid or supplemental ("medigap") coverage; or exchanging her FFS Medicare coverage for membership in the Medicare HMO. Depending on the Murats' income, savings, and state of residence, they may also qualify for a Medicare assistance program that pays for some combination of their Medicare premiums, deductibles, and co-insurance costs. Some older Americans may have additional health insurance options through the federal Department of Veterans Affairs or through their (or their spouses') present or previous employer or union.

Medicare is a federal insurance program run by the Centers for Medicare and Medicaid Services (CMS) that pays health professionals and organizations to provide acute health care for Americans who are 65 and older, disabled, or suffering from end-stage renal disease. As originally enacted, Medicare comprises two separate FFS plans (Part A and Part B), each of which pays predetermined amounts for specified health-related goods and services that are needed by its beneficiaries. More than 80% of older Americans are covered by both plans.

Medicare Part A uses regional insurance companies ("intermediaries") to pay hospitals, nursing homes, home-care agencies, and hospice programs for the Medicare-covered services they provide. Older Americans (and their spouses) who have had Medicare taxes deducted from their paychecks for at least 10 years are entitled to coverage through Part A without paying premiums. Others may be able to purchase Part A coverage (for $189 to $343 per month, depending on how long they had Medicare taxes deducted from their paychecks).

Medicare Part B uses other regional insurance companies ("carriers") to pay physicians, nurse practi-

Table 5.1—Health Insurance Coverage for Older Americans

	FFS Medicare		Supplemental Coverage		Medicare HMO Plan [b]
	Part A	Part B	Medicaid [a]	Medigap Policy	
Covers the cost of:					
Hospitals	100% [c]	—	$912	$912	100%
Postacute care in SNF	100% [d]	—	—	—	100%
Hospice	100% [e]	—	—	—	—
Home care ("medically necessary")	100%	100%	—	—	100%
Durable medical equipment	80% [f]	80% [f]	20%	20%	100%
Diagnostic laboratory tests	—	100%	—	—	100%
Diagnostic imaging tests	—	80%	20%	20%	100%
Physicians, nurse practitioners	—	80%	20%	20%	100%
Outpatient PT, OT, ST	—	80%	20%	20%	100%
Outpatient services, supplies	—	80%	20%	20%	100%
Emergency care	—	80%	20%	20%	100%
Ambulance services	—	80%	20%	20%	100%
Preventive services	—	[g]	20%	20%	[g, h]
Outpatient mental health care	—	50%	50%	50%	100%
Custodial care in nursing home	—	—	100%	—	—
Hearing, vision services	—	—	[i]	[i]	[i]
Outpatient medications	—	—	[i]	[i]	[i]
Additional costs to patient:					
Deductibles	$912 [j]	$110 [k]	—	[i]	[i]
Monthly premiums	—	$78	—	[i]	[i]

NOTE: FFS = fee for service; HMO = health maintenance organization; OT = occupational therapy; PT = physical therapy; SNF = skilled nursing facility; ST = speech therapy.

a Under the Balanced Budget Act of 1997, state Medicaid programs were given the option whether or not to pay deductibles and co-insurance costs.

b Some Medicare Advantage plans require members to pay deductibles and copayments.

c After the beneficiary or secondary insurer pays the deductible amount ($912).

d For the first 20 days of SNF care following a hospital stay of at least 3 days.

e Patient makes copayments of $5.00 per outpatient prescription and 5% of cost of respite care.

f When patient is receiving Medicare-covered home care.

g 100% of allowed cost of fecal occult blood test, Pap smear interpretation, prostate-specific antigen test, blood tests for diabetes and cardiovascular disease, and influenza and pneumococcal vaccinations; 80% of allowed cost of mammograms and clinical examination of breast and pelvis (no deductible applies); after the annual Part B deductible has been paid, 80% of allowed cost of a general physical examination at age 65, glaucoma screening, sigmoidoscopy or colonoscopy or barium enema, digital examination of rectum (men), measurement of bone mass, hepatitis B vaccination, and diabetic education and equipment.

h Some Medicare Advantage plans cover additional preventive services.

i Benefits and costs vary widely among medigap insurance plans and state Medicaid plans.

j Per benefit period (first 60 days following hospital admission).

k Annual.

tioners, social workers, psychologists, rehabilitation therapists, home-care agencies, ambulances, outpatient facilities, laboratory and imaging facilities, and suppliers of durable medical equipment for the Medicare-covered goods and services they provide. At age 65, people become eligible for Part B coverage if they are entitled to Part A coverage or if they are citizens or permanent residents of the United States. To obtain this coverage, eligible persons must enroll in Part B and pay premiums ($78 per month), usually by agreeing to have them deducted from their monthly Social Security checks.

Providers must choose whether to participate in the FFS Medicare program. For each Medicare-covered service performed, a participating provider will submit a claim to the Part B carrier, accept Medicare's fee for the service (80% of its preestablished "allowed" amount), and bill the patient or her secondary insurer for no more than a 20% co-insurance payment. For services not covered by Medicare, the provider may bill the patient, if the patient agrees in advance in writing. Providers who do not participate in Medicare can bill patients directly for up to 15% more than 95% of Medicare's allowed amounts. The patients pay the providers and then submit their requests to Medicare for partial reimbursement (ie, for 80% of 95% of the allowed amounts). Some providers choose to enter into "private contracts" with older patients. Under these contracts, Medicare (and medigap insurance plans) pay nothing, and patients pay providers the full amount of the fees specified by the contracts.

Neither Part A nor Part B of the Medicare program covers periodic physical examinations, outpatient medications, dental care, hearing aids, eyeglasses, foot care, orthopedic shoes, cosmetic surgery, care in foreign countries, or custodial long-term care at home or in nursing homes. Part B covers some preventive services (see Table 5.1).

Beneficiaries pay out-of-pocket for:

- monthly premiums for Part B ($78),
- annual deductible for Part B ($110),
- the deductible for Part A ($912 per benefit period, ie, the first 60 days following an admission),
- co-insurance payments (usually 20%) for goods and services for which Medicare or other insurance pays only a portion, and
- the full cost of those goods and services that are not covered by Medicare or other insurance, including outpatient prescription medications.

In 2003, the U.S. Congress passed and President George W. Bush signed a sweeping Medicare reform bill that included an option (Medicare Part D) for beneficiaries to purchase insurance coverage for prescription medications beginning in 2006. If Ms. Murat were to choose this option, she would pay annual premiums ($324), deductibles ($265), and co-insurance (25% of her remaining medication expenses or a copay depending on the plan); the plan pays 75% until the combined total equals $2000. The "gap" or "doughnut hole" is the time when there is no plan contribution once the $2000 annual threshold has been reached until a total of $3600 has been spent out-of-pocket for the year. Monthly premiums do not count toward the $3600. For more information, see www.medicare.gov.

Medicaid is a joint federal and state program that provides supplemental health insurance to people of all ages who have low incomes and limited savings. The exact criteria for Medicaid eligibility and the benefit packages provided by Medicaid programs vary considerably from state to state. Most programs pay Medicare Part B premiums, and some pay Medicare deductibles and co-insurance costs. Most important, Medicaid pays for long-term custodial care in nursing homes for those who qualify. Several states have begun offering fixed capitation payments to managed-care organizations that are willing to provide Medicaid and Medicare benefits to residents who are "dually eligible" (for Medicaid and Medicare).

Medigap supplemental plans fill some of the holes in the insurance coverage provided by Medicare Part A and Part B. Private insurance companies offer FFS medigap plans of ten types (A through J), classified according to the benefits they cover. For new Medicare beneficiaries at age 65, the premiums for A-level (basic) plans across the United States range from $40 to $125 per month. These policies cover a person's Part A and Part B co-insurance costs, for example, 20% of Medicare's allowed fees for durable medical equipment and providers' services. (In Minnesota, Wisconsin, and Massachusetts, A-level medigap policies are required by law to cover more than just the costs of Medicare co-insurance.) B-level plans cover Part A and Part B co-insurance, plus the Part A deductible ($912 per benefit period). Each successive level of medigap policy provides additional benefits and costs more. J-level plans cover co-insurance, deductibles, care in foreign countries, preventive services, and some of the cost of medications—at a cost of $175 to $400 per month. Consumers can obtain less expensive medigap coverage by purchasing plans that require the insured to pay high deductibles (F- and J-level plans only) or plans that cover the services of only selected providers and hospitals ("Medicare SELECT" policies). Medigap policies do not cover long-term care, dental care, eyeglasses, hearing aids, or private-duty nursing.

Within 6 months of their initial enrollment in Medicare Part B, beneficiaries are entitled to purchase any medigap policy on the market at advertised prices. After this open enrollment period, medigap insurers can refuse to insure individual beneficiaries or charge them higher premiums because of their past or present health problems.

Medicare HMOs hold contracts with CMS specifying that, for each Medicare beneficiary they enroll, they will provide at least the standard Medicare benefits in return for fixed monthly capitation payments. In order to attract enrollees, most Medicare HMOs also cover additional benefits and charge low or no premiums, deductibles, and copayments. The HMOs achieve cost savings by managing their enrollees' use of services within their networks of providers, with whom they negotiate price discounts in return for patient volume. Each January the HMOs have the option of changing their premiums, benefits, and provider networks—or of discontinuing their Medicare plans altogether.

Each November, beneficiaries covered by Medicare Part A and Part B have the option of joining any Medicare HMO operating in their area; they cannot be denied enrollment because of any health problems except end-stage renal disease. Enrollees must continue to pay their monthly Medicare Part B premiums, and they must obtain their health care from the HMO's provider network. They have the option of leaving the HMO at any time and going back to the FFS Medicare program. The primary advantages and disadvantages of each of Mrs. Murat's options are outlined in Table 5.2. Extensive information about all the options is available to consumers at each state's medical assistance office, at 1-800-MEDICARE (1-800-633-4227) or 1-877-486-2048 for hearing-impaired TTY users, and at the Medicare Personal Plan Finder (http://www.medicare.gov).

Table 5.2—Advantages and Disadvantages of Four Types of Health Insurance

Type of Insurance	Primary Advantages	Primary Disadvantages
FFS Medicare (Parts A, B, and D)	Traditional Medicare benefits, choice of any provider that participates in the Medicare program, partial coverage for prescription medications	Cost of co-insurance, deductibles, noncovered goods and services (eg, eyeglasses, hearing aids)
Medicaid	Coverage of co-insurance, deductibles, and some benefits* not covered by Medicare	Choice of providers restricted to a single network in some states
Medigap insurance	Coverage of co-insurance, deductibles, and some benefits** not covered by Medicare	Out-of-pocket monthly premiums range from $40 to $400, depending on the coverage provided by the policy purchased
Medicare Advantage plan (eg, HMO)	Traditional Medicare benefits plus coverage of additional goods and services**	Choice of providers restricted to a single network; potential for changes in premiums, copayments, deductibles, benefits, and providers at the discretion of the plan

NOTE: FFS = fee for service; HMO = health maintenance organization.

* Benefits vary from state to state.

** Benefits vary from plan to plan.

Managed Care

Mrs. Murat's provider of primary care, knowledgeable about her health and prognosis, can help her to choose the plan(s) that will cover the goods and services that she needs, both now and in the future. If she can obtain what she is likely to need from the HMO's network of providers, joining the HMO might be her best option, because it will allow her to obtain "free" eyeglasses, hearing aids, and preventive services and to avoid paying the usual Medicare premiums, deductibles, and co-insurance. Data about the quality of care and the satisfaction of other enrollees in all the local Medicare HMOs are available at the Medicare Personal Plan Finder.

In the event that she needs health care that is not available from the HMO's network, or if she is reluctant to change providers, retaining the flexibility of her traditional Medicare coverage (which covers her use of any provider that participates in the Medicare program) might be a better choice for Mrs. Murat, especially if she also qualifies for Medicaid or buys a medigap policy. Information from Medicare's information line or from the Medicare Personal Plan Finder would help her compare the prices and coverage of the medigap policies available in her area.

The recommendations of Mrs. Murat's primary care provider are likely to be influenced by the characteristics of the different plans Mrs. Murat is considering. For instance, if the primary care provider is not in the HMO's service network, the provider would point out to Mrs. Murat that her enrollment in the HMO would require her to select a new primary care provider. If the primary care provider is in the HMO's network, Mrs. Murat's enrollment would change (ie, probably reduce) the payment for her care. As shown in Table 5.3, the payments would depend on the type of HMO involved. If it is a group or independent practice association (IPA) model, the HMO may pay providers "discounted FFS," that is, less than Medicare Part B would pay for each service. Or it may pay primary providers a fixed capitation amount each month to cover specified services. If these services are limited to primary ambulatory care, the capitation amount will be relatively small. The HMO may reward primary providers with end-of-the-year bonus payments if they have limited their referrals to specialists and their admissions to hospitals. If the covered services also include specialty and inpatient care, the capitation amounts will be considerably larger, and the provider will have incentives to use these services judiciously because he or she will have to pay for them, at least in part.

Fee for Service

Under the Medicare FFS system, providers obtain the fairest possible reimbursement by understanding and following CMS's payment system, which is based on evaluation and management (E&M) codes (see Table 5.4).

For each Medicare-covered service provided, the provider submits to the regional Medicare carrier the appropriate E&M code and the international classification of disease (ICD) code that indicates the diagnosis for which the service was provided. Entries in the medical record, which are subject to audit, must document that the data collection and medical decision-making aspects of the service conform to standards established for the E&M code submitted. By providing and documenting services efficiently, providers can maximize their FFS reimbursements within the (tight) limits imposed by the Medicare fee schedules.

Table 5.3—How Medicare HMOs Pay Providers of Health Care

	Type of HMO		
	Staff Model	Group Model	IPA Model
Providers	Employees	One large group practice	Many small independent practices
Method of payments	Salary	FFS or capitation*	FFS or capitation*

NOTE: FFS = fee for service; HMO = health maintenance organization; IPA = independent practice association.

* The services covered by the capitation payments range from "primary care only" in some plans to "medications and all acute care" in others.

Table 5.4—Fee-for-Service Reimbursement by Medicare, Year 2005

E&M Service	E&M code	"Allowed" Amount ($)*	%	CMS Payment ($)**
Comprehensive office visit, new patient	99205	179	× 0.80 =	143
Detailed office visit, established patient	99213	55	× 0.80 =	44
Detailed office visit (mental health problem), established patient	99213	55	× 0.50 =	28
Comprehensive office consult	99245	230	x 0.80 =	184
Comprehensive inpatient consultation***	99255	201	× 0.80 =	161
Complex hospital admission	99223	161	× 0.80 =	129
Complex hospital follow-up visit	99233	81	× 0.80 =	65
Comprehensive nursing facility initial assessment	99303	111	x 0.80 =	89
Detailed nursing facility follow-up visit	99313	82	× 0.80 =	66
Comprehensive initial home visit	99345	205	× 0.80 =	164
Detailed follow-up home visit	99349	114	× 0.80 =	91
Home-health certification	G0180	77	x 0.80 =	62
Care plan oversight	99375	131	× 0.80 =	105

NOTE: E&M = evaluation and management; CMS = Centers for Medicare and Medicaid Services.

* For physicians who participate in Medicare; amounts vary by location (see http://www.cms.hhs.gov/physicians/mpfsapp/ for local rates and annual updates).

** For eligible services provided by nurse practitioners, payment is 85% of the amount shown.

*** Hospital or nursing facility consultation.

Regardless of the payment mechanism, the crucial question is whether the amount of payment suffices to support high-quality care. For example, if capitation rates are below the aggregate cost of the services they are intended to cover, the provider will feel pressure to take on more patients and limit the amount of service that each patient receives. Similarly, if FFS amounts are too small, the provider will feel pressure to schedule more visits and procedures and to reduce the time devoted to each patient. Each provider should, therefore, monitor carefully and continually the many changing elements in the practice environment (eg, payment schedules, covered services, expenses, patients' and families' expectations, population demographics) to help determine the numbers and types of services that are appropriate for each older patient.

INPATIENT CARE

Four months later, Mrs. Murat awakes dysarthric and unable to feel her left hand. Her face is asymmetric, and her left arm and left leg are weak. Her husband calls 911; the ambulance rushes her to the nearest emergency department, where the physician on duty diagnoses a right hemispheric stroke and admits her to the hospital.

Managed Care

If Mrs. Murat had joined the Medicare HMO, the HMO would pay for the ambulance, emergency, and physician services; in most cases, it would pay the hospital a prenegotiated lump sum or a per diem fee to cover all of her inpatient care. The amount of this lump sum would be determined by the diagnosis-related group (DRG) of her discharge diagnosis—in this case, stroke. If the admitting hospital had no contract with her HMO, Mrs. Murat would probably be transferred to a hospital in the HMO's provider network as soon as she was medically stable. Depending on the HMO's benefit package, she might be responsible for copayments and deductibles for some of these services.

Fee for Service

If Mrs. Murat had retained traditional Medicare as her only health insurance, she would have to pay Medicare's required deductibles ($110 per year under Part B for the ambulance and the emergency medical care, plus $912 under Part A for the hospital admission) and co-insurance amounts (20% of Medicare's allowed charges by physicians and the ambulance service). She would also have to pay any ambulance charges in excess of Medicare's approved fee. If she had supplemented her Medicare coverage, her Medicaid or private medigap coverage would cover some of these deductibles and co-insurance payments. She would not be transferred to another hospital for insurance reasons.

The hospital would submit its claim for emergency and inpatient care, which would be based on the DRG of her discharge diagnosis, to Medicare's Part A regional intermediary insurance company. The involved physicians and the ambulance service would submit their E&M coded claims to Medicare's Part B regional insurance carrier. The intermediary and the carrier would pay their shares of these costs and, if Mrs. Murat had supplemental coverage, they would forward requests for payment of the balances to the state Medicaid program or her medigap insurance company. Ultimately, CMS would reimburse the intermediary from the Medicare Part A Trust Fund and the carrier from the Medicare Part B Trust Fund.

POSTACUTE REHABILITATION

After 4 days of stabilization, evaluation, and rehabilitation, Mrs. Murat is deemed stable enough for discharge from the acute-care hospital. She has improved somewhat, but she is still mildly hemiparetic and dysarthric, and she is apathetic and easily fatigued. Because her days in the hospital are fewer than the average number of hospital days associated with the DRG of her discharge diagnosis (ie, 5.9 days) and because her discharge diagnosis is one of those listed in Table 5.5, CMS regards her "early" discharge as a "transfer." This permits CMS to reduce the amount it pays the hospital for her care. The consulting neurologist advises her and her husband that her progress during the next few weeks will determine her potential for functional recovery. Mr. Murat asks the neurologist to recommend a rehabilitation facility for his wife.

Managed Care

If she had joined the Medicare HMO, Mrs. Murat's insurance coverage would include postacute rehabilitative care, probably at a nursing home in the HMO's provider network rather than at a rehabilitation facility.

Some nursing homes concentrate such high-acuity patients in transitional (or postacute) care units and provide them with coordinated rehabilitative (physical, occupational, and speech), social, and nursing services. Most homes, lacking such units, offer only custodial care supplemented by rehabilitative services as needed. The HMO would also cover the provider's postacute services, but the Murats may be responsible for a deductible and copayments.

Fee for Service

If Mrs. Murat could participate in rehabilitative therapy, Medicare Part A would pay for 20 days of postacute rehabilitation, in either a rehabilitation facility or a transitional (postacute) care unit of a nursing home. Upon her admission to either type of postacute care unit, rehabilitation professionals would evaluate Mrs. Murat's functional status, establish a plan for her care, and certify her as needing one of 26 levels of intensity of care according to the resource utilization group system (RUGS). Her RUGS category would determine the daily rate that Medicare Part A would pay the facility for the first 2 weeks of her care as long as she was demonstrating progress in rehabilitation. After 2 weeks, a nurse would reevaluate her status, update her plan of care, and adjust her RUGS category and thereby adjust Medicare's payments to the facility for the next 2 weeks. Under this prospective payment system (PPS), the facility would be responsible not only for Mrs. Murat's nursing, rehabilitative, and social services, but also for the costs of her medications, laboratory tests, and visits to an emergency department not resulting in admission to the hospital.

Using nursing-home rates, Medicare Part B would pay 80% of the allowed charges for the postacute medical care performed by her provider. Any postacute care related to an inpatient surgical procedure would be the responsibility of the surgeon, who would receive a "global fee" to cover the surgery and all postoperative surgical care. The Murats would need to satisfy Medicare Part B's $110 annual deductible and then make 20% co-insurance payments for the provider's care. Their out-of-pocket expenses would be reduced or eliminated by any Medicare supplements in effect, such as Medicaid, medigap, or long-term-care coverage.

More than 3 million Americans have long-term-care insurance policies, but these policies pay for less than 2% of all nursing-home care. The high premiums for these policies, combined with consumers' uncertainty about needing long-term care in the future and their doubts about the policies' ability to cover the costs of long-term care in the future, have limited the growth of the long-term-care insurance sector. Many middle-aged Americans believe they will retain good health and independence into old age; they appear to

Table 5.5—Primary Diagnoses for Which "Early" Discharges from Hospitals Are Regarded as "Transfers" to Postacute Care

Primary Diagnosis	DRG Number	Hospital Days, National Average
Degenerative nervous system disorders	12	8.1
Specific cerebrovascular disorders, except transient ischemic attack	14	5.9
Seizure and headache with complications and comorbidities	24	5.0
Seizure and headache without complications and comorbidities	25	3.2
Chronic obstructive pulmonary disease	88	5.1
Simple pneumonia and pleurisy with complications and comorbidities	89	6.0
Simple pneumonia and pleurisy without complications and comorbidities	90	4.1
Amputation for circulatory system disorders, except upper limb and toe	113	12.3
Circulatory disorders with acute myocardial infarction and major complications, discharged alive	121	6.4
Circulatory disorders with acute myocardial infarction without major complications, discharged alive	122	3.7
Heart failure and shock	127	5.3
Peripheral vascular disorders with complications and comorbidities	130	5.7
Peripheral vascular disorders without complications and comorbidities	131	4.2
Major joint and limb reattachment procedures for lower extremity	209	5.1
Hip and femur procedures except major joint with complications and comorbidities	210	6.8
Hip and femur procedures except major joint without complications and comorbidities	211	4.9
Fractures of hip and pelvis	236	5.2
Pathological fractures and musculoskeletal and connective tissue malignancy	239	6.3
Cellulitis with complications and comorbidities	277	5.7
Cellulitis without complications and comorbidities	278	4.3
Diabetes mellitus	294	4.6
Nutritional and miscellaneous metabolic disorders with complications and comorbidities	296	5.2
Nutritional and miscellaneous metabolic disorders without complications and comorbidities	297	3.4
Kidney and urinary tract infections with complications and comorbidities	320	5.3
Kidney and urinary tract infections without complications and comorbidities	321	3.8
Red blood cell disorders	395	4.4
Organic disturbances and mental retardation	429	10.0
Extensive operating room procedure unrelated to principal diagnosis	468	13.0
Tracheostomy for face, mouth, and neck diagnoses	483	39.6

NOTE: DRG = diagnosis-related group.

be relying on a combination of good fortune, social insurance (ie, Medicaid), and their personal assets to see them through their later years. Those who are interested in long-term-care insurance can obtain information by reading "Choosing Long-Term Care: A Guide for People with Medicare" (CMS Publication No. 02223) or "A Shopper's Guide to Long-Term Care Insurance" (available from state insurance departments or the National Association of Insurance Commissioners, 2301 McGee St., Suite 800, Kansas City, MO 64108-3600).

HOME-HEALTH CARE

During the first 10 days of rehabilitative therapy, Mrs. Murat regains her ability to speak, and her left arm becomes stronger. During the following 8 days, however, she makes few additional gains. After 18 days, she is still unable to walk, cook, bathe, or dress herself without help. Her lack of continued progress toward functional independence will probably make her ineligible for coverage of additional rehabilitative services in either the HMO or the FFS Medicare program. The Murats will have to purchase any future physical therapy or occupational therapy on their own.

To obtain long-term care for her functional deficits, they will need to choose between a home-health agency and a custodial nursing home. If she returns home, neither the HMO nor the FFS Medicare program will be likely to pay for a home-health aide unless she is homebound and requires the services of a registered nurse or rehabilitation therapist. Local community agencies, however, may be able to offer assistance. The Murats could find information to help them choose a home-health agency by comparing the recent clinical performances of their local agencies—available at Home Health Compare (http://www.medicare.gov/HHcompare/home.asp).

Managed Care

If Mrs. Murat's condition made her homebound and dependent on skilled professional services, her HMO probably would pay a home-health agency a fixed fee to provide her with the services and equipment necessary to treat her primary diagnosis. The HMO would also provide her with the services of a primary care provider.

Fee for Service

In the FFS environment, if Mrs. Murat were homebound and dependent on skilled professional services, traditional Medicare Part A would pay any Medicare-certified home-health agency a fixed fee to provide her with the services and equipment necessary to treat her primary diagnosis. Medicare Part B would pay her primary care provider 80% of the allowed charges for house calls, office visits, and care plan oversight services. In addition, Medicare Part B will pay her provider for home-health certifications and recertifications. The Murats would be responsible for the annual Part B deductible ($110) and the 20% co-insurance payments, unless they had supplemental coverage through Medicaid, a medigap policy, or a long-term-care policy. (See also "Community-Based Care," p 118.)

PACE

If a health care organization in the area had contracted with CMS and the state Medicaid agency to create a Program for All-inclusive Care of the Elderly (PACE), it could provide community-based long-term care for "dually eligibles" (people eligible for both Medicare and Medicaid) whose disabilities qualified them for custodial care in a nursing home. (See also "Community-Based Care," p 118.) If she were eligible for Medicaid and she enrolled in PACE, Mrs. Murat would attend an adult day health care center several days each week and receive comprehensive outpatient, inpatient, acute, and long-term care from a salaried interdisciplinary team composed of a physician, a nurse practitioner, a nurse, a social worker, rehabilitation therapists, and other members of the PACE staff.

NURSING-HOME CARE

Three months after Mrs. Murat returns home, Mr. Murat, now 84 years old, suffers a myocardial infarction and is no longer able to care for his wife at home. Their daughter logs on to Nursing Home Compare (http://www.medicare.gov/NHcompare/home.asp) to look for a nursing home. After comparing the local facilities' nurse-to-resident ratios, results of recent quality-of-care inspections, and rates of pressure ulcers and behavior problems, she arranges for her mother to enter a high-quality nursing home in her neighborhood, at least until Mr. Murat recovers.

Managed Care

If Mrs. Murat had joined the Medicare HMO, one of the HMO's providers would provide her primary care in the nursing home. Unless she was covered by Medicaid or a long-term-care policy, however, she and her husband would be responsible for the nursing home's per diem charges for room, board, and other basic services, usually about $100 per day. After "spending down" their savings at this rate, the Murats might become sufficiently impoverished to qualify, if they had not qualified previously, for Medicaid coverage. If the Murats owned their house, some states would put a lien on it in order to recover some of its payments to the nursing home when the house was eventually sold.

Fee for Service

The FFS Medicare program would pay 80% of the allowed charges submitted by her provider for visits to the nursing home. The Murats would be responsible for the annual Medicare Part B deductible ($110) and the 20% co-insurance payments. Medicare would not cover any of the nursing home's per diem charges.

HOSPICE CARE

After residing in the nursing home for 6 months, Mrs. Murat suffers a massive stroke that leaves her physiologically stable, but in a persistent vegetative state. Her husband reports that she had always said she would not want to go on living in such a condition if there were little hope of recovery. Although she is unable to swallow thin liquids, her husband says she would not want to be fed through any sort of tube. Her physician says that, with oral feeding, she is likely to live for several weeks. With the understanding that she will receive palliative care without life-prolonging interventions, her husband agrees to enroll her in a hospice program.

Enrollment in hospice would require the traditional FFS Medicare program (Part A) to pay a Medicare-certified hospice program a daily fee that would cover all care of her terminal diagnosis, including home care, medications, equipment, respite, counseling, and social services even if she had enrolled in (and remained in) the Medicare HMO.

If she had remained in the FFS Medicare program, Part B would pay her primary care provider, 80% of the allowed charges for home or office visits and care plan oversight services. Mr. Murat would be responsible for the 20% co-insurance, for small copayments for outpatient prescription medications, and for respite care.

CHANGES IN THE FEDERAL FINANCING OF HEALTH CARE

The complex and evolving combinations of coverage and programs create difficult choices for older Americans and powerful incentives for the providers of their health care. The U.S. Congress and CMS continue to revise the Medicare program.

The Balanced Budget Act of 1997

In 1997, Congress passed, and President Bill Clinton signed, the Balanced Budget Act (BBA 97) through which they intended to limit future growth in the cost of the Medicare program, improve the quality of the health care it provides, and expand the number and variety of managed-care plans from which Medicare beneficiaries could choose. It authorized five types of "Medicare Advantage" (formerly called "Medicare Plus Choice") plans:

- Medicare HMOs (IPA, group, or staff model)—insurance companies that accept capitation payments from CMS and provide or purchase Medicare-covered health services;
- Preferred provider organizations (PPOs)—alliances of providers that accept capitation payments and deliver Medicare-covered health services to their enrolled patients;
- Provider-sponsored organizations (PSOs)—partnerships of physician groups and hospitals that accept capitation payments and deliver Medicare-covered health services to their enrolled patients;
- Private FFS plans—plans that may charge beneficiaries a premium, pay providers more liberally than the original Medicare FFS program does, and allow providers to charge their patients copayments of up to 15%;

- Medical savings accounts (MSAs)—accounts into which Medicare beneficiaries can make tax-deductible contributions and out of which they can withdraw funds to purchase routine health-related goods (including medications) and services (including long-term-care insurance) from any Medicare provider. Linked to the MSA is a catastrophic insurance policy that limits the individual beneficiary's expenses for health care to $6000 per year.

Perhaps because of the risks and uncertainties involved, very few PPOs, PSOs, private FFS insurance companies, or MSA providers have entered into Medicare Advantage contracts with CMS. Citing inadequate capitation payments and burdensome administrative requirements, many HMOs have withdrawn from the Medicare market, constricted their service areas (eliminating many rural counties), reduced the scope of the benefits they cover, and increased the premiums, deductibles, and copayments for which their enrollees are responsible. The total number of Medicare beneficiaries enrolled in Medicare Advantage plans declined from 6.4 million (17%) in 1999 to 4.6 million (11%) in 2003. As a result, nearly 2 million older Americans had to select new health plans and new health care providers. Between 2003 and 2005, the number of enrolled beneficiaries increased to 4.9 million.

Federal actuaries projected that BBA 97 would save the Medicare program $116 billion during 1998–2003 and extend the life of the Medicare Part A Trust Fund until 2023. The specific actions by which BBA 97 attempted to control costs include restricting Medicare benefits (eg, home care), reducing payments to providers (eg, hospitals and HMOs), and requiring CMS to begin risk-adjusting the capitation rates at which it paid managed-care plans.

CMS pays each managed-care plan a monthly county-specific capitation fee for each of its Medicare enrollees, an amount based on CMS's recent average adjusted per capita cost (AAPCC) for FFS Medicare beneficiaries in the county. The AAPCC amounts range from about $450 per month in many rural counties to more than $800 per month in some urban areas. Before BBA 97, the payment formulas adjusted these capitation amounts only for enrollees' age, sex, Medicaid enrollment status (yes or no), and living situation (nursing home or independent residence). BBA 97 required that CMS also begin adjusting capitation amounts according to enrollees' risk of requiring expensive health care. This results in higher capitation payments for high-risk enrollees and lower payments for low-risk enrollees.

The current risk-adjustment method is based on the diagnoses associated with beneficiaries' health care during a recent 12-month period. If a hospital or outpatient provider designated as a reason for providing a health care service a diagnosis included in CMS's list of 61 "selected significant disease" groups, CMS would increase the amount of its capitation payment for that beneficiary during the following year. For example, if a beneficiary received care for heart failure during the 12 months from July 2004 to June 2005, CMS would adjust its capitation payments for the beneficiary during 2006 to provide the extra funds typically needed to care for people who have heart failure. In order to make this risk-adjustment system cost-neutral, CMS offsets the diagnosis-related increases in capitation payments by reducing its capitation payments for beneficiaries who have not received care for diagnoses in the 61 disease groups during this 12-month period. CMS is incorporating this risk-adjustment method into its formula for computing its capitation rates gradually over several years. In 2004, 30% of the capitation amounts were determined by diagnoses; during subsequent years, this percentage will increase to 100%.

BBA 97 provisions for improving the quality of health care for older Americans include:

- the Quality Improvement System for Managed Care (QISMC),
- the Healthcare Employers' Data Information System (HEDIS), which requires Medicare Advantage plans to monitor and report to CMS their rates of compliance with selected processes and outcomes of health care (eg, mammography and immunization against influenza),
- the Medicare Health Outcomes Survey, which requires Medicare Advantage plans to contract with third parties to survey a sample of their members and report information to CMS about their health status, functional ability, and satisfaction with their recent health care.

CMS summarizes the information generated by all three systems and makes it available at the Medicare Personal Plan Finder to help older Americans make informed choices about Medicare's FFS program and its various managed-care options.

Balanced Budget Revision Act of 1999

Within the first 18 months of the enactment of BBA 97, the quality of health care for older Americans began to erode, and the decreases in the payments to providers proved to be steeper than projected. For example, Medicare payments for home-health care decreased by 45% between 1997 and 1999. In response, Congress passed the Balanced Budget Revision Act at the end of 1999. This legislation restored some

of the budget cuts made 2 years earlier, including $4.5 billion to Medicare Advantage plans.

Medicare Modernization Act of 2003

The contentious Medicare Prescription Drug Improvement and Modernization Act of 2003 required dramatic changes in the nature and scope of the Medicare program during the following years, including:

- The creation of an optional ("Medicare Part D") program covering prescription medications.
- Subsidies for employers who continue to provide their retirees with insurance that covers prescription medications.
- Elimination of coverage for prescription medications by Medicaid.
- Competition between traditional FFS Medicare and Medicare Advantage plans.
- Higher premiums for Medicare Part B to be paid by beneficiaries with higher incomes.
- Expanded coverage for preventive services.
- Increased reimbursement rates to providers and hospitals in rural areas.

The results of this act will be determined by the specific programs that it spawns and by subsequent legislative and administrative reactions during the years after its enactment.

The Future of Medicare and Medicaid

CMS is now conducting dozens of demonstration projects designed to improve the quality and outcomes of care for beneficiaries with chronic conditions. In most of these demonstrations, CMS is paying provider and managed-care contractors capitated monthly fees for providing case management or disease management services to beneficiaries with specified chronic conditions, such as heart failure, diabetes mellitus, or other "special needs." Many of these demonstrations are based on the principle of "pay for performance," which stipulates that CMS will pay the capitation fees only to the extent that the contractor attains pre-agreed standards of performance, eg, performing certain diagnostic tests, reducing Medicare's overall FFS payments, and satisfying beneficiaries with the services they provide.

The aging of the baby-boom generation, technology-driven increases in health care spending, and a decline in the number of workers per Medicare beneficiary will contribute to serious financial challenges for the Medicare program in the years ahead. Similarly, imminent sharp increases in the number of older Americans with serious disabilities will soon surpass states' ability to pay for their long-term care. To meet these challenges, the nation needs visionary leaders, committed professionals, and rapid major changes in its systems for providing and paying for health care.

REFERENCES

■ American Geriatrics Society. Information on the Medicare Prescription Drug, Improvement, and Modernization Act 2003 (Public Law No: 108-173). Available at http://www.americangeriatrics.org/policy/medicare_info.shtml (accessed October 2005).

■ Centers for Medicare and Medicaid Services, Department of Health and Human Services. Medicare Modernization Act. Available at http://www.cms.hhs.gov/medicarereform (accessed October 2005).

■ Centers for Medicare and Medicaid Services, Department of Health and Human Services. *Medicare: Resident and New Physician Guide: Helping Health Professionals Navigate Medicare.* 7th ed. Rockville, MD: US Government Printing Office; 2003.

■ Emmer S, Allendorf L. The Medicare Prescription Drug, Improvement, and Modernization Act of 2003. *J Am Geriatr Soc.* 2004;52(6):1013–1015.

■ Ettinger WH Jr. The Balanced Budget Act of 1997: implications for the practice of geriatric medicine. *J Am Geriatr Soc.* 1998;46(4):530–533.

■ Health Care Financing Administration. *2004 Guide to Health Insurance for People with Medicare.* Rockville, MD: US Government Printing Office; 2004. Pub. No. HCFA-02110. Available in regular and large print at http://www.Medicare.gov/publications/home.asp (accessed October 2005).

■ Health Care Financing Administration. *Medicare and You 2005.* Rockville, MD: US Government Printing Office; 2004. Pub. No. HCFA-10050. Available in regular and large print at http://www.Medicare.gov/publications/home.asp (accessed October 2005).

■ Medicare: The Official U.S. Government Site for People with Medicare. Available at http://www.medicare.gov (accessed October 2005).

APPROACH TO THE PATIENT

CHAPTER 6—ASSESSMENT

KEY POINTS

- Geriatric assessment is a multifaceted approach to the care of the older adult with the goal of promoting wellness and independent function.
- Assessment of function includes the physical, cognitive, psychologic, and social domains.
- Tools that are time efficient and valid are available to the clinician for use in a variety of settings to evaluate the older person's status in all these domains.
- Time tends to be a less important element than the skills of the clinician in facilitating successful communication with older patients.

Geriatric assessment is a multifaceted approach to the care of the older adult with the goal of promoting wellness and independent function. Function is defined broadly to encompass the physical, cognitive, psychologic, and social domains. The scope of the assessment of any individual domain depends on the site of care, the patient's level of frailty, time constraints, the goals of care, and the availability of a multidisciplinary team. The essential aspects of geriatric assessment should be performed routinely in all sites of care, whether the ambulatory setting, the emergency department, the hospital, the nursing home, or the home. Whenever possible, assessments should be performance based. A caregiver or family member who lives with the patient is often required to provide or to verify pertinent historical information about the older patient's day-to-day functioning.

Try This, a publication of the Hartford Institute for Geriatric Nursing, is a series of assessment tools in which each issue focuses on a topic specific to the older adult population. The content is directed to orient and encourage all nurses to understand the special needs of older adults and to use the highest standards of practice in caring for the elderly. Each of the more than 25 *Try This* issues is a 2-page document with a description of why the topic is important when caring for older patients, followed by an assessment tool that can be administered in 20 minutes or less. Each *Try This* is downloadable to a PDA or can be printed from the Hartford Institute for Geriatric Nursing Web site at http://www.hartfordign.org/resources/education/tryThis.html.

Topics include SPICES: An Overall Assessment Tool of Older Adults, the Katz Index of Independence in Activities of Daily Living, The Geriatric Depression Scale (GDS), Predicting Pressure Ulcer Risk, The Pittsburgh Sleep Quality Index, Assessing Pain In Older Adults, Fall Risk Assessment, Assessing Nutrition in Older Adults, Urinary Incontinence Assessment, Hearing Screening, Confusion Assessment Method, Caregiver Strain Index, Elder Abuse and Neglect Assessment, Beers' Criteria for Potentially Inappropriate Medication Use in the Elderly, Alcohol Use Screening and Assessment, The Geriatric Oral Health Assessment Index, Horowitz's Impact of Event Scale: An Assessment of Post Traumatic Stress in Older Adults, Preventing Aspiration in Oder Adults with Dysphagia, and Immunizations for the Older Adult. A special series focusing on assessment in those with dementia include topics such as Avoiding Restraints In Patients with Dementia, Assessing Pain in Persons with Dementia, Issues on Dementia, Brief Evaluation of Executive Dysfunction, Therapeutic Activity Kits, Recognition of Dementia in Hospitalized Older Adults, Wandering in the Hospitalized Older Adult, Communication Difficulties, Assessing and Managing Delirium in Persons with Dementia, and Decision Making and Dementia.

THE ROUTINE OFFICE VISIT

Efficient strategies are required to incorporate geriatric assessment into routine office practice. One such strategy entails rapid screening of targeted areas (Table 6.1), followed by comprehensive assessment in areas of concern. Many of the initial screens can be completed by trained office staff; some can be completed by the patients themselves while seated in the waiting area or at home prior to the visit. The use of a "rolling" assessment, which targets at least one area for screening during each office visit, should be considered. Finally, in the absence of specific target symptoms, parts of the routine examination, such as auscultation of the chest and palpation of the abdomen, can be replaced by aspects of geriatric assessment, such as observation of gait, balance, and transfers.

PATIENT-CLINICIAN COMMUNICATION

Because of the demands of a busy clinical practice, the time available for office visits is often constrained. Time tends to be less important, however, than the

Table 6.1—Rapid Screening Followed by Assessment and Management in Key Domains

Domain	Rapid Screen	Assessment and Management
Functional status	Answers "Yes" to one or more of the following: Because of a health or physical problem, do you need help to: (a) shop? (b) do light housework? (c) walk across a room? (d) take a bath or shower? (e) manage the household finances?	Assess all other activities of daily living listed in Table 6.3 Evaluate cognitive function and mobility using performance-based tests Assess social support Consider use of adaptive equipment
Mobility	"Timed Get Up and Go" test: unable to complete in less than 20 seconds	Treat underlying musculoskeletal or neurologic disorder Refer to physical therapy
Nutrition	Answers "Yes" to "Have you lost more than 10 lbs over the past 6 months without trying to do so?" OR body mass index $(kg/m^2) < 20$	See "Malnutrition," p 161
Vision	If unable to read a newspaper headline and sentence while wearing corrective lenses, test each eye with Snellen chart; unable to read greater than 20/40	See "Visual Impairment," p 140
Hearing	Unable to hear a 40-dB tone at 1000 or 2000 Hz in both ears or at either of these frequencies in one ear, as determined by use of a hand-held AudioScope	See "Hearing Impairment," p 145
Cognitive function	3-item recall: unable to remember all three items after 1 minute	Administer Folstein Mini–Mental State Examination
Depression	Answers "Yes" to "Do you often feel sad or depressed?"	Administer 15-item Geriatric Depression Scale (see the Appendix, p 458)

skills of the clinician in facilitating communication with older patients. Table 6.2 lists several simple strategies that may be used to enhance communication. (See also the table on communication in "Hearing Impairment," p 148.) To accommodate the high prevalence of sensory deficits among older adults, particular attention should be given to the environment of the examination room. The use of simple, inexpensive amplification devices with lightweight earphones can be especially effective, even for the severely hearing-impaired person. During the course of the interview, the clinician should go beyond the customary clinical inquiries by asking open-ended questions such as, "What would you like me to do for you?" Finding out what the patient wants can be a prime mechanism for solving potential problems, generating trust, and improving mutual satisfaction in the patient-clinician relationship.

PHYSICAL ASSESSMENT

The importance of a full, appropriately detailed physical examination cannot be overstated. Many older adults cannot see well enough to report signs of disease or have cognitive impairment that prevents them from being able to accurately report symptoms. The clinician cannot assume that "no news is good news" in the care of older adults.

Table 6.2—Effective Strategies to Enhance Communication

- Use a well-lit room and avoid backlighting.
- Minimize extraneous noise and interruptions.
- Carefully introduce yourself to establish a friendly relationship.
- Face the patient directly, sitting at eye level.
- Address the patient by his or her last name.
- Speak slowly.
- Inquire about hearing deficits and raise the volume and lower the tone of your voice accordingly.
- If necessary, write questions in large print.
- Allow sufficient time for the patient to answer.
- Touch the patient gently on the hand, arm, or shoulder during the conversation.

Functional Status

Functional status refers to the person's ability to perform tasks that are required for living. These tasks, usually referred to as activities of daily living (ADLs), are listed in Table 6.3. When assessing function, ask whether the patient is independent or requires the help of another person to complete the tasks. Bathing is typically the basic ADL with the highest prevalence of disability, and disability in bathing is often the reason why older adults receive home aide services. To identify patients with "preclinical" disability, that is, those who do not yet require personal assistance but who are at risk of becoming disabled, ask about

Table 6.3—Activities of Daily Living

Self-care	
Bathing	Toileting
Dressing	Grooming
Transferring from bed to chair	Feeding oneself

Instrumental	
Using the telephone	Doing laundry
Preparing meals	Doing housework
Managing household finances	Shopping
Taking medications	Managing transportation

Mobility
Walking from room to room
Climbing a flight of stairs
Walking outside one's home

perceived difficulty with the tasks and whether the patient has changed the way he or she completes the task because of a health-related problem or condition. Assess the use of any assistive devices, such as a cane or walker, as well as duration and circumstances of use.

Outside of a rehabilitation setting, performance-based testing of most of the self-care and instrumental ADLs is not practical. Hence, performance-based testing of functional status focuses primarily on mobility, including transfers, gait, and balance. Ask the patient to stand from the seated position in a hard-backed chair while keeping his or her arms folded. Inability to complete this task suggests lower extremity, or quadriceps, weakness and is highly predictive of future disability. Once he or she is standing, observe the patient walk back and forth over a short distance, ideally with the usual walking aid. Abnormalities of gait include path deviation; diminished step height or length or both; trips, slips, or near falls; and difficulty with turning. The tasks of rising from the chair, walking 10 feet (3 meters), turning around and returning to the chair, turning, and then sitting back down in the chair make up the "Timed Get Up and Go" test. Older adults who can complete this sequence of maneuvers in less than 10 seconds have intact mobility; those who take 20 seconds or longer require further evaluation.

An alternative assessment strategy is to measure gait speed as a predictor of future disability. A gait speed of 0.80 m per second allows for independent community ambulation; a speed of 0.60 m per second allows for community activity without the use of a wheelchair. These norms indicate that older adults who can walk 50 feet in your office corridor in 20 seconds or less should be able to walk independently in normal activities.

Balance can be tested progressively by asking the person to stand first with his or her feet side by side, then in semi-tandem position, and finally in tandem position. Difficulty with balance in these positions predicts an increased risk of falling. Although standardized instruments, such as the Tinetti Performance-Oriented Mobility Assessment, may be used to quantify impairments in gait and balance, a qualitative assessment is usually sufficient to make recommendations about the need for an assistive device, such as a cane or walker. When assessing gait and balance, particularly in older women, clinicians should observe for the use of proper footwear, that is, flat, hard-soled shoes. (Also see the Appendix, p 459, for falls-assessment guidelines.)

Finally, clinicians can often glean useful functional information by observing their older patients as they complete simple tasks, such as unbuttoning and buttoning a shirt or blouse, picking up a pen and writing a sentence, taking off and putting on shoes, touching the back of the head with both hands, and getting on and off an examination table.

Nutrition

Poor nutrition in older adults may reflect concurrent medical illness, depression, dementia, inability to shop or cook, inability to feed oneself, or financial hardship. Aside from visual inspection for signs of malnutrition, older adults should have their weight and height measured routinely. A low body mass index (ie, kg/m^2 <20) or an unintentional weight loss of more than 10 pounds in 6 months suggests poor nutrition and requires further evaluation. (See "Malnutrition," p 161.)

Vision and Hearing

Although visual impairment from cataracts, glaucoma, macular degeneration, and abnormalities of accommodation usually worsens with age, older persons are often unaware of their visual deficits. Asking about difficulty with driving, watching television, or reading may uncover a problem with vision. As a brief performance-based screen, an older patient can be asked to read (using corrective lenses, if applicable) a short passage from a newspaper or magazine, with the caveat that low literacy is not an uncommon problem among older persons. Significant impairment in vision can be confirmed through the use of a Snellen chart or Jaeger card; the inability to read greater than 20/40 is the standard criterion. (See "Visual Impairment," p 140.)

The high prevalence of hearing loss among older adults and its association with depression, dissatisfaction with life, and withdrawal from social activities make it an important target for assessment. Hearing loss is usually bilateral and in the high-frequency range. Hearing should be assessed routinely during the history-taking session and can be assessed more formally using a hand-held AudioScope. Inability to hear a 40-dB tone at 1000 or 2000 Hz in both ears or at either of these frequencies in one ear is considered abnormal and, in the absence of cerumen impaction, warrants a discussion about referral for formal audiometric testing. (See "Hearing Impairment," p 145.)

COGNITIVE ASSESSMENT

The prevalence of cognitive decline doubles every 5 years after the age of 65 and approaches 40% to 50% at age 90. Most patients with dementia do not complain of memory loss or even volunteer symptoms of cognitive impairment unless specifically questioned. Older adults with cognitive impairment, even in the absence of dementia, are at increased risk of accidents, delirium, medical nonadherence, and disability. Therefore, an important feature of every assessment of an older adult, especially those aged 75 years and older, is a brief cognitive screen.

Because short-term memory loss is typically the first sign of dementia, the best single screening question is recall of three words after 1 minute. Anything other than perfect recall should lead to further testing. An alternative strategy adds orientation to day of the week, month, and year to the three memory items. A cut-off of three or more errors has a sensitivity and specificity of nearly 90% for a diagnosis of dementia. The most commonly used instrument for formal testing of cognition is the Folstein Mini–Mental State Examination (MMSE), which assesses orientation, registration and recall, attention and calculation, language, and visual-spatial skills. Although scores on the MMSE need to be interpreted in the context of educational attainment, race, and age, scores lower than 24 generally warrant further evaluation for possible dementia.

An often overlooked area of cognition, which is essential for proper goal-directed behaviors, is executive function. The clock-drawing test is valuable because it assesses executive control and visual-spatial skills, two domains of cognition that are otherwise not tested or incompletely tested by the MMSE. In the clock-drawing test, the patient is asked to draw the face of a clock and to place the hands correctly to indicate 2:50 or 11:10. The clock-drawing test is combined with the three-item recall in the Mini-Cog Assessment Instrument for Dementia, a brief screening test that has been recently developed and validated. The Mini-Cog also has the advantage over the MMSE of being both very sensitive and specific when used with those patients whose native language is not English and those with less than a high school education.

Another useful question to assess executive function is asking the patient to name as many four-legged animals as possible in 1 minute. Fewer than 8 to 10 animals or repetition of the same animals is abnormal and suggests the need for further evaluation.

PSYCHOLOGIC ASSESSMENT

Although the prevalence of major depression among community-dwelling older adults is only about 1% to 2%, a large number of older adults suffer from significant symptoms of depression below the severity threshold of major depression as defined by the fourth edition of the *Diagnostic and Statistical Manual of Mental Disorders*. These subthreshold depressive symptoms, which often include somatic complaints such as poor sleep and fatigue, increase the risk of physical disability and slower recovery after an acute disabling event. They are also associated with a significant increase in the cost of medical services, even after accounting for the severity of chronic medical illness. Hence, clinicians should have a high index of suspicion for depressive symptoms and a low threshold for treatment. The best single question to ask is, "Do you often feel sad or depressed?" An affirmative response warrants further evaluation of other depressive symptoms, perhaps through the use of a standardized instrument such as the 15-item Geriatric Depression Scale (see the Appendix, p 458).

Anxiety and worries are also important symptoms in older adults and are often a manifestation of an underlying depressive disorder. Finally, because older adults are particularly likely to experience the loss of a loved one, special efforts should be made to recognize and manage the consequences of bereavement. (See "Depression and Other Mood Disorders," p 247.)

SOCIAL ASSESSMENT

The social assessment consists of several elements, including ethnic, spiritual, and cultural background, the availability of a personal support system, the need for a caregiver and his or her role, presence of caregiver burden, the safety of the home environment, the patient's economic well-being, the possibility of elder mistreatment, and the patient's advance directives. Although a comprehensive social assessment may not be feasible in a busy office practice, clinicians caring for older patients should be mindful of these aspects of an older patient's life. Some older adults, for example, may be illiterate, uneducated, or have a poor command of English, making it difficult for them to navigate through the complexities of the current health care system. Clinicians can uncover important clues to unmet needs by inquiring about the availability of help in case of an emergency. For frail older adults, particularly those who lack social support, referral to a visiting nurse may be helpful in assessing home safety and level of personal risk. (See "Psychosocial Issues," p 14, "Cultural Aspects of Care," p 46, "Elder Mistreatment," p 80.)

QUALITY OF LIFE

During the past decade, *quality of life* has been embraced as a convenient catchphrase to denote important patient outcomes other than death and traditional physiologic measures of morbidity. Although a gold standard for quality of life does not exist, most instruments designed to measure it include various aspects of physical, cognitive, psychologic, and social function. Perhaps the most commonly used instrument is the Short Form-36 Health Survey (SF-36), which includes 36 items organized into eight domains— physical function, role limitations due to physical health, role limitations due to emotional health, bodily pain, social functioning, mental health, vitality, and general health perceptions. The SF-36 has been tested extensively among community-living adults and hospitalized patients, but it may not be suitable for use among the oldest-old people, especially those who are frail, because of floor effects and insensitivity to clinically important changes in health status.

When assessing quality of life, ask about patient preferences regarding medical care and goals of care. Goals can be multiple, diverse, and sometimes conflicting. There is striking heterogeneity among older adults with respect to physiologic function, health status, belief systems, cultural and ethnic backgrounds, values, and personal preferences. The successful management of chronic conditions, such as diabetes mellitus, arthritis, and heart failure, requires that patients, families, and clinicians work collaboratively to define the specific problems, to elicit personal preferences, and to establish the goals of care. A patient's cultural and ethnic heritage has an important role in her understanding of her illness, its meaning in her life, and her response to it. It is crucial, therefore, for the clinician to have an appreciation of that heritage and the role it plays in the patient's understanding of health and illness. (See "Cultural Aspects of Care," p 46.) Treatment plans that include patient preferences have been shown to enhance adherence and increase satisfaction, and they have the potential to improve patient outcomes.

ASSESSING THE OLDER DRIVER

Evaluating the older driver presents a difficult challenge to the clinician. The automobile is the most important, and often the only, source of transportation for older people. Yet a variety of age-related changes, chronic conditions, and medications place the older adult at risk of automobile accidents. Although the absolute number of crashes involving older drivers is low, the number of crashes per mile driven and the likelihood of serious injury or death are higher than for any age group other than those aged 16 to 24 years.

To their credit, the vast majority of older people make prudent adjustments in their driving behaviors by avoiding rush hour or congested thoroughfares or by not driving at night or during adverse weather conditions. Nonetheless, impaired older adults who continue to drive represent an important safety hazard not only to themselves but also to other drivers, passengers, and pedestrians. Pertinent risk factors for automobile accidents include poor visual acuity (less then 20/40) and contrast sensitivity; dementia, particularly deficits in visual-spatial skills and visual attention; impaired neck and trunk rotation; and poor motor coordination and speed of movement. Alcohol and medications that adversely affect alertness, such as narcotics, benzodiazepines, antihistamines, antidepressants, antipsychotics, sedatives, and muscle relaxants, may impair driving skills and increase crash risk. Hence, caution is warranted when initiating or adjusting the dose of these medications, and patients should be warned about potential adverse effects on driving safety.

Any report of an accident or moving violation should trigger an assessment of the patient's driving capacity. Discuss safety concerns honestly with the older driver, and ideally with a spouse or other family member as well, particularly when the patient lacks insight into his or her driving limitations. Alternative modes of transportation should be considered. Recommendations to stop driving, however, should not be proffered lightly, because driving cessation can lead to a decrease in activity level and an increase in depressive symptoms. Referral for a formal driving evaluation by a skilled occupational therapist may be helpful in confirming unsafe driving behaviors or, perhaps, in suggesting interventions such as adaptive equipment to correct for specific physical disabilities. In the interest of public safety, clinicians should know their state's law on reporting impaired drivers. In most states, clinicians are encouraged, and in some states mandated, to report their concerns to the licensing agency. (See also the section on driving in "Legal and Ethical Issues," p 28.) An excellent reference is *The Physician's Guide to Assessing and Counseling Older Drivers* developed by the American Medical Association in cooperation with the National Highway Traffic Safety Administration, it was recently made available free of charge at http://www.ama-assn.org/ama/pub/category/10791.html.

COMPREHENSIVE GERIATRIC ASSESSMENT

Comprehensive geriatric assessment (CGA) is a process intended to determine a patient's medical, psychosocial, and functional capabilities and limitations, with the goal of developing an overall plan for treatment and long-term follow-up. Because CGA typically requires a highly trained team of geriatricians, geriatric nurse clinicians, physical and occupational therapists, geriatric psychiatrists, and social workers, it is expensive and time consuming. Success generally requires the geriatric team to take over the direct care of the patient. An extended period of intensive team involvement with ongoing care is essential to assure the efficacy of the intervention. When the geriatric team assumes a purely consultative role (ie, without a role in implementing the recommendations), CGA is unlikely to be successful in improving patient outcomes.

CGA has had its greatest success, in terms of improving function and reducing nursing-home placement and hospital readmissions, in inpatient geriatric units that are staffed by highly trained professionals. Accumulating evidence, however, suggests that preventive home visitation programs may also be beneficial. A meta-analysis of randomized trials demonstrated that these programs decrease nursing-home admissions and reduce functional decline if the interventions are based on CGA with extended follow-up, include multiple follow-up home visits, and target older adults at lower risk of death.

REFERENCES

- AGS position statement. Comprehensive geriatric assessment position statement. *Annals of Long-Term Care.* 2006;14(3):34-35. Also available at: http://www.americangeriatrics.org/products/positionpapers/cga.shtml

- Aminzadeh F, Byszewski A. Dalziel WB, et al. Effectiveness of outpatient geriatric assessment programs: exploring caregiver needs, goals, and outcomes. *J Gerontol Nurs.* 2005;31(12):19-25.

- Cohen HJ, Feussner JR, Weinberger M, et al. A controlled trial of inpatient and outpatient geriatric evaluation and management. *N Engl J Med.* 2002;346(12):905–912.

- Counsell SR, Callahan CM, Buttar AB, et al. Geriatric Resources for Assessment and Care of Elders (GRACE): a new model of primary care for low-income seniors. *J Am Geriatr Soc.* 2006;54(7):1136-1141.

- Gill TM, Kurland B. The burden and patterns of disability in activities of daily living among community-living older persons. *J Gerontol A Biol Sci Med Sci.* 2003; 58:70–75.

- Jones DM, Song X, Rockwood K. Operationalizing a frailty index from a standardized comprehensive geriatric assessment. *J Am Geriatr Soc.* 2004;52(11):1929-1933.

- McCusker J, Verdon J. Do geriatric interventions reduce emergency department visits? A systematic review. *J Gerontol A Biol Sci Med Sci.* 2006;61(1):53-62.

- Phibbs CS, Holty JE, Goldstein MK, et al. The effect of geriatrics evaluation and management on nursing home use and health care costs: results from a randomized trial. *Med Care.* 2006;44(1):91-95.

- Smeeth L, Fletcher AE, Stirling S, et al. Randomised comparison of three methods of administering a screening questionnaire to elderly people: findings from the MRC trial of the assessment and management of older people in the community. *BMJ.* 2001;323(7326):1403–1407.

- Studenski S, Perera S, Wallace D, et al. Physical performance measures in the clinical setting. *J Am Geriatr Soc.* 2003;51(3):314–322.

CHAPTER 7—CULTURAL ASPECTS OF CARE

KEY POINTS

- Cultural competence is a nuanced understanding of the role of culture in our lives.

- The culturally astute clinician remains alert to the differences among individual patients from a given culture and guards against stereotyping on the basis of ethnic or cultural affiliation.

- Communication and clinical care are enhanced when the patient and provider make an effort to negotiate a common understanding of causation, diagnosis, and treatment while maintaining respect for the beliefs and constructs of both individuals.

As the cultural diversity of older Americans continues to grow, it is increasingly important for clinicians caring for older adults to develop an approach to working with individuals from a broad range of cultural groups. The purpose of this chapter is to assist clinicians in developing and improving their skills during intercultural patient encounters. The chapter also appears in volume 1 of *Doorway Thoughts*, published by the American Geriatrics Society. Other chapters in *Doorway Thoughts* demonstrate how the general approach outlined here in each topic relates to working with patients in seven specific minority cultural groups. It is very important to keep in mind when using *Doorway Thoughts* that although the cultural information offered in each chapter is accurate *in general,* the beliefs, traditions, customs and preferences of individuals in all cultural groups vary widely. The astute clinician *never* assumes that any person's cultural background dictates his or her health choices or behavior. The culturally literate clinician remains alert to the differences among individual patients and families from a given culture and on guard against stereotyping an older person on the basis of his or her ethnic or cultural affiliation.

DOORWAY THOUGHTS IN CROSS-CULTURAL HEALTH CARE

The key concepts discussed in this chapter are "doorway thoughts"—factors that the culturally competent practitioner reflects upon before walking through the doorway of any examination, consultation, or hospital room. These factors can shape intercultural health care encounters and relationships for good or for ill. Cultural and historical facts and issues relating to the members of an entire minority group can be in play in any cross-cultural encounter or relationship. The practitioner should be sensitive to the possibility that these issues may affect their relationships with individual patients and families and may also affect patients' willingness or ability to understand, accept, and adhere to prescribed regimens.

The quality of any encounter between a clinician and a patient from different ethnic or cultural backgrounds depends on the clinician's skill and sensitivity. Questions about the individual patient's attitudes and beliefs should be worked naturally and carefully into the clinical interview. The clinician must remember that no culture is monolithic; attitudes and beliefs vary widely from one individual to another within a single cultural group. Prior familiarity with a patient's cultural background will not suffice, for it is inaccurate to assume that a person's outlook is inflexibly determined by his or her cultural heritage. The concepts presented here are intended to serve as guides in choosing appropriate questions, and not as a rigid list of cultural attributes or clinical scenarios.

PREFERRED TERMS FOR CULTURAL IDENTITY

The terms referring to specific cultural or ethnic groups can change over time, and individuals in any one group do not always agree on the terminology that is appropriate. It is important to learn what the individual patient's preferred term is for his or her cultural identity and to use that terminology in conversation with the patient, as well as in his or her health records.

FORMALITY

Attitudes regarding the appropriate degree of formality in a health care encounter differ widely among cultural groups. Learning what a new patient's preferences are with regard to formality and allowing that preference to shape the relationship is always advisable. Initially, a more formal approach is likely to be appropriate.

Addressing the Patient

The patient's correct title (eg, Dr., Reverend, Mr., Mrs., Ms., Miss) and his or her surname should be used unless and until he or she requests a more casual form of address. Another important issue is to determine the correct pronunciation of the person's name.

Addressing the Health Provider

It is also important to learn how the patient would prefer to address the clinician and to allow his or her preference to prevail. For example, in some cultures, trust in the clinician depends on his or her assuming an authoritative role, and informality would undermine the patient's trust. This is an aspect of the clinical relationship in which the clinician's personal preferences should be relinquished.

LANGUAGE AND LITERACY

- What language does this individual feel most comfortable speaking? Will a medical interpreter be needed?
- Does this patient read and write English? Another primary language? If so, which one(s)?
- If the patient is not literate, does he or she have access to someone who can assist at home with written instructions?

It is worthwhile to consider these questions early in the health care relationship to determine whether interpretation services are needed and to make certain that communication with the patient is effective. Even those who use English fluently may wish to discuss complicated issues in their native language. It is the clinician's responsibility to explain medical terms and to ask the patient for explanations of any cultural or foreign terms that are unfamiliar.

RESPECTFUL NONVERBAL COMMUNICATION

Body position and motion is interpreted differently from one cultural group to another. Specific hand gestures, facial expression, physical contact, and eye contact can hold different meanings for the patient and the clinician when their cultural backgrounds differ. The clinician should watch for particular body language cues that appear to be significant and that might be linked to cultural norms that are important to the patient, in order to cultivate sensitivity to the conditions that make the flow of communication feel easy and effective.

Conservative body language is an advisable choice early in a relationship with a patient or when in doubt about a patient's background or preferences; assume a calm demeanor, avoid expressive extremes such as very vigorous handshakes, a loud and hearty voice, many hand gestures or, on the other hand, an impassive facial expression, avoidance of eye contact, standing at a distance. Remain alert for signals that the person is comfortable or uncomfortable. Directly asking the patient questions about body language may also help. It is very important to avoid making negative judgments about a patient that are rooted in unconscious cultural assumptions about the meaning of his or her gestures, facial expressions, or body language.

The distance from others that individuals find comfortable varies, depending in part on their cultural background. The clinician should determine what distance seems to be the most comfortable for each patient and, whenever practicable, allow the patient's preference to establish the optimal distance during the encounter.

ELEPHANTS IN THE ROOM

Are there any issues that are critical to the success of the health care encounter that are present but that go unspoken? Remain alert for the possibility that such issues are indeed present. Examples include

- a lack of trust in health care providers and the health care system,
- a fear of medical research and experimentation,
- fear of medications or their side effects, and
- unfamiliarity or discomfort with the Western biomedical belief system.

In general, sensitivity to the possibility that such issues are in play is advised in all intercultural patient encounters.

HISTORY OF TRAUMATIC EXPERIENCES

Is the patient a refugee or survivor of violence or genocide? Are family members missing or dead? Have patients or family members been tortured? Such experiences could negatively affect the health care encounter without the clinician's knowledge unless relevant questions are included among standard questions about the patient's history.

It is important for clinicians to remember that in some historical periods and jurisdictions, health care providers have participated in torture and genocide. For example, during World War II, Nazi medical personnel were responsible in concentration camps for selecting individuals for gassing, supervising the gassing process, and administering lethal injections to inmates in "hospitals." The methods and tools of torture employed have sometimes resembled legitimate clinical procedures and tools. Patients who have survived such experiences may not feel safe in medical or governmental settings, and contact with all clinicians may invoke feelings of vulnerability, fear, panic, or anger. Great sensitivity is necessary in providing health care for these individuals.

ISSUES OF IMMIGRATION

Immigration Status

Some individuals may be residing in North America without the protection of appropriate immigration documents. Clinicians may wish to assure each patient that information given within the medical encounter will be kept in the strictest confidence.

History of Immigration or Migration

The history of the movements of a whole ethnic or cultural group can affect the attitudes and behavior of an individual in that group even when he or she has not immigrated to North America from another country. In addition, understanding the specific migration history of a person often provides insight into the key life transitions informing his or her outlook. Knowing how a person came to reside in North America can be important. The time and effort the clinician invests in learning more about a minority group's history and current situation can be repaid not only in a better relationship with the individual patient but also in an enhanced appreciation of the factors affecting clinical relationships with all patients from that group.

ACCULTURATION

Acculturation is defined as a process in which members of one cultural group adopt the beliefs and behaviors of another group. Acculturation of a group may be evidenced by changes in language preference, adoption of common attitudes and values, and gradual loss of separate ethnic identification. Although acculturation typically occurs when a minority group adopts the habits and language patterns of a dominant group, acculturation may also be reciprocal between groups.

It is essential to keep principles of acculturation in mind during any intercultural health encounter. Begin by determining how long a person has lived in North America and whether he or she was born here. However, remember that the degree to which the person is acculturated to Western customs and attitudes is the consequence of many factors, and not just of the number of years since he or she immigrated. Older adults who follow the traditions of their cultural group may have been born outside of the United States or Canada, may be recent arrivals to the continent, or may even be lifelong North American residents.

A patient's level of acculturation may greatly impact not only his or her health behavior but also preferences in end-of-life planning and decision making. Acculturation can also be an issue dividing family members, and a person's resistance to or ease of acculturation may be a matter of pride or shame and guilt. Developing sensitivity about the issues of acculturation for one's older minority patients is a key element in effective intercultural health care. Asking patients directly about their adherence to cultural traditions can be useful.

TRADITION AND HEALTH BELIEFS

People from non-Western cultural groups may not conceive of illness in Western terms. Some may have highly developed concepts of the causes of health and disease that are incompatible with the concepts that form the foundations of Western medicine. Non-Western paradigms include beliefs that illnesses have spiritual causation or are the result of imbalance among bodily humors, or that they are caused by a person's actions in past lives, to name but a few.

Patients may be making unexamined assumptions that are based on traditional beliefs, and these can cause confusion or create misunderstanding. The more the clinician knows about specific traditions, the more he or she can avoid such problems.

In addition, patients holding traditional beliefs may be using alternative remedies (eg, rituals, herbal preparations) that they do not mention, and questions about such practices should be included among other ques-

tions about the patient's history. It is unrealistic to expect that a patient will simply "adapt" to Western approaches to health and health care, just as it is impractical to expect the clinician to accept a new paradigm of wellness and disease. Clinical communication and efficacy will be enhanced when patients and providers make an effort to negotiate a common understanding of causation, diagnosis, and treatment for a specific health problem while maintaining respect for the beliefs and constructs of both individuals.

ATTITUDES TOWARD NORTH AMERICAN HEALTH SERVICES

Some minority patients may not feel comfortable in customary North American health care settings. Explanations for the discomfort, distrust, or uneasiness of some include lack of familiarity with Western practices, dissatisfying previous encounters with the health care system, or the belief that insensitivity or discrimination is inevitable for anyone in the cultural or ethnic group. Such feelings may result from having been stereotyped or treated insensitively or even unfairly by clinicians in the past. Sensitive exploration of these issues with patients is often both worthwhile and necessary. Generally, the clinician meeting a new patient from an ethnic or cultural minority group should be alert for signs of guardedness that signal an underlying lack of comfort or trust.

CULTURE-SPECIFIC HEALTH RISKS

Epidemiologic and medical research has identified numerous differences among ethnic and cultural populations with regard to specific health risks. The clinician who treats many patients from a specific group is advised to make every effort to stay abreast of the latest findings in relevant areas.

APPROACHES TO DECISION MAKING

The influence of specific cultures on approaches to health decision making has been the subject of many studies. Western bioethics emphasize individual autonomy in all health decisions, but for many other cultures, decision making is family or community centered. Autonomy principles allow competent persons to involve others in their health decisions or to cede those rights to a proxy decision maker. The clinician should ask patients if they prefer to make their own health decisions or if they would prefer to involve or defer to others in the decision-making process. Some may wish to assign the decision-making authority wholly to another individual or a group. In some cultures, the definition of family may include fictive kin. In families in which the degree of acculturation of the generations differs, the older person may defer to or depend on younger relatives, even though the tradition might suggest that the reverse would occur.

Establishing an understanding of each patient's decision-making preferences early in the clinical relationship will, in most instances, promote better communication and avoid the difficulties inherent in trying to address the issues at a time of crisis. When the patient's and clinician's cultural backgrounds differ, careful exploration of the issues is all the more important because the clinician cannot proceed as if he or she and the patient are starting from common assumptions.

ATTITUDES REGARDING DISCLOSURE AND CONSENT

Cultural attitudes toward truth telling and disclosure of terminal diagnoses vary widely. In some cultures, it is commonly believed that patients should not be informed of a terminal diagnosis, as this may be injurious to health or hasten death. Obtaining informed consent from patients with this belief may prove to be difficult. There is no consensus in bioethics concerning the rigorous application of full clinical disclosure in every situation. However, it is generally agreed that incorporating a patient's beliefs concerning disclosure and truth-telling into clinical planning whenever possible is desirable. Some patients may prefer not to know if they are terminally ill and ask that family members or other caregivers receive all diagnostic information and make all treatment decisions. It is advisable to explore each patient's preferences regarding disclosure of serious clinical findings early in the clinical relationship and to reconfirm these wishes at intervals.

GENDER ISSUES

Each culture has intricate traditions and structures with regard to gender roles. Societies seemingly based on the same patriarchal or matriarchal model may vary widely in their expressions of the model. A person's gender influences the sorts of experiences he or she has had, not only within the family but in the community and health care system as well. Another level of complexity may be added to health care encounters when an older adult's group struggles with conflicting traditional and contemporary views on gender roles. Cultural norms for men and women can profoundly influence their health behavior, and these norms for the genders vary widely from one culture to another. These norms also affect decision making, disclosure, and consent.

It is highly advisable for the clinician to explore each patient's attitudes regarding the interplay among gender, autonomy, and personal decision making early in the patient-provider relationship, to confirm his or her preferences at intervals, and to follow the individual patient's wishes whenever possible.

END-OF-LIFE DECISION MAKING AND CARE INTENSITY

Culture is an important influence in a person's formation of his or her attitudes toward supportable quality of life, approach to suffering, and beliefs about medical feeding, life-prolonging treatments, and palliative care. Some cultures value a direct struggle for life in the face of death, and both patients and families will expect an intensive approach to treatment. Other cultures ardently avoid direct confrontation of death and dying and will prefer to leave such decisions to the clinician. Still others will take a direct approach to death and dying but will reject too aggressive an approach.

Research has shown that clinicians and patients from shared cultural backgrounds have similar values in these areas; the implications of such findings for clinicians and patients from differing backgrounds are obviously important. Both clinicians and patients bring their own attitudes and beliefs to any clinical encounter. It is important for clinicians to be aware of their personal views and cultural set when discussing end-of-life plans with patients and to respect patients' beliefs and preferences even when they are different from their own.

In negotiating end-of-life decisions with a patient whose background is different from his or her own, the clinician must listen especially carefully to the patient's goals and concerns and exert every effort to avoid making culture-based assumptions that do not apply. For example, the assumption that "no one would want to live in that condition" or that "everyone would want treatment in this situation" is likely to be faulty. To ensure that end-of-life plans and decisions reflect an individual's rights and wishes, the clinician must strive to understand the patient's overall approach to life and death, and as far as possible provide care that is congruent with that approach.

ATTITUDES TOWARD ADVANCE DIRECTIVES

The use of advance directives and health care proxies has become more common in the past 20 years, but research indicates that the use of written directives may be more common among older persons in the dominant North American culture than among older persons in minority cultural groups. It is advisable in intercultural situations, when discussing attitudes and beliefs regarding written directives with a patient, to be sensitive to the possibility that some minority older persons will prefer to use alternatives—verbal directives or directives dictated to family members or others—and others will need to avoid any such discussion so as to observe proscriptions against talking about death. In view of the fact that preferences for care intensity may also differ according to cultural background, patients should also be given the opportunity to indicate the interventions they do want as well as those they do not want in any written or verbal directive used.

CULTURAL COMPETENCE: A FINAL WORD

There is no gold standard definition of cultural competence. Most definitions emphasize a careful coordination of individual behavior, organizational policy, and system design to facilitate mutually respectful and effective cross-cultural interactions.

Cultural competence combines attitudes, knowledge base, acquired skills, and behavior. It is an approach, not a technique. Cultural competence is not a form of "political correctness." Ideally, it is a nuanced understanding of the determining role that culture plays in all of our lives and of the impact culture has on every health care encounter, for both the clinician and the patient.

Cultural competence cannot be achieved exclusively by reading, but we hope that this chapter will provide clinicians who care for older adults from all minority groups with basic information and a foundation for further investigation. We would encourage clinicians to view each intercultural encounter as an opportunity to learn more, not only about the individual patient and his or her culture, but also about themselves. We also recommend that clinicians learn more about the impact of culture on health decisions by reading relevant publications, exploring Web sites, and attending workshops. We also urge clinicians to work with the entire interdisciplinary health care team, including administrators, to promote cultural competence in the health care organizations where they practice. Finally, we encourage clinician educators to develop their own teaching materials and educational programs designed to meet the needs of specific communities.

REFERENCES

■ American Geriatrics Society, Adler R, Kamel H. *Doorway Thoughts: Cross-Cultural Health Care for Older Adults.* Vol. 1. Boston, MA: Jones and Bartlett; 2004.

■ Brach C, Fraser I. Can cultural competency reduce racial and ethnic health disparities? A review and conceptual model. *Med Car Res Rev.* 2000;57 Suppl 1:181-217.

■ Whitifield K. *Closing the Gap: Improving the health of minority elders.* Washington, DC: Gerontological Society of America: 2004.

CHAPTER 8—PHYSICAL ACTIVITY

KEY POINTS

■ Promoting physical activity is one of the most important and effective preventive and therapeutic interventions in older adults.

■ The health benefits of physical activity accrue independently of other risk factors and are generally proportional to the amount of physical activity.

■ Clinical guidelines identify a role for physical activity in the management of numerous conditions, including cardiovascular and chronic lung disease, diabetes mellitus, hypertension, obesity, osteoporosis, knee osteoarthritis, and falls.

■ Adults should engage in a brisk walk, or an equivalently intense aerobic activity, for at least 10 minutes at a time, for a total of at least 30 minutes a day, on at least 5 days a week.

■ A useful clinical approach to promoting physical activity is to adopt the 5-A framework (assess, advise, agree, assist, and arrange).

Physical activity is defined as bodily movement produced by skeletal muscles that expend energy. Exercise is a subset of physical activity that involves a structured program designed to improve one or more components of physical fitness. The primary attributes of physical activity are type (mode), frequency, duration, and intensity. Promoting physical activity is one of the most important and effective preventive and therapeutic interventions in older adults. There is conclusive evidence that regular aerobic activity has large health benefits. Resistance training and balance training also have important health benefits in older adults. Flexibility training is important for maintaining the range of motion required to do physical activities.

PREVENTIVE HEALTH EFFECTS

Regular physical activity has beneficial effects on most, if not all, organ systems. Consequently, it prevents a large number of diseases. Physical activity reduces the risk of cardiovascular disease, high blood pressure, stroke, some lipid disorders, non-insulin-dependent diabetes mellitus, obesity, osteoporosis, colon cancer, and breast cancer. There is substantial evidence that physical activity also reduces the risk of fall injuries, sarcopenia, depression, and anxiety disorders. There is some evidence that physical activity reduces the risk of sleep problems, cognitive impairment, osteoarthritis, and back pain.

Consistent with its broad physiologic effects, regular physical activity decreases both cardiovascular and noncardiovascular mortality in older adults. The mortality benefit is large. Some studies report that inactive adults have mortality rates that are twice as high as those of active adults.

Observational studies consistently report that regular physical activity substantially delays the onset of functional limitations and loss of independence (disability). For example, an analysis of Established Population for Epidemiologic Studies of the Elderly (EPESE) data showed that inactive, nonsmoking women at age 65 have 12.7 years of active life expectancy, compared with 18.4 years of active life expectancy for highly active women. Higher levels of physical activity are associated with fewer years of disability preceding death.

The health benefits of physical activity accrue independently of other risk factors. For example, sedentary overweight smokers experience health benefits from increasing physical activity, even if they continue to smoke and do not lose weight.

The health benefits of physical activity are generally proportional to the amount of physical activity. When activity is performed above minimum thresholds for frequency, duration, and intensity, health benefit depends mainly upon the volume (energy expenditure) of aerobic activity. The dose-response relationship between physical activity and disease risk varies by disease in a manner that is incompletely understood. Cardiovascular disease risk decreases with volume of aerobic activity over a wide range of volume. Blood pressure shows little dose-response effect, as most of the effect of activity on blood pressure occurs at low levels of activity. The effect of activity on bone density is less related to volume of aerobic activity and more related to resistance training and high-impact activities.

ECONOMIC EFFECTS

Habitually active adults have lower medical expenditures. One study estimated direct medical expenditures in adults attributable to inactivity as being $330 per person in 1987 ($825 in 2002 dollars). Evidence is growing that medical expenditures decline in sedentary older adults who become more active. In one study comparing older adults who remained sedentary with sedentary older adults who became active 3 or more days each week, the active group was found to have a decline in medical expenditures averaging about $2200 a year. Data on the cost-effectiveness of promoting physical activity in older adults is promising but limited, and it varies by intervention. One study of subsidized exercise classes reported cost savings of around $175 per participant per year.

THERAPEUTIC EFFECTS

Physical activity has therapeutic benefits in the management of a wide variety of chronic conditions. Selected clinical guidelines for the use of physical activity in managing common chronic conditions are shown in Table 8.1. In addition, clinical practice guidelines identify a role for physical activity in the management of the following conditions: dementia, persistent pain, heart failure, syncope, reflex sympathetic dystrophy, possible venous thromboembolism, back pain, some sleep disorders, and constipation.

It is possible that physical activity will assume a prominent role in the management of mental health conditions in older adults. There is substantial evidence that both aerobic activity and resistance training improve symptoms of depression. Physical activity should be considered as an adjunct to medication and psychotherapy for older adults with depressive illness, pending more studies clarifying which patients can be prescribed activity as a substitute for medication and psychotherapy. Cognitive ability is positively correlated with higher levels of physical activity and fitness. Ongoing research is testing if, and how much, physical activity can improve cognitive function.

The therapeutic use of exercise to reverse low fitness, physical functional limitations, and disability has been carefully studied over the past 20 years. Randomized trials of exercise in sedentary older adults show that aerobic capacity, muscle strength, flexibility, and balance can be improved by appropriate forms of exercise. Several evidence-based reviews conclude that

Table 8.1—Selected Guidelines That Include Recommendations for Physical Activity

Topic	Guideline Source	Activity Recommendation
Cardiovascular disease	American Heart Association	Aerobic, strength, and flexibility training are recommended in the treatment of atherosclerotic cardiovascular disease. Both moderate and vigorous intensity aerobic activities are effective.
Hypertension	American College of Sports Medicine	"Dynamic aerobic training reduces resting BP in individuals with normal BP and HTN." "Resistance training performed according to ACSM guidelines reduces BP in normotensive and hypertensive adults."
Type 2 diabetes mellitus	American Diabetes Association	"To improve glycemic control, assist with weight maintenance, and reduce risk of CVD, we recommend at least 150 min/week of moderate-intensity aerobic physical activity . . . and/or at least 90 min/week of vigorous aerobic exercise. . . ." "In the absence of contraindications, people with type 2 diabetes should be encouraged to perform resistance exercise three times a week."
Falls	American Geriatrics Society, British Geriatrics Society, American Academy of Orthopaedic Surgeons	"Older people who have recurrent falls should be offered long-term exercise and balance training."
Osteoarthritis	American Geriatrics Society	Aerobic, strength, and flexibility training are recommended in the management of osteoarthritis.
Osteoporosis	American College of Sports Medicine	Weight-bearing aerobic activities, activities that involve jumping, and resistance exercise are recommended to preserve bone health in adults.
Major depression	Institute for Clinical Systems Improvement	"Among individuals with major depression, exercise therapy is feasible and is associated with significant therapeutic benefit, especially if exercise is continued over time."
Persistent pain	American Geriatrics Society	". . . there is strong evidence that participation in regular physical activity reduces the pain and enhances the functional capacity of older adults with persistent pain."
Dementia	American Academy of Neurology	"Walking and light exercise appear to reduce wandering, aggression and agitation...."
Heart failure	European Society of Cardiology	". . . regular exercise can safely increase physical capacity by 15–25%, improve symptoms and perception of quality of life in patients with stable class II and II heart failure (level of evidence B)."
Cholesterol	National Cholesterol Education Program Expert Panel (3rd Report)	"For management of atherogenic dyslipidemia, emphasis in management should be given to life-habit modification—weight control and increased physical activity."
Obesity	U.S. Preventive Services Task Force	"There is fair to good evidence that high-intensity counseling—about diet, exercise, or both—together with behavioral interventions aimed at skill development, motivation, and support strategies produces modest, sustained weight loss . . . in adults who are obese. . . ."

NOTE: ACSM = American College of Sports Medicine; BP = blood pressure; CVD = cardiovascular disease; HTN = hypertension.

SOURCES: (1) Fletcher GF, Balady GJ, Amsterdam EA, et al. Exercise standards for testing and training: a statement for healthcare professionals from the American Heart Association. *Circulation*. 2001;104:1694–1740, and Pollock ML, Franklin BA, Balady GJ, et al. Resistance exercise in individuals with and without cardiovascular disease: benefits, rationale, safety, and prescription. An advisory from the Committee on Exercise, Rehabilitation, and Prevention, Council on Clinical Cardiology, American Heart Association. *Circulation*. 2000;101:828–833. (2) Pescatello LS, Franklin BA, Fagard R, et al. American College of Sports Medicine position stand: exercise and hypertension. *Med Sci Sports Exerc*. 2004;36:533–553. (3) Sigal RJ, Kenny GP, Wasserman DH, et al. Physical activity / exercise and type 2 diabetes. *Diabetes Care*. 2004;27(10):2518–2539. (4) American Geriatrics Society, British Geriatrics Society, and American Academy of Orthopaedic Surgeons Panel on Falls Prevention. Guideline for the prevention of falls in older persons. *J Am Geriatr Soc*. 2001;49(5):664–672. (5) Exercise prescription for older adults with osteoarthritis pain: consensus practice recommendations: a supplement to the AGS Clinical Practice Guidelines on the management of chronic pain in older adults. *J Am Geriatr Soc*. 2001;49(6):808–823. (6) Kohrt WM, Bloomfield SA, Little KD, et al. American College of Sports Medicine position stand: physical activity and bone health. *Med Sci Sports Exerc*. 2004;36:1985–1996. (7) Institute for Clinical Systems Improvement (ICSI). *Major Depression in Adults in Primary Care*. 8th ed. Bloomington, MN: Institute for Clinical Systems Improvement (ICSI);2004:17–18. (8) AGS Panel on Persistent Pain in Older Persons. The management of persistent pain in older persons. *J Am Geriatr Soc*. 2002;50(6):S205–S224. (9) Doody RS, Stevens JC, Beck C, et al. Practice parameter: management of dementia (an evidence-based review). Report of the Quality Standards Subcommittee of the American Academy of Neurology. *Neurology*. 2001;56:1154–1166. (10) Remme WJ, Swedberg K. Guidelines for the diagnosis and treatment of chronic heart failure. *Eur Heart J*. 2001;22:1527–1560. (11) *Third Report on the National Cholesterol Education Program (NCEP) Expert Panel on Detection, Evaluation and Treatment of High Blood Cholesterol in Adults (Adult Treatment Panel III)*. National Institutes of Health, NIH Publication No. 01-3670, Washington, DC: May 2001. (12) U.S. Preventive Services Task Force. Screening for obesity in adults: recommendations and rationale. *Ann Intern Med*. 2003;139(11):930–932.

exercise has a beneficial effect on functional limitations (restrictions in basic physical actions such as walking). Although some exercise studies report only small improvements in functional limitations, most randomized trials prescribe just 3 or 4 days of exercise each week, for only 3 to 12 months. Generally, the benefits of exercise are most demonstrable in older adults with low fitness and clinically significant functional limitations. However, a study of relatively healthy older adults, using a highly sensitive physical performance measure of functional limitations, found that 6 months of aerobic exercise and strength training caused a 14% improvement in functional limitations. These results suggest that relatively healthy adults experience some functional gains with exercise. Other studies suggest that, after an initial boost in function due to exercise, exercisers show a decline in function, but have a slower rate of loss than nonexercisers. There are too few studies to determine whether physical activity in sedentary older adults has a beneficial effect on disability (ability to do activities of daily life such as personal care and work).

RECOMMENDED AMOUNTS OF PHYSICAL ACTIVITY

Aerobic Activity

An adult can achieve recommended levels of aerobic activity by doing either vigorous or moderate activity. The vigorous-intensity recommendation, developed in the 1980s, is to engage in at least 20 minutes of vigorous physical activity on 3 or more days each week. The moderate-intensity recommendation, published in 1995 by the Centers for Disease Control and Prevention (CDC) and the American College of Sports Medicine (ACSM), is that "every US adult should accumulate thirty minutes or more of moderate intensity physical activity on most, preferably all, days of the week." An alternative statement of the recommendation, which better communicates the meanings of some of its terms, is this: Adults should engage in a brisk walk, or an equivalently intense aerobic activity, for at least 10 minutes at a time, for a total of at least 30 minutes a day, on at least 5 days a week.

Several comments help to clarify these two recommendations. First, moderate-intensity physical activity is defined as aerobic activities that expend 3.0 to 6.0 METS (metabolic equivalents; ie, 4 to 7 kcal/min). The standard example of a moderate-intensity activity is brisk walking at 3 to 4 miles per hour. Vigorous activities, such as running, expend more than 6.0 METS. Many activities allow a broad range of intensity of effort, so they can be performed as either moderate or vigorous activities, including cycling, swimming,

backpacking, skiing, stair climbing, and volleyball. Second, only activity bouts of at least 10 minutes in duration count toward meeting either recommendation. Third, any physical activity, not just exercise, can count toward meeting the recommendations, including occupational activity, leisure-time activity, domestic activity such as gardening, and transportation activity. Fourth, daily physical activity is preferable, in part because there are beneficial acute effects of physical activity such as reduction in blood pressure. Daily activity is also recommended on the basis of the philosophy that the body is designed to be active every day. Finally, greater amounts of physical activity produce greater health benefits. It is inappropriate to cite the recommendations as meaning that "a person only needs 30 minutes a day."

Despite some evidence that vigorous activity has greater health benefit and some evidence that even low-intensity activities have benefit, the recommendations reflect consensus that moderate intensity is the minimum threshold for substantial health benefits. Despite the fact "more is better" and that a minimum of 60 minutes of moderate activity has been suggested, the recommendations reflect consensus that substantial health benefits accrue from 30 to 60 minutes of moderate activity.

Resistance Training

Adults should perform resistance training activities of the major muscle groups on 2 or 3 days each week, with at least 48 hours of rest in between. For all adults, ACSM recommends resistance training of moderate intensity that is sufficient to develop and maintain muscular fitness and fat-free mass. Selected adults may prefer high-intensity training instead. Dynamic resistance training (as opposed to static training) is recommended for most adults.

Flexibility Training

Activities that develop and maintain musculoskeletal flexibility and that are performed a minimum of twice a week are recommended. Unlike aerobic activities and resistance training, flexibility training by itself does not have substantial health benefits. It is recommended because regular physical activity requires an adequate range of motion, and flexibility training permits and facilitates the types of physical activity that have health benefit.

Balance Training

Unlike aerobic activity, resistance training, and flexibility training, balance training is not recommended for all adults. Balance training is currently recommended only for adults at increased risk of falls, as explained below.

PHYSICAL ACTIVITY LEVELS IN OLDER ADULTS

Older adults are the least active age group. In 2001, 11% of adults aged 65 and over reported strength training activities at least twice a week, and only 6% met both strength training and aerobic recommendations. However, trend data show increasing levels of physical activity in older adults over time. In 1990, 30% of adults aged 75 and over met either the strength training or aerobic recommendation, compared with 35% in 2000. In 1988, 41% of adults aged 70 and over were sedentary (reported no leisure-time physical activity), compared with 30% in 2002.

RECOMMENDING PHYSICAL ACTIVITY TO OLDER ADULTS

Preference for Moderate-Intensity Aerobic Activity

The vast majority of sedentary and insufficiently active older adults should gradually increase moderate aerobic activity, especially walking, so as to meet the recommendation for moderate intensity. Moderate exercise is associated with lower cardiovascular risk, lower risk of musculoskeletal injury, and, in comparison with vigorous exercise, a higher adherence to training. Most older adults prefer moderate-intensity activities. A target between 30 and 60 minutes of moderate activity on 5 to 7 days each week is appropriate for most older adults.

The traditional emphasis on walking for older adults is appropriate. The obvious advantages of walking are that it requires no special skills, equipment, or facilities. The risk of injury is relatively low. One study has reported that higher amounts of walking are not associated with a higher injury risk. Walking is the most common physical activity reported by older adults.

Importance of Resistance Training

Age-related decreases in skeletal muscle mass and quality, termed *sarcopenia*, contribute to functional limitations and dependence in older adults. Sarcopenia is more than just disuse atrophy, as even highly trained athletes lose muscle mass with age. The biologic mechanisms for sarcopenia are incompletely understood. Neurogenic mechanisms may involve the loss of

neurons for a variety of reasons, such as exposure to heavy metals, loss of blood supply, and mechanical damage. Denervated muscle fibers can be reinnervated by axonal sprouting of remaining motor neurons, but the process appears to be incomplete, so that cycles of denervation and reinnervation result in net loss of fibers. Myogenic mechanisms include the possibility that repair processes for contraction-induced muscle damage are impaired with aging. General mechanisms of cell damage may involve skeletal muscle, including damage of skeletal muscle mitochondria by free radicals.

Epidemiologic studies report that regular physical activity reduces age-related loss of muscle mass. Randomized controlled trials have demonstrated that resistance training increases muscle mass and thereby counteracts sarcopenia. Early studies of resistance training prescribed vigorous training similar to that prescribed for young adults. Subsequently, it has been demonstrated that less training has both physiologic effects on muscle function and health benefits. Larger gains in strength are typically reported by studies using weight machines. For older adults with good fitness, weight machines are usually the most feasible and safest training method. Randomized trails have also tested resistance training programs that use body weight or free weights, such as weight cuffs or dumbbells. These programs are more appropriate for adults with lower fitness levels, where lower amounts of weight provide adequate exercise stimulus. In theory, resistance in a home-based program can be adjusted on the basis of the progressive overload principle, and, given sufficient repetitions, strength should increase steadily. In practice, these programs typically report smaller gains in strength.

Other Considerations

With older adults, there is more emphasis on doing the minimum amount of all recommended types of activity: aerobic activities, resistance training, flexibility training, and (if at increased risk of falling) balance training. It is appropriate to encourage older adults to join exercise classes that mix aerobic, resistance, and flexibility training.

The traditional guidance to increase level of physical activity gradually over time is highly appropriate for older adults. Injury risk is minimized, and the experience is more pleasant. Focus group studies report that older adults view increasing physical activity as an extremely difficult task. It is appropriate to break this task up into stages, with intermediate goals. Adults with lower fitness should be permitted more time to adapt to each stage.

Older adults should be strongly encouraged to reduce sedentary behavior and get some activity each week, even if less than the minimum recommended. Illustrative of the dose-response relationship of activity and health, many studies show that levels of activity below minimum recommendations have health benefits in older adults.

For many older adults, exercise has a therapeutic role in one or more chronic conditions, as well as its traditional preventive role. Most commonly, integrating preventive and therapeutic recommendations involves essentially following public health recommendations, with specific preferences for modes of activity. For example, aquatic exercise classes are chosen for adults with arthritis, weight-bearing exercise is chosen for adults with osteoporosis, and rotation of exercise modes is chosen for adults with obesity to minimize risk of orthopedic injury. As chronic conditions become more severe, therapeutic considerations typically are the main determinants of the activity recommendation, such as pulmonary rehabilitation for adults with moderate to severe lung disease.

CONSIDERATIONS IN OLDER ADULTS WITH LOW FITNESS

For aerobic activities, a different definition of intensity is necessary for adults with low fitness. Intensity is defined, not as absolute energy expenditure in METS, but relative to the person's level of fitness, as judged by the heart-rate response to exercise. Moderate-intensity activity has a heart-rate response in the range of 55% to 69% of maximal heart rate (220 − age for men; 220 − [0.6 × age] for women), and vigorous intensity is the range greater than 69% of maximal heart rate. With this definition of intensity, unfit older adults need not do a brisk walk or equivalently intense activity to meet the moderate recommendation. Rather, the person should walk at a speed that causes a heart rate response in the range of moderate intensity.

Physical activity should be increased very gradually in adults with low fitness. Initially, short bouts of activity are appropriate. Activity bouts less than 10 minutes are acceptable. It is not necessary to specify a minimum heart rate.

Older adults in community-based long-term-care programs and residents of long-term-care facilities benefit from physical activity. Supervised classes of a few months' duration cause improvements in fitness and functional limitations, even in older adults who are physically frail or who have incontinence or mild dementia. Physical activity may improve sleep and decrease agitation. Exercise programs for nursing-home residents may include strength training, even high-intensity training. Randomized trials show strength training to be safe, increase strength, improve functional limitations, and increase amount of spontaneous activity.

OBESITY

The obesity epidemic has placed a great deal of attention on the role of physical activity in maintaining a healthy body weight. Public health recommendations advise that weight loss should be achieved by both reducing caloric intake and increasing energy expenditure. Possibly, regular physical activity during weight loss may be more important for older adults. Obesity increases the risk of many chronic diseases and of functional limitations in older adults, but it also has the beneficial effects of increasing bone and muscle mass. Weight loss is accompanied by loss of bone and muscle mass. Exercise during weight loss, particularly resistance training, should theoretically reduce loss of bone and muscle mass. For older adults advised to lose weight, a reasonable approach is to meet the moderate recommendations for 30 minutes or more and to limit caloric intake. Physical activity level then can be gradually increased as necessary to achieve and maintain a healthy weight.

OSTEOPOROSIS, FALLS, FRACTURES, AND BALANCE TRAINING

Regular physical activity by older adults has a modest effect in slowing age-related loss of bone mass. Evidence indicates that resistance and high-impact exercises are most beneficial. Weight-bearing aerobic activities can also provide the mechanical loading that maintains bone mass.

In older adults at increased risk for falling, randomized trials demonstrate that falls can be prevented by multicomponent interventions targeting factors such as sedative use, environmental hazards, and poor balance. Increasing physical activity is regarded as an effective component of falls prevention programs. Solid evidence of the effectiveness of exercise in falls prevention comes from a meta-analysis of a series of exercise studies in New Zealand, which reported that exercise reduces both falls and fall injuries by 35% to 45%. One meta-analysis of randomized trials reported that aerobic activity, resistance training, and balance training are all associated with reduced risk of falling. Balance training is specifically recommended in clinical practice guidelines for falls prevention in adults at increased risk. There is no experimental evidence that exercise reduces either total fractures or hip fractures. However, a meta-analysis of epidemiologic studies reported that physical activity reduces the risk of hip fracture by up to 50%.

A variety of balance training interventions have been studied. Some exercises focus on maintaining balance over a narrow base of support, such as a tandem stand or one-leg stand. Other exercises train dynamic balance, such as ability to do a tandem walk. Some programs have separate balance exercises. Others propose that some stretching and strengthening exercises be done in a manner that also improves balance. An example of the latter is the program described in the books *Exercise: A Guide from the National Institute on Aging* (http://www.niapublications.org/exercisebook/index.asp) and *Exercise: Getting Fit for Life* (http:www.niapublications.org/engagepages/exercise.asp).

Balance training is typically designed so that exercises are graduated in difficulty, and adults progress to more difficult exercise as training improves balance. For example, a tandem walk is easiest when holding on to a table and becomes progressively harder with arms in any position, arms close to the body, and arms close to the body while holding a weight.

Tai Chi Chuan is often mentioned as a form of exercise that improves balance and prevents falls. Although the original study of Tai Chi reported almost a 50% reduction in falls, a follow-up study reported a (nonsignificant) 25% reduction. A reasonable summary of the evidence is that Tai Chi remains a promising intervention that is popular, fun, and social, and it is appropriate for the balance training component of a falls prevention program.

THE RISKS OF PHYSICAL ACTIVITY

Although the benefits of physical activity far outweigh the risks, promoting physical activity should include strategies for minimizing risk. The main risk of physical activity is musculoskeletal injury. Several factors affecting musculoskeletal injury risk are modifiable and offer opportunities for risk management. The risk of injury is higher with vigorous exercise, with higher volume of exercise, and with obesity. The risk of injury is less with higher fitness, supervision, protective equipment such as bike helmets, and in well-designed exercise environments. The principle that physical activity should be increased gradually over time is widely regarded as critical for reducing risk of injury. Vigorous activity, such as running and participation in vigorous sports, should be recommended only to older adults who are accustomed to these activities or who have sufficient fitness, experience, and knowledge to perform vigorous activities and prevent injuries associated with them. ACSM recommends that older adults begin resistance training with one set of 10 to 15 repetitions of each exercise, rather than the 8 to 12 repetitions for younger adults. To complete more repetitions, training must begin with less resistance (relative to maximal strength), which should reduce injury risk.

The risk of both exercise-related myocardial infarction and sudden death is greatest in individuals who are the least active. Sedentary adults should avoid isolated bouts of vigorous activity and should increase activity gradually over time.

PROMOTING PHYSICAL ACTIVITY

A general clinical approach to promoting physical activity is shown in Figure 8.1. *Healthy People 2010* recommends that clinicians counsel physically inactive adults to increase their physical activity level. However, the U.S. Preventive Services Task Force regards the efficacy data on counseling as difficult to interpret. A wide variety of interventions have been studied, and the results are mixed. The U.S. Preventive Services Task Force has recommended high-intensity counseling about diet and exercise, together with behavioral interventions, for obese adults with a body mass index of 30 or greater.

One clinical approach to promoting physical activity is to adopt the 5-A framework (assess, advise, agree, assist, and arrange), which has been used in behavioral interventions such as smoking cessation. Because of the importance of physical activity, the clinician assesses an older patient's level of physical activity at least once a year and provides a specific recommendation about physical activity. The clinician and patient collaboratively agree on goals for physical activity. The clinician provides assistance. Counseling is one option; other options include self-help materials, referral to community programs, and referral to medically supervised programs.

Older adults typically feel overwhelmed by recommendations calling for substantial and immediate life-style changes. A stepwise approach is often appropriate. It allows the person to take small steps toward a tangible goal and feel rewarded upon meeting it, before moving on to the next, more ambitious goal.

Pedometers have become popular in promoting walking. Pedometers can be useful in providing feedback and monitoring progress toward physical activity goals. However, it is not appropriate to prescribe a universal step goal, such as 10,000 steps a day. Recommendations specify a minimum bout of 10 minutes, so many of the steps recorded by a pedometer do not count toward physical activity recommendations. Further, pedometers can miscount steps in older adults with slower gaits. However, some adults find step counters to be helpful in tracking activity levels and use them appropriately to ensure that every day includes an adequate amount of brisk walking. Some weight-management approaches use bouts of activity less than 10 minutes or low-intensity activity, or both,

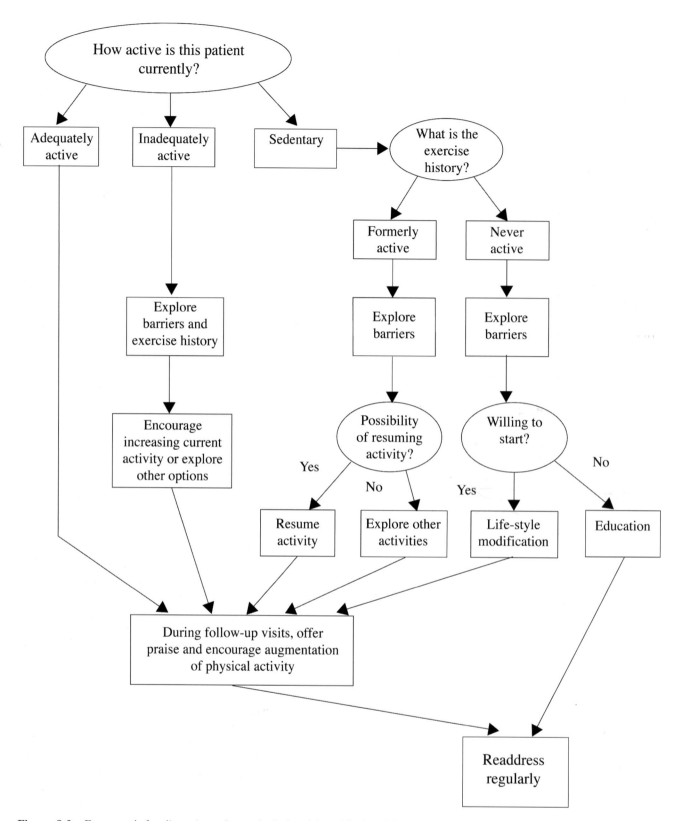

Figure 8.1—Framework for discussions about physical activity with the older patient.

SOURCE: Christmas C, Andersen RA. Exercise and older patients: guidelines for the clinician. *J Am Geriatr Soc.* 2000;48(3):321. Reprinted by permission of Blackwell Science, Inc.

to increase caloric expenditure. Pedometers can be useful in tracking progress to caloric expenditure goals.

Research highlights the importance of the physical and social environment in promoting physical activity. Studies report that people with access to recreational facilities are twice as likely to get recommended levels of physical activity. People are more likely to commute to work by bicycle or by walking if they live in a city center with a variety of destinations, such as grocery stores and restaurants, and have good access to public transportation. The medical care system should work in tandem with the community to promote environments that encourage physical activity. Clinicians should be aware that there are effective community-level interventions to promote physical activity. The Guide to Community Preventive Services identifies six recommended or strongly recommended community-level interventions proven effective in increasing physical activity. These are community-wide campaigns, prompts to increase usage of stairs, individually adapted behavior change programs implemented in groups of adults, school-based physical education, interventions that increase nonfamily social support such as programs that arrange walking groups, and enhanced access to recreational facilities (eg, parks and trails) combined with outreach to promote awareness of facilities.

REFERENCES

- Nelson ME, Layne JE, Bernstein MJ, et al. The effects of multidimensional home-based exercise on functional performance in elderly people. *J Gerontol A Biol Sci Med Sci.* 2004;59(2);154–160.

- Penninx BW, Messier SP, Rejeski WJ, et al. Physical exercise and the prevention of disability in activities of daily living in older persons with osteoarthritis. *Arch Intern Med.* 2001;161(19):2309–2316.

- Resnick B. A longitudinal analysis of efficacy expectations and exercise in older adults. *Res Theory Nurs Pract.* 2004;18(4):331–344.

- Resnick B, Orwig D, Magaziner J, et al. The effect of social support on exercise behavior in older adults. *Clin Nurs Res.* 2002;11(1):52–70.

- Tanasescu M, Leitzmann MF, Rimm EB, et al. Exercise type and intensity in relation to coronary heart disease in men. *JAMA.* 2002;288(16);1994–2000.

CHAPTER 9—PREVENTION

KEY POINTS

- The clinician has available a growing number of preventive services that have been shown to be effective in the care of older persons.

- It is important to consider all relevant issues in determining which conditions to screen for, the appropriate screening interval, and when (if ever) to discontinue screening in an older patient.

- Many factors need to be taken into account when recommending for or against screening for various cancers in the older person.

- Several system-based approaches can be employed for optimal implementation of preventive services (eg, trained office staff, computer reminders).

As the population ages and the average active life expectancy increases, issues of primary and secondary prevention become increasingly important. The prevalence of undetected, correctable conditions and comorbid diseases is high in older adults. Moreover, a growing number of older adults are highly motivated about disease prevention and health promotion. The clinician provides the information and opportunity for preventive care that helps older patients to maintain functional independence for as long as possible. Additionally, clinicians must understand the significant heterogeneity of the aging population. Recommendations for screening community-dwelling, cognitively and functionally intact individuals will necessarily be quite different from those dealing with functionally dependent and cognitively impaired nursing-home residents with multiple comorbidities.

Many findings from research on preventive care and the appropriate components of periodic health examinations are inconclusive. In addition, older persons are typically not included in clinical trials of preventive strategies, which has limited the clinician's ability to adjust guidelines for preventive practices for patients aged 65 and older on the basis of new scientific findings. Primary care clinicians are consequently compelled to rely on clinical judgment in planning the preventive care of their older patients.

A number of factors, including age, functional status, comorbidity, patient preference, socioeconomic status, and the availability of care, affect health care decisions of the older adult. Unlike chronologic age, physiologic age may be determined by self-rated health and overall medical condition. Classifications that are based on life expectancy, physiologic age, and functional status may facilitate medical decision making with older patients. For example, the clinician might strongly recommend fecal occult blood testing (FOBT) to a healthy, functionally independent patient; discuss the potential pros and cons of FOBT and offer the test to a chronically ill, partially dependent patient; and actually recommend against FOBT for a severely frail, demented patient. It is important to consider all relevant issues in determining which conditions to screen for, the appropriate screening interval, and when (if ever) to discontinue screening in an older patient.

The risks of screening and its follow-up diagnostics and treatments (eg, perforation from colonoscopy; impotence or incontinence from prostate surgery) need more emphasis when discussions regarding screening recommendations occur. Also, attention to all-cause mortality, as opposed to disease-specific mortality, must be taken into account. For example, finding a preventable cancer that might result in death in 5 to 10 years if not detected early is of no benefit (and can result in actual harm and considerable cost) in an individual whose life expectancy is less than 5 years. It is important, too, that the values, beliefs, and preferences of older patients be factored into discussions, as should issues regarding quality of life.

Attention to the underlying principles of primary and secondary prevention is important for patients of any age. Screening measures should be systematically performed when the prevalence and morbidity or mortality of the condition outweighs both the economic cost and potential consequences of a falsely positive or negative test result. Some recommendations may be applicable only to high-risk individuals, not to the general population. (See also the discussion of cancer screening in "Oncology," p 445, and definitions of terms used to assess screening tests in the Appendix, p 464.)

Increasingly important is the clinician's responsibility to counsel against the often grossly exaggerated and unproven claims of the anti-aging industry. The dollar costs and potential psychologic and physical damage associated with this burgeoning area are staggering and very worrisome.

RECOMMENDED PREVENTIVE SERVICES

A number of preventive services have been shown to be effective in the care of older persons and are widely endorsed. Table 9.1 summarizes these preventive activities, which are discussed below.

Screening

Obesity or Malnutrition

Routine measurement of height and weight can be used to calculate body mass index (BMI = kg/m^2). Obesity has been defined in men as a BMI $\geq$ 27.8 and in women as a BMI $\geq$ 27.3. An unintentional weight loss of 10 pounds in 6 months can indicate malnutrition or a serious occult illness. (See also "Malnutrition," p 161.)

Hypertension

The prevalence of hypertension increases with advancing age. The treatment of hypertension in older adults has been associated with a reduction in morbidity and mortality from left ventricular hypertrophy, heart failure, myocardial infarction, and stroke. However, older adults are more susceptible to adverse effects of antihypertensive therapy, such as hyponatremia, hypokalemia, depression, confusion, or postural hypotension. (See also "Hypertension," p 331.) This susceptibility is especially true for the oldest-old patients and those with multiple comorbidities and taking multiple medications.

Vision and Hearing Deficits

Uncorrected refractive errors, glaucoma, cataracts, and macular degeneration account for most undetected visual disorders. Routine screening with a Snellen chart is recommended by the U.S. Preventive Services Task Force (USPSTF). Undetected hearing loss can lead to social isolation and may indicate other underlying disorders. The USPSTF recommends periodically questioning older adults about their hearing and counseling them about the availability of hearing aid devices. The evidence for routine audiometry as a screening tool is unproven. (See also "Visual Impairment," p 140, and "Hearing Impairment," p 145.)

Depression

Depression is a disease with significant morbidity and mortality in the older age group. Treatment can be highly effective. The USPSTF recommends screening of the general adult population. Importantly, they add the recommendation that clinicians who do screen for depression have systems in place to assure accurate diagnosis, effective treatment, and follow-up. There are several reliable and valid depression screening instruments for older persons, including the Geriatric Depression Scale. (See the Appendix, p 458; see also "Depression and Other Mood Disorders," p 247).

Table 9.1—Evidence-Based Preventive Services Recommended for Older Adults

Preventive Activity	Frequency	Condition to Detect or Prevent
Screening		
Height and weight	at least annually	Obesity, malnutrition
Blood pressure	at least annually	Hypertension
Vision testing	annually	Visual deficits
Hearing ability	annually	Hearing impairment
Depression questionnaire	*	Depression
Alcoholism questionnaire	*	Alcoholism
Serum lipids (with prior MI, angina)	annually	Recurrent CAD
Abdominal ultrasonography (men aged 65–75 years who have ever smoked)	once	Abdominal aortic aneurysm
Bone density measurement	*	Osteoporosis
Glucose (with hypertension or hyperlipidemia)	*	Type 2 diabetes mellitus
Mammography	every 2–3 years	Breast cancer
Pap smear	at least every 3 years**	Cervical cancer
Fecal occult blood testing *and/or*	annually	Colorectal cancer
flexible sigmoidoscopy *or*	every 3–5 years	
colonoscopy	once	
Counseling to encourage:		
Smoking cessation	every visit	COPD, many cancers, CAD
Regular dental visits	annually	Malnutrition, oral cancers, edentulism
Low-fat, well-balanced diet	annually	Obesity, CAD
Adequate calcium intake	annually	Osteoporosis
Physical activity	annually	Immobility, CAD, osteoporosis
Injury prevention	annually	Injurious falls, motor vehicle crashes, burns, other injuries
Immunization		
Influenza vaccination	annually	Influenza
Pneumococcal vaccination	†	Pneumococcal disease
Tetanus booster	every 10 years	Tetanus
Chemoprophylaxis		
Aspirin therapy	daily	Recurrent MI, TIA, or stroke

Note: CAD = coronary artery disease; COPD = chronic obstructive pulmonary disease; MI = myocardial infarction; TIA = transient ischemic attack. For updates from the U.S. Preventive Services Task Force, see http://www.ahrq.gov/clinic/prevenix.htm (accessed November 2006).

* The optimal interval for screening is unknown.

** May stop screening at age 65 if patient has had regularly normal smears up to that age; if never tested prior to age 65, may stop after two normal annual smears.

† Vaccinate immunocompetent patients once at age 65; revaccination after 7–10 years may be appropriate.

Alcoholism

All older adults should be screened for alcohol abuse at least once and whenever a drinking problem is suspected. Screening questionnaires such as the CAGE (see Table 39.1, p 278) can be useful in detecting alcohol problems. (See also "Substance Abuse," p 274.)

Dyslipidemia

There is good evidence that in elderly persons with prior myocardial infarction or angina, correcting lipid abnormalities (ie, levels of low-density lipoprotein ≥ 130 mg/dL, of high-density lipoprotein ≤35 mg/dL, of triglycerides ≥200 mg/dL) lowers the risk of recurrent cardiac events. These persons should be screened for lipid abnormalities; treatment goals for those found to have dyslipidemia should be low-density lipoprotein levels of <100 mg/dL, high-density lipoprotein levels of >40 mg/dL, and tri-glyceride levels of <200 mg/dL. There is no evidence that screening older adults who are clinically free of coronary artery disease (CAD) or who have few cardiac risk factors for primary prevention of CAD is effective. (See also "Cardiovascular Diseases and Disorders," p 316.)

Abdominal Aortic Aneurysm

The USPSTF recommends one-time screening for abdominal aortic aneurysm (AAA) by ultrasonography in men aged 65 to 75 years who have ever smoked. Evidence shows that screening for AAA and surgical repair of large AAAs ($\geq$5.5 cm) in men aged 65 to 75 years who have ever smoked (current and former smokers) leads to decreased AAA-specific mortality. Because of the potential harms of screening and early treatment (including an increased number of surgeries with associated clinically significant morbidity and mortality), the USPSTF makes no recommendation for or against screening for AAA in men aged 65 to 75 years who have never smoked. Since women have a low prevalence of large AAAs, the USPSTF recommends against routine screening for AAA in women.

Osteoporosis

The USPSTF now recommends that women aged 65 and older be screened routinely for osteoporosis by the use of bone density measurements. For those at high risk for osteoporotic fractures, the task force recommends beginning screening at age 60. Clinician counseling regarding adequate calcium intake, smoking cessation, exercise, and avoidance of falls is also recommended. (See also "Osteoporosis and Osteomalacia," p 194.)

Breast Cancer

Despite considerable controversy regarding the efficacy of screening mammography, almost all government-sponsored groups, medical societies, and advocacy groups do recommend routine mammography for women aged 65 and older. How often to screen and at what age to stop remain unresolved. Mammography every 2 to 3 years for older women with an active life expectancy of 5 or more years is a reasonable guideline. For high-risk individuals, yearly screening is prudent. Medicare covers annual screening mammograms.

Clinician breast examination is not uniformly recommended for screening, and breast self-examination has not been shown to be efficacious.

(See also the section of breast cancer in "Oncology," p 448.)

Cervical Cancer

Approximately 40% of new cases of invasive cervical cancer and deaths from cervical cancer occur in women aged 65 years and over. The Papanicolaou smear is most cost-effective in older patients who have previously had incomplete screening. Between 4% and 8% of cervical cancers are found in the cervical stump in women who have undergone incomplete hysterectomy. Regular Pap smears every 1 to 3 years are recommended for all women who are or have been sexually active and who have a cervix. Medicare has covered triennial screening without age limit since 1990. The appropriate cut-off age for screening remains controversial, although most experts recommend cessation of screening after age 65 if the patient has had a history of regularly normal smears. In older women never previously screened, screening can cease after two normal Pap smears are obtained 1 year apart.

Colorectal Cancer

Although evidence is not yet definitive, screening for colorectal cancer by colonoscopy is the preferred method for older persons. The entire colon can be examined expeditiously by an experienced endoscopist and any appropriate biopsies can be obtained.

Medicare will pay for a screening colonoscopy every 10 years for all beneficiaries. In addition, Medicare provides coverage for annual FOBT and biennial flexible sigmoidoscopy. A double-contrast or air-contrast screening barium enema may be substituted for either a screening flexible sigmoidoscopy or a screening colonoscopy. When FOBT is recommended, instructions regarding proper diet, medication usage, and vitamin usage before and during stool collections and proper collection technique are crucial in order to avoid false positives and negatives. "Virtual" colonoscopy, a new method using thin-section, helical computed tomography, is currently under investigation as a screening tool for colorectal cancer.

Studies have refuted the concept that a low-fat, high-fiber diet plays a role in preventing colorectal cancer. Although epidemiologic data suggest that aspirin or nonsteroidal anti-inflammatory drugs may be protective against colorectal cancer, there is insufficient evidence to support the routine use of these medications for primary prevention. However, for individuals wanting to maximize prevention and having no contraindications, one aspirin daily is reasonable and justifiable. This does not replace screening, FOBT, sigmoidoscopy, or colonoscopy.

(See also the section on colon cancer in "Oncology," p 449.)

Counseling

Smoking Cessation

Smoking cessation at any age reduces rates of chronic obstructive pulmonary disease, many cancers, and CAD. All older adult smokers should be encouraged to and helped with smoking cessation at each office visit.

(See also "Substance Abuse," p 274, and "Respiratory Diseases and Disorders," p 300.)

Dental Care

Many common problems can be detected and effectively treated by regular dental visits, including periodontitis, xerostomia, and oral cancers. (See also "Oral Diseases and Disorders," p 294.)

Dietary Counseling

The importance of a well-balanced diet should be addressed routinely with older adults. An appropriate diet is high in fruits and vegetables and low in fat and salt, and it has adequate calcium content. Also, it is important not to overly restrict the diet of those who are underweight or frail. Restrictions in these situations can be counterproductive and lead to increased morbidity. (See also "Malnutrition," p 161.)

Physical Activity

Increasing evidence supports the importance of physical activity for both physical health and sense of well-being. Physical activity has been associated with greater mobility and lower rates of CAD and osteoporosis. Older adults should be counseled about an exercise program that balances modalities of flexibility (eg, stretching), endurance (eg, walking or cycling), strength (weight training), and balance (eg, Tai Chi or dance therapy). (See also "Physical Activity," p 51.)

Injury Prevention

The USPSTF recommends counseling older persons on measures to reduce the risk of falling (see also "Falls," p 187, "Gait Impairment," p 181, and the appendix, p 459 for details about preventing falls), safety-related skills and behaviors, and environmental hazard reduction. Safety-related behaviors include the regular use of seat and lap belts in automobiles, regular driving tests, and avoidance of alcohol use while driving or operating machinery. Environmental hazard reduction might include lowering hot-water temperature to prevent serious burns, installing smoke detectors, and, in homes of demented persons, installing alarms and automatic shut-off features on appliances, and removing or safely storing firearms. A home safety checklist or formal environmental assessment by a physical or occupational therapist can facilitate injury prevention.

Immunizations

Medicare covers the costs of influenza, pneumococcal, and tetanus immunizations.

OL Not approved by the U.S. Food and Drug Administration for this use.

Influenza Vaccine

The current influenza vaccine is a killed virus that is moderately immunogenic, with estimated efficacy rates of 70% for illness and 90% for mortality. Multiple evaluations of the vaccine's efficacy reveal that, although it incompletely protects against disease, it clearly reduces rates of respiratory illness, hospitalization, and mortality in the elderly age group. Annual vaccine administration must be provided because of antigenic drift and the short-lived (4 to 5 months) protection provided by the vaccine. Current recommendations are that all patients aged 65 or over or those under age 65 with underlying medical illnesses be immunized annually between October and mid-November, but any time from September to the end of influenza season is appropriate. Medical personnel and caregivers for high-risk patients should also be immunized. Potential adverse effects include fever, chills, myalgias, and malaise, but these are rare. Contraindications include anaphylactic egg hypersensitivity or allergic reactions following occupational exposure to egg protein. Live, attenuated influenza vaccines have been developed, appear to be more effective, and are likely to be approved for widespread use in the near future.

In outbreak situations, chemoprophylaxis can protect against influenza during the 2 weeks immediately after immunization until the antibody response is mounted, or in persons who cannot receive the vaccine. Zanamivir[OL] and oseltamivir, both neuraminidase inhibitors, are effective for influenza A and have activity against influenza B. These drugs differ greatly with regard to cost, adverse effects, mechanism of action, and mode of delivery. Zanamivir is administered via a disk-inhaler system, while oseltamivir is taken orally.

Treatment of influenza is also possible with both drugs and reduces the duration of illness by about 1 to 1.5 days, if started within 24 hours of symptom onset. Resistance to the neuraminidase inhibitors is not well characterized at this time.

Pneumococcal Vaccination

Pneumococcal vaccination is indicated for all persons aged 65 years or older and many persons under age 65 with comorbid conditions. If $\geq$ 5 years has elapsed since the first dose and the patient was vaccinated before the age of 65, repeat vaccination is indicated. Studies show that adverse events following revaccination are rare and mild. Thus, an unknown vaccination history should prompt administration of the pneumococcal vaccine. (*When in doubt, vaccinate!*) The vaccine does not prevent mucosal disease such as sinusitis and has unclear efficacy for preventing pneumonia. However, there is strong evidence that suggests that the vaccine reduces the risk of invasive disease (ie, bacteremia) and that it is cost-effective for older immune-competent adults.

Although the protective efficacy of the pneumococcal vaccine is estimated to be only 60% to 70% and studies have revealed mixed results regarding benefits in high-risk older adults, all patients aged 65 years and older should receive one dose of 0.5 mg IM. Studies suggest that people may benefit from revaccination every 7 to 10 years. Other than local soreness, adverse effects are usually minimal.

Tetanus Vaccination

More than 60% of tetanus infections occur in persons aged 60 years of age and older. There is evidence that the absorbed tetanus and diphtheria toxoids provide long-term protection 35 years after the primary series or booster. Older adults who have never been vaccinated should receive two doses, 0.5 mg IM 1 to 2 months apart, followed by an additional dose 6 to 12 months later. The optimal interval for booster doses is not established; the USPSTF and Canadian Task Force recommend booster vaccinations every 10 years. Local pain and swelling or, rarely, hypersensitivity may accompany vaccination. A neurologic or hypersensitivity reaction to a previous dose is an absolute contraindication.

OTHER PREVENTIVE SERVICES TO CONSIDER

A number of other preventive activities are recommended by assorted specialty organizations even though the evidence for effectiveness is lacking. Some of these preventive measures are listed in Table 9.2. In the face of unproven effectiveness for each of these procedures, clinicians must weigh the potential benefits of the preventive procedure against the potential risks of unnecessary treatment. Procedures that are particularly pertinent and controversial in the older adult population are discussed below.

Screening

Skin Cancer

The USPSTF recommends neither for nor against annual skin examination to detect early skin cancers because of a lack of research-proven effectiveness. However, the relatively low cost associated with annual

Table 9.2—Potentially Beneficial Services Lacking Evidence

Preventive Activity	Condition to Detect or Prevent
Screening	
Skin inspection	Skin cancer
Mental status examination	Dementia
Blood glucose	Diabetic complications
Thyrotropin	Hypo- and hyperthyroidism
PSA *or* digital rectal examination *or* both	Prostate cancer
Serum lipids (without apparent CAD)	MI, angina
Nutritional supplementation, vitamins, antioxidants	Cancer, atherosclerosis
Chemoprophylaxis	
Aspirin therapy	Initial MI or stroke, or colon cancer

NOTE: CAD = coronary artery disease; MI = myocardial infarction; PSA = prostate-specific antigen.

skin examinations and the low costs and morbidity associated with treatment (eg, excision, cryotherapy) of false positives makes the decision to screen considerably less weighty for skin cancer than for prostate cancer. The USPSTF does recommend counseling high-risk patients (those who are light-skinned or with a past history of skin cancer) to avoid sun exposure and to use protective clothing when outdoors. (See also "Dermatologic Diseases and Disorders," p 284.)

Dementia

Although routinely screening for dementia in the general older population is not recommended by the USPSTF, clinicians should be alert to detect new cases as early as possible since a combination of medications, education, and counseling can benefit patients and their families.

For primary prevention, aggressively controlling cardiovascular and cerebrovascular risk factors (eg, hypertension, hyperlipidemia) may be helpful for both vascular and Alzheimer's dementias. There is some evidence that staying mentally active (eg, reading, pursuing new areas of learning, working crossword puzzles) may be beneficial in prevention as well. Estrogen and nonsteroidal anti-inflammatory agents are not efficacious in Alzheimer's prevention. Statins are currently under investigation and cannot at this time be routinely recommended for prevention of Alzheimer's disease. (See also "Dementia" p 204.)

Diabetes Mellitus

The increased prevalence of diabetes mellitus with age and the consequent morbidity burden warrants consideration for screening. Routine screening of asymptomatic adults for diabetes is not recommended by the USPSTF; however, the USPSTF does recommend screening for type 2 diabetes in those individuals with hyperlipidemia, as a method to improve an individual's risk estimates for coronary heart disease. (See also "Diabetes Mellitus," p 349.)

Thyroid Disease

The prevalence of subclinical and clinical hyperthyroidism and hypothyroidism increase with advancing age. The USPSTF does not recommend routine screening but acknowledges that screening may be performed on the basis of the high prevalence of the disease and the likelihood that its symptoms will be overlooked in older adults. The preferred test is the immunometric assay that is sensitive to thyrotropin. (See also "Endocrine and Metabolic Disorders," p 337.)

Prostate Cancer

Randomized controlled trials of screening by prostate-specific antigen or digital rectal examination, currently in progress, should provide valuable information on the efficacy of these modalities. Until the results of those trials are known, however, patients should be counseled about the implications of an elevated prostate-specific antigen level or a mass detected by digital rectal examination and the potential adverse effects (surgery, incontinence, impotence) of treating false or even true positives. The American College of Physicians supports selective testing in 50- to 69-year-old men, provided that optimistic assumptions are used and the risks, benefits, and uncertainties are understood. With evidence currently available, it is difficult to justify screening in men aged of 70 and over. Medicare covers the cost of prostate cancer screening. (See also "Prostate Disease," p 389.)

Nutritional Supplementation

For a discussion of vitamin and mineral supplements and antioxidants, see "Malnutrition," p 161.

Chemoprophylaxis: Aspirin Therapy

Aspirin therapy up to 500 mg per day has not been consistently shown to reduce myocardial infarction or cardiovascular mortality. The adverse bleeding effects of aspirin increase with age, although the absolute serious adverse-effect rate of dosages ≤325 mg per day is low. Older adults with risk factors for myocardial infarction or stroke may be more appropriate for prophylaxis with aspirin. (See also "Cardiovascular Diseases and Disorders," p 316.)

See also the section on infective endocarditis in "Infectious Diseases" (p 311) for the use of antibiotics to prevent infective endocarditis and prosthetic device infections in at-risk patients.

PREVENTIVE SERVICES NOT INDICATED IN OLDER ADULTS

Table 9.3 lists services that have been shown not to be effective in preventing certain conditions or their adverse outcomes. There is excellent evidence that the general screening modality of the annual complete history and physical examination is not any more effective for improving outcomes than a more targeted approach of individual screening, counseling, immunoprophylaxis, and chemoprophylaxis. Current evidence does not support specific screening for lung, pancreatic, ovarian, bladder, or hematologic malignancies for the general population. However, promising new screening modalities, such as helical low-density computed tomography of the chest for lung cancer and homocystinemia for heart disease, are being actively developed and investigated.

Recent evidence has demonstrated that the risks of estrogen-progestin combinations significantly outweigh any potential benefits and therefore should not be recommended. (See the section on estrogen replacement therapy in "Endocrine and Metabolic Disorders," p 347.)

DELIVERY OF PREVENTIVE SERVICES

A well-organized systems-based approach using various personnel, sites, and communication methods may narrow the gap between the knowledge of age-appropriate practice recommendations and the implementation of preventive measures. Lack of time and inadequate reimbursement are only two of the

Table 9.3—Preventive Services That Have Been Demonstrated Not to Be Beneficial

Annual complete history and physical examination
Screening for specific diseases
   Lung cancer
   Pancreatic cancer
   Ovarian cancer
   Bladder cancer
   Hematologic malignancies
Routine laboratory testing
   Annual complete blood cell count
   Annual blood chemistry panel
   Annual electrocardiogram
   Annual chest radiography
Chemoprophylaxis
   Hormone replacement therapy

barriers faced by clinicians. Overcoming these barriers commonly involves the assistance of paramedical personnel and the use of technology. A nurse or trained office assistant may be able to adequately explain a screening procedure such as FOBT and its implications in terms of follow-up diagnostic testing. Reminders can be used to prompt clinicians to offer selected screening tests and improve adherence to recommendations. Mailed or computer-generated reminders can be used to enhance screening rates for procedures such as mammography, colorectal cancer screening, and influenza vaccination. Automated telephone technology may be useful to deliver behavioral interventions for improving medication adherence, dietary modification, and physical activity among sedentary persons. Primary and secondary preventive services may be provided at a variety of sites, including ambulatory clinics, assisted-living and long-term-care facilities, mobile vans, and supermarket-based pharmacies.

The implementation and evaluation of novel approaches for preventive practice are clearly warranted if progress is to be made in this increasingly important field. The more the primary care clinician is able to rely upon others to help explain and perform preventive maneuvers, the greater the likelihood that the patient adherence will improve as well.

REFERENCES

■ Agency for Healthcare Research and Quality. Preventive Services. Available at http://www.ahrq.gov/clinic/prevenix.htm (accessed November 2006).

■ Kelley CG, Daly BJ, Anthony MK, et al. Nurse practitioners and preventive screening in the hospital. *Clin Nurs Res.* 2002;11(4):433–449.

■ Momeyer MA, Luggen AS. Geriatric nurse practitioner guideline: periodontal disease in older adults. *Geriatr Nurs.* 2005;26(3):197–200.

■ Resnick B. Promoting health in older adults: a four-year analysis. *J Am Acad Nurse Pract.* 2001;13(1):23–33.

■ Resnick B. Health promotion practices of the old-old. *J Am Acad Nurse Pract.* 1998;10(4):147–153.

■ Walter LC, Covinsky KE. Cancer screening in elderly patients: a framework for individualized decision making. *JAMA.* 2001;285(21):2750–2756.

CHAPTER 10—PHARMACOTHERAPY

KEY POINTS

■ Age-associated changes in body composition, metabolism, and pharmacodynamics make benzodiazepine use by older adults especially hazardous.

■ Risk factors associated with inappropriate prescribing and overprescribing include having more than one prescriber, poor record keeping, and the use of more than one pharmacy.

■ Recent evidence suggests that underprescribing of indicated medications for older patients is a bigger problem than the prescribing of inappropriate medications.

■ Cardiovascular drugs, diuretics, nonsteroidal anti-inflammatory drugs (NSAIDs), hypoglycemics, atypical antipsychotics, and anticoagulants are the drug classes most often associated with preventable adverse drug events.

■ Collaboration with pharmacists and access to up-to-date drug information can help the clinician to minimize the total number of medications and doses prescribed to individual patients and to avoid important drug-drug and drug-disease interactions.

People aged 65 years or older are prescribed the highest proportion of medications in relation to their percentage of the U.S. population. Currently, approximately 13% of the U.S. population is aged 65 years or older; this age group purchases 33% of all prescription drugs. By the year 2040, approximately 25% of the US population is expected to be 65 years or older, purchasing 50% of all prescription drugs.

Drugs are the most common treatment for acute and chronic diseases. They are also used to prevent many of the diseases and disorders of older adults. Successful pharmacotherapy requires the correct drug at the correct dosage, for the correct disease or condition, for the correct patient. Unfortunately, achieving these goals is not simple or easy. Many other factors come into play, including the patient's other disease states, other medications, adherence, beliefs, functional status, physiologic changes due to aging and disease, and ability to afford the medication. The basic principle of prescribing for older patients—briefly, start low, go slow—is repeated often. However, even the best clinicians who carefully adhere to this principle will encounter patients who have negative outcomes from one or more of their medications.

The principles of pharmacotherapy have not changed significantly during the past 20 years, but drug treatment has become more complex. More drugs are available every year, some with a new pharmacologic profile or mechanism of action. In addition, clinicians must contend with expanded indications for available agents, both those that are approved by the U.S. Food and Drug Administration (FDA) and those that are off-label. Clinicians also must be responsive to frequent changes in the managed-care formulary, coverage by Medicare Part D, the scientific advances in the understanding of drug-drug interactions (ie, the cytochrome P-450 system), the change of many drugs from prescription to nonprescription, and the boom in an unregulated third class of medications called *nutriceuticals,* ie, nutritional supplements, alternative medicines, and herbal preparations. Finally, very little information is available about the use of these unregulated medications in older patients—particularly, sick older patients on other medications.

AGE-ASSOCIATED CHANGES IN PHARMACOKINETICS

Pharmacokinetic studies define the time course of a drug and its metabolites throughout the body with respect to four parameters: absorption, distribution, metabolism, and elimination. The effects of aging on each parameter have been studied, and the resulting generalizations have been incorporated into the principles of prescribing for the older patient.

Absorption

Aging does not affect drug absorption via the gastrointestinal tract to any clinically significant degree. The rate of absorption may be slowed with age, but the extent of absorption remains unchanged. Consequently, the peak serum concentration of a drug in the older patient may be lower and the time to reach it delayed, but the overall amount absorbed (*bioavailability*) does not differ in younger and older patients. Exceptions include drugs that undergo an extensive first-pass effect (eg, nitrates); they tend to have higher serum concentrations or increased bioavailability, because less drug is extracted by the liver as a consequence of decreased liver size and blood flow.

Factors that have a greater impact on drug absorption include the way a medication is taken, what it is taken with, and a patient's comorbid illnesses. For example, the absorption of many fluoroquinolones (eg, ciprofloxacin) is reduced when they are taken with divalent cations such as calcium, magnesium, and iron that are found in antacids, sucralfate, dairy products, or vitamins. Enteral feedings interfere with the absorption of some drugs (eg, phenytoin). An increase in gastric pH from proton-pump inhibitors, H_2 antagonists, or antacids may increase the absorption of some drugs, such as nifedipine and amoxicillin, and decrease the absorption of other drugs, such as the imidazole antifungals, ampicillin, cyanocobalamin, and indinavir. Agents that promote or delay gastrointestinal motility, such as stimulant laxatives and metoclopramide, can, in theory, affect a drug's absorption by increasing or decreasing the time spent in the segment of the intestinal tract necessary for dissolution or absorption. Another mechanism that can increase or decrease drug absorption is the inhibition or induction of enzymes in the gastrointestinal tract (discussed on p 71, in the section on drug interactions).

Distribution

Distribution refers to the locations in the body a drug penetrates and the time required for the drug to reach those locations. Distribution is expressed as the volume of distribution (Vd), with units of volume (eg, liters) or volume per weight (eg, L/kg).

Age-associated changes in body composition can alter drug distribution. In older patients, drugs that are water soluble (*hydrophilic*) have a lower volume of distribution, because older people have less body water and lean body mass. Drugs affected include ethanol and lithium. Digoxin, which distributes and binds to skeletal muscle, has been reported to have a reduced volume of distribution in older patients because of the reduced muscle mass of older adults. Drugs that are fat soluble (*lipophilic*) have an increased volume of distribution in older patients because they have greater fat stores than do younger people. Thus, it takes longer for an older patient taking a lipophilic drug to reach a steady-state concentration and longer for the drug to be eliminated from the body. Examples of fat-soluble drugs include diazepam, flurazepam, thiopental, and trazodone.

The extent to which a drug is bound to plasma proteins also influences its volume of distribution. Albumin, the primary plasma protein to which drugs bind, is often decreased in older patients; thus, a higher proportion of drug is unbound (free) and pharmacologically active. Drugs that bind to albumin and have an unbound fraction that is increased in elderly patients include ceftriaxone, diazepam, lorazepam, phenytoin, valproic acid, and warfarin. Normally, additional unbound drug is eliminated; however, age-related decreases in the organ systems of elimination may result in the accumulation of unbound drug in the body. Phenytoin provides an example of the way an increase in unbound drug can lead to an unnecessary and potentially harmful dosage increase. A patient with a low serum albumin (≤3 g/dL) whose phenytoin dose is increased because his or her total phenytoin concentration is subtherapeutic may develop symptoms and signs of phenytoin toxicity after a dosage increase because the concentration of free phenytoin is increased.

Metabolism

The liver is the most common site of drug metabolism, but metabolic conversion also can occur in the intestinal wall, lungs, skin, kidneys, and other organs. Aging affects the liver by decreasing hepatic blood flow as well as by decreasing hepatic size and mass. Consequently, in the older patient the metabolic clearance of drugs by the liver may be reduced. Drug clearance is also reduced with aging for drugs that are subject to the phase I pathways or reactions, which include hydroxylation, oxidation, dealkylation, and reduction. Most drugs metabolized through phase I pathways may be converted to metabolites of lesser, equal, or greater pharmacologic effect than the parent compound (eg, diazepam). Drugs metabolized through the phase II pathways are converted to inactive compounds through glucuronidation, conjugation, or acetylation (eg, lorazepam). Medications subject to phase II metabolism are generally preferred for older patients, because their metabolites are not active and will not accumulate.

Age and gender differences also have been reported. For example, oxazepam is metabolized faster in elderly men than in elderly women. The reason is unknown. Nefazodone concentrations have been reported to be 50% greater in older women, but no differences were found between older men and younger persons.

In drug metabolism, factors other than aging can exaggerate or override the effects of aging. For example, hepatic congestion due to heart failure decreases the metabolism of warfarin, resulting in an increased pharmacologic response. Smoking stimulates monooxygenase enzymes and increases the clearance of theophylline even in older patients.

Elimination

Elimination refers to a drug's final route(s) of exit from the body. For most drugs, this involves elimination by the kidney as either the parent compound or as a metabolite or metabolites. Terms used to express elimination are a drug's *half-life* and its *clearance*.

A drug's half-life is the time it takes for its plasma or serum concentration to decline by 50%, for example, from 20 µg/mL to 10 µg/mL. Half-life is usually expressed in hours. Steady state is reached when the amount of drug entering the systemic circulation is equal to the amount being eliminated. For a drug administered on a regular basis, 95% of steady state in the body is achieved after five half-lives of the drug.

Clearance is usually expressed as volume per unit of time (eg, L/hour or mL/minute) and represents the volume of plasma or serum from which the drug is removed (ie, cleared) per unit of time. Clearance may also be expressed as volume per weight per unit of time (L/kg/hour). Half-life and clearance can also refer to metabolic elimination.

The effects of aging have been studied to a greater extent on kidney function than on liver function. Glomerular filtration declines as a consequence of decreased kidney size, renal blood flow, and functioning nephrons. On average, kidney function begins to decline when people reach their mid-30s, with an average decline of 6 to 12 mL per minute per 1.73 m² per decade. Follow-up studies (conducted in men only) over 10 to 15 years found three normally distributed groups: those whose creatinine clearance declined to the extent that it was clinically significant; a second group whose creatinine clearance declined to the extent that it was statistically but not clinically significant; those whose creatinine clearance did not change. Renal tubular secretion also declines with age.

Serum creatinine does not accurately reflect creatinine clearance in elderly patients. Because of the age-related decline in lean muscle mass, the older person's production of creatinine is reduced. The decrease in glomerular filtration rate counters the decreased production of creatinine, and serum creatinine stays within the normal range, not revealing the change in creatinine clearance.

The conservative approach in treating the older patient is to calculate the appropriate dosage for renally eliminated medications as if the patient's kidney function actually has declined with aging. Measuring a patient's 24-hour creatinine clearance would be the most accurate way to determine the appropriate dosage, but this is time consuming and requires an accurate 24-hour urine collection. An 8-hour collection time has been shown to be accurate but has not been widely accepted.

To initially estimate a patient's creatinine clearance (CrCl), the clinician can use the Cockroft and Gault equation (see below).

$$CrCl = \frac{(140 - age) \times weight}{72 \times serum\ creatinine}$$

Weight in kg; serum creatinine in mg/100 mL; 85% less in women.

The equation is widely applied, but it has limitations. First, not all patients experience a significant age-related decline in renal function, and for them, the equation would underestimate creatinine clearance. Second, for patients whose muscle mass is reduced beyond that of normal aging, the creatinine clearance would be overestimated. This would apply to patients whose serum creatinine is less than normal, ie, <0.7 mg/dL. It has been suggested that 1 mg/dL be substituted for a low serum creatinine. However, normalizing the serum creatinine has not been shown to be a precise estimate, and it generally underestimates the actual creatinine clearance.

In cases in which the patient's kidney function may be impaired but estimates of function are uncertain, the clinician should consider the following:

- Avoid drugs that depend on renal elimination and for which accumulation would result in toxicity (eg, imipenem).

- If the use of such an agent cannot be avoided, obtain an accurate measure of kidney function (eg, an 8- or 24-hour creatinine clearance).

- Monitor serum or plasma concentrations of the drug (eg, aminoglycosides).

AGE-ASSOCIATED CHANGES IN PHARMACODYNAMICS

The pharmacodynamic action of a drug—that is, its time course and intensity of pharmacologic effect—may change with the increasing age of the patient. An excellent example of such pharmacodynamic changes in older patients has been demonstrated with the benzodiazepines. Older people have more sedation and lower performance than younger people on a psychomotor test after a single dose of triazolam. These differences are attributed to pharmacokinetic changes, ie, to significantly higher plasma triazolam concentrations that are due to reduced clearance in elderly people. However, nitrazepam (an intermediate-acting benzodiazepine similar to lorazepam) has a different pattern: The pharmacokinetics of nitrazepam were found to be no different in young and older adults after a single 10-mg dose; yet, 12 hours and 36 hours after a 10-mg dose, older adults made significantly more mistakes on a psychomotor test than when they had taken placebo. Younger persons did not demonstrate significant impairment at any time. In addition, even with short-term use, young and elderly patients may experience impaired balance and posture after a single dose of a benzodiazepine.

It is uncertain whether the age-associated pharmacokinetic changes of morphine account for the increased level and prolonged duration of pain relief experienced by older patients. In older adults, morphine has a smaller volume of distribution, higher plasma concentrations, and longer clearance than in younger adults. Older patients achieve pain relief at least equivalent to that of younger patients at half the intramuscular dose, and their pain relief lasts longer. Thus, the dose or frequency, or both, of morphine given intramuscularly or by intravenous infusion should be lower, at least initially, in older patients.

Pharmacodynamic and pharmacokinetic changes, alone or together, generally result in an increased sensitivity to medications by older adults. In some patients, particularly those who are frail, the use of lower doses, longer intervals between doses, and longer periods between changes in dose are ways to successfully manage drug therapy and decrease the chances of medication intolerance or toxicity. Disease- and drug-specific monitoring are also necessary to ensure a successful outcome.

OPTIMIZING PRESCRIBING

Optimizing drug therapy for older adults means achieving the balance between overprescribing and underprescribing of beneficial therapies. Overprescribing of drug therapies not only refers to the use of multiple medications but also implies a lack of appropriateness in medication selection, dosage, or use. One survey found that 40% of nursing-home residents had an order for at least one potentially inappropriate medication. Analyses of national medication use surveys in the ambulatory setting have consistently shown that >20% of older patients received at least one potentially inappropriate medication, with at least one potentially inappropriate medication prescribed at approximately 8% of office visits. Furthermore, nearly 4% of office visits and 10% of medical hospital admissions resulted in a prescription for one or more medications classified as "never" or "rarely appropriate" for older patients. The potential consequences of overprescribing include adverse drug events (ADEs), drug-drug interactions, duplication of drug therapy, decreased quality of life, and unnecessary costs.

The factors associated with inappropriate prescribing or overprescribing are listed in Table 10.1. Simply limiting the number of medications for a given patient, however, is not always possible or desirable. For example, a patient with heart failure may be appropriately treated with three or four drugs: a diuretic, an angiotensin-converting enzyme (ACE) inhibitor, a β-blocker, and perhaps digoxin. If this patient has hyperlipidemia and diabetes mellitus, another two or three medications could be required. Hence, such a patient would be taking five to seven indicated medications for major medical conditions alone.

The underprescribing of medications to older adults is also of concern. Underprescribing may result

Table 10.1—Factors Associated With Inappropriate Prescribing or Overprescribing

Patient Factors

Advanced age

Female gender

Lower educational level

Rural residence

Belief in using "a pill for every ill"

Multiple health problems

Use of multiple medications

Use of multiple pharmacies

System Factors

Multiple prescribers for individual patient

Poor record keeping

Failure to review a patient's medication regimen at least annually

from an effort to avoid overprescribing, a complex medication regimen, or adverse effects. It may also result from the thinking that older adults will not benefit from medications intended as primary or secondary prevention, or from aggressive management of chronic conditions, such as hypertension and diabetes mellitus.

Medications often cited as underprescribed in older adults include ACE inhibitors and β-blockers for heart failure and at discharge after an acute myocardial infarction (MI), aspirin within 24 hours and at discharge after an acute MI, warfarin for atrial fibrillation, HMG–CoA reductase inhibitors for primary prevention of cardiovascular events, gastroprotective agents for patients at high risk of NSAID-induced gastrointestinal bleeding, and narcotic analgesics for pain control.

Underprescribing was recognized by the Centers for Medicare and Medicaid Services (CMS), which implemented quality indicators in 1998 to measure the use of recommended medications before discharge for acute MI, stroke, and pneumonia in hospitalized patients with fee-for-service Medicare. Comparison of data from 1998–1999 to 2000–2001 found that the percentage of patients receiving appropriate care had improved for the nation as a whole in the management of these conditions, but the prescribing of an ACE inhibitor in heart failure had declined. In spite of this overall improvement, between 16% and 29% of patients did not receive appropriate pharmacotherapy before discharge after their MI.

Investigators from the Assessing Care of Vulnerable Elders (ACOVE) project developed explicit medication quality indicators divided into four categories: prescribing indicated medications; avoiding inappropriate medications; education, continuity, and documentation; and medication monitoring. These indicators were applied to "vulnerable" older adults enrolled in

two managed care organizations and the results were reported as the percentage of eligible patients who met the indicator or "pass rate." The prescribing of indicated medications category had an overall pass rate of 50% (range 11% to 94% for the 17 indicators); avoiding the prescription of inappropriate medications had an overall pass rate of 97% (range 79% to 100% avoidance across the 9 indicators). The overall pass rate for education, continuity, and documentation indicators was 81% (range 10% to 99% for the 8 indicators). The 9 indicators for medication monitoring had an overall pass rate of 64% (range 22% to 80%). These results suggest that the prescribing of inappropriate medications is less of a problem than the underprescribing of indicated medications and the failure to monitor medications, document information about medications, maintain continuity, and educate patients.

ADVERSE DRUG EVENTS

An ADE is defined as an injury resulting from the use of a drug. Preventable ADEs are among the most serious consequences of inappropriate drug prescribing among older adults. An adverse drug reaction (ADR) is a type of ADE; it refers to harm that is directly caused by a drug at usual doses. For a listing of risk factors for ADEs in older patients, see Table 10.2.

ADEs are estimated to be responsible for 5% to 28% of acute geriatric medical admissions; the estimated annual incidence rate is 26 per 1000 beds for hospitalized patients. It has been estimated that in the nursing home, for every dollar spent on medications, $1.33 in health care resources is spent on the treatment of drug-related morbidity and mortality. A cohort study of all long-term-care residents in 18 nursing homes in Massachusetts demonstrated that ADEs are common and often preventable in nursing homes. During the 28,839 resident-months of observations, 546 ADEs were identified. Overall, 51% of these ADEs were judged to have been preventable. Most of the errors occurred at the ordering and monitoring stages. A cohort study of residents of two long-term-care facilities found the overall rate of ADEs

Table 10.2—Risk Factors for Adverse Drug Events in Older Patients

- Age > 85 years
- Low body weight or body mass index
- ≥ 6 Concurrent chronic diagnoses
- An estimated creatinine clearance < 50 mL per minute
- ≥ 9 Medications
- ≥ 12 Doses of medications per day
- A prior adverse drug reaction

to be 9.8 per 100 resident months. Atypical antipsychotics, anticoagulants, and diuretics were the drug classes most frequently associated with ADEs.

In the ambulatory setting, the ADE rate has been reported to be 50.1 per 1000 person-years, and the preventable ADE rate to be 13.8 per 1000 person-years. Cardiovascular drugs, diuretics, NSAIDs, hypoglycemics, and anticoagulants are the drug classes most often associated with preventable ADEs. Again, errors occurred most often at the time of prescribing or were related to inadequate monitoring. The majority of ADEs ($\geq$95%) experienced by older patients are considered to be predictable.

A common pathway for ADEs and polypharmacy has been described as the "prescribing cascade." One form of this cascade occurs when a medication results in an ADE that is mistaken as a separate diagnosis and treated with more medications, which puts the patient at risk of additional ADEs and more medications. Examples that have been studied include metoclopramide-induced parkinsonism and the subsequent prescribing of antiparkinson medications, and calcium channel blockers that result in peripheral edema and the subsequent use of diuretics.

DRUG INTERACTIONS

A drug-drug interaction (DDI) is defined as the pharmacologic or clinical response to the administration of a drug combination that differs from that anticipated from the known effects of each of the two agents when given alone. Drug-drug interactions are important because they may lead to ADEs. The likelihood of DDIs increases as the number of medications a patient takes increases. Among prescription drugs, cardiovascular and psychotropic drugs are most commonly involved in DDIs. A positive correlation exists between the number of potential DDIs and the number of adverse effects experienced by hospitalized older patients. The most common adverse effects are neuropsychologic (primarily delirium), arterial hypotension, and acute kidney failure. Drug combinations that are reported to result in increased risk of hospitalization for older patients are shown in Table 10.3. Drugs commonly involved in DDIs in long-term care are listed in Table 10.4. Risk factors associated with DDIs include the use of multiple medications, receiving care from several prescribing clinicians, and using more than one pharmacy.

Drug interactions can take many forms. For example, absorption can be enhanced or diminished (as described above), drugs with similar or opposite pharmacologic effects can result in exaggerated or impaired effects, and drug metabolism may be inhibited or induced. Research focusing on the cytochrome P-450 system has proposed or studied in vivo or in vitro numerous DDIs involving the different P-450 isozymes. The effect of aging on the cytochrome P-450 system and the clinical implications for prescribing have not been completely determined. Cross-sectional data have shown that cytochrome P-450 content declines incrementally, once in the fourth decade and again after age 70. In vitro microsomal activity of cytochrome (CYP) 3A4 is not altered by aging, but in vivo age- and gender-related reductions in drug clearance have been found for CYP3A4 substrates erythromycin, prednisolone, verapamil, alprazolam, nifedipine, and diazepam. CYP3A4 accounts for 30% of the P-450 content in the liver and is also prominent in the intestinal tract. This

Table 10.3—Most Common Drug-Drug Adverse Effects Identified Upon Hospitalization

Combination	Risk
ACE inhibitor + diuretic	Hypotension; hyperkalemia
ACE inhibitor + potassium	Hyperkalemia
Antiarrhythmic + diuretic	Electrolyte imbalance; arrhythmias
Benzodiazepine + antidepressant	Confusion, sedation, falls
Benzodiazepine + antipsychotic	Confusion, sedation, falls
Benzodiazepine + benzodiazepine	Confusion, sedation, falls
Calcium channel blocker + diuretic	Hypotension
Calcium channel blocker + nitrate	Hypotension
Digitalis + antiarrhythmic	Bradycardia, arrhythmias
Diuretic + digitalis	Arrhythmias
Diuretic + diuretic	Dehydration, electrolyte imbalance
Diuretic + nitrate	Hypotension
Nitrate + vasodilator	Hypotension

NOTE: ACE = angiotensin-converting enzyme.

SOURCE: Data from Doucet J, Chassagne P, Trivalle C, et al. Drug-drug interactions related to hospital admissions in older adults: a prospective study of 1000 patients. *J Am Geriatr Soc.* 1996;44(8):944–948.

Table 10.4—Dangerous Drugs Involved in Drug-Drug Interactions in Long-Term Care

Medication	Interacting Medications
Angiotensin-converting enzyme inhibitors	Potassium supplements, potassium-sparing diuretics
Digoxin	Antiarrhythmics, verapamil
Quinolones	Theophylline, warfarin
Warfarin	Sulfa drugs, macrolides, quinolones, nonsteroidal anti-inflammatory drugs, phenytoin

SOURCE: Data from the American Society of Consultant Pharmacists. Multidisciplinary Medication Management Project. Top Ten Dangerous Drug Interactions in Long-Term Care. Available at http://www.scoup.net/M3Project/topten/#1 (accessed October 2005).

isozyme is involved in the metabolism of more than 50% of drugs on the market and can be induced by drugs such as rifampin, phenytoin, and carbamazepine, and inhibited by many drugs, including the macrolide antibiotics, nefazodone, itraconazole, ketoconazole, as well as grapefruit juice. The isozyme CYP2D6 is involved in the metabolism of 25% to 30% of marketed drugs and has been associated with only minimal age-related changes. CYP2D6 is involved in the metabolism of many psychotropic drugs and can be inhibited by many agents. In addition, approximately 10% of white people are deficient in this isozyme and have reduced ability to clear and increased sensitivity to CYP2D6 substrates. Clinically, these patients and those taking CYP2D6 inhibitors (eg, quinidine, paroxetine, fluoxetine) cannot convert codeine and tramadol to their active metabolites and have a reduced analgesic response to these agents.

For DDIs involving herbal preparations, see "Complementary and Alternative Medicine" (p 74).

DRUG-DISEASE INTERACTIONS

Drug-disease combinations common in older patients can affect drug response and lead to adverse drug events. Obesity and ascites alter the volumes of distribution of lipophilic and hydrophilic drugs, respectively. Patients with dementia may have increased sensitivity or paradoxical reactions to drugs with central nervous system or anticholinergic activity. In patients with renal insufficiency or impaired hepatic function caused by cirrhosis or hepatic congestion the detoxification and excretion of drugs is impaired.

PRINCIPLES OF PRESCRIBING

Principles of prescribing for older patients are shown in Table 10.5. This basic approach applies primarily to medications used to treat chronic conditions for which an immediate, complete therapeutic response is not necessary. A dosage adjustment may still be needed for medications used to treat conditions requiring an immediate response (eg, when prescribing antibiotics for a patient with impaired kidney function).

Overprescribing can be prevented by reviewing a patient's medications on a regular basis and each time a new medication is started or a dosage is changed. The importance of maintaining accurate records of all medications taken by the patient cannot be overemphasized. It is crucial to document in the patient's record what other prescribers have given the patient and what the patient is self-prescribing. Many patients do not consider vitamins, herbal preparations, or over-the-counter medications (even aspirin) to be medications,

so clinicians must be specific when they inquire about use of other medications. Medications that have been newly approved by the FDA should be used cautiously in treating older patients. Such drugs are likely to be more expensive, and information about their use in older patients is often limited.

It is best if the patient brings all medications to the review, including over-the-counter medications, vitamins, and any herbal preparations or other types of supplements (a "brown-bag" evaluation). Examining the containers and labels and asking what each medication is for and how and when it is taken can provide insight into the patient's understanding and adherence to his or her medication regimens. When there is no longer an indication for their continued use medications should be discontinued. Any new complaints or worsening of an existing condition should prompt the consideration of whether it could be drug-induced. When considering treatment for a new medical condition, nonpharmacologic approaches should always be considered first. If a drug therapy is still indicated, select within the class to minimize the risk of an ADE.

When initiating therapy, the basic principle should be to start low go and go slow. Ongoing consideration should be given to decreasing dosages of medications that are particularly likely to cause adverse effects. Although the FDA requires that labeling for new drugs regarding dosing in older patients not be extrapolated from another patient population (eg, patients with kidney impairment), it does not require that a drug be studied explicitly in older adults. Older adults are used in studies of phase I and II dose tolerability and pharmacokinetic and pharmacodynamic actions of many new drugs, but the older adults chosen for these studies are usually healthy and free of concomitant illnesses. Much of what is known about medications and how to use them in sick older patients, particularly those who are frail, is learned only after a drug has been available for several years.

OPTIMIZING ADHERENCE TO MEDICATION

Nonadherence and underadherence to medication regimens is a huge and often unrecognized problem in drug treatment. It is estimated that nonadherence among elderly people may be as high as 50%. Patients may be reluctant to admit that they are not taking medications or not following directions. If nonadherence is suspected, the clinician needs to consider the patient's financial, cognitive, and functional status, as well as his or her beliefs about and understanding of medications and diseases. Adherence to a medication

Table 10.5—Principles of Prescribing for Older Patients

The basics:

- Start with a low dose.
- Titrate the dose upward slowly, as tolerated by the patient.
- Try not to start two drugs at the same time.

Determine the following before prescribing a new medication:

- Is the medication necessary? Are there nonpharmacologic ways to treat the condition?
- What are the therapeutic end points and how will they be assessed?
- Do the benefits outweigh the risks of the medication?
- Is one medication being used to treat the adverse effects of another?
- Is there one medication that could be prescribed to treat two conditions?
- Are there potential drug-drug or drug-disease interactions?
- Will the new medication's administration times be the same as those of existing medications?
- Do the patient and caregiver understand what the medication is for, how to take it, how long to take it, when it should start to work, possible adverse effects that it might cause, and what to do if they occur?

At least annually:

- Ask the patient to bring in all medications (prescription, over-the-counter, supplements, and herbal preparations) to the office; for new patients, conduct a detailed medication history.
- For prescription medications, determine whether the label directions and dose match those in the patient's chart; ask the patient how each medication is being taken.
- Ask about medication side effects.
- Note who else is prescribing medications for the patient, and what the medications are and their indications.
- Look for medications with duplicate therapeutic, pharmacologic, or adverse effect profiles.
- Screen for drug-drug and drug-disease interactions.
- Eliminate unnecessary medications; confer with other prescribers if necessary.
- Simplify the medication regimen; use the fewest possible number of medications and doses per day.
- Always review any changes with the patient and caregiver; provide the changes in writing.

regimen is a team effort and should include input from medicine, pharmacy, nursing, social work, and the patient and/or family. Adherence may be improved by use of aids such as pill boxes, a change in the treatment plan, increased access to the medication through a change in prescription plan, patient education about the benefit of the medication, or family reminders.

Prescription drug costs have increased substantially, and supplemental prescription drug benefit plans are expensive. Some plans still may leave a patient with a copayment that he or she cannot afford or with only a fixed dollar amount for the year. Clinicians should avoid prescribing expensive new medications that have not been shown to be superior to less expensive generic alternatives.

Cognitive impairment may also cause nonadherence, because patients may forget to take medications or confuse them. Simplifying the regimen and involving a caregiver to oversee medication management can be helpful approaches. Medication trays or drug calendars also may help with organization, and they are very useful for patients who have difficulty remembering when they last took a medication.

The older patient's ability to read labels, open containers, or pour medications or even a glass of water may be impaired, so functional assessment can be useful. Some patients may need additional education or reinforcement about the purpose of a medication, especially those used to treat conditions that are usually asymptomatic, such as diabetes mellitus and hypertension. Older patients also may need reassurance regarding the safety and possible adverse effects of certain medications, particularly newly prescribed medications or those associated with serious adverse events, such as warfarin.

REFERENCES

- Fick DM, Cooper JW, Wade WE, et al. Updating the Beers criteria for potentially inappropriate medication use in older adults: results of a U.S. consensus panel of experts. *Arch Intern Med.* 2003;163(22):2716–2724.

■ Goulding MR. Inappropriate medication prescribing for elderly ambulatory care patients. *Arch Intern Med.* 2004;164(3):305–312.

■ Gurwitz JH, Field TS, Harrold LR, et al. Incidence and preventability of adverse drug events among older persons in the ambulatory setting. *JAMA.* 2003;289(9):1107–1116.

■ Murray MD, Callahan CM. Improving medication use for older adults: an integrated research agenda. *Ann Intern Med.* 2003;139(5 Pt 2):425–429.

■ Rollason V, Vogt N. Reduction of polypharmacy in the elderly: a systematic review of the role of the pharmacist. *Drugs Aging.* 2003;20(11):817–832.

CHAPTER 11—COMPLEMENTARY AND ALTERNATIVE MEDICINE

KEY POINTS

■ The use of complementary and alternative medicine appears to be on the rise in all adult age groups, including the elderly population.

■ Stress-reduction techniques may benefit many conditions prevalent among older patients, including falls, osteoporosis, osteoarthritis, high blood pressure, obesity, insomnia, depression, irritability related to the menopause, diabetes mellitus, and certain effects of cancer.

■ Saw palmetto is commonly used to reduce the symptoms associated with benign prostatic hyperplasia, and in at least one well-conducted study it has been shown to exert effects similar to those of standard pharmacologic treatments.

■ Though many herbal and biologic preparations offer promise, they are largely of unproven benefit and their contents are unregulated by government agencies, making their use very challenging to endorse and guide.

Complementary and alternative medicine (CAM), as currently defined by the National Center for Complementary and Alternative Medicine (NCCAM) of the National Institutes of Health, refers to "a group of diverse medical and health care systems, practices, and products that are not presently considered to be part of conventional medicine." Although some scientific evidence exists regarding certain CAM therapies, for most there are key questions that are yet to be answered through well-designed research studies—questions such as whether they are safe and whether they work for the diseases or medical conditions for which they are used.

NCCAM conceptualizes the diversity of CAM modalities as follows:

■ Mind-body interventions, such as meditation, prayer, relaxation, and art, dance, and music therapies

■ Biologically based therapies, such as herbal preparations, botanicals, and dietary supplements

■ Manipulative and body-based methods, such as chiropractic, therapeutic massage, and osteopathic manipulation

■ Energy therapies such as Reiki, therapeutic touch, and bioelectromagnetic-based therapies

■ Whole medical systems, such as traditional Chinese medicine, Ayurvedic medicine, homeopathy, and naturopathic medicine, which incorporate many or all of the above-noted therapies.

The list of what is considered to be CAM is continually evolving, as therapies that are proved to be safe and effective become adopted into conventional health care and as new approaches to health care emerge.

The use of CAM is widespread. The National Health Interview Survey (NHIS) selected a nationally representative sample of over 31,000 U.S. adults. Sixty-two percent of those interviewed noted some use of 27 different CAM modalities during the previous 12 months when CAM was defined to include prayer for health reasons. Most CAM use is complementary, that is, in addition to mainstream interventions; only a minority of CAM use serves as an alternative to conventional treatment. Approximately 60% of CAM users in the United States do not discuss their use of CAM modalities with their health care providers. This is of particular concern in the care of older adults because of the increased risk for adverse interactions between conventional drugs and various CAM biologic agents. Moreover, aging impacts the metabolism of numerous prescription and over-the-counter medications, and possibly that of many herbal preparations, botanicals, and dietary supplements. Age-related alterations in hepatic and renal function contribute importantly to these phenomena, both in the absence and presence of disease.

HEALTH CARE FOR THE AGING POPULATION

The aging of the baby-boomer generation is contributing to the already established largest group of health care consumers—older adults. Among the most common health challenges in aged men are diseases of the circulatory, musculoskeletal, and connective tissue and of the genitourinary systems. In aging women, the most common health challenges are musculoskeletal, circulatory, and mental health disorders. Demographic considerations assure that the need of the expanding aging population for medical services will continue to increase, and it is logical to predict that specific interest in, and use of, CAM modalities will expand as well.

The use of CAM by older persons is beginning to be more closely studied, in part to help design safer and more efficacious treatments specific to the needs of those older than 65 years. In one small study, 30% of adults surveyed aged 65 and older (N = 311) reported using alternative medicine, and 19% visited an alternative medicine provider. The CAM modalities used most commonly by the older adults in this study were herbal preparations and chiropractic, both of which can cause problems in this population. Of note, CAM use can vary, depending on a particular geographic region as well as ethnic group.

In a study reported in 2003, which was conducted in three ethnically diverse groups of community-dwelling elderly persons (N = 525) in southern California, 251 respondents (47.8%) reported CAM use. The differences in predominant patterns of CAM use among the three groups—Asian, Hispanic, and white non-Hispanic—suggested that differing sociocultural beliefs influence the frequency and pattern of CAM use. Another such example can be found in the large variety of home remedies used by older black Americans, which can be related to regional customs in the United States. CAM use by black Americans is viewed as a combination of European, Native American, and African customs. In addition, Native American and black American groups also view spirituality as integral to the prevention of illness and maintenance of health. Knowledge of patients' spiritual beliefs can assist providers to provide sensitive, culturally specific care. Recognition of the individual patient's cultural heritage may augment communication and trust between providers and patients about CAM, resulting in improved, comprehensive health care. (See also "Cultural Aspects of Care," p 46.)

CURRENT ISSUES: SAFETY AND EFFICACY

Currently in the United States, a wide variety of CAM modalities are available from practitioners, or as self-care practices. These span the spectrum from indigenous health practices that are centuries old to CAM modalities that are licensed and provided by a trained practitioner. However, most CAM practices have not been regulated, and licensure and certification can vary among practices and by geographic location. There are numerous anecdotal reports or claims of the efficacy and safety of diverse CAM modalities, yet there is a general lack of product and practice standardization and a dearth of credible scientific information supporting these practices. There is substantial potential for adverse reactions with the use of herbal preparations and of botanical and dietary supplements in older adults (Table 11.1). Nonetheless, most consumers are satisfied, and few malpractice or wrongful injury lawsuits are filed.

CAM USE FOR MANAGING ILLNESS IN OLDER PERSONS

Musculoskeletal Disorders

The incidence of osteoporosis and nontraumatic fractures of the wrist, spine, and hip increase with age in women and men. Phytoestrogen and soy products are increasingly used to prevent or treat osteoporosis in postmenopausal women, although there is little evidence confirming their benefits. Dehydroepiandrosterone (DHEA), a widely used dietary supplement, is the most abundant adrenal steroid in humans. Circulating DHEA levels decline progressively with age. Small-scale trials of DHEA supplementation in older persons have produced conflicting results regarding its effects on bone density, and further studies are needed to determine its utility in preventing or treating osteoporosis in older people.

Osteoarthritis is one of the most common chronic diseases affecting older men and women. In one recent study, almost half (47%) of the patients with osteoarthritis aged 55 to 75 years reported using some CAM modality. Because the personal experience of pain can increase the levels of associated suffering, addressing any negative beliefs and emotions that the patient may be struggling with is as important as addressing the physical symptoms. CAM techniques specifically focused to provide stress relief, such as relaxation breathing and music therapy, may be of benefit as adjunctive therapy. Gentle movement and stretching techniques, such as those in yoga, Tai Chi, and warm-water aquatics, can provide an alternative to more vigorous exercise regimens. Other CAM modalities that are chosen by osteoarthritis patients include acupuncture, massage, chiropractic manipulation, glucosamine supplements, Reiki, and prayer. Large multicenter trials are under way to assess the separate

Table 11.1—Safety Issues Related to Dietary Supplements Used by Older Adults

Supplement	Adverse Effects	Interacts With:
Coenzyme Q10	Infrequent nausea, emesis, epigastric pain, headaches > 300 mg/day linked to increased liver transaminase	Warfarin
Dehydroepiandrosterone (DHEA)	Women: weight gain, voice changes, facial hair, headaches Men: prostatic hypertrophy, possible increase in hormone-sensitive tumors	Calcium channel blockers, sildenafil
Echinacea	Allergic reactions, hepatitis, asthma, vertigo, anaphylaxis (rare)	Immunosuppressants
Ginkgo biloba	All rare: serious bleeding, seizures, headaches, dizziness, vertigo	Anticoagulants
Glucosamine	Nausea, diarrhea, heartburn	Hypoglycemic drugs (reduces effectiveness)
Omega-3 fatty acids	Belching, halitosis, blood glucose elevations	Antiplatelets, anticoagulants, antihypertensives
SAM-e	Nausea, vomiting, diarrhea, anxiety, restlessness	Tricyclics and selective serotonin-reuptake inhibitors
Saw palmetto	All rare: constipation, diarrhea, decreased libido, headaches, hypertension, urine retention	None described
St. John's wort	Nausea, allergic reactions, dizziness, headache, photosensitivity (rare)	Anticoagulants, antivirals, selective serotonin-reuptake inhibitors

and combined effects of glucosamine, chondroitin sulphate, and acupuncture in the treatment of pain associated with osteoarthritis of the knee. Herbal preparations, including capsaicin cream and Phytodolor, may have limited but unproven efficacy in reducing pain and improving motility; they are thought to exert effects mechanistically in much the same way as conventional nonsteroidal anti-inflammatory treatments. (See also "Musculoskeletal Diseases and Disorders," p 396, and "Persistent Pain," p 131.)

Lower back pain is one of the most difficult health challenges for which CAM modalities are used, particularly, therapeutic massage, acupuncture, mind-body relaxation, and energy modalities. One study reported that the combined use of massage, self-care relaxation, and acupuncture may be more effective than the use of any of these modalities separately. (See also "Back and Neck Pain," p 410.) A meta-analysis of randomized trials of acupuncture for lower back pain found it to be superior to various control modalities, but a significant placebo effect was found.

Cardiovascular Disorders

Cardiovascular disease affects at least 60% to 70% of the population older than 65 years. Of particular relevance is the higher incidence of cardiovascular disease occurring in obese patients or those with type 2 diabetes mellitus. Increased individual and public health efforts to prevent disease and identify those older adults at risk of developing disease should contribute to decreases in morbidity and mortality.

Healthy diet and aerobic exercise are the first recommendations to manage high blood pressure and dyslipidemia. A heart-healthy diet includes limiting sodium intake, refined sugar, and saturated fat while increasing amounts of complex carbohydrates, fruits, and vegetables. In the Dietary Approach to Stop Hypertension (DASH) trial, nearly 70% of participants following the healthy diet decreased both systolic and diastolic blood-pressure measurements. In addition, recent studies suggest that diets including essential fatty acids may lower blood pressure, increase levels of high-density lipoproteins, and lower levels of triglycerides and low-density lipoproteins. Examples of essential fatty acids are omega-3 and omega-6 acids. The omega-3 fatty acids can be found in fresh deep-water fish and in flaxseed oil. Omega-6-linoleic acid is found in raw nuts and seeds. For further reduction of the risk of developing hypertension and obesity, aerobic exercise, such as swimming or brisk walking, is advised for at least 30 minutes three times a week. Recent reports suggest that even mild to moderate increases in physical activity, such as walking slowly or gardening, have beneficial cardiovascular effects. Increased blood pressure can also be associated with inadequate sleep. The use of stress-management techniques, such as relaxation breathing, music therapy, and meditation, may reduce blood pressure in hypertensive patients and improve sleep quality in aging patients. (See also "Hypertension," p 331;

"Physical Activity," p 51; and "Sleep Problems," p 229.)

Neurologic and Emotional Disorders

Depression is one the most common and debilitating major public health problems, and its incidence increases with advancing age. Although depression is more common in women, increasing attention is focused on the issue of depression in men, in whom it is more often unrecognized or untreated. There is an alarming prevalence of depression and suicide in widowed men aged 70 years and over. CAM use by the aging patient may assist in the management of mild to moderate depression. However, adequate treatment of severe depression may involve psychotherapy and psychotropic medication to prevent further morbidity and mortality. Recent research suggests that depression is also a systemic disease and is associated with an increased incidence of sleep disorders, osteoporosis, obesity, insulin resistance, and immune dysfunction. The impact of CAM modalities on these outcomes is unclear.

A healthy diet can be one of the first recommendations to assist with improving mood. Dietary intake that includes complex carbohydrates can improve serotonin levels. Increasing essential fatty acids and protein intake may increase alertness and mood. Of equal importance is discontinuing excess alcohol, caffeine, and tobacco, which can contribute to depression and irritability.

Aerobic exercise is also prescribed as a treatment for mild to moderate depression in aged patients. Exercise in combination with antidepressants can yield faster, more lasting results than either alone.

The botanical known as St. John's wort has received considerable attention and remains widely used. A large multicenter study failed to show the efficacy of this agent in patients with major depression of mild to moderate degree. Whether St. John's wort will prove to be efficacious in patients with mild symptoms of depression, social phobia, and seasonal affective disorder remains to be determined. The adverse effects of St. John's wort include gastrointestinal upset, fatigue, dizziness, headache, dry mouth, and photosensitivity. St. John's wort interacts with the hepatic P-450 enzyme system that induces the metabolism of many drugs, thus causing clinically significant adverse interactions and potential therapeutic failure with various antiretroviral, anticoagulant, immunosuppressant, antidepressant, and chemotherapeutic drugs.

S-adenosylmethionine (SAM-e) is a naturally occurring compound that is necessary for the brain to adequately produce dopamine and serotonin. This compound is currently marketed as an antidepressant.

In one promising study involving 195 patients, taking 400 mg of SAM-e daily was found to lessen depressive symptoms.

See also "Depression and Other Mood Disorders" (p 247).

Some studies have investigated the use of supplements for treatment of dementia from Alzheimer's disease and vascular insufficiency. *Ginkgo biloba* extract (EGb 761) has shown some benefit in improving cognitive ability and memory impairment in Alzheimer's patients, in some, but not all studies. Brain tissue studies and spinal fluid abnormalities in Alzheimer's patients also offer reasonable rationale for supplementing with various antioxidants, including vitamins A, C, and E and selenium, though evidence of their effect has yet to be demonstrated in clinical trials. (See also "Dementia," p 204.)

Studies have shown that Parkinson's disease patients have reduced brain levels of glutathione, an antioxidant involved in neuroprotective functions. Parkinson's patients also have deficiencies in coenzyme Q10. Supplementation with these two naturally occurring substances has been shown to slow the progression of disease and reduce the severity of symptoms in very small unblinded clinical trials. Patients with Parkinson's disease may also benefit from a combination of dietary food additions containing higher amounts of coenzyme Q10, as found in salmon, sardines, and mackerel. Acupuncture, music therapy, and physical therapy are used by Parkinson's patients to attempt to reduce disabilities and improve cognitive, emotional, and social functioning. (See also "Neurologic Diseases and Disorders," p 423.)

Sleep disorders are common in older persons, affecting both sleep quality and quantity. Studies suggest that abnormalities in slow-wave and rapid-eye-movement sleep may also be linked to psychologic, endocrine-metabolic, and immune system dysfunctions. Nutritional and exercise modifications are among the safest recommendations when working with the elderly patients. Milk contains tryptophan, which is a precursor of serotonin. Having warm milk before bedtime or eating other tryptophan-containing foods such as bananas, brown rice, and turkey may be helpful in relieving depression-associated sleep difficulties. Chamomile is an herbal tea that is also known for its relaxing properties. Evidence suggests that use of valerian root or melatonin may also promote improved sleep quality. Aerobic exercise in the early evening has been shown to contribute to improved sleep quality. However, exercise later in the evening can be too stimulating and counteract restful sleep. Other CAM modalities for improving sleep used by older patients include aromatherapy combined with a warm bath and relaxing music. (See also "Sleep Problems," p 229.)

Urogynecologic Disorders

Menopause is now seen more as a natural progression of aging than as a pathologic process. This perspective lends itself to the use of behavioral, nutritional, and exercise interventions as well as nonpharmacologic supplements to manage some of the symptoms associated with menopause. More than 30% of menopausal women report using one or more CAM modalities, such as acupuncture, natural and plant estrogens, and other herbal preparations, despite a lack of scientific evidence of efficacy. This number is likely to increase because of the expanding population of aged women and increasing concerns about the long-term safety of conventional estrogens. (See also the section on estrogen replacement therapy in "Endocrine and Metabolic Disorders," p 347.) Of particular importance is the necessity to use caution when recommending phytoestrogen to women with hormone-dependent cancers. Phytoestrogen has yet to be proven conclusively to be an agonist or antagonist of the estrogen receptor. Black cohosh is an herb that has shown some benefit for managing hot flushes, mood disturbances, and sleep disorders. Both aerobic exercise and mind-body relaxation techniques are also helpful in decreasing irritability, restlessness, and anxiety.

Symptomatic benign prostatic hyperplasia affects more than 40% of men aged 70 and older. During the past several years, men have increasingly begun to self-treat this condition with the herbal compound known as saw palmetto, which has become the fifth leading medicinal herb consumed in the United States. Saw palmetto and other supplements (eg, pygeum) have been studied and need further, more rigorous scientific investigation to confirm initial efficacy claims. In one study, older men averaging 65 years of age with moderate benign prostatic hyperplasia were evaluated for 3 months. The efficacy of saw palmetto was found to exceed that of placebo treatment and to be similar to that of standard pharmacologic treatment. (See also "Prostate Disease," p 389.)

Diabetes

Type 2 diabetes mellitus, a major public health problem, is associated with increased incidence of obesity, hypertension, dyslipidemia, and macro- and microvascular disease. Normal aging is associated with increased insulin resistance and glucose intolerances, and increased risk of developing type 2 diabetes. In one survey, approximately 50% to 60% of diabetic patients reported the use of CAM interventions, including folk remedies in ethnic populations. There is considerable interest in examining the potential benefit of using various CAM biologic agents (eg, chromium, vitamin C, other dietary antioxidants) or other modali-

ties (eg, stress-reduction techniques) in combination with dietary modifications, exercise, and weight management. Acupuncture has shown some benefit in managing the pain associated with diabetic neuropathy. (See also "Diabetes Mellitus," p 349.)

Cancer

Approximately 30% to 50% of cancer patients in one survey noted that they were using CAM interventions to manage their specific cancer. Cancer CAM therapies purportedly can be used to strengthen the body's innate immune systems as well as to manage the adverse effects of conventional treatments, such as chemotherapy and radiation. One of the most important benefits for many cancer patients who use CAM modalities is the experience of being more empowered while dealing with the challenges of cancer. This has been substantiated by numerous studies examining various indices of health-related quality of life. The CAM therapies most frequently used are herbal preparations, exercise, and spiritual and energy modalities (such as qi gong, therapeutic touch, Reiki, polarity, healing touch, or Johrei).

Controversy remains regarding the role of diet as a possible risk factor for developing breast cancer. Of particular importance is the link between obesity and increased estrogen levels that may contribute to de novo breast cancer and recurrence after early-stage disease. High-fiber, low-fat diets with fruits, vegetables, whole grains, fish, and legumes are associated with a decreased risk of disease. Biologic agents, herbal preparations, and vitamins have all been tried by patients; however, most of these modalities have not had much scientific study. In addition, life-style changes to include exercise and stress management have been helpful with managing mood and energy changes associated with breast cancer.

Prostate cancer usually develops slowly in older men, and CAM use in combination with conventional treatment has been reported to reduce associated discomforts and improve the quality of life. Risk of death in this population is higher from heart disease than from prostate cancer per se. Until recently, the botanical mixture known as PC-SPES had been used as a CAM dietary supplement that in early small-scale trials was found to lead to decreases in serum prostate-specific antigen levels and pain, plus improved quality of life. However, in June 2002 several lots of PC-SPES were found to be adulterated with diethylstilbestrol, warfarin, and other undeclared prescription ingredients. As a result, PC-SPES was removed from the market. At present, exercise and healthy diet remain the safest CAM recommendations to assist with the management of side effects and improvement of quality of life in these patients. (See also "Prostate Disease," p 389.)

Lung cancer has been linked not only to smoking but also to excesses in dietary intake of dairy products, red meats, and saturated fats, though these associations have been questioned. In addition, preliminary research has suggested that ingestion of vitamin A by those who smoke may be harmful, whereas vitamin A intake in those who do not smoke may be beneficial. Dietary changes as well as mind-body interventions may assist lung cancer patients to manage emotional distress and the adverse effects of treatment. Cancer patients using relaxation and stress-management techniques have been able to manage cravings when pursuing tobacco cessation. These mind-body techniques are also effective in managing the emotional and physical distress associated with the adverse effects of treatment.

Currently, there are no herbal preparations or botanic supplements that appear to be useful in the prevention or management of patients with colon cancer. A fiber-rich diet has been postulated to possibly prevent the onset of colon cancer; however, studies are inconclusive. Lutein, which is present in broccoli, carrots, oranges, and spinach, was found in one study to be beneficial for colon cancer prevention.

See also "Oncology" (p 442).

SAFETY OF CAM MODALITIES

There are several important concerns regarding the safety of the use of CAM modalities by elderly persons. They often assume that the use of dietary supplements and related biologic products, which are among the most popular CAM therapies, are both safe and effective because these products are characterized as "natural." Under the Dietary Supplement Health and Education Act (DSHEA) of 1994, the U.S. Food and Drug Administration is not empowered to evaluate or regulate dietary supplements, and the industry is not required to prove that the advertised ingredients provide the health benefits or safety they claim. Multiple studies have found that dietary supplements often can contain little, none, or more of what the product labels claim, as well as contaminants or adulterants with unlisted products and prescription drugs.

There is little information related to possible differences in the pharmacokinetics and pharmacody-

namics of various CAM biologic agents in elderly persons; as a result, proper dosage adjustments for these compounds are unknown. Coupled with the increased likelihood of elderly persons' use of multiple medications, there is an increased risk for adverse herbal-drug interactions in older persons. Without the knowledge of what these products contain in their entirety, or the consequences of their use, consumers and health care professionals must increase communication while continued research is conducted to provide accurate evaluations. It is imperative that practitioners ask patients specifically about their use of dietary supplements and biologic products and look at the ingredients in those supplements.

CAM use in the United States continues to increase in all age groups. The life stressors experienced by older adults, including depression, cognitive decline, chronic pain, musculoskeletal changes, and sleep disorders, may be ameliorated by CAM interventions. Given the particular concerns inherent in managing the health challenges of the aging population, more research to establish the safety and efficacy of CAM modalities commonly used by older persons is imperative.

REFERENCES

- Barnes PM, Powell-Griner E, McFann K, et al. Complementary and alternative medicine use among adults: United States, 2002. Advance data from the Vital and Health Statistics; No. 343. Hyattsville, MD: National Center for Health Statistics; 2004.

- Fink S. International efforts spotlight traditional, complementary, and alternative medicine. *Am J Pub Health.* 2002; 92(11):1734–1739.

- Foster DF, Phillips RS, Hamel MB, et al. Alternative medicine use in older Americans. *J Am Geriatr Soc.* 2000;48(12):1560–1565.

- Kaptchuk TJ. Acupuncture: theory, efficacy, and practice. *Ann Intern Med.* 2002;136(5):374–383.

- Najm W, Reinsch S, Hoehler F, et al. Use of complementary and alternative medicine among the ethnic elderly. *Altern Ther Health Med.* 2003; 9(3):50–57.

CHAPTER 12—ELDER MISTREATMENT

KEY POINTS

- Elder mistreatment affects almost 4% of adults aged 65 and over.

- Screening for elder mistreatment by clinicians is important and is most effective when conducted in a sensitive manner.

- Indicators of elder mistreatment range from dramatic (eg, bruising, fractures) to subtle (eg, withdrawn behavior, dehydration).

The term *elder mistreatment* (EM) as defined by the National Research Council in its report on elder mistreatment refers to "(a) intentional actions that cause harm or create a serious risk of harm (whether or not harm is intended) to a vulnerable elder by a caregiver or other person who stands in a trust relationship to the elder or (b) failure by a caregiver to satisfy the elder's basic needs or to protect the elder from harm." The authors of the American Medical Association (AMA) *Diagnostic and Treatment Guidelines on Elder Abuse and Neglect* describe EM as acts of omission or commission that result in harm or threatened harm to the health or welfare of an older adult. EM is a syndrome that may manifest itself in a variety of ways. It may take the form of physical abuse, emotional abuse, intentional or unintentional neglect, financial exploitation, or abandonment, or it may be a combination of these. Research suggests that the national incidence of EM is approximately 450,000 annually, with a prevalence range of 700,000 to 1.2 million older adults, accounting for approximately 4% of those aged 65 years or older. Given these estimates, routine screening for EM is an appropriate part of primary care for elderly people.

Research conducted in the context of a longitudinal aging cohort study sought to determine the mortality of EM. In a pooled logistic regression analysis that adjusted for demographics, chronic disease, functional status, social networks, cognitive status, and depressive symptoms, the risk of death was found to remain elevated for cohort members experiencing either EM or self-neglect. To date, no intervention studies have evaluated the impact of screening on health outcomes, and such studies are needed. However, screening for EM appears warranted, given the findings of case studies and longitudinal studies that document risk factors, as well as the information in the databases from the adult protective services organizations across the country.

RISK FACTORS AND PREVENTION

Risk factors for EM are known to include poverty, dependency of the elderly person for caregiving needs, age, race, functional disability, frailty, and cognitive impairment. Some factors may really be proxies for other variables. For example, lower socioeconomic status is often associated with fewer resources to meet caregiving demands.

Frail, debilitated older persons may need a level of care that at times exceeds caregiver ability. In particular, the demented person who exhibits disturbing behaviors, such as hitting, spitting, or screaming, poses immense challenges to caregivers. Caregiver stress may give way to any of the forms of EM, and a careful assessment of caregiver stress may identify opportunities to prevent EM. Table 12.1 lists factors that indicate a risk for the development of inadequate or abusive caregiving.

HISTORY

An interdisciplinary approach to assessment and care planning is optimal. Comprehensive interdisciplinary geriatric assessment (see "Assessment," p 41) that includes the physical, psychosocial, and financial domains of the older adult should detect potential or any alleged EM.

The EM history, provided by both the older person and caregiver(s), is conducted in privacy so that the patient and the caregiver(s) can speak freely and

Table 12.1—Risk Factors for Inadequate or Abusive Caregiving

- Cognitive impairment in patient, caregiver, or both
- Dependency of the caregiver on the elderly patient, or vice versa
- Family conflict
- Family history of
    - abusive behavior
    - alcohol or drug misuse or abuse
    - mental illness
    - mental retardation
- Financial stress or lack of funds to meet new health demands
- Isolation of the patient or the caregiver, or both
- Living arrangements inadequate for the needs of the ill person
- Stressful events in the family, eg:
    - death of a loved one
    - loss of employment

frankly. Studies suggest that the different cultures of racial and ethnic groups define abuse and neglect very differently; thus, cultural sensitivity is important (see "Cultural Aspects of Care," p 46). The older patient or caregiver from a different culture than the clinician's may be offended by some EM screening questions. Carefully worded EM questions will avoid alienating the patient or caregiver and closing down any further opportunity to help the patient and family.

If the patient's responses to EM questions indicate that mistreatment may be occurring, progressively focused follow-up questions are indicated. For example, the clinician might first ask, "Is there any difficult behavior in your family you would like to tell me about?" If the answer is positive, the questions to follow then might be, "Has anyone tried to hurt or hit you?" "Has anyone made you do things that you did not want to do?" "Has anyone taken your things?" Obtaining such information requires clinical interviewing skills similar to those needed when asking about sexual orientation, alcoholism, or substance abuse.

Private interviews with caregivers may detect not only abusive or neglectful behavior but also signs of stress, isolation, or depression in the caregiver, in which case help for the caregiver can also be provided. Caregivers may be reluctant to discuss their own problems in the presence of the person who depends on their care. Because caregivers may range from registered professionals to well-intended neighbors, it is important to know and to document the level of skill the caregiver has, as well as his or her understanding of the situation. The caregiver's level of understanding is an essential factor for evaluating the intentionality underlying any mistreatment of a dependent older person. For example, a registered nurse in a nursing home is held to a different level of accountability than a frail spouse providing care in the home setting.

Identification of shortcomings in the patient's care may be the most elusive aspect of a comprehensive assessment. The symptoms and signs of incomplete, inadequate, or neglectful caregiving may be subtle (eg, when a patient fails to do as well as expected on a given regimen) or attributable to the patient's physical or emotional disorders (eg, weight loss in a patient with a history of depression).

Effective assessment is that which detects EM without directing undue suspicion on well-meaning caregivers or undermining a family's ability to care for an elderly person with appropriate support and counseling.

Examples of symptoms and signs that indicate a particularly high level of risk for EM are listed in Table 12.2. A number of assessment instruments have been developed in order to help clinicians screen for and assess EM, though none have been fully validated yet, and research is ongoing.

Table 12.2—Screening for Elder Mistreatment: Key Indicators

General
   Clothing: inappropriate dress, soil or disrepair
   Hygiene
   Nutritional status
   Skin integrity

Abuse
   Anxiety, nervousness, esp. toward caregiver
   Bruising, in various healing stages, esp. bilateral or on inner arms or thighs
   Fractures, esp. in various healing stages
   Lacerations
   Repeated emergency department visits
   Repeated falls
   Signs of sexual abuse
   Statements about abuse by the patient

Neglect
   Contractures
   Dehydration
   Depression
   Diarrhea
   Failure to respond to warning of obvious disease
   Fecal impaction
   Malnutrition
   Medication under- or over use or otherwise inappropriate
   Poor hygiene
   Pressure ulcers
   Repeated falls
   Repeated hospital admissions
   Urine burns
   Statements about neglect by the patient

Exploitation
   Evidence of misuse of patient's assets
   Inability of patient to account for money and property or to pay for essential care
   Reports of demands for money or goods in exchange for caregiving or services
   Unexplained loss of Social Security, pension checks
   Statements about exploitation by the patient

Abandonment
   Evidence that patient is left alone unsafely
   Evidence of sudden withdrawal of care by caregiver
   Statements about abandonment by the patient

SOURCE: Data in part from Fulmer T. Elder abuse and neglect assessment. *Try This.* May 2002;2(15):2.

PHYSICAL ASSESSMENT

Key signs of mistreatment are physical indicators that are incongruent with the patient's history; examples are bruises and welts in unusual places or in various stages of healing. Bilateral bruises on the upper torso are rarely the result of falls and warrant follow-up. Other indications of possible EM include frequent, unexplained, or inconsistently explained falls and injuries, multiple emergency department visits, delays in seeking treatment, inconsistent follow-up, or constant switching among doctors. The clinician needs to search for unusual patterns or marks, such as bruises on inner arms or thighs; cigarette, rope, chain, or chemical burns; lacerations and abrasions on the face, lips, and eyes; or marks occurring in areas of the body usually covered by clothes. The presence of head injuries, hair loss, or hemorrhages beneath the scalp as a consequence of hair pulling are significant markers. Cachectic states may be the result of malnutrition that is a consequence of neglect. Unusual discharges, bruising, bleeding, or trauma around the genitalia or rectum raise concern of possible sexual abuse, prompting gynecologic and rectal examination.

The behavior of the patient when in the presence of the suspected abuser may be significant. An EM victim may avoid eye contact, or dart his or her eyes continuously. He or she may sit a distance away from an abusive caregiver, cringe, back off, or startle easily as if expecting to be struck. The caregiver may be nervous and fearful, or quiet and passive. The patient may defer excessively to the caregiver, who may invariably answer for the patient or even try not to allow a private interview with or examination of the patient. Dubious explanations may be given to explain the patient's injuries.

The emergency department is an important setting for EM assessment. The emergency department may see elderly persons in crisis, and every effort should be made not to simply treat and release patients whose situation merits further assessment. Astute emergency personnel can identify cases where there may be serious safety problems in the caregiving situation.

PSYCHOLOGIC ASSESSMENT

EM is not invariably or entirely physical. Psychologic abuse or neglect is generally more difficult than outright physical abuse to detect and confirm, but it can be equally dangerous to the dependent older person. The behavior of both the patient and the caregiver may provide important clues about the quality of their relationship and of the care the older person is receiving. Factors that suggest a poor or deteriorating social and emotional situation are an important focus of assessment for EM.

Psychologic abuse includes taunting, name-calling, the promotion of regressive behaviors by infantilization, making painful jokes at the expense of the patient, or other activities that are demeaning. The caregiver's style of communication will provide important clues. Impatience, irritability, and demeaning statements may indicate a pattern of verbal abuse. However, psychologic neglect or mistreatment by the caregiver may take more subtle forms. For example, failing to provide social or emotional stimulation, or restricting or preventing the patient's normal activities may result in the patient's total social isolation.

The patient's demeanor and emotional status may suggest the presence of psychologic neglect or abuse. For example, ambivalence or high levels of anxiety, fearfulness, or anger toward the caregiver indicate the need for further assessment. Unexpected depression or uncharacteristic withdrawal also merits follow-up. Other high-risk behaviors include lack of adherence with treatment recommendations, frequent requests for sedating medication, or frequently canceled appointments.

Cognitive impairment, dementia, and depression have been shown to be prevalent in older adults referred for evaluation for possible EM. It is therefore appropriate to check any older adult presenting with cognitive impairment, dementia, or depression for symptoms and signs of neglect or mistreatment. Aggressive behaviors associated with dementia may trigger abusive responses in caregivers. (See also "Behavioral Problems in Dementia," p 213.)

FINANCIAL ASSESSMENT

Financial mistreatment includes unauthorized use of the older adult's funds, possessions, or property. Fiscal neglect consists of the failure to use the older adult's funds and resources for his or her needs. Signs that the elderly patient is being mistreated financially include:

- a recent marked disparity between the patient's living conditions or appearance and his or her assets,
- a sudden inability to pay for health care or other basic needs,
- an unusual interest on the part of caregivers in the patient's assets.

SELF-NEGLECT

For some elderly persons, especially those who live in isolation or who choose to accept and endure mistreatment, self-neglect may be an issue. Successful management in such cases will require an assessment of the patient's capacity to understand the risks and benefits of the situation, as well as consequences of allowing circumstances to persist. (See sections on decisional capacity in "Legal and Ethical Issues," p 21.) These are complex situations, but the patient's right to autonomy and self-determination must be honored. Paternalistic viewpoints regarding what the older person "should" do need to be avoided. In self-neglect cases, the clinician may need support when coming to terms with the requirement to respect the decisionally capable older person's wishes when this involves his or her choosing to continue in an abusive or neglectful situation. (The clinical dilemma resembles that confronting clinicians who treat battered women.) Intervention contrary to the decisionally capable patient's choice is generally inappropriate, although this may be uncomfortable for the clinician. (See also the section on autonomy versus protectionism in "Legal and Ethical Issues," p 26.)

THE ROLE OF THE OLDER PERSON

The relationship of the older person with caregivers can be very complex, and dysfunctional relations between a dependent older person and a caregiver may not be the fault entirely of the caregiver. To approach such situations with the idea that the older person is inevitably the victim infantilizes the person and is unfair to caregivers. Situations in which elderly persons are mistreated can be arrayed along a spectrum from victimization to mutual abusiveness to relationships where the older person can be viewed as a witting cause of the mistreatment. Moreover, there are cases where the older person and his or her caregivers are making the best of a tragic situation.

To determine the best possible approach for ameliorating if not solving a dysfunctional caregiving relationship, the clinician makes every effort to determine the facts in the situation and fathom the motives of the people involved. Consultation with social workers, psychologists, or psychiatrists may be useful. Legal reporting requirements are not limited in any way by these considerations. If an elderly man hits his son and the son strikes back, clinicians in most states are required to report the latter hitting.

INSTITUTIONAL MISTREATMENT

EM in the setting of home care by family or friends has been the focus of much of the discussion so far, but detecting and intervening to prevent EM in the institutional setting is also important. Several factors in this setting could aggravate the problem, including poor working conditions, low salaries, inadequate staff training and supervision resulting in poor motivation, and prejudiced attitudes. Disruptive or insulting behavior by the older adult may also be a factor; resident behaviors can at times be provocative.

The Omnibus Budget Reconciliation Act of 1987 set a new standard for care in nursing homes. (See "Nursing-Home Care," p 112.) The clinician who is alert to the possibility of abuse and neglect in any institutional setting plays an important role in protecting vulnerable older patients. Equally important is the clinician's readiness to use the resources available through the institution itself or through state regulatory agencies to investigate and intervene, where appropriate. In cases of suspected institutional EM, the challenge is to balance the rights of staff members with the rights of patients. State departments of public health are usually responsible for investigating nursing-home abuse and neglect cases.

INTERVENTION

The clinician who suspects EM can use the following questions to guide intervention:

- How safe is the patient if I send him or her back to the current setting, or does he or she need to be removed to a safe environment?
- What services or resources are available locally to support the care of this older person?
- Are there any caregivers who have health problems of their own that need attention?
- Does this situation need the expertise of others (eg, in medicine, nursing, social work), and if so, who would best serve the patient's needs?

Successful intervention in cases of EM can become complex. Among the factors governing the clinician's course of action are these:

- the exact nature and degree of the EM,
- whether the patient can or will cooperate with evaluation and intervention, and
- whether the caregiver(s) can or will cooperate with evaluation and intervention.

Procedures and interventions are laid out in two algorithms developed under AMA auspices (see the AMA guidelines listed in the references at the end of this chapter). Both algorithms take into account the issues highlighted above, especially the patient's safety, willingness to accept help, and capacity to understand and cooperate with the health care team.

Local resources in support of interventions for EM vary, but information is readily available. (See, eg, resources listed in the Appendix, p 466.) Consultation with the social work staff of the hospital, nursing home, or local health department may be a useful early step. Each state's Adult Protective Services (APS) will yield relevant information as well as direct assistance. In addition, the AMA Web site also provides a convenient starting point in the search for information and resources (http://www.ama-assn.org), as does the National Center on Elder Abuse (http://www.elderabusecenter.org).

THE MEDICAL-LEGAL INTERFACE

It is important to know state laws applicable to cases of EM; 46 states have a reporting mechanism for EM, either through APS or state agencies associated with aging. Clinicians need to be familiar with the reporting mandates that apply in their area. In some states, neglect by others must be reported, but reports of self-neglect are not required. Adult children can be charged with neglect of the elderly parent if a caregiving relationship can be proven and it can also be proven that care has been precipitously withdrawn without substitute services. In states where self-neglect is reportable, this is usually the largest intake category. Finally, states may mandate reports for self-neglect but may not provide any services unless the older adult agrees to accept them.

Clinicians are in a key position to assess and report suspected EM, and most states require such reporting. Although clinicians are appropriately wary of acting precipitously, they should be willing to enlist the help of government agencies and the courts when EM is clearly dangerous for an elderly patient. Penalties may be assessed against a nonreporter in some regions. Reports of EM are confidential, and, as is the case with child abuse reporting, the clinical reporter is protected from litigation unless it can be proven that the report was made maliciously. The home page for the National Center on Elder Abuse (cited above) provides one means for reporting information; in addition, published articles include tables that review all 50 states and the procedures expected in each (see the resources listed in the Appendix, p 466). The AMA guidelines also provide clinical algorithms for reporting suspected EM cases.

Especially when a case is to be reported, photographs and body charts may be required to document the findings on physical examination. Risk management personnel can provide guidance in documentation and assist the clinician when evidence suggests that there may be a need for police or court action. In any case where the clinician is called to court to discuss his or her findings, documentation is an important part of testimony. EM cases are often extremely complicated, and it is likely that experts in several fields will need to work with clinicians and administrators to avoid under- or over-reporting of EM and to provide the best outcomes for the victims of EM.

REFERENCES

- Dyer CB, Pavlik VN, Murphy KP, et al. The high prevalence of depression and dementia in elder abuse or neglect. *J Am Geriatr Soc.* 2000;48(2):205–208.

- Fulmer T, Guadagno L, Bitondo Dyer C, et al. Progress in elder abuse screening and assessment instruments. *J Am Geriatr Soc.* 2004;52(2):297–304.

- Lachs MS, Williams CS, O'Brien S, et al. The mortality of elder mistreatment. *JAMA.* 1998;280(5):428–432.

- National Center on Elder Abuse at The American Public Human Services Association (Formerly the American Public Welfare Association) in Collaboration with Westat, Inc. *The National Elder Abuse Incidence Study; Final Report: September 1998.* Washington, DC: National Aging Information Center; 1998.

- National Research Council. *Elder Mistreatment: Abuse, Neglect, and Exploitation in an Aging America.* Bonnie RJ, Wallace RB, eds. Washington, DC: National Academies Press; 2003.

- Pavlou MP, Lachs MS. Could self-neglect in older adults be a geriatric syndrome? *J Am, Geriatr Soc.* 2006;54(5):831–842.

CHAPTER 13—HOSPITAL CARE

KEY POINTS

- Persons aged 65 years or older make up 13% of the population and account for 36% of acute-care hospital admissions and nearly half of hospital expenditures for all adults.

- Older hospitalized patients should be routinely assessed for a limited number of common geriatric problems regardless of the admission diagnosis.

- Specific system changes in providing care to hospitalized older adults have resulted in improved patient outcomes.

Older people are at disproportionate risk of becoming seriously ill and requiring hospital care, whether it is in an emergency department, on a medical or surgical ward, or in a critical-care unit. Persons aged 65 years or older, who make up only 13% of the U.S. population, account for 36% of acute-care hospital admissions and nearly half of hospital expenditures for adults. The impact of older adults on acute hospital care will increase rapidly with the aging of the population: the proportion of the U.S. population aged 65 years or older is expected to increase to as much as 19% by 2025, with those aged 85 years or older increasing most rapidly.

Hospital use rates vary as much as threefold for Medicare beneficiaries with the same illnesses across different regions of the United States. There is no evidence that these differences in practice patterns are explained by differences in disease rates or severity.

Hospital use and the use of hospital resources is much lower among patients enrolled in capitated insurance plans than among those enrolled in fee-for-service plans; this difference in resource use has not been systematically linked to differences in patient outcomes.

During hospitalization, older patients tend to receive less costly care than do younger patients. In the large Study to Understand Prognoses and Preferences for Outcomes and Risks of Treatments (SUPPORT), for example, seriously ill patients in their 80s were found to have received fewer invasive procedures and less resource-intensive, less costly hospital care than similar younger patients received. This preferential allocation of hospital services to younger patients was not based on differences in patients' severity of illness or general preferences for life-extending care and is consistent with evidence regarding outpatient care. Differences in the aggressiveness of care have not been shown to explain differences between older and younger patients in survival or other outcomes. The best guides to assessment and management in the care of any older hospitalized patient are the clinical circumstances and the patient's preferences, irrespective of the patient's age.

Seriously ill older adults also vary widely in their preferences for life-sustaining treatments. On the basis of findings of SUPPORT, it has been recognized that even though fewer older patients prefer aggressive care than do younger patients, many older patients want cardiopulmonary resuscitation and care that is focused on life extension. Moreover, patients' families and physicians commonly underestimate older patients' desires for aggressive care. Thus, in providing care for acutely ill older persons, it is essential to determine individual preferences for the site of care and to define with the patient the goals of care.

ASSESSING AND MANAGING HOSPITALIZED OLDER PATIENTS

Many of the serious illnesses disproportionately experienced by older patients require hospital care for optimal management. The benefits of hospitalization can be remarkable: correcting serious physiologic derangements, repairing vascular obstructions and broken bones, using highly technical biomedical advances in the treatment of life-threatening illnesses. The hospital can also be a place where older patients are exposed to unintended hazards: deteriorating functional status, adverse drug reactions, and cognitive decline. A systematic approach to assessing and managing older hospitalized patients offers the best chance of reducing the risk and consequences of these common hazards.

An initial comprehensive assessment of the hospitalized older patient includes an evaluation of function at the level of the organ system, the whole person, and the person's environment. This assessment can identify needs for which targeted interventions may improve function or reduce risk for adverse outcomes. This approach complements the traditional medical assessment by highlighting problems that are common in hospitalized older patients, and it is similar in concept to comprehensive geriatric assessment conducted in other settings. (See "Assessment," p 41.)

Table 13.1 lists 10 hazards and opportunities that are commonly overlooked in elderly hospitalized patients. These problems are selected on the basis of their importance in relation to other clinical issues, the quality of relevant evidence, and their specificity to older adults. Other important problems (eg, prevention of deep-vein thrombosis, the effects of alcohol or tobacco use, ameliorating pain, and advance directives) are not specific to older adults, and some problems specific to elderly patients (eg, age-related decline in renal function) are widely recognized. (See also "Substance Abuse," p 274, "Palliative Care," p 125, "Legal and Ethical Issues," p 20, "Kidney Diseases and Disorders," p 367, "Perioperative Care," p 92.) Table 13.2 shows where assessment for these common geriatric problems can be incorporated into the routine of a hospital admission history and physical examination.

Two types of evidence suggest that these interventions are useful. First, for each problem, there is compelling evidence (cited below) supporting the proposed intervention, either because the efficacy of the

Table 13.1—Commonly Encountered Hazards and Opportunities to Address During an Elderly Patient's Hospital Stay

Problem	Possible Interventions
Functional impairments	Physical therapy, occupational therapy, assessment of social environment
Immobility and falls	Avoidance of restraints, encouragement of ambulation in hospital, physical therapy
Sensory impairment	Eyeglasses, hearing aids
Depression	Pharmacotherapy, cognitive therapy, or both
Cognitive impairment	Evaluation of dementia or delirium, assessment of social environment
Suboptimal pharmacotherapy	Modification of prescriptions
Atrial fibrillation	Warfarin or treatment to maintain sinus rhythm, or both
Nutrition	Supplementation of water, calories, protein; assessment of social environment
Mistreatment and social support	Early involvement of family and social services in discharge planning
Influenza, pneumonia vaccine	Vaccination against influenza, pneumococcus, or both

Table 13.2—Systematic Assessment of the Older Patient at Admission to the Hospital

Step	Assessments to Include
Past medical history	■ Ask about vaccination history
Medications review	■ Assess indications for each drug, appropriateness of dosing, potential interactions ■ Determine patient's or caregiver's method for assuring adherence (eg, pill boxes)
Social history	■ Ask about help needed (and who provides) for ADLs and IADLs ■ Ask about social support ■ Ask if patient feels free and safe
Review of systems	■ Ask about weight loss in preceding 6 months ■ Ask about dietary change ■ Ask about anorexia, nausea, vomiting, diarrhea ■ Ask about problems with memory or confusion ■ Ask about falls or difficulty walking ■ Ask about difficulties with vision or hearing
Physical examination	■ Take pulse (confirm arrhythmias with electrocardiography) ■ Assess for loss of subcutaneous fat, muscle wasting, edema, ascites ■ Screen for cognitive function with Mini-Cog or MMSE* ■ Assess vision and hearing ■ Use a depression screen

NOTE: ADLs = activities of daily living; IADLs = instrumental activities of daily living; Mini-Cog = Mini-Cog Assessment Instrument for Dementia; MMSE = Mini–Mental State Examination.

* See Borson S, Scanlan J, Brush M, et al. The Mini-Cog: a cognitive "vital signs" measure for dementia screening in multi-lingual elderly. *Int J Geriatr Psychiatry*. 2000;15(11):1021–1027; and Folstein MF, Folstein SE, McHugh PR. Mini-Mental State Examination. Available at http://www.minimental.com (accessed October 2005). See also "Dementia," p 204.

intervention is well established (eg, warfarin to prevent stroke associated with atrial fibrillation), or because the associated problem is common, often overlooked, and ameliorable with a safe and inexpensive intervention. Second, systematic approaches to the evaluation and management of acutely ill older adults can improve patient outcomes and reduce hospital costs.

Functional Impairments

Once hospitalized, older patients are at high risk for loss of independence and institutionalization. Among hospitalized medical patients aged 70 years or older, ~15% decline during hospitalization in their ability to perform basic self-care activities of daily living (ADLs), another ~20% are discharged without recovering their baseline prehospitalization abilities, and 15% of those admitted from home are discharged to a nursing home. Loss of personal independence is often hastened by the combined effects of the acute illness that led to hospitalization and underlying chronic illnesses and impairments. In addition, many older patients have lost their "bounce"—their ability to adapt and maintain the homeostasis of their physiologic, psychologic, and social systems in the face of the acute insults to these systems by illness and hospitalization. Functional decline during hospitalization and failure to recover baseline function have been independently associated with increasing age, lower preadmission function in instrumental activities of daily living (IADLs), and several admission characteristics, including cognitive impairment, symptoms of depression, and malnutrition. Optimal care for the hospitalized older patient requires the clinician to manage acute illness and simultaneously intervene when necessary to promote or maintain independent functioning.

The ability to perform ADLs and IADLs is necessary if the older adult is to live independently, and functional dependence is associated with worse quality-of-life outcomes, shortened survival, and increased resource use. The older patient's ability to perform ADLs and IADLs, determined at the time of admission, will serve as a useful baseline. If functional dependence is identified, the causes can be explored (eg, dependence in IADLs is often associated with dementia), and strategies to maintain and improve functional capacity can be initiated (eg, physical and occupational therapy). These strategies may be best implemented effectively for many patients by ward staff without consultation or referral. Social work consultation and early involvement of family or other caregivers is often necessary to plan postdischarge care for those older patients who are functionally dependent. (See also "Rehabilitation," p 101; "Psychosocial Issues," p 14.)

Immobility and Falls

Walking facilitates the performance of virtually all ADLs and IADLs. The ability to walk briskly and the habit of regularly walking 1 mile or more daily are associated with prolonged survival. Immobility during hospitalization, however, leads rapidly to deconditioning and subsequent difficulty walking. The major risk for deconditioned hospital patients of walking is falling, which can lead to serious injury. Falls and fall-related injuries in hospitalized patients are associated with cognitive impairment, new medications and multiple medications, environmental factors in the hospital, and abnormalities of gait, balance, and lower-extremity strength, as well as with multiple chronic medical conditions and depression.

It is helpful to assess the patient's gait, balance, lower-extremity strength, ability to get up from bed, cognition, and mood during the initial physical examination. Persons able to walk independently should be encouraged to do so frequently during hospitalization. Those able to walk but unable to do so safely and independently can receive assistance from hospital staff while walking several times daily. Formal physical therapy may yield additional benefits. The initial physical examination is also a good time to assess a patient's risk for falls by inquiring about a history of falls and by a careful musculoskeletal and neurologic examination. Interventions that reduce falls in other settings may also prevent falls in the hospital. Prudent preventive strategies include avoiding restraints and tethers, providing walking assistance for those who walk with difficulty, and providing physical therapy for those with weakness or gait abnormalities. If significant soft-tissue and bony abnormalities of the feet are discovered, a referral for podiatric care is appropriate. (See "Falls," p 187; "Gait Impairment," p 181; "Physical Activity," p 51; "Rehabilitation," p 101; and "Diseases and Disorders of the Foot," p 416.)

Sensory Impairment

Most hospitalized elderly patients have impaired vision or hearing, and these sensory impairments are risk factors for falls, incontinence, delirium, and functional dependence. Although most visual and hearing impairments are readily corrected by eyeglasses or hearing aids, these appliances are often forgotten in the hospital.

Hospitalized older patients can be screened for sensory impairment by routinely asking if they have difficulty with seeing or hearing and whether they use eyeglasses or hearing aids. Physical examination including a test of visual acuity (eg, with a pocket card of the Jaeger eye test) and the whisper test of hearing, in which a short, easily answered question is whispered in each ear, is the next appropriate step in evaluation. For people with visual or hearing impairments, it is important to provide the appropriate assistive devices (eyeglasses or hearing aids brought from home), and staff may need to be instructed in the use of appliances to communicate more effectively. (See "Hearing Impairment," p 145, and "Visual Impairment," p 140.)

Depression

Depressive symptoms in hospitalized older patients are common, prognostically important, and potentially ameliorable. Major or minor depression occurs in roughly one third of hospitalized patients aged 65 years or older but is often undiagnosed. The presence of depressive symptoms is associated with increased risk for dependence in ADLs, nursing-home placement,

and shortened long-term survival, even after controlling for baseline function and the severity of acute and chronic illness.

It is important to consider depression in all hospitalized older patients. Simply asking whether they feel down, depressed, or hopeless, or whether they have lost interest or pleasure in doing things, is a good place to start. A positive response to any one of these questions is likely sensitive to the diagnosis of depression (based on evidence from outpatients) and can be followed up by a formal assessment for an affective disorder. In hospitalized older patients, the presence of 3 or more of 11 depressive symptoms has been found to be 83% sensitive and 77% specific for a diagnosis of major depression.

Detection is the first and most important step in the management of depression. Psychotherapeutic interventions (environmental, behavioral, cognitive, and family) are safe and often effective in the initial management of patients with suspected depression. It is rarely necessary to begin pharmacotherapy during hospitalization for a medical or surgical condition, but follow-up shortly after discharge is critical. If pharmacotherapy is initiated, selective serotonin-reuptake inhibitors are often preferred because approximately 50% of older hospitalized patients have a contraindication to tricyclic antidepressants. (See "Depression and Other Mood Disorders," p 247.)

Cognitive Impairment

Delirium is present in 10% to 15% of hospitalized older patients on admission, and it develops in up to 30% during the course of hospitalization. Delirium arising during the course of hospitalization is a predictor of prolonged hospital stay. Delirium is also associated with increased rates of in-hospital death and nursing-home placement. In patients who develop delirium, chronic cognitive impairment may worsen. Symptoms of delirium commonly persist for months following hospital discharge. Roughly one third of cases of delirium can be prevented by appropriately managing six risk factors for delirium: cognitive impairment, sleep deprivation, immobility, visual impairment, hearing impairment, and dehydration. The diagnosis of delirium should be considered when any of the following is observed: fluctuation in mental status or behavior, inattention, disorganized thinking, and altered consciousness. The Confusion Assessment Method (CAM) is a useful screen for delirium. Prudent measures to prevent or ameliorate delirium include: avoiding medicines associated with delirium whenever possible; treating infection and fever; detecting and correcting metabolic abnormalities; frequently orienting patients with cognitive or sensory impairment; and avoiding excessive bed rest, room changes, and restraints. (See "Delirium," p 220.) Prevention is the best strategy: a recent randomized trial examined the effect of systematic assessment for established delirium in hospitalized elderly patients on a medical service, with multidisciplinary care provided to delirious patients. Patients in the intervention arm had no better outcomes than those assigned to usual care.

Underlying cognitive impairment consistent with dementia is present on admission in 20% to 40% of hospitalized older patients, and it commonly goes undetected. Preexisting cognitive impairment is a risk factor for delirium, falls, use of restraints, and nonadherence with therapy. Also, there is intrinsic value in identifying previously undiagnosed dementia so that appropriate evaluation and management strategies can be implemented after discharge. Cognitive function can be assessed by the use of an established test of cognitive function, such as the Mini–Mental State Examination (MMSE) or the Mini-Cog test. The diagnosis of dementia should be considered in those with a score of 24 or less on the 30-point MMSE. When dementia is a possibility, it is important to exclude reversible causes and to identify those patients for whom pharmacologic therapy and family-oriented interventions are warranted. (See "Dementia," p 204.)

Suboptimal Pharmacotherapy

The number of drugs prescribed to hospitalized patients is directly proportional to their age. Moreover, hospitalization is a period of rapid turnover in drug therapies for older patients: One study found that 40% of drugs prescribed before admission were discontinued during hospitalization and 45% of drugs prescribed at discharge were started during hospitalization. Although older patients are at increased risk for inappropriate drug therapy, adverse drug effects, and drug-drug interactions, they may also be undertreated when effective therapies are not used or are used in inadequate doses. In one study 88% of older hospitalized patients were found to have had at least one or more clinically significant drug problem, and 22% had at least one potentially serious and life-threatening problem. Consultation by clinical pharmacists can improve appropriate prescribing and improve the older patient's adherence to prescribed therapy.

A hospital admission is an ideal time to completely review a patient's medication regimen and to discontinue those that are unnecessary or have low therapeutic value (eg, sedative hypnotics). During hospitalization and at discharge, a medication review is useful to identify prescribing errors in six common categories: inappropriate choice of therapy, incorrect dosage, incorrect schedule, drug-drug interactions, therapeutic duplication, and allergy. (See "Pharmacotherapy," p 66.)

Atrial Fibrillation

Nonvalvular atrial fibrillation is present in 5% or more of hospitalized older patients, often as an incidental finding. Consistent and compelling evidence from randomized trials shows that the risk of stroke in people with atrial fibrillation can be reduced approximately two thirds by treatment with warfarin (eg, from 4.5% per year to 1.4% per year). Moreover, the beneficial effect of warfarin is maintained in persons aged 75 years or older and in those with other risk factors for stroke. Nonetheless, many older patients with atrial fibrillation are discharged from hospital without warfarin therapy, even when warfarin is indicated. Failure to prescribe warfarin is likely due to underestimation of the benefit of therapy, overestimation of its potential risk, and the difficulty of implementing, monitoring, and modifying therapy to minimize adverse effects.

In every hospitalized older patient, the history and physical examination can be targeted to identify the presence of chronic or paroxysmal atrial fibrillation. When atrial fibrillation is diagnosed, it is important to exclude valvular disease and hyperthyroidism as causes. In the absence of a strong contraindication, anticoagulation therapy is indicated to prevent stroke, usually with warfarin (see "Perioperative Care," p 92, and anticoagulation information in the Appendix, p 453). In a large randomized trial, the long-term effects of ventricular rate control and anticoagulation were compared with rhythm control (in which an attempt is made to convert patients to and maintain them in normal sinus rhythm). Adverse drug effects were less frequent with rate control and anticoagulation, and mortality at 5 years was somewhat lower (23.8% versus 21.3%, $P = .08$). New joint guidelines from the American Academy of Family Physicians and the American College of Physicians recommend rate control with anticoagulation as the preferred strategy for most patients. (See also the section on atrial fibrillation in "Cardiovascular Diseases and Disorders," p 327.)

Nutrition

Serious deficiencies of macronutrients and micronutrients are common in hospitalized older patients. Key macronutrients are protein, calories, salt, water, and fiber. On admission, severe protein-calorie malnutrition is present in approximately 15% of patients aged 70 years or older, and moderate malnutrition is present in another 25%. Moreover, 25% of older patients suffer further nutritional depletion during hospitalization. Even after controlling for the underlying illness, its severity, and comorbid illnesses, malnutrition is associated with increased risk for death, dependence, and institutionalization.

In addition to other deficiencies of vitamins and electrolytes that may develop with protein-calorie malnutrition, vitamin-D deficiency is especially common among older hospitalized patients. In one large hospital, nearly two thirds of medical inpatients aged 65 years or older were found to be deficient in vitamin-D; vitamin-D deficiency was nearly as common in inpatients without a risk factor for vitamin-D deficiency and in those taking multivitamins as in other patients. These data regarding the high prevalence of vitamin-D deficiency in hospitalized older patients complement evidence that vitamin D and calcium supplementation reduce by half the incidence of nonvertebral fractures in men and women aged 65 years or older. (See "Osteoporosis and Osteomalacia," p 194, and "Malnutrition," p 161.)

One review examined the evidence from randomized controlled trials of the benefits of oral nutritional supplements for older adults at risk of malnutrition. (Of the almost 2500 subjects included in the review, 22% were from studies of hospitalized patients.) Nutritional supplementation was found to be associated with reduced mortality and shortened length of hospital stay, although the reviewers call for additional research to substantiate these findings, because most of the studies included in their analysis were of poor quality. Beyond prescribing supplements, clinicians should assess malnourished older hospitalized patients for remediable factors such as difficulty chewing, or insufficient time or encouragement to eat. (See "Eating and Feeding Problems," p 167.)

The maintenance of water and electrolyte balance requires special attention in older adults during and after fluid administration because of their decreased capacity to achieve and maintain homeostasis. Initial efforts can be directed toward achieving normovolemia and correcting electrolyte abnormalities. Subsequent efforts to maintain fluid and electrolyte balance are based on estimates of daily metabolic requirements. The intracellular volume is about 25% to 30% of body weight for men aged 65 to 85 years weighing between 40 and 80 kg (88 to 176 lb) and about 20% to 25% of body weight for women in the same age and weight ranges. The daily metabolic requirements, as a proportion of intracellular volume, can be estimated as follows: water in L, 10%; energy in 1000 kcal, 10%; protein in g, 0.3%; sodium in mol, 0.3%; and potassium in mol, 0.2%. Thus, for a 75-year-old woman weighing 60 kg (intracellular volume 12 to 15 L), the daily maintenance requirements are 1.2 to 1.5 L of water and nutrients providing 1200 to 1500 kcal, 36 to 45 mmol of sodium, and 24 to 30 mmol of potassium. Administration of fluids and electrolytes must be adjusted on the basis of daily physical examination and of serum values of electrolytes and renal function, as needed.

Mistreatment and Social Support

Hospitalization of older adults is sometimes precipitated by mistreatment, which includes physical or psychologic abuse, neglect, self-neglect, exploitation, and abandonment. Elder mistreatment was not recognized in the medical literature until 1975; it is now estimated to affect 700,000 to 1.2 million Americans annually. In a large prospective cohort study, the annual incidence of referral to protective services for mistreatment was found to be approximately 1% among adults aged 65 years or older. Those referred for abuse, neglect, or exploitation were found to have a lower rate of survival over 13 years of follow-up (9%) than those referred for self-neglect (17%) and those not referred (40%). Most older adults referred to protective services because of physical abuse have been seen in hospital emergency departments, and many emergency visits lead to hospitalization.

Universal screening for mistreatment has been recommended and can be implemented by asking each older patient, "Do you feel safe returning to where you live?" (The sensitivity and specificity of this and other screening approaches are unknown.) Further questions can explore the living situation and specific settings or aspects of mistreatment. It is important to consider the diagnosis of mistreatment when there are physical or psychologic stigmata, such as unexplained injury, dehydration, malnutrition, social withdrawal, or recalcitrant depression or anxiety. When mistreatment is suspected, most states require that Adult Protective Services or the equivalent state agency be contacted. (See "Elder Mistreatment," p 80.)

Influenza and Pneumococcus Vaccines

All adults aged 65 years or older should be asked at the time of admission to the hospital whether they have received influenza or pneumococcal vaccination. During the fall and winter months, influenza vaccination can be administered to those who have not already received it. Pneumococcal vaccination can be administered to older hospitalized patients who do not recall having received it in the past 10 years. (See also "Prevention," p 63.)

SYSTEMS OF CARE FOR OLDER HOSPITAL PATIENTS

Nurses Improving Care for Health System Elders

Recognizing the need to improve the care of older adults in hospitals, leaders in geriatric nursing created the Nurses Improving Care for Health System Elders (NICHE) program in 1992. NICHE has evolved into a national geriatric nursing program that has been implemented in more than 160 hospitals in the United States and Canada. NICHE is a program of The John A. Hartford Foundation Institute for Geriatric Nursing at New York University, with the goal of achieving systematic nursing change that will benefit hospitalized older patients. The focus of NICHE is on programs and protocols that are dominantly under the control of nursing practice; in other words, areas in which nursing interventions have a substantive and positive impact on patient care.

NICHE is unlike other programs in that it does not prescribe how institutions should modify geriatric care; rather, it provides the materials and services necessary to stimulate and support the planning and implementation process. NICHE enables an institution to: 1) assess staff perceptions and knowledge regarding quality of geriatric care and the gaps and needs in this area, 2) modify nursing care practice to better meet the needs of older patients, particularly the gaps identified, and 3) evaluate the effectiveness of the interventions.

When NICHE is implemented, hospitals report: 1) enhanced nursing knowledge and skills regarding treatment of common geriatric syndromes, 2) greater patient satisfaction, 3) decreased length of stay for elderly patients, 4) reduced readmission rates, 5) increased length of time between readmissions, and 6) reduced costs associated with hospital care for the elderly.

In conjunction with a team of nationally recognized geriatric nursing leaders, NICHE has created a variety of "tools" to improve geriatric care. Hospitals are asked to complete a "NICHE Ready Sheet" to assess their "readiness" for NICHE. Once an institution is committed to the NICHE model of improving care, a comprehensive assessment process is then conducted to determine: 1) what nurses working in the hospitals know about basic principles of caring for older adults and 2) whether these principles are used in practice.

One instrument, the Geriatric Institutional Assessment Profile (GIAP), was designed to help hospitals define how well they incorporate best practice standards of care. The GIAP addresses six major dimensions: 1) knowledge of institutional policies, 2) institutional obstacles to best practice, 3) conflict over appropriate care, 4) clinical knowledge of selected content matter, 5) personal liability for inadequate practice, and 6) perceptions of support in the workplace. GIAP results help guide a hospital's performance improvement. Items for each of the six dimensions in the GIAP focus on the management of four geriatric syndromes that frequently affect elderly hospitalized

patients: pressure ulcers, incontinence, confusion, and sleep disturbances. These geriatric syndromes are benchmarks for best practice and provide a baseline from which a hospital can assess current practice and measure subsequent improvement in care of older adults. Once the GIAP has been completed, the data are analyzed and gauged against a standard for best practice. Such national benchmarking against other NICHE institutions helps to provide an empirical basis for mentoring and improving care at the institutional level. Once the data have been analyzed, institutions select a specific model to guide their program.

The Geriatric Resource Nurse Model

The Geriatric Resource Nurse (GRN) model originally began at Beth Israel Hospital in Boston and was further developed at Yale-New Haven Hospital. The GRN model is based on the following beliefs:

- Primary nurses know the most about the patterns and problems of older patients who are admitted to their units.

- Primary nurses serving as GRNs are more likely to integrate new behaviors into practice because of the unit-based visibility and regular feedback available.

- A GRN program can recognize nursing expertise that later may be reflected in a clinical ladder program for primary nurses.

Geriatric Resource Nurses are unit based RNs who gain enhanced skills in care of older adults through a continued education program developed in the NICHE hospital by an advanced practice geriatric nurse. GRNs carry a usual caseload of patients while serving as the unit's resource on geriatric best practices. A geriatric advanced practice nurse works closely with the GRNs through clinical rounds and activities such as geriatric nursing interest group conferences. When possible, the GRN model uses a geriatrician to consult on complex geriatric care problems. Alternatively when a geriatrician is unavailable, primary care and internal medicine physicians are invited to consult. This highly popular model has been adopted in numerous NICHE sites.

For additional information about the NICHE model, see www.hartfordign.org.

Geriatric Evaluation and Management (GEM) Units

GEM units for elderly patients who have stabilized during an acute hospitalization were developed and pioneered in Veterans Affairs medical centers. These units incorporate comprehensive geriatric assessment (including screening for geriatric syndromes, and assessment for and treatment of functional, cognitive, affective, and nutritional problems) with interdisciplinary team-based care. A multicenter randomized trial demonstrated improved ADL function and physical performance, relative to usual hospital care, for veterans assigned to GEM units. Some measures of health-related quality of life were also superior for patients treated on GEM units. These units did not affect mortality and were cost-neutral after consideration of both initial hospitalization costs and the costs of care after discharge.

Acute Care for Elders (ACE) Units

ACE is designed to help acutely ill older patients to maintain or achieve independence in ADLs and IADLs. This approach has been adapted in many acute-care hospitals in which acutely ill elderly patients are admitted to an ACE unit. The four components of this intervention are as follows:

- a prepared environment to promote mobility and orientation (eg, with carpeting, raised toilet seats, low beds, clocks, calendars, and pictures to promote orientation);
- patient-centered care with nursing-initiated protocols for independent self-care, nutrition, sleep hygiene, skin care, mood, and cognition;
- planning to go home, with early social work intervention to mobilize family and other resources at home; and
- medical care review to promote optimal prescribing.

In a randomized trial involving 651 medical patients aged 70 years or older in a university teaching hospital, ACE was found to be associated with greater independence in ADLs at discharge, less frequent nursing-home discharge, and somewhat shorter and less expensive hospitalization. In a second randomized trial involving 1531 community-dwelling adults aged 70 years or older in a community teaching hospital, ACE was found to be associated with substantial differences in the satisfaction of patients, family members, physicians, and nurses but with only modest differences in ADL function. These findings demonstrate that ACE is a promising approach to improving outcomes and reducing hospital costs for acutely ill older general medical patients, but the effects of ACE on patient outcomes are likely sensitive to factors dependent on the function of the interdisciplinary team.

The Hospital Elder Life Program (HELP)

HELP involves a multicomponent intervention to prevent delirium in hospitalized older patients. The intervention consists of protocols to manage six risk factors for delirium: cognitive impairment, sleep deprivation, immobility, visual impairment, hearing impairment, and dehydration. Elderly patients receiving this intervention are not segregated on a special hospital ward or unit. In a prospective controlled study, the incidence of delirium was found to be reduced by one third, from 15.0% to 9.9%. The intervention was also associated with significant improvement in the degree of cognitive impairment among patients with cognitive impairment at admission and a reduction in the rate of use of sleep medications among all patients. Among the other risk factors, there were trends toward improvement in immobility, visual impairment, and hearing impairment. The intervention was not associated with a reduction in the severity, duration, or recurrence of delirium, and the effects of the intervention on other outcomes have not yet been reported. Nonetheless, these findings suggest that primary prevention of delirium is probably the most effective treatment strategy.

ALTERNATIVES TO AND TRANSITIONS FROM HOSPITAL CARE

It is often assumed that older adults would prefer to be treated for acute illness at home rather than in the hospital whenever possible. The safety and feasibility of this approach for acutely ill older adults who would usually be hospitalized has been demonstrated. This approach, sometimes called the *home hospital*, requires intensive resources for medical and nursing care at home that are not yet widely available.

Older adults' preferences for home rather than hospital care vary widely. In a study of community-dwelling older persons, virtually all preferred care in the site that would provide the higher probability of survival. When home care and hospital care provide equivalent probabilities of survival, roughly half of patients prefer care in each site, with those preferring home care being more likely to be white, better educated, living with a spouse, deeply religious, and dependent in two or more ADLs. The major difference perceived by older patients between home care and hospital care was feeling safer in the hospital than at home.

Almost one quarter of hospitalized patients aged 65 and older are discharged to another institution. Although it is labor-intensive, meticulous discharge planning may maximize the probability that patients maintain the clinical and functional benefits achieved by hospitalization, and probably reduces the risk of early readmission and the use of emergency services. Discharge planning ideally begins at hospital admission, with a projection of medical, nursing, rehabilitative, and functional support required by the patient at the time of discharge. The following items should be communicated to patients (or their caregivers) who are being discharged directly home: follow-up appointments; warning symptoms or signs to watch for with instructions on whom to contact; clinical disciplines (eg, nursing, physical therapy) contracted for provision in the home; and a reconciled medication list, with clarification of which prehospital medications are to be continued. Patients being discharged to other care venues should be oriented with respect to the nature of the institution, the identity of a new primary care provider, and the expected frequency of provider visits. If the provider at the receiving institution differs from the hospital clinician, then clear and prompt communication is essential. Some items of information (critical but pending study results, nuances of goals of care or family dynamics) call for direct communication between sending and receiving clinicians. Otherwise, a concise and prompt discharge summary containing the following will suffice: summary of hospital course with care provided; a list of problems and diagnoses; baseline physical functional status; baseline cognitive status; medication list (with termination dates for time-limited drugs such as antibiotics); allergies; tests results still outstanding; follow-up appointments; and information related to goals, preferences, and advance directives.

REFERENCES

■ Cohen HJ, Feussner JR, Weinberger M, et al. A controlled trial of inpatient and outpatient geriatric evaluation and management. *N Engl J Med*. 2002;346(12):905–912.

■ Coleman EA. Falling through the cracks: challenges and opportunities for improving transitional care for persons with continuous complex care needs. *J Am Geriatr Soc*. 2003;51(4):549–555.

■ Counsell SR, Holder CM, Liebenauer LL, et al. Effects of a multicomponent intervention on functional outcomes and process of care in hospitalized older patients: a randomized controlled trial of Acute Care for Elders (ACE) in a community hospital. *J Am Geriatr Soc*. 2000;48(12):1572–1581.

■ Mezey M, Kobayashi M, Grossman S, et al. Nurses improving care to health system elders (NICHE): Implementation of Best Practice Models. *J Nurs Admin*. 2004;34(10):451–457.

■ Siegler EL, Mirafzali S, Foust JB. *An introduction to Hospitals and Inpatient Care*. New York: Spring Publishing Company; 2003.

■ Silverstein H, Maslow K. *Improving Care for Hospitalized Elders with Dementia*. New York: Springer Publishing Company; 2005.

CHAPTER 14—PERIOPERATIVE CARE

KEY POINTS

■ Operative therapy is an important option for many health problems that affect older persons.

■ The overall complication rates of surgery on older persons are below 3%.

■ Risk indices and practice guidelines for common cardiac, pulmonary, and neuropsychiatric problems assist in decision making and management of older surgical patients.

■ Comprehensive preoperative assessment and attentive perioperative management can be helpful in minimizing complications of older persons with chronic medical problems and functional impairments.

OVERVIEW OF OPERATIVE THERAPY FOR OLDER PERSONS

Surgery is a common form of treatment for older persons; currently more than 55% of all operative procedures are done in patients aged 65 or over, and the proportion is expected to grow. Many of the chronic conditions that increase in prevalence with advancing age—cataracts, arthritis, vascular occlusions, and cancers—are amenable to surgery. Over half of all malignancies occur in patients aged 65 or over, and the primary treatment for many tumors is surgical. Advances in surgical, anesthetic, and medical care have lowered surgical risks and shifted the risk-benefit ratio to favor surgery in increasingly older patients with more complex conditions. Nevertheless, although older patients account for just over half of all surgical procedures, they suffer three quarters of the postoperative mortality and also the disproportionate majority of postoperative morbidity as well. For this reason, physicians are commonly asked to perform preoperative evaluations to reduce the risks of complications and death and to optimize patient outcomes.

Many of the changes of normal aging physiology impact the perioperative management of the elderly surgical patient. For example, altered body composition, diminished kidney function, and decreased liver blood flow and enzyme activity all contribute to changes in the pharmacokinetics of drugs. Cardiac and vascular stiffening complicate fluid management and optimization of intravascular volume. Both volume overload and volume depletion occur commonly and are poorly tolerated by many older persons. Stiffening of the thoracic cage and decrements in ciliary function contribute to decreases in pulmonary reserve and heightened risk of postoperative pneumonia. Because of decreased thermoregulation, the older surgical patient is at particular risk for perioperative hypothermia. Finally, by mechanisms that are not yet fully elucidated, changes in the brain that accompany aging make older individuals exquisitely susceptible to postoperative cognitive changes. The cumulative effect of multiple organ systems with limited physiologic reserve results in "homeostenosis," a condition that greatly increases the risk of iatrogenic events. (See "Biology," especially p 9.)

It is well recognized that the aging process is extremely variable from person to person and that within a person not all organ systems age at the same rate, producing dramatic heterogeneity even among healthy elderly persons. Older individuals may have accumulated several chronic conditions that may impact on the perioperative care, either directly or through the medications they use to treat those conditions. The heterogeneity in physiologic aging combined with the potential for multiple accumulated comorbidities means older patients require a more complex and individualized preoperative evaluation. They often benefit from a multidisciplinary approach to perioperative care and recovery.

PREOPERATIVE ASSESSMENT AND MANAGEMENT

Cardiovascular System

It is estimated that 25% to 30% of postoperative deaths are from cardiac causes, and the rate of postoperative cardiac events is directly related to age. Cardiac risk assessment is the most fully developed and widely investigated portion of the preoperative medical assessment. Several schemes are available to help calculate cardiac risk, and decision trees have been well described to guide risk assessment and management. The American Society of Anesthesiologists (ASA) classification of patient physical status relies heavily on clinical judgment and is not specific for cardiovascular morbidity and mortality (see Table 14.1). This system has been used by anesthesiologists for years and has consistently been shown to be useful in predicting postoperative outcomes. An early cardiac risk index by Goldman and colleagues was published in the 1970s, a time when surgery on frail 80- and 90-year-olds was uncommon. The American College of Cardiology and the American Heart Association (ACC/AHA) Guideline for Perioperative Cardiovascular Evaluation for Noncardiac Surgery is widely employed to help stratify risk and direct management. This algorithm takes into account clinical predictors, functional status, and surgical risk and is available on the web at http://www.acc.org/clinical/guidelines/perio/update/periupdate_index.htm.

Because of increasing recognition of the benefit of medical therapy to reduce preoperative cardiac events in patients with clinical risk factors and mounting evidence of little benefit of noninvasive stress testing and invasive therapies to reduce preoperative cardiac events, the trend is now moving away from special preoperative cardiac testing and more toward treating with medical therapies on the basis of clinical judgment. A coronary artery revascularization prophylaxis study demonstrated in a prospective and randomized controlled trial that in patients undergoing elective repair of abdominal aneurysm or surgical therapy for peripheral arterial disease who have coronary artery disease (CAD) amenable to revascularization, revascularization either by coronary artery bypass grafting (CABG) or angioplasty resulted in a delay until a proposed vascular surgery but otherwise no difference

Table 14.1—ASA Classification of Physical Status

Class	Description
I or P1	A normal healthy patient
II or P2	A patient with mild systemic disease
III or P3	A patient with severe systemic disease
IV or P4	A patient with severe systemic disease that is a constant threat to life
V or P5	A moribund patient who is not expected to survive without surgery
VI or P6	A declared brain-dead patient whose organs are being harvested for donor purposes

NOTE: There is no additional information to help further define these categories.

SOURCE: Data from American Society of Anesthesiologists. ASA Physical Status Classification System. Available at http://www.asahq.org/clinical/physicalstatus.htm (accessed October 2005).

in postoperative death, myocardial infarction, stroke, dialysis, loss of limb, or survival up to 2.6 years in comparison with medical therapies, even in high-risk groups. It should be noted that patients with indications that have been shown to clearly benefit from CABG (ie, known left main disease, unstable angina, and multivessel disease with low ejection fraction) were excluded from randomization. Also, risk of perioperative myocardial infarction is markedly elevated when the surgical procedure is performed within the first 6 weeks after angioplasty and stenting. It seems clear that revascularization should not be performed simply to "get someone through a surgical procedure" and that this approach may be in fact harmful. The preoperative cardiac evaluation is therefore is quite simplified in the geriatric age group (see Figure 14.1).

The evidence base supporting the use of perioperative β-blockers, particularly in patients aged 65 or over with known CAD or risk factors for CAD, appears well established. This means the majority geriatric patients undergoing surgery are likely to derive benefit from perioperative β-blocker usage unless there is a clear contraindication to this. Growing interest in the use of both aspirin and so-called statin medications (HMG CoA reductase inhibitors) is based on evidence of benefit of these therapies from nonrandomized studies in high-risk patients. In a prospective but nonrandomized study of over 5000 patients undergoing CABG, those patients taking aspirin within 48 hours of their surgery had nearly a 50% reduced risk of myocardial infarction and stroke, almost three quarters the rate of kidney failure, and no increase in the risk of bleeding or gastritis. A case-control study of patients undergoing elective peripheral vascular surgery found that current users of statin medications had an 80% reduction in the odds of postoperative death in comparison with nonusers. Randomized trials of both of these therapies are needed to further investigate their utility in reducing postoperative cardiac complications.

The greatest risks associated with valvular heart disease include heart failure and endocarditis. Prophylactic antibiotics are recommended to prevent bacterial endocarditis in selected patients undergoing specific procedures. The highest risk for endocarditis is among patients with prosthetic cardiac valves, complex congenital heart disease, and surgically constructed systemic-pulmonary shunts or conduits, or a previous history of endocarditis. Patients at moderate risk are those with other congenital cardiac malformations, acquired valvular dysfunction, hypertrophic cardiomyopathy, and mitral valve prolapse with regurgitation or thickened leaflets, or both. Endocarditis prophylaxis is recommended for patients undergoing procedures that involve the respiratory, biliary or intestinal mucosa, prostate surgery, cystoscopy, or urethral dila-

tion. For the most recent guidelines of the American Heart Association, see their Web site: http://www.amhrt.org.

Respiratory System

Postoperative pulmonary complications have been reported to prolong the hospital stay by an average of 1 to 2 weeks in the elderly age group. The in-hospital mortality rate for those with postoperative respiratory failure is around 40%, versus 5% for those without respiratory failure. Possible patient-related factors for development of pulmonary complications postoperatively include smoking, general health status, age, obesity, chronic obstructive pulmonary disease (COPD), neurologic status, cardiovascular status, and intravascular volume shifts. Procedure-related risk factors include the site of the incision, length of the surgery, and type of anesthesia. The risk of pulmonary complications increases as the incision approaches the diaphragm; upper abdominal and thoracic procedures carry the greatest risk (10% to 40%).

A recent investigation of over 160,000 veterans undergoing noncardiac surgery established a clinical prediction model for postoperative pneumonia. Patients were assigned points based on the type of operation, age decile, functional status, and selected clinical conditions (weight loss, administration of general anesthesia, impaired sensorium, history of stroke, level of blood urea nitrogen, and transfusion of greater than 4 units of blood). Individual points were summed to create a score, and the study sample could be divided into five risk classes according to these scores. Pneumonia rates were 0.2% among those with 0 to 15 risk points, 1.2% for those with 16 to 25 risk points, 4.0% for those with 26 to 40 risk points, 9.4% for those with 41 to 55 risk points, and 15.3% for those with more than 55 risk points. As an example, an 82-year-old woman (17 points) with some functional limitations (6 points) who was undergoing an open cholecystectomy (10 points) under general anesthesia (4 points) would have a score of 37 points and fall into the category of those patients with 9.4% risk of postoperative pneumonia. This tool may be useful in guiding perioperative respiratory care, including encouragement of coughing, deep breathing exercises, incentive spirometry, and early mobility to reduce the risk of respiratory problems.

Whether age independently increases the risk of postoperative pulmonary complications is not clear. Chronologic age is less predictive of pulmonary complications following surgery than the presence of coexisting conditions. Patients with COPD have a threefold higher risk of postoperative pulmonary complications. Even among those with severe COPD, age has not been shown to be an independent risk factor for

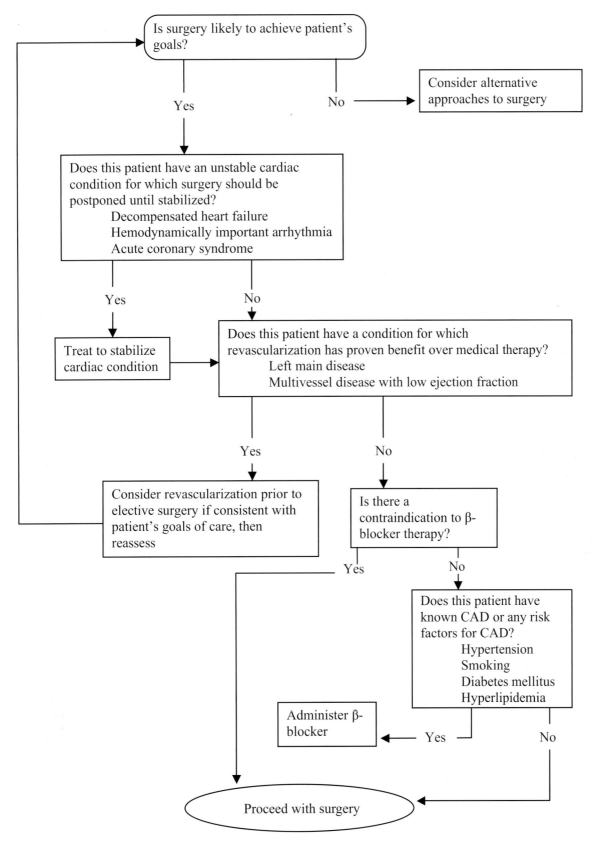

Figure 14.1—Approach to geriatric preoperative cardiac care.
CAD = coronary artery disease.

pulmonary complications. The use of perioperative pulmonary function tests in patients with known lung disease is largely discouraged but may be useful in evaluating dyspnea or wheezing when the diagnosis is unknown.

Thromboembolic complications, including pulmonary embolism, are common during the perioperative period. Since these complications can be serious and difficult to treat, attention is focused on prophylaxis. The most commonly used prophylactic regimens for patients over age 60 who are having general surgery are low-dose unfractionated heparin or low-molecular-weight heparin administered subcutaneously. More details regarding prophylactic anticoagulant regimens are found in the Appendix (p 453).

When a patient who is being treated with anticoagulants is being prepared for an operative intervention, the anticoagulants can be safely withheld for 5 doses preoperatively and then resumed the evening after surgery. This strategy may not be safe for those patients on warfarin therapy because of an artificial heart valve. In these high-risk patients, while warfarin is being withdrawn, intravenous heparin can be administered, holding it 6 hours before the operation and restarting postoperatively, continuing it until a therapeutic level of anticoagulation is achieved with warfarin. Low-molecular-weight heparins should be held for 12 hours before an operation and resumed 24 hours after the procedure, especially if spinal anesthesia is used. There is no standard for the management of antiplatelet agents. Traditionally, aspirin has been withheld for a week before surgery, but more recent data suggest that this practice is not needed to reduce bleeding complications. A large but nonrandomized study found dramatically lower rates of myocardial ischemia, gut ischemia, stroke, and kidney failure when aspirin is continued in the perioperative period in patients undergoing CABG. Importantly, in this study, the risk of bleeding and need for transfusions were not found to be increased in the patients who continued their aspirin. Randomized studies are needed to confirm the potential benefit of initiating or continuing aspirin in high-risk patients undergoing surgical procedures. For now, whether to continue, discontinue, or initiate aspirin is not clear.

Kidneys and Metabolism

As mentioned previously, renal and glomerular blood flow decreases with age. Concomitantly, there is a loss of muscle mass with age, such that an apparently normal serum creatinine may by misinterpreted as indicating normal kidney function. Glomerular filtration could be more accurately estimated by calculating the creatinine clearance using the Cockroft-Gault equation (see the section on elimination in "Pharmacotherapy," p 68) or relying on the MDRD (Modification of Diet in Renal Disease study) method that some laboratories use to automatically calculate glomerular filtration rate. Since many drugs administered during the perioperative period may require dosage adjustments with diminished renal function, accurate estimation of glomerular filtration rate is important.

Also, because of decrements in the ability of the kidney to appropriately retain salt or to maximally concentrate or dilute urine in response to intravascular volume, the use of intravenous fluids needs to be monitored very carefully. Volume resuscitation is best achieved with normal saline or blood (if appropriate), since half-normal saline or water are hypotonic and more readily diffuse to the extravascular tissues. The combination of pain in a patient who is receiving nothing by mouth and receiving intravenous D5 half-normal saline inevitably produces hyponatremia in this setting. See also the section on acute tubular necrosis in "Kidney Diseases and Disorders," p 367.)

Neuropsychiatric Concerns

Delirium is a common and morbid event in the postoperative period. The type of surgery appears to be an important determinant of delirium, with incidence rates ranging from about 4% or 5% in cataract or urologic procedures to rates reported to be as high as 50% or 60% in some series of patients with infrarenal abdominal aortic aneurysm repair or hip fracture surgery. Both preoperative and intraoperative factors have been evaluated as risk factors for delirium. Preoperative factors in patients undergoing noncardiac surgery that predispose to postoperative delirium include: age 70 years or over, cognitive impairment, limited physical function, a history of alcohol abuse, abnormal serum sodium, potassium or glucose, intrathoracic surgery, and abdominal aneurysm surgery. The most important intraoperative factor found to be associated with delirium is intraoperative blood loss. Patients with a postoperative hematocrit <30% had an increased risk of delirium (odds ratio = 1.7, 95% confidence interval 1.1 to 2.7) irrespective of the presence or absence of preoperative risk factors. When preoperative risk factors are present, the clinician can identify patients at greatest risk for developing delirium and can be especially vigilant about correcting fluid, electrolyte and metabolic derangements, optimizing replacement of blood loss, maintaining circadian rhythms by getting patients out of bed during the day and minimizing sleep interruptions at night, and cautious drug prescribing. (See also the section on postoperative delirium in "Delirium," p 224.)

Avoiding Iatrogenic Complications

Untoward effects of well-intentioned interventions are common among older hospitalized persons. Some of the more common pitfalls to be avoided include restricting mobility, excessive use of catheters, inattention to nutrition and hydration status, and inappropriate use of medications. Few disease states benefit from bed rest. It is important to maintain mobility and function as much as possible by encouraging time out of bed and avoiding restraints. The risks of skin breakdown, muscle atrophy, joint stiffness, and bone loss can be reduced by preserving mobility. Although bladder catheters can sometimes be critical in accurately measuring urine output, there is a substantial risk of infection with prolonged use of an indwelling catheter. These can also contribute to restricted mobility and should be removed as soon as possible. Restricted diets and lack of access to water can contribute to compromise in nutrition and hydration. Conversely, continued administration of intravenous fluids after the patient is able to maintain hydration orally can result in volume overload and impaired oxygenation. A regular review of medication administration can avoid unnecessary drug use and inappropriate dosing.

POSTOPERATIVE MANAGEMENT OF SELECTED MEDICAL PROBLEMS

Surgery in elderly persons often results in destabilization of chronic, coexistent medical conditions. Additionally, because of the diminished physiologic reserve common in older persons, new medical problems may arise in the postoperative period. Some of the most common medical issues to contend with postoperatively are discussed here.

Cardiovascular Problems

The most common cardiovascular problems that arise in older persons after surgery are hypertension, rhythm disturbances, and heart failure. Postoperative hypertension should initially prompt a search for a noncardiovascular cause, such as pain or urinary retention. Next, it is important to assess volume status, review fluid administration records, and note whether antihypertensive medications were mistakenly omitted before the procedure. To treat uncontrolled essential hypertension, parenteral formulations are available in several classes of medications: β-blockers, calcium channel blockers, angiotensin-converting enzyme inhibitors, and drugs that block both α- and β-adrenergic receptors. Topical agents, such as topical nitroglycerin, could also be considered useful in this setting.

Cardiac rhythm disturbances are concerning because they can lead to myocardial ischemia and heart failure. Supraventricular tachycardia, commonly seen in older persons, is associated with a history of prior supraventricular dysrhythmias, asthma, heart failure, and premature atrial complexes on a preoperative electrocardiogram. This rhythm disturbance is also more common in patients who have had vascular, abdominal, or thoracic procedures. Early restoration of sinus rhythm, or at least controlling the ventricular rate, can be attempted with an infusion of adenosine, a β-blocker, or a calcium channel blocker. If the rhythm is atrial fibrillation, conversion to sinus rhythm can be attempted with electrical cardioversion or by an infusion of amiodarone. Since spontaneous reversion to sinus rhythm often occurs within 6 weeks of the operation, long-term use of an anti-dysrhythmic like amiodarone may not be necessary. Persistent atrial fibrillation beyond 24 to 48 hours is associated with an increased risk of thromboembolism, and consideration should be given to anticoagulation therapy to reduce the risk of stroke.

Cardiac reserve is often compromised among older persons, especially those with longstanding hypertension or CAD. Heart failure may develop as a result of excessive fluid administration, or new cardiac ischemia or a rhythm disturbance. It can be extremely challenging to ensure optimal ventricular filling pressures on the basis of the clinical assessment of volume status in older persons by physical examination and standard laboratory parameters alone. Although some have recommended the use of pulmonary artery catheters in high-risk patients, studies have not shown a mortality benefit for this intervention.

Kidney and Electrolyte Disorders

Impaired preoperative kidney function increases the risk of postoperative kidney failure. The impaired reserve makes the aging kidney more susceptible to the effects of even transient reduction of cardiac output or brief exposure to nephrotoxic medications. When kidney damage has been sustained, early clinical manifestations include oliguria, isosthenuria, and an increase in serum creatinine. When impaired renal blood flow is the cause, the urine sodium will typically be less than 40 mEq/L and the urine-to-plasma creatinine ratio will be greater than 10:1. In contrast, if acute tubular necrosis is the mechanism of injury, the urine sediment may have granular or epithelial cell casts, and the urine sodium will be greater than 40 mEq/L with a urine-to-plasma creatinine ratio of less than 10:1. When acute tubular necrosis is suspected, vigorous efforts should be made to preserve kidney function by holding all potentially nephrotoxic medications and meticulously maintaining a euvolemic state. The indications for dialysis are no different in the perioperative period and include hypervolemia, hyperkalemia, metabolic acidosis, or encephalopathy. Another important mechanism of postoperative kidney failure is obstructive nephropathy, especially in older men with prostatic hyperplasia. The partial outflow obstruction combined with immobility and exposure to medications with anticholinergic effects compromising detrusor function all conspire to precipitate acute urinary retention. In addition to oliguria and an increase in serum creatinine, the bladder will typically be palpable because of distention. Treatment consists of insertion of a bladder catheter to reduce the risk of hydronephrosis and impaired kidney function. (See also the section on acute tubular necrosis in "Kidney Diseases and Disorders," p 372.)

Gastrointestinal Concerns

Constipation is quite common postoperatively, as a consequence of the combined effects of altered diet, immobility, and usually narcotic and other constipating medication use. At times, ileus and obstipation may be severe and produce significant anorexia, nausea, and even vomiting. The role of postoperative iron therapy to treat anemia is unproven and likely also contributes. Given the common co-occurrence of these risk factors for constipation in the postoperative period, a reasonable approach is to simultaneously order a stool softener and a mild stimulant laxative (eg, senna) every time a narcotic prescription is ordered, particularly if the patient has a history of constipation or it is reasonably anticipated that mobility will be reduced for more than 1 day. Prunes or prune juice, applesauce, and bran can all also have promotility effects. Table 14.2 lists the many medications useful in preventing and managing constipation.

Postoperative diarrhea should raise concern for fecal impaction and antibiotic-associated or *Clostridium difficile* diarrhea in the setting of recent antibiotic use. Checking manually for fecal impaction and sending stool specimens for leukocytes and *C. difficile* toxin may be appropriate. Management must focus carefully on volume resuscitation and treating the underlying cause.

Finally, nausea is not uncommon in the postoperative period, often as a result of narcotic, anesthetic, and other medications or slowed gut motility. See the section on nausea in "Palliative Care" (p 128) for a discussion on approach to management.

Managing Common Endocrine Abnormalities

Type 2 diabetes mellitus is a common comorbid condition of many older persons undergoing surgery. Usually, given the long half-life of oral hypoglycemic

agents and the nothing-by-mouth status for surgery, oral diabetes drugs are held the day of surgery. It may be especially important to hold metformin, given the potential additional risk of metabolic acidosis from this drug during a time of stress. To optimize glucose control, an intravenous solution containing glucose can be administered at a constant rate while blood glucose by finger stick assay is closely monitored, administering subcutaneous insulin as necessary to control glucose levels until the patient is able to resume eating. A type 2 insulin-using diabetic patient should have her insulin held on the day of surgery and receive sliding-scale insulin. Once the patient is able to advance her diet, usually half the outpatient dose of diabetes drugs are administered the first day of oral intake, with additional sliding-scale insulin coverage as needed, and then full doses are resumed as the patient consumes a usual diet. Notably, there is currently no evidence that rigorous control of blood glucose in the perioperative period provides benefit in terms of recovery of function, reduction of infections, or wound healing; thus, "permissive moderate hyperglycemia" may be prudent until adequate oral intake is ensured.

Patients taking supplemental corticosteroids require special consideration during the perioperative period. Those taking more than 20 to 30 mg of prednisone daily for more than a week or with known adrenal insufficiency should be given "stress doses" of steroids perioperatively. A single measure of cortisol, if elevated, is useful to assess the hypothalamic-pituitary axis (HPA) in patients who chronically use steroids when the function of the HPA is in question. If the cortisol level is not high, a 30-minute ACTH test may be useful. The dose of steroids to use is debated, but some authorities advise the equivalents of 25 mg of hydrocortisone the day of surgery only for minor procedures, 50 to 75 mg hydrocortisone equivalents daily (for example, hydrocortisone 20 mg intravenously every 8 hours) for 1 to 2 days for moderate surgical stress, and 100 to 150 mg hydrocortisone equivalents daily (for example, hydrocortisone 50 mg intravenously every 8 hours beginning within 2 hours of surgery) continuing for 2 to 3 days postoperatively, and then transitioned to the usual steroid regimen for high surgical stress. Other authorities simply recommend continuation of usual doses of steroids for elective, uncomplicated surgeries, or doubling or tripling the outpatient dose by giving hydrocortisone intravenously up to 100 to 150 mg daily for higher risk or anticipated complicated operations.

Delirium and Postoperative Cognitive Decline

Delirium is one of the most common postoperative complications. In a randomized study, a multicom-

Table 14.2—Medications That May Relieve Constipation

Medication	Onset of Action	Starting Dosage	Site and Mechanism of Action
Bulk laxatives			
Methylcellulose (Citrucel),* psyllium (Metamucil)*	12–24 h (up to 72 h)	1–2 rounded tsp or packets qd–tid with water or juice	Small and large intestine; holds water in feces; mechanical distention
Polycarbophil (FiberCon,* others)	12–24 h (up to 72 h)	1250 mg qd–qid	Small and large intestine; holds water in feces; mechanical distention
Osmotic laxatives			
Lactulose (Cephulac)	24–48 h	15–30 mL qd–bid	Colon; osmotic effect
Polyethylene glycol (MiraLax)	48–96 h	17 g pwd qd (~1 tbsp) dissolved in 8 oz water	Gastrointestinal tract tract; osmotic effect
Sorbitol 70%*	24–48 h	15–30 mL qd–bid	Colon; delivers osmotically active molecules to colon
Saline laxatives			
Magnesium citrate (Citroma*)	0.5–3 h	120–240 mL × 1	Small and large intestine; attracts, retains water in intestinal lumen
Magnesium hydroxide (Milk of Magnesia*)	30 min–3 h	30 mL qd–bid	Osmotic effect and increased peristalsis in colon
Sodium phosphate or biphosphate emollient enema (Fleet*)	2–15 min	14.5-oz enema × 1, repeat prn	Colon, osmotic effect; potential hyperphosphatemia in patients with renal insufficiency
Stimulant laxatives			
Bisacodyl tablet (Dulcolax*)	6–10 h	5–15 mg × 1	Colon; increases peristalsis
Bisacodyl suppository (Dulcolax*)	0.25–1 h	10 mg × 1	Colon; increases peristalsis
Senna (Senokot*)	6–10 h	2 tabs or 1 tsp qhs	Colon; direct action on intestine; stimulates myenteric plexus; alters water and electrolyte secretion
Surfactant laxative (stool softener)			
Docusate (Colace*)	24–72 h	100 mg qd–bid	Small and large intestine; detergent activity; facilitates admixture of fat and water to soften feces

* Over-the-counter medication.

NOTE: bid = twice a day; h = hour(s); min = minute(s); oz = ounces; prn = as needed; pwd = powder; qd = every day; qhs = each bedtime; qid = four times a day; tid = three times a day; tbsp = tablespoon; tsp = teaspoon.

ponent intervention, focusing on reducing sleep interruptions, minimizing medications and immobility, enhancing sensory input, and reducing dehydration was found to reduce the rate of developing delirium by one third over standard care for hospitalized medical patients. This approach, though not specifically studied in the postoperative setting, is likely to be beneficial in the postoperative phase as well. See "Delirium" (p 220) for descriptions of risk factors for delirium and a reasonable approach to diagnosis, evaluation, and treatment. For the postoperative geriatric surgical patient, undertreated pain, constipation, electrolyte abnormalities, and perioperative myocardial infarction must be particularly considered.

Postoperative cognitive decline can be subtle or dramatic and is considered to be a syndrome distinct from delirium characterized by abnormalities in learning and memory. It has been reported most commonly after cardiac surgery but is experienced by patients undergoing procedures that do not involve extracorporal circulation. Although the symptoms are often short-lived, they persist for many months in 10% to 30% of patients. Efforts to define the cause of the syndrome have not yet been successful; studies have not been able to demonstrate links with hypotension, hypoxemia, or type of anesthesia. Lacking a better understanding of the pathophysiology, treatment efforts are supportive.

Pain Management

Management of postoperative pain remains a challenge, particularly in the patient with dementia, delirium, or both. The key points to the evaluation and management of acute pain are quite similar to those discussed in "Persistent Pain" (p 131), and Table 19.1, Common Pain Behaviors in Cognitively Impaired Elderly Persons (p 134), provides a useful guide to the tools to assist in assessment of postoperative pain in cognitively impaired patients. The oldest-old and cognitively impaired patients appear to be at highest risk for undertreatment of pain, so they deserve particular attention. Undertreatment of pain, at least in nondemented individuals, appears in fact to be a more powerful predictor of the development of postoperative delirium than narcotic use.

Most postsurgical pain will require therapy with narcotic analgesia. Cognitively intact patients may have improved pain relief and overall lower use of narcotics if drugs are administered by patient-controlled analgesia (PCA) pump. Individuals with less severe pain may be able to tolerate scheduled acetaminophen (not to exceed 4 g a day) with only as-needed use of narcotic analgesics, if they are able to ask for them. Patients who are unable to communicate effectively and have pain should be given standing orders for narcotic analgesics, with guidelines as to when to hold the medications, combined with frequent assessment of medication effect. Nonsteroidal anti-inflammatory medications are best avoided in this setting. Recall that narcotic analgesics may precipitate constipation; thus, concomitant use of stool softeners and laxatives is generally advised. See the Web site for *Geriatrics At Your Fingertips* for comprehensive, up-to-date information on pain medications and dosing at http://www.geriatricsatyourfingertips.org.

Nonpharmacologic therapies, such as ice packs, heating pads, massage, and relaxation techniques, are also useful adjuncts to therapy.

Planning for Transitions

Older patients can be aided by anticipating and planning for transitions in care. Well before the time of discharge, it is important to understand how the patient will get help if he or she returns home. Watching a patient transfer, walk, and perform activities of daily living will help guide choices about appropriate discharge destination and home services that would be required to maximize a safe transition.

The time of transition is also treacherous in terms of medication errors. Carefully review with the patient (or her caregiver) her diagnoses, the summary of her hospital course, what specific medications she should take at home, and which of her old medicines she should discontinue. Include any special instructions about dosing and timing of the medication; also assess whether she will be able to obtain and administer her medications appropriately. It is useful to make sure that she (or her caregiver) understands the basics about how to manage her disease and the treatments and the need for the follow-up appointments; it should also be clear who is responsible for scheduling these appointments. Because geriatric patients tend to be more complex, it may be useful to facilitate the transition by communicating directly with the next care provider, especially for those patients who are being discharged to another institutional setting.

REFERENCES

■ Arozullah AM, Khuri SF, Henderson WG, et al. Development and validation of a multifactorial risk index for predicting postoperative pneumonia after major noncardiac surgery. *Ann Intern Med.* 2001;135(10):847–857.

■ Bailes BK. Perioperative care of the elderly surgical patient. *AORN J.* 2000;72(2):186–207.

■ Eagle KA, Berger PB, Calkins H, et al. ACC/AHA guideline update for perioperative cardiovascular evaluation for noncardiac surgery—executive summary. *Circulation.* 2002;105(10):1257–1267. Also available at: http://www.acc.org and http://www.americanheart.org (both accessed October 2005).

■ Mamaril ME. Nursing considerations in the geriatric surgical patient: the perioperative continuum of care. *Nurs Clin North Am.* 2006; 41(2):313–328.

■ Smetana GW. Preoperative pulmonary evaluation. *N Engl J Med.* 1999;340(12):937–944.

CHAPTER 15—REHABILITATION

KEY POINTS

- The World Health Organization conceptual model of functioning and disability provides a useful framework for geriatric rehabilitation by taking into account the complex interactions of body functions and structures, health conditions, individual activities and participation in life situations, and environmental and personal factors.

- A Medicare-certified inpatient rehabilitation hospital program must demonstrate that a certain percentage of patients have at least one of thirteen conditions and receive 3 hours of therapy per day.

- Since rehabilitation treatments require active patient participation and long-term self-management, the patient and family are core members of the rehabilitation team.

- Factors that influence recovery after a hip fracture include prior mobility and functional status, comorbid conditions, cognitive status, and social support.

- Optimal rehabilitation outcomes depend on comprehensive assessment of the patient, coordinated interdisciplinary team management, multifaceted interventions, and access to appropriate and high-quality care.

OVERVIEW

Rehabilitation is a critical component of geriatric health care because disabling conditions in the elderly population are common. Although these conditions drastically influence quality of life, they often improve with treatment. Chronic disease almost always underlies disability in older adults; for example, stroke occurs most often in people with other vascular diseases, and hip fractures occur most often in people with osteoporosis and gait disorders. Worsening disability also occurs in progressive chronic diseases like osteoarthritis, Parkinson's disease, or amyotrophic lateral sclerosis or in the context of deconditioning from inactivity during acute illness. To provide the best functional recovery possible, those providing geriatric rehabilitation must

- use systematic approaches to assess the causes of disability,
- be familiar with the advantages and disadvantages of all potential sites of care,
- understand the role of multidisciplinary teams and care plans,

- adapt care to comorbidities and disabilities, and
- be familiar with the basic requirements for rehabilitation of common geriatric conditions.

This chapter is designed to provide an overview of these key issues.

CONCEPTUAL MODEL FOR GERIATRIC REHABILITATION

Geriatric rehabilitation services can be organized around a conceptual model of disability in order to assess the status and needs of the patient, match treatments with specific conditions, and evaluate rehabilitation outcomes. The recently revised World Health Organization (WHO) *International Classification of Functioning, Disability, and Health* (ICF) provides a useful framework. See the WHO Web site (available at http://www3.who.int/icf/beginners/bg.pdf) for an ICF guide and a discussion of the ICF model of disability (Figure 15.1). The ICF has two main domains: "Health Condition" and "Contextual Factors." Disability and functioning are viewed as outcomes of interactions between health conditions (diseases, disorders, injuries) and contextual factors, which range from a person's most immediate environment, like furniture in the room, to the more general environment, like access to public transportation. Personal factors include a person's age, race, gender, educational background, personality, fitness, and life style.

In the WHO model, interventions can be designed to modify a person's impairments, limitations in activities, and restrictions in participation. For example, a treatment plan may be developed to improve a person's strength (impairment level), but the significance of this intervention is due to its effect on his or her physical mobility (activity) and ultimately the person's ability to return to social or physical roles (participation). The effects of gains in strength and physical mobility on participation could be modified by the person's motivation or social support. For example, if a man improves in strength and balance but his family and friends continue to "do everything for him" and do not encourage independent function, he may remain dependent. The physical environment is another powerful modifier. Even the person who achieves improved function cannot regain prior work or household roles if physical barriers to access in the community are not removed or adapted by such means as ramps or modified bathrooms. In summary, the interaction of disease and disability is particularly complex in older adults. The ICF model is useful for structuring comprehensive rehabilitation care for older patients.

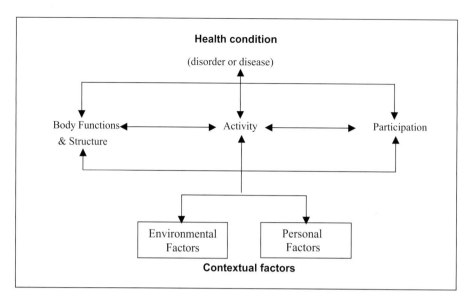

Figure 15.1—Current understanding of interactions among the components of the disability model of ICF.

The new edition of the International Classification of Functioning, Disability and Health (ICF) differs substantially from the 1980 version in its stress on health and functioning, rather than on disability. Previous models conceived of disability as beginning where health ended. The new model synthesizes the medical and social models of disability, providing a coherent view of its biological, individual, and social aspects.

SOURCE: World Health Organization, *Towards a Common Language for Disability and Health: ICF.* Geneva: World Health Organization; 2002:9. Reprinted with permission of the World Health Organization (WHO) and all rights are reserved by the Organization.

SITES OF REHABILITATION CARE

Rehabilitation services are offered in both inpatient and community-based sites. Inpatient care may be provided in rehabilitation centers (freestanding hospitals or units attached to acute hospitals) or nursing facilities (Medicare skilled nursing facilities). Outpatient rehabilitation services can be provided in hospital-based or independent clinics, in day hospital settings, or in the home. The patient's eligibility, the particular services provided, and costs vary across sites of care. The balance of advantages and disadvantages for the individual patient are important factors for the clinician to consider in recommending a site or sites of rehabilitation care.

Sites of Care: Coverage and Services

A Medicare-certified inpatient rehabilitation hospital program must demonstrate that a certain percentage of their patients have at least one of thirteen conditions, and that at least a certain percentage of patients receive 3 hours of therapy per day. Patients must be seen by a physician on a daily basis, have 24-hour rehabilitation nursing care, and be managed by a interdisciplinary team of skilled nurses and therapists. Medicare prospective reimbursement is now based on case-mix groups using the Functional Independence Measure (FIM).

The Medicare-approved skilled nursing facility must provide 24-hour nursing care. Dietary, pharmaceutical,

dental, and medical social services are also available. Physicians must supervise patient care and can visit the patient infrequently, but they must be available 24 hours a day on an emergency basis. Therapy services are available, but multidisciplinary coordination may not occur. In this setting, maintenance of function without progress may be the goal of care. Reimbursement is based on prospective payment according to the resource utilization groups (RUG III) classification, which is based on the Minimum Data Set (MDS 2).

Medicare provides home-health benefits to patients who require intermittent or part-time skilled nursing care and therapy services and who are homebound, defined flexibly to include individuals who "occasionally leave the home." These services must be prescribed and recertified every 60 days by a physician. There is no prior hospitalization requirement or limit on the number of visits a person may receive. Medicare provides care in 60-day episodes. As long as patients continue to remain eligible for home-health services, they may receive an unlimited number of medically necessary episodes of care. Home-health services provide skilled nursing and home-health aides, therapy services, medical social services, and supplies. Even though physicians must certify the patient for services, they are rarely involved in the supervision of care, and multidisciplinary coordination of care may not be available.

The escalating expenditures for Medicare's postacute care benefits from $2.5 billion in 1986 to more than $30 billion in 1996 led to the Balanced Budget Act (BBA) of 1997, which mandated prospective payment systems rather than fee-for-service reimbursement. In skilled nursing facilities, the BBA mandated the implementation of a per diem prospective payment system covering all costs (routine, ancillary, and capital) related to the services furnished to the patients under Part A of the Medicare program. Per diem payments for each admission are case-mix adjusted by the use of a resident classification system (RUG III) that is based on data from patient assessments (the MDS 2) and relative weights developed from staff time data. Home-health care reimbursement is now under a prospective payment system. Payment rates are based on relevant data from patient assessments conducted by clinicians using the Outcome and Assessment Information Set (OASIS). The OASIS was originally developed to assess quality of care in home health. The OASIS is lengthy, encompassing sociodemographic, environmental, support system, health status, and functional status attributes; it is required for reimbursement by Medicare for home-health services. For each 60-day episode of care, national payment rates vary, depending on the intensity of care required. Home-health agencies receive less than the full 60-day episode rate if they provide only a minimal number of visits to beneficiaries.

Sites of Care and Outcomes

The effect of site of care on rehabilitation outcomes is not well established. A study of outcomes among persons with stroke and hip fracture examined rates of discharge to home and recovery of function that were based on use of inpatient or nursing rehabilitation services. When controlling for case-mix differences, the researchers found that stroke but not hip fracture patients were more likely to be discharged home and to recover activities of daily living (ADLs) if treated in an inpatient rehabilitation setting. Nursing homes with high volumes of Medicare patients were found to influence stroke outcomes more than traditional nursing homes. Overall, there were no differences in outcomes for hip fracture patients by site of care. In another study, stroke patients treated under managed care were found to be more likely to receive rehabilitation in skilled nursing facilities than in inpatient rehabilitation hospitals. Patients in fee-for-service setting improved more in ADLs during the treatment phase, but there were no differences in ADLs between groups 1 year later. At 1 year, the patients in managed care were 2.4 times more likely to reside in nursing homes. On the other hand, a recent observational cohort study of the effect of rehabilitation site on recovery from stroke suggests that rehabilitation at inpatient facilities, in comparison with skilled nursing facilities, produces more rapid recovery and higher proportions of patients who achieve independence as measured by the Functional Independence Measure, even after accounting for baseline differences in patient populations between the sites of care.

The effect on outcomes of site of rehabilitation care for a more broad range of conditions has also been studied in a sample of consecutive patients enrolled from 52 hospitals in three cities with five targeted conditions (chronic obstructive pulmonary disease, heart failure, hip procedures, hip fractures, and stroke). Using case-mix adjustment models, these researchers found that patients who were discharged to nursing homes fared worst and those who were sent home with home-health or to rehabilitation hospitals did best. This type of observational study is vulnerable to bias, despite adjusting the analyses, since patient prognosis for recovery may influence discharge site; those with poor prognosis are more likely to go the nursing home, and those with better prognosis for recovery go to inpatient or home-health settings. Nevertheless, site of care may be an important factor in recovery.

The effect of prospective payment on postacute rehabilitation has been examined. Patients discharged from acute-care settings with one of five diagnoses that commonly use rehabilitation services were followed for patterns of postacute services before and after prospective payment. The transition to prospective payment appeared to result in an increase in the proportions of patients receiving no rehabilitation services, in a decrease in home-health services, and in stable or slightly increased inpatient services. This study found no consistent effects of these changes on clinical outcomes. Another study found decreases in intensity and duration of rehabilitation services in skilled facilities after prospective payment was initiated. The clinician who advocates for an appropriate site of rehabilitation care on the basis of severity of impairments, functional status, and social support might improve the outcomes of many patients.

Each site of care has advantages and disadvantages from the patient's perspective. Inpatient care is the most intense but may not be endurable for frail elderly patients, since it requires 3 hours per day of active (and fatiguing) therapy. Skilled nursing offers 24-hour care for those who cannot care for themselves or do not have a full-time caregiver. Outpatient services have clear advantages and disadvantages. Patients often prefer to return to their own homes but may not have the care support they need. Participation in day hospital or outpatient clinic requires transportation, which can be costly and time consuming.

In summary, clinicians must be familiar with the services provided in a wide range of rehabilitation settings and with the advantages and disadvantages of each. The clinician is responsible for recommending the best match between patient needs and program services. However, under certain insurance plans, decisions about location of services may be heavily influenced by costs. More systematic evaluation of rehabilitation outcomes that is based on the structures and processes of care offered by various settings is essential if we are to have more rational use of rehabilitation programs in the future. The Centers for Medicare and Medicaid Services (CMS) is currently monitoring the quality of patient care using information from the patient assessments. A research study of preventive rehabilitation ("Prehab") using a home-health approach in high-risk community-dwelling older adults demonstrated reduced frequency of functional decline.

TEAMS AND ROLES

Numerous health professionals are required to meet the rehabilitation needs of older adults. Coordinating this care is the function of the interdisciplinary care team; team members must be able to define roles, share tasks, and communicate within and outside the team. Team building and improving team function are important issues for geriatric rehabilitation service providers. All health professionals who work with older adults should have a basic understanding of the roles and functions of various team members. The primary goal of interdisciplinary team management is to ensure that patients receive comprehensive assessments and interventions for the disabling illness and associated comorbid conditions, as well as for the specific impairments and environmental factors that may affect activities and participation. The team must establish common goals and a cohesive treatment plan.

The patient and the family are core members of the rehabilitation team; their expectations and preferences must be integrated into the care plan. Rehabilitation, unlike many other interventions, requires active patient participation. If the patient is the leader in decision making, he or she gains a sense of control and responsibility. Patient self-management is now an essential part of the effective management of chronic disease. Chronic disease self-management incorporates self-monitoring, knowledge about disease, and personal control over prevention and management practices.

For information on Geriatric Interdisciplinary Team Training, see www.gitt.org.

IMPACT OF COMORBID CONDITIONS

In the elderly patient, comorbid diseases and conditions may interrupt or delay treatment and often require adaptations in the care plan. Many of the illnesses that can interfere with rehabilitation of the older adult are predictable in this high-risk population and are potentially preventable. A systematic approach to assessment, prevention, and management of comorbid conditions can improve the patient's chance of receiving maximal benefit from rehabilitation services. Table 15.1 highlights common causes in older patients of delayed or interrupted rehabilitation and describes measures that can be taken to reduce their impact on rehabilitation.

Older adults with reduced mobility are at high risk for skin breakdown, which can interfere with recovery and require extensive treatment. Immobility or altered weight bearing can precipitate pressure ulcers that heal poorly. Clinicians should monitor pressure and weight-bearing areas and be prepared to modify footwear, wheelchairs, and bedding as needed. (See also "Pressure Ulcers," p 238.) Since thromboembolic events are also common with reduced mobility, their prevention should be a routine part of care. (See also the discussions of thromboembolism in "Respiratory Diseases and Disorders," p 300, and "Perioperative Care," p 92.)

Incontinence is prevalent among older patients; causes include detrusor hyperactivity, obstruction, neurogenic bladder, immobility, and cognitive deficits. Indwelling catheters increase the risk of infection and are rarely appropriate. A structured approach to the assessment and treatment of bladder problems should be a basic component of any rehabilitation service. (See also "Urinary Incontinence," p 171.)

The risk of pneumonia is increased by inactivity and disordered swallowing, as well as underlying lung disease. The prevention of aspiration pneumonia involves difficult tradeoffs. Routine radiologic screening for aspiration has precipitated a marked increased awareness of this problem, but the clinical relevance of modest amounts of aspiration detected radiologically is unknown. Conservative measures such as changing food consistency with liquid thickeners and cohesive food substances and lowering head position while eating may help alleviate the problem. Sometimes aspiration risk is addressed by discontinuing all oral feeding and placing an enteral feeding tube. This approach eliminates the fundamental human pleasure of eating and may not be successful, since oral secretions or refluxed gastric contents can still be aspirated. (See also "Eating and Feeding Problems," p 167.) Upper gastrointestinal bleeds may occur during rehabilitation as a consequence of stress or medications and may not be preceded by typical symptoms. (See also "Gastrointestinal Diseases and Disorders," p 357.)

Mental functioning is critical for rehabilitation, which requires the ability to follow commands and learn. Since older adults who have been acutely ill are

Table 15.1—Methods to Reduce the Impact of Selected Comorbidities on Rehabilitation

Confusion
  Screening for toxic or metabolic contributors (eg, medications, hypoxia, electrolyte disturbance)
  Sensory aids
  Planned reassessment for improvement if confusion limits rehabilitation potential

Deep-vein thrombosis and pulmonary embolism
  Mobilization
  Hydration
  Compression stockings
  Intermittent pneumatic compression
  Coumadin
  Low-molecular-weight heparin

Depression or apathy
  Screening for depression
  Treatment with medications, counseling, support groups

Kidney or bladder infection
  Avoidance, removal of indwelling catheter
  Check of postvoid residual
  Frequent toileting
  Rarely helpful: prophylactic antibiotics

Pneumonia
  Mobilization
  Treatment of chronic obstructive pulmonary disease, as needed
  Influenza vaccination
  Incentive spirometry
  Screening, precautions for aspiration*

Seizures
  Prevention of recurrence with anticonvulsants, carbamazepine, or valproic acid

Skin breakdown
  Mobilization
  Positioning
  Pressure-relieving mattresses
  Early care with dressings

Spasticity
  Physical therapy to control
  Muscle relaxants
  Botulinum toxin (trials ongoing)

Upper gastrointestinal bleeding
  Avoidance of nonsteroidal anti-inflammatory drugs and use of acetaminophen for pain
  Hematocrit monitoring
  Consideration of prophylactic agents

* See text for controversies.

SOURCE: Data in part from Studenski SA, Duncan P, Maino JH. Principles of rehabilitation in older patients. In: Hazzard WR, Blass JP, Ettinger WII, et al., eds. *Principles of Geriatric Medicine and Gerontology.* 4th ed. New York: McGraw-Hill; 1999.

at increased risk for delirium, clinicians should assess mental status and screen for easily reversible causes in their older patients. (See also "Delirium," p 220.) Depression is endemic in newly disabled persons and can manifest as low motivation; formal screens for depression and early intervention are essential. (See also "Depression and Other Mood Disorders," p 247.) Seizures can develop after stroke, and spasticity can develop during stroke recovery. Interventions for spas-

ticity such as physical therapy or muscle relaxants have offered only modest benefit; some trials of botulinum toxin have suggested promising results but others have had no effect. (See also the section in stroke in "Neurologic Diseases and Disorders," p 425.)

Certain comorbid conditions common in elderly patients, including diabetes mellitus, heart disease, peripheral vascular disease, musculoskeletal disorders, sensory impairments, and dementia, require ongoing adaptations in rehabilitation. Activity level is a powerful factor in glucose metabolism; diabetic patients are therefore likely to experience changes in glucose levels and medication requirements during rehabilitation. Increased caloric intake during recovery may also affect their medication needs. Therapy personnel should know how to assess diabetic control, use a glucometer, and intervene for hypoglycemia. (See also "Diabetes Mellitus," p 349.) Most abnormal gaits increase the energy requirements of walking; an abnormal gait in a patient with coronary artery disease may cause coronary symptoms to worsen. Persons with poor cardiac output may have extreme exercise limitations. Medication adjustments for heart diseases may be necessary but can cause adverse effects of their own, such as orthostatic hypotension. Patients with one vascular disease often have others; peripheral vascular disease is common, often associated with insensitive or painful feet and high risk of skin breakdown. Treatment of painful peripheral neuropathy and other persistent pain syndromes may foster increased activity and avoid pressure ulcers (see also "Persistent Pain," p 131.) Musculoskeletal status should be monitored to avoid overuse syndromes involving increased demand on vulnerable joints. For those with vision and hearing impairment, corrections must be provided and teaching approaches adapted accordingly. In patients with dementia, rehabilitation progress is still possible, but carryover may be decreased and the need for supervision and cueing increased.

REHABILITATION APPROACHES AND INTERVENTIONS

The primary goals of rehabilitation treatment are restitution of function, compensation for and adaptation to functional losses, and prevention of secondary complications. Ultimately, rehabilitation should maximize the person's potential for participation in social, leisure, or work roles. Many strategies can be used to achieve these goals. Restitution of physical function usually depends on therapeutic exercises to improve flexibility, strength, motor control, and cardiovascular endurance. Although exercise has been shown to improve strength, endurance, and balance in well-defined populations of disabled older adults, there is still uncertainty about whether these gains translate into changes in mobility, ADLs, participation, or a reduction in falls. (See also "Physical Activity," p 51.) In stroke, speech and language therapy can be used to treat aphasia. Cognitive rehabilitation might improve alertness and attention. However, the research evidence is insufficient to demonstrate that speech and language therapy, or cognitive rehabilitation, improve functional deficits.

Therapeutic modalities such as massage, heat, cold, and ultrasound are used to decrease pain and muscle spasm. These and other pain management strategies may contribute to increased function and tolerance for further rehabilitation. There is little research evidence supporting objective benefits from modalities, but patients commonly report symptomatic relief. (See also "Persistent Pain," p 131.)

Equipment for mobility, dressing and bathing assistance, orthotic and prosthetic devices, and splints all can augment or replace the function of impaired body parts and thereby reduce limitations in activities and participation. For example, an ankle orthosis can prevent foot drop and improve safety and speed of walking. A wheelchair can provide mobility for community activities.

Repeated practice of task-specific activities such as bed mobility, transfers, and walking can improve functional mobility. Upper extremity function improves with specific functional training activities, such as grasps, reaches, and fine manipulations. Balance training may improve balance and reduce the risk of falls. Older adults may benefit from retraining in instrumental ADLs, such as cooking, managing finances, or driving a car.

Contextual factors, both environmental and personal, should be addressed to minimize restrictions on a person's activities and participation. For example, motivation may be addressed by collaborative goal setting, patient and family education, detection and management of depression, and use of support groups. Environmental modifications such as grab bars and raised toilet seats in the bathroom or curb cutouts on public streets can promote independent functioning.

To maintain function and enhance health status after rehabilitation, patients and families should assume responsibility for long-term self-management. Rehabilitation goals include a prevention program for worsening disability, including reintegration into social programs such as senior center programs, and health and wellness programs.

COMPREHENSIVE ASSESSMENT

Comprehensive assessment of rehabilitation patients is necessary for appropriate clinical management and for the evaluation of outcomes. The treatment plan should be guided by the results of the initial assessment. The primary components of any assessment include patient demographics, social support, place of residence prior to illness, medical comorbidities, severity of current illness, and the patient's prior functional status. Impairments such as deficits in range of motion and flexibility, strength, sensory functions, balance, cognition, and depression should always be assessed. In conditions such as stroke, there should be an evaluation of swallowing and language function. The patient's functional status is assessed with standardized measures of ADLs (eg, FIM, the Barthel ADL Index), and measures of instrumental ADLs. The patient's participation or quality of life is assessed with generic measures like the SF-36 Health Survey (available at http://www.sf-36.org) or disease-specific measures like the Stroke Impact Scale or the Harris Hip Questionnaire.

STROKE

Stroke is a major cause of mortality and morbidity in the United States, particularly among persons aged 55 years and over. Acute stroke occurs in more than 700,000 people each year, and 80% or more are likely to survive, many with residual neurologic difficulties. Stroke-related deficits are severe in approximately one third of the survivors. Many patients with mild and moderate stroke become independent in ADLs, but other more complex dimensions of health status may still be affected. As stroke survival continues to increase, the need for comprehensive stroke rehabilitation will rise. Rehabilitation programs must address a broad range of stroke-related disabilities, including those in basic ADLs, instrumental ADLs, participation, and integration into health and wellness programs.

Goals of Rehabilitation

The overall goals of rehabilitation for the elderly stroke patient include restitution of function, compensation for or adaptation to functional losses, and prevention of secondary complications. Specific objectives include:

- preventing or recognizing and managing comorbid illness and medical complications,
- assessing each patient comprehensively, using standardized assessments,
- matching the patient's needs to the program capabilities,
- training the patient to maximize independence in ADLs and instrumental ADLs,
- facilitating the patient's and family's psychosocial coping and adaptation,
- preventing recurrent stroke and other vascular conditions such as myocardial infarction, and
- assisting the patient in reintegrating into the community.

Rehabilitation for older adults with stroke is complex because of the heterogeneity of causes, symptoms, severity, and recovery. Stroke patients present with varying symptoms, depending on the site and size of the brain lesions. The most common type of neurologic deficit is hemiparesis, but other deficits may include sensory impairment, aphasia, dysarthria, cognitive impairment, motor incoordination, hemianopsia, visual-perceptual deficits, depression, dysphagia, and bowel and bladder incontinence. The degree of initial recovery and the time needed to reach maximal recovery is affected by the number of deficits. For example, individuals who have hemiparesis, hemianopsia, and sensory deficits are less likely to ambulate independently and require longer to regain skills than do those with hemiparesis only.

Stroke patients usually experience some degree of recovery. This recovery is most dramatic in the first 30 days but may continue more gradually for months. In the Framingham study, improvement in motor function and self-care was found to slow 3 months after stroke but to continue at a reduced pace throughout the first year. Language and visual-spatial function was recovered over 12 months, but cognitive function improved only during the first 3 months.

Approach to Management

Guidelines for rehabilitation following stroke have been updated by a team sponsored by the Department of Veterans Affairs and the Department of Defense (available at http://www.oqp.med.va.gov/cpg/STR/STR_base.htm). The guidelines offer algorithms for initial assessment and rehabilitation referral, followed by management in inpatient or community settings. The guidelines assess the quality of evidence for a series of recommendations. Recommendations considered to have a "good" evidence base are highlighted. Many important issues in management have not yet been assessed in clinical trials and thus do not meet standards for a "good" evidence base. Yet, management recommendations may still be considered appropriate care, since a lack of evidence should not be considered to indicate a lack of benefit. The guidelines emphasize that better clinical outcomes are achieved when patients with acute stroke are treated in a setting that provides coordinated, multidisciplinary stroke-related evaluation and services. Recent studies have confirmed that adherence to guidelines promotes better outcomes. Coordinated care reduces 1-year mortality, improves functional independence, and increases satisfaction with care. Benefits are not restricted to any particular subgroup of patients. Stroke severity should be systematically assessed, using the NIH Stroke Scale

(available at http://www.strokecenter.org/trials/scales/nihss.html).

In general, therapy should be started early, but later supplementary interventions may also be beneficial. For persons who have completed acute poststroke rehabilitation, a structured, supervised, progressive therapeutic program in the home has been shown to produce gains in endurance, balance, and walking capacity, but no change in motor control. The benefits of this program are probably due to the aggressive intervention on deconditioning and mobility. There is less evidence to support specific therapeutic interventions for stroke.

There are several philosophical approaches to physical rehabilitation following stroke. Neurophysiologic approaches based on the theories of Bobath and Brunnstrom and on proprioceptive neuromuscular facilitation traditionally are used to restore motor control. These approaches consider the patient to be the recipient of therapy and the therapist to be the decision maker in charge of problem solving. There is no convincing evidence that any one specific technique is superior to another. New therapeutic interventions for restitution of motor function are in development. Constraint-induced movement therapy discourages the use of the unaffected extremity and encourages active use of the hemiparetic extremity, with a goal of improved motor recovery. Results in patients with chronic stroke impairment suggest potential gains beyond usual therapy. A large randomized clinical trial of constraint-induced therapy is now under way. Treadmill walking with partial body weight support using a harness connected to an overhead system may improve gait velocity, balance, and motor recovery. Speech and language therapy are often provided for stroke patients with aphasia. However, there is no universally accepted treatment. Although a recent Cochrane report states that the evidence does not support a finding of either clear effect or lack of effect, the Veterans Affairs guidelines support "good" evidence for follow-up evaluation and treatment by the speech language professional for long-term residual communication difficulties. The guidelines also support "good" evidence for cognitive retraining for attention or visual-spatial perceptual deficits and compensatory training for short-term memory deficits. The same guidelines find "good" evidence for medication treatment for depression and emotional lability. Spasticity can develop gradually after stroke and can inhibit function and interfere with hygiene. Most interventions have been disappointing, but investigational trials of botulinum toxin type A [OL] injection for hand spasticity have been encouraging.

The patient who has had a stroke is at high risk for recurrence: up to 7% to 10% annually. The rehabilitation phase is an appropriate time to ensure that assessment and treatment for stroke prevention has occurred. Assessments for significant carotid stenosis and for atrial fibrillation should be completed. Indications for carotid endarterectomy and anticoagulation with warfarin should be reviewed. Antiplatelet medications such as aspirin alone or in combination with dipyridamole or clopidogrel should be considered in many patients. Treatment with angiotensin-converting enzyme inhibitors[OL] and statins[OL] has also demonstrated reductions in risk of stroke. Other risk factors to be targeted include hypertension control and smoking.

In summary, the evidence for specific interventions for stroke rehabilitation is weak. The collective benefits of well-organized multidisciplinary care, including secondary prevention, are well established. (See also the section on cerebrovascular diseases in "Neurologic Diseases and Disorders," p 423.)

HIP FRACTURE

Epidemiology and Surgical Care

Each year in the United States, about 250,000 people have a hip fracture. The risk of fracture is higher in women, in nursing-home residents, and in persons with dementia. Mortality is about 5% during the initial hospitalization but nears 25% in the year following fracture. Recovery to the prior level of function occurs in about 75% of survivors, but their overall mobility will be more limited; up to half of those with recovery will still require an assistive device. About half of patients will have an initial decline requiring transient long-term care, and about 25% will still be in long-term care 1 year later.

For medically stable patients, surgical repair is recommended 24 to 72 hours after the fracture. This early repair has been associated with a reduction in 1-year mortality as well as with lower incidence of complications like pressure ulcers and delirium. However, delay of surgery is warranted to allow a medically unstable patient to improve sufficiently to tolerate the procedure. The surgical approach is determined by the location of the fracture, the presence or absence of displacement, and the prefracture mobility. One third of hip fractures occur at the femoral neck, and the other two thirds are intertrochanteric, occurring lateral to the femoral neck. Prefracture mobility is used as a guide to determine the goal of surgical treatment and to allow the risks and benefits of each surgical procedure to be considered.

Femoral neck fractures without any displacement can be surgically corrected with simple screws. However, femoral neck fractures with any degree of displacement are at increased risk for nonunion or avascular necrosis and therefore are usually treated with a prosthetic femoral head (hemiarthroplasty). Patients with significant underlying boney acetabular disease and a displaced femoral neck fracture may benefit from complete hip arthroplasty. Patients are usually allowed to bear weight immediately after repair of a femoral neck fracture, no matter which technique has been used.

For intertrochanteric fractures, the treatment of choice is open reduction and internal fixation with a compression screw or similar device. Provided there is little or no displacement, immediate weight bearing is usually allowed. However, displaced or comminuted intertrochanteric fractures commonly remain unstable, even after surgical fixation. Therefore, full weight bearing is often not allowed for up to 6 weeks or until the stability of the fracture is assured. Factors that influence recovery should be assessed, including prior mobility and functional status, comorbid conditions, cognitive status, and social support. Other information includes type of injury and repair as well as pain status. Mobility performance can be systematically assessed with numerous instruments, including one developed specifically for hip fracture (Harris Hip Questionnaire).

See also "Perioperative Care" (p 92).

Rehabilitation of Hip Fracture

Rehabilitation of hip fracture includes pain management, mobilization, and prevention of complications, such as delirium and thromboembolic events. The most important factors influencing recovery appear to be how soon mobilization is initiated and how frequently therapy is provided. Delay in mobilization is often driven by surgical recommendation, with proper healing of the fracture taking precedence over mobility. Partial weight bearing is difficult for many older patients to achieve; they are either up on their feet or not. Prolonged inactivity is clearly associated with poorer functional outcomes, and early weight bearing has been shown to be associated with low rates of surgical failure. Accelerated rehabilitation with rapid mobilization, coordinated planning, early discharge, and community follow-up has been associated with a 17% reduction in costs and no detriment to rates of recovery. Intensity of service clearly affects outcome, as those who receive more than once-daily physical therapy during initial rehabilitation are more likely to be discharged directly to home than those who receive physical therapy once a day or less.

Prevention of Recurrence

Persons who have had a hip fracture often have other comorbidities, such as osteoporosis and balance problems, that place them at risk for further fractures. Efforts to diagnose and treat osteoporosis, improve balance, and reduce injury risk are a key part of treatment planning during rehabilitation. (See also "Osteoporosis and Osteomalacia," p 194.) The use of hip protectors has been extensively studied, with varying results. For those living in an institutional setting, there may be some benefit. For patients living in the community, hip protectors do not appear to decrease the incidence of hip fractures. As a recent study demonstrates, adherence remains a major issue. Only 38% of community-dwelling women in the study found the hip protectors to be acceptable and agreed to participate. At the end of 1 year, only about half the participants were still wearing the hip protectors daily.

TOTAL HIP AND KNEE ARTHROPLASTY

Natural History

In the United States, joint arthroplasty is the most common elective surgical procedure performed; approximately 280,000 are done annually. The primary indications for joint replacement are progressive pain and mobility limitation despite conservative care. The most common diagnosis associated with the need for joint replacement is osteoarthrosis, followed by rheumatoid arthritis. The long-term results of joint replacement have generally been excellent and include significant pain relief and improved function. Continued success rates in the 90% range are seen 10 to 15 years after joint replacement. The most common reason for failure of the hip or knee replacement is loosening of the implant. Joint infection is another major concern; infection affects 0.2% to 1.1% of total hip and 1% to 2% of total knee replacements. Deep infections often necessitate removal of the implant, long-term antibiotics until there is no sign of infection, then ultimate replacement with another implant. (See also "Infectious Diseases," p 304, especially the section on prosthetic device infections, p 312.)

Assessment

Plain radiographs are the usual method for determining the severity of joint damage at both the hip and knee. Loss of cartilage is shown by joint-space narrowing, and often osteophyte formation is also present.

Management

Anticoagulation to prevent thromboembolism and good pain control are the major goals during the immediate postoperative period for both hip and knee arthroplasty. (See also "Perioperative Care," p 92, and anticoagulation information in the Appendix, p 453.) It is recognized that patients who have undergone a major orthopedic procedure like total hip or knee arthroplasty are at particularly high risk for both symptomatic and asymptomatic venous thromboembolism (VTE). Recent guidelines for the prevention of VTE suggest the routine use of low-molecular-weight heparin, fondaparinux, or adjusted-dose warfarin. Pain control in the initial postoperative period is often achieved with narcotics dispensed orally, intravenously, or by patient-controlled analgesia pumps. For both hip and knee arthroplasty, early mobilization is the standard of care, and weight bearing often begins on the second postoperative day. Patients at low risk can often be discharged from the acute care hospital within 5 days. For those at high risk, defined as being older than 70 years or having two or more comorbid conditions, early inpatient rehabilitation has been shown to improve functional outcomes and decrease total length of stay. Age alone should not be used as a criterion for eligibility for joint replacement, as even persons older than 80 years who are in good health with stable chronic conditions have excellent results.

To decrease the risk of dislocation after total hip arthroplasty, patients are taught to avoid motions such as deep squats and crossing their legs. To prevent excessive hip flexion, a raised toilet seat is recommended for the first few months after surgery. Rehabilitation focuses on strengthening especially the abductors, which are weakened by the surgical approach, as well as on progressive range-of-motion and gait training. Recently, orthopedic surgeons have been examining the use of a minimal incision, less than 10 centimeters, for total hip arthroplasty. This approach may lead to quicker recovery and return to function but is still being studied.

After total knee replacement, recovery of range of motion is the key to return of function and is often aided by the use of a continuous passive motion machine (CPM). Its use has been shown to decrease the need for postoperative manipulation and, combined with physical therapy, has increased active range of motion and shortened length of stay. Surgeons have also applied the concept of minimal incisions to the total knee replacement operation and with significantly more success. This operation, in the hands of an experienced surgeon, has been shown to decrease blood loss and length of stay. Postoperative swelling is common and interferes with regaining motion. However, thigh-high compression stockings, the CPM, and possibly cryotherapy can be used to manage swelling.

AMPUTATION

Epidemiology

More than 50,000 people undergo lower extremity amputation each year in the United States. Most of these people have systemic vascular disease, with or without diabetes mellitus. Those with diabetes often have other end-organ disease, such as blindness, end-stage renal disease, and peripheral neuropathy. Mortality in this group approaches 50% at 2 years and 70% at 5 years. For up to one fifth of patients, amputation of the contralateral extremity is needed within the first 2 years after the initial amputation. The majority of dysvascular amputees have such a burden of comorbid disease that the prosthesis is largely used for limited mobility, such as transfers and ambulation within the home.

Assessment

Key factors to assess include the patient's prior functional status, stability of comorbid conditions, cognition, and upper extremity use, as well as the condition of the stump and other lower extremity. Successful prosthetic ambulation is associated with independent prior ambulation, ability to bear weight on the contralateral leg, stable medical status, and ability to follow directions. Blindness and end-stage renal disease do not necessarily preclude rehabilitation. A systematic approach to monitoring amputee status has been incorporated into an instrument, the Prosthetic Profile of the Amputee.

Rehabilitation for Amputation

Rehabilitation starts in the preoperative stage, when the patient begins with strength and flexibility exercises and receives teaching about the recovery process. Amputation surgery generally aims to preserve the knee, since the below-the-knee amputee has a much lower energy requirement of walking than does the above-the-knee amputee. This decision must be weighed against risks of poor wound healing with more distal amputation.

Postoperative rehabilitation includes efforts at early mobilization, prevention of contractures, wound healing, and shaping of the stump. Poor wound healing delays rehabilitation in about 25% of cases. Prostheses vary in weight, socket type, style of foot, and suspensions. The older amputee benefits from a prosthesis that is lightweight, stable, and easy to use. Prosthetic rehabilitation involves progressive ambulation, teaching about prosthesis and stump care, and monitoring for stump injury.

Last, phantom limb pain is common after amputation, with an estimated incidence of 60% to 80%, and pain management influences progress with rehabilitation. Treatment remains difficult, and clear evidence-based guidelines are lacking. As tricyclic

<hr>

OL Not approved by the U.S. Food and Drug Administration for this use.

antidepressants[OL] and sodium channel blockers[OL], like carbamazepine[OL], are generally effective for neuropathic pain, they are often used for phantom pain despite the lack of well-controlled trials. A number of other medication regimens, using such agents as opiates[OL] and anesthetic blocks[OL], have also had success in small trials. Two recent trials of memantine showed no benefit in the treatment of phantom limb pain.

MOBILITY AIDS, ORTHOTICS, ADAPTIVE METHODS, AND ENVIRONMENTAL MODIFICATIONS

Assistive devices, orthotics, adaptive methods, and environmental modifications are effective for elderly patients with disabilities and handicaps. It is important to identify the underlying causes of disability before prescribing a device or modification, because medical or surgical treatment for individual diseases and impairments may be more effective or may enhance the usefulness of these approaches.

Mobility Aids

Canes typically support 15% to 20% of the body weight and are to be used in the hand contralateral to the affected knee or hip. The tips, handles, materials, and lengths of canes vary. As the number of tips increases, the degree of support also increases, but the cane becomes heavier and more awkward to use. The cane tip is fitted with a 5-cm diameter rubber tip with a concentric ring to prevent slipping. The handle of the cane may be curved or have a pistol grip; the pistol grip offers more support but is less aesthetically pleasing to some people. Canes can be made of a variety of materials, but most are made of wood or lightweight aluminum. The length of the cane is important for stability. Some canes are adjustable, but wooden canes must be cut to size. One of three methods may be used to evaluate the proper cane length: measuring the distance from the distal wrist crease to the ground when the patient is standing erect, measuring the distance from the greater trochanter to the ground, or measuring the distance between the ground 15 cm in front of and to the side of the tip of the shoe and the elbow flexed at 30 degrees.

Crutches can support full body weight but are seldom recommended for older persons. Problems with crutches include the large amount of arm strength required, the risk of brachial plexus injury, and the necessity to use an unnatural gait pattern.

A walker is prescribed when a cane does not offer sufficient stability. A walker can completely support one lower extremity but cannot support full body weight. Walker types include pick-up and wheeled walkers. The pick-up walker is lifted and moved forward by the patient, who then advances before lifting the walker again; the result is a slow, staggering gait. It requires strength to repeatedly pick up the walker and cognitive ability to learn the necessary coordination. A wheeled walker allows for a smoother, coordinated, and faster gait and takes advantage of overlearned gait patterns. It is more likely to be correctly used by persons with cognitive impairment. The most commonly used type is the two-wheeled walker, which brakes automatically with increased downward pressure. Four-wheeled walkers are rarely used because they are less stable and more difficult to control, although they are occasionally useful for persons with Parkinson's disease. Three-wheeled walkers may offer some advantages in ease of turning but are not yet in common use. The Merry Walker Ambulation Device has a seat and bars all the way around. It is the same size as a wheelchair and is best reserved for those with severe balance problems. It is also useful for severely demented patients.

Patients who cannot safely use or are unable to ambulate with an assistive device will require a wheelchair. A wheelchair must be fitted according to the patient's body build, weight, disability, and prognosis. Incorrect fit may result in poor posture, joint deformity, reduced mobility, pressure ulcers, circulatory compromise, and discomfort. For the elderly patient with only one functional arm, the wheelchair may be lowered to allow for foot propulsion. Patients with lower extremity amputations may have the wheels set posteriorly to compensate for a change in the center of gravity. Motorized wheelchairs may be used by mentally alert persons with bilateral upper extremity weakness or severe cardiopulmonary disease who lack the endurance to push a wheelchair. Motorized scooters offer less trunk support than motorized wheelchairs but are more acceptable to some people. Motorized scooters and wheelchairs increase patients' mobility but increase their risk of deconditioning, as they might otherwise push a wheelchair or ambulate. The use of a wheelchair commonly requires home modifications, including ramps and widened doorways. Cars may need to be adapted with lifts.

Orthotics, Adaptive Methods, and Environmental Modifications

Orthotics are exoskeletons designed to assist, resist, align, and stimulate function. Orthotics are named by the use of letters for each joint that the device involves in its structure. Thus, an AFO is an ankle and foot orthotic device used to support weak calf or pretibial muscles (eg, for a stroke patient with lower extremity weakness).

Adaptations to facilitate dressing may be necessary for patients with problems such as frequent soiling or diminished flexibility, coordination, and endurance. Their clothing should be easy to clean, and tops should fit easily over the head or fasten in the front and allow for freedom of movement. Fastening clothes is commonly a problem for elderly persons. Hooks and loops or Velcro are usually easier to use than buttons, and they may be sewn on to replace buttons and zippers. When buttons are necessary, button hooks with customized grips may be used, or the buttons can be sewn on with elastic thread, which may eliminate the need to manipulate the buttons. Donning shoes and socks is particularly difficult for elderly persons with decreased agility. Longer, looser socks (eg, tubular socks) are easier to don. For patients who find that reaching the feet to put on shoes is a problem, a long-handled shoehorn may be useful. Elastic shoelaces eliminate the need for tying and untying.

Environmental modifications can have a major impact on the elderly person's ability to function independently or with minimal assistance at home. A variety of assistive devices, such as reachers, special utensils, and adapted telephones, can reduce the difficulty of performing daily tasks and have a significant impact on a person's quality of life.

The bathroom is a common place for falls. Any older person with impaired balance or lower extremity weakness should have bars installed near the toilet and tub or shower. Raised toilet seats and bathtub benches are available to assist those with lower extremity weakness. These are also useful for persons with arthritis of the hips or knees because they reduce biomechanical stress on the joint. Long-handled bath brushes, hand-held shower, and "soap on a rope" may be helpful for persons with upper extremity impairment.

REFERENCES

- Gill TM, Baker DI, Gottschalk M, et al. A program to prevent functional decline in physically frail, elderly persons who live at home. *N Engl J Med.* 2002; 347(14):1068–1074.

- Gillespie WJ. Extracts from "clinical evidence": hip fracture. *BMJ.* 2001; 322(7292):968–975.

- Nikolajsen L, Jensen TS. Phantom limb pain. *Br J Anaesth.* 2001;87(1):107–116.

- Ottenbacher KJ, Smith PM, Illig SB, et al. Trends in length of stay, living setting, functional outcome and mortality following medical rehabilitation. *JAMA.* 2004;292(14):1687–1695.

- Wells JL, Seabrook JA, Stolee P, et al. State of the art in geriatric rehabilitation: part II: clinical challenges. *Arch Phys Med Rehab.* 2003;84(6):898–903.

CHAPTER 16—NURSING-HOME CARE

KEY POINTS

- Currently there are 17,000 U.S. nursing homes with 1.8 million beds, 1.6 million residents, and 2.4 million discharges each year.

- The typical nursing-home physician is an internist or family physician who devotes 2 hours or less per week to nursing-home care.

- The Omnibus Budget Reconciliation Act of 1987 requires a periodic comprehensive assessment of all nursing-home residents, sets minimum staffing requirements, and fosters residents' rights by limiting the use of restraints and psychoactive medications.

- The care of nursing-home residents has become more complex over the past several years, commensurate with an increasing level of medical acuity in an environment constrained by lack of resources.

Nursing homes have evolved dramatically over the past several years, responding to a variety of government and market-driven forces. The almshouse, common at the turn of the century, has been transformed into a highly regulated institution for persons with severe physical and mental disabilities. Nursing homes, more than ever, present the clinician with a set of unique and complex care issues, many of which are best understood in the context of population needs, government policy, and reimbursement and staffing patterns.

THE NURSING-HOME POPULATION

The average nursing-home resident is characterized by significant impairments in physical and instrumental activities of daily living (ADLs). Overall, the level of disability in the nursing home has increased over the past decade and exceeds that found in persons receiving home care. Among nursing-home residents, 22.3% require assistance with one or two ADLs, and 74.9% require assistance with three or more. In addition to impairments of ADLs, 81% of nursing-home residents are impaired in their ability to make daily decisions; two thirds have orientation difficulties or memory problems, or both, and over half (54%) have either bowel or bladder incontinence. Hearing and visual impairments are found in 36% and 39% of residents, respectively. Dementia remains the most commonly occurring condition in the nursing home, with estimates ranging from 50% to 70%. Behavioral problems,

understandably, are also common, occurring in at least one third of nursing-home residents. Such behaviors include verbal and physical abuse, social inappropriateness, resistance to care, and wandering. Communication problems are noted in 60% of residents; 44% have difficulty with both being understood and understanding others. Depression is diagnosed in 20% of nursing-home residents.

Almost half of all nursing-home residents are aged 85 years or over, with fewer than 9% under the age of 65. The majority are women (72%), white (89%), and unmarried (60% widowed) with limited social supports. The percentage of black residents in U.S. nursing homes has increased in recent years (9%), approaching national population norms. In fact, black Americans 65 to 74 years of age are more likely than white Americans to be admitted to a nursing home. Nonetheless, other nonwhite populations, such as Hispanic Americans, Asian Americans, and Native Americans, are underrepresented in nursing homes despite even higher disability rates in these groups. Older adults with developmental disabilities constitute another unique population that is requiring increasing nursing-home care as their elderly parents die. These persons often require specialized care that many nursing homes have difficulty providing (see "Mental Retardation," p 280).

NURSING-HOME AVAILABILITY AND FINANCING

Currently there are 17,000 U.S. nursing homes with 1.8 million beds, 1.6 million residents, and 2.4 million discharges (ie, to home, hospital, or secondary to death). Of these facilities, 65% are proprietary (for-profit), with voluntary nonprofit (25%) and government nursing homes (10%) accounting for the remainder. The average nursing home operates 107 beds, and a minority (8%) have more than 200 beds. A little more than half of all nursing homes (56%) are part of a chain.

By age 65 a person's risk of nursing-home admission before death is estimated at 46%; one third have lifetime risk of nursing-home stays of 90 days or less. The risk of nursing-home admission rises steeply with age; approximately 20% of persons aged 85 years and over reside in nursing homes versus 1.4% of those aged 65 to 74 years. Barring breakthroughs in the treatment of dementia, the number of persons 65 years and older using nursing homes will double by the year 2020. Interestingly, the occupancy rates in nursing homes nationally have declined over the past several years and now stand at 88%. This decline has generally been attributed to the availability of other long-term-care options, such as assisted living, but there are likely other causal social and financial variables that have yet to be articulated. The availability and use of home-care services for Medicare-eligible patients have not been found to consistently reduce nursing-home admissions.

Postacute care is increasingly being offered in nursing-home settings, a response to the higher care needs of older persons occurring in conjunction with declining lengths of hospital stays. Though the types of postacute services and programs vary significantly from one locale to another (ie, dialysis, orthopedic, ventilator, postoperative, rehabilitative, or wound care), they remain distinct from the standard nursing-home services by integrating the features of acute medical, long-term-care nursing, and rehabilitative settings. The challenge in postacute care is that of accommodating to patients with varying degrees of disease severity, functional dependence, and comorbidities. Some limited studies suggest that, for selected patient populations, postacute care in the nursing home achieves outcomes equal to or better than postacute care in acute hospitals. Definitions as to what constitutes postacute care, however, vary widely, as do regulatory standards, thus making comparison studies difficult.

Despite the significant disability associated with most nursing-home residents, the population remains quite heterogeneous. Short stayers (3 months or less) currently account for 25% of all nursing-home admissions, 50% will spend at least 1 year in the nursing home, and 21% will reside in the nursing home almost 5 years. Many short-stay residents are admitted for rehabilitation, and some enter nursing homes for terminal care. Interestingly, improvement in function for the longer-stay nursing-home residents is quite common, which reflects the heterogeneity of this population. The number of nursing-home admissions has risen since 1994, reflecting the dynamic nature of this sector of the long-term-care continuum.

Nursing-home expenditures currently total $90 billion and are projected to increase to $150 billion by 2007. Public expenditures constitute 62% of all nursing-home spending (Medicaid 48%, Medicare 12%, other 2%), with private spending constituting 38% of the total (31% out of pocket, 5% health insurance, 2% other private funds). On admission to a nursing home, almost one third of residents are eligible for Medicaid, and another third eventually qualify as financial resources are depleted. Under the new prospective payment system enacted as part of the Balanced Budget Act of 1997, Medicare payments to skilled nursing facilities are no longer cost-based, but are predicated on the person's functional needs and rehabilitative potential. Although the prospective payment system has not conclusively limited access to skilled nursing care for Medicare beneficiaries, it has definitely forced nursing homes to be more diligent with regard to their admission policies. Not unexpectedly, physical, occupational, and speech therapies are commonly prescribed in the nursing home, with half of all nursing-home admissions receiving at least 90 minutes of these rehabilitation services, according to one study. The prospective payment system requires nursing-home staff to carefully document gains in function to ensure reimbursement. Interestingly, declines in Medicare spending on home-health care since enactment of prospective payment may eventually force some individuals into nursing homes for lack of affordable home-care options. (See "Financing, Coverage, and Costs of Health Care," p 29.)

STAFFING PATTERNS

It is generally conceded that the current nursing-home population is "sicker" and more disabled than nursing-home residents were in the past. Studies have confirmed the correlation between the provision of quality care to total nursing hours and the ratio of professional nurses (ie, registered nurses) to nonprofessional nursing staff. An Institute of Medicine report in 2001 recommended increasing nurse staffing levels to enhance the quality of nursing-home care and has spurred Congress to debate the merits of mandatory minimum staffing ratios. The Centers for Medicare and Medicaid Services (CMS) has refused to institute regulatory changes that would be based on current evidence but has rather called for additional research in this area. Even if significantly higher staffing ratios eventually are mandated, the financial resources to achieve them remain elusive. Recruiting and retaining staff, particularly nursing assistants who constitute the bulk of the nursing-home workforce, also continues to be difficult. Turnover rates for registered nurses and licensed practical nurses also are very high, at more than 50% per year. Turnover rates have been associated with increased rates of hospitalization for nursing-home residents and have been linked to the organizational culture within the nursing facility.

Staffing issues are also pertinent to physicians practicing in nursing homes. The typical nursing-home physician is a primary care internist or family physician who devotes 2 hours or less per week to nursing-home care. Many physicians avoid nursing-home practice because of perceptions of excessive regulations, paperwork, limited reimbursement, and aversion to the long-term-care environment. A paucity of credible role models for physicians in training has greatly contributed to this lack of interest and involvement in long-term-care issues. Closed staff models are thought to deliver a higher intensity and quality of care in part because of the integration of the physician into the nursing facility culture, which ultimately facilitates interdisciplinary communication and treatment. Limited evidence suggests that hospitalization rates for nursing-home residents may be lower in facilities that employ a limited number of committed physicians. One study has demonstrated that the quality of drug use in the nursing home is positively correlated with enhanced nurse-physician communication and with regular multidisciplinary team discussions.

FACTORS ASSOCIATED WITH NURSING-HOME PLACEMENT

Although there is a significant chance of being admitted to a nursing home with increasing age, other factors, such as low income, poor family supports (especially lack of spouse and children), and low social activity have been associated with institutionalization. Cognitive and functional impairments have also predicted nursing-home placement, often permanently. Interestingly, for patients with dementia, education and caregiver support have been shown to delay the need for nursing-home placement for up to 1 year. Not surprisingly, older adults with more positive attitudes toward nursing homes are more likely to use skilled nursing facilities than are adults with less favorable dispositions. The range of long-term-care services that are now available (ie, skilled nursing, home care, assisted living) further increases the complexity of placement decisions, as the relative value and merits of available options have not been empirically tested. The use of formal (ie, paid-for) community services does not necessarily reduce the likelihood of nursing-home placement for patients with severe disabilities.

THE INTERFACE OF ACUTE AND LONG-TERM CARE

The majority of nursing-home admissions derive from acute-care hospitals. Conversely, nursing-home residents have high rates of hospitalization, ranging upward of 549 admissions per 1000 nursing-home beds per year. A 2001 survey by the Centers for Disease Control and Prevention noted that nursing-home residents constitute 2% to 3% of all emergency department visits. Infection is the most common reason for transfer of nursing-home residents to short-stay hospitals, accounting for one quarter of all such admissions. Studies to date suggest that nurse practitioners and physician assistants, who act in concert with the primary care physician, provide more intensive care in the nursing home, enhance satisfaction with care, and often decrease hospitalization rates while maintaining cost neutrality. Unfortunately, the transition from acute to long-term care is often complicated by suboptimal information transfer. Illegible or nonexistent transfer summaries, omission of prescribed medications, and the lack of documentation of advanced directives, psychosocial information, and behavioral issues are but a few of the information gaps commonly reported. (See also the section on transitions from hospital care in "Hospital Care," p 91, and "Perioperative Care," p 100.)

QUALITY ISSUES

Extensive nursing-home reforms enacted in 1987 (in the Omnibus Budget Reconciliation Act of 1987) significantly changed the landscape of long-term care. In addition to setting training guidelines and minimum staffing requirements and bolstering residents' rights, including limiting the use of restraints and psychoactive medications, the law required a periodic comprehensive assessment of all nursing-home residents. This assessment, known as the Minimum Data Set (MDS), focuses specifically on clinical issues with relevance to quality care. If any real or potential problems are identified with any of these issues, the health care team must review accompanying resident assessment protocols that outline standard diagnostic and therapeutic approaches to the specific problems in question. The protocols are, in essence, practice guidelines that the team, including the primary care physician, is encouraged to use. In addition to comprehensive assessments, the physician must also clearly document the need for all medications, particularly psychoactive agents. Unnecessary drugs are defined as those that are given in excessive doses, for excessive periods of time, without adequate monitoring, without adequate indications for use, or in the presence of adverse consequences that indicate the need for dose reduction or discontinuation. In addition to these generic instructions, specific types of drugs have been banned (ie, usage will warrant a citation from the state survey inspection team unless a clear rationale is documented in the chart) from use in the nursing home on the basis of criteria developed by a group of experts. Although some evidence exists to suggest that the 1987 act and subsequent mandates have resulted in a decreased prevalence of pressure ulcers and reduced use of restraints, their impact on the quality of care overall has been difficult to quantify. Interestingly, recent surveys indicate that only a minority of physicians ever review the MDS or related care plans. A new set of quality indicators based on MDS items has been instituted nationally in an effort to hasten efforts to improve quality. With this system, nursing facilities are able to compare their individual performance with regional and national norms to help guide their efforts to improve the quality of care (see http://www.cms.hhs.gov). Future versions of the MDS will likely include additional quality-of-life measures relating to personal preferences and activities.

A host of variables interact in nursing homes to determine the level of quality achieved. These include staffing levels, reimbursement rates, and processes of care extant in the nursing home. Although surveys of nursing facilities are mandated every 15 months, there is much debate as to whether the survey process can adequately identify quality practices and engender lasting improvements when deficiencies in care are found. The survey process, based on a deterrent regulatory paradigm, has been criticized for its inconsistencies, disassociation between outcome and process, surveyor subjectivity, and a failure to discriminate between trivial and important quality issues. The percentage of nursing-home residents receiving inadequate care or experiencing physical harm has declined to 20%, according to a recent General Accounting Office report. This figure, however, remains unacceptably high.

MEDICAL CARE ISSUES

The care of nursing-home residents has become more complex over the past several years, commensurate with an increasing level of medical acuity in an environment continually constrained by lack of adequate resources. Comprehensive, ongoing assessment within an interdisciplinary framework provides the practitioner the opportunity to restore function, whenever possible, and almost always to enhance quality of life.

Clinical challenges abound in the nursing home, created, in part, by the atypical and subtle presentation of illness so characteristic of patients with profound physical and psychologic frailty. In addition, limited access to biotechnology, frequent dependence on nonphysicians such as nurses and nurse assistants for patient evaluation, and the high prevalence of cognitive impairment in a setting of intense regulatory oversight all complicate the medical decision-making process. Families of nursing-home residents often remain an integral part of the overall care plan and may require specific educational and psychosocial supports. Ethical and legal concerns are also very common, particularly those regarding end-of-life, feeding, hydration, and resident rights issues. (See "Legal and Ethical Issues," p 20.) Finally, the heterogeneity among nursing-home residents precludes a uniform care plan, but rather demands an individualized, thoughtful, and reasoned approach to each person in the nursing-home setting.

Problems in nursing homes that commonly require unique diagnostic and treatment strategies include infections, falls, malnutrition, dehydration, incontinence, behavioral disturbances, the use of multiple medications, and prevention and screening. (See "Infectious Diseases," p 304; "Falls," p 187; "Malnutrition," p 161; "Urinary Incontinence," p 171; "Behavioral Problems in Dementia," p 213;

"Pharmacotherapy," p 66; and "Prevention," p 59.) For example, determining the risks and benefits of tube feedings for frail nursing-home patients must be predicated not only on underlying illness but also on the resident's and the family's value system, the resources available in the nursing facility, and staff acceptance of the intervention. Given that the evidence for and against enteral feeding in nursing-home patients is controversial (ie, benefits are not well established, with up to one fourth of residents with chewing and swallowing problems able to have their feeding tubes removed), the practitioner must continue to individualize therapy. (See "Eating and Feeding Problems," p 167.) Many of the problems commonly encountered in the nursing home result when multiple comorbidities interact with a host of environmental factors, all of which may only be partially remediable. Unfortunately, expectations of family, as well as state regulators, often do not account for these complexities and commonly engender "risk-averse" behavior that is counter to autonomy and optimum quality of life.

PHYSICIAN PRACTICE IN THE NURSING HOME

Physicians have traditionally had limited involvement in nursing homes. Perceptions of excessive regulations, paperwork, and limited reimbursement raise further disincentives to nursing-home practice. In reality, the medical care of nursing-home residents is both challenging and fulfilling, requiring excellent clinical skills as well as sensitivity to a variety of ethical, legal, and interdisciplinary issues. Medical interventions, whether they be curative, preventive, or palliative, demand an individualized approach that recognizes the complex interplay among resident, family, and staff needs. Further, the evidence upon which to base treatment may be nonexistent.

The comorbidity present in most nursing-home residents commonly creates the need for multiple drug therapies, with attendant complications. Even though residents receiving more than nine medications (one third of all nursing-home residents) are flagged by state survey teams as reflecting potential quality concerns, the use of multiple medications cannot always be avoided. The most common health conditions found in the nursing home for persons aged 65 years and older, following dementia, are heart disease, hypertension, arthritis, and stroke. The approaches to these and other illnesses have evolved dramatically in recent years and complicate treatment decisions where cost-effectiveness is increasingly looked upon as a desirable goal. Clear documentation of the rationale for a given medication or intervention is the best way to protect against potential scrutiny; frequent discussion with the facility's consultant pharmacist is also helpful. (See "Pharmacotherapy," p 66.)

Physicians who schedule and structure their visits to the nursing home will benefit from the resultant efficiencies and secondarily will be more fully integrated into the health care team. Nurse practitioners and physician assistants have become increasingly involved in the primary care of nursing-home residents. Studies suggest that nurse practitioners and physician assistants who act in concert with the primary care physician as a coordinated team provide more intensive care to the nursing-home resident and may decrease hospitalization rates while maintaining cost neutrality. Information regarding physician responsibilities and Omnibus Budget Reconciliation Act mandates can be found at the Web site of the American Medical Directors Association (http://www.amda.com). Such responsibilities encompass ongoing comprehensive assessment and coordination of care in order to assure patient autonomy and safety as well as optimization of physical and psychosocial function. (See Table 16.1.)

Several studies have documented misdiagnoses, inappropriate interventions, and poor preventive care practices in nursing homes. In an often-cited study of Maryland nursing homes, for example, only 11% of patients with four common types of infection were found to have received even a minimal evaluation (eg, failure to obtain a urine sample when treated for a urinary tract infection). In a study of nursing-home patients with nonmalignant pain, 25% were found to be receiving no analgesics. Intensive research is currently being directed to understand the processes necessary to integrate validated care guidelines into nursing homes in an effort to improve quality of care.

Certain care strategies that have been developed may enhance care quality. The commonly employed special care units, though conceptually attractive, have not consistently been shown to enhance quality of care apart from the involvement of individual professionals. Specific consultation services in the nursing home, however, may improve care practices and patient outcomes, as shown by a randomized controlled trial of an effort to reduce falls in a group of Tennessee nursing-home residents. In addition, interactive educational programs for physicians and nursing staff may improve practice, as has been demonstrated in programs to promote appropriate psychoactive drug use.

Understanding each nursing-home resident's preference for care in the context of his or her underlying value system will undoubtedly improve overall quality. Interestingly, fewer than one in eight nursing-home residents have discussed preferences with their health care providers. In addition, there is often a lack of follow-up of do-not-resuscitate discussions in the hospital when the patient is subsequently admitted to the nursing home. Sixty percent of nursing-home residents

Table 16.1—The Physician's Responsibilities in the Nursing Home

- Comprehensive admission assessment, including history and physical examination, and review of available medical records.
- Development of a plan of care in concert with interdisciplinary team members, the resident, and the family that is consistent with the resident's needs and goals.
- Periodic monitoring of chronic health problems at appropriate intervals, using diagnostic testing, consultation, and pharmacologic and nonpharmacologic interventions as warranted.
- Prompt and thorough assessment of acute medical problems or change in function, instituting change in the medical treatment plan as indicated.
- Communication with interdisciplinary team members, the resident, and the family concerning new diagnoses and treatment plans.
- Periodic review, in concert with the consultant pharmacist, of all medications with regard to ongoing need, adverse effects, appropriate laboratory monitoring, and potential interactions.
- Optimization of quality of life and function, with special attention to cognition, mobility, falls, skin integrity, nutrition, and continence.
- Determination of each resident's decision-making capacity and assistance in establishing advance directives.
- Physical attendance to each resident, with documentation in the medical record in accordance with all state and federal guidelines.

have orders for cardiopulmonary resuscitation, and almost 90% desire hospitalization for acute illness. When ethical dilemmas do present themselves, the availability of institutional ethics committees can provide important guidance. The multidisciplinary nature of these committees ensures a spectrum of opinion and insight critical for nursing-home residents, and they are particularly relevant to end-of-life issues. (See also "Legal and Ethical Issues," p 20.)

THE ROLE OF THE NURSE PRACTITIONER

The increasing numbers of nurse practitioners (NPs) in health care in the United States has brought exciting change to the practice setting. Geriatric nurse practitioners (GNP's) are a vital, albeit small, component of the nurse practitioner movement. The estimated 3500 GNP's in the country make up about 5% of all nurse practitioners, the largest percentage of whom operate in the adult and family nurse practitioner role.

The utilization of GNP's in nursing homes is more popular than ever, as studies have repeatedly demonstrated the efficacy and quality of care provided. There are numerous ways in which a physician, NP, and long-term care facility can choose to organize their operations. The model selected will determine how the relationship between these three entities will function, including the division of responsibility, division of power, method of payment, and method of reimbursement. Each model is associated with its own profile of advantages and disadvantages.

The Nurse Practitioner as Nursing-Home Employee

Some institutions choose to retain NPs as full-time employees, paying them a regular salary to serve as a complement to regular physician care. The physician is paid on a fee-for-service basis. This arrangement increases the influence the nursing facility has on the NP, connecting him or her more to the facility than to the physician with whom he or she works. This has its positives and negatives; it allows the two individuals to work more as equals without dealing with financial matters, but it also introduces a third party to their relationship to cause complications where they do not exist in other arrangements.

The Teaching Nursing Home

This model uses both fee-for-service and full-time, salaried NPs. Regardless of how the NP is paid, however, he or she will receive joint appointments to a school of nursing and to the teaching nursing home. The key element of this model is that the NP is expected to do a great deal of active in-service training of other staff members. In fact, in some cases, the NP will spend up to 50% of his or her time performing training activities and participating in specialized team functions (eg, wound care, pain management). However, it is important to note that most of these activities are nonreimbursable under Medicare, so it is vital under this model to clearly define the role of the NP and the amount of nonreimbursable activity that he or she is to perform.

The Private Practice Model

The most popular model is one in which the NP is salaried by the physician; NPs provide care to nursing facilities on a fee-for-service basis. In some cases, the NP works with a group of physicians, while in others, the NP is the direct employee of an individual. This method has the advantage of simplicity and ease of communication, eliminating the third party from the physician–NP relationship.

Other Models

Most other models involve health maintenance organizations and other forms of managed care. Under this format, either the physician and the NP work in a team

of two, or the NP provides primary care while the physician provides follow-up.

Financial Considerations

The most important financial issue regarding the use of NPs also applies to the payment of physicians: striking a balance between productivity and effective care. If a nursing facility hires a physician or NP, then the facility obviously will have somewhat more control over the operations of its employees. However, a direct salary payment schedule reduces the incentive for a physician or NP to see as many patients as possible. The facility can therefore be hurt, because a certain number of visits per day is required in order to receive reimbursement for the employee's salary.

For this reason, many long-term-care facilities choose to employ physicians and NPs on a fee-for-service basis, accepting a separate bill for each patient treated. The problem is that such payment system can lead to troubles of its own, such as "blitzes of service," where a physician and nurse practitioner claim to see 50 or more patients in a single day. In such cases, patients are clearly not receiving an appropriate level of care. Moreover, the nursing home may suffer financially from such acts; Medicare will often recognize these blitzes for what they are and deny reimbursement. Therefore, it is vital that the nursing facility find the right balance between productivity and adequate care.

Other Medicare reimbursement issues are especially significant in the case of nurse practitioners. Because the role of the NP is often vaguely defined and varies among different institutions, there is a tendency for the NP to accumulate considerable hours in nonreimbursable activities, including in-service training of other staff members. Administrators and other staff members commonly view an NP as a kind of clinical expert, able to dispense knowledge and resources about any condition or problem that might arise. The end result is that the facility must be prepared to absorb the cost of all this assistance, which is not reimbursable under Medicare.

In addition, Medicare provides a stringent set of regulations that must be strictly observed in order for nursing facilities to receive reimbursement for care provided. Personal visits after the initial visit must alternate between the NP and the physician, and the physician must sign all rehabilitation orders. In fact, all NP orders must be countersigned by the physician within 24 hours in order to be eligible for reimbursement. Unfortunately, this can cause a number of handicaps for the NP and for the nursing facility interested in providing effective care. Additional state regulations may further complicate this process; in New York State, NPs may not perform an initial assessment of a patient, and the physician must conduct a "meaningful review" of each patient's records every 3 months. Constant and systematic communication between the NP and the physician is the surest way of overcoming these restrictions.

The Collaborative Practice Agreement

The best way to avoid many of these difficulties is for the physician and the NP to agree upon and sign a collaborative practice agreement at the outset of their professional relationship, spelling out the specifics of that relationship in a way that both parties are comfortable with. A collaborative practice agreement should document responsibilities of both individuals relating to charting, coverage agreements, and peer review, and should provide a system for resolving disputes. Many administrators and physicians prefer to begin with a restrictive agreement in the beginning, to be altered and made more liberal as the NP earns a greater degree of trust. Finally, a collaborative practice agreement should enumerate in the most detailed fashion possible the duties and assigned role of the nurse practitioner. This will avoid confusion on the part of the physician, NP, and nursing facility, and allow all concerned to provide the most effective and efficient care possible.

THE ROLE OF THE MEDICAL DIRECTOR

The quality of physician practice in the nursing home is, in many ways, determined by the medical director. The medical director, in concert with the medical staff, sets quality standards for the nursing home and operationalizes these through specific policies and procedures. The medical director must ensure compliance with all relevant state and federal guidelines and work with the nursing-home administrator and director of nursing to foster effective team care and continuing staff education. The medical director of a nursing home works closely with all disciplines and must be constantly aware of the unique interplay between laws, regulations, organization, and delivery of medical care. Certification for medical directors following completion of a formal course is now offered through the American Medical Directors Association.

REFERENCES

- Dimant J. Roles and responsibilities of attending physicians in skilled nursing facilities. *J Am Med Dir Assoc.* 2003;4(4):231–243.

- Dimant J. The role of the consultant in long-term care facilities. *J Am Med Dir Assoc.* 2003;4(5):274–280.

- Kane RA. Definition, measurement, and correlates of quality of life in nursing homes: toward a reasonable practice, research, and policy agenda. *Gerontologist.* 2003;43(Spec No. 2):28–36.

- Katz PR, Mezey M, Kapp M, eds. Physician practice in long-term care: workforce shortages and implications for the future. In: *Advances in Long-Term Care.* Vol. 5. New York: Springer Publishing Co.; 2003.

- Mezey M, Burger SG, Bloom HG, et al. Experts recommend strategies for strengthening the use of advanced practice nurses in nursing homes. *J Am Geriatr Soc.* 2005;53(10):1790–1797.

CHAPTER 17—COMMUNITY-BASED CARE

KEY POINTS

- Home care has changed dramatically since the introduction of prospective payment for services; the number of recipients has declined by 20%, and many home-health agencies have closed because of financial constraints, limiting access to home-care services in some areas.

- Primary care providers often find home care rewarding; reimbursement charges for home visits have improved, making home visits more financially viable for clinicians.

- Community-based services that do not require a change of residence (adult day care, day hospitals, home hospitals, PACE, telemedicine) may be a useful alternative to inpatient services. However, the availability of these services strongly depends on financial reimbursement.

- Community-based services requiring a change of residence (assisted living, group homes, adult foster care, and continuing-care retirement communities) offer a wide range of services. These are regulated at the state level and vary considerably in availability, cost, and services provided.

HOME CARE

The 2000 U.S. census data revealed that almost 10 million older adults living in the community require help with activities of daily living (ADLs). For a large number of these people, home care has the potential to improve their quality of life and avoid unnecessary institutionalization.

Under a cost-based reimbursement system, home care grew rapidly in the 1980s and 1990s. This growth coincided with the initiation of the prospective payment system (diagnostic related groups or DRGs) for hospitals that resulted in patients' being discharged sooner from hospitals, which increased the need for home services. New technologies created the possibility of providing therapies in the home that were previously available only in hospitals or nursing homes. Because of an explosive increase in costs, Congress placed limits on Medicare spending as mandated in the 1997 Balanced Budget Act, which led to the development of a prospective payment system (PPS) for home-care services. Since the PPS was enacted, the number of recipients of home-care services and the number of visits for patients receiving home care have declined by more than 20%. Many home-care agencies have adjusted to these changes and developed more efficient, targeted home care, but hundreds have closed because of the financial pressures. Rural agencies have closed at a higher rate than urban ones. The Outcome and Assessment Information Set (OASIS) is a tool meant to set fees for Home Health Related Groups (HHRGs). The OASIS instrument is completed by the home-health agency and tracks several domains of patients' functional status and medical needs. Like the DRGs, the HHRGs provide the basis for reimbursement to the agencies and are based on severity of the patient's illness, disabilities, and nursing needs; they include an adjustment for location in the United States. The instrument is also intended to provide a uniform means of measuring quality of care across all home-care agencies.

Like other sectors of our health care system, home-care agencies are charged with developing cost-effective high-quality care despite diminishing reimbursement. Another major challenge facing home-care agencies is recruiting and retaining qualified nurses and aides. Developing community-wide systems of care between hospitals, home care, nursing homes, and practitioners' offices may help meet these challenges and ensure that patients receive timely and appropriate care.

The Primary Care Provider's Role in Home Care

The primary care provider's role in home care is to serve as a member of an interdisciplinary team that is generally composed of nurses, therapists (speech, physical, occupational, and respiratory), social workers, personal care aides, home medical equipment suppliers, and, most importantly, informal caregivers. The physician is, by law, responsible for the patient's care plan. The primary care provider determines the patient's health care needs; develops, certifies, and recertifies the plan of care; and confers regularly with team members to address patient care issues and to handle documentation and other administrative matters. The change to a PPS makes it even more important for physicians to be attentive to the development, certification, and recertification of the plan of care. In particular, the PPS requires physicians to certify the level of need for individual therapy services; the amount of therapy services will partly determine the HHRG assignment. Patients requiring more than ten rehabilitation or therapy visits during a 60-day period will be assigned a higher HHRG level. Changes in patient condition within the 60-day episodic payment period will require recertification by the physician. The shift to prospective payment may encourage some home-health agencies to reduce services to lower costs. The advent of prospective payment makes it even more critical for the physician to certify that the patient requires services and to ensure that the appropriate quantity and quality of services are being provided.

Physicians are reimbursed for certification of the home-care plan and for oversight of complex cases in skilled home care and hospice. Table 17.1 lists the billing codes and requirements for these services. The documentation requirements for billing allow activities over multiple days in a month to be combined. Nurse practitioners and physician assistants may also bill for home-care services under Medicare regulations adopted in January 1998. Table 17.2 lists codes and reimbursement for home visits. When visits become prolonged, time codes can be used that justify an enhanced reimbursement. Reimbursement can vary in different localities, particularly where health maintenance organizations act as intermediaries for Medicare.

House calls can add an important dimension to the clinician's knowledge of the patient's circumstances and environment. Home evaluation can identify additional problems not readily apparent in office-based assessment. Barriers to maximal functioning can be identified and addressed. House calls have the additional benefit of reducing the burden of transportation for patients who have difficulty getting outside the home. Changes in Medicare have increased reimbursement for home visits, making home visits more financially feasible for clinicians.

Patient Assessment

Homebound patients have significant functional impairment. Comprehensive geriatric assessment is par-

Table 17.1—Codes, Reimbursement, and Requirements in Home-Care Certification

Codes	Reimbursement*	Requirements**
G0179	$ 51.39	Physician recertification for Medicare-covered home-health services. This includes reviewing and signing Home Health Care Plan of Care (form 485), contacts with agency personnel, review of reports per 60-day certification period. Documentation (copy of form 485) must be present in patient medical record.
G0180	$ 66.44	Physician certification for Medicare-covered services. As above, the physician affirms the implementation of the care plan and affirms that it meets the patient's needs as documented in form 485, and a copy exists in patient record.
G0181	$112.25	Physician supervision of a patient receiving Medicare-covered services requiring complex and multidisciplinary care involving regular physician involvement or revision of care plans, review of subsequent reports of patient status, review of diagnostic tests, and discussions with family. This must be 30 minutes or more within a calendar month. Documentation must be present in the patient medical record or log.
G0182	$118.46	Same as G0180 but with a patient in a Medicare-approved hospice program.

* Reimbursement may vary with different health maintenance organizations and will change with continued enactment of the Balanced Budget Act.

** The patient is not present for these activities.

Table 17.2—Billing Codes and Reimbursement for Home Visits

New Patients		Established Patients		
Codes	Reimbursement	Codes	Reimbursement	Requirements
99341	$ 54.00	99347	$ 41.00	Problem-focused history and examination, straightforward medical decision making
99342	$ 81.00	99348	$ 69.00	Expanded problem-focused history and physical examination with medical decision making of low complexity. Generally 30 minutes spent with patient or family.
99343	$121.00	99349	$107.00	Detailed history and examination; medical decision making of moderate complexity. Typically about 45 minutes.
99344	$158.00	99350	$156.00	Comprehensive history and examination with medical decision making of moderate complexity. Time about 60 minutes.
99345	$193.12			Above plus medical decision making of high complexity. Time about 75 minutes.

SOURCE: Data from the 2005 American Medical Association Current Procedures and Terminology (CPT) booklet.

ticularly valuable in this setting to establish a baseline, monitor the course of illness, and evaluate effects of intervention. However, assessment in the home has some important differences from assessment in the office.

During a home visit, the patient's actual environment can be assessed to determine whether the home is safe and supportive, given the particular patient's abilities and disabilities. Performance-based functional assessment can focus on the practical aspects of performing ADLs by direct observation of the environment for bathing, dressing, and transferring. Difficulties can be identified, and the assessor can evaluate the caregiver's abilities to address the patient's needs. The caregiver's needs for counseling, training, support, and education can also be identified and addressed.

Environmental modifications can be recommended to improve function. For example, modifications of the bathtub, a hand-held shower, a shower seat, grab-bars, and a bedside commode can improve the patient's quality of life and functioning. Barriers to wheelchairs and walkers such as door sills can be identified and removed. Chair lifts and outdoor ramps can help patients circumvent stairs. Occupational therapy consultation can be particularly useful in identifying other personal care and assistive devices for performing ADLs and housekeeping chores. A number of home safety checklists are available to help a reviewer assess the home. Additional technological additions to improve home safety, including necklace or wrist radio devices to call for help, can be considered. Some types of emergency response systems require that a person push a button by a specified time each day to avoid triggering an emergency response or telephone call to check on the owner of the device.

Health care providers are finding that home diagnostics, including radiology and electrocardiography, are available in most areas, and hand-held laboratory devices are becoming more common. These home diagnostics allow for a much more comprehensive medical evaluation to take place in the home.

Developing an Office-Based House-Call Program

Medical care in the home may be provided as part of an ongoing office-based program, as an extension of hospitalization through a postacute care program, or as a freestanding entity. Regardless of the method chosen, it is important that the organization of the home-care program be well conceived to maximize effectiveness and efficiency and to remain financially viable. Current regulations allow house calls to be provided by physicians, nurse practitioners, and physician assistants. Regardless of the primary care medical provider, appropriate links to other providers of home-based services are necessary to develop an interdisciplinary team. Consistency and familiarity among all members of the interdisciplinary team are essential to a smoothly functioning house-call program.

Home Care Patient Criteria

To qualify for Medicare home-care benefits, a patient must meet two criteria to establish homebound status. First, the patient must be absent from the home for reasons other than obtaining medical treatment infrequently (three times or fewer per month) or for short periods of time. Second, leaving home must require considerable and taxing effort on the part of the patient or the caregiver, or both—for example, if the patient is bedbound or has a severe mobility impairment.

Patients who are likely to be good candidates for house calls are those with mobility impairments that make transportation to the office difficult; those with disruptive behaviors; patients with terminal illnesses; and patients with multiple medical, psychiatric, and social problems. House calls are needed for some patients a limited amount of time, but others require house visits on an ongoing basis. Home visits may be particularly useful when adequate therapy is either not effective or inconsistently effective. A diagnostic home visit may reveal caregiver burnout, elder mistreatment, or the use of medications from other sources that may be interfering with the expected response. (See also "Pharmacotherapy," p 66; "Elder Mistreatment," p 80.)

Financial Considerations

House calls are now more financially feasible for clinicians; documentation remains the key to receiving requested remuneration. There are no specific restrictions on the number of visits as long as there is sufficient justification in the progress notes. As with most documentation, it is necessary that the primary care provider identify historical data, physical examination findings, diagnostic test results, and an assessment that reflects all the active diagnoses. Further, an evaluation of the patient's functioning, caregiver issues, and documentation of the medical plan of care are important elements to include in the house-call progress note.

Caregiver Support

Family caregivers provide most of the care received by patients in the community. In the United States, three out of four caregivers are women, either wives or daughters. Caregiving is often intense, time consuming, and stressful. The caregiver's physical and emotional health may be affected, resulting in depression and a worsening of his or her own health problems. Attention to caregiver support and issues are essential to help the patients continue to provide care. Caregiver support groups may be particularly helpful (see the resources listed in the Appendix, p 466).

For discussions of specific issues concerning caregiving, see "Psychosocial Issues" (p 16), "Dementia" (p 204), "Behavioral Problems in Dementia" (p 213), "Elder Mistreatment" (p 80), and "Depression and Other Mood Disorders" (p 247).

Limitations of Home Care

Most elderly adults would prefer to remain in their own home, but certain situations and conditions arise that make institutional care a more appropriate choice than in-home care. For example, caregivers may not be available to adequately address the needs of the patient. Relatively unstable medical situations requiring frequent laboratory testing, respiratory interventions, or intravenous medications may make institutional care a better choice than home care for some patients. Caregiver burnout and caregiver stress may prevent continued safe care for the patient in the home.

Further, the home environment itself may be a barrier to continuing in-home care. Unsafe neighborhoods, ongoing household social disruptions from alcohol or drug use, and inadequate room for equipment or environmental modifications may make in-home care a poor or risky option.

Finally, home care may be prohibitively expensive for the patient. It is not always the least expensive alternative, and out-of-pocket expenses may make on-going home care unaffordable. Insurance coverage is more likely to cover care that is rendered in a nursing facility or other institutional setting.

Ethics and Decisions About Institutionalization

Two ethical themes arise commonly in home care. The first is the balance between patient autonomy and patient safety. The second involves issues surrounding elder mistreatment and neglect.

Respect for patient autonomy often dictates that the patient remain in the home as a result of the patient's (or surrogate decision maker's) choice. Conflict arises when a patient's medical care or safety cannot be adequately maintained in the home, yet the patient insists on staying at home. It is difficult to balance respect for patient autonomy with the desire to prevent patient neglect. In some situations, the outcome is likely to be terminal, regardless of whether the patient is maintained at home or in an institution. In such situations, a hospice referral may help provide additional services in the home and support for both the patient and family. In situations in which there is a clearly neglectful or abusive situation, Adult Protective Services should be contacted (see "Elder Mistreatment," p 80, and "Legal and Ethical Issues," p 20).

COMMUNITY-BASED SERVICES NOT REQUIRING A CHANGE IN RESIDENCE

Adult Day Care

Adult day care is a community-based option that provides a wide range of social and support services in a congregate setting. Adult day care has become increasingly common. Providers of adult day care may offer a variety of services, ranging from simple nonskilled custodial care to more advanced skilled services. The availability of a registered nurse allows for on-site health services, clinical assessment and monitoring, and assistance with medication management. Adult day care is used commonly for patients with dementia who need supervision and assistance with their ADLs while primary caregivers work. Adult day care may also serve as a form of respite for caregivers. Most adult day care centers are community based, either in churches or community centers. In general, custodial adult day care is not covered by Medicare, though some costs may be covered by Medicaid or other insurers.

Day Hospitals

Day hospitals provide a broad range of skilled nursing care services, including parenteral antibiotics, chemotherapy, and intensive rehabilitation. The majority of programs are housed in chronic care hospitals or rehabilitation centers. This arrangement allows for the provider to take advantage of in-house professional expertise and resources, while allowing the patient to return to his or her own home or alternative living site after day treatment is complete. Services are covered under Medicare, with similar requirements to those surrounding home-health care.

Day hospitals are most often used for two groups of patients: those needing multidisciplinary rehabilitation and those with psychiatric illnesses. A systematic review of day hospital care found no significant differences between day hospitals and alternative sources of care with respect to death, disability, or use of health services, but that among patients receiving care in a day hospital, there is a trend toward less functional decline and less hospital and institutional care.

Program of All-Inclusive Care for the Elderly

The Program of All-Inclusive Care for the Elderly (PACE) is a capitated model of care that pools funds from Medicare and Medicaid to provide acute and long-term care to frail older people. (See also "Financing, Coverage, and Costs of Health Care," p 37.) Participants in the PACE program must meet state-defined requirements regarding their need for a nursing-home level of care. The goal of the program is to keep the participant in the community for as long as it is medically, socially, and financially feasible. The system, designed to be seamless, uses an interdisciplinary team of health care providers who know the patient and caregivers well and who provide care across the spectrum of hospital, home, alternative living situations, and institutional care. Integrated financing allows the program to provide traditional coverage of acute, rehabilitative, home, and institutional care. It also allows for adult day care, respite care, transportation, medication coverage, rehabilitation including maintenance physical and occupational therapy, hearing aids, eyeglasses, and a variety of other benefits. The program, at the discretion of the interdisciplinary team, has the flexibility to pay for nonmedical costs in unusual circumstances (eg, paying a person's electric or gas bill). Care by the interdisciplinary team provides for the complex social as well as for the medical needs of the participant. PACE has been described as one of the few truly integrated systems of care in the United States. Although the effectiveness of PACE has not been directly tested by a randomized controlled trial, research has shown that PACE provides high-quality care, albeit with significant site-to-site variation.

In 1997, legislation was passed that changed the status of PACE from a demonstration program to a permanent provider under Medicare. PACE is an optional program under state Medicaid. As of November 2003, 29 programs in 17 states were operational, and 50 more were in various stages of development. It is anticipated that the program will continue to expand.

Capitated financing for PACE is provided through Medicare and, in participating states, Medicaid. The Medicare rate-setting method for PACE has traditionally been based on the average cost of providing care to Medicare beneficiaries in a given geographic area, which is multiplied by a frailty adjuster. This method is likely to change in the near future. Each state determines the Medicaid rate of capitation.

Social Health Maintenance Organizations

The first generation Social Health Maintenance Organization (SHMO) project started in the middle 1980s with the intention of developing innovative, integrated, acute, and long-term care for Medicare beneficiaries. The four initial sites offered a variety of services and a system of care that focused on assessment and case management and that offered additional home and community-based services. Unlike the PACE program, the SHMOs serve not only low-income frail seniors but also healthier, more affluent, nondisabled Medicare recipients. The first round of the SHMO demonstration found that outcomes for participants were similar to those for control persons without any clear cost savings. One of the original four sites elected to drop out of the demonstration in 1994; an additional four sites for the second generation (SHMO II) were approved in 1996. It was hoped that SHMO II would provide a greater degree of effectiveness and integration through a variety of modifications to SHMO I, including more emphasis on personnel with geriatrics expertise, geriatric practice guidelines, and education of nongeriatrician practitioners on the essentials of geriatric care. Only one SHMO II, the Health Plan of Nevada, was actually implemented in the second phase of this program. A recent report from the Centers for Medicare and Medicaid Services concluded that there was no consistent evidence that SHMOs improved patient outcomes. There was evidence in a small subset of medically frail patients that hospital use was reduced. This begs the question of whether targeting a more frail population would result in the SHMOs' having a more positive impact on beneficiaries.

Telemedicine

The growth of telemedicine in home care has not paralleled its increasing availability and affordability. Although telemedicine has been used successfully in radiology, where it has been reimbursed, it has not been used to a great extent in other areas of medicine. Telemedicine has been used in some capitated health care programs in prisons and mental health centers. There are also a number of demonstration studies utilizing telemedicine in remote areas that include real-time clinician-patient encounters and that store and forward recordings of patients which are later reviewed by a physician or other provider. Some home-health agencies are beginning to use telemedicine to monitor patients, because the PPS has created financial incentives to limit the number of home visits. Telemedicine may have particular applicability in rural settings and other areas where access to health care providers is limited.

Telemedicine involves the transmission of data to the primary care provider, who can then evaluate and make decisions regarding the patient's health care. Systems vary considerably. For example, some systems are relatively disease specific. One example is an automated scale, blood-pressure cuff, and heart-rate monitor for patients with heart failure. More elaborate telemedicine systems allow for audio and video two-way communication, distance electrocardiography, distance auscultation through the use of an onsite stethoscope that can transmit breath, heart, and abdominal sounds, and camera lenses that allow for detailed examination of the skin and eyes. System costs vary considerably, ranging from approximately $1500 for simple audio and video systems to $20,000. In the future they are likely to become more affordable and useful, because broadband eliminates the need for expensive lines and allows for quicker transmission of data than do telephone connections. In certain situations telemedicine is Medicare reimbursable in rural areas. Some states are providing coverage through Medicaid.

Home Hospital

The home hospital focuses on providing more complex care at home to older people who would have been hospitalized for an acute-care need. Patients receiving home-hospital care have access to nurses and physicians on a regular basis and for episodic care through an on-call system that allows problems to be addressed promptly. The concept may be viewed as an evolution of home care, which it resembles, though it is more intense. Studies conducted outside of the United States suggest that care is comparable for selected patients and that patient satisfaction is high. (See also "Hospital Care," p 84.)

Community-Based Services Requiring a Change of Residence

Assisted Living

More than 800,000 people live in assisted-living facilities, and the number is expected to grow rapidly as our population ages. Even though these facilities are based on a social (not medical) model, they are caring for more frail people with significant medical needs. The transitional nature of assisted living is suggested by the average length of residency, about 2 years in 2002. The most common reason for discharge is need for nursing-home care.

Assisted-living residences are characterized by some level of coordination or provision of personal care services, social activities, health-related services, and supervision services that are provided in a home-like atmosphere that maximizes autonomy and privacy. The services provided under assisted living vary considerably, both within states and between states.

One national survey of assisted-living facilities found a range of privacy options, from private rooms to apartment units; about half would not admit residents with moderate to severe cognitive impairment; about two thirds did not have a registered nurse on staff but did provide 24-hour staff oversight, housekeeping, two meals, and personal assistance with ADLs. One example of the difference between state licensing requirements is in the area of medication administration. Depending on licensing requirements, medication administration and management may be directed by nonskilled, skilled, or fully licensed nursing staff.

In states where regulations do not require skilled care in assisted-living facilities, home-health skilled care is often provided as an external or independent service to the individual patient who happens to be living in an assisted-living facility. In this context, the boundary between assisted-living and skilled nursing facilities often becomes blurred. Because care in assisted living is generally less costly than in a nursing home, there has been a trend to use assisted living as a lower-cost alternative to nursing-home care. Part of the reason assisted-living care is usually less expensive is that there are fewer regulations governing assisted-living facilities. However, because these facilities are coming to care for more people with increasing disability and more medical needs, the pressure to regulate them has increased.

Costs for assisted-living residences vary greatly and depend on the size of units, services provided, and location. A survey in 2001 found that 48% of residences charge an average between $1,000 and $2,000 in monthly rent and fees. Another 23% charge between $2,000 and $3,000, and 9% charge more than $3,000 each month; 16% of assisted-living facilities charge less than $1,000.

Assisted living is covered in a growing number of long-term-care insurance policies. The Health Insurance Association of America reports that all 11 of the leading insurance companies that sell long-term-care insurance offer assisted-living coverage. However, the majority of people in assisted-living residences or their families pay for care themselves because most elderly Americans do not carry long-term-care insurance.

Assisted living is not covered by Medicare, but certain services are paid under Supplementary Security Income and Social Services Block Grant programs. Thirty-eight states reimburse or plan to reimburse for assisted-living services as a Medicaid service. In addition, states have the option to pay for assisted living under Medicaid by including services in the state's Medicaid plan or petitioning the U.S. Department of Health and Human Services for a waiver.

Group Homes

Group homes (including domiciliary care, single-room occupancy residences, board-and-care homes, and some congregate living situations) are houses or apartments in which two or more unrelated people live together. Group homes vary in types of residents and often serve patients with chronic mental illness or dementia. Residents share a living room, dining room, and kitchen but usually have their own bedrooms. Advantages of this arrangement include a lower cost of living and socialization with peers. Independence and functional status are supported through the interdependence and relationships of the residents. Resident-to-staff ratios may be higher than in other supported-living environments. Opportunities for socialization are increased, reducing social isolation. Most group homes are run as for-profit businesses, and some states require licensing.

Adult Foster Care

Foster care homes generally provide room, board, and some assistance with ADLs by the sponsoring family or by paid caregivers, who customarily live on the premises. Perhaps the longest experience with adult foster care is in the state of Oregon, where it is used as an alternative to long-term care and institutionalization. Adult foster care has the advantages of maintaining frail elderly people in a more home-like environment. Regulations for foster care vary by state, and some states require licensing. Some states provide coverage of adult foster care through their Medicaid programs.

Sheltered Housing

Sheltered housing is funded through the Older Americans Act and is offered as an option for housing subsidized through section 8, Housing and Urban Development programs for seniors and disabled residents. Often these arrangements are sheltered homes offering personal care assistance, housekeeping services, and meals. Programs may be supplemented by social work services and activities coordinators. Charges to clients are based on a sliding scale, which may cost up to 30% of income.

Continuing-Care Retirement Communities

More affluent seniors may choose a continuing-care retirement community (CCRC). CCRCs usually have a variety of living options, ranging from apartments or condominiums, to assisted living, and skilled nursing-home care. Often, residents enter the more independent living areas and progress through assisted living and into skilled care as they age.

Three financial models are common: the all-inclusive model, which provides total health care coverage, including long-term care; the fee-for-service model in which payments match the level of care; and the modified coverage model, which covers long-term care to a predetermined maximum. Most CCRCs require an entry fee, which may or may not be refundable, plus a variable monthly fee to pay for rent and supportive services. Monthly fees vary, depending upon the level of care being provided. Funding is largely private, though some facilities have Medicare- or Medicaid-funded beds for skilled care.

See also "Financing, Coverage, and Costs of Health Care" (p 29).

REFERENCES

- Bodenheimer T. Long-term care for frail elderly people—the On Lok model. *N Engl J Med.* 1999;341(17):1324–1328.

- Citro J, Hermanson S, Consumer Team, Public Policy Institute Research Group. *Assisted Living in the United States.* Washington, DC: American Association of Retired People (AARP); 1999.

- Dick K, Frazier SC. An exploration of nurse practitioner care to homebound frail elders. *J Am Acad Nurse Pract.* 2006;18(7):325–334.

- Field MJ, Grigsby J. Telemedicine and remote patient monitoring. *JAMA.* 2002;288(4):423–425.

- Levine SA, Boal J, Boling PA. Home care. *JAMA.* 2003;290(9):1203–1207.

- Quaglietti S. Anderson B. Developing the adult NP's role in home care. *Nurse Pract.* 2002;27(3):14, 81–82.

CHAPTER 18—PALLIATIVE CARE

KEY POINTS

- For many older persons, dying is characterized by inadequately treated physical distress, fragmented care systems, poor to absent communication among doctors, patients, and families, and enormous strains on family caregiver and support systems.

- Geographic variations in practice patterns and services available, religious beliefs, economic status, medical differences, gender, and cognitive status all affect the experiences of the dying person.

- Pain assessment is especially challenging in patients with poor communication skills, and the clinician must be sensitive to nonverbal clues.

- Loss of appetite is almost a universal symptom at the end of life; often it is more distressing to loved ones than to the patient.

- The patient's self-report is the only reliable measure of dyspnea, one of the most distressing symptoms experienced by many dying persons.

In the United States the overwhelming majority of deaths occur among the elderly population. Older persons typically die slowly of chronic diseases, with multiple coexisting problems, progressive dependency on others, and heavy care needs that are met mostly by family members. Many of these deaths become protracted processes that must be negotiated by clinicians, patients, and family members, who must make difficult decisions about the use or discontinuation of life-prolonging treatments. There is abundant evidence that the quality of life during the dying process is often poor. For many older persons, dying is characterized by inadequately treated physical distress, fragmented care systems, poor to absent communication among doctors, patients, and families, and enormous strains on family caregiver and support systems.

Although most Americans spend the majority of their final months at home, in most parts of the country their deaths actually occur in the hospital or nursing home. The experience of dying, however, varies greatly from one part of the nation to another. In Portland, Oregon, for example, only 35% of adult deaths occur in hospitals, but in New York City more than 80% occur in hospitals, a difference associated in part with differences in regional hospital bed supply and the availability of community supports for the dying. Social and medical differences also account for some patterns. The need for institutionalization or paid caregivers in the last months of life is much higher among poor people and women. Similarly, elderly persons suffering from cognitive impairment and dementia are much more likely than cognitively intact elderly persons to spend their last days in a nursing home.

OVERALL CARE NEAR DEATH

The Hospitalized Elderly Longitudinal Project (HELP) attempted to characterize the last 6 months of life and dying in very old persons. It used a prospective study design, providing a retrospective characterization of the last 6 months of the lives of 1266 patients aged 80 and older. Results showed that patients tended to overestimate their chances of survival near the end of life. Patients who died within 1 year of enrollment had significant functional impairment in activities of daily living and expressed strong preferences for not being resuscitated and for comfort care. The number of patients reporting severe pain increased toward the end of life, with one in three reporting severe pain within 3 months of death. These results highlight the need for physicians to talk with their patients early about their preferences, as well as to provide better symptom control and palliative measures at the end of life.

Part of the challenge in providing excellent end-of-life care stems from the inability to adequately predict end of life. Through active research, we hope to be better able to predict death and thus better target efforts at palliation and facilitate setting of goals and expectations of care with patients and their families.

PALLIATIVE CARE AND HOSPICE

Palliative care, as defined here, seeks to prevent, relieve, reduce, or soothe the symptoms of disease or disorder without effecting cure. It attends closely to the emotional, spiritual, and practical needs and goals of patients and of those close to them. Palliative care is generally restricted to those who are at imminent risk of dying, as best as can be estimated, but is also important to those who are extremely ill or who are living with serious complications at the end stages of chronic disease.

Hospice as a Medicare health care benefit was established in 1982 by the federal government. Initially, hospice coverage was made available through an expanded Medicare benefit; now it is supported through a Medicare or Medicaid benefit, and it is also a benefit of most commercial insurances. The benefit is a highly regulated, fully capitated health care system, which is now implemented through more than 3000 hospice services, most nonprofit, and is dedicated to providing comprehensive palliative care for patients with all types of terminal illnesses and their families. Hospice is primarily a home-care program, with access to inpatient beds for the management of acute problems. Hospice receives one of four daily rates for reimbursement that are based on four levels of care: home care, inpatient level of care, continuous care, and respite care. The services hospice provides are summarized in Table 18.1.

Access to hospice is based on two conditions:

- A licensed physician must certify that he or she believes that the patient has a life expectancy of 6 months or less if the disease runs its expected course.
- The patient or proxy must elect hospice and thereby agree that the care plan with respect to the terminal illness will be managed by the hospice program.

The patient must be recertified on a regular basis. If the physician cannot state that life expectancy is still anticipated to be 6 months or less, then the patient must be discharged from hospice. The patient may revoke the hospice benefit at any time.

The referring physician must certify that the prognosis is 6 months or less and decide whether to remain the physician of record or refer the patient to the hospice medical director. If the referring physician remains the physician of record, he or she continues to direct the care of the patient, becomes part of the hospice interdisciplinary team, must coordinate treatment decisions related to the terminal illness with the case manager (primary nurse), and may bill under Part B of Medicare or Medicaid.

See also "Financing, Coverage, and Costs of Health Care" (p 29).

COMMUNICATING BAD NEWS

The vast majority of Americans want to be told if they have a life-threatening illness. The ability to deliver bad

Table 18.1—Hospice Services

- Care provided by an interdisciplinary team: nurse, social worker, chaplain, aides, volunteers, physical therapist, music therapist
- Case management by a hospice nurse
- Access to a hospice physician
- Drugs at no cost, as long as they are related to the terminal diagnosis and are palliative, as determined by the hospice plan of care
- Tests and other treatments at no cost, as long as they are related to the terminal diagnosis and are palliative, as determined by the hospice plan of care
- Durable medical equipment
- Bereavement services for 13 months after a death

news in an effective manner is an essential skill for physicians. However, physicians receive little formal training in communication skills, and as a result they may feel unprepared to deliver bad news. Others may fear that the news will adversely affect the patient and the family or the physician-patient relationship. A systematic approach to delivering bad news can foster collaboration among the patient, the family, and clinicians. Effective discussions can improve the patient's and the family's ability to plan for the future, set realistic goals, and support one another emotionally.

A six-step framework for communicating bad news can be used as a guide for these difficult conversations.

Step 1: Preparation

Discussions of bad news require careful preparation. Before delivering bad news to a patient, plan what will be discussed, ensure the medical facts, and ensure that all needed confirmation is available. Establishing the proper physical context is also important. Ideally, bad news should be delivered in person in a private area in which there will be no interruptions. Allot adequate time for discussions, minimize interruptions, and determine whether any support staff, family, or friends that the patient may want on hand are available.

Step 2: Establishing the Patient's Understanding

Begin the discussion by exploring the patient's knowledge of the illness. Patients with a thorough understanding of their illness require a different approach than an uninformed or less sophisticated patient. Useful questions to elicit this information include the following: "What do you understand about your illness?" "When you first had symptom *x*, what did you think it might be?" "What have other doctors told you about your condition or procedures that you have had?"

Step 3: What the Patient Wants to Know

Although the majority of Americans say they want to be fully informed about their illnesses, a substantial minority may not want to know the full details or may prefer to have another family member informed. Data suggests that this may be particularly true for certain ethnic groups. (See also "Cultural Aspects of Care," p 46.) Just as patients have the right to be told the truth, they also have the right to decline to learn unwanted information. Thus, it is crucial to establish how much each patient wants to know. Helpful questions to ask include the following: "If this condition turns out to be something serious, do you want to know?" "Would you like me to tell you the full details of your condition? If not, is there somebody else you would like me to talk to?"

Step 4: Telling the Patient

Once the physician has established the patient's understanding of the illness and willingness to hear bad news, it is time to tell the patient. Deliver information in a sensitive, straightforward manner, avoiding technical language or euphemisms. Frequently check for understanding and clarify difficult concepts and terms. Phrasing that includes a "warning shot" helps brace and prepare patients for the bad news. For example: "Mr. X, I feel bad to have to tell you this, but the growth turned out to be cancer." "The report is back, and it's not as we had hoped. It showed that there is cancer in your colon."

Step 5: Responding to Feelings

The responses of patients and families are both unpredictable and diverse. Active listening, encouraging the expression of emotion, and acknowledging patient's emotions are all important and helpful. Useful probes to help elicit an understanding of the patient's emotions include the following: "What does this news mean to you?" "What worries you the most?" "You appear angry. Can you tell me what you are feeling?" "Tell me more about how you are feeling about what I just said."

Step 6: Planning and Follow-Up

Finally, the physician should organize an immediate therapeutic plan that includes specific references to the patient's concerns and incorporates the patient's agenda. The plan should include an appointment for a follow-up visit; a discussion of additional tests, referrals, and sources of support; and information as to how you can be reached if additional questions arise. The physician also needs to ensure that the patient will be safe when he or she leaves the office.

PAIN

For assessing and treating pain, see "Persistent Pain" (p 131), which also includes a section on pain in cognitively impaired patients, and the section on postoperative pain management in 'Perioperative Care" (p 99).

PALLIATION OF NONPAIN SYMPTOMS

Constipation

Constipation is one of the most common and distressing symptoms seen in terminally ill patients. Constipation is a universal adverse effect of opioids, and it is exacerbated by the immobility and poor fluid intake that accompanies most serious and life-threatening illnesses. Other unwanted side effects of opioids generally diminish over time, but constipation can be expected to persist, requiring ongoing bowel management as long as opioid therapy is used. Patients on opioids should receive prophylactic laxatives consisting of a stool softener (eg, docusate sodium) and a bowel stimulant (eg, senna, bisacodyl) unless diarrhea has already been a problem. If these measures fail, then an osmotic laxative (eg, sorbitol, lactulose) should be added. Any time there has been no bowel movement within 4 or more days, an enema should be considered. Patients presenting with constipation should be evaluated for bowel obstruction or fecal impaction. If impaction is present, the patient should be disimpacted

manually or with enemas before laxative therapy is initiated. See also the section on postoperative gastrointestinal problems in "Perioperative Care" (p 98), especially Table 14.2.

Nausea and Vomiting

The incidence of nausea and vomiting is estimated to be between 40% and 70% in patients with advanced cancer. Symptoms may be caused by disease or its treatment, so it is first important to clarify the cause of the nausea and vomiting. Emesis is mediated centrally by the chemoreceptor trigger zone in the area postrema, in the floor of the fourth ventricle. Peripherally, emesis is mediated in the gut and in the vestibular apparatus. Various receptors are involved in the mediation of emesis (eg, serotonin [5-hydroxytryptamine or 5-HT], dopamine, histamine, acetylcholine), and the selection of an appropriate antiemetic agent should therefore seek to identify the likely cause, the pathway that is mediating symptoms, and the neurotransmitters involved (see Table 18.2).

Dopamine antagonists like haloperidol[OL], metoclopramide, or droperidol act primarily on the chemoreceptor trigger zone. Serotonin antagonists such as ondansetron or granisetron act in synergy with dopaminergic antagonists in the chemoreceptor trigger zone and additionally act peripherally in the gut. Muscarinic blockers such as scopolamine or meclizine are useful for patients with disturbed vestibular function. Prokinetic agents like metoclopramide can potentiate cholinergic activity in the gastrointestinal tract and

Table 18.2—Treatment of Nausea and Vomiting

Site	Involved Receptors	Common Causes	Medications
Chemoreceptor trigger zone in the vomiting center	Dopamine Serotonin H_1	Drugs: opioids, digoxin, estrogen, cefotaxime Biochemical disorders: hypercalcemia, uremia Toxins: tumor-produced peptides, infection, radiotherapy, abnormal metabolites	Butyrophenones: eg, haloperidol[OL]; droperidol; phenothiazines: eg, prochlorperazine Prokinetic agents: eg, metoclopramide Serotonergic antagonists: eg, ondansetron, granisetron
Gut	Serotonin H_1	Gastric irritation (eg, drugs: alcohol, iron, mucolytics, expectorants; blood), tumors (external compression, intestinal obstruction), constipation, liver capsule stretch, peritoneal inflammation, gastric distension, stasis (eg, opioids), upper bowel, genitourinary, and biliary stasis	Serotonin antagonists, antihistamines, prokinetic agents
Vestibular apparatus	Muscarine Acetylcholine H_1	Toxic action of drugs: aspirin, opioids Motion sickness: Ménière's disease, labyrinthitis Local tumors: acoustic neuroma, brain tumors, bone metastases to base of skull	Antihistamines: eg, meclizine
Cerebral cortex		Raised intracranial pressure	Dexamethasone

[OL] Not approved by the U.S. Food and Drug Administration for this use.

are useful if the cause is gastroparesis. Antihistamines (eg, hydroxyzine[OL], dimenhydrinate) may be useful adjuvant agents when combined with either serotonergic or dopaminergic agents, although their side effects (eg, sedation, urinary retention, delirium) may limit their use in frail older adults. It is believed that these agents act on H_1 receptors in the vomiting center, vestibular afferents, and the gut. Serotonin-receptor blockers, including ondansetron, granisetron, and dolasetron, are very effective for radiotherapy- or chemotherapy-induced emesis. They do not reverse nausea mediated by dopamine pathways (eg, those that are opioid induced). Finally, corticosteroids possess intrinsic antiemetic properties and enhance the effect of other antiemetics. Corticosteroids are also useful for nausea and vomiting that is associated with increased intracranial pressure.

Diarrhea

Diarrhea, a relatively uncommon complaint of terminally ill patients, affects 7% to 10% of patients with cancer being admitted to hospice. Diarrhea is defined as the passage of more than three unformed stools within a 24-hour period. The clinician should be alert to the possibility of fecal impaction that presents as watery diarrhea, particularly in immobile older adults on opioids. Initiate the treatment of impaction with manual disimpaction and tapwater enemas, followed if unsuccessful by high colonic enemas. Laxatives should not be administered until the impaction is cleared because of the risk of bowel perforation. Untreated fecal impaction can be life threatening. Another common cause of diarrhea in palliative medicine is an excess of laxative therapy, especially after laxatives doses have been increased to clear an impaction. This will respond to temporary cessation of laxatives and reintroduction at a lower dosage. Radiotherapy involving the abdomen and pelvis causes diarrhea, peaking during the second or third week of therapy. This typically responds to cholestyramine 4 to 12 g three times a day. Diarrhea caused by fat malabsorption (eg, pancreatic insufficiency or small bowel disease) will respond to pancreatic enzymes such as pancreatin. Diarrhea following ileal resection also responds to cholestyramine.

Anorexia and Cachexia

Loss of appetite is almost a universal symptom of patients with serious and life-threatening illness. Anorexia in patients who are actively dying and who do not express a desire to eat should not be treated. Symptoms of dry mouth can be alleviated with ice chips, popsicles, moist compresses, or artificial saliva. Lemon glycerin swabs should not be used, because they irritate dry and cracked mucosa. Megestrol acetate and corticosteroids[OL] have been found to enhance appetite, cause weight gain (primarily fat), and improve quality of life in some patients with anorexia. These agents, however, have not been found to prolong survival, improve function, or improve treatment tolerance of cancer therapies and are associated with their own adverse effects. Dronabinol is used for nausea, vomiting, and anorexia. In general, patients should be encouraged to eat whatever is most appealing without regard to dietary restrictions.

Delirium

Delirium, agitation, and confusion are common in elderly terminally ill patients and are often distressing to both patients and family members. Initial efforts should be directed at identifying potentially reversible causes (eg, infection, impaction, uncontrolled pain, urinary retention, hypoxia). Antipsychotics like haloperidol[OL] or risperidone[OL] in low doses are effective treatments for both hypoactive and hyperactive delirium. Actively dying patients who are nonambulatory and who experience terminal delirium often appear less distressed with use of sedating antipsychotics, such as chlorpromazine. Because benzodiazepines are often associated with paradoxical agitation and a worsening of the delirium in older adults, their use should be carefully considered. (See also "Delirium," p 220.)

Depression

Depression is under-recognized and undertreated both in older adults and terminally ill patients. It may be underdiagnosed because of the clinician's mistaken belief that it is either a normal consequence of aging or appropriate in the context of a terminal illness. Because of the underlying illness, standard vegetative symptoms described in the fourth edition of the *Diagnostic and Statistical Manual of Mental Disorders* (insomnia, anorexia, weight change) are often not reliable indicators. Instead, the clinician should watch for change in mood, loss of interest, and suicidal ideation. Suicidal ideation should be openly discussed, including any symptoms that are contributing to the patient's suffering, which may be influencing his or her consideration of suicide. Aggressive treatment of symptoms, antidepressant therapy, and psychiatric consultation are all appropriate initial responses. Continued discussion with the patient about the wish to hasten death often reveals a change of mind as time passes.

Standard antidepressant therapy is effective, but most agents have a delayed onset of 2 to 6 weeks.

[OL] Not approved by the U.S. Food and Drug Administration for this use.

Psychostimulants (methylphenidate[OL], dextroamphetamine[OL]) are well tolerated, safe, and effective treatments for medically ill depressed persons. Additionally, they have a rapid onset and beneficial effect on energy, mood, appetite, and mental alertness. Methylphenidate can be started at 2.5 mg in the early morning hours, can be given concurrently with standard antidepressants, and should be avoided in the evening hours. Finally, electroconvulsive therapy is an effective, safe method of rapidly treating depression and should be used for those who are severely depressed. The American Psychiatric Task Force Report states that electroconvulsive therapy be considered a first-line therapy when rapid response is needed. The presence of space-occupying central nervous system lesions is an important contraindication. (See also "Depression and Other Mood Disorders," p 247.)

Dyspnea

Dyspnea, the subjective experience of breathlessness, is one of the most distressing symptoms experienced by dying patients. Patient self-report is the only reliable measure of dyspnea, as respiratory rates and laboratory tests often do not correlate with breathlessness. Physicians may mistakenly fear that treating dyspnea in patients close to the end of life is associated with unacceptably high risks, leading some to withhold treatment and others to dose medications inadequately, which will not alleviate the patient's suffering.

There can be many causes of breathlessness (eg, anxiety, airway obstruction, bronchospasm, hypoxemia, pneumonia), so symptomatic management should begin immediately, while the underlying cause is being sought. Treatment should not be delayed in the pursuit of disease-modifying interventions. Like pain, dyspnea is mediated through the interaction of complex pathophysiologic processes with poorly defined psychologic factors. At a physiologic level, dyspnea results from the interplay of chemoreceptors in the respiratory tract and central nervous system, upper airway receptors that sense the mechanical effect of airflow or the temperature changes that accompany it, stretch receptors in chest wall skeletal muscles, irritant receptors in the airway epithelium, and C fibers located in the alveolar wall and blood vessels. The experience of dyspnea, however, depends on the modulation of these physiologic events by psychologic factors, and as a consequence, the patient's perception of dyspnea may not correlate well with objective signs, such as respiratory rate, pulmonary congestion, hypoxia, or hypercarbia.

The optimal therapy for dyspnea is to treat its underlying cause. When this is not possible, one of a number of agents that have been evaluated for the treatment of intractable dyspnea might be used. Oxygen is considered by many to be an important component of any regimen, although caution must be used for patients retaining carbon dioxide. Although oxygen is usually considered beneficial only when oxygen saturation falls below 90%, there are some circumstances when oxygen may reduce dyspnea when this saturation value is exceeded. Cool air moving across the face (eg, from fans or an open window) may also treat dyspnea by stimulating the second branch of the fifth cranial nerve (V2), which has a central inhibitory effect on the sensation of breathlessness.

In addition to oxygen, several centrally acting agents have been evaluated for the treatment of intractable dyspnea. Benzodiazepines may be beneficial in controlling the anxiety associated with dyspnea, but these agents have not been found to improve breathlessness in randomized controlled trials involving nonanxious persons with chronic obstructive pulmonary disease. The fact that respiratory depression can occur following the administration of benzodiazepines in normal adults suggests that these medications should be used only in breathless patients with an accompanying component of anxiety. Studies with phenothiazines, and the phenothiazine antihistamine promethazine, have shown mild improvement in dyspnea with their use. However, anticholinergic and sedative adverse effects may limit the use of these agents in elderly patients.

The most widely used centrally active agents for the treatment of dyspnea are opioids. Opioids are believed to act via a number of different mechanisms, although their predominant effect appears to be a reduction in the central respiratory responsiveness to carbon dioxide, resulting in a decrease in respiratory drive. The increase in Pco_2 that often accompanies this respiratory suppression can occasionally limit this approach in dyspnea management because of somnolence induced by the hypercarbia and by a decreased respiratory response to hypoxia. Opioids also appear to act centrally by decreasing the perception of dyspnea and peripherally on opioid receptors in the lung, perhaps by decreasing ventilatory response to, and oxygen cost of, exercise without affecting respiratory drive. Randomized controlled trials have shown both oral and parenteral formulations to be effective. Anecdotal evidence supports the use of nebulized morphine for intractable dyspnea, but studies supporting this approach are lacking. The advantages of nebulized morphine include the avoidance of systemic absorption and the resulting constipation, hypotension, sedation, respiratory depression, and hypercapnia; rapid and efficient absorption because of the large surface area of the lung parenchyma; and the ease of administration. Randomized controlled trials employing nebulized morphine

---

[OL] Not approved by the U.S. Food and Drug Administration for this use.

have not demonstrated consistent benefit, and this route of administration should be reserved for patients who experience intolerable adverse effects from opioids administered by other routes.

Cough

Cough is a common symptom whose prevalence has been reported in the palliative care literature as ranging from 29% to 83%. Normal cough maintains the patency and cleanliness of the airways and thus should be treated only when distressing to the patient. Cough can be caused by the production of excessive amounts of fluids (eg, blood, mucus), inhalation of foreign material, or stimulation of irritant receptors in the airway. Additionally, patients with neuromuscular disorders may be unable to swallow saliva because of the involvement of bulbar cranial nerves, with the result that saliva causes coughing as it trickles into the larynx or trachea.

Underlying causes of cough should be sought and treated (eg, diuretics for heart failure, antibiotics for infection, anticholinergics for aspiration of saliva resulting from motor neuron disease); however, resolution of the underlying cause may be impossible. Opioids can be useful in these situations.

Dextromethorphan is structurally related to opioids and has central cough-suppressant action with few sedative effects. Codeine and dihydrocodeine, usually in the form of elixirs, are also good first-line choices. Methadone syrup may also be helpful when taken as a single dose because of its longer duration of action.

Cough due to an irritated pharynx because of local infection or malignancy may be helped by nebulized anesthetics. Nebulized lidocaine up to four times daily has been reported, anecdotally, to offer relief.

See also the section on intensive care for critically ill patients in "Respiratory Diseases and Disorders" (p 300).

REFERENCES

- Buckman R. *How to Break Bad News: A Guide for Health Care Professionals.* Baltimore, MD: The John Hopkins University Press; 1992.

- Doyle D, Hanks GWC, Macdonald N, eds. *Oxford Textbook of Palliative Medicine.* 2nd ed. Oxford, England: Oxford University Press; 1998.

- Jacox A, Carr DB, Payne R, et al. *Management of Cancer Pain. Clinical Practice Guideline No. 9.* Rockville, MD: US Department of Health and Human Services, Public Health Service, Agency for Health Care Policy and Research. March 1994. AHCPR Pub. No. 94-0592/3.

- Mitchell SL, Morris JN, Park PS, et al. Terminal care for persons with advanced dementia in the nursing home and home care settings. *J Palliat Med.* 2004;7(6):808–816.

- Morrison RS, Meier DE, eds. *Geriatric Palliative Care.* New York: Oxford University Press; 2003.

- Standards and Accreditation Committee, Medical Guidelines Task Force. *Medical Guidelines for Determining Prognosis in Selected Non-Cancer Diseases.* 2nd ed. Arlington, VA: National Hospice Organization; 1996.

- SUPPORT Principal Investigators. A controlled trial to improve care for seriously ill hospitalized patients: The Study to Understand Prognoses and Preferences for Outcomes and Risks of Treatment (SUPPORT). *JAMA.* 1995;274(20):1591–1598.

CHAPTER 19—PERSISTENT PAIN

KEY POINTS

- Pain requires a thorough assessment to determine its source, severity, and impact on the functioning and well-being of the patient.

- Multiple pain scales are available to help quantify the severity of pain. The selection of a pain scale is based on the cognitive and communication abilities of the patient.

- A stepped approach to the treatment of pain is advised; local therapies, such as heat, cold, or massage, should be considered to alleviate the

need for or reduce the amount of systemic therapies that have greater risk of toxicity.

- Tolerance generally develops to the respiratory depression, fatigue, and sedation effects of opioid analgesics but not to the constipating effect.

Pain, defined as an unpleasant sensory and emotional experience, is common in older persons aged 65 and older. Studies have revealed that 25% to 50% of community-dwelling older adults and 45% to 80% of nursing-home residents have substantial pain. It is also believed to be commonly undertreated. This is due to several factors: some older adults tend to minimize or not report their symptoms, and others are unable to report their pain because of language or cognitive impairments. Also, clinicians may inadequately assess pain or undertreat it with ineffective therapies or encounter intolerable adverse effects with more effective therapies. This chapter describes the evaluation and treatment of persistent pain. Chronic or persistent pain, in contrast to acute pain, is pain lasting 3 to 6 months or more after the original injury has healed, pain that is associated with a chronic medical condition, or pain that recurs at intervals of a month to years.

Persistent pain is complex, involving an amalgamation of physical, social, and psychologic factors. Untreated, it can result in difficulty performing activities of daily living, cognitive dysfunction, depression, anxiety, social isolation, appetite impairment, and sleep disorders. Lastly, patients with chronic pain accrue greater health care costs than do patients who are pain-free.

ASSESSMENT

A major barrier to effective pain treatment is inadequate assessment. A thorough assessment is necessary to formulate a plan to successfully treat persistent pain. This assessment should include an examination of physical, emotional, and social function, recognizing the considerable impact that each of these domains has on the experience of pain and suffering. Since there are no blood tests or imaging modalities to measure pain objectively, clinicians must rely on the patient's or caregiver's description of the pain and on the findings of a thorough physical examination. The goal of the assessment is to identify the source of the pain so that it can be treated with the most effective, targeted, and specific treatment known. The evaluation of older persons is complicated by several challenges, including under-reporting of symptoms by many older persons, the existence of multiple medical comorbidities exacerbating the pain and impairing the function of the patient, and the increased prevalence of cognitive impairment as people age.

Initial evaluation begins with a complete history of the pain, including inquiry about the character of the pain, the course of its onset, its duration, and its location. Patients should be asked what relieves and exacerbates their pain. The patient's functional status needs to be carefully evaluated to determine his or her ability to perform activities of daily living and instrumental activities of daily living. The patient's cognitive state, participation in social activities, mood, and quality of life are all components of a complete evaluation.

Pain intensity can be quantified using pain intensity scales. Three commonly used validated scales are the Numeric Rating Scale, the Faces Pain Scale, and the Verbal Descriptor Scale. These scales are referred to as unidimensional because they ask the patient to rate the intensity of a single characteristic of the symptom, in this case the intensity of the pain. The patient is asked to rate his or her pain by assigning a numerical value (with zero indicating no pain and 10 representing the worst pain imaginable), a verbal description ("no pain" to "pain as bad as it could be"), or a facial expression corresponding to the pain. The choice of scale depends on the presence of a particular language or sensory impairment. For example, if the patient does not speak English well, the faces scale may be the best choice because it relies on pictures rather than words or numbers. The same scale should be used at follow-up examinations to evaluate how the pain has changed since the initial assessment. Scales such as the McGill Pain Questionnaire and the Pain Disability Scale measure pain in a variety of domains, including the intensity, location, and affect. Although long, scales measuring multiple domains can provide a wealth of information about the patient's unique experience of pain.

Before the physical examination, the patient can describe the location of the pain using a drawing of a human figure, called a pain map. The patient is asked to indicate the locations on the figure that corresponds to their own pain. Pain maps can enhance patient-clinician communication. If the patient's pain pattern is erratic and diffuse and therefore nonsensical anatomically, referral to a mental health specialist may be appropriate.

The physical examination should include a careful examination of the reported site of the pain and any part of the body that may be a source of referred pain. Experts suggest that the initial evaluation should include a complete musculoskeletal examination, recognizing the common finding of a musculoskeletal disorder such as fibromyalgia, osteoarthritis, and myofascial pain as either the primary source of pain or an exacerbating process. Accurate diagnosis of these disorders is a critical part of formulating the correct therapeutic plan (see the section, below, on treatment). Fibromyalgia is an under-recognized but not uncommon disorder in older adults. It is typically characterized by multiple tender points, sleep disturbance, fatigue, generalized pain (often with a strong axial component), and morning stiffness. (See also the section on fibromyalgia in "Musculoskeletal Diseases and Disorders," p 400.) Myofascial pain is present in the vast majority of patients with persistent pain and is diagnosed by the presence of taut bands of muscles and trigger points (ie, pain that may radiate distally upon application of firm pressure to a muscle, as opposed to tender points, in which radiation of pain is absent).

Pain syndromes can be divided into at least three types: nociceptive, neuropathic, and mixed or unspecified. Nociceptive pain describes pain due to the activation of nociceptive sensory receptors by noxious stimuli resulting from inflammation, swelling, and injury to tissues. It can be defined further as either somatic or visceral pain. Somatic pain is well localized in skin, soft tissue, and bone. It is commonly described as throbbing, aching, and stabbing. Visceral pain, due to cardiac, gastrointestinal, and lung injury, is not well localized and difficult to describe. Patients describe visceral pain as crampy, tearing, dull, and aching. Neuropathic pain derives from the irritation of components of the central or peripheral nervous system. Patients typically report burning, numbness with "pins and needles" sensations, and shooting pains. Common causes of neuropathic pain include post-herpetic neuralgia, post-stroke central pain, and phantom limb pain experienced following amputation. Nociceptive pain is often adequately treated with common analgesics. Neuropathic pain responds unpredictably to opioid analgesia; it may respond well to nonopioid therapies such as anticonvulsants, tricyclic antidepressants (TCAs), and antiarrhythmic medications. Confusion between neuropathic pain and myofascial pain is possible, as patients may describe both as "burning." Careful physical examination will help to differentiate these disorders (ie, taut bands and trigger points with myofascial pain and allodynia or hyperalgesia with either disorder), although both may exist in the same patient. Mixed or unspecified pain is described as having characteristics of both nociceptive pain and neuropathic pain. An example of a mixed pain syndrome is chronic headaches of unknown causes. It may be necessary to treat these patients with trials of different medications or with combinations of medicines. Older adults often have mixed pain syndromes. Lower back pain, for example, is often a combination of spinal malalignment, myofascial pathology, and neurologic impingement.

ASSESSING AND TREATING PAIN IN COGNITIVELY IMPAIRED PERSONS

While they are able to speak, patients with mild to moderate dementia are often able to self-report pain and localize it. Patients with severe cognitive impairment who are unable to verbally express pain pose a challenge to the clinicians who care for them. Not only are they unable to describe the pain and request analgesia, but clinicians are hesitant to administer pain medications, fearing that drugs will worsen the patients' mental status. Clinicians must rely on observing the patient for possible pain-related behaviors as well as observations noted by the patient's caregivers. Table 19.1 lists common pain behaviors in cognitively im-

paired older adults. Validated scales such as the Hurley Discomfort Scale and the Checklist of Nonverbal Pain Indicators have been developed; however, these require trained evaluators to complete properly. Experts suggest providing empiric analgesic therapy during procedures and conditions known to be painful. Trials of analgesia should also be considered for patients exhibiting pain-related behaviors.

TREATMENT

Fundamental Approaches to Pain Treatment

A comprehensive review of nonpharmacologic therapies for persistent pain is beyond the scope of this chapter; however, specific therapies are worth mentioning. Many of the strategies mentioned below are appropriate suggestions for all patients' treatment plans.

Patient education and involvement in treatment decisions are an important part of all treatment plans for persistent pain. Patients should be taught how to take medications properly and how to use assessment instruments. They can be given information on the use of nonpharmacologic treatments such as heat and cold application, massage therapy, and transcutaneous electrical nerve stimulation. Cognitive behavioral therapy may be particularly useful in helping patients learn to cope with the stresses of persistent pain. When possible, family members and caregivers should be included in the therapy.

Regular physical activity has been shown to improve mood, boost functional status, and stabilize gait. Referral to the Arthritis Foundation or community resources such as the YMCA for exercise classes can be considered for many patients. Others who are frail may require closely monitored rehabilitation services. The goals should include improvements in flexibility, strength, endurance, and function, with reduction in pain and improved quality of life.

Patients with persistent pain that do not respond to first-line treatment efforts should, if possible, be referred to a pain clinic that is geared toward interdisciplinary team treatment. Suboptimal treatment response should not be viewed as a permanent state, but as an opportunity for input from specialists who have additional expertise in treating these difficult problems.

See also "Complementary and Alternative Medicine" (p 74).

Pharmacologic Therapy

Individual analgesics, with their starting doses and common adverse effects, are listed in Table 19.2.

Table 19.1—Common Pain Behaviors in Cognitively Impaired Elderly Persons

Behavior	Examples
Facial expressions	Slight frown; sad, frightened face Grimacing, wrinkled forehead, closed or tightened eyes Any distorted expression Rapid blinking
Verbalizations, vocalizations	Sighing, moaning, groaning Grunting, chanting, calling out Noisy breathing Asking for help Verbal abusiveness
Body movements	Rigid, tense body posture, guarding Fidgeting Increased pacing, rocking Restricted movement Gait or mobility changes
Changes in interpersonal interactions	Aggressive, combative, resists care Decreased social interactions Socially inappropriate, disruptive Withdrawn
Changes in activity patterns or routines	Refusing food, appetite change Increase in rest periods Sleep, rest pattern changes Sudden cessation of common routines Increased wandering
Mental status changes	Crying or tears Increased confusion Irritability or distress

NOTE: Some patients demonstrate little or no specific behavior associated with severe pain.

SOURCE: AGS Panel on Persistent Pain in Older Persons. The management of persistent pain in older persons. *J Am Geriatr Soc.* 2002; 50(6 Suppl): S211. Reprinted with permission

Pharmacologic therapy for patients with persistent pain should be viewed not as an end, but as a means to promote improved function and enhance adherence with rehabilitation efforts. When initiating pharmacologic therapy in older adults, it is important to consider the balance of risks and benefits of the treatment. If appropriate, nonsystemic therapies should be tried first. For example, patients that primarily have knee pain might respond to intra-articular corticosteroid injections, avoiding the need for systemic analgesics. Patients with myofascial pain often respond to local modalities such as massage, gentle stretching exercises, ultrasound, and trigger-point injections. Topical preparations such as capsaicin or ketamine gel [OL] or lidocaine patches might be effective as primary or adjunctive therapy in the treatment of patients with neuropathic or myofascial pain syndromes. If these modalities are ineffective and a decision is made to begin systemic therapy, patients will need to be monitored closely to ensure that the treatment is effective and adverse effects are mini-

[OL] Not approved by the U.S. Food and Drug Administration for this use.

mized. Choice of initial dose and rate of titration depends on the individual patient's physiology, which varies considerably in older persons. As a general rule, when starting opioid therapy it is prudent to start with the lowest dose possible and to titrate slowly. That said, patients who are in a pain crisis should not have medications withheld. Rather, they need to be monitored closely to ensure that the dose can be safely and adequately escalated.

Mild to moderate pain can commonly be treated with acetaminophen or cautious use of nonsteroidal anti-inflammatory drugs (NSAIDs). Acetaminophen has been shown to provide adequate analgesia for many mild to moderate pain syndromes, particularly musculoskeletal pain. No more than 4 g of acetaminophen every 24 hours should be administered to patients with normal hepatic and renal function, given the risk of hepatotoxicity. Caution should be taken with treating patients at risk for liver dysfunction, particularly those who have a history of heavy alcohol intake. In these patients, the dose should be lowered by 50%, or acetaminophen should be avoided. Because acetaminophen is commonly contained in many over-the-counter and prescription products, knowledge of all medications that a patient is taking is critical to avoiding acetaminophen toxicity. NSAIDs are effective drugs for the treatment of mild to moderate pain and may be useful when acute exacerbations of pain are not controlled with acetaminophen. However, significant adverse effects, including renal dysfunction, gastrointestinal (GI) bleeding, platelet dysfunction, fluid retention, and precipitation of delirium limit their use in the treatment of older persons' chronic pain. COX-2 inhibitors were developed to decrease the risk of GI bleeding by acting on a more selective receptor, but the risk for renal complications, including hypertension, remains the same as with other NSAIDs, and the degree to which longer term GI toxicity is reduced is not clear. Several studies have confirmed high cardiovascular risks associated with COX-2 inhibitors, which is now believed to be a class effect. Though one is currently still on the market, the COX-2s certainly should be considered with caution if at all in older individuals. Misoprostol, a prostaglandin analog, or a proton-pump inhibitor may be used to reduce the risk of NSAID-induced GI bleeding, but this does not reduce the risks of renal disease, hypertension, fluid retention, or delirium. Alternatively, nonacetylated salicylates such as salsalate and trisalicylate may have less renal toxicity and antiplatelet activity than other NSAIDs and therefore may be preferable in older persons, though evidence supporting this theory is sparse.

Moderate to severe pain or pain that requires chronic treatment often requires opioid medications to

Table 19.2—Systemic Pharmacotherapy for Persistent Pain Management

Drug	Starting Dose*	Usual Effective Dose (Maximum Dose)	Titration	Comments
		NONOPIOIDS		
Acetaminophen (Tylenol)	325 mg q 4 h– 500 mg q 6 h	2–4 g/24 h (4 g/24 h)	after 4–6 doses	Reduce maximum dose 50%–75% in patients with hepatic insufficiency, history of alcohol abuse
Anticonvulsants				
Carbamazepine[OL] (Tegretol)	100 mg qd	800–1200 mg/24 h (2400 mg/day) in divided doses	after 3–5 days	Monitor liver enzymes, CBC, BUN/Creat., electrolytes. Approved only for trigeminal neuralgia and glossopharyngeal neuralgia; not approved for any other types of pain
Clonazepam[OL] (Klonopin)	0.25–0.5 mg hs	0.05–0.2 mg/kg/day (20 mg)	after 3–5 days	Monitor sedation, memory, CBC
Gabapentin[OL] (Neurontin)	100 mg hs	300–900 mg tid (3600 mg)	after 1–2 days	Monitor sedation, ataxia, edema. Approved for post-herpetic neuralgia; not approved for any other types of pain
Pregabalin (Lyrica)	25 mg tid	100 mg tid (200 mg tid)	may not be necessary; precise recommendations pending	Schedule C-V. Dizziness and somnolence are the most troubling adverse effects. Adjust dosage when CrCl < 60 mL/min
Baclofen[OL] (Lioresal)	5 mg	5–20 mg bid–tid (200 mg)	after 3–5 days	Monitor muscle weakness, urinary function; avoid abrupt discontinuation because of CNS irritability
Choline magnesium trisalicylate (Tricosal, Trilisate)	500–750 mg q 8 h	2000–3000 mg/24 h (same)	after 4–6 doses	Long half-life may allow qd or bid dosing after steady state is reached. In frail patients or those with diminished hepatic or renal function, it may be important to check salicylate levels during dose titration and after steady state is reached
Corticosteroids (prednisone) (eg, Deltasone, Liquid Pred, Orasone)	5 mg qd	variable (NA)	after 2–3 doses	Use lowest possible dose to prevent chronic steroid effects; anticipate fluid retention and glycemic effects
Mexiletine[OL] (Mexitil)	150 mg	150 mg tid–qid (variable)	after 3–5 days	Avoid use in patients with conduction block, bradyarrhythmia; monitor ECG
Salsalate (eg, Disalcid, Mono-Gesic, Salflex)	500–750 mg q 12 h	1500–3000 mg/24 h (3000 mg/24h)	after 4–6 doses	In frail patients or those with diminished hepatic or renal function, it may be important to check salicylate levels during dose titration and after steady state is reached
Tricyclic antidepressants:** desipramine[OL] (Norpramin), nortriptyline[OL] (Aventyl, Pamelor)	10 mg hs	25–100 mg hs (variable)	after 3–5 days	Significant risk of adverse effects in older patients; anticholinergic effects

(table continued on next page)

[OL] Not approved by the U.S. Food and Drug Administration for this use.

Drug	Starting Dose*	Usual Effective Dose (Maximum Dose)	Titration	Comments
OPIOIDS				
Hydrocodone (eg, Lorcet, Lortab, Vicodin, Vicoprofen)	5 mg q 4–6 h	5–10 mg (see comments)	after 3–4 doses	Useful for acute recurrent, episodic, or breakthrough pain; daily dose limited by fixed-dose combinations with acetaminophen or NSAIDs
Hydromorphone (Dilaudid, Hydrostat)	2 mg q 3–4 h	variable (variable)	after 3–4 doses	For breakthrough pain or for around-the-clock dosing
Morphine, immediate release (eg, MSIR, Roxanol)	2.5–10 mg q 4 h	variable (variable)	after 1–2 doses	Oral liquid concentrate recommended for breakthrough pain
Morphine, sustained release (eg, MSContin, Kadian)	15 mg q 12 h	variable (variable)	after 3–5 days	Usually started after initial dose determined by effects of immediate-release opioid; toxic metabolites of morphine may limit usefulness in patients with renal insufficiency or when high-dose therapy is required; continuous-release formulations may require more frequent dosing if end-of-dose failure occurs regularly
Oxycodone, immediate release (OxyIR)	5 mg q 4–6 h	5–10 mg (see comments)	after 3–4 doses	Useful for acute recurrent, episodic, or breakthrough pain; daily dose limited by fixed-dose combinations with acetaminophen or NSAIDs
Oxycodone, sustained release (OxyContin)	10 mg q 12 h	variable (variable)	after 3–5 days	Usually started after initial dose determined by effects of immediate-release opioid
Tramadol (Ultram)	25 mg q 4–6 h	50–100 mg (300 mg/24 h)	after 4–6 doses	Mixed opioid and central neurotransmitter mechanism of action; monitor for opioid side effects, including drowsiness and nausea. Exert caution when used with another serotonergic drug, and observe for symptoms of serotonergic syndrome. Lowers seizure threshold.
Transdermal fentanyl (Duragesic, Duragesic 12)	25 μg/h patch q 72 h	variable (variable)	after 2–3 patch changes	Usually started after initial dose determined by effects of immediate-release opioid; currently available lowest dose patch (12.5 μg/h) recommended for older patients or for patients who require 60 mg per 24-h oral morphine equivalents; peak effect of first dose takes 18–24 h. Duration of effect is usually 3 days, but may range from 48 h to 96 h

NOTE: ASA = acetylsalicylic acid; bid = twice daily; BUN = blood urea nitrogen; CBC = complete blood cell count; CNS = central nervous system; CrCl = creatinine clearance; Creat. = serum creatinine; CV = cardiovascular; DEA = U.S. Drug Enforcement Agency; ECG = electrocardiogram; FDA = U.S. Food and Drug Administration; GI = gastrointestinal; h = hour; hs = at bedtime; NA = not applicable; NSAIDs = nonsteroidal anti-inflammatory drugs; q = each, every; qd = daily; qid = four times daily; tid = three times daily.

* Oral dosing unless otherwise specified.

** Amitriptyline is not recommended.

SOURCE: Adapted from AGS Panel on Persistent Pain in Older Persons. The management of persistent pain in older persons. *J Am Geriatr Soc.* 2002; 50(6 Suppl): S214–S215. Reprinted with permission. For comprehensive, regularly updated information on drugs for pain, see the online version of *Geriatrics At Your Fingertips* at http://www.geriatricsatyourfingertips.org (accessed October 2005).

provide sufficient relief. In general, continuous pain should be treated with 24-hour pain medications in long-acting or sustained-release formulations after opioid requirements are estimated on the basis of an initial trial of a short-acting agent. These may be combined with fast-onset medications with short half-lives to cover breakthrough pain. A typical patient requires approximately 5% to 15% the daily dose offered every 2 hours orally for breakthrough pain. In general, different opioids provide similar analgesic efficacy. Cost and route of delivery can help guide the choice of medication.

Opioids are metabolized by the liver and excreted by the kidney. In kidney failure, the active metabolites of morphine, including morphine-6-glucuronide and morphine-3-glucuronide, can accumulate, which places the patient at increased risk for prolonged sedation. The dosing intervals should be increased or the dose lowered to reduce this risk. Some experts and limited data suggest that oxycodone is safer in kidney failure because its metabolism results in fewer active metabolites, but this remains controversial.

Barriers to Using Opioids in Older Persons

Older persons may have concerns about addiction and tolerance that keep them from accepting adequate treatment for their pain. Patients may fear that taking opioid therapy for their current level of pain will result in the pain medicines' losing their effectiveness in the future when pain becomes more severe. They may fear addiction to the medicines. In fact, fear of addiction is a major obstacle to prescribing medications to older adults. A frank discussion of these concerns may help to alleviate these fears.

Physical dependence is an expected change in a patient's physiology that occurs while a patient is receiving chronic, continuous opioid medications. If opioids are discontinued suddenly, a patient who is physically dependent will experience a withdrawal syndrome that may include restlessness, tachycardia, hypertension, fever, tremors, and lacrimation. Symptoms of withdrawal can be avoided by tapering opioids carefully over days to weeks. *Tolerance* refers to a change in physiology resulting in the need to increase opioid medicines over time to achieve adequate analgesic effect. Experts note that tolerance to analgesia, as opposed to tolerance to sedation and respiratory depression, develops slowly in stable disease. If a rapid titration of medicines is required to reduce pain, the cause of the pain should be evaluated, including searching for new pathologies and exacerbation of known sources of pain, as well as consideration of nonphysical factors. Of note, there is limited cross-tolerance between different opioids. Therefore,

when switching a patient from one opioid to another (eg, morphine to oxycodone), the clinician should reduce the dose to 50% to 65% of the equivalent dose.

Psychological *dependence*, or true *addiction*, refers to a psychiatric state defined by compulsive drug seeking and drug using with disregard for adverse social, physical, and economic consequences. It is very rare for patients who have chronic pain to become addicted to opioids. Addiction must be distinguished from *pseudo-addiction*, which refers to a patient with significant unrelieved pain who adopts behaviors similar to those of truly addicted patients while seeking relief from suffering, but generally with less prominent disregard for adverse social, physical, and economic consequences.

Adverse Effects of Opioids

The most common adverse effect of opioid treatment is constipation. Opioid-induced constipation is due to multiple mechanisms, including dehydration, decreased GI tract secretions, and decreased motility of the GI tract. Although tolerance develops fairly rapidly to other adverse effects of opioids, such as respiratory depression and sedation, constipation usually complicates opioid use for the duration of treatment. Therefore, education regarding the probable need for a laxative is recommended for all patients at the time opioid therapy is initiated. Many experts recommend starting therapy with a stimulant laxative (such as bisacodyl or senna); however, these should be avoided in any patient with signs or symptoms of bowel obstruction. Bulking agents such as fiber and psyllium should be avoided in patients who are inactive and who have poor oral intake, given the risk of causing stool impaction and obstruction. All patients should be encouraged to exercise, as they are able, and to stay well hydrated.

Nausea and vomiting are common side effects of opioids. They have a direct effect on the part of the brain associated with the sensation of vomiting called the *chemoreceptor trigger zone*. Other common causes of nausea and vomiting in patients taking opioids include gastroparesis, constipation, and metabolic disorders such as renal and hepatic failure. Although the nausea and vomiting is usually self-limited to the first few doses, some patients experience chronic nausea. After evaluation for reversible causes of nausea such as constipation, some patients benefit from changing to an alternative opioid. Others may need to be treated with chronic antiemetics, accepting the high prevalence of adverse effects in older adults treated with these medications, including drowsiness, delirium, and anticholinergic effects.

Older persons may experience sedation, fatigue, and mild cognitive impairment with opioid treatment.

These changes commonly occur during dose adjustment. Patients commonly overcome the fatigue and sedation over days to weeks as they become tolerant to the medication. They need to be warned of the risks of increased falls and asked not to drive or operate heavy equipment when the medication is initiated. A small subset of patients treated with opioids experience incessant fatigue that limits their function significantly. A limited course of a stimulant such as low-dose methylphenidate could reasonably be tried in this situation. Rotation to a different opioid is an alternative strategy used to alleviate opioid-induced fatigue.

Respiratory depression is a feared complication of opioid therapy. Older persons and persons with a history of lung dysfunction are at particular risk when opioid doses are increased too rapidly. Naloxone, an opioid receptor antagonist, can reverse opioid-induced respiratory depression; however, when it is given to a patient who has been treated chronically with opioids, it can precipitate a pain crisis and acute withdrawal symptoms. Experts suggest withholding naloxone unless the patient's respiratory rate decreases to less than 8 breaths per minute or the oxygen saturation drops to below 90%. When it is needed, naloxone should be titrated carefully, using the lowest dose possible.

Nonopioid Medication to Treat Persistent Pain

Nonopioid or adjuvant medications can be used as the sole agent or in combination with opioids. These medications may be particularly useful in treating patients with neuropathic pain or mixed pain syndromes.

Tricyclic antidepressants (TCAs) are the most extensively studied medications for neuropathic pain, though none of the TCAs has been approved for the treatment of pain. Their efficacy in the treatment of post-herpetic neuralgia and diabetic neuropathy has been exhibited in numerous placebo-controlled studies. However, they are associated with significant anticholinergic adverse effects in older persons, including constipation, urinary retention, dry mouth, cognitive impairment, tachycardia, and blurred vision. Of note, desipramine[OL] and nortriptyline[OL] may have fewer adverse effects than amitriptyline[OL].

Clinical depression in patients with persistent pain requires treatment to effect optimal analgesia and quality of life. Other classes of antidepressants (eg, selective serotonin-reupake inhibitors) have generally been less studied than TCAs as analgesics, but older adults typically tolerate these agents better than TCAs when they are used in antidepressant doses. Duloxetine, an inhibitor of norepinephrine and

serotonin uptake, is approved as both an antidepressant and for the treatment of pain from diabetic neuropathy.

Antiepileptic drugs such as carbamazepine (approved for some types of neuropathic pain), gabapentin, and clonazepam[OL] are commonly used as treatments for neuropathic pain. Gabapentin has demonstrated clinical efficacy in the treatment of post-herpetic neuralgia, and it has considerably fewer adverse effects than TCAs, though its cost is substantially more. The main side effects of gabapentin are sedation and dizziness, which frequently limit dose escalation.

Corticosteroids are useful adjuvants to treat pain associated with swelling, inflammation, and tissue infiltration, as well as neuropathic pain. In addition to their analgesic properties, they also may increase appetite and improve energy. Adverse effects occurring with short-term use of steroids include psychosis, fluid retention, hair loss, loss of skin integrity, hyperglycemia, and immunosuppression. Intravenous bisphosphonates may substantially reduce pain from malignant bone metastases.

Medications to Avoid in Older Persons

Several medications should not be administered to older persons. Propoxyphene (Darvon) is an older opioid medication used to treat mild to moderate pain. However, research and clinical experience has shown that the drug may accumulate in older persons and cause ataxia and dizziness as well as tremulousness and seizures. It has also never been shown to be a more effective analgesic than placebo. Meperidine (Demerol) is metabolized to normeperidine, a substance that has no analgesic properties but that can accumulate in patients with decreased kidney function and cause tremulousness, myoclonus, and seizures. Neither of these medications is recommended for use in older persons.

Tramadol (Ultram) has combined mechanisms of opioid-receptor binding and norepinephrine- and serotonin-reuptake inhibition. It can lower the seizure threshold and is therefore not recommended for patients with a history of seizures or taking other medications that could lower the seizure threshold. Caution should also be exercised in patients taking other medications with serotonergic properties to avoid serotonin syndrome (myoclonus, agitation, abdominal cramping, hyperpyrexia, hypertension, and potentially death).

Mixed agonist-antagonists such as nalbuphine and butorphanol also have the potential to cause restlessness and tremulousness and therefore should be avoided in older persons. Because of high risks of GI and renal toxicity and substantial risk of delirium in older individuals, NSAIDs should be used cautiously. As mentioned previously, COX-2 inhibitors have been shown to in-

---

[OL] Not approved by the U.S. Food and Drug Administration for this use.

crease the risk of cardiovascular events, in addition to the risks associated with the nonselective NSAIDs.

REFERENCES

■ AGS Panel on Persistent Pain in Older Persons. The management of persistent pain in older persons. *J Am Geriatr Soc*. 2002;50(6 Suppl): S205–S224.

■ Herr K, Coyne PJ, Key T, et al. Pain assessment in the nonverbal patient: position statement with clinical practice recommendations. *Pain Manag Nursing*. 2006;7(2):44–52.

■ Weiner DK, Herr K, Rudy TE. *Persistent Pain in Older Persons: An Interdisciplinary Guide for Treatment*. New York: Springer Publishing Company; 2002.

SYNDROMES

CHAPTER 20—VISUAL IMPAIRMENT

KEY POINTS

- Visual impairment affects 20% to 30% of persons aged 75 and over.
- Cataracts and refractive error are common; both are correctable, and correction improves quality of life.
- Age-related macular degeneration (ARMD) is common; the wet form, the major complication of ARMD leading to blindness, may respond to laser surgery or intravitreal anti-angiogenesis injection. Antioxidant multivitamins may slow progression to the wet form.
- Glaucoma is common and no longer requires elevated intraocular pressure to meet diagnostic criteria. Screening for glaucoma should take place every 1 to 2 years after age 50, and more often in high-risk individuals.

Visual impairment, defined as visual acuity less than 20/40, increases exponentially with age such that 20% to 30% of the population aged 75 years or older is affected. Blindness, visual acuity of 20/200 or worse, affects 2% of the population aged 75 years and older. Those aged 65 and over make up 12% of the total U.S. population, but 50% of the blind population. Refractive error, cataract, age-related macular degeneration, diabetic retinopathy, and glaucoma are the most common causes of blindness. The respective order of importance varies according to the region and race surveyed. As the baby boomers age, the elderly population is expected to nearly double by the year 2030, and the prevalence of these conditions will surge.

Visual impairment has considerable impact on the medical system and the older age group. Chronic eye conditions represent one of the most common reasons for office-based visits to the physician among those aged 65 and over. Of all office visits by older persons, 14% are to ophthalmologists, one of the highest rates of all specialty visits. Falls and car crashes, each associated with impaired vision in elderly persons, consume considerable medical resources. Moreover, impaired vision has been linked to a significant deterioration in the quality of life and the activities of daily living of older persons.

The American Academy of Ophthalmology recommends a comprehensive eye examination every 1 to 2 years for persons aged 65 and over. The U.S. Preventive Services Task Force recommends annual vision testing. Prophylactic and therapeutic ocular manage-ment can effectively alter the course of various conditions causing visual impairment. About one third of all new cases of blindness can be avoided with effective use of available ophthalmologic services.

REFRACTIVE ERROR AND CATARACT

The leading cause of visual impairment worldwide is refractive error and cataract, for which eyeglasses and surgical cataract extraction, respectively, are mainstays of treatment. Despite the considerable successes of these therapeutic options, many populations do not receive adequate treatment for these problems.

Refractive error may be categorized as emmetropia (neutral refraction), ametropia, or presbyopia. Three forms of ametropia exist: myopia (nearsightedness), hyperopia (farsightedness), and astigmatism (distorted vision). Typically, older patients demonstrate increasing hyperopia, unless a cataract is present, which can induce a myopic shift. Although contact lens wear and laser refractive surgery are available for myopic and hyperopic refractive errors, these alternative forms of treatment traditionally have been used more by younger persons. After the age of approximately 40, emmetropic persons begin to develop progressive presbyopia, impaired ability to focus at near objects that is caused by gradual hardening of the lens and decreased muscular effectiveness of the ciliary body. Reading glasses or bifocal eyeglasses may be prescribed.

Approximately 20% of persons aged 65 years and over and 50% aged 75 years and over have a cataract, a vision-reducing lens opacity. Cataracts may be associated with increased glare, decreased contrast sensitivity, and decreased visual acuity. Several risk factors have been reported: decreased vitamin intake, light (ultraviolet B) exposure, smoking, alcohol use, long-term corticosteroid use, and diabetes mellitus. The most important risk factor is increased age.

Cataract extraction is one the most successful surgeries in medicine (90% of patients achieve vision of 20/40 or better). Approximately 1.5 million cataract procedures are performed each year in the United States alone. In inner cities and underdeveloped countries such as India, the demand for surgery has surpassed available resources.

Cataract extraction is safe and can be completed in less than 15 minutes under local or topical anesthesia. The surgery involves the sonographic breakdown and aspiration of the lens (phacoemulsification). An artificial implant (intraocular lens) is placed in the capsular bag that is the only remnant of the native lens retained. A secondary laser procedure (capsulotomy) may be necessary to ablate subsequent capsular opacification that may develop in 15% or more of patients.

AGE-RELATED MACULAR DEGENERATION

Age-related macular degeneration (ARMD) is the most common cause of blindness in older persons throughout the developed world. Increased age is the most important risk factor, although a genetic predisposition also contributes. Other risk factors include smoking and hypertension. Fair-skinned persons are at greater risk of developing this disease than those who are black, in whom pigment may serve as a protective element.

ARMD may be classified into two forms, dry and wet. The dry form is much more common and is characterized by deposits of drusen under the macula. Drusen, submacular yellow deposits composed of by-products of metabolism, do not typically cause vision loss but are a marker for the wet form of ARMD, which is characterized by angiogenesis or choroidal neovascularization (CNV). The presence of larger, more numerous drusen conveys the greatest risk for the development of CNV. The Age-Related Eye Disease Study found that the risk of development of CNV could be decreased by 25% when patients with high-risk drusen are treated with high-dose oral multivitamin therapy. Combination multivitamins containing beta-carotene 25,000 IU, vitamin E 400 IU, vitamin C 500 mg, and zinc 80 mg are available. This vitamin therapy, however, is contraindicated in smokers because of the risk of lung cancer in smokers who take beta-carotene supplements.

Patients with the dry form of ARMD should be examined periodically by an ophthalmologist. Patients who develop sudden distortion or vision loss, signaling the development of CNV, require urgent evaluation. Severe vision loss or central visual blindness is usually caused by the wet form of ARMD defined by the presence of CNV. Less commonly, geographic atrophy within the macular region may explain severe vision loss. CNV is marked by the presence of subretinal fluid and blood with or without a gray-green membrane (Figure 20.1). The natural history of CNV is progressive subfoveal growth and leakage with associated fibrotic scarring and central blindness.

Laser therapy for CNV has been beneficial, but only under very special circumstances, when membranes are well defined (ie, the margins of the lesion

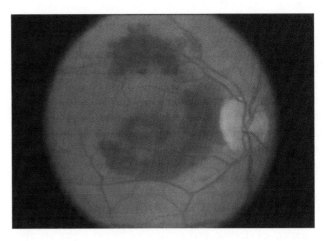

Figure 20.1—Choroidal neovascularization in a patient with the wet form of age-related macular degeneration demonstrating a gray-green membrane associated with subretinal hemorrhage.

are clearly delineated) and extra- or juxtafoveal. Photodynamic therapy (PDT) using porphyrin-derived dyes has been shown to be useful in those patients with subfoveal CNV in whom conventional laser therapy will destroy the fovea. According to the Treatment of Age-Related Macular Degeneration with Photodynamic Therapy Study (TAP), 43% of patients receiving photodynamic therapy sustained moderate visual loss (>15 letters from baseline) after 1 year of follow-up versus 57% of patients not receiving the photoactivated dye laser treatment. Moreover, 16% of those receiving photoactivated dye laser treatment sustained an improvement in visual acuity, but only 7% in the placebo group showed improvement. These benefits continued after 2 years of follow-up but required as many as five sessions of PDT. Although the benefits are not overwhelming, PDT is a relatively safe alternative that is the most effective procedure available for delaying visual loss in patients with wet ARMD and CNV that is not occult.

A great deal of excitement has been generated regarding angiogenesis inhibition. Specifically, various types of inhibitors to vascular endothelial growth factor (VEGF) have already been approved by the Food and Drug Administration (FDA) for treatment of diseases such as colorectal cancer and the wet form of ARMD; several additional indications await completion of the FDA review process. Serial intravitreal injections (9 per year) of pegaptanib sodium, an anti-VEGF aptamer or mRNA oligonucleotide that acts as an antagonist to VEGF, has been approved by the FDA for the treatment of all subtypes of wet ARMD. Similar to PDT, the injections do not typically improve vision but reduce the risk of vision loss. Another approved anti-angiogenesis inhibitor, ranibizumab, is a fragment antibody that exhibits broad-spectrum inhibition of VEGF. This intravitreal pharmacotherapy requires monthly injections.

A concerted effort to find a candidate gene for ARMD has been for many years unsuccessful until recently, when multiple centers uncovered a 30% to 50% association of a mutation in the complement factor H (CFH) gene with various forms of ARMD. CFH is a regulator of complement activation, the mutation of which may lead to increased inflammation and leakage and the development of ARMD.

DIABETIC RETINOPATHY

Duration of disease and control of blood sugar are the most important variables in the development and progression of diabetic retinopathy. After 10 years, 70% of those with type 2 diabetes demonstrate some form of retinopathy, and nearly 10% show proliferative disease. Diet control, exercise, and proper glucose management with frequent daily glucose testing and the use of oral hypoglycemics or insulin, or both, are crucial in maintaining glycosylated hemoglobin levels lower than 7%. The Diabetic Control and Complications Trial demonstrated that tight blood-sugar control in those with type 1 diabetes results in a long-lasting decrease in the rate of development and progression of diabetic retinopathy. The United Kingdom Prospective Diabetes Study validated these results in an older population with type 2 diabetes. Tight blood-pressure control (≤140/80) with either β-blockers or angiotensin-converting enzyme inhibitors was also found to be an important factor in decreasing microvascular complications, such as the need for retinal laser therapy. Other systemic risk factors, including kidney function and serum cholesterol, may also influence the course of diabetic retinopathy and should be optimized. Angiotensin-converting enzyme inhibitors have been found to decrease progressive nephropathy in diabetic patients and may have similar benefits to the retina.

Type 2 diabetic patients require baseline ophthalmologic screening at diagnosis of systemic disease. Subsequent follow-up will depend on the grade of retinopathy; however, even patients without retinopathy should be evaluated annually. Nonproliferative diabetic retinopathy, the earliest stage of retinopathy, may first be manifested by retinal microaneurysms. Intraretinal hemorrhages and exudates, with or without associated macular edema, may ensue. Progressive ischemia characterized by increasing hemorrhages, venous caliber changes or intraretinal microvascular abnormalities or both, and capillary nonperfusion on fluorescein angiography characterize the preproliferative stage of diabetic retinopathy. About 40% of patients with preproliferative retinopathy de-

velop proliferative diabetic retinopathy (PDR) within 1 to 2 years, characterized by neovascularization or new blood vessel growth of the retina or disc, or both.

Visual loss in diabetic patients may occur as a result of macular nonperfusion or macular edema. The Early Treatment Diabetic Retinopathy Study demonstrated the benefit of focal or grid laser photocoagulation in stabilizing and improving vision in diabetic patients with clinically significant macular edema (Figure 20.2). Neovascularization (Figure 20.3) may cause severe visual loss or blindness in the setting of PDR as a result of vitreous hemorrhage or tractional retinal detachment. PDR is amenable to treatment by panretinal laser photocoagulation to inhibit the growth stimulus for neovascularization. The Diabetic Retinopathy Study demonstrated an 11% incidence of severe visual loss in patients treated with panretinal photocoagulation but a 26% incidence in those who did not receive laser during a 2-year follow-up. Nonclearing vitreous hemorrhage or tractional macular

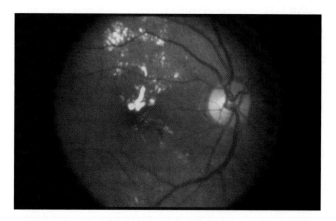

Figure 20.2—Intraretinal edema and exudate in the superior macular region consistent with clinically significant macular edema in a patient with type 2 diabetes mellitus.

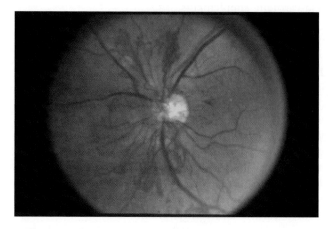

Figure 20.3—Florid neovascularization of the disc in a patient with high-risk proliferative diabetic retinopathy.

detachment may be addressed surgically by pars plana vitrectomy, membrane peeling, and endolaser.

GLAUCOMA

Glaucoma is the second most common cause of blindness worldwide and, in the United States, the most common cause of blindness in black Americans. It affects more than 2.25 million Americans aged 40 years or over and results in more than 3 million office visits each year. The financial burden is considerable because of the prevalence and chronicity of this disease and the debilitation that results. Federal costs are reported to reach as high as $1 billion for glaucoma-related Medicare and Medicaid payments and disability.

The definition of glaucoma, now defined as characteristic optic nerve head damage and visual field loss, has undergone a considerable evolution. Elevated intraocular pressure (IOP) is no longer considered an absolute criterion, although it is a very important risk factor. There are many different types of glaucoma, of which primary open-angle glaucoma (POAG) is the most common. Adults over age 50 should have screening for glaucoma every 1 to 2 years. Older adults with a positive family history of glaucoma, black origin, or other risk factors may need more frequent screening.

POAG is a chronic disease most commonly affecting older patients. Aqueous may access the filtration site, but the network is "clogged," resulting in impaired passage out of the angle. Slow aqueous drainage leads to chronically elevated IOPs. This is in contrast to acute angle-closure glaucoma, in which the entry site is suddenly blocked off, IOP rises precipitously, and the patient presents with considerable redness and pain with acute vision loss. Pain may be so severe as to cause headache, nausea, and vomiting. Emergent ophthalmologic referral is required to reverse the angle closure and reduce the IOP through the use of aqueous suppressants, miotics, and laser iridotomy. Conversely, the IOP rise in POAG is slow and much less severe. Patients with POAG are asymptomatic and may suffer substantial field loss before consulting an ophthalmologist, which underscores the importance of regular ophthalmologic screening of the older adult.

Development of POAG is most likely multifactorial and polygenic. Initial pedigrees were found to demonstrate linkage to the 1q locus. Subsequent investigations have more precisely defined the GLC1A gene that encodes for myocilin, the trabecular meshwork-induced glucocorticoid response protein. Several other chromosomal loci, including those mapped to chromosomes 2, 3, 7, and 10, have also been found to be associated with the development of glaucoma.

The management of POAG may be approached by the ophthalmologist in a stepwise manner. A variety of IOP-lowering medications, both local and systemic, exist. Mechanisms of action include decreased aqueous production or increased aqueous outflow (see Table 20.1). Various eyedrop formulations are available; prostaglandin analogs that increase uveal-scleral outflow and α_2-adrenergic agonists that decrease aqueous production are two relatively new and effective drugs. In the face of visual field progression despite maximal medications or intolerance to medications, argon laser trabeculoplasty (application of laser energy to the trabecular meshwork) can be effective in lowering IOP in approximately 50% of patients for 3 to 5 years after treatment. Intraocular surgery involves the creation of a fistula or filtration site to allow an alternative route of aqueous egress (trabeculectomy). Adjunctive antimetabolite use with 5-fluorouracil[OL] or mitomycin-C[OL] has increased the success of this procedure in those patients at high risk of failure because of fibrosis and scarring of the filtration site. Alternative surgeries for glaucoma include drainage devices or aqueous shunts. Drainage devices, which are made of a foreign material such as plastic, shunt fluid from the anterior chamber to the subconjunctival space. Ciliary body destructive procedures with cryotherapy or laser (cyclocryoablation or cyclophotocoagulation) may be used in eyes with a poor visual prognosis.

ANTERIOR ISCHEMIC OPTIC NEUROPATHY

Anterior ischemic optic neuropathy (Figure 20.4) may result in acute vision or field loss. Microvascular

Table 20.1—Adverse Effects of Selected Eyedrops for Glaucoma

Class	Adverse Effects
Aqueous suppressants:	
α-Agonists (eg, brimonidine)	Allergic conjunctivitis
β-Blockers (eg, timolol)	Bradycardia, dyspnea, asthma, heart failure exacerbations
Carbonic anhydrase inhibitors (eg, dorzolamide)	Blurriness
Aqueous outflow facilitators:	
Epinephrine (eg, dipivefrin)	Palpitations, angina, cystoid macular edema
Miotics (eg, pilocarpine)	Brow arch, blurriness, nyctalopia
Prostaglandins (eg, latanoprost)	Pain, redness, increased eyelashes, iris pigmentation, cystoid macular edema

[OL] Not approved by the U.S. Food and Drug Administration for this use.

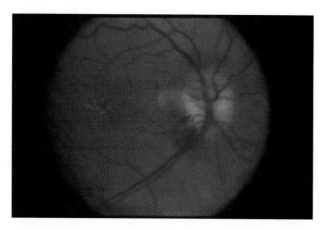

Figure 20.4—Pallid swelling of the optic nerve head in a patient with anterior ischemic optic neuropathy.

occlusion of the blood supply to the optic nerve may be attributed to atherosclerotic vascular disease or inflammation in the setting of giant cell (temporal) arteritis. The former, the nonarteritic form, typically affects patients with vasculopathic risk factors such as diabetes mellitus and hypertension; the latter, the arteritic form, tends to occur in elderly patients with a history of myalgias, headaches, and weight loss. An elevated Westergren erythrocyte sedimentation rate and a positive temporal artery biopsy are diagnostic. Systemic corticosteroid treatment is crucial to avoid visual loss in the other eye.

MISCELLANEOUS

Red eye in elderly patients may be classified by cause, benign or malignant. Malignant causes are typically associated with significant pain and vision loss and include corneal ulceration identified by the presence of a white corneal infiltrate. Emergent corneal scraping by an ophthalmologist to exclude an infection and the need for fortified antibiotic treatment is indicated. The presence of a corneal abrasion in the absence of an infiltrate or ulcer is prognostically much more favorable and may be diagnosed with fluorescein staining and treated with patching. Anterior or posterior uveitis is relatively unusual in the older adult population. Suspicion should be aroused by the symptom of photophobia with vision loss; urgent ophthalmologic referral is required. Treatment may include corticosteroid eye drop therapy, which can be complicated by cataract and increased IOP, and which is best prescribed by an ophthalmologist. Systemic investigations to exclude autoimmune diseases, systemic infections, and occult malignancies may be necessary.

Benign causes of red eye may include blepharitis or dandruff of the eye lashes. Treatment includes lid hygiene, topical antibiotics, and gentle scrubbing with nontearing baby shampoo twice daily. Less commonly, viral conjunctivitis associated with mucus discharge and matting of the eyelids, especially in the morning, may be noted and may be treated supportively with warm compresses and education to limit spread of the infection to the other eye or to contacts.

Allergic conjunctivitis is a common benign condition affecting older adults and causing red, itchy eyes. Advise patients to avoid known precipitants (eg, pet dander). Management of allergic conjunctivitis includes systemic antihistamines, topical antihistamines or decongestants, and ophthalmic corticosteroids. Patients should be cautioned about side effects of topical ophthalmics.

The use of ophthalmic corticosteroids in older adults merits comment. Indications include inflammatory conditions of the eye; risks include secondary ocular infections, cataract formation, glaucoma, and corneal thinning. Because of the risks, the prescription of ophthalmic corticosteroids is best limited to practitioners with training and experience in their use.

Tears serve several important functions, including corneal lubrication, debris clearance, and immune protection. With age, tear production decreases, and older patients are prone to develop dry-eye syndrome or keratitis sicca, characterized by redness, foreign body sensation, and reflex tearing. Management includes tear replacement with artificial tears during the day and an ointment at bedtime. Temporary and permanent punctal plugs may be employed to retard tear egress through the nasolacrimal drainage system in more severe cases. Keratitis sicca may be associated with autoimmune disease; conditions such as Sjögren's syndrome should be excluded.

Lid abnormalities are a common problem for older persons. Because of the gradual loss of elasticity and tensile strength that develops with age, secondary degenerative changes may take place. Blepharochalasis (drooping of the brow) and blepharoptosis (drooping of the eyelid) may cause cosmetic deformity and, if severe, may impair vision. Lid ectropion or entropion, eversion and inversion of the lid margins, respectively, can disrupt the ocular surface and cause discomfort for the patient. Various surgical procedures are available to address these problems.

Herpes zoster ophthalmicus, or shingles, is a painful reactivation of varicella zoster virus that not uncommonly affects older persons. Dermatomal distribution of weeping vesicles affecting the ophthalmic division of the trigeminal nerve is the classic presentation. Ocular involvement may be signaled by lesions on the tip of the nose (Hutchinson's sign) and may include dendritic keratopathy or uveitis. Oral acyclovir may shorten the course of disease. Trifluridine eyedrops are indicated with herpetic, dendriform corneal ulcers. Post-herpetic neuralgia may be quite debilitating; various local ointments (eg, capsaicin, lidocaine[OL]) or systemic medications (eg, corticosteroids[OL], tricyclic antidepressants[OL]) may be helpful. (See also "Dermatologic Diseases and Disorders," p 284.)

LOW-VISION REHABILITATION

Despite considerable advancements in the medical treatment of ocular conditions, many patients, especially those with the wet form of ARMD, may ultimately sustain permanent visual loss. Visual training and the provision of visual aids are indispensable services available to the patient with low vision (visual acuity <20/60).

Patients with low vision may develop useful adaptive skills with proper instruction. Eccentric viewing by ARMD patients with central macular pathology uses the principle of off-center fixation. The patient can benefit from formal training to find and use the most effective eccentric viewing points. Instruction in scanning and tracking and other skills may help the patient integrate his or her visual environment.

Various low-vision aids are available to improve one's ability to see both near and far. The fine detail required for reading is the most common indication for visual aids. Improved lighting is a simple modification that can enhance visualization of print. Selection of reading material using bold, enlarged fonts and accentuated black-on-white contrast may also be helpful. Magnification also is commonly employed. Various

---

[OL] Not approved by the U.S. Food and Drug Administration for this use.

devices such as high-plus spectacles, hand-held magnifiers, stand magnifiers, and closed-circuit television can also enhance reading. Distance magnification may be achieved with the use of telescopic devices that can be hand-held for spot viewing or spectacle mounted for continuous viewing. Talking devices, which are computers used to create voice synthesis such as those used at stoplights, or Braille may be especially helpful for those who have lost vision altogether.

REFERENCES

- Comer GM, Ciulla TA, Heier JS, et al. Future pharmacological treatment options for nonexudative and exudative age-related macular degeneration. *Expert Opin Emerg Drugs.* 2005;10(1):119–135.

- Gandhewar RR, Kamath GG. Acute glaucoma presentations in the elderly. *Emerg Med J.* 2005;22(4):306–307.

- Jain A, Sarraf D, Fong D. Preventing diabetic retinopathy through the control of systemic risk factors. *Curr Opin Ophthalmol.* 2003;14(6):389–394.

- Rowe S, MacLean CH, Shekelle PG. Preventing visual loss from chronic eye disease in primary care: scientific review. *JAMA.* 2004;291(12):1487–1495.

- Bressler NM; Treatment of Age-Related Macular Degeneration with Photodynamic Therapy (TAP) Study Group. Photodynamic therapy of subfoveal choroidal neovascularization in age-related macular degeneration with verteporfin: two-year results of 2 randomized clinical trails—TAP Report 2. *Arch Ophthalmol.* 2001;119(2):198–207.

CHAPTER 21—HEARING IMPAIRMENT

KEY POINTS

- Hearing loss is among the most common chronic diseases among older persons: 10% of persons aged 65 to 75 years and 25% of those older than 75 years have hearing loss.

- Treatment of hearing loss and attention to communication strategies can improve the hearing-impaired person's quality of life.

- Important issues when considering hearing aids for an older person with hearing loss are the nature and degree of hearing loss, the person's ability to manipulate the aid and adapt to its use, and the social support and financial resources available to him or her.

Hearing loss is the fourth most common chronic disease among elderly persons. Hearing impairment is often assumed to be benign, but it has profound effects on quality of life. The psychologic effects of hearing loss include family discord, social isolation, loss of self-esteem, anger, and depression. Epidemiologic studies suggest an association between hearing loss and cognitive impairment, and between hearing loss and reduced mobility. Hearing loss can also affect an older person's interaction with clinicians, making history taking and patient education difficult. Treatment of hearing loss and attention to communication strategies can improve the hearing-impaired person's quality of life by facilitating interaction with family, friends, and caregivers. Studies indicate that hearing aid use can relieve symptoms of depression that are associated with hearing loss.

NORMAL HEARING AND AGE-RELATED CHANGES IN THE AUDITORY SYSTEM

The normal ear is an efficient transducer of sound energy into nerve impulses. Sound energy is transmitted through the external ear to the tympanic membrane and the auditory ossicles. The malleus, incus, and stapes in series transmit vibrations to the oval window of the cochlea. Fluid waves within the cochlea stimulate the outer hair cells of the scala tympani. These cells stimulate the inner hair cells, which generate sensory potential. In turn, an excitatory postsynaptic potential is generated. When threshold is reached, impulses are sent via cochlear neurons to the cochlear nuclei and then to auditory pathways elsewhere in the brain.

Age-related changes in the auditory system can interfere with its function. The walls of the external ear canal become thin. Cerumen becomes drier and more tenacious, increasing the likelihood of cerumen impaction. The eardrum becomes thicker and appears duller than in younger persons. Degenerative changes of the ossicular joints occur but generally do not interfere with sound transmission to the cochlea. Cochlear changes include loss of sensory hair cells and fibrocytes in the organ of Corti, stiffening of the basilar membrane, calcification of auditory structures, and cochlear neuronal loss. Changes in the stria vascularis include thickening of capillaries, decreased production of endolymph, and decreased Na+ K+ ATPase activity. These degenerative changes occur to varying degrees in different individuals. It currently is not possible to fully correlate the degree of hearing loss with histologic changes in the aging ear.

Changes in central auditory processing also occur with aging. One study found that when competing speech stimuli are presented to each ear, the right ear has a 5% to 10% advantage over the left ear in younger persons. (The effect of right- and left-handedness was not assessed; all the participants were right-handed.) In persons aged 80 to 89 years, this difference increases to more than 40%. This difference may be related to a loss of efficiency of interhemispheric transfer of auditory information through the corpus callosum.

EPIDEMIOLOGY OF HEARING LOSS

The prevalence of hearing loss increases with age. Ten percent of adults aged 65 to 75 years and 25% of those older than 75 years have hearing loss. In nursing homes, estimates of prevalence vary from 50% to 100%, depending on the criteria used to define hearing loss.

Hearing loss can be caused by pathology in the external ear canal, the middle ear, the inner ear, the auditory nerve, central auditory pathways, or a combination of these.

Conductive hearing loss is due to disease in the external ear, such as ceruminosis, or foreign body in the canal, or to middle-ear pathology, such as otosclerosis, cholesteatoma, tympanic membrane perforation, or middle-ear effusion.

Sensorineural hearing loss is most often caused by cochlear disease. Noise is the most common factor in cochlear damage. Hearing loss is less common among persons in quiet rural environments than among people in industrialized communities. Other causes of hearing loss include ototoxic medications, genotype, vascular disease, and, rarely, occupational and environmental chemical exposures. Smokers have higher rates of hearing loss than nonsmokers. Autoimmune disease and auditory nerve tumors are rare causes of sensorineural hearing loss. Neuronal loss can affect the brain stem and cortical ascending auditory pathways, including the cochlear nuclei, superior olivary complex, lateral lemniscus, inferior colliculi, and medial geniculate complex. The resulting deficits in central auditory processing can affect perception of sound and the ability to understand speech.

PRESBYCUSIS

Most hearing loss in elderly persons is categorized as presbycusis (literally, "older hearing"). Presbycusis is a sensorineural, usually symmetrical hearing loss that may have central components. Presbycusis can be classified as sensory, neural, strial, cochlear conductive, combined, or indeterminate, depending on cochlear pathology. Many persons with presbycusis can be helped by amplification.

Sensory presbycusis is often slowly progressive, beginning with the higher frequencies of 8000 Hz, 6000 Hz, and 4000 Hz. It may also involve the 3000 and 2000 Hz range, which is the higher portion of the range of frequencies in human speech. Persons with this type of hearing loss often have trouble hearing in the presence of background noise but will be able to hear adequately in quiet settings. Amplification often helps these patients, since speech discrimination is satisfactory. This loss of auditory acuity can begin as early as the 20s but may not become clinically evident until later decades. Sensory presbycusis is attributed to a loss of sensory hair cells in the basal end of the cochlea.

Strial presbycusis is considered a metabolic form of hearing loss. The stria vascularis maintains high potassium concentrations in the endolymph. Strial presbycusis, pathologically defined as atrophy of 30% or more of the stria vascularis, is a form of cochlear dysfunction. This disorder typically begins between the ages of 20 and 60 and is characterized by mild to moderate hearing loss in most frequencies. Persons with strial presbycusis usually have good speech discrimination and do well with amplification.

Neural presbycusis is due to a cochlear neuronal loss of 50% or more compared with the normal number in neonates. Despite preserved pure-tone thresholds, which are not affected until more than 90% of cochlear neurons have been lost, patients with neural presbycusis show very poor speech discrimination. Successful use of amplification is difficult in this form of presbycusis.

Cochlear conductive presbycusis is caused by changes in cochlear mechanics produced by mass or stiffness changes or spiral ligament atrophy. Speech discrimination may also be impaired. Pathologically, this form is defined by the absence of histologic changes seen in the other forms of presbycusis.

Most presbycusis is probably a mixture of these forms. Audiogram results and speech discrimination scores will depend on the extent of injury to various components of the cochlea.

DIAGNOSIS OF HEARING LOSS

Partly because of the slowly progressive nature of hearing loss, many older persons are unaware of their hearing deficit. In some cases, the stigma of wearing a hearing aid causes the patient to deny the problem. The hearing loss may be brought to medical attention by family members, who complain that the patient does not hear them or plays the television or radio too loud. Clinicians may notice that the patient does not respond when spoken to out of his or her field of view, or seems to misunderstand questions. Hearing loss can also be misunderstood as cognitive impairment. Caregivers and clinicians may not recognize the presence of hearing loss or may assume it is a benign component of aging.

Screening programs to identify hearing loss are important. Fitting hearing aids early in the course of hearing loss may help the person adjust to their use, and treatment can reduce psychologic morbidity. A handheld otoscope with a tone generator can be used by primary care providers to screen for the presence of hearing loss at selected frequencies (0.5, 1, 2, and 4 KHz) and two loudness levels (25 and 40 dB HL). This device should be used in a quiet environment. When set at 40 dB HL, testing at 1 and 2 KHz has a sensitivity of 94% and a specificity between 82% and 90% for detecting hearing loss. The Hearing Handicap Inventory for the Elderly—Screening Version is a 10-item questionnaire that asks about difficulty with communication in various settings. It can be useful to determine the impact that hearing loss has on a patient's daily activities. When a screening test is consistent with hearing loss and the patient is willing and able to pay for a hearing aid, referral to an audiologist should be discussed. The patient's ear canals should be examined before referral to exclude the presence of obstruction. Cerumen impaction can cause a clinically significant hearing loss, as much as 40 dB.

The otolaryngologist will further evaluate the hearing loss and identify treatable causes. An asymmetrical hearing loss demands thorough investigation. Auditory nerve tumors are rare, but tumors of the posterior pharynx can obstruct the eustachian tube, causing a middle-ear effusion with conductive hearing loss.

The audiologist will assess hearing to determine the presence and the type of hearing loss. A comprehensive audiologic assessment consists of pure-tone thresholds for both air and bone conduction, speech-recognition thresholds, speech discrimination, and middle-ear function. This information, along with the medical evaluation, will be used to determine treatment for the patient. Audiologists recommend and fit hearing aids and provide auditory rehabilitation.

TREATMENT OF HEARING LOSS

Some causes of hearing loss are amenable to medical or surgical treatment. Paget's disease of the bone can affect the middle ear, causing conductive loss, or the inner ear, leading to sensorineural loss. This loss sometimes responds to bisphosphonates. Otosclerosis or tympanosclerosis may be correctable with surgery. Sudden hearing loss may be autoimmune in nature and sometimes responds to corticosteroids or immunosuppressant therapy. The majority of older persons with hearing loss are treated with communication strategies or amplification, or both. Hearing aids often improve ability to understand speech, particularly soft speech and conversational loud speech.

Strategies to Enhance Communication

Hearing-impaired persons should be encouraged to let others know about their hearing loss and to suggest strategies that will help them communicate more easily (Table 21.1). In addition to using these strategies, clinicians should provide options for patients with hearing loss, such as sign language interpreters, the use of pen and paper, or assistive devices. Office and hospital staff should be alerted to a patient's hearing loss. Background noise from the environment can interfere with hearing and should be reduced as much as possible.

Table 21.1—Strategies to Improve Communication with Hearing-Impaired Persons

- Obtain the listener's attention before speaking.

- Eliminate background noise as much as possible.

- Be sure the listener can see the speaker's lips; for example:

  Speak face-to-face in the same room.

  Do not obscure the lips with hands, mustaches, or other objects.

  Make certain that light shines directly on the speaker's face, not from behind the speaker.

- Speak slowly and clearly, but avoid shouting.

- Speak toward the better ear, if applicable.

- Change phrasing if the listener does not understand at first.

- Spell words out, use gestures, or write them down.

- Have the listener repeat back what he or she heard

- **Ask the listener what is the best way to communicate with him or her.**

Lipreading can be a useful adjunct to listening, but it requires thoughtfulness on the part of the speaker. When speaking to a hearing-impaired person who lip-reads, it is important to face him or her and obtain the person's attention before speaking; a gentle touch on the hand or arm will usually suffice. Speak each word clearly and distinctly. Shouting not only distorts lip movements so they are harder to read, but the speaker may sound angry even when not. Use complete sentences. Single words are hard to lip-read because the listener often needs cues from context to identify meaning. It is helpful to make certain the person knows the topic of conversation. Use appropriate language for the listener's educational level. Unlike deaf persons who have been deaf all or most of their lives, most older persons with hearing loss do not know sign language. Sometimes amplification and lip-reading are not enough. Gestures can aid communication even with cognitively impaired patients.

For patients with hearing impairment, it can also be helpful to write words down. For those with both hearing and visual impairment, large printing with a marker pen or a laptop computer screen with magnified print may be necessary. These patients may benefit from correction of the visual problem, if possible (eg, cataract removal or use of eyeglasses). In any case, providing written instructions to those who can read improves understanding and retention of important information.

Be alert to misunderstandings. If a reply does not make sense, try repeating what was said, using different words. Have the patient repeat what he or she heard, since misunderstandings are common.

Hearing Aids

Hearing aids are the most common form of amplification. Many factors need to be considered in deciding whether to fit the patient with a hearing aid. In addition to the nature and degree of hearing loss (Table 21.2), the patient's motivation and ability to adapt to its use and physically manipulate the aid (Table 21.3), the degree of his or social support, and his or her ability to afford the expense (Table 21.4) must be considered.

In general, two hearing aids are more beneficial than one. The first aid provides the most gain; the second one helps with speech discrimination and with localizing the source of sounds. However, the presence of asymmetrical hearing loss or significant difficulty in understanding competing speech stimuli may mean that the use of a single hearing aid is more appropriate.

Not everyone benefits from a hearing aid. The pattern of sensorineural damage may be such that speech discrimination is poor even with amplification. Some patients are unable to tolerate the presence of the hearing aid in the ear. Patients with dementia may remove and dispose of the aid. It is important to be sure that the aid can be returned during an initial trial period, usually 30 days, without having to pay the full cost. It is equally important not to give up on the aid too soon, because the audiologist often can adjust it to

Table 21.2—Effects and Rehabilitation of Hearing Loss, by Degree of Loss

Degree of Loss	Loss in db HL	Sounds Difficult to Hear	Effect on Communication	Amplification or Other Assistance Needed
Mild	25–40	Whisper	Difficulty understanding soft speech or normal speech in presence of background noise	Hearing aid needed in specific situations
Moderate	41–55	Conversational speech	Difficulty understanding any but loud speech	Frequent need for hearing aid
Severe	56–80	Shouting, vacuum cleaner	Can understand only amplified speech	Amplification needed for all communication
Profound	≥ 81	Hair dryer, heavy traffic, telephone ringer	Difficulty understanding amplified speech; may miss telephone calls	May need to supplement hearing aid with lip-reading, assistive listening devices, sign language

SOURCE: Data in part from *A Report on Hearing Aids: User Perspectives and Concerns*. Washington, DC: American Association of Retired Persons; 1993:2.

Table 21.3—Advantages and Disadvantages of Hearing Aid Styles

Style	Degree of Hearing Loss	Advantages	Disadvantages
CIC	Mild to moderate	Almost invisible Less occlusion of ear canal allows more natural sound Easier to use with headphones and telephone	Dexterity may be a problem Small size may limit available features May cost more than canal or ITE aids Shorter battery life
Canal	Mild to moderate	More cosmetic than larger aids Telecoil available in some models May be able to use with headphones	Dexterity may be a problem Small size may limit available features
ITE	Mild to severe	Ease of handling Comfortable fit Available options: telecoil, directional microphone More power than CIC or canal aid	More conspicuous than CIC or canal aid May be difficult to use with headphones
BTE	Mild to profound	Greatest power Available options: telecoil, direct audio input, directional microphone Earmold can be changed separately	More conspicuous May be more difficult to insert than ITE Difficult to use with headphones
Body aid	Severe to profound	Greatest separation of microphone from receiver reduces feedback	Most conspicuous Body-level microphone is subject to noise from clothing Microphone is on chest, but speech isusually directed at ear level
Bone conduction aid	Mild to severe	Bypasses middle ear; used if ear canal is unable to tolerate aid or earmold	Receiver causes pressure on the scalp, which can be uncomfortable; does not correct sensorineural loss

NOTE: BTE = behind the ear; CIC = completely in the canal; ITE = in the ear.

Table 21.4—Costs of Assistive Listening Devices and Hearing Aids

Type of Technology	Cost	Comments
Assistive listening devices (personal amplifiers, telephone amplifiers, television listening devices)	$150–$200	Useful for specific situations (see text for details)
Hearing aids		
Analog	$750–$1,100	Smaller aids are more expensive
Analog programmable	$1,150–$1,600	Smaller aids are more expensive
Digital, low end	$1,150–$1,500	Similar to analog aid, but with better sound quality
Digital, mid-range	$1,600–$2,300	Some sound processing included, eg, a second program, feedback control, telecoil
Digital, premium	$2,300–$3,000	Multiple features available, eg, background noise suppression, feedback management, multiple programs, telecoil
Bone conduction	$400–$900	Available as all-in-one headpiece or as body aid; used only if in-the-ear aid or earmold is not tolerated

NOTE: Assistive listening devices and hearing aids are not covered by Medicare.

improve comfort and sound quality. The audiologist should provide counseling for its optimal use.

Many different styles of hearing aids are available (Table 21.3). Behind-the-ear aids hang behind the ear and are connected directly to an earmold. The earmold is custom made to fit each patient's ear. Some behind-the-ear aids can be connected to assistive listening devices via a "boot," which fits over the end of the aid to provide direct audio input. Body aids are worn on the belt or in a pocket or a harness, and they are connected to a custom-made earmold by a wire. These are rarely used. All in-the ear aids and canal aids have cases that are custom fit to the user. The smaller hearing aids may have remote controls. Selection of aid style for each individual depends on the degree of hearing loss, available features, and the person's dexterity and motivation.

The telecoil is an induction coupling coil that can be built into the hearing aid. It detects the magnetic field produced by telephones compatible with hearing aids. The telecoil is used to listen to the telephone with less distraction from noise in the same room. It can also be used with many assistive listening devices. The amount of coupling, and therefore the volume of the signal, depends on the angle of the telecoil with respect to the magnetic field. Users may need to experiment to find the right angle. Strongly magnetic devices such as computer monitors often produce interference, which also depends on the angle and the distance of the telecoil from the device. These drawbacks aside, the telecoil is a useful feature and can be added to hearing aids at a relatively small cost. Consumers with moderate to severe hearing loss should be encouraged to consider purchasing an aid with a telecoil.

The choice of analog or digital hearing aids depends on the individual. Analog aids are less expensive than digital aids and may provide acceptable sound quality. However, newer digital technology has allowed improved sound quality, reduced size, and increased ability to customize the amplification of the aid to the needs of the user. Programmable aids are adjusted for each individual while he or she is wearing the aid. Often, two or more programs are available within a single aid. Using a computer, the audiologist can adjust to gain, response in different frequency ranges, and loudness balance for each program. One program may be most useful in the presence of background noise, whereas another works better in a quiet environment, and a third works with a telecoil. Persons with Ménière's disease can have their aids reprogrammed to accommodate fluctuating hearing loss. Some hearing aids automatically adjust the volume to increase amplification of soft sounds while avoiding uncomfortable loudness, reducing the need for the user to manipulate the aid. A study comparing different methods of limiting loudness suggested that users with mild to moderate hearing loss were more likely to prefer compression-limiting or wide dynamic range compression circuitry to peak-clipping circuitry, though the absolute differences in user preference and speech comprehension between these methods were small.

Background noise is a significant problem for hearing-aid users. Traditional hearing aids amplify sound indiscriminately, so that noises from papers rattling or water running can be very distracting. The use of multiple microphones in the hearing aid, combined with digital signal processing, can decrease background noise. This can significantly improve the wearer's ability to understand speech and increase user satisfaction with the aid.

Unfortunately, the cost of hearing aids is often a significant barrier to their use and may affect the purchaser's choice of features (Table 21.4). Medicare and the majority of private health insurance companies typically do not pay for hearing aids, although they may provide coverage for audiometric evaluation for

hearing aids. Medicaid may provide coverage for hearing aids, but the reimbursement may be below the provider's cost. Federal programs such as the Department of Veterans Affairs may pay for hearing aids, depending on the recipient's eligibility for services.

Assistive Listening Devices

For some persons with hearing impairment, a personal amplifier may be more useful than hearing aids. These pocket-sized devices are considerably less expensive than hearing aids and are harder to misplace. Headphones stay on the head better than earbuds and provide sound to both ears. The volume and microphone placement of the amplifier should be adjusted to find the best combination for a given user. Every health care facility should have at least one or two of these devices available, as they are not personalized and can be used by different people.

Adaptive equipment can facilitate telephone use. State agencies for deaf and hard-of-hearing persons may provide amplified telephones, vibrating and flashing ringer alert devices, and text telephones (TTY) at no cost to hearing-impaired persons. This equipment is available from electronics and telephone equipment stores.

Many other assistive devices are available. Television listening devices can spare others from overly loud volume levels. FM loop systems can be used for groups of people with FM receivers or telecoil switches in their hearing aids. Wireless FM transmitters and receivers are also available for indoor or outdoor use. Infrared group listening devices are primarily useful indoors. Vibrating and flashing devices such as alarm clocks and timers, smoke alarms, doorbell alerts, and motion sensors can improve the hearing-impaired person's convenience and safety. These items can be purchased through the agencies mentioned above or from catalog retailers of assistive listening devices.

Cochlear Implants

For persons with severe to profound hearing loss who gain little or no benefit from hearing aids yet who are motivated to participate in the hearing world, cochlear implants can provide useful hearing. A cochlear implant is an electronic device that bypasses the function of damaged or absent cochlear hair cells by providing electrical stimulation to cochlear nerve fibers. A receiver-stimulator and an intracochlear electrode array are surgically implanted. A headset is worn behind the ear. The headset microphone transmits signals to the speech processor, which filters and digitizes the sound into coded signals. The coded signals are sent to the cochlear implant, which then stimulates auditory nerve fibers in the cochlea. Nerve signals are then sent through the auditory system to the brain. Patients must be able to tolerate general anesthesia and to participate in extensive pre-implant testing and post-implant training. The procedure is covered by most Medicare carriers and insurance companies. In general, outcomes of cochlear implantation in persons aged 65 and older have been comparable to those of younger adults, with patients obtaining excellent results by both audiologic and quality-of-life measures. Meningitis is a rare complication of cochlear implants.

REFERENCES

- American Academy of Audiology: Consumer Guides. Frequently asked questions about hearing aids. Available at: http://www.audiology.org/consumer/guides/hafaq.php (accessed October 2005).

- Department of Otolaryngology—Head and Neck Surgery, University of Washington Medical Center. Cochlear implants. Available at: http://depts.washington.edu/otoweb/patients/pts_specialties/pts_hear-n-bal/pts_hear-n-bal_cochlear-implant.htm (accessed October 2005).

- Iezzoni LI, O'Day BL, Killeen M, et al. Communicating about health care: observations from persons who are deaf or hard of hearing. *Ann Intern Med.* 2004;140(5):356–362.

- Yueh B, Shapiro N, MacLean CH, et al. Screening and management of adult hearing loss in primary care: scientific review. *JAMA.* 2003;289(15):1976–1985.

CHAPTER 22—DIZZINESS

KEY POINTS

- The classification of dizziness into vertigo and nonvertiginous dizziness (presyncope, disequilibrium, and lightheadedness) may be useful in guiding the clinician in patient evaluation; however, precise classification is often difficult, and multiple causes of the same symptoms are common.

- Common causes of the spinning sensation of vertigo include benign positional vertigo, labyrinthitis, and Ménière's disease.

- Presyncope, the sensation of near fainting, implies impaired cerebral perfusion. Most older adults with presyncope have symptoms related to orthostatic blood-pressure changes or vagally mediated changes rather than cardiac causes.

- Multiple factors can contribute to disequilibrium, a feeling of unsteadiness. vestibulopathies, neuropathies, and visual and musculoskeletal problems. Nondescript lightheadedness may suggest depression, anxiety, or other emotional problems.

- Most dizziness resolves within days to several months. Despite the increased risk of falls, chronic or recurrent dizziness has not been found to be associated with increased mortality, hospitalization, or functional decline but is associated with syncope, depression, and worse self-rated health.

- Key physical examination steps include checking for orthostatic hypotension, performing the head-hanging (Dix-Hallpike) test, and observing gait. If the cause is not identified, a brief vestibular evaluation including other maneuvers for nystagmus is merited.

- Treatment options for dizziness vary with cause.

Dizziness accounts for an estimated 7 million clinic visits in the United States each year and is one of the most common symptoms of patients referred to neurology and otolaryngology practices. Among older persons, the reported prevalence ranges from 13% to 38%. Several factors make dizziness a challenging symptom to evaluate and manage. First, precise classification of the cause is often difficult. Second, patients and clinicians alike may worry about a serious cardiac or neurologic cause. Third, specific therapy is not available for many patients with dizziness. Fourth, like other geriatric syndromes such as delirium and falls, dizziness may be related to multiple potentially causative factors at least half of the time.

CLASSIFICATION

Drachman popularized a symptom-oriented approach, classifying dizziness as vertigo (rotational sensation), presyncope (impending faint), disequilibrium (loss of balance without head sensation), or lightheadedness (ill-defined, not otherwise classifiable). Although some sensations correspond more often than not to at least a general etiologic category (eg, vertigo suggests vestibular dysfunction at least 80% to 90% of the time), these four sensations remain nonspecific, occurring with many different disorders. Following is a brief delineation of the sensations and the most common corresponding causes.

Vertigo

The three most common specific peripheral vestibular disorders are benign positional vertigo (BPV), labyrinthitis, and Ménière's disease. BPV is episodic and aggravated or brought on by changes in position, such as turning, rolling over, getting in and out of bed, or bending over. BPV spells are often brief (5 to 15 seconds) and milder than the severe vertiginous attacks seen with disorders such as labyrinthitis and Ménière's disease. Labyrinthitis (sometimes called vestibular neuronitis) occurs acutely, lasts for several days, and resolves spontaneously. Ménière's disease is characterized by repeated episodes of tinnitus, fluctuating hearing loss, and severe vertigo accompanied eventually by a progressive sensorineural hearing loss. The frequency and severity of vertigo may improve as hearing impairment worsens.

Central vestibular disorders account for a minority of cases of vertigo; these include cerebrovascular disease, brain tumors, multiple sclerosis, and rarer central causes. In vertigo of vascular origin, dizziness has been reported as the presenting symptom less than 20% of the time. Much more commonly, it is preceded or accompanied by other neurologic deficits in the distribution of the posterior circulation. Indeed, verifying a transient ischemic attack as the cause of vertigo can be difficult in the absence of other neurologic deficits, since isolated vertigo is nonspecific and there is no good noninvasive diagnostic test of the vertebrobasilar circulation.

Tumors are found in less than 1% of dizzy patients and are slightly more prevalent (2% to 3%) among older patients referred to neurologists. The most common tumor associated with dizziness is an acoustic neuroma, for which cochlear symptoms (tinnitus and hearing loss) rather than dizziness predominate. Dizziness with unilateral cochlear symptoms suggests acoustic neuroma; bilateral symptoms in older persons typically represent presbycusis rather than a tumor.

Nonvertiginous Dizziness

Presyncope is the sensation of near fainting. This chapter does not deal with full loss of consciousness or syncope, which requires a different diagnostic approach. (See "Syncope," p 156.) Presyncope reflects diminished cerebral perfusion. Cardiac causes of presyncope can be electrical (tachy- or bradyar-rhythmias) or structural (especially aortic outflow obstruction). Vascular causes of syncope are typically not ischemic events but are less serious, reversible conditions, such as orthostatic hypotension or temporary reactions due to vagal stimulation. Most presyncopal patients presenting with dizziness have symptoms attributable to postural change (with or without orthostatic hypotension) rather than more serious cardiac causes. Postural symptoms without orthostatic blood-pressure changes are particularly common in elderly persons. Likewise, orthostatic blood-pressure changes in the absence of symptoms are also quite common. Finally, certain stimuli (eg, micturition, defecation, coughing) can precipitate vagally mediated autonomic changes. Thus, the elderly man who rises to urinate in the middle of the night, the older person straining to have a bowel movement, or the pulmonary patient having paroxysms of coughing can experience lightheadedness or even frank syncope.

Disequilibrium is a sensation of being unsteady when standing or, in particular, walking. Balance depends not only on the vestibular system but also on the visual and somatosensory systems. Thus, multiple factors can contribute to imbalance, including chronic vestibulopathies, visual problems (eg, errors of refraction, cataract, loss of binocular vision, macular degeneration), musculoskeletal disorders (eg, arthritis, muscle weaknesses), and somatosensory or gait deficits (eg, neuropathies, previous strokes, cerebellar disease, Parkinson's disease, dementia).

Lightheadedness is a vaguer sensation best reserved as a descriptor for patients who do not experience one of the three more discrete types of dizziness sensations—vertigo, presyncope, or disequilibrium. In the vernacular of patients, these latter three sensations may be experienced as "spinning," "fainting," or "falling." Although any cause of dizziness may occasionally produce a nondescript "lightheaded" type of sensation, the two most prominent considerations are psychiatric (primarily depressive, anxiety, or somatoform disorders) or idiopathic causes, which together account for up to a third of all cases of dizziness.

Among other causes, prescription drug toxicity is an important contributing factor to dizziness in older patients. The use of at least three to five medications is a risk factor for dizziness among older adults, as are drugs that cause orthostatic hypotension, most commonly cardiovascular, antihypertensive, and psychotropic medications. Three purported causes particularly germane to elderly patients—cervical arthritis, visual disorders, and carotid sinus hypersensitivity—are seldom reported as causes in published series of dizzy patients. In part, this may be due to their common occurrence among older persons without dizziness as well as the fact that confirming these factors as the actual cause of dizziness can be difficult.

PROGNOSIS

Dizziness usually resolves within days to several months, but about one fourth of patients may experience chronic or recurrent symptoms. A 1-year prospective study of 102 patients found that dizziness due to psychiatric disorders, disequilibrium, or a vestibulopathy other than BPV or labyrinthitis was more likely to persist. Among 1087 community-dwelling older persons, chronic dizziness (ie, a month or longer) was reported by 24% and at 1-year follow-up was not associated with mortality, hospitalization, or functional status decline. Chronic dizziness, however, was associated with an increased risk of falling (relative risk of 1.4) and syncope (relative risk of 2.3), as well as worse self-rated health and depression.

EVALUATION

A brief, focused evaluation coupled with simple follow-up rather than initial diagnostic testing or referral is warranted in most patients. As mentioned, symptoms gradually improve in most patients. Moreover, specialized testing only occasionally reveals unsuspected diagnoses. More than 75% of the cases in which a diagnosis can be established are diagnosed by history and physical examination alone, with the history contributing most of these diagnoses.

History

As with many common symptoms, history is the single most useful part of the evaluation. The clinician must establish early on whether dizziness stems from a serious or benign cause. Although it is best to elicit the patient's own description of the event without prompting, four questions are particularly helpful:

- Is the dizziness characterized by one of three key sensations: spinning, fainting, or falling?
- Is there a positional effect on the dizziness and related symptoms? With BPV, the effect is almost always one of transient dizziness with change of head position, lying down, or sitting up. The most common cause of presyncope is an orthostatic change in blood pressure, in which case the patient reports that dizziness occurs on assuming a more upright position (supine to sitting, or sitting to standing). Disequilibrium is manifested only when the patient is walking or standing.
- What associated symptoms are experienced along with the dizziness? Syncope is a particularly important symptom to inquire about, since actual loss of consciousness targets that very small subset of dizzy patients in whom

early cardiac evaluation might be contemplated. Tinnitus or hearing changes, or both, are associated with certain vestibular disorders such as Ménière's disease or the rare acoustic neuroma. Nausea and, in particular, vomiting suggests vertigo rather than a nonvertiginous cause of dizziness. A central cause would not commonly present with isolated dizziness but instead would be expected to produce "neighboring" neurologic symptoms as well. Psychogenic causes, such as depression, anxiety, or somatoform disorders, typically have fatigue, insomnia, pain, or other physical and emotional symptoms in addition to dizziness.

- What medications is the patient taking? One should be particularly suspicious of new medications that were started around the time that symptoms of dizziness began.

Physical Examination

A focused physical examination would include the following steps.

- Measure the blood pressure and pulse while the patient is supine and again after standing for 2 to 3 minutes to detect orthostatic changes.
- Perform the head-hanging (Dix-Hallpike) test (described below).
- Perform a brief cardiovascular (murmurs, abnormal rhythm) and neurologic (cerebellar or focal deficits) examination.
- Observe the patient walk and turn (look for balance or gait difficulties).

Dizziness correlates best with postural hypotension when the latter is defined as a drop (eg, 20% decrease) in mean blood pressure, which is one third systolic plus two thirds diastolic, rather than a drop in systolic pressure only.

A screening vestibular examination is warranted in cases in which the cause of dizziness is not obvious. The four elements of a brief vestibular examination can be performed in about a minute and have in common the detection of nystagmus:

- **Primary position:** Have the patient look straight ahead and look for nystagmus.
- **Gaze-evoked:** Have the patient look to the right, left, up, and down, holding each position for 5 to 10 seconds. Deviations of 30 to 45 degrees of eye movement are sufficient to detect pathologic nystagmus; extreme gaze may accentuate physiologic nystagmus. More than three to five beats of nystagmus is abnormal.

- **Dix-Hallpike test:** With the patient seated on the examination table, help him or her lie down quickly with one ear turned toward the table. Help the patient up to a sitting position and repeat the maneuver with the other ear facing the table. Although hyperextending the patient's neck over the edge of the table has traditionally been recommended, this is not always possible and may not be necessary in many patients. The Dix-Hallpike test is positive in about half of patients with BPV—usually those with symptoms of recent onset. The occurrence of nystagmus (and often vertigo) that lasts 10 to 30 seconds after a few seconds of latency indicates a positive response.

- **Head-shaking:** Have the patient close his or her eyes, rapidly shake the head back and forth for 10 seconds, and then open his or her eyes. Look for nystagmus.

Nystagmus due to peripheral causes usually beats horizontally. Vertical nystagmus (ie, upward or downward beating) is uncommon and should prompt early evaluation (eg, neuroimaging, formal vestibular testing, neurology or otolaryngology referral) for central causes.

Diagnostic Testing

Simple laboratory tests, including complete blood cell counts, electrolytes, glucose level, serum creatinine, thyroid function, and serologic tests for syphilis, have a very low yield. Audiometry may be helpful in the patient with cochlear symptoms, such as tinnitus or asymmetric hearing loss. Abnormal audiograms may indicate Ménière's disease or, rarely, a cerebellopontine angle tumor such as acoustic neuroma. However, the most common abnormal audiometric finding in elderly patients is high-frequency hearing loss due to presbycusis; this represents a coincidental finding rather than a diagnostic explanation of dizziness.

Vestibular testing most commonly involves electronystagmography (ENG), which has important limitations. Sensitivity is variable, and it cannot readily distinguish between central and peripheral causes. In a community-based study of older persons, 80% of dizzy persons and 79% of persons in the control group were found to have at least two ENG abnormalities. Other tests include brain-stem auditory evoked responses, rotatory chair, and dynamic posturography. The latter two tests may substitute for or augment ENG in special situations, while testing for brain-stem auditory evoked responses is occasionally indicated if clinical

evaluation, audiometry, or ENG suggest a central vestibulopathy.

Neuroimaging is occasionally warranted in the evaluation of the dizzy patient. This expensive and relatively low-yield testing should usually be reserved for patients with "red flags" (cerebellar or focal neurologic symptoms, vertical nystagmus). Although a computed tomography scan is the procedure of choice for strokes (because of cost and availability), magnetic resonance imaging (MRI) is better able to image posterior fossa structures. A community-based study of persons aged 65 and older found a similar prevalence of MRI abnormalities in the dizzy and nondizzy groups, prompting the authors to conclude that routine MRI is unlikely to identify a specific cause of dizziness. Neither electroencephalography nor lumbar puncture is typically useful in evaluating dizziness, and noninvasive carotid studies are warranted only if other neurologic symptoms suggest transient ischemic attacks.

An electrocardiogram is commonly obtained in older patients with cardiovascular risk factors but has a low diagnostic value in patients with a normal cardiac examination and nonsyncopal dizziness. Other tests helpful in evaluating syncope, ischemia, or valvular disease (Holter and event monitors, echocardiography, stress testing, tilt tables, and electrophysiologic studies) have not been shown to be useful in evaluating isolated dizziness.

Psychiatric disorders should be considered when the dizziness is nondescript (eg, lightheadedness), persistent and unexplained, or associated with multiple other somatic or emotional symptoms. Although brief case-finding instruments for depression are available, a single question about depressed mood has a sensitivity of 85% to 90% for detecting major depression. (See "Depression and Other Mood Disorders," p 247.)

MANAGEMENT

Although well-proven therapies for dizziness are limited, the natural history is nonetheless often favorable. In up to half of patients, dizziness spontaneously resolves or substantially improves within 2 weeks. In some cases, dizziness is an associated symptom of viral or other self-limited illnesses. Other times, it results from dehydration or a medication adverse effect. The two most common causes of peripheral vertigo—labyrinthitis and BPV—typically resolve within days or weeks, respectively. Types of dizziness for which specific management strategies may be helpful are discussed briefly below.

- **Acute vertigo attacks:** Attacks that occur with peripheral vestibular disorders such as labyrinthitis and Ménière's disease may benefit from meclizine and, if needed, a benzodiazepine. However, meclizine probably is overprescribed for chronic vestibulopathies and nonvertiginous dizziness.

- **Benign positional vertigo:** BPV usually can be treated with simple reassurance, since symptoms are typically mild and usually improve within weeks to several months. For severe or persistent symptoms, the patient may be educated about home habituation exercises or the canalolith repositioning (liberatory) maneuvers developed by Epley and Semont (see Figure 22.1).

- **Ménière's disease:** Attacks that are frequent or disabling may benefit from prophylactic treatment with salt restriction or diuretic therapy, or both. Occasional patients may require referral to otolaryngology for consideration of surgery.

- **Orthostatic hypotension:** Correct reversible causes.

- **Disequilibrium:** Advise the elderly patient with chronic disequilibrium to take measures to prevent falls, including the use of a cane, walker, or other assistive device, if necessary.

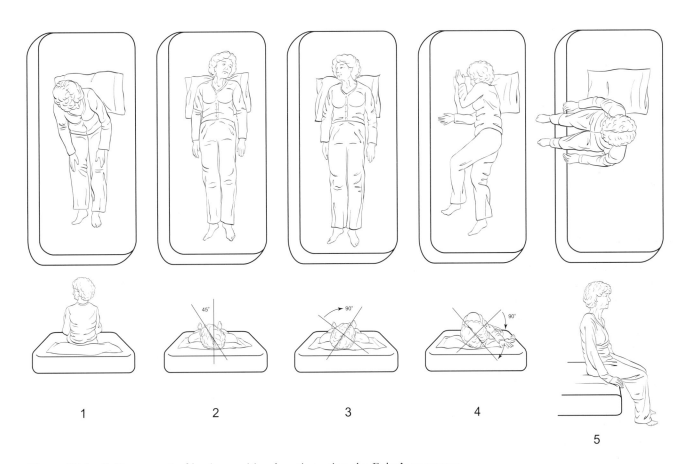

Figure 22.1—Self-treatment of benign positional vertigo using the Epley's manuever.

Perform the maneuver three times a day until free of positional vertigo for 24 hours. Use the positions shown here when the right ear is affected. Reverse all positions (left instead of right) when the left ear is affected. The affected ear is the ear that when turned downward during the Dix-Hallpike maneuver triggers vertigo or nystagmus, or both.

Each maneuver consists of the following steps (numbered to match the illustration):

1. Sit on the bed with a pillow far enough behind you to be under your shoulders when you lie back. Turn your head 45 degrees to the left.

2. Holding your head in the turned position, lie back quickly so that your shoulders are supported on the pillow and your head is reclined on the bed. Hold this position for 30 seconds.

3. Remain prone on the bed and turn your head 90 degrees to the right. Hold this position 30 seconds.

4. Turn your head and body another 90 degrees to the right; you should now be looking down at the bed. Hold this position for 30 seconds.

5. Sit up, facing to the right.

SOURCE: Data from Radtke A, Neuhauser H, von Brevern M, et al. A modified Epley's procedure for self-treatment of benign paroxysmal positional vertigo. *Neurology* 1999;53(6):1358–1360.

- **Psychogenic dizziness:** Psychogenic dizziness may be related to depressive or certain anxiety (eg, panic) disorders. Consider a trial of selective serotonin-reuptake inhibitors. In an open-label study involving 60 patients with dizziness, selective serotonin-reuptake inhibitors[OL] produced improvement in 63% of participants, many who had previously failed vestibular suppressants or benzodiazepines.

- **Chronic vestibulopathy:** Vestibular rehabilitation (a type of physical therapy exercise program) may be beneficial in persons with persistent dizziness.

Finally, when managing a patient with dizziness, it is important to remember that half of patients may have two or more potential causative or contributory factors for their symptoms. In community and clinic-based studies of older persons, Tinetti and colleagues have found several factors associated with dizziness, including depressive or anxiety symptoms, impaired vision or hearing, the use of multiple medications, abnormal balance or gait, postural hypotension, diabetes mellitus, and past myocardial infarction. A multifactorial intervention targeting such factors might reduce the frequency or severity of dizziness in older patients. For example, an elderly patient may have a complex type of dizziness variably described as feeling faint when standing, unsteadiness when walking, and a nagging lightheadedness unrelated to position. Upon evaluation, the patient is found to have orthostatic hypotension related to one or more medications, depression, and disequilibrium due to a peripheral neuropathy and macular degeneration. Identifying potentially remediable factors, such as orthostasis and depression, may at least partially ameliorate the dizziness. In addition, it is important to consider safety issues specific to dizziness including falls (see "Falls" p 187).

REFERENCES

- Barreire SO. Spin cycle: evaluation and management of dizziness and vertigo. *Adv Nurse Pract.* 2005;13(3):22–27; quiz 28.

- Colledge N, Lewis S, Mead G, et al. Magnetic resonance brain imaging in people with dizziness: a comparison with non-dizzy people. *J Neurol Neurosurg Psychiatry.* 2002;72(5):587–589.

- Hoffman R, Einstadter D, Kroenke K. Evaluating dizziness. *Am J Med.* 1999;107(5):468–478.

- Johnson MA. When the report is dizziness. *Geriatr Nurs.* 2006;27(1):41–44.

- Kao AC, Nanda A, Williams CS, et al. Validation of dizziness as a possible geriatric syndrome. *J Am Geriatr Soc.* 2001;49(1):72–75.

- Parnes LS, Agrawal SK, Atlas J. Diagnosis and management of benign paroxysmal positional vertigo (BPPV). *Can Med Assoc J.* 2003;169(7):681–693.

- Sloane PD, Coeytaux RR, Beck RS, et al. Dizziness: state of the science. *Ann Intern Med.* 2001;134(9 Pt 2):823–832.

- Tinetti ME, Williams CS, Gill TM, et al. Dizziness among older adults: a possible geriatric syndrome. *Ann Intern Med.* 2000;132(5):337–344.

- Tinetti ME, Williams CS, Gill TM. Health, functional, and psychological outcomes among older persons with chronic dizziness. *J Am Geriatr Soc.* 2000;48(4):417–421.

CHAPTER 23—SYNCOPE

KEY POINTS

- The incidence of syncope increases with age.

- In older adults, the cause of syncope is often multifactorial. In nearly one in five cases, the cause of syncope is not determined, but these cases generally have a favorable prognosis.

- Though many diagnostic procedures are available to search for the cause of syncope, most of them are expensive and have a low yield unless findings from the history or physical examination suggest a particular cause.

- The absence of cardiac disease strongly suggests that the cause of syncope is not cardiac.

- Bradycardia is the single most common cardiac cause of syncope.

- The treatment of syncope focuses on treating the underlying disorder and often with geriatric patients requires treatment of multiple possible underlying causes.

Syncope—a sudden, transient loss of postural tone and consciousness not due to trauma and with spontaneous full recovery—is common. Annually it accounts for approximately 3% of emergency department visits and 2% to 6% of hospital admissions. The incidence of syncope doubles among those aged 70 and older, and rates among those 80 and older is three to four times that seen among younger persons. Approximately 80% of the patients hospitalized for syncope are aged 65 or older. Syncope is a clinically important condition that is commonly difficult to evaluate. Its potential causes range from those that are benign and self-limited to those that are life threatening. In the older adult, the cause of syncope may also be multifactorial, adding to the diagnostic difficulty. Because it encompasses a wide range of potential causes (see Table 23.1 for the most common causes), the diagnostic evaluation of syncope can be complex and expensive. Although a wide variety of diagnostic tools can be employed, in many cases the patient's history provides the best clues to the cause and help direct the work-up.

NATURAL HISTORY

Syncope is generally caused by a reduction in cerebral perfusion. Hemodynamic disturbances that can decrease cerebral perfusion include alterations in systemic blood pressure or an increase in cerebral vascular resistance. Common causes of transient decreases in blood pressure include the following:

- Cardiac arrhythmias, such as atrial fibrillation with a rapid ventricular response, ventricular tachycardia, sick sinus syndrome with sinus pauses, and atrioventricular block
- Alterations in the peripheral vasculature due to arterial vasodilation or increased venous pooling
- Cardiopulmonary obstruction, such as that due to pulmonary emboli, aortic stenosis, hypertrophic obstructive cardiomyopathy, and atrial myxoma

Syncope can also occur as a consequence of an increase in cerebrovascular resistance. In hyperventilation syndrome and panic attacks, cerebrovascular vasoconstriction can occur without a change in systemic vascular resistance. In this situation, syncope can occur as a result of the relative decrease in cerebral blood flow without systemic hypotension. In rare instances, localized atherosclerotic disease can predispose a person to syncope by decreasing cerebral perfusion without a decrease in systemic blood pressure (vertebral basilar insufficiency and subclavian steal).

Syncope occurs most commonly while a person is standing. The effects of gravity cause up to a third of the blood volume to pool in the lower extremities when a person assumes the standing position. Unopposed, this reduces cardiac output by reducing venous return and decreases cerebral blood pressure. A number of reflex pathways involving the autonomic and endocrine systems are responsible for rapid compensation of the gravitational effects of standing. The baroreceptor reflex is triggered by carotid and aortic baroreceptors, which act to increase autonomic sympathetic tone, resulting in peripheral vasoconstriction and an increase in heart rate. Increased sympathetic activity of the renal nerve leads to stimulation of renin release from the juxtaglomerular apparatus. The activation of the renin-angiotensin system leads to direct vasoconstriction by the action of angiotensin II and the secretion of aldosterone from the adrenal cortex to retain sodium, thereby raising the extracelluar fluid volume. A postural change to a standing position also rapidly reduces the level of atrial natriuretic factor, which is a vasodilator and inhibitor of the renin-angiotensin system. The reduction in atrial natriuretic factor facilitates vasoconstriction, and the activity of the volume effects of the renin-angiotensin contributes to vasoconstriction.

In aging, many of these reflex mechanisms are less responsive. The cardiac response to β-adrenergic stimulation (cardiac acceleration and increased contractility) decreases with advancing age. As a result of this and perhaps other mechanisms, the baroreflex (increasing heart rate and vasoconstriction) is also less effective with advancing age. In addition, comorbid conditions that can affect postural responses, such as diabetes mellitus, are prevalent among elderly persons. Medications such as α-blockers, β-blockers, and tricyclic antidepressants may also impair postural reflexes. The effects of age-related decline in adaptive reflexes, comorbid conditions, and medications may combine, becoming factors in syncopal events in the elderly person. Because older persons have a decreased ability to increase heart rate in response to sympathetic stimulation, blood volume maintenance and vasoconstriction become more important in maintaining postural blood pressure. Thus, the elderly person may be particularly sensitive to the effects of dehydration and vasodilator drugs.

Table 23.1—Common Causes of Syncope in Elderly Persons

Arrhythmia

Aortic stenosis

Carotid sinus hypersensitivity

Hypoglycemia

Myocardial infarction

Orthostatic hypotension

Postprandial hypotension

Psychogenic causes

Pulmonary embolism (large)

Vasovagal faint

The prognosis of syncope depends on the underlying cause. The major issue is whether a cardiac cause is responsible. The 1-year mortality for patients with cardiac causes for syncope averages 18% to 33% (deaths are due to underlying disease, not syncope), whereas syncope due to noncardiac causes has a much more favorable prognosis, a 1-year mortality of approximately 6%. In one third to one half of syncopal patients, no cause can be found. The prognosis for these patients is intermediate but generally favorable.

EVALUATION OF THE PATIENT WITH SYNCOPE

History

The clinical history obtained from the patient and, if possible, from witnesses to the event may provide a diagnosis in up to 50% of cases in which a diagnosis can be established. First, it is important to establish whether the patient suffered a true syncopal event, as opposed to dizziness (disequilibrium) or lightheadedness. Key elements to obtain from the history follow:

- Was there a precipitant? Could the patient's activities around the time of the event have triggered it? Such activities include eating, urinating, coughing, using medication, and experiencing emotional stress. Syncope occurring during physical exertion should raise the possibility of myocardial ischemia or aortic stenosis. A history of syncope after turning motions of the head should raise the possibility of carotid sinus hypersensitivity.

- Were there prodromal symptoms before the event? Symptoms of chest pain, palpitations, or shortness of breath suggest a cardiac or pulmonary cause. Diaphoresis, presyncope, and gastrointestinal symptoms, such as nausea or vomiting, can be associated with vasovagal syncope. Sudden onset of syncope with less than 5 seconds of warning is characteristic of syncope due to a cardiac arrhythmia.

- What medications are being used? It is important to establish how medications were taken with relationship to meals and other activities, and whether there have been recent changes in the medication regimen. Specifics about dosage times should be obtained.

- What did witnesses observe? They should be queried about the duration of the event and the appearance of the patient during the event. Patients with cardiac causes of syncope are generally flaccid in tone and motionless while unconscious, unless the event lasts for more than 15 seconds, when myoclonic jerks and truncal extension may be seen. In contrast, increased body motion, tone, and head turning to one side with loss of consciousness are more common with seizure activity.

- Are there significant comorbid conditions? A history of coronary artery disease or its associated symptoms is particularly important. Approximately 5% of myocardial infarctions present as syncope. Sustained ventricular tachycardia resulting in syncope is most common in patients with prior myocardial infarction. Patients with diabetes mellitus are at increased risk for coronary atherosclerosis as well as autonomic dysfunction predisposing to syncope.

Table 23.2 summarizes the characteristics of three classes of syncope.

Physical Examination

A physical examination should focus on elements raised by the history. It is estimated that of those patients in whom a cause of syncope can be established, 20% are identified by features found during physical examination. The blood pressure should be measured in both arms, as well as postural changes in the blood pressure. The pulse should be taken with the patient in the supine and standing positions. Blood pressure with the patient in the standing position should be obtained after 1 minute of standing and repeated after the patient has been standing for 3 minutes. Although any definition of postural hypotension is arbitrary, a decrease in systolic blood pressure of more than 20 mm Hg is the definition used most frequently.

The character of the carotid pulse should also be assessed for the delayed upstroke and low volume characteristic of significant aortic stenosis. The presence of a carotid bruit, a history of cerebrovascular disease, and recent myocardial infarction are relative contraindications to carotid sinus massage. Even in the absence of contraindications, carotid sinus massage should be performed only under continuous electrocardiographic monitoring (to detect induced atrioventricular [AV] block or other arrhythmias) in a setting where resuscitation equipment is available.

The physical examination of the patient with syncope should include cardiac examination for evidence of murmurs characteristic of valvular abnormalities or extra heart sounds suggestive of cardiomyopathy. Examination of the stool for occult blood and neurologic examination for focal deficits are also important.

An electrocardiogram (ECG) is indicated for all patients presenting with syncope. Though ECG estab-

Table 23.2—Characteristics of Three Classes of Syncope

Phase	Cardiac Arrhythmia	Vasovagal	Seizure
Prior to event	Occurs in any position	Aborted if person lies flat	Any position
	Less than 5 seconds' warning	Seconds' to minutes' warning	No warning or prodrome
	Precipitant absent	Precipitant present	—
	Palpitations rare	—	—
	—	Nausea, diaphoresis common	—
	—	Visual changes	—
During event	Flaccid tone	Motionless, relaxed tone	Rigid tone
	Pulse absent, faint	Slow, faint pulse	Rapid pulse, elevated blood pressure
	Blue, ashen	Pale color	—
	Incontinence rare	—	—
	—	Dilated, reactive pupils	Tonic eye deviation common
	—	—	Frothing at mouth
Recovery	Rapid and complete	Fatigue common after event	Slow, incomplete recovery
	—	No retrograde amnesia	Disorientation
	—	Diaphoresis and nausea common	—
	—	—	Focal neurologic findings

lishes a diagnosis in only 5% of those with syncope, approximately 50% have an abnormal ECG. Abnormalities on an ECG may provide clues for further cardiovascular evaluation; a normal ECG is associated with a more favorable prognosis. Key features to assess on an ECG include evidence of acute or remote myocardial infarction. Conduction abnormalities, especially block in the AV node or below, and pre-excitation, such as Wolff-Parkinson-White, may be detected as well; inappropriate sinus bradycardia may also be found. A prolonged QT interval can predispose a person to ventricular arrhythmias, including torsade de pointes.

Ambulatory Electrocardiographic Monitoring

An ambulatory ECG recording can establish or exclude many causes of syncope if the patient experiences syncopal or presyncopal symptoms during the recording. Unfortunately, the occurrence of symptoms during ambulatory ECG monitoring is relatively rare in most patients with syncope that remains unexplained after a history, physical examination, and ECG. On average, studies examining the diagnostic yield of ambulatory ECG report an arrhythmia correlating with symptoms in approximately 4% of patients. In another 15% of patients studied, an arrhythmia was excluded by the presence of symptoms during the recording, but without evidence of an arrhythmia; in approximately 14% of patients, arrhythmias were found to be present but without concomitant symptoms. These patients may

represent a diagnostic dilemma. However, certain arrhythmias, even asymptomatic ones, such as nonsustained ventricular tachycardia, second- and third-degree AV block, and sinus pauses in excess of 3 seconds, are rare in persons without heart disease. Their presence, even if asymptomatic, in a patient with a history of syncope indicates the need for further evaluation.

Ambulatory loop recorders that may be worn for a many days or weeks at a time are commonly used to capture ECG recordings of symptoms that occur infrequently. These devices constantly record an ECG tracing on a 5- to 10-minute loop; the patient presses a button to stop the recording after an event has occurred and then transmits this by telephone to a monitoring center. Among patients who are able operate the recorder, the diagnostic yield is approximately 25%. However, many elderly patients are unable or unwilling to capture and transmit these recordings.

Implantable Loop Recorders

Subcutaneous implantable loop recorders have been developed; these devices are placed in the prepectoral region under local anesthesia. The devices have long-term memories and a battery life of approximately 14 to 18 months. Generally, no patient intervention is required for the device to store recordings, but the patient can also trigger the device to record and retain an ECG if symptoms occur. Implantable loop recorders have recently been shown to be efficient and cost-effective in establishing a cause in selected patients with an ejection fraction >35% and symptoms not consistent with a neural cause of syncope.

Echocardiography

Two-dimensional echocardiography has a low yield in the absence of features suggestive of heart disease by history, physical examination, or ECG. It is most useful in confirming a specific diagnosis suspected by other assessment. However, unsuspected findings on echocardiography are reported in approximately 5% to 10% of unselected patients. Thus, echocardiography has been advocated for the evaluation of syncope. Occult coronary artery disease is also prevalent among elderly persons, and stress testing is often employed to screen for this. In some patients, particularly those with the suggestion of structural cardiac abnormalities and ischemia by history, physical examination, or ECG, it is efficient to perform stress echocardiography as a single procedure.

Tilt-Table Testing

Head-up tilt-table testing results in pooling of blood in the lower extremities and, in susceptible individuals, may trigger syncope mediated by neurocardiogenic mechanisms. Tilt-table testing is useful for patients suspected of having vasovagal syncope and those with unexplained syncope who are not suspected of having a cardiac cause. In tilt-table testing, the patient reclines on a table that then slowly rotates the patient from supine to head up slowly and passively. The patient is secured on the surface, usually with straps and a foot rest, to minimize muscle contraction and maximize venous pooling in the extremities. The patient is continuously monitored for symptoms and with an electrocardiograph and blood-pressure monitor. The test is considered positive if the patient has a cardioinhibitory or vasodepressor response to tilting, or both. Various protocols are available for this testing, and some may include administration of intravenous medications. The sensitivity and specificity of tilt-table testing vary considerably, depending on the protocol used and the patient population. A positive tilt-table result occurs in approximately 11% of normal elderly persons. Thus, a positive tilt-table result alone does not ensure that a vasovagal event is the cause. It is generally recommended that men over the age of 45 and women over the age of 55 have stress testing prior to tilt-table testing so that a positive result on a tilt-table test does not delay diagnosis of coronary ischemia when that is the true culprit.

Responses to tilt testing performed for syncope evaluation tend to differ by age among persons without significant structural heart disease. Those aged 65 and older tend to have far higher rates of symptoms due to pure vasodilatation without significant change in heart rate than do individuals aged 35 or younger. In contrast, individuals aged 35 or younger tend to have more profound cardioinhibitory responses characterized by profound bradycardia or asystole induced by tilt testing than do those aged 65 and older. The different pattern of responses induced by tilt studies between younger and older persons suggests that different mechanisms for neurocardiogenic syncope predominate at different ages. Exaggerated autonomic response is common in younger persons, whereas attenuated autonomic responses become predominant with advancing age.

Electrophysiologic Studies

Guidelines suggest that invasive electrophysiologic (EP) testing should be employed in the evaluation of patients with structural heart disease with unexplained syncope. There is also agreement that EP testing should not be employed in situations where the results of the test would not influence subsequent treatment or in which a cause of the syncope has been established. The role of EP testing in patients with recurrent syncope with no structural heart disease and negative tilt-table studies remains undefined. EP testing is most sensitive for detecting ventricular arrhythmias in the setting of ischemic heart disease and is less sensitive for the detection of ventricular arrhythmias in dilated nonischemic cardiomyopathies. The sensitivity of EP testing for detecting most bradyarrhythmias is also low.

Neurologic Testing

Neurologic testing, including imaging of the head by computed tomography or magnetic resonance imaging and electroencephalographic recording, is appropriate in situations when focal neurologic signs or symptoms are present or when the history suggests seizure.

TREATMENT

The treatment of syncope depends on the underlying cause. When a single underlying cause is established, that is where therapeutic interventions should be concentrated. This is particularly important for cardiac causes. Myocardial ischemia causing syncope may require revascularization (percutaneous or surgical) or aggressive medical therapy. Valvular heart disease causing syncope, particularly aortic stenosis, is typically managed surgically. Treatment of symptomatic supraventricular tachyarrhythmias, such as atrial flutter or fibrillation, may involve antiarrhythmic drug therapy or electrophysiology ablation procedures. Significant ventricular tachyarrhythmias are often treated with implanted defibrillators or antiarrhythmic drugs. Most bradyarrhythmias causing syncope require pacemakers, unless drug side effects or metabolic disturbances are the principal factors.

Orthostatic hypotension is common among older adults and often responds to modifications in drug regimens. In particular, avoidance of vasodilator drugs may help. An important measure is to ensure that patients have adequate volume by reducing or discontinuing diuretics and, if necessary, liberalizing salt intake. Other nonpharmacologic measures that may help include the use of waist-high compression stockings, squatting, and sleeping in a head-up position. Avoidance of excessively warm environment and activities associated with straining (Valsalva) may also be beneficial. If autonomic dysfunction is present and hypertension, heart failure, and hypokalemia are not concerns, then low-dose fludrocortisone may be effective.

When vasovagal syncope occurs as the result of a specific trigger (eg, sights, smells), avoidance is best if this is feasible. A number of pharmacologic therapies have been proposed, including β-blockers, clonidine, paroxetine, midodrine, and others. The pharmacologic approach to the treatment of vasovagal syncope remains somewhat controversial and may require sequential trials of several agents.

Carotid sinus hypersensitivity is best treated by avoiding stimulating factors (tight collars or rapid neck motions). If these measures are ineffective, pacemaker implantation may be useful.

Postprandial hypotension may be improved by avoidance of alcohol and large carbohydrate meals.

Caffeine consumption and remaining recumbent following meals may also help.

When syncope in the geriatric patient has several causes, addressing a single factor in isolation may be only partially effective, and a broader approach addressing several contributing causes is required. Careful review of medications, as well as discontinuation of medications that increase the risk of syncope, is always an early step.

For patients with recurrent syncope without an identifiable cause, care must be taken to help them avoid harming themselves or others if they remain at risk for syncope. The issue of driving may need to be addressed. Guidelines from the American Heart Association recommend that driving be restricted for several months and that, if the patient remains recurrence free, driving be resumed. However, physicians should be aware that many states have laws regarding driving with a history of syncope.

REFERENCES

- Garcia-Civera R, Ruiz-Granell R, Morell-Cabedo S, et al. Selective use of diagnostic tests inpatients with syncope of unknown cause. *J Am Coll Cardiol.* 2003;41(5):787–790.

- Kurbaan AS, Bowker TJ, Wijesekara N, et al. Age and hemodynamic responses to tilt testing in those with syncope of unknown origin. *J Am Coll Cardiol.* 2003;41(6):1004–1007.

- Soteriades ES, Evans JC, Larson MG, et al. Incidence and prognosis of syncope. *N Engl J Med.* 2002;347(12):878–885.

CHAPTER 24—MALNUTRITION

KEY POINTS

- Aging is associated with changes in body composition such that well-standardized nutrient requirements for younger or middle-aged adults cannot be generalized to older persons.

- The Mini-Nutritional Assessment—Short Form is a brief and simple instrument useful for nutritional screening in geriatric patients.

- Identification of the presence of protein-energy undernutrition or obesity can be facilitated by determining a patient's body mass index.

- Many drugs have anorexia as a major adverse effect or can reduce nutrient availability in the older adult.

- Various appetite stimulants and trophic agents are being used in older patients and are the focus of intensive investigation.

Older persons suffer a burden of malnutrition that spans the spectrum from under- to overnutrition. Nutritional problems accompany many of the chronic disease processes that afflict older persons. Moreover, age-related changes in physiology, metabolism, and function may alter the older person's nutritional requirements. Better understanding among clinicians of the aging process and of nutritional screening, assessment, and interventions could potentially improve the health and independence of older persons.

AGE-RELATED CHANGES

Body Composition

Aging is associated with notable changes in body composition: bone mass, lean mass, and water content all decrease, while fat mass increases. The increase in total body fat is commonly accompanied by greater intra-abdominal fat stores. The consequence of these changes in body composition is that well-standardized nutrient requirements for younger or middle-aged adults cannot be generalized to older persons. The aging process also affects organ functions, although the degree of change observed is highly variable among individuals. Decline in organ functions may affect nutritional assessment and intervention.

Energy Requirements

Reduced basal metabolic rate in older persons reflects loss of muscle mass. The basal metabolic rate is the principal determinant of total energy expenditure; energy expenditure in relation to physical activity is the most variable component. The Harris-Benedict equations may be used to predict basal energy expenditure. A simple method for estimating the total daily energy needs of the older patient is based on body weight alone (Table 24.1). In any determination of energy needs for older persons, care must be taken to avoid overfeeding while still meeting basal requirements.

Macronutrient Needs

Modified food guide pyramids for older persons based upon the USDA food guide pyramid have been released See http://nutrition.tufts.edu/consumer/pyramid.html). The food selections are more relevant to the target audience, and appropriate intakes of water, fiber, and supplements of calcium, vitamin D, and vitamin B_{12} are highlighted. The new USDA food pyramid (http://www.mypyramid.gov) released in 2005 may offer opportunity to further tailor recommendations for older persons.

The Food and Nutrition Board of the Institute of Medicine has released macronutrient guidelines that recommend a prudent diet, with 20% to 35% calories as fat and reduced intakes of cholesterol, saturated fat, and trans-fatty acids. Carbohydrates should constitute 45% to 65% of total calories; complex carbohydrates are the preferred fiber source. More specifically, the recommended fiber intake for those aged 60 years and

Table 24.1—Nutritional Requirement Calculations

Estimation of energy needs on basis of body weight

25–30 kcal/kg body weight /day

For the obese individual, use a reduced compromise body weight that approximates 120% of ideal.

Estimation of energy needs using the Harris-Benedict equation for basal energy expenditure (BEE)

Male BEE = 66 + (13.7 × weight in kg) + (5 × height in cm) – (6.8 × age)

Female BEE = 655 + (9.6 × weight in kg) + (1.8 × height in cm) – (4.7 × age)

Adjust BEE with empiric stress factors (1.00 for nonstressed and 1.5 for stressed) to estimate total energy expenditure of ill elderly patients.

Estimation of protein needs on basis of body weight

Protein = (0.8 to 1.5) g / kg body weight / day

For the obese individual, use ideal body weight.

NOTE: 1 lb = 0.453 kg; 1 in = 2.54 cm.

over is 30 g for men and 21 g for women. Protein intake is recommended at 0.8 g per kg of body weight per day at approximately 10% to 35% of total calories. With stress or injury, protein requirements are typically estimated at 1.5 g per kg of body weight per day, but underlying renal or hepatic insufficiency may warrant protein restriction (Table 24.1).

Micronutrient Requirements

Revisions of the Dietary Reference Intakes include recommended dietary allowances (RDAs) with more specific guidelines for older persons; those for the group aged 71 years and older are shown in Table 24.2.

Fluid Needs

Dehydration is the most common fluid or electrolyte disturbance in older persons. Normal aging is associated with a decreased perception of thirst, impaired response to serum osmolarity, and reduced ability to concentrate urine following fluid deprivation. A decline in fluid intake can also result from disease states that reduce mental or physical ability to recognize or express thirst, or that result in decreased access to water. In general, fluid needs of older persons can be met with 30 mL per kg of body weight per day or 1 mL per kcal ingested. Fluid needs may be altered during episodes of fever or infection, as well as with diuretic or laxative therapy. Common signs of dehydration are decreased urine output, fever, constipation, mucosal dryness, skin turgor changes, and confusion. Altered fluid status (overhydration or underhydration) may affect anthropometric and biochemical measures, resulting in inaccurate assessments.

Table 24.2—Micronutrients: Recommended Dietary Allowances for Persons Aged 71 and Older

Nutrient	Men	Women
Calcium (mg)*	1200	1200
Phosphorus (mg)	700	700
Magnesium (mg)	420	320
Vitamin D (µg)*	15	15
Fluoride (mg)*	4	3
Thiamin (mg)	1.2	1.1
Riboflavin (mg)	1.3	1.1
Niacin (mg)	16	14
Vitamin B_6 (mg)	1.7	1.5
Folate (µg)	400	400
Vitamin B_{12} (µg)	2.4	2.4
Pantothenic acid (mg)*	5	5
Biotin (µg)*	30	30
Choline (mg)*	550	425
Vitamin C (mg)	90	75
α-Tocopherol (mg)	15	15
Selenium (µg)	55	55

*Adequate intakes, not recommended dietary allowances.

SOURCES: Data from: Standing Committee on the Scientific Evaluation of Dietary Reference Intakes, Food and Nutrition Board, Institute of Medicine, *Dietary Reference Intakes for Calcium, Phosphorus, Magnesium, Vitamin D, and Fluoride.* Washington, DC: National Academy Press; 1997. Standing Committee on the Scientific Evaluation of Dietary Reference Intakes, Institute of Medicine, *Dietary Reference Intakes for Thiamin, Riboflavin, Niacin, Vitamin B6, Folate, Vitamin B12, Pantothenic Acid, Biotin, and Choline.* Washington, DC: National Academy Press; 1999. Standing Committee on the Scientific Evaluation of Dietary Reference Intakes, Food and Nutrition Board, *Dietary Reference Intakes for Vitamin C, Vitamin E, Selenium, and Beta Carotene, and Other Carotenoids.* Washington, DC: National Academy Press; 2000. Available at http://www.nal.usda.gov/fnic/etext/000105.html (accessed October 2005).

NUTRITION SCREENING AND ASSESSMENT

Anthropometrics

Anthropometric measurements are a mainstay of nutritional assessment of older persons. An unintended weight loss of 10 pounds in the preceding 6 months is a useful indicator of morbidity. This degree of weight loss is predictive of functional limitations, health care charges, and need for hospitalization. The Minimum Data Set (MDS) used by Medicare-certified nursing homes defines weight loss as 5% or more in the past month or 10% or more in the past 6 months. Body mass index (BMI)—weight in kilograms / (height in meters)^2—has received increasing attention. National Institutes of Health guidelines regarding body size classification have been released (Table 24.3). BMI is a useful measure of body size and indirect measure of body fatness that does not require the use of a reference table of ideal weights. The risk threshold for low BMI is set at 18.5. Other anthropometric tools include skin-fold and circumference measurements, but their practical application has been limited because of the difficulty of achieving acceptable reliability among trained personnel.

Table 24.3—Body Size Classification

Body Size	Body Mass Index (kg/m^2)
Underweight	< 18.5
Normal weight	18.5–24.9
Overweight	25–29.9
Obesity	≥ 30
Extreme obesity	≥ 40

NOTE: 1 lb = 0.453 kg; 1 in = 2.54 cm.

SOURCE: Data from: NHLBI Obesity Education Initiative Expert Panel. *Clinical Guidelines on the Identification, Evaluation, and Treatment of Overweight and Obesity in Adults: The Evidence Report.* Bethesda, MD: National Institutes of Health, National Heart, Lung and Blood Institute; September 1998: xiv. Pub. No. 98-4083.

Nutritional Intake

Generally, inadequate nutritional intake has been defined as average or usual intake of servings of food groups, nutrients, or energy below a threshold level of the RDA. The limited reliability of accurately assessing dietary intake measures is well known, so thresholds of 25% to 50% below the RDA have generally been selected. A study found reduced energy intake (less than 50% of calculated maintenance energy requirements) in 21% of a sample of hospitalized older persons. This subset of patients had higher rates of in-hospital mortality and 90-day mortality than did those above the threshold of energy intake. The MDS uses a different measure: intake of less than 75% of food provided is the threshold to trigger nutritional assessment in nursing homes. Surveys of nutritional status conducted among chronically institutionalized older persons suggest that 5% to 18% of nursing-home residents have energy intakes below their recommended average energy expenditure.

Energy intakes of men and women aged 65 to 98 years have been estimated in a nationwide food consumption survey. Investigators report that 37% to 40% of the men and women studied had energy intakes lower than two thirds of the RDA, and many reported skipping at least one meal each day. Estimated intakes by consumption surveys, however, may be unreliable because some studies suggest that older persons under-report energy intakes by 20% to 30%.

Food security issues are prevalent contributors to inadequate nutritional intakes among older persons. It is important to ascertain whether limitations in resources, transportation, or functionality may limit access to food or ability to prepare food.

Laboratory Tests: Albumin, Prealbumin, Cholesterol

Serum albumin has been recognized as a risk indicator for morbidity and mortality. Hypoalbuminemia lacks specificity and sensitivity as an indicator of malnutrition; however, it may be associated with injury, disease, or inflammation. As a negative acute phase reactant, it is subject to cytokine-mediated decline in synthesis and to increased degradation and transcapillary leakage. It is thought that albumin synthesis does not decrease with age; however, longitudinal studies of serum albumin suggest a modest decline in levels with aging that may be independent of disease. The prognostic value of hypoalbuminemia may be largely due to its utility as a proxy measure for injury, disease, or inflammation. In the community setting, hypoalbuminemia has been associated with functional limitation, sarcopenia, increased health care use, and mortality. In the hospital setting, it has also been associated with increased length of hospital stay, complications, readmissions, and mortality. Other protein markers of nutritional status are being investigated. Prealbumin has received the most attention, because it has a considerably shorter half-life than albumin and may therefore more adequately reflect short-term changes in protein status. Unfortunately, prealbumin otherwise appears to suffer the same limitations as albumin as an indicator of nutritional status.

Serum cholesterol has also been linked to nutritional status. Low cholesterol levels (<160 mg/dL) are often detected in persons with serious underlying disease, such as malignancy. Poor clinical outcomes have been observed among hospitalized and institutionalized older persons with hypocholesterolemia. A study of community-dwelling older persons found that those in the lowest quartile of serum cholesterol did not differ from others in their nutrient intakes. It appears likely, again, that acquired hypocholesterolemia is a nonspecific feature of poor health status that is independent of nutrient or energy intakes, and that it may better reflect a proinflammatory condition. Of interest is the observation that community-dwelling older persons with both hypoalbuminemia and hypocholesterolemia exhibit the highest rates of adverse functional and mortality outcomes in comparison with those with hypoalbuminemia or hypocholesterolemia alone.

Drug-Nutrient Interactions

Drugs may modify the nutrient needs and metabolism of older persons. Certain drugs, such as digoxin and phenytoin, even at therapeutic levels, can cause anorexia in the older person. Additional agents that have anorexia as a major potential adverse effect include selective serotonin-reuptake inhibitors, calcium channel blockers (dihydropyridines), H_2 receptor antagonists, proton-pump inhibitors, narcotic analgesics, furosemide, potassium supplement, ipratropium bromide, and theophylline. Many drugs are known to interfere with taste and smell (see "Oral Diseases and

Disorders," Table 42.2, p 299) and others may reduce the availability of specific nutrients (Table 24.4).

Multi-Item Tools for Nutrition Screening

The nutritional status of the older person can be influenced by a variety of factors (Table 24.5). The absence of single assessment measures that are valid indicators of comprehensive nutritional status has prompted the development of multi-item tools. Older persons in acute- or chronic-care facilities have been extensively studied to identify indicators and predictors of nutritional status, while those in the community setting have been studied less. Nutrition screening tools for older persons have been widely disseminated, and health professionals are beginning to use such tools for a variety of purposes. Their effectiveness remains to be demonstrated; specifically, we need to learn whether these tools can identify undernourished individuals whose problems are amenable to intervention.

The Nutrition Screening Initiative is a collaborative effort of the American Dietetic Association, the American Academy of Family Practitioners, and the National Council on Aging, Inc. Three interdisciplinary tools to

Table 24.4—Drug-Nutrient Interactions

Drug	Reduced Nutrient Availability
Alcohol	Zinc, vitamins A, B_1, B_2, B_6, folate, vitamin B_{12}
Antacids	Vitamin B_{12}, folate, iron, total kcal
Antibiotics, broad-spectrum	Vitamin K
Colchicine	Vitamin B_{12}
Digoxin	Zinc, total kcal (via anorexia)
Diuretics	Zinc, magnesium, vitamin B_6, potassium, copper
Isoniazid	Vitamin B_6, niacin
Levodopa	Vitamin B_6
Laxatives	Calcium, vitamins A, B_2, B_{12}, D, E, K
Lipid-binding resins	Vitamins A, D, E, K
Metformin	Vitamin B_{12}, total kcal
Mineral oil	Vitamins A, D, E, K
Phenytoin	Vitamin D, folate
Salicylates	Vitamin C, folate
SSRIs	Total kcal (via anorexia)
Theophylline	Total kcal (via anorexia)
Trimethoprim	Folate

NOTE: SSRI = selective serotonin-reuptake inhibitor.
SOURCE: Modified from Silver AJ. Malnutrition. In: Beck JC, ed. *Geriatric Review Syllabus: A Core Curriculum in Geriatric Medicine.* 1st ed. New York: American Geriatrics Society; 1989:100.

Table 24.5—Risk Factors for Poor Nutritional Status

Alcohol or substance abuse

Cognitive dysfunction

Decreased exercise

Depression, poor mental health

Functional limitations

Inadequate funds

Limited education

Limited mobility, transportation

Medical problems, chronic diseases

Medications

Poor dentition

Restricted diet, poor eating habits

Social isolation

screen for nutrition risk were developed by the Nutrition Screening Initiative to aid in the evaluation of the nutritional status of older persons. The DETERMINE checklist was created to raise public awareness about the importance of nutrition to the health of older persons (see the Appendix, p 463 and http://www.aafp.org/nsi.xml). This self-report questionnaire is composed of 10 items and is intended to identify potential risks, but not to diagnose malnutrition. The Level I screen, intended for use by health care professionals, incorporates additional assessment items regarding dietary habits, functional status, living environment, and weight change, as well as measures of height and weight. The Level II screen, for use by more highly trained medical and nutrition professionals and suggested for use in the diagnosis of malnutrition, contains all the items from Level I with additional biochemical and anthropometric measures, as well as provision for more detailed evaluation of depression and mental status, as indicated (see http://www.aafp.org/nsi.xml).

The Mini-Nutritional Assessment tool was developed to evaluate the risk of malnutrition among frail older persons and identify those who may benefit from early intervention. More extensive cross validation studies among healthy older persons have since been completed. This assessment tool requires administration by a trained professional and is composed of 18 items. The assessment includes questions about BMI, mid-arm and calf circumferences, weight loss, living environment, medications, dietary habits, clinical global assessment, and self-perception of health and nutrition status. A shortened screening version that contains only six items, the short form Mini-Nutritional Assessment (MNA-SF), is now available (see http://www.mna-elderly.com/clinical-practice.htm).

NUTRITION SYNDROMES

Undernutrition

Attempts to subdivide the group of nutritional syndromes characterized by loss of weight have been challenging. The nomenclature used implies that these syndromes are distinct, when in practice it is often quite difficult to distinguish one from another, and the syndromes commonly overlap. The presence (cachexia) or absence (wasting) of cytokine-mediated response to injury or disease is at times used, but in examples such as the weight loss from AIDS, there appears that some, but not all, of the loss is the result of inflammation. Some authors note that with cachexia, resting energy expenditure is increased whereas with wasting it is decreased, but this measure is not generally available to most practicing clinicians. Even more confusing are the terms *semi-starvation* and *protein-energy undernutrition*, both of which imply that nutritional interventions would be the appropriate correction of the underlying problem, but as will be discussed in the following section, data to support this implication are weak.

Obesity

The growing prevalence of obesity in America extends to older persons in their 60s and 70s. According to National Health and Nutrition Examination Surveys (NHANES), the prevalence of obesity (BMI $\geq$30) has climbed from 14% to 31% between the years 1976 and 2000. Trends were similar for all age, gender, and racial or ethnic groups (see Table 24.6).

Excess body weight and modest weight gain ($\geq$5 kg or greater) in middle age may be associated with medical comorbidities in later life that include hypertension, diabetes mellitus, cardiovascular disease, and osteoarthritis. Adverse outcomes associated with obesity include impaired functional status, increased health care resource use, and increased mortality. A BMI of $\geq$35 is associated with increased risk for functional decline among older persons. Many homebound older persons are now found to be obese. Of interest, poor diet quality and micronutrient deficiencies are relatively common among obese older persons, especially obese older women living alone. Change (increase or decrease) in body weight may be even more strongly correlated with mortality and comorbid conditions like cardiovascular disease or functional limitation. The National Institutes of Health has suggested: "Age alone should not preclude weight loss treatment for older adults. A careful evaluation of potential risks and benefits in the individual patient should guide management." The focus must be on achieving a more healthful weight to promote improved health, function, and quality of life. A combination of prudent diet,

Table 24.6—Prevalence of Overweight and Obesity Among Older Persons: NHANES 1976–80, 1988–94, and 1999–2000

Age (*years*) and Gender	Overweight (%)			Obese (%)		
	1976–80	1988–94	1999–2000	1976–80	1988–94	1999–2000
Men 65–74	54.2	68.5	77.2	13.2	24.1	33.4
Men ≥ 75	—	56.5	66.4	—	13.2	20.4
Women 65–74	59.5	60.3	70.1	21.5	26.9	38.8
Women ≥ 75	—	52.3	59.6	—	19.2	25.1

SOURCE: Data from National Center for Health Statistics, *Health, United States, 2002* (Hyattsville, MD: Centers for Disease Control and Prevention, National Center for Health Statistics; 2002), table 70.

behavior modification, and activity or exercise may be appropriate for selected candidates. For frail obese older persons, the emphasis may better be placed not on weight reduction, but on preservation of strength and flexibility.

NUTRITIONAL INTERVENTIONS

Oral Nutrition and Supplements

Preventing undernutrition is much easier than treating it. Food intake can be enhanced by catering to food preferences as much as possible and avoiding therapeutic diets unless their clinical value is certain. Patients should be prepared for meals with appropriate hand and mouth care, and they should be comfortably situated for eating. Those needing assistance with eating should be helped. Placing two or more patients together for meals can increase sociability and food intake. Foods should be of appropriate consistency, prepared with attention to color, texture, temperature, and arrangement. The use of herbs, spices, and hot foods helps to compensate for loss of the sense of taste and smell often accompanying old age and to avoid the excessive use of salt and sugar (see "Oral Diseases and Disorders," p 294). Hard-to-open individual packages should be avoided. Adequate time should be taken for leisurely meals. Title III C of the Older Americans Act has provided for congregate and home-delivered meals for older persons, regardless of economic status. This service is available in most parts of the country, although in some locations there is a waiting list. Adequate access to nutritious and appetizing food should be assured for patients of various cultural backgrounds and in all settings.

Dietary supplements have been widely used in an effort to enhance nutrient intake. Food intake is often decreased by the use of such supplements, but there is usually an increase in overall nutritional intake owing to the nutrient quality and density of the supple-ments. Standard supplements contain macro- and micro-

nutrients and are available in liquid and bar forms. They are selected on the basis of the patient's preference and chewing ability and on their cost.

There is also growing interest in the use of micronutrient supplements in health promotion. A wide variety of vitamin and mineral supplements are now commonly available in supermarkets and drugstores. New recommendations for older persons include higher intake of calcium and vitamin D to prevent osteoporosis (see Table 24.2). Immune function may be improved by supplementation of protein, vitamin E, zinc, and other micronutrients. Whether the effects of antioxidants are beneficial is the subject of controversy; it has been suggested that they may help in preventing age-related cataracts and macular degeneration and that naturally occurring dietary antioxidants may reduce cardiovascular disease and mortality. Vitamin E supplementation has not been shown to slow the progression of Alzheimer's disease or prevent cardiovascular disease, and it may be associated with higher risk of hemorrhagic stroke. DNA damage from micronutrient deficiencies may be factors in cancer promotion. Since approximately 50% of older persons may also take self-prescribed dietary supplements, it is imperative that the clinician obtain information about the older patient's use of all supplements. The appropriateness and safety of each supplement should be evaluated, since consumers are often unaware of potential risks and adverse effects of many over-the-counter supplements, and solid evidence in favor of these purported benefits are currently lacking.

Drug Treatment for Undernutrition Syndromes

A number of agents have been suggested to promote increased appetite or to serve as anabolic aids. Appetite stimulants include the antidepressant mirtazapine [OL], the serotonin and histamine antagonist cyproheptadine[OL], the progestin megestrol[OL] and the cannabinoid dronabinol[OL]. Anabolic aids include human growth hormone, testosterone, and oxandrolone. However, the use of all these drugs for the treatment of undernutrition syndromes is not FDA approved, and side

[OL] Not approved by the U.S. Food and Drug Administration for this use.

effects in older persons are an issue. In adition, the small amount of research that has been done on the anabolic aids has not demonstrated clinically meaningful benefits to date.

ETHICAL AND LEGAL ISSUES

In the nursing home, unacceptable weight loss, as defined by the Omnibus Budget Reconciliation Act of 1987, is any loss greater than or equal to 5% in the past month or 10% in the past 6 months. The MDS is a functionally based assessment tool performed on admissions to long-term-care facilities that are receiving payments from the Centers for Medicare and Medicaid Services. Sections of the MDS that are related to nutritional status include those assessing cognitive function, mood and behavior, physical function, health condition, oral and nutritional status, dental status, skin condition, and special treatments and procedures, including restorative care for eating and swallowing. Resident Assessment Protocols ensure prompt identification of problems focused on by the MDS. Standards of care dictate that:

- a resident maintain acceptable parameters of nutritional status such as body weight and protein levels, unless the resident's clinical condition demonstrates that this is not possible, and
- a resident receive a therapeutic diet when there is a problem.

Adequate nutrition and hydration should always be provided to the elderly patient unless:

- a fully competent older person refuses invasive nutritional support after having been fully apprised of the potential consequences and states this in written form with witnesses, or
- the terminally ill older person has executed a

legally binding living will or medical directive that precludes artificial feeding in the event of terminal illness or impending death.

Standards of care and ethical principles also maintain that artificial feeding may be withheld or terminated in accordance with a patient's advance directive (known as *advance care plan* in some contexts), with careful consideration of additional comorbidities and futility. Appropriate counseling of the patient and surrogate regarding the consequences of withholding feeding is obligatory. After total cessation of nutrition, several weeks may ensue before death. In this setting, palliative care, including emotional support, is extremely important and complex (see "Palliative Care," p 125, "Legal and Ethical Issues," p 20; "Eating and Feeding Problems," below).

REFERENCES

- DiMaria-Ghalili RA, Amella E. Nutrition in older adults. *Am J Nurs.* 2005;105(3):52–62.

- Flegal, KM, Carroll MD, Ogden CL, et al. Prevalence and trends in obesity among US adults, 1999–2000. *JAMA.* 2002;288(14):1723–1727.

- Institute of Medicine, Food and Nutrition Board. *Dietary Reference Intakes for Energy, Carbohydrate, Fiber, Fat, Fatty Acids, Cholesterol, Protein, and Amino Acids (Macronutrients).* Washington, DC: National Academy Press; 2002.

- Kedziera P, Coyle N. Hydration, thirst, and nutrition. In Ferrell Br, Coyle N, eds. *Textbook of Palliative Nursing, 2nd ed.* NY: Oxford University Press; 2006:239–247.

- Sullivan DH, Johnson LE. Nutrition and aging. In Hazzard WR, Blass JP, Halter JB, et al, eds. *Principles of Geriatric Medicine and Gerontology, 5th ed.* NY: McGraw Hill; 2003:1151–1169.

CHAPTER 25—EATING AND FEEDING PROBLEMS

KEY POINTS

- Several age-related changes in older persons contribute to a slowed ability to swallow.
- Dementia is the most common cause of oral dysphagia.
- Most healthy people aspirate without any important clinical consequences.

- Aspiration pneumonia is believed to occur when contaminated oral secretions arrive in the lungs in a high enough inoculum to overcome host defenses.
- No studies demonstrate that feeding tubes reduce the occurrence of aspiration, but rather, many studies identify feeding tubes as major risk factors for aspiration.

- The assessment of swallowing function is controversial. Data correlating specific findings from any type of swallowing examination with clinically meaningful outcomes are lacking.

Swallowing is an important and complex task that can be affected by both normal aging and by diseases that are common in older persons. Treatment of eating and feeding problems varies, depending on the identified cause or causes and contributing factors.

SWALLOWING IN HEALTH AND DISEASE

Swallowing and Aging

Swallowing can be divided into three phases on the basis of anatomy. First is the preparatory or oral phase, which includes the complex activities of mastication and propelling the food bolus to the back of the mouth toward the pharynx. This stage is under voluntary control. The second or pharyngeal phase is involuntary and involves the initiation of the swallow reflex with propulsion of the food bolus past the laryngeal vestibule and into the esophagus. Execution of the oral and pharyngeal phases of swallowing requires the complex coordination of five cranial nerves and a large number of small muscles in the head and neck, with regulation from cortical input to the medullary swallow center, all in the appropriate sequence, usually within 1 second. The third stage of swallowing is the esophageal phase, during which food is propelled down the esophagus by the action of skeletal muscle proximally and smooth muscle distally; this phase is regulated by its own intrinsic innervation.

Normal aging is associated with several alterations in eating. With advanced age, there is a diminution of the taste sensation, but not of taste discrimination (an older person may be able to distinguish sweet from salty but may need to add more salt to food to taste it sufficiently). Further, olfactory function declines with advancing age, further impairing taste sensation. Salivary function is not clearly reduced with aging, but xerostomia is a common complaint of older persons, usually owing to the adverse effects of medication. Loss of teeth greatly reduces chewing efficiency (ie, the need to chew for a longer period of time and with more chewing strokes to achieve the same level of food maceration), which is only partly ameliorated with dental prostheses. Sarcopenia, or age-related loss of lean muscle mass, may contribute to loss in chewing efficiency and to pharyngeal muscle weakness demonstrated on videofluoroscopic deglutition examination of asymptomatic older persons. Whether aging alone contributes to esophageal dysmotility (so-called

presbyesophagus) remains a subject of debate. Esophageal function is probably well preserved, except, perhaps, in very advanced age. In total, these changes with age result in a prolonged duration of each swallow. Further, many diseases that produce dysphagia are more common in older persons.

Dysphagia

Dysphagia, or difficulty swallowing, can occur when a disease affects any level of swallowing function. Dysphagia is usually classified as oral, pharyngeal, or esophageal. Oral dysphagia occurs when there is difficulty with the voluntary transfer of food from the mouth to the pharynx. This might be diagnosed, for example, when scrambled eggs are discovered in the cheeks of a demented patient shortly before lunch. The most common cause of oral dysphagia is dementia.

In pharyngeal dysphagia, reflexive transfer of the food bolus from the pharynx to initiate the involuntary esophageal phase of swallowing while simultaneously protecting the airway from misdirection of food is difficult. The affected person may notice coughing, choking, or nasal regurgitation while eating and localize the symptoms to the throat. The most common cause of pharyngeal dysphagia is stroke, but any disease that impairs the swallowing center in the brain stem or the cranial nerves involved (eg, Parkinson's disease, central nervous system tumor), the oropharyngeal striated muscle (eg, myasthenia gravis, amyotrophic lateral sclerosis), or the local structures involved (eg, retropharyngeal abscess, tumor) may lead to pharyngeal dysphagia. Treatment of both oral and pharyngeal dysphagia involves treatment of the underlying disorder and devising an individualized, often labor-intensive, feeding program.

Esophageal dysphagia presents with the sensation that food has gotten "stuck" after a swallow. Dysphagia for both solids and liquids suggests an esophageal motility disorder (eg, achalasia, scleroderma), whereas progressive dysphagia for solids suggests a mechanical obstruction (eg, cancer, esophageal ring, stricture from mucosal irritation). None of these diseases is unique to the geriatric population, though older persons tend to take more medications and are therefore more likely to experience medication-induced esophagitis (which manifests initially as odynophagia, followed by dysphagia). Common causes of medication-induced esophagitis in older persons are potassium, nonsteroidal anti-inflammatory agents, alendronate, and tetracycline-related antibiotics. (See also the section on dysphagia in "Gastrointestinal Diseases and Disorders," p 357.)

Aspiration

The misdirection of pharyngeal contents into the airway is termed *aspiration*. Generally, there are two major sources of aspiration: oropharyngeal flora or gastric contents. Despite this relatively straightforward definition, however, controversy persists over the definition of *aspiration pneumonia*. Aspiration pneumonia is believed to occur when bacteria arrive in the lungs from the pharynx in a large enough inoculum to overcome host defenses. Pneumococcal pneumonia arises from aspiration of this organism from a colonized oropharynx, however, and is usually not considered an aspiration pneumonia. Aspiration of gastric contents, or Mendelson's syndrome, usually results in a chemical pneumonitis, and the usefulness of antibiotics in this situation is questionable. Most often, local host defense mechanisms clear the lung of the offending aspirate, without serious clinical impact. It is well established that many healthy individuals episodically aspirate without any important clinical consequences.

Neither aspiration of contaminated oral contents nor of gastric contents is prevented by placement of a feeding tube. Tube feeding is universally cited as a risk factor for major aspiration, and some patients who have never previously aspirated begin to do so after placement of a feeding tube. A 1996 review found no evidence that tube feeding of any sort would reduce the risk of aspiration pneumonia. A common misconception is that jejunostomy tube feeding has lower rates of associated aspiration of gastric contents than gastrostomy does; however, there is no evidence to support this misconception. A single nonrandomized prospective comparison of hand with tube feeding in patients with oropharyngeal aspiration found that hand feeding (personal assistance with oral intake) results in lower rates of pneumonia. No prospective randomized trials comparing hand with tube feeding to reduce aspiration have been published. An active area of clinical research is focused on the role of substance P in swallowing and aspiration and the potential benefit of angiotensin-converting enzyme inhibitors (which prevent the breakdown of substance P) in patients who aspirate, but to date this research is inconclusive.

Assessment of Oropharyngeal Dysphagia

Several tools may be used to assess swallowing function when oropharyngeal dysphagia is clinically suspected. The most common are the full bedside evaluation, of which there are many variations, and the videofluoroscopic deglutition examination (VDE), a variant of the modified barium swallow. There is considerable controversy regarding the relative efficacy of these tools.

VDE is usually performed by a speech-language pathologist who videotapes the patient swallowing several consistencies of barium-impregnated foods while the patient maintains various head positions. This may permit identification of the food consistency or compensatory mechanisms that minimize fluoroscopic evidence of aspiration. Depending on the results of the VDE, the therapist may recommend swallow therapy or diet modifications, or both. Swallow therapy may be compensatory (eg, turn head toward weaker side while swallowing), indirect (eg, exercises to improve the strength of the involved muscles), or direct (ie, exercises to perform while swallowing, such as swallowing multiple times per bolus). Dietary recommendations generally consist of altering bolus size or consistency of food or of restricting foods of certain consistencies.

Data conflict regarding the usefulness of VDE and subsequent treatment recommendations and derive from small, historically controlled studies rather than larger prospective randomized trials. A systematic review of studies of dysphagia secondary to stroke published by the Agency for Health Care Policy and Research (now the Agency for Healthcare Research and Quality) concluded that evidence was insufficient to recommend one type of swallowing study over another and that data correlating specific findings from any type of examination with clinically meaningful outcomes are lacking.

FEEDING

When an older person experiences difficulty eating, the two main therapeutic approaches are careful feeding by hand or tube. The first requires extraordinary patience and is labor intensive; the latter is an invasive intervention associated with its own risks. Data about either approach are limited, and randomized comparisons have not been done. The role of dietary supplements, if any, in augmenting the caloric intake of hand-fed persons has not been clearly defined. One systematic review suggested a mortality benefit to the use of oral protein and energy supplements in acutely hospitalized or community-dwelling persons older than age 65 years, though the quality of the studies reviewed was not optimal. Functional status does not appear to be improved with oral nutritional supplements in any of the studies evaluating this outcome. (See Table 25.1 for details about the composition of specific feeding solutions.)

The number of percutaneous endoscopic gastrostomy (PEG) feeding tubes placed in patients aged 65 years and older has grown at an astonishing rate over the past decade. Low procedure-related complication rates are often cited; however, long-term studies reveal substantial mortality among tube-fed patients. Despite the popularity of feeding tubes, a

Table 25.1—Composition of Commonly Used Tube-Feeding Solutions

Trade Name	Calories (kCal/mL)	Protein (g/L)	Carbohydrate (g/L)	Sodium (mEq/L)	Osmolarity (mOsm/kg)	Comments
Ensure HP	0.95	50	150	53	610	Useful when caloric requirements are less
Ensure Plus HN	1.50	63	199	52	650	Useful for fluid-restricted patients
Jevity 1.2	1.20	56	175	59	450	Good source of fiber
Nepro	2.00	70	215		635	Designed for patients with renal failure
Osmolite	1.06	37	151	28	300	Standard feeding solution
Pulmocare	1.50	63	106	57	475	Designed to reduce CO_2 production
Two Cal HN	2.00	84	217	57	690	Useful for fluid-restricted patients

review of the literature from 1966 to 1999 found no studies demonstrating improved survival, reduced incidence of pneumonia or other infections, improved symptoms or function, or reduced pressure ulcers with the use of feeding tubes of any type in demented persons who have eating difficulties. Median survival after placement of a feeding tube is well under a year, but it is unknown whether this results from tube feeding or if the need for tube feeding is a marker that death is near.

Complications described with feeding tubes are numerous and include an increased risk of aspiration pneumonia, metabolic disturbances, diarrhea, and local cellulitis. Monitoring for these complications should be meticulous. A study employing a large administrative data set found that 1-year mortality was higher in 5266 nursing-home residents with chewing or swallowing difficulties who were fed with a tube than in those who were not, even when statistically accounting for potential confounding variables. A second study by the same authors of 1386 nursing-home residents with recent progression to severe cognitive impairment found no improvement in 2-year survival in the group who were tube fed, again adjusting for potential confounders. No prospective randomized studies comparing tube and hand feeding have been published, and information on quality-of-life outcomes is sorely needed.

Placement of a PEG or jejunostomy bypasses the oropharynx and the esophagus and allows nutrients and medications to be instilled directly into the stomach or the jejunum and be absorbed by a functioning gut. There is little evidence to support the use of feeding tubes in most debilitating chronic diseases, and in particular the wealth of data demonstrate that their use has no clinical benefit in patients with oropharyngeal dysphagia from dementia. It is clear that neither gastrostomy nor jejunostomy feeding tubes reduce aspiration in comparison with a program of hand feeding, but no randomized trials comparing these interventions have been published. The only disease for which feeding tubes have been shown to be of clinical benefit to the patient is esophageal obstruction, such as from malignancy. For most other disease states, their utility remains unproved.

Contraindications to gastrostomy include the inability to pass an endoscope into the stomach, uncorrectable coagulopathy, massive ascites, peritonitis, and bowel obstruction. After successful placement of a gastrostomy, tube feedings of commercially available canned nutritional supplements can be initiated either as slow gravity boluses over 30 to 60 minutes or as a continuous drip. The feeding tube should be flushed with water before and after each feeding or at least four times a day in cases of continuous feedings.

Consideration of feeding tube placement requires careful examination of the data, with a focus on whether there is evidence of clinical benefit to support this invasive and potentially burdensome approach.

Not all feeding problems, of course, are related to dysphagia, and many contributing factors are quite amenable to therapy. Other approaches to consider in older persons who demonstrate eating or feeding problems are evaluation for depression, elimination of unduly restrictive diets, consideration of individual food preferences, consideration of the environment in which the person eats to improve socialization and reduce disruptive stimuli, examination of the condition of the oral cavity, determination of the needs for personal assistance with feeding, and reduction or elimination of medications that may cause inattention, xerostomia, movement disorders, or anorexia. Small studies have documented improved clinical outcomes in nursing-home residents with the use of flavor enhancers, increased food variety, and attention to the meal ambiance.

REFERENCES

■ Finucane TE, Christmas C, Travis K. Tube feeding in patients with advanced dementia. *JAMA*. 1999;282(14): 1365–1370.

- Marik PE, Kaplan D. Aspiration pneumonia and dysphagia in the elderly. *Chest.* 2003;124(1):328–336.

- Mitchell SL, Kiely DK, Lipsitz LA. Does artificial enteral nutrition prolong the survival of institutionalized elders with chewing and swallowing problems? *J Gerontol A Biol Sci Med Sci.* 1998;53(3):M207–M213.

- Simmons S, Schnelle J. Feeding assistance needs of long-stay nursing home residents and staff time to provide care. *J Am Geriatr Soc.* 2006;54(6):919–924.

- Simmons S, Patel A. Nursing home staff delivery of oral liquid nutritional supplements to residents at risk for unintentional weight loss. *J Am Geriatr Soc.* 2006;54(9):1372–1376.

CHAPTER 26—URINARY INCONTINENCE

KEY POINTS

- Of persons aged 65 years and over, 15% to 30% in the community and at least 50% in long-term care are incontinent.

- Especially in older persons, incontinence may not reflect abnormal micturition physiology. Continence also depends on the ability to toilet oneself and the absence of medical conditions, medications, or other factors that cause or contribute to lower urinary tract dysfunction or affect volume status and urine excretion.

- The multifactorial nature of urinary incontinence requires a comprehensive diagnostic evaluation with a careful search for all possible causes and precipitants beyond the genitourinary tract.

- Correction of medical illnesses, medications, and other precipitating factors are crucial for improving continence.

Urinary incontinence (UI) is a multifactorial syndrome produced by a combination of genitourinary pathology, age-related changes, and comorbid conditions that impair normal micturition or the functional ability to toilet oneself, or both.

PREVALENCE AND IMPACT

The prevalence of UI increases with age and affects women more than men (2:1) until age 80, after which men and women are equally affected. Of persons aged 65 years and over, 15% to 30% in the community and at least 50% in long-term care are incontinent. UI may cause morbidity, including cellulitis, pressure ulcers, urinary tract infections, falls with fractures, sleep deprivation, social withdrawal, depression, and sexual dysfunction. UI is not associated with increased mortality. UI impairs quality of life, affecting the older person's emotional well-being, social function, and general health. Incontinent persons often manage to maintain their activities, but with an increased burden of coping, embarrassment, and poor self-perception. Caregiver burden is higher with incontinent older persons, which can contribute to decisions to institutionalize. Estimated annual UI-related costs total more than $26 billion.

THE PATHOPHYSIOLOGY OF INCONTINENCE

Normal Micturition

The detrusor contracts via parasympathetic nerves from spinal cord levels S2 to S4 (sacral micturition center). Urethral sphincter mechanisms include proximal urethral smooth muscle (which contracts by sympathetic stimulation from spinal levels T11 to L2), distal urethral striated muscle (which contracts via cholinergic somatic stimulation from the sacral micturition center), and musculofascial urethral supports. In women, these tissues form a two-layered "hammock" that supports and compresses the urethra when abdominal pressure increases. Micturition is coordinated by the central nervous system: Parietal lobes and thalamus receive and coordinate detrusor afferent stimuli; frontal lobes and basal ganglia provide signals to inhibit voiding; and the pontine micturition center integrates these inputs into socially appropriate voiding with coordinated urethral relaxation and detrusor contraction until the bladder is empty. Urine storage is under sympathetic control (inhibiting detrusor contraction and increasing sphincter tone), and voiding is parasympathetic (detrusor contraction and relaxation of sphincter tone).

Incontinence in Older Persons

Especially in older persons, incontinence may not reflect abnormal micturition physiology. Continence also depends on the ability to toilet oneself—requiring physical function, cognition, motivation, and toilet availability—and the absence of medical conditions, medications, or other factors that affect lower urinary tract function, volume status, and urine excretion. Table 26.1 and Table 26.2 list the mechanisms by which these conditions may impair continence. Evaluation and correction of these factors are crucial in the care of older persons with UI.

Age-related changes in the lower urinary tract (Table 26.3) are found in both continent and incontinent older persons. Why some older persons develop UI and others do not remains unclear; differences in lower urinary tract and other compensatory mechanisms may play a role.

Risk Factors

Risk factors in community-dwelling older persons include advanced age, parity, depression, transient ischemic attacks and stroke, heart failure, fecal incontinence and constipation, obesity, chronic obstructive lung disease, chronic cough, diabetes mellitus, impaired mobility, and impaired activities of daily living. Among institutionalized older persons, UI is associated with impaired mobility, depression, stroke, diabetes mellitus, and Parkinson's disease; at least one third have multiple conditions. Although moderate to severe dementia is associated with UI, even severely demented persons remain continent if they have mobility for transfers. Thus, UI in demented persons may not be caused by dementia but may be a multifactorial epiphenomenon with treatable causes.

Urge Incontinence

Urge UI is the most common type in older persons. It is characterized by abrupt urgency, frequency, and nocturia; the volume of leakage may be small or large. Urge UI is associated with uninhibited bladder contractions—detrusor overactivity (DO)—that may be age related, idiopathic, secondary to lesions in central inhibitory pathways (eg, stroke, cervical stenosis), or due to local bladder irritation (infection, bladder stones, inflammation, tumors). Because DO is found in healthy, continent older persons, failure of lower urinary tract and functional compensatory mechanisms may play an important role in urge UI. Distinctions between neurogenic DO (due to central nervous system lesions) and idiopathic DO are commonly blurred in the older person with comorbidity. Less common causes of urge UI are interstitial cystitis (urge UI with otherwise unexplained pelvic pain) and spinal cord injury, which results in impaired detrusor compliance (excessive pressure response to filling), detrusor-sphincter dyssynergia, or both. Stress maneuvers may trigger DO; with such stress-related urge UI, leakage occurs after a several-second delay following the stress maneuver.

Table 26.1—Medications Commonly Associated With Incontinence

Medication	Effect on Continence
Alcohol	Frequency, urgency, sedation, delirium, immobility
α-Adrenergic agonists	Outlet obstruction (men)
α-Adrenergic blockers	Stress leakage (women)
Angiotensin-converting enzyme inhibitors	Associated cough with stress or stress-induced urge leakage
Anticholinergics: Antiarrhythmics (Norpace) Antidiarrheals (Lomotil) Antihistamines Antiparkinsonian (Artane) Antispasmodics (Bentyl)	Impaired emptying, retention, delirium, fecal impaction
Antidepressants	Anticholinergic effects, sedation
Antipsychotics	Anticholinergic effects, sedation, immobility, rigidity
Calcium channel blockers	Impaired detrusor contractility, retention, pedal edema causing nocturnal diuresis (dihydropyridine agents)
Loop diuretics	Polyuria, frequency, urgency
Narcotic analgesics	Urinary retention, fecal impaction, sedation, delirium
Nonsteroidal anti-inflammatory drugs	Pedal edema causing nocturnal enuresis
Sedative hypnotics	Sedation, delirium, immobility
Thiazolidinediones	Pedal edema causing nocturnal enuresis

SOURCE: Data from Dubeau CE. Interpreting the effect of common medical conditions on voiding dysfunction in the elderly. *Urol Clin North Am.* 1996;23(1):11–18.

Table 26.2—Comorbidities Commonly Associated With Incontinence

Comorbidity	Effect on Continence
Cardiovascular disease	
Arteriovascular disease	Detrusor underactivity or areflexia from ischemic myopathy or neuropathy
Heart failure	Nocturnal diuresis
Metabolic disease	
Diabetes mellitus	Detrusor underactivity due to neuropathy, DO, osmotic diuresis; altered mental status from hyper- or hypoglycemia; retention and overflow from constipation
Hypercalcemia	Diuresis, altered mental status
Vitamin-B_{12} deficiency	Impaired bladder sensation and detrusor underactivity from peripheral neuropathy
Neurologic disease	
Cerebrovascular disease, stroke	DO from damage to upper motor neurons; impaired sensation to void from interruption of subcortical pathways; impaired function and cognition
Delirium	Impaired function and cognition
Dementia	DO from damage to upper motor neurons; impaired function and cognition
Multiple sclerosis	DO, areflexia, or sphincter dyssynergia (dependent on level of spinal cord involvement)
Normal-pressure hydrocephalus	DO from compression of frontal inhibitory centers; impaired function and cognition
Parkinson's disease	DO from loss of inhibitory inputs to pontine micturition center; impaired function and cognition; retention and overflow from constipation
Spinal cord injury	DO, areflexia, or sphincter dyssynergia (dependent on level of injury)
Spinal stenosis	DO from damage to detrusor upper motor neurons (cervical stenosis); DO or areflexia (lumbar stenosis)
Psychiatric disease	
Affective and anxiety disorders	Decreased motivation
Alcoholism	Functional and cognitive impairment; rapid diuresis and retention in acute intoxication
Psychosis	Functional and cognitive impairment; decreased motivation
Other organ system diseases	
Gastrointestinal disease	Retention and overflow UI from constipation; fecal and urinary incontinence commonly coexist
Musculoskeletal disease	Mobility impairment; DO from cervical myelopathy in rheumatoid arthritis and osteoarthritis
Peripheral venous insufficiency	Nocturnal diuresis
Pulmonary disease	Exacerbation of stress UI by chronic cough

NOTE: DO = detrusor overactivity; UI = urinary incontinence.
SOURCE: Data from Dubeau CE. Interpreting the effect of common medical conditions on voiding dysfunction in the elderly. *Urol Clin North Am.* 1996;23(1):11–18.

Table 26.3—Age-Related Changes Potentially Resulting in Urinary Incontinence

Change	Predisposition	Type of Urinary Incontinence
Atrophic vaginitis and urethritis	Decreased urethral mucosal seal, irritation, UTI	Urge and stress UI
Benign prostatic hyperplasia	Prostatic hyperplasia or outlet obstruction or both with frequency, urgency, nocturia, DO	Urge or "overflow" UI
Decreased ability to postpone voiding	Frequency, urgency, nocturia	New or worsening urge, stress, mixed UI
Decreased detrusor contractility	Decreased flow rate, elevated postvoid residual, hesitancy	"Overflow" UI, DHIC
Decreased total bladder capacity	Frequency, urgency, nocturia	New or worsening urge, stress, mixed UI
DO (~20% of healthy, continent persons)	Frequency, urgency, nocturia	Urge and mixed UI, DHIC
Increased postvoid residual (< 50 mL)	Frequency, nocturia	New or worsening urge, stress, mixed UI
More urine output later in the day	Nocturia	Nocturnal UI

NOTE: DHIC = detrusor hyperactivity with impaired contractility; DO = detrusor overactivity; UI = urinary incontinence; UTI = urinary tract infection.

DO may coexist with impaired detrusor contractility (detrusor hyperactivity with impaired contractility, or DHIC), characterized by urge UI with an elevated postvoid residual (PVR) volume in the absence of outlet obstruction. DHIC accounts for most established UI in frail older persons. Women with DHIC can be misdiagnosed with stress UI if weak DHIC contractions are not detected, and men misdiagnosed with outlet obstruction because of the similarity of the symptoms (urgency, frequency, weak flow rate, and elevated PVR).

Stress Incontinence

Stress UI, the second most common type of UI in older women, results from failure of the sphincter mechanisms to preserve outlet closure during bladder filling. Leakage is due to impaired pelvic supports or, less commonly, failure of urethral closure. The latter occurs with trauma, scarring from anti-incontinence surgery, severe urethral atrophy in women, and post-prostatectomy in men. Unlike the episodic leakage of "genuine" stress UI, this leakage is typically continual and can occur while the person is sitting or standing quietly. Many women may have mixed UI, with both stress and urge symptoms.

Bladder Outlet Obstruction and Detrusor Underactivity

So-called "overflow" UI results from detrusor underactivity (impaired contractility), bladder outlet obstruction, or both. Leakage is typically small in volume but continual. The PVR volume is high, and symptoms may include dribbling, weak urinary stream, intermittency, hesitancy, frequency, and nocturia. Associated urge and stress UI may occur. Rarely, continual leakage is due to extraurethral incontinence (eg, vesicovaginal fistula).

Outlet obstruction is the second most common cause of UI in older men; most obstructed men, however, are not incontinent. Causes include benign prostatic hyperplasia, prostate cancer, and urethral stricture. In women, obstruction is uncommon and usually due to previous anti-incontinence surgery or a large cystocele that kinks the urethra.

Detrusor underactivity causing urinary retention and UI occurs in only 5% to 10% of older persons. Intrinsic causes are replacement of detrusor smooth muscle by fibrosis and connective tissue (eg, from chronic outlet obstruction). Neurologic causes include peripheral neuropathy (diabetes mellitus, vitamin B_{12} deficiency, alcoholism) or damage to the spinal detrusor afferents by disc herniation, spinal stenosis, tumor, or degenerative neurologic disease.

ASSESSMENT AND MANAGEMENT

UI is like many geriatric syndromes, in that its multifactorial nature requires a comprehensive diagnostic evaluation, with a careful search for all possible causes and precipitants beyond the genitourinary tract. UI management is similar to that for other chronic conditions, using a stepped approach over time. Table 26.4 provides a framework for evaluating and managing common types of UI over several visits. The sections below describe techniques.

History

The clinician must ask the patient about UI symptoms because 50% of affected persons do not volunteer UI symptoms. Sudden, compelling urgency suggests DO, and leakage with cough, for example, is sensitive for stress UI. Leakage with minimal maneuvers or continual urine dripping suggests intrinsic sphincter damage. Frequency, nocturia, slow urine stream, hesitancy, interrupted voiding, straining, and terminal dribbling are common with DO, DHIC, bladder outlet obstruction, detrusor underactivity, many medical conditions, and volume overload. Symptom scores (eg, the American Urological Association symptom score for benign prostatic hyperplasia) are useful as severity measures but lack specificity. Assess UI characteristics such as frequency, volume, timing, and precipitants (eg, medications, caffeine, alcohol, physical activity, cough), and associated factors (bowel and sexual function, medical conditions and medications with temporal relation to UI). Inquire how patient and caregiver quality of life are affected with respect to activities of daily living, social role, emotional and interpersonal (eg, sexual) relations, self-concept, general health perception, and the most bothersome aspect.

Physical Examination

The general examination must include cognition and functional status. Cardiovascular examination focuses on volume status (peripheral edema, heart failure). Abdominal palpation for bladder distension is insensitive. Neurologic evaluation should include cervical signs (limited lateral rotation and lateral flexion, interossei wasting, and Hoffman's or Babinski's sign). Assess rectum for masses, prostate nodules or firmness, and tone (at rest and volitional, tightening around examiner's finger). Prostate sizing by digital examination is inaccurate (see "Prostate Disease," p 389). Check sacral root integrity by perineal sensation, anal "wink" (lightly scratch the perianal area and look for anal sphincter contraction), and bulbocavernosus reflex (lightly touch the clitoris or glans and look for rectal contraction). Assess vaginal mucosa and pelvic support

Table 26.4—Stepped Approach to Urinary Incontinence Evaluation and Management

Measures to Take	Comments, Examples
Visit 1: Initial screening and behavioral interventions	
Screen for UI in all adult patients	Ask "Have you had any problems with bladder or urine control?" If yes, then ask: "Do you leak urine when you lift something, cough, or sneeze?" "Do you have sudden urge to urinate and then leak urine before you can reach the bathroom?" "Do you ever leak urine with any physical activity or warning?"
Conduct brief UI history, pertinent past medical history, and review of systems	Review lower urinary tract symptoms Target system review at medical conditions and functional impairments associated with UI Review all medications and fluid intake Ask about UI impact on quality of life
Evaluate for any pathologic conditions (eg, UTI, malignancy)	Ask about bleeding, pelvic pain, dysuria, sudden UI onset Screen for neurologic syptoms
Perform physical examination	Assess patient's mobility, volume status (including checking for pedal edema) Perform rectal examination—note sphincter strength with voluntary contraction. Perform pelvic examination and note any signficant pelvic organ prolapse (consider gynecology referral if past the introitus); check pelvic muscle contraction during manual examination Perform clinic stress test, if possible Include PVR, if time allows (see visit 2)
Urinalysis	Flags: hematuria, glycosuria (see text, p 176, regarding pyuria and bacteriuria)
General management and behavioral therapy	Physical therapy for patients with impaired mobility; bedside commode Volume management (eg, adjust intake, diuretics, compression hose, foot elevation) See text (p 177) for behavioral therapies
Medication review	See Table 26.1
Ask patient to complete a 2- to 3-day bladder diary	For sample bladder diary see http://www.healthinaging.org/public_education/bladder_control.php
Visit 2 (4–8 weeks): Detailed evaluation and treatment	
Review completed bladder diary	See text (p 176)
Re-review UI and lower urinary tract symptoms	Review fluid intake for volume and caffeine, which can contribute to UI Assess response to therapy aimed at transient factors
Evaluate further	Ideally, PVR should be assessed in all patients; it should always be done in men and in persons with diabetes mellitus, neurologic disorders, significant pelvic prolapse, or taking medications that impair detrusor contractility; may be done by catheterization or ultrasound by provider or referral Perform clinical stress test, if possible and not done previously
Refine treatment	Review and reinforce general management and behavioral therapy Consider antimuscarinic medication for patients with urge UI (see text, p 176)
Consider referral for further evaluation and treatment	Referral for biofeedback- or electrical stimulation-assisted pelvic muscle exercises for women with mixed or stress UI Other indications: persistent pelvic pain, hematuria, urinary retention, elevated PVR (> 200–300 mL, possibly lower in men); persistent postprostatectomy UI; bothersome pelvic prolapse (or try pessary); patient requests surgical consultation for stress UI or possible bladder outlet obstruction; diagnosis remains uncertain
Visit 3 (4–6 weeks after visit 2): Treatment evaluation and referral	
Evaluate response to therapy	Review behavioral management and response to medications Titrate medications on basis of UI, adverse effects, and (especially if UI has worsened) PVR
Consider referral for further evaluation and treatment	Indications: same as above, plus failure to respond to empirical therapy

NOTE: PVR = postvoid residual; UI = urinary incontinence; UTI = urinary tract infection.

SOURCE: Adapted with permission from: American Geriatrics Society Urinary Incontinence Education Initiative Editorial Board: Goode PS, Chair, Brown J, DuBeau C, et al. Evaluating and treating older adult urinary incontinence: a step-wise approach for primary care providers. See http://www.americangeriatrics.org/jasper_test/education/ui_index.shtml (accessed October 2005).

(see "Gynecologic Diseases and Disorders," p 376). Check uncircumcised men for phimosis, paraphimosis, and balanitis.

Testing

Laboratory tests include renal function and urinalysis. Pyuria and bacteriuria on urinalysis may represent asymptomatic bacteriuria (see the section on urinary tract infection in "Infectious Diseases," p 309). Urine cytology and cystoscopy are indicated if hematuria or pelvic pain is present. Tests for glucose, calcium, and vitamin B_{12} levels are optional.

A bladder diary provides baseline UI severity, the timing and circumstances of UI and typical voided volume, voiding frequency, and the total day and nocturnal urine output (for a sample diary see http://www.healthinaging.org/public_education/bladder_control.php). In institutions, have staff record the patient's continence status (dry, damp, soaked) every 2 hours. If nocturnal diuresis occurs, seek causes (eg, pedal edema, heart failure, or use of an alcohol "nightcap"). UI occurrence at a typical time of day suggests an association with medication, beverages, or activity.

Postvoiding residual volume (PVR) measurement is recommended. Men with a PVR volume >200 should be screened for hydronephrosis.

A clinical stress test is best done with the bladder full, the patient relaxed, and using a single vigorous cough. It is specific for stress UI if leakage is instantaneous but insensitive if the patient cannot cooperate, is inhibited, or if bladder volume is low. If results are negative, consider repeating the test with the patient standing. On urine flow rate testing (if available), a peak flow ≥12 mL/sec with voided volume ≥150 mL excludes bladder outlet obstruction. Routine urodynamic testing is usually not needed. Precise diagnosis is most important when surgical treatment is being considered for stress UI or outlet obstruction, because surgery is ineffective for DO, DHIC, and detrusor weakness that present with similar symptoms. Geriatric UI is multifactorial, and lower urinary tract pathology is rarely the only cause. A focus on urodynamic diagnosis detracts from more relevant precipitants. Moreover, some treatments are effective for several types of UI (see the section, below, on specific treatment strategies). Urodynamics also should be considered if the diagnosis is unclear or if empiric therapy has failed. Cystometry measures bladder proprioception, capacity, detrusor stability, and contractility; carbon dioxide cystometry may be unreliable. Simultaneous measurement of abdominal pressure is necessary to exclude abdominal straining and detect

DHIC. Fluoroscopic monitoring, abdominal leak-point pressure, or profilometry tests detect and quantify stress UI. Pressure-flow studies are the criterion standard for obstruction.

Management

Correction of medical illnesses, medications, and other precipitating factors alone often improves continence. Relieving the most bothersome aspects of UI for the patient is key. A stepped strategy moving from the least to more invasive treatments should be used, with behavioral methods tried before medication, and both tried before surgery. Treatment that simply decreases the number of UI episodes may not be sufficient for persons most bothered by the timing of UI, nocturia, or leakage with exercise. Cure often requires multiple visits. Evidence for the efficacy of UI treatment is summarized in Table 26.5, Table 26.6, and Table 26.7.

General management suggestions include avoiding high fluid intake (>2L/day), caffeinated beverages, and alcohol, and minimizing evening intake if nocturnal UI is bothersome. Constipation should be reduced. If pads and protective garments are used, they should be chosen on the basis of the patient's gender and the type and volume of UI. Because these products are expensive, some patients may not change pads frequently enough. Medical supply companies and patient advocacy groups publish illustrated catalogs for product selection.

SPECIFIC TREATMENT STRATEGIES

Urge Incontinence

Behavioral treatment for urge UI employs two principles: frequent voluntary voiding to keep bladder volume low, and retraining of central nervous system and pelvic mechanisms to inhibit detrusor contractions and leakage. Cognitively intact persons can use bladder retraining, with timed voiding while awake and suppression of urgency by relaxation techniques (for patient handouts see http://www.healthinaging.org/public_education/bladder_control.php). The initial toileting frequency can be every 2 hours or based on a bladder diary (using the shortest interval between voids). When the urgency occurs, the patient is instructed to stand still or sit down, contract the pelvic muscles, and concentrate on making the urgency decrease and pass: to take a deep breath and let it out slowly, or to visualize the urgency as a wave that peaks and then falls. Once in control of the urgency, the patient should walk slowly to a bathroom and void. After 2 days without leakage, the time between sched-

---

OL Not approved by the U.S. Food and Drug Administration for this use.

Table 26.5—Efficacy of Behavioral and Pharmacologic Treatments for Urge Incontinence

Treatment	Target Population	Efficacy	Evidence*
Behavioral			
Bladder training	Cognitively intact	≥ 35% decrease in UI episodes over controls; patient's perception of cure at 6 months RR 1.69 [1.21 to 2.34]	A
Prompted voiding	Dependent, cognitively impaired	Average reduction 0.8–1.8 episodes daily; cure rare	A
Habit training	Able to complete voiding record	≥ 25% decrease in episodes in one third of patients	B
Scheduled toileting	Unable to toilet independently	30%–80% decrease in episodes, study quality fair	C
Pelvic muscle exercises	Women	Up to 80% decrease in episodes; motivated patients	A
Pharmacologic			
All antimuscarinics	Unresponsive to behavioral treatment alone	WMD in daily UI episodes 0.6 (95% CI, 0.4 to 0.8); RR dry mouth 2.56 (95% CI, 2.24 to 2.92)	A
Darifenacin	Unresponsive to behavioral treatment alone	7.5 or 15 mg daily: 68% and 73% respectively, median reduction in weekly UI episodes (vs 56% with placebo), dry mouth 19% and 31% respectively, constipation 14% (both doses)	
Oxybutynin	Unresponsive to behavioral treatment alone	ER: 71% mean reduction weekly UI episodes, cure rate 23%, dry mouth 30%	A
Solifenacin	Unresponsive to behavioral treatment alone	5 or 10 mg daily: 61% and 52% respectively, mean reduction daily UI episodes (vs 28% with placebo), dry mouth 8% and 23% respectively, constipation 4% and 9% respectively	
Tolterodine	Unresponsive to behavioral treatment alone	ER: 69% mean reduction weekly UI episodes, cure rate 17%, dry mouth 22%	A
Trospium	Unresponsive to behavioral treatment alone	20 mg bid: 59% mean reduction daily urge UI episodes (vs 44% with placebo), cure rate 21%, dry mouth 22%, constipation 10%	

* Evidence strength: A = randomized controlled studies; B = case-control studies; C = case descriptions or expert opinion.

NOTE: CI = confidence interval; ER = extended release; RR = relative risk; UI = urinary incontinence; WMD = weighted mean difference.

SOURCES: Data from Fantl JA, Newman DK, Colling J, et al. *Urinary Incontinence in Adults: Acute and Chronic Management.* Clinical Practice Guideline No. 2, 1996 Update. Rockville, MD: US Department of Health and Human Services, Public Health Service, Agency for Health Care Policy and Research; March 1996. AHCPR Pub. No. 96-0682; Abrams P, Cardozo L, Khoury S, et al., eds. *2nd International Consultation on Incontinence.* Plymouth, UK: Health Publication Ltd; 2002; Cochrane Library (accessed July 2003); Diokno A, Appell RA, Sand PK, et al. Prospective, randomized, double-blind study of the efficacy and tolerability of the extended-release formulations of oxybutynin and tolterodine for overactive bladder: results of the OPERA trail. *Mayo Clin Proc.* 2003;78:687–695; Zinner N, Gittelman M, Harris R, et al. Trospium chloride improves overactive bladder symptoms: a multicenter phase III trial. *J Urol.* 2004;171:2311–2315; Cardoza L, Lisec M, Millard R, et al. Randomized, double-blind placebo controlled trial of the once daily antimuscarinic agent solifenacin succinate in patients with overactive bladder. *J Urol.* 2004;172:1919–1924; Haab F, Stewart L, Dwyer P. Darifenacin, an M3 selective receptor antagonist, is an effective and well-tolerated once-daily treatment for overactive bladder. *Eur Urol.* 2004;45:420–429.

uled voids is increased by 30 to 60 minutes until the person voids every 3 to 4 hours without leakage. Although marginal benefit is unproven, many experts believe biofeedback can improve teaching and outcomes. Successful bladder retraining usually takes several weeks; patients need reassurance to proceed despite any initial failure.

For cognitively impaired patients, behavioral methods include habit training (timed voiding, with the interval based on a person's usual voiding schedule), scheduled voiding (timed voiding usually every 2 to 3 hours), and prompted voiding. Prompted voiding has three components: regular monitoring with encouragement to report continence status, prompting to toilet on a scheduled basis, and praise and positive feedback when the person is continent and attempts to toilet. Persons most likely to respond to prompted voiding are those with who void four or fewer times in 12 daytime hours and who toilet correctly over 75% of the time in an initial trial. These methods require training, motivation, and continued effort by patients and caregivers; special attention and staff reinforcement are needed in institutionalized settings to ensure continued treatment success.

When behavioral methods alone are not sufficient, bladder-suppressant medications can be added. The combination of behavioral and drug therapy has higher efficacy than either alone. There are now five available antimuscarinic agents. The oxybutynin (immediate-release 2.5 to 5mg mg two to four times daily; extended-release 5 to 20 mg once daily; topical patch 3.9 mg applied to abdomen, thighs, or buttocks twice weekly); tolterodine (immediate-release 1 to 2 mg twice daily, extended-release 2 to 4 mg once daily); trospium 20 mg twice daily; darifenacin 7.5 to 15 mg once daily; and solifenacin 10 to 20 mg once daily.

Table 26.6—Efficacy of Behavioral and Pharmacologic Treatments for Stress and for Mixed Urge and Stress Incontinence

Treatment	Target Population	Efficacy	Evidence*
Behavioral			
PME	Women	56%–95% decrease in episodes	A
PME and biofeedback	Women	50%–87% improvement	A
	Men, postprostatectomy	RR for continued UI vs no treatment 0.74 [0.6 to 0.93]	A–C
PME and vaginal cones	Women	No data in postmenopausal women	—
Electrical stimulation	Women, stress ± urge UI	No marginal benefit over behavioral therapy alone	A
Bladder retraining	Mixed UI, cognitively intact	≥ 50% decrease in episodes in 75% of patients	A
Prompted voiding	Mixed UI, dependent, cognitively impaired	Average reduction 0.8–1.8 episodes daily	A
Habit training	Mixed UI, voiding record available	≥ 25% decrease in episodes in one third of patients	B
Scheduled toileting	Mixed UI, unable to toilet independently	30%–80% decrease in episodes	C
Pharmacologic			
Duloxetine[OL]	Women	All UI episodes reduced 64% versus 41% with placebo	A
Estrogens	Women	Oral ineffective, especially when combined with a progestin; scant data on topical forms	A–B

* Evidence strength: A = randomized controlled studies; B = case-control studies; C = case descriptions or expert opinion.

NOTE: PME = pelvic muscle exercises; UI = urinary incontinence.

SOURCES: Data from Fantl JA, Newman DK, Colling J, et al. *Urinary Incontinence in Adults: Acute and Chronic Management.* Clinical Practice Guideline No. 2, 1996 Update. Rockville, MD: US Department of Health and Human Services, Public Health Service, Agency for Health Care Policy and Research; March 1996. AHCPR Pub. No. 96-0682; Abrams P, Cardozo L, Khoury S, et al., eds. *2nd International Consultation on Incontinence.* Plymouth, UK: Health Publication Ltd; 2002; Cochrane Library (accessed July 2003); Goode PS, Burgio KL, Locher JL, et al. Effect of behavioral training with or without pelvic floor electrical stimulation on stress incontinence in women. *JAMA.* 2003;290:345–352.

Overall, they have similar efficacy, with some variation in adverse events (See Table 26.5). Lack of response to one agent does not preclude response to another.

Anticholinergic side effects can be bothersome (eg, constipation and compensatory fluid intake for xerostomia may exacerbate UI) but also potentially dangerous. Chronic xerostomia predisposes the patient to caries and tooth loss. Visual changes and cognitive impairment present safety issues. Although there are a growing number of case reports regarding cognitive effects, outcome studies of cognitive impairment from these agents are still under way. The PVR should be monitored if UI worsens; if high, then UI may improve when the dose is lowered. Patients with DHIC may tolerate bladder-suppressant medications if initial dose is low and titration is slow and based on symptom response; the PVR should be monitored.

These agents also differ in metabolism, drug interactions, and ease of use. Trospium should be given once daily in persons with renal insufficiency, and it needs to be taken on an empty stomach. Tolterodine is metabolized by the cytochrome P-450 pathways and interacts with drugs that induce 2D6 (eg, fluoxetine) or are metabolized by 3A4 (eg, erythromycin, ketoconazole). There are case reports of interactions between bladder relaxants and cholinesterase inhibitors,

and caution should be used if drugs in the two classes are to be used together.

Other agents (propantheline, dicyclomine, imipramine, hyoscyamine, calcium channel blockers, and nonsteroidal anti-inflammatories) have scant efficacy data. Flavoxate is ineffective. Vasopressin was found to decrease nocturnal voids in a small randomized trial in healthy older persons, yet its expense and risk of heart failure and hyponatremia argue against routine use.

Sacral nerve neuromodulation by an implanted S3 electrode may decrease severe refractory DO, but reimplantation is required in one third of patients. Augmentation cystoplasty surgery has high morbidity and is reserved for patients with profound DO (usually younger persons with poorly compliant bladders from neurologic disease).

Stress Incontinence

Pelvic muscle exercises (PME) strengthen the muscular components of urethral support and are the cornerstone of noninvasive treatment for stress UI. PME, like strength training, employ a small number of isometric repetitions at maximal exertion. Unfortunately, professional and lay misinformation about PME abounds; persons who report failing PME trials may have used inadequate methods. PME requires motivated patients

Table 26.7—Efficacy of Surgical Treatments for Stress Incontinence

Treatment	Target Population	Efficacy	Evidence*
Retropubic suspension	Women	Short term cure 69%-88%, 5 years 70%; cure or improvement 84%;** complications 18% (range 6%–57%)	A–B
Needle suspension	Women	More likely to fail than open suspension (29% failed vs 16%, RR 2.00 [95% CI, 1.47 to 2.72]), with no differences in complications (23% vs 16%) if first UI surgery. May be as effective as anterior vaginal repair (36% failed vs 39%, RR 0.93 [0.68 to 1.26]). Limited data comparing with suburethral slings.	A
Anterior vaginal repair (colporrhaphy)	Women	Less effective than open suspension (year 1 failure rate 29% vs 14%; long-term 41% vs 17%), with more repeat operations (23% vs 2%, RR 8.87 [95% CI, 3.28 to 23.9])	A–B
Vaginal sling	Women with stress UI, ISD, hypermobility	Short term-cure rates with TVT similar to open abdominal retropubic suspension; complications 9%. Gore-Tex slings may have higher complications than rectus fascia slings. Limited long-term results	B–C
Marshall-Marchetti-Krantz (open suspension)	Women	Scant data in older or frail women; in younger women up to 88% success rate	C
Periurethral bulking injections	Women with ISD	Cure 50% (range 8%–100%), cure or improvement 67%	B
	Men with ISD	Cure 20% (range 0%–66%), cure or improvement 42%	B
Artificial sphincter	Women with ISD	Cure 77%, cure or improvement 80%; revision rate 40%–50%; less data than with men	B
	Men with ISD	Cure 66% (range 33%–88%), cure or improvement 85% (range 75%–95%); revision rate 40%–50%	B

* Evidence strength: A = randomized controlled studies; B = case-control studies; C = case descriptions or expert opinion.

** Subjective cure may be less because of persistent or de novo urge incontinence or voiding difficulty.

NOTE: CI = confidence interval; ISD = intrinsic sphincter deficiency; RR = relative risk; TVT = tension-free vaginal tape; UI = urinary incontinence.

SOURCES: Data from Fantl JA, Newman DK, Colling J, et al. *Urinary Incontinence in Adults: Acute and Chronic Management.* Clinical Practice Guideline No. 2, 1996 Update. Rockville, MD: US Department of Health and Human Services, Public Health Service, Agency for Health Care Policy and Research; March 1996. AHCPR Pub. No. 96-0682; Abrams P, Cardozo L, Khoury S, et al., eds. *2nd International Consultation on Incontinence.* Plymouth, UK: Health Publication Ltd; 2002; Cochrane Library (accessed July 2003).

and instruction and monitoring by health professionals, although simple instruction booklets alone have been shown to have moderate benefit. PME instruction should focus on isolation of pelvic muscles; avoidance of buttock, abdomen, or thigh muscle contraction; moderate repetitions of a strong, slow-velocity contraction sustained for 6 to 8 seconds, performed in sets of 8 to 12 contractions three or four times a week and continued for at least 15 to 20 weeks (the patient handout at http://www.healthinaging.org/public_education/bladder_control.php should be amended to decrease initial contraction frequency). The marginal benefit of adding biofeedback or weighted vaginal cones is uncertain, yet many experts feel that biofeedback helps instruction. Adjunctive electrical stimulation does not increase efficacy.

Pessaries may benefit women with stress UI exacerbated by bladder or uterine prolapse. (See "Gynecologic Diseases and Disorders," p 380.)

In numerous epidemiologic and intervention studies, oral estrogen was not found to be effective for the treatment of stress or mixed UI, especially when combined with progestins. Further studies are needed to evaluate topical estrogen (cream, vaginal tablet, or slow-release ring). α-Adrenergic agonists stimulate urethral smooth muscle contraction, but no pure α-agonists are currently available. The α-agonist and anticholinergic actions of imipramine [OL] have been used for mixed UI, yet efficacy data are scant and anticholinergic effects are marked. Duloxetine[OL] is a novel norepinephrine- and serotonin-reuptake inhibitor that increases sphincter contraction; early short term data suggest efficacy for both stress and mixed UI. However, the dose for incontinence is twice the dose used to treat depression and neuropathic pain, with concomitant higher rates of adverse effects such as nausea. (The manufacturer has put the application for this indication in the United States on hold. The drug does have approval for this indication in Europe and is approved in the United States for depression and pain.)

Surgery provides the highest cure rates for stress UI in women, yet there are few data to assist in procedure and patient selection for older women, especially if they have mixed UI, poor detrusor con-

[OL] Not approved by the U.S. Food and Drug Administration for this use.

tractility, prior failed anti-incontinence surgery, and comorbidity. The standard procedure has been bladder neck suspension (eg, transvaginal colposuspension). Suburethral slings and tension-free vaginal tape (synthetic sling inserted at midurethra without tension) are increasingly used; complication rates can exceed 10%. Periurethral injection of collagen, Teflon, or autologous fat is a short-term (≤1 year) alternative, usually requiring a series of injections. Anterior colporrhaphy and needle suspensions are less effective and not recommended. Artificial sphincters are used for severe sphincter damage (eg, from surgical scarring).

Postprostatectomy stress UI is more common in older men. Overall, UI rates decline over 6 to 12 months, regardless of PME therapy. Although preoperative PME improves early postoperative UI rates, there is no difference from controls at 1 year. No drugs are known to be effective. Artificial sphincter replacement can be effective but requires manual dexterity and cognition, and it has high revision rates (up to 40%); urodynamics should assist patient selection, as outcomes are worse with severe DO and poor detrusor compliance. Early short-term reports suggest that suburethral sling placement may offer benefit.

Bladder Outlet Obstruction

A range of medical and surgical alternatives are available for prostatic obstruction (see "Prostate Disease," p 389). Obstruction should be considered as a diagnosis in women with previous vaginal or urethral surgery; treatment by unilateral suture removal or urethrolysis (remobilization of adhesions) may restore continence. Pessaries may improve urethral kinking due to pelvic organ prolapse; otherwise, prolapse repair surgery can be considered.

Detrusor Underactivity

Treatment is supportive. Drugs that impair detrusor contractility and increase urethral tone should be decreased or stopped, and constipation should be treated. Bethanechol chloride is ineffective except possibly for patients with overflow UI who must remain on anticholinergic agents (eg, antidepressant or antipsychotic medications). Intermittent clean catheterization is effective for willing and able patients. Sterile intermittent catheterization is preferred for frailer patients and those in institutionalized settings. In some cases bladder emptying may improve with double voiding or simply unhurried voiding.

Catheters and Catheter Care

Indwelling catheters cause significant morbidity, including polymicrobial bacteriuria (universal by 30 days),

febrile episodes (1 per 100 patient days), nephrolithiasis, bladder stones, epididymitis, chronic renal inflammation and pyelonephritis, and meatal damage. External collection devices also cause bacteriuria, infection, penile cellulitis and necrosis, and urinary retention and hydronephrosis if the condom twists or its external band is too tight.

Indwelling catheters should be reserved for the following situations: short-term decompression of acute retention; chronic retention that cannot be managed surgically or medically; wounds that need protection from urine; a terminally ill or severely impaired patient who cannot tolerate garment changes, or when there is persistent patient preference for catheter management despite risks. The passage of the 1990 Omnibus Budget Reconciliation Act has resulted in more appropriate and decreased catheter use in long-term care but with an increased prevalence of UI.

Several general principles guide safe and effective catheter care. Bacteriuria and infection are reduced by closed drainage systems. Topical meatal antimicrobials, catheters with antimicrobial coating, collection bag disinfectants, and antimicrobial irrigation are not effective. Although antibiotics decrease bacteriuria and infection, routine use induces resistant organisms and secondary infections such as *Clostridium difficile* colitis. Bacteriuria is universal in catheterized patients and should not be treated unless there are clear symptoms. Routine cultures should not be done because of the changing flora and failure to predict infection. In symptomatic patients, cultures should be done after the old catheter is removed and a new catheter is placed. Institutionalized patients with catheters should be kept in separate rooms to decrease cross-infection.

With acute urinary retention, decompression should continue at least 7 days, followed by a voiding trial after catheter removal (never clamping). Prophylactic antibiotics are recommended only with short-term catheterization in high-risk patients (eg, those with prosthetic heart valves). For men with chronic obstruction, suprapubic catheters can avoid meatal and penile trauma, and intraurethral stents, if available, may be another alternative (but sometimes at a cost of increased urgency and frequency).

Risk factors for catheter blockage include alkaline urine, female gender, poor mobility, calciuria, proteinuria, copious mucin, *Proteus* colonization, and preexistent bladder stones. Changing the catheter every 7 to 10 days may decrease blockage in such patients. In the absence of risk factors, catheters need not be changed routinely as long as monitoring is adequate. If patients cannot be monitored, changing catheters every 30 days is reasonable. Persistent leakage around the catheter can be caused by irritation by a large Foley balloon, catheter diameter that is too large, bacteriuria, constipation or impaction, improper catheter positioning, or catheter materials.

Clean intermittent catheterization is an alternative for willing patients with sufficient dexterity. Strict sterility is not necessary, although good handwashing and regular decontamination of the catheters is needed. Bacteriuria can be minimized by a frequency of catheterization that keeps bladder volume <400 mL. Stiffer catheters are easier to insert.

Resources, including Web site addresses, of use to clinicians treating patients with UI are listed in the Appendix (p 476).

REFERENCES

■ Diokno A, Appell RA, Sand PK, et al. Prospective, randomized, double-blind study of the efficacy and tolerability of the extended-release formulations of oxybutynin and tolterodine for overactive bladder: results of the OPERA trail. *Mayo Clin Proc.* 2003;78(6):687–695.

■ Dowling-Castronovo A, Bradway CW. Urinary incontinence. In: Mezey M, Fulmer T, Abraham I, eds. *Geriatric Nursing Protocols for Best Practice, 2nd Ed.* New York: Springer Publishing Company, Inc.; 2003:83–98.

■ Goode PS, Burgio KL, Locher JL, et al. Effect of behavioral training with or without pelvic floor electrical stimulation on stress incontinence in women. *JAMA.* 2003; 290(3):345–352.

■ Schnelle JF, Kapur K, Alessi C, et al. Does an exercise and incontinence intervention save healthcare costs in a nursing home population? *J Am Geriatr Soc.* 2003, 51(2):161–168.

■ Schnelle JF, Smith RL. Quality indicators for the management of urinary incontinence in vulnerable community-dwelling elders. *Ann Intern Med.* 2001;135(8 Pt 2):752–758.

■ Simmons SF, Ouslander JG. Resident and family satisfaction with incontinence and mobility care: sensitivity to intervention effects? *Gerontologist.* 2005;45(3):318–326.

■ Wagner TH. Subak LL. Evaluating an incontinence intervention in nursing home resident [editorial]. *J Amer Geriatr Soc.* 2003, 51(2):275–276.

CHAPTER 27—GAIT IMPAIRMENT

KEY POINTS

■ Gait disorders are common in older adults and are a predictor of functional decline.

■ The cause of gait impairment in older adults is usually multifactorial; a full assessment must therefore consider a number of different causes, as determined from a detailed physical examination as well as functional performance evaluation.

■ Interventions, ranging from medical to surgical to exercise, are effective and reduce the extent of the disorder, although residual impairment is often present.

Gait disorders are commonly associated with falls and disability in older adults. This chapter reviews the epidemiology of gait impairments, comorbidities that contribute to these disorders, and office-based clinical assessments and interventions to reduce their functional impact.

EPIDEMIOLOGY

Limitations in walking increase with age. At least 20% of noninstitutionalized older adults admit to difficulty with walking or require the assistance of another person or special equipment to walk. In some samples of noninstitutionalized older adults aged 85 and over, the incidence of limitation in walking can be over 54%. Age-related gait changes such as decrease in speed are most apparent past age 75 or 80, but the majority of gait disorders appear in connection with underlying diseases, particularly as disease severity increases. For example, advanced age (>85 years), three or more chronic conditions at baseline, and the occurrence of stroke, hip fracture, or cancer predict catastrophic loss of walking ability.

Determining that a gait is disordered is difficult because there are no clearly accepted general standards of normal gait for older adults. Some believe that slowed gait speed suggests a disorder; others believe that deviations in smoothness, symmetry, and synchrony of movement patterns suggest a disorder.

Longitudinal studies suggest that certain gait-related mobility disorders progress with age and that this progression is associated with morbidity and mortality. Gait or postural disorders, as measured by the Unified Parkinson's Disease Rating Scale (UPDRS) (including abnormalities in rising from a chair and turning), increased variably in most (79%) of a sample of nondemented Catholic clergy (mean age 75) who were followed for up to 7 years. This increase was more common in the older age groups and was associated with a higher mortality rate. The increased UPDRS score may represent increased parkinsonian-like signs with age but likely also represents an increasing burden of associated disease and inactivity.

CONDITIONS THAT CONTRIBUTE TO GAIT IMPAIRMENT

Impaired gait may not be an inevitable consequence of aging but rather a reflection of the increased prevalence and severity of age-associated diseases. These diseases, both neurologic and non-neurologic, are the major contributors to impaired gait. In addition, attributing a gait disorder to one disease in an older adult is particularly difficult because similar gait abnormalities are common to many diseases. (For a glossary of gait abnormalities, see Table 27.1.)

Patients in primary care consider pain, stiffness, dizziness, numbness, weakness, and sensations of abnormal movement to be the most common contributors to their walking difficulties. The most common conditions found in primary care that are thought to contribute to gait disorders are degenerative joint disease, acquired musculoskeletal deformities, intermittent claudication, impairments following orthopedic surgery and stroke, and postural hypotension. Usually, more than one contributing condition is found. In a group of community-dwelling adults older than age 88, joint pain was by far the most common contributor, followed by multiple causes such as stroke and visual loss. Factors such as dementia and fear of falling also contribute to gait disorders. The disorders found in a neurologic referral population include frontal gait disorders (usually related to normal-pressure hydrocephalus and cerebrovascular processes), sensory disorders (also involving vestibular and visual function), myelopathy, previously undiagnosed Parkinson's disease or parkinsonian syndromes, and cerebellar disease. Known conditions causing severe gait impairment, such as hemiplegia and severe hip or knee disease, are commonly not mentioned in these neurologic referral populations. Thus, many gait disorders, particularly those that are classical and discrete (eg, those related to stroke and osteoarthritis) and those that are mild or may relate to irreversible disease (eg, vascular dementia), are presumably diagnosed in primary care and treated without a referral to a neurologist. Other less common contributors to gait disorders include metabolic disorders (related to renal or hepatic disease), central nervous system tumors or subdural hematoma, depression, and psychotropic medications. Case reports also document reversible gait disorders due to clinically overt hypo- or hyperthyroidism and B_{12} and folate deficiency.

Factors that contribute to slowed gait speed are also considered contributors to gait disorders. These factors are commonly disease associated (eg, cardiopulmonary or musculoskeletal disease) and include reductions in leg strength, vision, aerobic function, standing balance, and decreased physical activity, as well as joint impairment, previous falls, and fear of falling. Combining these factors may result in an effect greater than the sum of the single impairments (as when combining balance and strength impairments). Furthermore, the effect of improved strength and aerobic capacity on gait speed may be nonlinear, that is, for very impaired individuals, small improvements in strength or aerobic capacity yield relatively larger gains in gait speed, whereas these small improvements yield little gait speed change in healthy older persons.

Although older adults may maintain a relatively normal gait pattern well into their 80s, some slowing occurs, and decreased stride length thus becomes a common feature in descriptions of gait disorders of older adults. Some authors have proposed the emergence of an age-related gait disorder without accompanying clinical abnormalities, that is, essential "senile" gait disorder. This gait pattern is described as broad-based with small steps, diminished arm swing, stooped posture, decreased flexion of the hips and knees, uncertainty and stiffness in turning, occasional difficulty initiating steps, and a tendency toward falling. These and other nonspecific findings (such as the inability to perform tandem gait) are similar to gait patterns found in a number of other diseases, and yet

Table 27.1—Glossary of Gait Abnormalities

Term	Description
Circumduction	Outward swing of leg in semicircle from the hip
Equinovarus	Excessive plantar flexion and inversion of the ankle
Festination	Acceleration of gait
Foot drop	Loss of ankle dorsiflexion secondary to weakness of ankle dorsiflexors
Foot slap	Early, frequent audible foot-floor contact with steppage gait compensation
Genu recurvatum	Hyperextension of the knee
Propulsion	Falling forward
Retropulsion	Falling backward
Scissoring	Hip adduction such that the knees cross in front of each other with each step
Steppage gait	Exaggerated hip flexion, knee extension, and foot lifting
Trendelenburg gait	Shift of the trunk over the affected hip, which drops because of hip abductor weakness
Turn en bloc	Moving the whole body while turning

the clinical abnormalities are insufficient to make a specific diagnosis. This "disorder" may be a precursor to an as-yet-undiagnosed disease (eg, related to subtle extrapyramidal signs) and is likely to be a manifestation of concurrent, progressive cognitive impairment (eg, Alzheimer's disease or vascular dementia). "Senile" gait disorder thus may reflect a number of potential diseases and is generally not useful in labeling gait disorders in older adults.

Subclinical as well as clinically evident cerebrovascular disease is increasingly recognized as a major contributor to gait disorders (see the section below on assessment). Nondemented persons with clinically abnormal gait (particularly unsteady, frontal, or hemiparetic gait) followed for approximately 7 years were found to be at higher risk of developing non-Alzheimer's, particularly vascular, dementia. Of note, those with abnormal gait at baseline may not have met criteria for dementia but already had abnormalities in neuropsychologic function, such as in visual-perceptual processing and language skills. Gait disorders with no apparent cause (also termed *idiopathic* or *senile* gait disorder) are associated with a higher mortality rate, primarily from cardiovascular causes. These cardiovascular causes are likely linked to concomitant, possibly undetected, cerebrovascular disease.

ASSESSMENT

A potentially useful approach to assessing contributors to a gait impairment (see Table 27.2) categorizes these deficits according to the sensorimotor levels that are affected.

Disorders that are the result of pathology of the low sensorimotor level can be divided into peripheral sensory and peripheral motor dysfunction, including myopathic or neuropathic disorders that cause weakness and musculoskeletal diseases. These disorders are generally distal to the central nervous system. With peripheral sensory impairment, unsteady and tentative gait is commonly caused by vestibular disorders, peripheral neuropathy, posterior column (proprioceptive) deficits, or visual impairment. With peripheral motor impairment, a number of classical gait patterns emerge. Examples of these patterns include Trendelenburg gait (weight shifts over the weak hip, which drops because of hip abductor weakness), antalgic gait (avoidance of weight bearing and shortening of stance on one side because of pain), and foot drop (due to ankle dorsiflexor weakness, early, frequently audible foot-floor contact with steppage gait compensation, ie, excessive hip flexion). These gait impairments are the result of body segment and joint deformities, pain, and focal myopathic and neuropathic weakness. Note that if the gait disorder is limited to this low sensorimotor level (ie, the central nervous system is intact), the person adapts well to the gait disorder, compensating with an assistive device or learning to negotiate the environment safely.

At the middle level, the execution of centrally selected postural and locomotor responses is faulty, and the sensory and motor modulation of gait is disrupted. Gait may be initiated normally but stepping patterns are abnormal. Diseases causing spasticity (eg, those related to myelopathy, B_{12} deficiency, and stroke), parkinsonism (idiopathic as well as drug induced), and cerebellar disease (eg, alcohol induced) are examples of those that cause this type of impairment. Gait abnormalities appear when the spasticity is sufficient to cause leg circumduction and fixed deformities (eg, equinovarus), when the Parkinson's produces shuffling steps and reduced arm swing, and when the cerebellar ataxia increases trunk sway sufficiently to require a broad base of gait support.

At the high or central level the gait impairments become more nonspecific. Lesions in the frontal lobe account for most of the gait abnormalities at this level. The severity of the frontal-related disorders runs a spectrum from gait ignition failure (ie, difficulty with initiation) to frontal disequilibrium, where unsupported stance is not possible. Cerebrovascular insults to the cortex, as well as to the basal ganglia and their interconnections, may contribute to gait ignition failure and apraxia.

Dementia and depression are also thought to contribute to an abnormal gait at this level. With increasing severity of the dementia, particularly in patients with Alzheimer's disease, frontal-related symptoms also increase. Gait impairments in this category have been given a number of overlapping descriptions, including *gait apraxia*, *marche à petits pas*, and *arteriosclerotic parkinsonism*.

There is likely to be more than one disease or impairment present that contributes to a gait disorder; one example is the longstanding diabetic patient with peripheral neuropathy and a recent stroke who is now very fearful of falls. Certain disorders may actually involve multiple parts of the nervous system, such as Parkinson's disease affecting cortical and subcortical structures. Drug and metabolic causes (eg, from sedatives, tranquilizers, and anticonvulsants) may involve both central and peripheral nervous systems; phenothiazines, for example, can cause central sedation and extrapyramidal effects.

History and Physical Examination

A careful medical history will help elucidate the multiple factors contributing to the older patient's gait impairment. A brief systemic evaluation for evidence of subacute metabolic disease (eg, thyroid disorders),

Table 27.2—Abnormalities of Gait and Associated Findings, by Sensorimotor Level

Sensorimotor Level	Type of Impairment	Condition or Disease	Physical Findings	Gait Abnormality*
Low	Peripheral sensory dysfunction	Peripheral neuropathy, proprioceptive deficits	Loss of position sense, touch	Possible steppage gait
		Vestibular disorders		May weave, fall to one side
		Visual impairment	Visual loss	Tentative, uncertain, uncoordinated
	Peripheral motor dysfunction	Extremity (body segment and joint) deformities Pain Focal myopathic, neuropathic weakness	Pain-related avoidance of weight bearing on affected side Limited flexion in painful extremity (especially knee) and may lead to loss of joint range and contracture Decreased lumbar lordosis	Shortened stance phase on affected side Trendelenburg gait Painful limb may buckle with weight bearing Unequal leg length can produce trunk and pelvic motion abnormalities (including Trendelenburg gait)
			Stooped posture Pelvic or hip girdle weakness	Pelvic girdle weakness can lead to exaggerated lumbar lordosis and lateral trunk flexion (Trendelenburg and waddling gait)
			Proximal muscle weakness Distal muscle weakness	Proximal weakness can produce waddling gait Weak ankle dorsiflexors result in foot drop or slap or steppage gait
Middle	Postural and locomotor impairment	Cerebellar ataxia	Poor trunk control, incoordination or other cerebellar signs	Wide-based with increased trunk sway, irregular stepping, staggering, especially on turns
		Parkinsonism	Rigidity Bradykinesia Trunk flexion	Small shuffling steps, hesitation, festination, propulsion, retropulsion, turning en bloc, absent arm swing
		Hemiplegia or hemiparesis	Arm and leg weakness, spasticity Equinovarus Genu recurvatum	Leg circumduction Loss of arm swing Foot drag or scrape
		Paraplegia or paraparesis	Leg weakness, spasticity	Bilateral leg circumduction, scraping feet, possibly also scissoring
High	Central nervous system (esp frontal) disorder	Cautious gait Mild Alzheimer's disease	May have fear of falling	Normal to widened base, shortened stride, decreased velocity, en bloc turns
		Cerebrovascular disease Normal-pressure hydrocephalus	May have evidence of other atherosclerotic disease, cognitive impairment, weakness and spasticity, and urinary incontinence	Range of findings may include difficulty initiating gait and shuffling gait, preservation of upright posture and arm swing, leg apraxia (can imitate gait movements in non-weight-bearing position), freezing (especially with attention diversion)

NOTE: For descriptions of gait abnormalities, see Table 27.1.

acute cardiopulmonary disorders (eg, myocardial infarction), or other acute illness (eg, sepsis) is warranted because an acute gait disorder may be the presenting feature of acute systemic decompensation in an older adult. The physical examination should include an attempt to identify motion-related factors, for example, by provoking both vestibular and orthostatic responses. Blood pressure should be measured with the patient both supine and standing to exclude orthostatic hypotension. Vision screening, at least for acuity, is essential. The neck, spine, extremities, and feet should be evaluated for pain, deformities, and limitations in range of motion, particularly regarding subtle hip or knee contractures. Leg-length discrepancies such as may occur with a hip prosthesis and either as an antecedent or subsequent to lower back pain can be measured simply as the distance from the anterior superior iliac spine to the medial malleolus. A formal neurologic assessment is critical, to include assessment of strength and tone, sensation (including proprioception), coordination (including cerebellar function), station, and gait. The Romberg test screens for simple postural control and whether the proprioceptive and vestibular systems are functional. Some investigators have proposed one-legged stance time less than 5 seconds as a risk factor for injurious falls, although even relatively healthy adults aged 70 and older may have difficulty with one-legged stance. Given the importance of cognition as a risk factor, assessing cognitive function is also indicated.

Laboratory and Imaging Assessments

Depending upon the history and physical examination, further laboratory and diagnostic imaging evaluation may be warranted. Complete blood cell count, chemistries, and other metabolic studies may be useful only where systemic disease is suspected. Head or spine imaging, including radiography, computed tomography, or magnetic resonance imaging (MRI) are not indicated unless there are neurologic abnormalities by history and physical examination, either preceding or of recent onset, that are related to the gait disorder. However, cerebral white matter changes, often considered to be vascular (termed *leukoaraiosis*), have been increasingly associated with nonspecific gait disorders. Periventricular high signal measurements on MRI as well as increased ventricular volume, even in apparently healthy older adults, are associated with gait slowing. White matter hyperintensities on MRI correlate with longitudinal changes in balance, and the periventricular frontal and occipitoparietal regions appear to be most affected. Age-specific guidelines for and the sensitivity, specificity, and cost-effectiveness of these work-ups remain to be determined.

Performance-Based Functional Assessment

Technologically oriented assessments involving formal kinematic and kinetic analyses have not been applied widely in clinical assessments of balance and gait disorders in older adults. Comfortable gait speed and a related measure, distance walked (as measured by the 6-minute walk test), are powerful predictors of a number of important outcomes, such as disability, institutionalization, and mortality. Gait speed is faster in individuals who are taller, who have a lower disease burden, and who are more active and less functionally disabled. It has been suggested that slow (impaired) walkers can be defined as those who walk at a speed <0.6 m/sec and fast walkers (unimpaired) walkers walk at >1.0 m/sec. A number of timed and semi-

quantitative balance and gait scales have been proposed as a means to detect and quantify abnormalities and to direct interventions. Fall risk, for example, may be increased with more abnormal gait and balance scale scores. Perhaps the simplest battery in the clinical setting is the Timed Get Up and Go (TUG), a timed sequence of rising from a chair, walking 3 meters, turning, and returning to sit in the chair. One study suggests a TUG score of 14 seconds or higher as an indicator for fall risk. Other investigators have found limitations in TUG in the presence of cognitive impairment and difficulty in completing the test due to immobility, safety concerns, or refusal. Another functional approach that may be useful clinically is the Functional Ambulation Classification scale, which rates the use of assistive devices, the degree of human assistance (either manual or verbal), the distance the patient can walk, and the types of surfaces the patient can negotiate.

INTERVENTIONS TO REDUCE GAIT DISORDERS

Even if a diagnosable condition is found on evaluation, many conditions causing a gait disorder are, at best, only partially treatable. Functional improvement becomes the treatment goal. Achievement of premorbid gait patterns may be unrealistic, but improvement in measures such as gait speed is reasonable as long as gait remains safe. Comorbidity, disease severity, and overall health status tend to strongly influence treatment outcome.

Many of the older reports dealing with treatment and rehabilitation of gait disorders in older adults are retrospective chart reviews and case studies. Gait disorders presumably secondary to B_{12} deficiency, folate deficiency, hypothyroidism, hyperthyroidism, knee osteoarthritis, Parkinson's disease, and inflammatory polyneuropathy show improvement as a result of medical therapy. A variety of modes of physical therapy for diseases such as knee osteoarthritis and stroke also result in modest improvements in function but continued residual disability. For example, a combined aerobic, strength, and functionally based group exercise program was found to increase gait speed approximately 5% in patients with knee osteoarthritis. The focus is on strengthening the extensor groups (especially knee and hip) and stretching commonly shortened muscles (such as the hip flexors). A recent review suggests that the effects of conventional physical therapy in the treatment of Parkinson's gait disorders are unclear, but that cueing, specifically audio and visual, can improve gait speed. Other studies suggest an incremental reduction of gait impairment with the use of a body-weight support and a treadmill to provide task-specific gait training following total hip arthroplasty, in Parkinson's disease, and particularly in hemiparetic stroke patients. However, a Cochrane review found no statistically significant effect favoring treadmill training with or without body support over conventional training to improve gait speed or disability in stroke patients. Note that the Cochrane review found a small but clinically important trend (an improvement of 0.24 m/sec in the body-weight support plus treadmill group) in those who could walk independently.

A few studies of group exercise have demonstrated improvements in gait parameters such as gait speed. Generally, the most consistent effects are with varied types of exercise provided in the same program. A 12-week combined program of leg resistance, standing balance, and flexibility exercises was found to increase usual gait speed 8% in minimally impaired life-care community residents. A similar varied 16-week format with more intensive individual support and prompting in selected demented older adults (mean MMSE 15) resulted in a 23% improvement in gait speed. A number of these studies note improvement in functional, gait-oriented measures (although not strictly gait "disorder" measures), such as the distance walked in 6 minutes by knee osteoarthritis patients undergoing either an aerobic or resistance training program.

Modest improvement and residual disability are also the result of surgical treatment for compressive cervical myelopathy, lumbar stenosis, and normal-pressure hydrocephalus. Few controlled prospective studies and virtually no randomized studies address the outcome of surgical versus nonsurgical treatment for these disorders. A number of problems plague the available series: outcomes such as pain and walking disability are not reported separately, the source of the outcome rating is not clearly identified or blinded, the criteria for classifying outcomes differ, the outcomes may be subjective and subject to interpretation, the follow-up intervals are variable, the subjects who are reported in follow-up may be a highly select group, the selection factors for conservative versus surgical treatment between studies differ or are unspecified, and there is publication bias (only positive results are published). Many of the surgical series include all ages, although the mean age is usually above 60 years old. A few studies document equivalent surgical outcomes with conservative, nonsurgical treatment.

Many older adults with lumbar stenosis have reduction in pain and improvement in maximal walking distance following laminectomies and lumbar fusion surgery, although they have continued residual disability. In a somewhat younger cohort (mean age 69) and after an average of 8 years of follow-up after surgery for lumbar stenosis, approximately half reported that they were unable to walk two blocks and many of them attributed their decreased walking ability to their back problem. Part of the problem in determining long-term lumbar stenosis surgical outcomes are other mobility-influencing comorbidities, such as cardiovascular or musculoskeletal disease. Nevertheless, some improvement can be found in selected patients older than 75 (mean age 78); one uncontrolled study found that the 45% of patients with preoperative "severe" limitation of ambulatory ability wound up with either "minimal" or "moderate" limitation postoperatively after an average of 1.5 years of follow-up. Studies involving cervical stenosis gait outcomes in older adults are limited, although significant improvement in walking speed following cervical myelopathy decompression can be expected in most patients.

In a noncontrolled study post-shunt for normal-pressure hydrocephalus (follow-up interval not specified), walking speed was found to have increased more than 10% in 75% of the patients and more than 25% in over 57% of the patients. Although there may be initial improvement following shunt placement, long-term results are often disappointing (eg, 65% of post-shunt patients have initial improvement in their gait disorder, but only 26% maintain this improvement by 3-year follow-up). The poor long-term outcomes may be related to concurrent cerebrovascular and cardiovascular disease, a common cause of mortality in these cohorts. Post-shunt gait outcomes may be better in those in whom the gait disturbance precedes cognitive impairment and in those who respond with improvement in gait speed following a trial of cerebrospinal fluid removal.

Outcomes for hip and knee replacement surgery for osteoarthritis are better, although some of the same methodologic problems exist. Sizable gains in pain relief, gait speed, and joint motion occur, although residual walking disability continues for a number of reasons, including residual pathology on the operated side and symptoms on the nonoperated side. For total knee replacements, despite rehabilitation postoperatively, some residual weakness, stiffness, and slowed or altered gait may remain. Simple function may be maintained following knee replacement, such as maintaining the ability to safely clear an obstacle, but usually at the expense of additional compensation by the ipsilateral hip and foot.

Finally, the use of orthoses and other mobility aids will help reduce the gait disorder. Although there are few data supporting their use, lifts (either internal or external) to correct for limb length inequality may be provided in a conservative, gradually progressive manner. Other ankle braces, shoe inserts, shoe body and sole modifications, and their subsequent adjustments are part of standard care for foot and ankle weakness, deformities, and pain but are beyond the scope of this review. In general, well-fitting walking shoes with low heels, relatively thin firm soles, and, if feasible, high, fixed heel collar support are recommended to maximize balance and improve gait. Mobility aids such as canes and walkers reduce load on a painful joint and increase stability. Note that light touching of any firm surface like walls or "furniture surfing" provides feedback and enhances balance. (See also "Rehabilitation," p 101, and "Diseases and Disorders of the Foot," p 416.)

REFERENCES

■ Alexander NB. Gait disorders in older adults. *J Am Geriatr Soc.* 1996;44(4):434–451.

■ Liston R, Mickelborough J, Bene J, et al. A new classification of higher level gait disorders in patients with cerebral multi-infarct states. *Age Ageing.* 2003;32(3):252–258.

■ Van Hook FW, Demonbreun D, Weiss BD. Ambulatory devices for chronic gait disorders in the elderly. *Am Fam Physician.* 2003;67(8):1717–1724.

■ Verghese J, Lipton RB, Hall CB, et al. Abnormality of gait as a predictor of non-Alzheimer's dementia. *N Engl J Med.* 2002;347(22):1761–1768.

CHAPTER 28—FALLS

KEY POINTS

■ A fall is one of the most common events threatening the independence of older adults. Complications resulting from falls are the leading cause of death from injury in men and women aged 65 and older.

■ The causes of a fall often involve a complex interaction among factors intrinsic to the individual (age-related declines, chronic disease, acute illness, medications), challenges to postural control (environment, changing position, normal activities), and mediating factors (risk-taking behaviors, underlying mobility level).

■ For patients presenting with a fall, important components of the history include the activity of the faller at the time of the incident, the occurrence of prodromal symptoms (lightheadedness, imbalance, and dizziness), the location of the fall, and the time of the fall.

■ A systematic review of interventions to reduce the incidence of falls by elderly persons revealed several that were likely to be effective.

PREVALENCE AND MORBIDITY

A fall is one of the most common events threatening the independence of older persons. A fall is considered to have occurred when a person comes to rest inadvertently on the ground or a lower level. Most discussions in the literature of falls by older persons do not include falls associated with loss of consciousness (eg, syncope, seizure) or with over-whelming trauma. The majority of falls are not associated with syncope.

The incidence of falls increases with age and varies according to living status. Each year, between 30% and 40% of community-dwelling persons aged 65 years and older fall. Among those with a history of a fall in the previous year, the annual incidence of falls is close to 60%. In the long-term-care setting each year, about half of all persons fall.

Complications resulting from falls are the leading cause of death from injury in men and women aged 65 and older. The death rate attributable to falls increases with age, with white men aged 85 years and older having the highest death rate (>180 deaths per 100,000 population). Most falls result in an injury of some type, usually minor soft-tissue injuries, such as bruises and scrapes; however, 10% to 15% result in fracture or other serious injury. In general, falls are associated with subsequent declines in functional status, greater likelihood of nursing-home placement, increased use of medical services, and the development of a fear of falling. Of those elderly persons who fall, only half are able to get up without help, thus experiencing the "long lie." Long lies are associated with lasting declines in functional status.

The true cost of falls in health care dollars is difficult to ascertain. It has been estimated that in the United States the lifetime costs of fall-related injuries for persons aged 65 and older is $12.6 billion. Since many falls result in injury, there is a significant use of emergency department facilities among fallers. Studies from the early 1990s indicate that each year almost 8% of persons aged 70 and older go to emergency departments because of a fall-related injury, and close to a third of these people are admitted to the hospital for a median length of stay of 8 days.

CAUSES

Falls, incontinence, delirium, and other geriatric syndromes result from the accumulated effects of impairments in multiple domains. The falls of older people are rarely due to a single cause. Rather, there is often a complex interaction among factors intrinsic to the individual (age-related declines, chronic disease, acute illness, medications), challenges to postural control (environment, changing positions, normal activities), and mediating factors (risk-taking behaviors, underlying mobility level).

Multiple prospective cohort studies of risk factors for falls have been published over the past decade. Across these studies, many risk factors were found to be consistently associated with falls. These included age, cognitive impairment, female gender, past history of a fall, lower extremity weakness, gait problems, foot disorders, balance problems, hypovitaminosis D, psychotropic drug use, arthritis, and Parkinson's disease. These studies differed significantly in the types of risk factors evaluated, the types of population studied (eg, past fall history was sometimes an entry criterion), and the outcome (one fall, two or more falls, injurious falls). The multiple risk factors found across the studies highlights the multifactorial nature of falls and suggests that there may also be unique circumstances surrounding falls that are not accounted for in the studies. In general, the risk of falling increases with the number of risk factors, although some persons with no risk factors experience falls.

Successful prevention of falls begins with a knowledge of the age-related changes that increase the risk of falls. Thus, with aging, there are declines in the visual, proprioceptive, and vestibular systems. For example, the visual system demonstrates reductions in visual acuity, depth perception, contrast sensitivity, and dark adaptation. The proprioceptive system loses sensitivity in the lower extremities. The vestibular system demonstrates a loss of labyrinthine hair cells, vestibular ganglion cells, and nerve fibers.

Despite these age-related changes in sensory systems, it has been difficult to quantify the age-related changes in postural control that are independent of disease. In general, when postural stability is tested in young and old persons with no apparent musculoskeletal or neurologic impairment, age-related differences in measured sway are found to be most pronounced when moderately severe perturbations of stance are administered, such as changing the support surface, changing body position, altering the visual input, or moving the support surface horizontally or rotationally. This occurs because these perturbations stress the redundancy of the sensory systems in their ability to maintain postural stability. In addition, there may be other age-related changes in the central nervous system that affect postural control, including the loss of neurons and dendrites, and the depletion of neurotransmitters, such as dopamine, within the basal ganglia.

Since it is difficult to find elderly persons without at least subtle neurologic findings, studies have been unable to determine whether some of the young-old differences may be due to these factors. Some of the most striking postural control differences between young and old persons relate to the order or grouping of muscle activation patterns. Thus, in response to perturbations of the support surface, older persons tend to activate the proximal muscles, such as the quadriceps, before the more distal muscles, such as the tibialis anterior. This strategy may not be an efficient way to maintain postural stability. Similarly, in the elderly person there may be greater co-contraction of antagonistic muscles, and the onset of the muscle activation and associated joint torque may be delayed. Finally, the ability to recover balance upon a postural disturbance may be compromised by an age-related decline in the ability to rapidly develop joint torque by using muscles of the lower extremity. All of these strategies potentially impair maintenance of upright posture.

Another important physiologic contributor to the successful maintenance of upright posture is the regulation of systemic blood pressure. The failure to perfuse the brain, which accompanies hypotension, increases the risk of a fall, usually in association with syncope. In addition to the age-related declines in baroreflex sensitivity to hypotensive stimuli manifested as a failure to cardio-accelerate, everyday stresses such as changing posture, eating a meal, or suffering an acute illness may result in hypotension. Since many elderly persons have a resting cerebral perfusion that is compromised by vascular disease, even slight reductions in blood pressure may produce cerebral ischemic symptoms, such as falls. Finally, with aging, there is a reduction in total body water, which places older persons at increased risk of dehydration with acute illness, diuretic use, or hot weather. Since there is a progressive decrease in basal and stimulated renin levels, as well as a decrease in aldosterone production with aging, dehydrating stresses may lead to orthostatic hypotension and a fall.

A number of age-related chronic conditions deserve special mention because of their association with fall risk. Parkinson's disease, in particular, increases the risk of falls through several mechanisms, including the rigidity of lower extremity musculature, the inability to correct sway trajectory because of the slowness in initiating movement, hypotensive drug effects, and, in some cases, cognitive impairment. Another common disease contributing to falls is osteoarthritis. When present in the knee, osteoarthritis may affect mobility, the ability to step over objects and maneuver, and the tendency to avoid complete weight bearing on a painful joint.

One of the most easily modified risk factors for falls that has been repeatedly demonstrated in observational studies is medication use. Individual classes of medications, such as the benzodiazepines, antidepressants (including selective serotonin-reuptake inhibitors), and antipsychotic drugs, have been associated with an increased risk of hip fracture. An increased risk of falling has also been found to be associated with recent changes in the dose of a medication and the total number of prescriptions.

The relative importance of environmental factors to the risk of falling appears to be much less than intrinsic factors in the individual; however, the interaction between environmental factors and intrinsic factors has not been well quantified. Well-designed intervention studies have focused on improving the risk-factor profile of the person or have combined individual interventions with environmental manipulation, making it difficult to isolate the contributions of the environmental factors. Nevertheless, attention to safety hazards in the home environment would appear to be worthwhile, and one intervention study targeting environmental factors was successful in reducing falls.

DIAGNOSTIC APPROACH

The evaluation and management of falls in the geriatric patient may differ according to the clinical setting (home, hospital, nursing home). Table 28.1 highlights some of the differences that might be considered according to setting.

History and Physical Examination

Many falls never come to clinical attention for a variety of reasons: The patient may never mention the event, there is no injury at the time of the fall, the clinician may fail to ask the patient about a history of falls, or the patient or the clinician may make the invalid assumption that falls are an inevitable part of the aging process. In institutional settings, despite attention to falls and even incident reporting, not all falls come to the attention of the nursing staff. The treatment of injuries resulting from falls commonly fails to include an investigation of the cause of the fall.

In the clinical evaluation of the noninstitutionalized geriatric patient who is not specifically being seen for a problem with falling, it is still important that an assessment of fall risk be integrated into the history and physical examination. (See Figure 28.1 for an overview of falls assessment and management in all older persons.) The most important point in the history is the previous history of a fall, since this is a strong risk factor for future falls. For patients presenting with a fall, important components of the history include the activity of the faller at the time of the incident, the occurrence of prodromal symptoms (lightheadedness, imbalance, dizziness), the location of the fall, and the time of the fall. Loss of consciousness is associated with injurious falls and should raise important considerations, such as orthostatic hypotension or cardiac or neurologic disease. (See "Syncope," p 156.) Information on previous falls should be collected to identify patterns that may help target strategies to reduce risk factors. A complete medication history should focus specifically on the use of vasodilators, diuretics, and sedative hypnotics because these agents have been associated with increased risk of falls. In addition to inquiring about the circumstances surrounding the fall, the clinician taking the history should attempt to identify environmental factors that may have contributed. Thus, information on lighting, floor covering, door thresholds, railings, and furniture may add important clues.

The physical examination of the person who has fallen should focus on risk factors. Much of the examination duplicates that of a gait assessment (see "Gait Impairment," p 181.) Footwear may also be an important factor to consider. In one small study to test the effect of various shoe types on balance in older men, shoes with thin, hard soles were found to produce the best results, even though they were perceived as less comfortable than thick, soft, mid-soled shoes, such as running shoes.

Probably the most important part of the physical examination is an assessment of integrated musculoskeletal function, which can be accomplished by performing one or more of the following tests of postural stability.

A simple maneuver called the *functional reach test* is a practical way to test the integrated neuromuscular base of support and has predictive validity for falls by elderly men. This test is performed with a leveled yardstick secured to a wall at the height of the acromion. The person being tested assumes a comfortable stance without shoes or socks and stands so that his or her shoulders are perpendicular to the yardstick. He or she makes a fist and extends the arm forward as far as possible along the wall without taking a step or losing balance. The total reach is measured along the yardstick and recorded. Inability to reach 6 inches or more is cause for concern and merits further evaluation. In its initial description, the functional reach correlated with other physical performance measures, such as walking speed ($r = 0.71$), tandem walk using an ordinal scale ($r = 0.67$), and standing on one foot measured as number of seconds that a one-footed stance could be maintained ($r = 0.64$).

Table 28.1—The Role of Setting in the Assessment and Management of Falls Risk

Characteristic	Home	Hospital	Nursing Home
How falls come to clinical attention	Patient or family reports or clinician queries patient	Nurse, other staff witnesses fall or finds patient on floor	Nurse, other staff witnesses fall or finds resident on floor

Assessment of falls risk	Age
	Past history of fall
	Cognitive impairment
	Female gender
	Lower extremity weakness
	Gait problems, foot disorders
	Balance problems
	Hypovitaminosis D
	Psychotropic drug use
	Arthritis
	Parkinson's disease
		Age
		Past history of a fall
		Impaired mental status
		Special toileting needs
		Impaired mobility
		Visual impairment
			Using MDS data:
			  Age ≥87 years
			  Past history of fall
			  Male gender
			  Unsteady gait
			  Wandering
			  Walking aid
			  ADLs deterioration
			  Transfer independence
			  Wheelchair independence

Management	Muscle strengthening or balance training individual prescribed by clinician Tai Chi Home hazard assessment prescribed for those with history of falls Multidisciplinary, multifactorial health and environmental risk-factor screening or intervention programs for: ■ unselected community-dwelling older people ■ older people with a history of falling ■ older people selected because of known risk factors	No proven interventions have been reported Many risk assessments have reasonable sensitivity and specificity to be of potential value in targeting high-risk patients if a proven intervention is developed	No proven interventions have been reported Since nursing-home residents are a very high-risk population, applying universal precautions may be more appropriate than relying on individual assessments

NOTE: ADL = activities of daily living; MDS = Minimum Data Set.

Another useful test of integrated strength and balance is the Get Up and Go test, which can be performed with or without timing. It consists of observation of an individual standing up from a chair without using the arms to push against the chair, walking across a room, turning around, walking back, and sitting down without using the arms. This test can demonstrate muscle weakness, balance problems, and gait abnormalities.

Laboratory and Diagnostic Tests

There is no standard diagnostic evaluation of a person with a history of falls or with a high risk of falling. Obviously, laboratory tests for hemoglobin, serum urea nitrogen, creatinine, or glucose levels can help to exclude such causes of falling as anemia, dehydration, or hyperglycemia with hyperosmolar dehydration. There is no proven value of routinely performing Holter monitoring of persons who have fallen. Because data demonstrate that carotid sinus hypersensitivity contributes to falls and even hip fracture, some have advocated performing carotid sinus massage with con-tinuous heart rate and phasic blood-pressure measurement in persons with unexplained falls. Similarly, the decision to perform echocardiography, brain imaging, or radiographic studies of the spine should be driven by the findings of the history and physical examination. Echocardiography should be reserved for those with cardiac conditions believed to contribute to the maintenance of blood flow to the brain. Spine radiographs or magnetic resonance imaging may be useful in patients with gait disorders, abnormalities on neurologic examination, lower extremity spasticity, or hyperreflexia to exclude cervical spondylosis or lumbar stenosis as a cause of falls.

TREATMENT AND PREVENTION

Multiple studies of preventive interventions have been conducted over the past decade, including programs to improve strength or balance, educational programs, optimization of medications, and environmental modifications in homes or institutions. Some interventions have targeted single risk factors; others have attempted to address multiple factors.

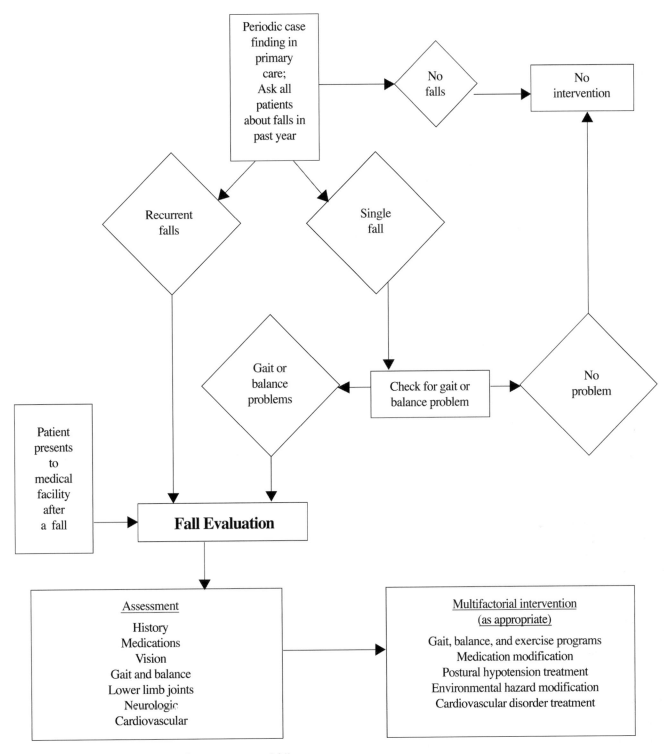

Figure 28.1—The assessment and management of falls.

SOURCE: American Geriatrics Society, British Geriatrics Society, and American Academy of Orthopaedic Surgeons Panel on Falls Prevention. Guideline for the prevention of falls in older persons. *J Am Geriatr Soc.* 2001;49(5):666. Reprinted by permission of Blackwell Science, Inc.

A Cochrane Collaboration systematic review of interventions to reduce the incidence of falling in elderly persons was performed. This review considered only studies that included elderly persons of either sex who were living in the community or in institutional care, randomized to an intervention versus control or into one of two interventions. As of the February 2005 update of this systematic review, 62 individual trials meeting the inclusion criteria were identified. Of the 62 studies, 47 reported the effect of interventions in persons living in the community, eight were set in long-term-care institutions or in nursing homes, and four studies were in rehabilitation or geriatric assessment wards in hospitals. Three further studies included participants with specific conditions from a range of residential settings. Interventions were grouped into ten groups:

- Exercise or physical therapy
- Modification of home hazards
- Cognitive-behavioral intervention
- Medication withdrawal or adjustment
- Nutritional or vitamin supplementation
- Hormonal and other pharmacologic therapies
- Referral for correction of visual deficiency
- Cardiac pacemaker insertion for syncope-associated falls
- Multidisciplinary, multifactorial, health, and environmental risk-factor screening and intervention
- System modifications to prevent falls in high-risk hospital patients

Results from this systematic review suggested interventions that were likely to be beneficial:

- A program of muscle strengthening and balance training, individually prescribed at home by a trained health professional (three trials, 566 participants, pooled relative risk [RR] 0.80, 95% confidence interval [CI], 0.66 to 0.98)
- A 15-week Tai Chi group exercise intervention (one trial, 200 participants, risk ratio 0.51, 95% CI, 0.36 to 0.74)
- Assessment and modification of home hazards that is professionally prescribed for older people with a history of falling (three trials, 374 participants, relative hazard 0.66, 95% CI, 0.54 to 0.81)
- Multidisciplinary, multifactorial, health and environmental risk factor screening or intervention programs, both for unselected community-dwelling older people (data pooled from four trials, 1651 participants, pooled RR

0.73, 95% CI, 0.63 to 0.85), and for older people with a history of falling or selected because of known risk factors (data pooled from five trials, 1176 participants, pooled RR 0.86, 95% CI, 0.76 to 0.98)

- Withdrawal of psychotropic medications (1 trial, 93 participants, relative hazard 0.34, 95% CI, 0.16 to 0.74)
- Cardiac pacing for fallers with cardioinhibitory carotid sinus hypersensitivity (1 trial, 175 participants, weighted mean difference −5.20, 95% CI, −9.40 to −1.00)

In contrast, many interventions were reviewed as being of unknown effectiveness:

- Group-delivered exercise interventions (nine trials, 2177 participants)
- Nutritional supplementation (one trial, 50 participants)
- Vitamin D supplementation, with or without calcium (three trials, 679 participants)
- Modification of home hazards in association with advice on optimizing medication (one trial, 658 participants) or in association with an education package on exercise and reducing fall risk (one trial, 3182 participants)
- Pharmacologic therapy with raubasine-dihydroergocristine, a European drug not listed in U.S. formularies (one trial, 95 participants)
- Falls prevention programs in institutional settings
- Interventions using a cognitive-behavioral approach alone (two trials, 145 participants)
- Modification of home hazards for older people without a history of falling (one trial, 530 participants)
- Hormone replacement therapy (one trial, 116 participants)
- Individual lower limb strength training (one trial, 222 participants)
- Correction of visual deficiency (one trial, 276 participants)

More data are needed to confirm whether strategies apparently effective in significantly reducing the number of older people sustaining falls are also effective in reducing more serious sequelae of falls, such as fractures or other injuries.

Interventions that target risk factors for falls in three domains—medications, mobility, and medical conditions—constitute a practical approach for clinicians who are treating older patients with a high risk for or a history of falling (see Table 28.2).

Table 28.2—Preventing Falls: Selected Risk Factors and Suggested Interventions

Factors	Suggested Interventions
Medication-related factors	
Benzodiazepines, sedative-hypnotics, or antipsychotics, antidepressants	Taper and discontinue medications, as possible Address sleep and mood problems with nonpharmacologic interventions (see "Sleep Problems," p 229) Educate regarding appropriate use of medications and monitoring for adverse effects
Recent change in dose or number of prescription medications or use of ≥ 4 prescription medications or use of other medications associated with fall risk	Review medication profile and modify, as possible Monitor response to medications and to dose changes
Mobility-related factors	
Presence of environmental hazards (eg, improper bed height, cluttered walking surfaces, lack of railings, poor lighting)	Improve lighting, especially at night Remove floor barriers (eg, loose carpeting) Replace existing furniture with safer furniture (eg, correct height, more stable) Install support structures (eg, railings and grab bars, esp. in bathroom) Use nonslip bath mats
Impaired gait, balance, or transfer skills	Refer to physical therapy for comprehensive evaluation and rehabilitation Gait training Balance or strengthening exercises If able to perform semi-tandem stance, refer for Tai Chi, yoga, or postural awareness Provide training in transfer skills Prescribe appropriate assistive devices Recommend protective hip padding Install environmental changes (eg, grab bars, raised toilet seats) Recommend appropriate footwear (eg, good fit, nonslip)
Impaired leg or arm strength or range of motion, or proprioception	Strengthening exercises (eg, use of resistive rubber bands, putty) Resistance training 2–3 times/wk to 10 repetitions with full range of motion, then increase resistance Tai Chi Physical therapy
Medical factors	
Parkinson's disease, osteoarthritis, depressive symptoms, impaired cognition, other conditions associated with increased falls	Optimize medical therapy Monitor for disease progression and impact on mobility and impairments Determine need for assistive devices Use bedside commode if frequent nighttime urination
Postural hypotension: drop in systolic blood pressure ≥ 20 mm Hg (or ≥ 20%) with or without symptoms, either immediately or within 3 min of standing	Review medications potentially contributing and adjust dosing or switch to less hypotensive agents; avoid vasodilators and diuretics if possible Educate on activities to decrease effect (eg, slow rising, ankle pumps, hand clenching, elevation of head of bed) and slow rising from recumbent or seated position Prescribe pressure stockings (eg, Jobst) Liberalize salt intake if appropriate Caffeinated coffee (1 cup) or caffeine 100 mg with meals for postprandial hypotension Consider medication to increase pressure (if hypertension, heart failure, and hypokalemia not serious): ■ midodrine 2.5–5 mg three times a day ■ fludrocortisone 0.1 mg once to three times a day
Vision or hearing impairment	Refraction Cataract extraction Good lighting Home safety evaluation Mobility training for visually impaired Cerumen removal Audiological evaluation with hearing aid, if appropriate

SOURCE: Adapted from Reuben DB, Herr KA, Pacala JT, et al. *Geriatrics At Your Fingertips, 2006,* 8th ed. New York: American Geriatrics Society; 2006: Table 39. Reprinted with permission.

Hip Protectors

Many geriatric clinicians are beginning to consider the use of hip protectors to reduce fall-related hip fractures. Systematic reviews of the topic have concluded that there is no evidence that hip protectors are effective in reducing hip fractures in studies in which randomization was by individual patient within an institution or among patients living at home. Earlier studies that found benefits with hip protectors randomly assigned groups of patients to an intervention based on setting (such as by ward in a nursing home) and were potentially susceptible to bias on this basis; more recent studies have randomized individual patients, which is less susceptible to bias. This suggests that there may be unintended "co-interventions" that occur when whole units or facilities participate in trials and are allocated to use hip protectors, and that these co-interventions may benefit residents of these facilities. In addition, the apparent lack of efficacy of hip protectors may be due in part to low adherence rates.

At least a dozen types of hip protectors are commercially available. Many of these hip protectors have not been tested in either the laboratory or in clinical trials, yet they are being promoted by manufacturers. Despite these concerns, until the results from studies with higher rates of adherence are available, it is not unreasonable for clinicians to consider the use of hip protectors in patients at high risk of hip fractures who are willing to use them. Most of the published trials used Safe Hip.

Clinical Guidelines

For elderly patients who have sustained a fall, a multifactorial approach that is based on data about risk factors and a multidimensional assessment of the patient and that targets interventions on the basis of these findings is appropriate. For elderly persons who have no history of falling, it is reasonable to use traditional multidimensional geriatric assessment with targeted interventions as risk factors are identified. For a summary of the recommendations of the expert panel on falls prevention assembled by the American Geriatrics Society, the British Geriatrics Society, and the American Academy of Orthopaedic Surgeons, see the Appendix (p 459).

References

- American Geriatrics Society, British Geriatrics Society, and American Academy of Orthopaedic Surgeons Panel on Falls Prevention. Guideline for the prevention of falls in older persons. *J Am Geriatr Soc.* 2001;49(5):664–672.

- Colon-Emeric C, Schenck A, Gorospe J, et al. Translating evidence-based falls prevention into clinical practice in nursing facilities: Results and lessons from a quality improvement collaborative. *J Am Geriatr Soc.* 2006;54(9):1414–1418.

- Fletcher PC, Hirdes JP. Risk factors for falling among community-based seniors using home care services. *J Gerontol A Biol Sci Med Sci.* 2002;57(8):M504–M510.

- Gillespie L, Gillespie W, Robertson M, et al. Interventions for preventing falls in elderly people. *Cochrane Database Syst Rev.* 2003;4:CD00340; 2005 update.

- Kron M, Loy S, Sturm E, et al. Risk indicators for falls in institutionalized frail elderly. *Am J Epidemiol.* 2003;158(7):645–653.

- Robertson MC, Devlin N, Gardner MM, et al. Effectiveness of economic evaluation of a nurse delivered home exercise programme to prevent falls. 1: randomised controlled trial. *BMJ.* 2001;322(7288):697–701.

CHAPTER 29—OSTEOPOROSIS AND OSTEOMALACIA

Key Points

- Osteoporosis is a common, preventable, and treatable disorder in older adults. Osteomalacia, though less common, is also treatable and preventable; it should be considered in older adults with myalgias, fatigue, proximal muscle weakness, and fractures.

- Measurement of bone mineral density is recommended routinely in women aged 65 and older, and in others with risk factors for osteoporosis.

- Secondary osteoporosis should be excluded in men and women with osteoporosis. Common causes of secondary osteoporosis include medications, hypogonadism, hyperthyroidism, hyperparathyroidism, and osteomalacia.

- Prevention of osteoporosis includes adequate calcium and vitamin D intake, weight-bearing exercise, and consideration of bisphosphonates, which continue to be first-line pharmacologic treatment. Consider raloxifene for high-risk patients.

- Because osteoporosis is a result of unbalanced bone formation and resorption, and associated fractures usually involve a fall, optimal prevention and treatment also include strategies to minimize bone resorption and to reduce falls, as well as measures to reduce risk factors, especially smoking, low physical activity, and poor diet.

DEFINITION OF OSTEOPOROSIS

Osteoporosis was defined previously by a consensus panel as a "disease characterized by low bone mass and microarchitectural deterioration of bone tissue leading to enhanced bone fragility and a consequent increase in fracture incidence." According to this definition, the diagnosis of osteoporosis requires the presence of a fracture. The World Health Organization now defines osteoporosis by bone mineral density (BMD) measurement, which allows diagnosis and treatment of osteoporosis prior to incident fracture. If a woman has a BMD measurement at any site <2.5 standard deviations below the young adult standard (a T score of <−2.5), the diagnosis of osteoporosis can be made. Further, women with osteopenia (low bone mass, with a T score of ≥−2.5 but <−1) and normal bone mass (with a T score of ≥−1) can also be identified. Thus, the clinician can make the diagnosis of osteoporosis and begin the appropriate therapy before fracture occurs. In addition, women with osteopenia can be placed on a preventive regimen and then followed carefully for further bone loss. Specific standards for definitions of osteoporosis have not been established for men or for racial and ethnic groups other than white persons, although it appears that similar standards apply to men and to Hispanic women.

EPIDEMIOLOGY AND IMPACT OF OSTEOPOROSIS

In 1990 more than 1.25 million hip fractures were reported worldwide in women, and 500,000 in men. In the United States, the estimated numbers of hip and vertebral fractures in women annually are more than 250,000 and 500,000, respectively. To this number must be added fragility fractures in men, which occur at about one third the rate seen in women. Thus, approximately 1 million Americans suffer fragility fractures each year, at a cost of more than $14 billion. The consequences of osteoporosis include diminished quality of life, decreased independence, and increased morbidity and mortality. The pain and kyphosis, height loss, and other changes in body habitus that occur as a result of vertebral compression fractures erode quality of life for both women and men. In addition, the functional status of patients who have had vertebral crush fractures may also decrease. These patients may be unable to bathe, dress, or walk independently. Increased mortality is related primarily to hip fractures; 20% higher mortality rates are seen in older adults in the year after hip fracture. In addition, approximately 50% of women with hip fracture do not fully recover prior function. Thus, in older adults, it is important to prevent as many fractures as possible.

BONE REMODELING AND BONE LOSS IN AGING

Bone is able to repair itself by actively remodeling, a coupled process (also called *bone turnover*) of bone resorption followed by bone formation; bone remodeling continues throughout life. Local signals, not yet fully understood, bring osteoclasts to specific areas of bone where resorption is initiated and resorption cavities are formed. Once osteoclasts have completed the resorption process, osteoblasts move into the area and begin to lay down osteoid and, later, to calcify the matrix. Under optimal conditions, once bone remodeling is completed in a specific area, the resorption spaces are completely filled with new bone. However, after menopause in women, and with aging in men and women, the remodeling cycle becomes unbalanced, and bone resorption increases more than formation does, resulting in net bone loss. The majority of treatments for osteoporosis act to inhibit bone resorption rather than to increase bone formation.

Bone mass changes over the life span of an individual. In women, bone mass increases rapidly from the time of puberty until approximately the mid-20s to mid-30s, at which time bone mass peaks. Once bone mass peaks, a few years of stability are followed by a slow rate of bone loss, beginning well before the onset of menopause. After menopause, the rate of bone loss is quite rapid—as much as 7% per year—for up to 7 years, as a consequence of estrogen deficiency. In later life, bone loss continues, albeit at a slower rate, generally 1% to 2% per year; however, some older women may lose bone density at a higher rate. Data strongly suggest that terminating bone loss at any time will decrease fracture risk. It has been estimated that a 14% increase in bone density in 80-year-old women would halve the hip fracture risk. This 14% increase would also be realized if bone loss were prevented in 70-year-old women.

Although studies thus far have focused mostly on women, it is well documented that men lose bone with age. Cross-sectional studies have detected a slower rate of bone loss in men than in women, but in a longitudinal study the rates of bone loss in men were found to equal those of older women, although men start from a higher bone mass. It is estimated that men aged 30 to 90 years lose approximately 1% per year in the radius and spine; some men with risk factors lose as much as 6% per year. These data suggest that older men lose bone at rates similar to those of older women; however, vertebral fracture rates in men are lower.

Both men and women lose predominantly cancellous bone, which is concentrated in the vertebral spine. Cortical bone accounts for 45% to 75% of the mechanical resistance to compression of the vertebral spine, and men actually gain cortical bone through periosteal bone deposition. Men also increase the cross-sectional area of their vertebrae by 15% to 20%, increasing maximal load levels until the age of 75. The increased bone strength seems to be reversed by thinning of the cortical ring by age 75, the age at which men begin to present with vertebral fractures. Although bone loss at the hip has not been extensively studied in men, in cross-sectional analyses healthy men were found to lose 40% of femoral neck BMD between the ages of 20 and 90 years.

PATHOGENESIS OF OSTEOPOROSIS

Estrogen Deficiency in Women

The pathogenesis of osteoporosis in women is complex. Factors that affect the level of peak bone mass, the rate of bone resorption, and the rate of bone formation need to be considered. Peak bone mass appears to be 75% to 80% genetically determined, although which genes are involved is not clear. A number of candidate genes that may be important to osteoporosis are being explored currently: vitamin D receptor, estrogen receptor, transforming growth factor, interleukin-6, interleukin-1 receptor 2, type I collagen genes, and collagenases. Several factors may work to increase bone resorption in older women. After menopause, and with estrogen deficiency, a variety of factors that act locally on bone may lead to increased bone resorption. Factors thought to play a role in the bone loss of estrogen deficiency include interleukin-1, interleukin-1 receptor antagonist, interleukin-6, and tumor necrosis factor, as well as their binding proteins and receptors.

Calcium Deficiency and Secondary Hyperparathyroidism

The mechanism by which older men and women continue to lose bone is likely related to calcium deficiency, which produces secondary hyperparathyroidism. Parathyroid hormone (PTH) is a potent stimulator of bone resorption when chronically elevated. Aging skin and decreased exposure to sunlight reduce the conversion of 7-dehydrocholesterol to cholecalciferol (vitamin D_3) by ultraviolet light, and the result is vitamin-D insufficiency in older adults. Vitamin-D insufficiency, in turn, reduces the absorption of calcium. Further, older adults tend to ingest inadequate amounts of vitamin D and calcium. As a result of decreased serum levels of calcium, PTH—acting to maintain serum levels of calcium—increases, which leads to increased bone resorption. In one study, older women (mean age 79 years) hospitalized with a hip fracture had lower 25(OH)D levels and higher PTH, higher bone resorption, and lower bone formation than women in the control group (mean age 77 years). Further, data from the Study of Osteoporotic Fractures indicate that women with low fractional absorption of calcium are at increased risk of hip fracture. (See also "Endocrine and Metabolic Disorders," p 337, for more on disorders of calcium metabolism.)

Androgens in Men

Androgens are important determinants of peak bone mass in men. Bone accretion is closely related to sexual maturity, and men who have abnormal puberty or delayed puberty have reduced bone mass. In addition, men with estrogen deficiency or resistance have decreased bone mass and lack of epiphyseal closure. Several studies have demonstrated that late-onset hypogonadism can also play a role in osteoporosis in men. Although it is evident that severe male hypogonadism can cause osteoporosis, the effect of moderate decreases in testosterone levels in aging men on rates of bone loss is uncertain. One study found that more than 60% of men presenting with hip fracture had low testosterone levels, compared with about 20% of men in the control group.

Changes in Bone Formation

In men and women, osteoblast activity appears to decrease with aging, compounding the bone loss that results from increased resorption seen with aging and, for women, with menopause. Growth factors, such as transforming growth factor B and insulin-like growth factor 1, may be impaired with estrogen deficiency or with aging, resulting in decreased osteoblast function.

DIAGNOSIS OF OSTEOPOROSIS AND PREDICTION OF FRACTURE

Risk Factors

Risk factors for osteoporosis and osteoporotic fracture have been identified and have been used to determine who should be placed on preventive or therapeutic regimens. Risk factors, however, are mediocre predictors of low bone density and fractures, and it is more useful to identify modifiable risk factors and to implement change as part of a treatment or preventive program. Table 29.1 lists modifications of risk factors of osteoporosis; all of these risk factors should be addressed by the clinician as part of the routine care of an older adult. Risk factors can also be used to identify women younger than 65 years of age who should have BMD screening.

Secondary Causes

The diagnosis of idiopathic or primary osteoporosis is made by bone density measurement prior to fracture or by incident fracture. Exclusion of other diseases that may present as fracture or with low bone mass is important in the evaluation of women and men with osteoporosis, since different treatment would be required. The major secondary causes of osteoporosis are listed in Table 29.2, along with laboratory tests used to exclude each disease. These laboratory tests should be considered for patients who present with acute compression fracture or who present with a diagnosis of osteoporosis by BMD measurement. The most common causes of secondary osteoporosis in women are primary hyperparathyroidism and glucocorticoid use. Men are more likely to have a secondary cause of osteoporosis than women; as many as 50% of osteoporotic men may have a secondary cause. The most commonly reported secondary causes of osteoporosis in men are hypogonadism and malabsorption syndromes, including gastrectomy. Medications that might have a detrimental effect on bone should be given with adjusted doses or discontinued. In older adults, glucocorticoids and thyroid hormone are used

Table 29.1—Modifications to Reduce the Risk of Osteoporosis

Exercise: Encourage regular, weight-bearing exercise

Nutrition: Encourage

- adequate intake of calcium and vitamin D
- lower intake of animal protein

Medications that may increase risk of osteoporosis—use with caution:

- anticonvulsants
- cyclosporine
- glucocorticoids
- long-term heparin
- methotrexate
- thyroid hormone replacement (dose dependent)

Smoking cessation

OL Not approved by the U.S. Food and Drug Administration for this use.

Table 29.2—Screening for Secondary Osteoporosis*

Disease	Recommended Laboratory Tests
Cushing's disease	**Electrolytes**, 24-hour urinary cortisol
Hyperthyroidism	**Thyroid-stimulating hormone**, thyroxine levels
Hypogonadism (men only)	**Bioavailable testosterone**
Multiple myeloma	**Complete blood cell count, serum electrophoresis**, urine electrophoresis
Osteomalacia	**Alkaline phosphatase**, 25(OH)D
Paget's disease	**Alkaline phosphatase**
Primary hyperparathyroidism	**Calcium**, parathyroid hormone levels

* Bolded items are recommended routinely.

quite commonly; accordingly, the effects these medications may have on the already increased risk of fracture should be considered when they are prescribed for older adults.

Glucocorticoids result in bone loss primarily through the direct suppression of bone formation, although they also further reduce sex hormone levels and cause secondary hyperparathyroidism through their effects on intestinal calcium absorption. The prevalence of vertebral fractures in people taking glucocorticoids for 1 year is estimated to be 11%. The rate of trabecular bone loss is dose dependent and generally occurs in the first 6 months of therapy. Although inhaled corticosteroids have not been as well studied, high doses of high-potency inhaled steroids may also result in bone loss. The best strategy for older adults who require long-term glucocorticoid therapy is to maximize bone health by a variety of interventions. It is important to use the lowest possible dose of glucocorticoids, to assure adequate calcium and vitamin D intake (see the treatment section, below). Further, alendronate OL, risedronate, and intermittent etidronate OL have been shown to successfully prevent bone loss that is due to glucocorticoid therapy when they are initiated at the same time as the steroids (see the treatment section, below).

Bone Density Measurement

BMD, or bone mass measurement, is the best predictor of fracture. The relative risk of fracture is 10 times greater in women in the lowest quartile of BMD than in women whose BMD is in the highest quartile.

Bone density of the hip, spine, wrist, or calcaneus may be measured by a variety of techniques. The preferred method of BMD measurement is dual-energy radiographic absorptiometry (DXA). BMD of the hip, anterior-posterior spine, lateral spine, and wrist can be measured with this technology. Other methods of measuring BMD, include quantitative computed tomography, heel ultrasonography, single radiographic absorptiometry of the heel, and radiographic absorptiometry. Quantitative DXA is the best predictor of hip fracture and is equal to the wrist in predicting fractures at other sites; the relative risk of fracture for each decrease in standard deviation in BMD is 2.6. In the Study of Osteoporotic Fractures, heel ultrasonography was found to be slightly worse that DXA of the hip in predicting hip fracture in women 65 years and older. The National Osteoporosis Foundation, in conjunction with numerous specialty organizations including the U.S. Preventive Services Task Force, recommends BMD testing for all women aged 65 years and older, regardless of risk-factor status; there are no data to determine the frequency of screening or the age to stop screening for osteoporosis in women. For women between 60 and 64 years of age, the presence of additional risk factors, particularly low body weight and no estrogen replacement therapy, makes their risk of osteoporosis and fracture comparable to that of women over 65 years. Indications for BMD testing are listed in Table 29.3. The cost for DXA testing is between $200 and $300, and Medicare and Medicaid will cover the cost if indications for its use (eg, estrogen deficiency) are met.

BMD testing may also be used to establish the diagnosis and severity of osteoporosis in men, and it should be considered for men with low-trauma fractures, radiographic criteria consistent with low bone mass, or diseases known to place a person at risk of osteoporosis. Data relating BMD to fracture risk are derived from studies of women, but data suggest that similar associations may be valid for men. Data from several studies indicate that patients with hip fractures are often not evaluated and treated for osteoporosis. The diagnosis of osteoporosis should be considered in any older adult with a fracture, and evaluation is indicated if treatment would be considered for the individual patient.

Biochemical Markers of Bone Turnover

Serum and urine biochemical markers can estimate the rate of bone turnover (remodeling) and may provide additional information to assist the clinician. A number of markers have been developed that reflect collagen breakdown (or bone resorption) and bone formation. Several markers have been associated with increased hip fracture risk, decreased bone density, and bone loss in older adults. In addition, markers of bone resorption and formation decrease in response to antiresorptive treatment. The use of markers in clinical practice, however, is controversial because of the substantial overlap of marker values in women with high and low

Table 29.3—Indications for Bone Mineral Density Testing*

Postmenopausal women with multiple risk factors** for osteoporosis

Postmenopausal women who present with fractures

Men with conditions† indicating high risk for osteoporosis

Women and men with osteoporosis who have been on treatment for prolonged periods

All women ≥ 65 years old

* In persons who would consider treatment for osteoporosis.
** Early menopause, white or Asian race, low body weight, no current use of estrogen therapy, sedentary, smoking, alcohol abuse, primary hyperparathyroidism, hyperthyroidism, glucocorticoid use.
† Hypogonadism and glucocorticoid use are the two most common.

bone density or rate of bone loss. Further, few studies have compared the response of a particular marker (or combination of markers) and bone density with therapy in order to determine the magnitude of decrease of a biochemical marker necessary to prevent bone loss or, more importantly, fracture. Two markers of bone resorption, deoxypyridinoline cross-links and cross-linked N-telopeptides of type I collagen, and one formation marker, bone alkaline phosphatase, may be used in clinical practice to provide an early assessment of treatment efficacy. A decrease from baseline levels in the level of these markers after 3 to 6 months of therapy indicates successful treatment.

PREVENTION AND TREATMENT OF OSTEOPOROSIS

The Role of Exercise

Exercise is an important component of osteoporosis treatment and prevention, although exercise alone is not adequate to prevent the rapid bone loss associated with estrogen deficiency in early menopause. Among exercisers in the Rancho Bernardo cohort, those who reported strenuous or moderate exercise had higher BMD at the hip than did those who reported mild or less-than-mild exercise. Similar associations were seen for lifelong regular exercisers and hip BMD. In a randomized study of women ≥10 years postmenopausal, the group receiving calcium supplementation plus exercise had less bone loss at the hip than did those assigned to calcium alone. Further, the effectiveness of high-intensity strength training in maintaining femoral neck BMD as well as in improving muscle mass, strength, and balance in postmenopausal women has been demonstrated, suggesting that resistance training would be useful to help maintain BMD and to reduce the risk of falls among older adults.

Marked decrease in physical activity or immobilization results in a decline in bone mass; accordingly, it is important to encourage older adults to be as active as possible. Weight-bearing exercise, such as walking, can be recommended for all adults. Older people should be encouraged to start slowly and gradually increase both the number of days as well as the time spent walking each day. (See "Physical Activity," p 56.)

Calcium and Vitamin D

Calcium and vitamin D are required for bone health at all ages. In order to maintain a positive calcium balance, the current recommendations for calcium intake for postmenopausal women and men aged 65 years and older is at least 1200 mg per day of elemental calcium. The amount of vitamin D required is between 400 and 800 IU per day. In older adults, regardless of climate or exposure to sunlight, a daily supplement of ≥400 IU per day of vitamin D is recommended because skin changes that occur with aging result in less efficient use of ultraviolet light by the skin to synthesize vitamin-D precursors. Calcium plus vitamin D at different doses have been shown to increase or maintain bone density in postmenopausal women and to prevent hip as well as all nonvertebral fractures in older adults. The dietary intake of calcium for postmenopausal women in the United States averages 500 to 700 mg per day; thus, most American women require calcium supplementation to ensure adequate intake. (See Table 29.4 for information on the calcium contained in selected foods.)

Pharmacologic Options

The dosing, relative costs, and special considerations for the medications used to prevent and treat osteoporosis are provided in Table 29.5.

Bisphosphonates

Alendronate has been approved for osteoporosis prevention (women) and treatment (men and women). Women with osteoporosis who were treated with alendronate and compared with women on placebo were found to have increased bone density of the spine and hip, as well as decreased vertebral fracture rate. The Fracture Intervention Trial examined the effect of alendronate on postmenopausal women with severe osteoporosis, with or without vertebral fracture at baseline. Regardless of the presence of vertebral fractures at baseline, alendronate was found to decrease the vertebral fracture rate. In addition, alendronate resulted in a 50% reduction in hip fractures. A study in women aged 60 to 85 years indicated that an even lower dose of alendronate might be effective in older women. Further, data indicate that once-weekly dosing with alendronate (70 mg) is as effective in increasing

Table 29.4—Calcium-Containing Foods

Food	Serving Size	Calcium (mg) per serving
Dairy Products		
Milk	1 cup	290–300
Yogurt	1 cup	240–400
Swiss cheese	1 ounce (1 slice)	250–270
American cheese	1 ounce (1 slice)	165–200
Ice cream	½ cup	90–100
Cottage cheese	½ cup	80–100
Parmesan cheese	1 tablespoon	70
Powdered non-fat milk	1 teaspoon	50
Other		
Sardines in oil with bones	3 ounces	370
Calcium-fortified orange juice	1 cup	300
Canned salmon with bones	3 ounces	170–210
Broccoli	1 cup	160–180
Tofu (soybean curd)	4 ounces	145–155
Turnip greens	½ cup, cooked	100–125
Kale	½ cup, cooked	90–100
Cornbread	2 ½-inch square	80–90
Egg	1 medium	55
Other fortified foods (bread, cereal, fruit juices)	1 serving	Varies: read label

Table 29.5—Medications Used to Prevent and Treat Osteoporosis

Medication	Dosage	Cost	Special Considerations
Bisphosphonates			
Alendronate	10 mg/d or 70 mg/week; 5 mg/d or 35 mg/week for prevention	$$$$$	Adherence to dosing instructions required (Table 29.6); used in men and women to prevent glucocorticoid-induced osteoporosis
Ibandronate	150 mg/month; IV dosage 3 mg q 3 months	$$$$	Must be taken fasting with water, standing upright and taking nothing by mouth for at least 60 minutes after taking; do not use if CrCl is <30 mL/min
Risedronate	5 mg/d or 35 mg/week	$$$$$	Adherence to dosing instructions required (see Table 29.6)
Selective estrogen receptor modulator			
Raloxifene	60 mg/d	$$$$$	May prevent breast cancer
Calcitonin			
Nasal spray	200 IU/d	$$$$$	Metered spray; 1 spray gives daily dose; alternate nostrils each day to reduce side effects
Injectable (subcutaneously or intramuscularly)	50–100 IU 3 to 5 times/week	$$$$	Injectable still useful, depending on patient
Estrogen	See text	$	Not recommended as first-line choice
Parathyroid hormone (teriparatide)	20 μg/d (injection)	$$$$$	For use in patients who are at high risk for fractures

NOTE: $ = approximately $10 per month.

spine BMD over 1 year as is daily dosing (10 mg) in postmenopausal women with osteoporosis (age range 42 to 95 years). Alendronate has also been approved for the prevention of osteoporosis in early postmenopausal women. The daily dose for prevention is lower—5 mg—than that for treatment of osteoporosis—10 mg. If treatment with alendronate alone is not effective (bone loss of >4% or fracture within 3 months of initiation), combining raloxifene or estrogen replacement therapy with alendronate, which has an additive effect on bone density, may be indicated. In women with lesser degrees of osteoporosis, alendronate has not been shown to prevent hip fracture. Alendronate is approved to treat osteoporosis in men and in glucocorticoid-induced osteoporosis. The optimal duration of treatment with bisphosphonates is unclear; however, one study indicated that the greatest increase in vertebral bone mass occurred during the first 5 years of treatment, and benefit was maintained for 10 years without undue risk.

The major adverse effects of alendronate are gastrointestinal, including abdominal pain, dyspepsia, esophagitis, nausea, vomiting, and diarrhea. Musculoskeletal pain may also occur. Esophagitis, particularly erosive esophagitis, may be seen most commonly in patients who do not take the medication properly. The absorption of oral bisphosphonates is very poor; thus, it is extremely important to provide specific and detailed instructions for patients receiving any bisphosphonate therapy (Table 29.6).

Table 29.6—Instructions for Administration of Bisphosphonates

- Take first thing in the morning before eating or drinking anything else
- Take with at least 8 ounces of plain tap water
- Take while upright in a chair or standing, and remain upright after ingestion
- Do not eat or drink anything for 30 minutes after taking the medication (60 minutes for ibandronate)

Risedronate, another bisphosphonate, is approved for osteoporosis prevention and treatment (women only). In a 3-year study of postmenopausal women with ≥1 vertebral fracture at baseline, the cumulative incidence of new vertebral fractures was reduced by 41% (95% CI, 18% to 58%) in the group receiving risedronate (5 mg per day) rather than placebo. In addition, the incidence of nonvertebral fractures also decreased by 39% (95% CI, 6% to 61%) in the treatment group. BMD of the hip and spine increased significantly in the risedronate group. In the same study, 2.5 mg per day of risedronate was ineffective and discontinued after the first year of the study. Withdrawals because of side effects and any upper gastrointestinal adverse events were similar in the risedronate and placebo groups. In older women (70 to 79 years) with osteoporosis, risedronate decreased the risk of hip fracture by 40% compared with placebo (all participants received adequate calcium and vitamin D) with a relative risk of 0.6 (95% CI, 0.4 to 0.9). In women at least 80 years of age, risedronate did not significantly reduce hip fracture incidence; however, these women were selected primarily on the basis of clinical risk factors rather than on BMD criteria. This study demonstrates that even in older women, BMD measurement and assessment of previous vertebral fractures are needed to identify those for whom the treatment will be the most effective.

Another bisphosphonate approved for the treatment and prevention of osteoporosis in postmenopausal women, ibandronate is the first drug in this class that can be taken daily or monthly. Adverse events and cost are comparable to those of the other bisphosphonates. Decreased vertebral fractures in women with a history of osteoporotic vertebral fractures have been found with daily doses. Neither dosing schedule has been found to reduce the risk of fractures in women without a history of previous fractures or to reduce the risk of hip or nonvertebral fractures.

Selective Estrogen Receptor Modulators

The selective estrogen receptor modulators are agents that act as estrogen agonists in bone and heart but act as estrogen antagonists in breast and uterine tissue. These medications have the potential to prevent osteoporosis or cardiovascular disease without the increased risk of breast or uterine cancer. Tamoxifen, an agent used to treat breast cancer, has beneficial effects on bone, as reported in several studies, but it also has stimulatory effects on the uterus. Thus, tamoxifen is not indicated for osteoporosis treatment or prevention.

Raloxifene has been approved for the treatment and prevention of osteoporosis in postmenopausal women. Comparison of raloxifene with placebo in postmenopausal women with osteoporosis found that raloxifene decreases bone turnover and maintains hip and total body bone density. There were no differences between groups in breast abnormalities or endometrial thickness. Most importantly, data demonstrate that raloxifene (60 mg per day) reduces incident vertebral fractures by about 60%, despite only modest increases in bone density. In this study raloxifene did not significantly reduce nonvertebral, hip, or wrist fractures. Reported adverse effects with raloxifene include flu-like symptoms, hot flushes, leg cramps, and peripheral edema.

Another important finding with raloxifene was reduced risk of breast cancer in women who participated in the Multiple Outcomes of Raloxifene Trial. When women receiving raloxifene were compared with women receiving placebo, the relative risk of developing breast cancer for women receiving raloxifene was 0.24 (95% CI, 0.13 to 0.44). In the same study, raloxifene did not increase the risk of endometrial cancer but did increase the risk of venous thromboembolic disease. In other studies, raloxifene

decreased total and low-density lipoprotein cholesterol and lipoprotein (a) levels without affecting high-density lipoprotein cholesterol or triglyceride levels. Thus, in clinical trials to date, raloxifene appears to benefit several organ systems, although further study is required with regard to cardiovascular diseases and breast cancer prevention.

Calcitonin

Calcitonin is a hormonal inhibitor of bone resorption, and is approved for the treatment of osteoporosis in women. It is available as a subcutaneous injection and as a nasal spray. The nasal spray has fewer reported side effects and greater patient acceptance, but it may be less effective. Calcitonin has been shown to increase bone density in the spine and reduce vertebral fractures. In epidemiologic studies, calcitonin has been shown to reduce the incidence of hip fractures, although in clinical trials, hip bone density has not been found to increase. Results of a 5-year study demonstrated that the incidence of vertebral fractures in women receiving 200 IU per day of nasal spray calcitonin was lower than that of women on placebo. The reduction in hip fracture incidence was not statistically significant in the group receiving calcitonin compared with the placebo group. Dosages of 100 and 400 IU per day were studied as well, but they did not reduce incidence of vertebral fractures. In the same study, BMD changes at 3 years and changes in markers of bone turnover in the treatment and placebo groups were found not to be significantly different. Although there are no direct comparisons, calcitonin appears to be less effective than other antiresorptive drugs. There is some evidence that calcitonin produces an analgesic effect in some women with painful vertebral compression fractures.

Estrogen Replacement Therapy

Estrogen replacement therapy (ERT) is an option for osteoporosis prevention (approved by the Food and Drug Administration; indication for treatment has been withdrawn); however, it is not recommended as a first-line choice. In case-control and cohort studies, ERT has been associated with a 30% to 70% reduction in hip fracture incidence. Multiple studies have demonstrated that postmenopausal estrogen use prevents bone loss at the hip and spine when initiated within 10 years of menopause. However, in a cross-sectional study, BMD in women who began hormone replacement therapy (HRT) after age 60 years was not significantly different from that of women who began HRT within 2 years of menopause. In the Postmenopausal Estrogen/Progestin Intervention trial, older women, women with low initial BMD, and women who had not previously used HRT gained more bone than did young women, women with higher baseline BMD, and women who had previously used HRT. Incident vertebral fractures were decreased in a small study of postmenopausal women using a transdermal estradiol preparation. Recent prospective data from the Women's Health Initiative (WHI) also demonstrated that postmenopausal women who took hormone replacement therapy for approximately 7 years had a decreased risk of hip fracture; however, the dose and preparation of hormone therapy used also increased the risk of breast cancer, heart disease, stroke, and deep-vein thrombosis. Given the WHI findings, recent U.S. Preventive Services Task Force guidelines advise against the routine use of estrogen plus progesterone for the prevention of chronic conditions in postmenopausal women. The estrogen-only arm of WHI was also stopped 1 year ahead of schedule and demonstrated an increased risk of stroke but not of coronary heart disease or breast cancer. Estrogen alone decreased hip fracture risk (relative risk 0.61 [95% CI, 0.41 to 0.91]). Previously, HRT was recommended for prevention of osteoporosis; however, given the results of the WHI and the availability of other effective medications for osteoporosis prevention and treatment, the Food and Drug Administration changed its indication for estrogen and estrogen-progestin products. "When these products are being prescribed solely for the prevention of postmenopausal osteoporosis, approved non-estrogen treatments should be carefully considered. Estrogens and combined estrogen-progestin products should only be considered for women with significant risk of osteoporosis that outweighs the risks of the drug."

See also the section on hormone replacement therapy in "Endocrine and Metabolic Disorders" (p 337).

Parathyroid Hormone

The synthetic form of PTH, teriparatide, although leading to increased bone resorption when continuously elevated, can increase bone mass, trabecular connectivity, and mechanical strength when administered intermittently. Teriparatide is approved for the treatment of osteoporosis in postmenopausal women and in men at high risk of fractures. A history of one or more osteoporotic fractures, a very low BMD, or poor tolerance or lack of response to previous osteoporosis medications indicate a high risk of fractures. Teriparatide should not be used as a first-line therapy for osteoporosis.

Investigational Agents

Other bisphosphonates currently under investigation for the treatment and prevention of osteoporosis include pamidronate, zoledronate, and tiludronate. New selective estrogen receptor modulators are also being tested for use in osteoporosis treatment.

The use of fluoride to treat osteoporosis is appealing because fluoride results in a large increase in vertebral bone density; however, the increase in BMD has not been consistently associated with a decrease in vertebral fractures. In fact, in one study, the group receiving fluoride therapy had a higher rate of appendicular fractures. Slow-release fluoride therapy has been associated with an increase in vertebral BMD, as well as decreased incidence of vertebral fractures. Further studies are required before slow-release fluoride can be recommended for the treatment of osteoporosis.

The use of 3-hydroxy-3-methylglutaryl coenzyme A reductase inhibitors (statins) may also affect bone. This class of medication is commonly prescribed for the management of hypercholesterolemia and stimulates bone formation in animals. Preliminary epidemiologic data suggest that the use of statins is associated with decreased incidence of fracture. However, recent data from the WHI Observational Study indicated that neither fracture risk nor BMD is altered by statin use.

Strontium ranelate increases bone formation and decreases bone resorption in animals. A randomized, placebo-controlled study in postmenopausal women with osteoporosis (at least one vertebral fracture plus lumbar spine T score <-2.5) at baseline demonstrated that strontium ranelate increases BMD and decreases the incidence of vertebral fractures at the highest dose tested (2 g per day). At this dosage, bone alkaline phosphatase increases and urinary excretion of N-telopeptides of type I collagen decreases.

WORKING WITH THE PATIENT

Establishing and maintaining an optimal regimen usually requires considerable discussion with individual patients and is much easier if patients are well informed. The use of educational materials can be quite helpful, as can the efforts of a nurse or other office personnel. Effective prevention and treatment of osteoporosis is possible if the patient and clinician work together in a sustained fashion.

The osteoporosis patient's adherence to the medication regimen is important. Baseline and follow-up BMD measurements (every 1 to 2 years) are important to assess response to therapy; these measurements may also improve adherence by providing visual information regarding the effectiveness of the therapy. Another way to inform patients about their response to therapy is to measure markers of bone resorption. In particular, adequate estrogen and bisphosphonate therapy will almost certainly decrease the levels of urine or serum markers of bone resorption within 3 to 6 months.

MANAGEMENT OF VERTEBRAL FRACTURES

Most vertebral fractures are asymptomatic and are diagnosed by spinal radiographs. Over time, one may notice decreased height, increased kyphosis, or simply the fact that clothes no longer fit the person properly. Many older adults have chronic back pain due to the changes in the spine that occur with vertebral compression. In the case of symptomatic vertebral compression fractures, adequate pain control is essential. The pain usually lasts 2 to 4 weeks and can be quite debilitating. Nonsteroidal anti-inflammatory drugs and calcitonin can be tried; narcotics are commonly required to control the pain. Physical therapy is an important part of osteoporosis treatment programs for the management of acute and chronic pain, as well as for patient education. The physical therapist can provide postural exercises, alternative modalities for pain reduction, and information on changes in body mechanics that may help prevent future fractures. (See also "Persistent Pain," p 131.) Support groups for patients with osteoporosis are also important. Newer treatments for vertebral fractures involve the injection of bone cement into the collapsed vertebra (vertebroplasty) or use of a balloon tamp into the fractured vertebrae (kyphoplasty). Although these methods have not been studied in randomized controlled trials, case reports suggest that they decrease pain and improve quality of life and function. Long-term benefits and complications have not yet been demonstrated; therefore, further study is required before these procedures are used routinely.

OSTEOMALACIA

Osteomalacia, an impairment of bone mineralization, is much less common than osteoporosis and can be definitively diagnosed only by bone biopsy. The clinical syndrome associated with osteomalacia consists of pain, myopathy, and fracture. The most common cause of osteomalacia in older adults is vitamin-D deficiency as a result of inadequate intake. In addition, excessive use of phosphate-binding antacids, chronic use of anticonvulsants, chronic kidney failure, hepatobiliary disease, and malabsorption syndromes may also result in osteomalacia. The use of high-dose etidronate and

fluoride may cause osteomalacia, albeit rarely. The symptoms of osteomalacia may be subtle, and thus the diagnosis may be delayed. Patients typically complain of diffuse bone pain and tenderness, proximal muscle weakness, and generalized fatigue. A characteristic waddling gait may result from the hip pain and thigh weakness. Laboratory studies typically demonstrate an elevated alkaline phosphatase, low phosphate, low or normal calcium, and low 25(OH)D levels. Plain radiographic films may show osteopenia or characteristic pseudofractures, most commonly in the proximal femur.

Osteomalacia is managed by treating the underlying cause. If vitamin-D deficiency is diagnosed, repletion can be accomplished with oral vitamin D, 1000 IU per day. Hypophosphatemia is corrected by the use of neutral phosphate salts, 500 mg four times daily. Patients on long-term anticonvulsant therapy may be supplemented with 400 to 800 IU of vitamin D daily. Osteomalacia due to hepatobiliary disease or chronic kidney failure is managed with supplemental 25(OH)D and $1,25(OH)_2D$, respectively.

REFERENCES

- Bauer DC, Ettinger B, Nevitt MC, et al. Risk for fracture in women with low serum levels of thyroid-stimulating hormone. *Ann Intern Med*. 2001; 134(7):561–568.

- Bellantonio S, Fortinsky R, Prestwood K. How well are community-living women treated for osteoporosis after hip fracture? *J Am Geriatr Soc*. 2001;49(9):1197–1204.

- Bonnick SL, Shulman L. Monitoring osteoporosis therapy: bone mineral density, bone turnover markers, or both? *Am J Med*. 2006;119(4 Suppl 1):S25–31.

- Cauley JA, Robbins J, Chen Z, et al. Effects of estrogen plus progestin on risk of fracture and bone mineral density: the Women's Health Initiative randomized trial. *JAMA*. 2003; 290(13):1729–1738.

- Gass M, Dawson-Hughes B. Preventing osteoporosis-related fractures: an overview. *Am J Med*. 2006;119(4 Suppl 1):S3–S11.

- McClung MR, Geusens P, Miller PD, et al. Effect of risedronate on the risk of hip fracture in elderly women. *N Engl J Med*. 2001;344(5):333–340.

- Orwoll E, Ettinger M, Weiss S, et al. Alendronate for the treatment of osteoporosis in men. *N Engl J Med*. 2000;343(9):604–610.

CHAPTER 30—DEMENTIA

KEY POINTS

- Alzheimer's disease, vascular dementia, and dementia with Lewy bodies are the most common forms of degenerative dementias seen in late life.

- Cholinesterase inhibitors and N-methyl-d-aspartate antagonists may be modestly helpful in reducing the rate of decline in Alzheimer's dementia.

- Behavioral symptoms may occur with any type of dementia and tend to respond best to a combination of environmental modifications and symptomatic medication management.

Dementia is a general term used to describe a series of disorders that cause significant decline in two or more areas of cognitive functioning. One of these areas must be severe enough to cause functional decline. Of those who suffer from dementia, most have Alzheimer's disease (AD), which affects an estimated 4 million people in the United States. The pain and anguish of the disorder also afflicts millions more caregivers and relatives, who must cope with the patient's progressive and irreversible decline in cognition, functioning, and behavior. Both caregivers and patients may misinterpret the initial symptoms of dementia as normal age-related cognitive losses, and clinicians may not recognize early signs or may misdiagnose them. However, dementia and aging are not synonymous. As people age, they usually experience such memory changes as slowing in information processing, but these kinds of changes are benign. By contrast, dementia is progressive and disabling and not an inherent aspect of aging.

Diagnostic and treatment advances have benefited many patients. Early and accurate diagnosis of dementia and its cause may minimize costly use of medical resources and give patients and their relatives time to anticipate future medical, financial, and legal needs. Sustained reversal of the progressive cognitive decline of dementia is not currently possible, but psychosocial and pharmacologic treatments may improve such associated conditions as depression, psychosis, and agitation. (See also "Psychosocial Issues," p 14, "Legal and Ethical Issues," p 20, "Financing, Coverage, and Costs of Health Care," p 29.)

EPIDEMIOLOGY AND SOCIETAL IMPACT

Dementia is a disease of late life, generally beginning after age 60 years. AD represents the most common type of dementia, accounting for approximately two thirds of all cases and affecting 6% to 8% of those aged 65 and over. The disease prevalence doubles every 5 years after age 60; an estimated 30% or more of those who are aged 85 or older have AD. Vascular dementia is thought to be the second most common, causing an estimated 15% to 25% of cases. In recent years, dementia associated with Lewy bodies has received increased attention, and although the exact prevalence is not known, estimates suggest that it may be as common as vascular dementia. Frontotemporal dementia is also a more recent diagnostic category of dementia and represents a smaller percentage of cases, with a younger age of onset than other dementias. Neurodegenerative diseases such as Huntington's disease, Parkinson's disease, or other metabolic causes such as head injury and alcoholism account for other dementia syndromes.

Dementia has a major impact on society. The total costs approach $100 billion annually if the costs of medical and long-term care, home care, and lost productivity for caregivers are included. Medicare, Medicaid, and private insurance pay much of the direct cost, but families caring for patients with dementia must bear the greatest burden of expense.

The financial costs of dementia are only one aspect of the total burden. The emotional toll is immense for both patients and their families. Nearly half of primary caregivers of patients with dementia experience psychologic distress, particularly depression. An accurate economic assessment of the problem underestimates the true cost of the disease to society unless the quality of life of both patients and caregivers is included in the analysis.

RISK FACTORS AND PREVENTION

The two greatest risk factors for AD are age and family history. Studies that account for death from other causes suggest that by age 90 years, nearly half of persons with first-degree relatives (ie, parents, siblings) with AD develop the disease themselves. Rare forms of familial AD beginning before age 60 have been associated with genetic mutations on chromosomes 1, 14, and 21. Most commonly, AD begins late in life; for such late-onset cases, the apolipoprotein E gene (*APOE*) on chromosome 19 influences risk.

The *APOE* gene has three alleles, *APOE*2*, *APOE*3*, and *APOE*4*. Everyone inherits one allele from each parent, so that six common genotypes are possible (2/2, 2/3, 3/3, 2/4, 3/4, and 4/4). Approximately 3% of the general population has the 4/4 genotype, 20% has the 3/4 genotype, and most persons have the 3/3 genotype. The *APOE*4* allele increases risk and decreases age of onset in a dose-related fashion, whereas the *APOE*2* allele may have a protective effect. Thus, the 2/3 genotype has a lower risk for AD than the 3/4 genotype; the AD risk is higher for the 3/4 genotype, and highest for the 4/4 genotype. The *APOE*4* allele may be less common in black Americans.

Using *APOE* genotyping as a prognostic test for asymptomatic persons is not recommended until results from further studies are available. *APOE*4* is neither necessary nor sufficient to cause AD, and cognitively normal centenarians who are homozygous for *APOE*4* have been reported. The asymptomatic person who learns that his or her genotype is 3/3 or 2/3 may be falsely reassured, whereas the person who learns that his or her genotype is 3/4 may be falsely alarmed. *APOE* genotyping may be useful only in increasing the diagnostic confidence for AD if a patient already has dementia.

Other possible risk factors include a previous head injury, female sex, and fewer years of educational achievement. Head trauma is thought to disrupt neuronal synapses. Research suggests that education may delay the onset of dementia, which may represent a confounding variable of socioeconomic status or a factor that truly provides protection by supplying a cognitive "reserve." Risk factors for vascular dementia include hypertension, hyperlipidemia, diabetes mellitus, smoking, age, male sex, and perhaps homocysteine levels. These factors are thought to increase risk by predisposing individuals to impairment in cognition through ischemic mechanisms, although there is new evidence linking some vascular risk factors to Alzheimer's pathology.

The prevention of dementia, especially AD, has been the subject of recent research. Drugs associated with reduced risk in epidemiologic studies include nonsteroidal anti-inflammatory drugs, statins, and possibly antioxidants. Research in normal elderly persons shows a possible protective effect of physical and intellectual activity on the risk for cognitive decline. The onset of dementia may also be delayed by the treatment of hypertension. Table 30.1 lists both risk and protective factors for dementia.

ASSESSMENT METHODS

Most cases of dementia can be diagnosed on the basis of a general medical and psychiatric evaluation. It is important for primary care clinicians to be alert to the early symptoms, as dementia is often undetected until severe symptoms or an adverse event flags its presence. If a patient or family member expresses concerns about cognitive decline, a mental status assessment and probably a dementia evaluation are indicated. There are

Table 30.1—Risk Factors and Protective Factors for Alzheimer's Disease

Definite	
Protective Factors	Risk Factors
Unknown	Age
	Family history
	APOE*4 allele
	Down syndrome

Possible	
Protective Factors	Risk Factors
Nonsteroidal anti-inflammatory drugs	Other genes
Antioxidants	Head trauma
Intellectual activity	Lower educational achievement
Physical activity	Late-onset depression
Statins	

now consensus guidelines available for the clinical diagnosis and treatment of most types of dementia.

The informant interview and office-based clinical assessment are the most important diagnostic tools for dementia. Both the patient and a reliable informant should be interviewed to determine the patient's current condition, medical and medication history, patterns of alcohol use, and living arrangements. Useful informant-based instruments, such as the Functional Activities Questionnaire, can help determine whether lapses in memory or language use have occurred and assess the patient's ability to learn and retain new information, handle complex tasks, and demonstrate sound judgment. Any changes are best determined by comparing present with previous performance, since functional decline and multiple cognitive deficits confirm the diagnosis.

A comprehensive physical examination includes a brief neurologic and mental status evaluation. Brief quantified screening tests of cognitive function, such as the Folstein Mini–Mental State Examination or the Mini-Cog Assessment Instrument for Dementia, may be useful, particularly if they demonstrate change over a 6-month or 1-year follow-up period. A laboratory evaluation, generally including a complete blood cell count, blood chemistries, liver function test, rapid plasma reagent test, and thyrotropin stimulating hormone and vitamin B_{12} levels, is also recommended. In addition, the history or physical examination may indicate the need for other laboratory tests. It is important to conduct cognitive and functional assessments in the patient's native language, if at all possible. In the face of cognitive decline, it is common for dementia patients to retain the greatest fluency in their language of origin.

Although brain imaging studies are optional, specialists may recommend them. They may be considered if:

- onset occurs at an age below 65 years;
- the condition is postacute, that is, symptoms have occurred for less than 2 years;
- there is evidence of focal or asymmetrical neurologic deficits;
- the clinical picture suggests normal-pressure hydrocephalus (ie, onset has occurred within 1 year, gait disorder is present, unexplained incontinence is present); or
- there is a history of a recent fall or other head trauma.

In general, a noncontrast computed tomography head scan is adequate to exclude intracranial bleeding, space-occupying lesions, and hydrocephalus. If vascular dementia is suspected, magnetic resonance imaging (MRI) is often performed, but white matter changes revealed by T2 weighted MRI images generally are not related to dementia and should not be overinterpreted. In cases of unclear diagnosis, a repeat assessment in 6 months will confirm the presence or absence of progressive cognitive decline. Functional brain imaging studies such as positron emission tomography often show the characteristic parietal and temporal deficits in AD or the widespread irregular deficits in vascular dementia and may be useful when the diagnosis is uncertain after routine testing.

Cognitive tests are influenced by educational level. Affected patients with more years of education may have normal scores while patients with less education may have low scores and no decline in function. In addition, it has been shown that tests that are most sensitive to language performance may have cultural differences that lead to an overinterpretation of dementia in minority patients. Poor performance on cognitive tests may result in an increased rate of dementia diagnoses among patients in ethnic minority groups, even though the actual rate of dementia determined in systematic cross-cultural studies does not appear to be different across populations. One way to improve the accuracy of assessment is to evaluate changes in everyday memory function by evaluating a person's performance of daily living skills, either by direct observation or obtaining information from reliable family members.

The practical utility of cognitive measures is that they provide a quantitative baseline against which to compare future assessments. Neuropsychologic testing is helpful in distinguishing normal aging from dementia, as well as identifying deficits that point to a specific diagnosis, and it is recommended when the diagnosis is unclear. In general, the diagnosis of dementia is a clinical one, and laboratory assessment is used to identify uncommon treatable causes and common treatable comorbid conditions.

DIFFERENTIAL DIAGNOSIS OF DEMENTIA

Dementia can be defined as an acquired syndrome of decline in memory and other cognitive functions sufficient to affect daily life in an alert patient. Diagnosis then requires further investigation to identify the cause of the dementia by determining chronology of symptoms along with the pattern and extent of deficits. A general discussion of the most common dementias is provided below, and an overview of diagnostic features is provided in Table 30.2.

Table 30.2—Diagnostic Features of Dementia Syndromes

Feature	Mild Cognitive Impairment	Alzheimer's Disease	Vascular Dementia	Lewy Body Dementia	Fronto-temporal Dementia
Onset	Gradual	Gradual	May be sudden or stepwise	Gradual	Gradual, age < 60
Cognitive domains, symptoms	Primarily memory	Memory, language, visuospatial	Depends on anatomy of ischemia	Memory, visuospatial, hallucinations, fluctuating symptoms	Executive: disinhibition, apathy, language, +/- memory
Motor symptoms	Rare	Rare early, apraxia later	Correlates with ischemia	Parkinsonism	None
Progression	Unknown, 12% per year proceed to AD	Gradual, over 8 to 10 years	Stepwise with further ischemia	Gradual, but faster than AD	Gradual, but faster than AD
Laboratory tests	Normal	Normal	Normal	Normal	Normal
Imaging	Possible global atrophy, small hippocampal volumes	Possible global atrophy, small hippocampal volumes	Cortical or subcortical changes on MRI	Possible global atrophy	Atrophy in frontal and temporal lobes

NOTE: AD = Alzheimer's disease; MRI = magnetic resonance imaging.

Cognition in aging is now understood to be a continuum ranging from mild changes in normal aging to the significant impairments that define dementia. Although studies are not conclusive, it appears that normal aging involves some mild decline in memory, usually requiring more effort and time to recall new information. However, this decline does not impair functioning and is usually well compensated with lists, calendars, and other memory supports.

With early identification of cognitive deficits, a disorder now referred to as *mild cognitive impairment* has been identified. These patients do not have dementia but do have significant impairment in memory without deficits in other cognitive domains and no overt functional impairment. Some research suggests that these individuals convert to AD at a rate of about 12% per year. There is disagreement among experts if this is a unique disorder or merely an early prodrome to AD that has been identified with earlier diagnosis of memory impairments. Studies are under way to determine what if any interventions may be beneficial in this condition.

AD is characterized by gradual onset and progressive decline in cognitive functioning; motor and sensory functions are spared until late stages. Memory impairment is a core symptom of any dementia, and in AD it is present in the earliest stages. Typically, AD patients demonstrate difficulty learning new information and retaining it for more than a few minutes. In later disease stages their ability to learn shows even greater compromise, and patients are unable to access older, more distant memories. Aphasia, apraxia, disorientation, visuospatial dysfunction, and impaired judgment and executive functioning are also present. The initial stages of AD are characterized by normal motor, sensory, and cerebellar functioning. If focal motor or sensory signs, except fluent aphasia and apraxia, are present, a diagnosis of vascular dementia or mixed vascular dementia with AD is likely.

Vascular dementia refers to cognitive deficits most often associated with vascular damage in the brain. Cognitive and neurologic impairments should correlate anatomically with the areas of ischemia, although the often diffuse nature of vascular disease may make this correlation difficult to identify. A history of "small strokes," unless accompanied by a clear demonstration of focal signs of motor or sensory impairment, may not necessarily constitute vascular dementia. Cerebrovascular disease, however, does appear to contribute to the severity of cognitive symptoms in AD.

In recent years dementia with Lewy bodies has received increased attention. For a diagnosis of dementia with Lewy bodies, both dementia and at least one of the following must be present: detailed visual hallucinations, parkinsonian signs, and alterations of alertness or attention. The diagnosis may overlap with AD and the dementia associated with Parkinson's disease. Poor visuospatial abilities are also often out of proportion to other cognitive deficits. The chronology of symptoms and pattern of cognitive deficits allow differentiation between dementia with Lewy bodies and AD or the dementia associated with Parkinson's disease. Parkinsonian signs, particularly a "pill rolling" tremor that develops prior to cognitive impairment, generally indicate Parkinson's disease rather than AD. When parkinsonian rigidity and bradykinesia are present during the onset of dementia, a diagnosis of dementia with Lewy bodies should be considered.

Frontotemporal dementia is a disease often seen in patients with younger onset of cognitive symptoms; these patients present most often with executive and language dysfunction and significant behavioral changes. These include disinhibition and hyperorality, and they often have had a profound effect on the patient's social functioning. Memory deficits are often not as pronounced in these patients in the early stages as they are in patients with other dementias. The language impairments in frontotemporal dementia may be detected in neuropsychologic tests such as the Boston Naming Test and may progress even early in the course of illness in excess of other cognitive impairments. It is important to recognize the difference between frontotemporal dementia and AD with "frontal" symptoms. The latter refers to social disinhibition and behavioral impulsivity that may occur with AD. In these patients the behavioral problems occur much later in the course of illness, after a memory problem is already clearly evident. In contrast, the patient with frontotemporal dementia will display social disinhibition prior to prominent memory decline.

Common to all types of dementia, cognitive impairment eventually has a profound effect on the patient's daily life. Difficulties in planning meals, managing finances or medications, using a telephone, and driving without getting lost are not uncommon. Such functional impairments may first alert others that a problem is emerging. Numerous functions are maintained in patients with dementia of mild to moderate severity, including such activities of daily living as eating, bathing, and grooming. Many patients remain socially appropriate during the early disease stages.

Behavior and mood changes are common, including personality alterations, irritability, anxiety, or depression. During the middle and late stages of the disease, delusions, hallucinations, aggression, and wandering may develop. These behaviors are extremely troubling to caregivers and often result in family distress and nursing-home placement. Although the course of dementia is variable, the progression of dementia often follows a sequential clinical and functional pattern of decline (see Table 30.3).

Table 30.3—The General Progression of Dementia

Stage 1: No cognitive impairment

Unimpaired individuals experience no memory problems, and none are evident to a health care professional during a medical interview.

Stage 2: Very mild cognitive decline

Individuals at this stage feel as if they have memory lapses, especially in forgetting familiar words or names or the location of keys, eyeglasses, or other everyday objects. However, these problems are not evident during a medical examination or apparent to friends, family, or coworkers.

Stage 3: Mild cognitive decline

Early-stage Alzheimer's can be diagnosed in some, but not all, individuals with these symptoms.

Friends, family, or coworkers begin to notice deficiencies. Problems with memory or concentration may be measurable in clinical testing or discernible during a detailed medical interview. Common difficulties include:

- Word- or name-finding problems noticeable to family or close associates
- Decreased ability to remember names when introduced to new people
- Performance issues in social or work settings noticeable to family, friends, or coworkers
- Reading a passage and retaining little material
- Losing or misplacing a valuable object
- Decline in ability to plan or organize

Stage 4: Moderate cognitive decline (mild or early-stage Alzheimer's disease)

At this stage, a careful medical interview detects clear-cut deficiencies in the following areas:

- Decreased knowledge of recent occasions or current events
- Impaired ability to perform challenging mental arithmetic—for example, to count backward from 100 by 7s
- Decreased capacity to perform complex tasks, such as marketing, planning dinner for guests, or paying bills and managing finances
- Reduced memory of personal history

The affected individual may seem subdued and withdrawn, especially in socially or mentally challenging situations.

Stage 5: Moderately severe cognitive decline (moderate or mid-stage Alzheimer's disease)

Major gaps in memory and deficits in cognitive function emerge. Some assistance with day-to-day activities becomes essential. At this stage, individuals may:

- Be unable during a medical interview to recall such important details as their current address, their telephone number, or the name of the college or high school from which they graduated
- Become confused about where they are or about the date, day of the week, or season
- Have trouble with less challenging mental arithmetic; for example, counting backward from 40 by 4s or from 20 by 2s
- Need help choosing proper clothing for the season or the occasion
- Usually retain substantial knowledge about themselves and know their own name and the names of their spouse or children
- Usually require no assistance with eating or using the toilet

Stage 6: Severe cognitive decline (moderately severe or mid-stage Alzheimer's disease)

Memory difficulties continue to worsen, significant personality changes may emerge, and affected individuals need extensive help with customary daily activities. At this stage, individuals may:

- Lose most awareness of recent experiences and events as well as of their surroundings
- Recollect their personal history imperfectly, although they generally recall their own name
- Occasionally forget the name of their spouse or primary caregiver but generally can distinguish familiar from unfamiliar faces
- Need help getting dressed properly; without supervision, may make such errors as putting pajamas over daytime clothes or shoes on wrong feet
- Experience disruption of their normal sleep-waking cycle
- Need help with handling details of toileting (flushing toilet, wiping, and disposing of tissue properly)
- Have increasing episodes of urinary or fecal incontinence
- Experience significant personality changes and behavioral symptoms, including suspiciousness and delusions (for example, believing that their caregiver is an impostor); hallucinations (seeing or hearing things that are not really there); or compulsive, repetitive behaviors such as hand wringing or tissue shredding
- Tend to wander and become lost

Stage 7: Very severe cognitive decline (severe or late-stage Alzheimer's disease)

This is the final stage of the disease when individuals lose the ability to respond to their environment, the ability to speak, and, ultimately, the ability to control movement.

- Frequently individuals lose their capacity for recognizable speech, although words or phrases may occasionally be uttered.
- Individuals need help with eating and toileting, and there is general incontinence of urine.
- Individuals lose the ability to walk without assistance, then the ability to sit without support, the ability to smile, and the ability to hold their head up. Reflexes become abnormal and muscles grow rigid. Swallowing is impaired.

SOURCE: Excerpted from http://www.alz.org/AboutAD/Stages.asp and reproduced with permission of the Alzheimer's Association. Copyright 2004 Alzheimer's Association, www.alz.org, 800.272.3900.

Dementia recognition may be complicated by the presence of either delirium or depression. Delirium has been defined as an acquired impairment of attention, alertness, and perception. Delirium and dementia are in some ways similar: both are characterized by global cognitive impairment. Delirium can be distinguished by an acute onset, cognitive fluctuations throughout the course of a day, impaired consciousness and attention, and altered sleep cycles. In hospitalized patients, delirium and dementia often occur together. The presence of dementia increases the risk for delirium and accounts in part for the high rate of delirium in elderly patients. A delirium episode in an older person, therefore, should alert the clinician to search for dementia once the delirium clears. (See also "Delirium," p 220.)

Symptoms of depression and dementia often overlap, presenting additional diagnostic challenges. Patients with primary dementia commonly experience symptoms of depression, and such patients may minimize cognitive losses. By contrast, patients with primary depression may demonstrate decreased motivation during the cognitive examination and express cognitive complaints that exceed objectively measured deficits. Patients with primary depression, moreover, usually have intact language and motor skills, whereas patients with primary dementia may show impairment in these domains. As many as half of elderly patients who present with reversible dementia and depression become progressively demented within 5 years. (See also "Depression and Other Mood Disorders," p 247.)

TREATMENT AND MANAGEMENT

The primary treatment goals for patients with dementia are to enhance quality of life and maximize functional performance by improving cognition, mood, and behavior. Both pharmacologic and nonpharmacologic treatments are available, and the latter should be emphasized. Patients with dementia often develop significant behavioral symptoms that are a challenge to both family and professional caregivers. Any acute change requires an evaluation for undiagnosed medical problems, pain, depression, anxiety, sleep loss, or delirium. Other factors that may contribute to behavioral symptoms include interpersonal or emotional issues. Addressing such issues, treating underlying medical conditions, providing reassurance, and attending to the possible need for changes in the patient's environment may reduce agitation. (See "Behavioral Problems in Dementia," p 213.) The use of pharmacologic treatments for behavioral problems is recommended only after nonpharmacologic ones prove ineffective, or there is an emergent need for them (eg, risk of danger, extreme patient distress).

Nonpharmacologic Treatment

Cognitive Enhancement

Reality orientation and memory retraining have been proposed as possible psychotherapeutic techniques to restore cognitive impairment. Although memory retraining may provide modest, transient benefit, it can also cause frustration for both patients and caregivers. Given that new learning is a skill lost very early in the course of AD, an overemphasis on quizzing or retraining may lead to anxiety and self-depreciation. In general, a preferred approach is to provide support to accommodate lost skills.

Individual and Group Therapy

Emotion-oriented psychotherapy, such as "pleasant events" and "reminiscence" therapy, and stimulation-oriented treatment, including art and other expressive recreational or social therapies, exercise, and dance, are examples of psychosocial treatments that may influence depressive symptoms. Patient support groups may be helpful, but only when patients are mildly impaired. Well-controlled trials have not demonstrated efficacy for these approaches, but preliminary studies and clinical experience suggest their usefulness for some behavioral and mood symptoms in patients and family members.

Regular Appointments

One approach to ensuring optimal health care for patients with dementia is to schedule regular patient surveillance and health maintenance visits every 3 to 6 months. During such visits the clinician should address and treat comorbid conditions, evaluate ongoing medications, and consider initiating drug-free periods. In addition, it is useful to check for sleep and behavioral disturbances and provide guidance on proper sleep hygiene. Caregiver well-being should also be regularly assessed.

Communication With Family and Caregivers

Working closely with family members and caregivers will help establish a therapeutic alliance. Education of family and caregivers about diagnosis, clinical course, treatment options, and management strategies is critical. Information about community resources as well as strategies for managing challenging behavioral symptoms can allow families to cope more effectively. Relatives are often helpful sources of information about cognitive and behavioral changes, and generally they take the primary responsibility for implementing and monitoring treatment. Often they are responsible for medical and legal assistance as well. However, early identification of dementia can allow the affected individual to participate in treatment decision and future planning. Subjects to pursue with family include medical and legal advance directives (also called *advance care plans* in some contexts). It is often best for a trusted relative to cosign important financial transactions and attend to paying bills. (See "Legal and Ethical Issues," p 20.)

Discussion about long-term-care placement options should be initiated early rather than late, to provide the individual or family members time to complete the arrangements and begin to adjust emotionally. Eventually, almost 75% of patients with dementia need admission to a long-term-care facility and remain for a long time. Caregivers often express concern about their own memory lapses, which should be addressed with counseling or neuropsychologic assessment. Caregiver distress is often reduced with support-group participation, which may relieve common feelings of anger, frustration, and guilt. Respite care is another community resource that offers caregivers relief. Psychosocial support may enhance quality of life for patients and family and even delay nursing-home placement. (See the resources section in the Appendix, p 466.)

Environmental Modification

Patients with dementia can be extremely sensitive to their environment; in general, a moderate level of stimulation is best. When they experience overstimulation, increased confusion or agitation may result, whereas too little stimulation may cause withdrawal. Familiar surroundings will maximize existing cognitive functions, and predictability through daily routines is often reassuring. Other helpful orientation and memory measures include conspicuous displays of clocks, calendars, and to-do lists. Links to the outside world through newspapers, radios, and televisions may benefit some mildly impaired patients. Simple sentence structure and repeated reminders about conversation content also may enhance communication.

Attention to Safety

Door locks or electronic guards prevent wandering, and many families benefit from registering with Safe Return through the Alzheimer's Association. (See the resources section in the Appendix, p 466.) Patient name tags and medical-alert bracelets will assist in locating lost patients.

Cognitive impairment affects driving skills, and the visuospatial and planning disabilities of many even mildly demented patients may make them unsafe drivers. Discussions about driving are best initiated early in treat-ment. In California and some other states, physicians must report patients with dementia to the health department, which forwards the information to the motor vehicle department for further assessment. Patients with advanced dementia definitely should not drive, but clinicians disagree about driving by mildly demented patients. Referral for an independent driving assessment is recommended if there is any concern regarding safety. Certainly, when a patient has a history of traffic accidents or significant spatial and executive dysfunction, driving abilities should be carefully scrutinized. (See also the section on the elderly driver in "Assessment," p 45.)

Pharmacologic Treatment

General Issues

When prescribing medications for older patients with dementia, the clinician should consider several factors. Patients in the upper age groups vary in their response, so that treatments need to be individualized. In addition, age is associated with decreased renal clearance and slowed hepatic metabolism. Older patients often take several medications simultaneously, so drug interactions and side effects are likely. Drugs with anticholinergic effects present a particular problem for patients with dementia because they may worsen cognitive impairment and lead to delirium. Another group of problem drugs that may worsen cognition include those causing central nervous system sedation. The best strategy, in light of such factors, is to start with low doses and increase dosing gradually ("start low and go slow"). The goal is to identify the lowest effective dose, thus minimizing side effects, and still avoid subtherapeutic dosing. Before initiating any treatment, conduct a thorough medical examination to identify and treat any underlying medical conditions that might impair cognition.

Cholinesterase Inhibitors

The primary treatments available for stabilizing cognitive function in AD are cholinesterase inhibitors. Currently, four cholinesterase inhibitors approved by the U.S. Food and Drug Administration (FDA) for patients with AD of mild to moderate severity are available: tacrine (rarely prescribed because of its side effects), donepezil, rivastigmine, and galantamine. In 2006, donepezil was also approved for patients with advanced dementia, and rivastigmine was approved for Parkinson's disease dementia. By slowing the breakdown of the neurotransmitter acetylcholine, these medications are thought to facilitate memory function because of the association of acetylcholine and memory. Clinical trials show that these drugs may modestly improve cognition and activities of daily living in patients with AD of mild to moderate severity. Studies of patients with dementing disorders other than AD are also becoming available. Data indicate that cholinesterase inhibitors may be helpful in managing the hallucinations associated with dementia with Lewy bodies, and preliminary data indicates a potential role in vascular dementia as well. There appears to be no role for cholinesterase inhibitors in treating frontotemporal dementia.

Donepezil is the most widely prescribed cholinesterase inhibitor. The recommended starting dosage is 5 mg per day; after 4 to 6 weeks of treatment, an increase to 10 mg daily is recommended. For patients experiencing gastrointestinal side effects such as nausea and diarrhea, a slower titration may reduce side effects. Rivastigmine is started at 1.5 mg by mouth twice daily for 2 weeks and then doubled no faster than every 2 weeks, to a maximum of 6 mg twice daily. Galantamine is prescribed in initial doses of 4 mg by mouth twice daily for at least 4 weeks, then 8 mg twice daily for at least 4 weeks, and then increased to a maximum of 12 mg twice daily. An extended-release formulation is also now available that permits the option of once-daily dosing. Although the higher doses are more efficacious for all agents, they are more likely to cause such cholinergic effects as nausea, diarrhea, and insomnia, especially if the dose is increased too rapidly. Such adverse effects also may worsen the patient's behavior. Other cholinesterase inhibitors and cholinergic receptor antagonists are currently under development. Direct comparisons among them have not been conducted.

Memantine

Memantine, an N-methyl-d-aspartate antagonist, has been used in Europe for many years. This drug is thought to have neuroprotective effects by reducing glutamate-mediated excitotoxicity. Recently completed clinical trials in the United States support the efficacy of this medication in moderate to severe stages of AD. Memantine now has FDA approval for the treatment of moderate to severe AD. The recommended dosing for memantine in the management of Alzheimer's type dementia involves 5 mg by mouth once daily, which may then be increased on a weekly basis in 5-mg increments to 10 mg per day, dosed as 5 mg by mouth twice daily, then up to 15 mg per day dosed as 5 mg by mouth in the morning then 10 mg by mouth in the evening, and finally arriving at a target dose of 20 mg per day dosed as 10 mg twice daily after a 4-week titration period. The most common side effects noted with memantine are constipation, dizziness, and headache. Memantine has been used safely in conjunction with cholinesterase inhibitors, and one study in 2004 has suggested additional benefits, but this area awaits further research.

Other Cognitive Enhancers

Ongoing studies are assessing a variety of other agents in AD, including antioxidants and *Ginkgo biloba* extract. In a trial including over 300 patients with moderately severe AD, treatment with vitamin E (α-tocopherol) or the selective monoamine oxidase-B inhibitor selegiline (approved for Parkinson's disease treatment) was found to lower rates of functional decline. The use of these agents, however, was not associated with evidence of cognitive improvement, but this study involved patients with moderate to severe dementia, so effects on cognition earlier in the illness remain unknown. Results from a randomized placebo-controlled trial of the use of vitamin E and donepezil in mild cognitive impairment showed some short-term benefit from donepezil in delaying conversion to AD but no effect of vitamin E. High-dose vitamin E supplementation was associated with increased mortality in a meta-analysis and should be prescribed with caution.

Extract from the leaf of the ginkgo tree has been promoted primarily in Europe for peripheral vascular disease as well as "cerebral insufficiency." Other studies in Europe and the United States have explored its use in AD. One 52-week double-blind, placebo-controlled study of ginkgo leaf extract in treating AD seemed to show small but statistically significant improvement in some cognitive measures. However, global measures did not improve in the small, limited study. Uncommonly, *G. biloba* has been linked to an increase of bleeding. More research is needed before ginkgo can be recommended.

Many patients also use over-the-counter preparations for cognitive enhancement. A complete review of medications includes questions about over-the-counter medications being used.

Antidepressants

Antidepressant drug treatment is generally considered for AD patients with depressive symptoms, including depressed mood, appetite loss, insomnia, fatigue, irritability, and agitation. (See "Depression and Other Mood Disorders," p 251.) Anecdotal evidence exists that selective serotonin-reuptake inhibitors may be helpful in managing the disinhibitions and compulsive behaviors associated with frontotemporal dementia.

Psychoactive Medications

Behavioral symptoms of dementia—paranoia, agitation, and irritability—are best managed by nonpharmacologic strategies, such as reducing overstimulation. However, when medications are required, identify the target symptoms and select therapy accordingly.

Cholinesterase inhibitors have been demonstrated to have modest effects on controlling behavioral symptoms. Antipsychotics can be used to manage delusions, hallucinations, and paranoia as well as some of the irritability associated with dementia. The antipsychotics have been associated with extrapyramidal (eg, rigidity, tremor) symptoms in dementia with Lewy bodies, and only very small doses of atypical antipsychotic medications should be considered for treating these patients. However, the FDA recently issued a "black box" warning that atypical antipsychotics have been associated with an increase in mortality among elderly patients with dementia who are being treated for behavioral disorders. This warning arose from an analysis of placebo-controlled trials performed with olanzapine, aripiprazole, risperidone, or quetiapine in elderly dementia patients with behavioral disorders. These trials showed a 1.6- to 1.7-fold increase in mortality in the drug-treated groups over that in the placebo-treated patients. Specific causes of death revealed that most were due either to heart-related events (eg, heart failure, sudden death) or infections (mostly pneumonia). More information is available at: http://www.fda.gov/cder/drug/infopage/antipsychotics/default.htm. Data on the use of drugs such as carbamazapine and valproic acid in managing irritability and agitation suggest that they may be included as options for drug therapy. Avoid the use of benzodiazepines and medications with anticholinergic effects. Finally, antidepressants with sedating effects such as mirtazapine and trazodone can be considered in the management of insomnia.

Other Resources

Most primary care clinicians successfully treat and manage most patients with dementia, but referral to a specialist is sometimes necessary. When the presentation or history is atypical or complex, particularly when the onset begins before age 60, consultation with a specialist in treating dementia patients (eg, geriatric psychiatrist, neurologist) can be useful. Geriatric specialists with psychology or psychiatry training can assist with behavioral management, particularly when patients are agitated, psychotic, or violent. They are also helpful when patients are suicidal or suffer from major depression or when individual or family therapy is indicated for patients or caregivers.

A neurologist can be helpful for patients with parkinsonism, focal neurologic signs, unusually rapid progression, or abnormal neuroimaging findings. Neuropsychologic consultation may clarify diagnostically complex cases, and clinical psychologists can provide psychotherapy, especially for caregivers. Social workers may provide counseling and contact with community resources. Guidance on physical and group

activity can be sought from physical therapists, and occupational therapists can assess the patient's functional level and suggest approaches to maximize functioning. Nurses can make management suggestions and guide behavior management, feeding, and other care issues. Wills, conservatorships, estate planning, and other legal matters are best addressed with the assistance of an attorney. Because most dementias are progressive, patients with early dementia should be offered an opportunity to plan for future incapacity and illness. (See "Legal and Ethical Issues," p 20.)

Community support can be informal, when neighbors or friends help out, or formal, such as home-care or family service agencies, the aging or mental health networks, or adult day care centers. Available specialized services include adult day care and respite care, home-health agencies that can provide skilled nursing, help lines of the Alzheimer's Association, and outreach services offered by Area Agencies on Aging and Councils on Aging, which are mandated and funded under the federal Older Americans Act. Food services for the homebound are available from meals-on-wheels, and many senior citizens' centers, church and community groups, and hospitals offer transportation options.

Organizations providing information and referral for dementia patients and families are listed in the resources section of the Appendix (p 474).

REFERENCES

- Birks J. Cholinesterase inhibitors for Alzheimer's Disease. *Cochrane Database Sys Rev.* 2006;25(1).

- Borson S, Scanlan JM, Watanabe J, et al. Improving identification of cognitive impairment in primary care. *Int J Geriatr Psychiatry.* 2006:21(4):349–355.

- Boustani M, Peterson B, Hanson L, et al; US Preventive Services Task Force. Screening for dementia in primary care: a summary of the evidence for the US Preventive Services Task Force. *Ann Intern Med.* 2003;138(11):927–937.

- Doody RS, Stevens JC, Beck C, et al. Practice parameter: management of dementia (an evidence-based review). Report of the Quality Standards Subcommittee of the American Academy of Neurology. *Neurology.* 2001;56(9):1154–66.

- Knopman DS, Dekosky ST, Cummings JL, et al. Practice parameter: diagnosis of dementia (an evidence-based review). Report of the Quality Standards Subcommittee of the American Academy of Neurology. *Neurology.* 2001;56(9):1143–1153.

- Sink KM, Holden KF, Yaffe K. Pharmacological treatment of neuropsychiatric symptoms of dementia: a review of the evidence. *JAMA.* 2005;293(5):596–607.

KEY POINTS

- The need to express basic needs such as hunger, thirst, or fatigue, which the patient cannot adequately communicate in dementia, may precipitate a behavioral disturbance.

- Delirium secondary to an underlying condition such as dehydration, urinary tract infection, or medication toxicity is a common cause of abrupt behavioral disturbances in patients with dementia.

- Medication effects on behavioral disturbances in dementia tend to be modest and should be implemented only after environmental and nonpharmacologic techniques have been employed.

- Antipsychotic medications may reduce agitation, and antidepressants may be helpful if symptoms of depression are evident in the patient with a behavioral disturbance.

Most dementias are associated with a range of neuropsychiatric and behavioral disturbances, with as many as 80% to 90% of patients developing at least one distressing symptom over the course of their illness. The development of behavioral disturbances or psychotic symptoms in dementia often precipitates nursing-home placement. These disturbances are potentially treatable, and it is vital that clinicians anticipate and recognize them early. If these symptoms become apparent, it is essential to perform a thorough evaluation of contributing factors, identify the target symptoms of treatment, and implement appropriate interventions for the patient and caregiver.

Research that compares different treatment strategies for the behavioral and psychologic symptoms of dementia is growing in response to the great need for evidence-based treatment guidelines. It is possible to draw some conclusions from randomized controlled trials of studies of medications for the treatment of depression and psychosis, but this area is still lacking rigorous studies of elderly adults with dementia. Interventions using behavioral treatment modalities have also been studied, but often in small samples and using varying methods. These studies have allowed for recommendations in many areas; however, many aspects of treatment must still draw on case reports and clinical experience.

CLINICAL FEATURES

Particularly as the dementia progresses, psychiatric symptoms may develop that take on a variety of characteristics resembling discrete mental disorders such as depression or mania; however, the course and features are more difficult to predict, and treatments are less reliably effective than when these disorders occur in younger adults without dementia. Depressive symptoms are common and often manifest as apathy or a lack of interest in previously enjoyable activities. This depressive syndrome may also include a loss of interest in self-care, eating, or interacting with peers. A propensity for irritability and impulsivity may also occur. If these features become progressive, overt hostility or violence may ensue. It is at this juncture that patients may be characterized as "agitated," reflecting a loss of the ability to modulate their behavior in a socially acceptable way. This may involve verbal outbursts, physical aggression, resistance to bathing or other care needs, and restless motor activity such as pacing or rocking. This type of overlap across symptoms, where some are associated with a depressive disorder but others such as hostility are considered atypical, often creates a significant challenge in diagnostic labeling. In this situation, the fairly nonspecific term *agitation* is commonly employed to describe the patient, but it may best be accompanied by additional description as to whether the problem is accompanied by simple irritability, vocal or physical aggression, or motor disturbances.

In many cases the presence of agitation may occur concomitantly with evidence of paranoia or delusional thinking, such as a false belief that caregivers are plotting to steal one's possessions or incur harm. When delusions occur, the patient is then characterized as suffering from "psychotic" symptoms. False perceptions such as hallucinations are another type of psychotic symptom that may accompany episodes of agitated behavior. One way to conceptualize this complex condition is to consider the term *agitation* as a descriptor for the presence of abnormal behavior such as aggression, while the presence of psychosis (eg, paranoid delusions) reflects the abnormal perceptions and beliefs that may lead to the agitated behavior. Depending on the degree of communication deficits in a given patient, the ability to discern the presence of psychosis is variable, and in many cases agitated behaviors may occur in the absence of clear evidence as to whether delusions or other psychoses may be precipitating the disturbance. Antipsychotic medications are commonly used in the management of agitated behaviors, with the presumption that disturbed perceptions may be underlying the problem.

Occasionally a behavioral syndrome occurs that includes features of hyperactivity, euphoric mood, and grandiose beliefs that resemble a manic episode associated with bipolar affective disorder. The features of this "manic-like" syndrome are described later in this chapter, and much like other mood symptoms in dementia, the features are similar but less predictable than those seen in younger adults and treatment strategies are more challenging. One key feature of the manic-like syndromes seen in dementia patients is the tendency to develop additional symptoms outside the typical course of a bipolar manic episode, such as agitated behaviors, defiance, and confusion.

Among the behavioral complications of dementia, the most severe disruptions in caregiving occur when patients develop physical behaviors such as hitting or wandering, or develop paranoid delusions that lead to hostility and altercations with the caregiver. Caregivers, both professional and family, may use the word *agitation* to describe a variety of behaviors and psychologic symptoms. The clinician must consider agitation to be a nonspecific complaint and pursue further history of the problem, including a description of specific behaviors and the time course, frequency, and severity with which they occur. Environmental precipitants such as excessive stimuli or a change in the environment such as a new roommate may induce behavioral problems. The presenting complaint may relate to internal cues such as pain, hunger, thirst, or other needs that the patient is not able to express.

The complaints from family caregivers and professional caregivers in a nursing home or assisted-living facility often arise from behavioral complications occurring during daily care that involve a resistance to bathing, dressing, or other routines. Family members may feel more overwhelmed than professional caregivers do and may consequently attribute more overall distress to these episodes. This type of overt resistance to care is most often seen in later stages of dementia, but it is important to note that behavioral problems may also be a first sign of an incipient cognitive decline in earlier stages as well. Neuropsychiatric symptoms such as apathy, poor self-care, or paranoia may be the first indication of dementia before cognitive decline is recognized, such that an evaluation for dementia in any older patient who presents with new behavioral or emotional symptoms may reveal a previously undetected dementia syndrome.

ASSESSMENT AND DIFFERENTIAL DIAGNOSIS

Comprehensive assessment includes a history both from the patient and from an informant or other source. The information should include a clear description of the behavior: its temporal onset, course, associated circumstances, and its relationship to key environmental factors, such as caregiver status and recent stressors. The problem behaviors and symptoms should be then considered in the context of the patient's family, past, personal, social, and medical history.

A differential diagnosis of the disturbance should proceed on the basis of findings from a comprehensive geriatric evaluation. The first step is to decide whether the disturbance is a symptom of a new or a preexisting medical condition or a medication adverse effect. Disturbances that are new, acute in onset, or evolving rapidly are most often due to a medical condition or medication toxicity. An isolated behavioral disturbance in a demented patient can be the *sole* presenting symptom for acute conditions such as pneumonia, urinary tract infection, arthritis, pain, angina, constipation, or poorly controlled diabetes mellitus. Additionally, the need to satisfy basic physical needs, such as hunger, sleepiness, thirst, boredom, or fatigue, which the patient cannot adequately communicate, may precipitate a behavioral disturbance. Medication toxicity due to new or existing medications might also present as behavioral symptoms alone. Treatment or stabilization of the medical or physical cause is often sufficient to resolve the disturbance. Older adults with dementia may require several weeks longer to recover from routine medical problems than those who are cognitively intact.

The second step is to consider whether the behavioral disturbance is related to an environmental precipitant. These include disruptions in routine, time change (eg, with daylight savings time or travel across time zones), changes in the caregiving environment, new caregivers, a new roommate, or a life stressor (eg, death of a spouse or family member). Other common environmental precipitants include overstimulation (eg, too much noise, crowded rooms, close contact with too many people), understimulation (eg, relative absence of people, spending much time alone, use of television as a companion), and the disruptive behavior of other patients. For many disturbances, correcting an environmental precipitant or removing the stressor commonly improves the symptoms.

Another consideration is whether the disturbance results from stress in the patient-caregiver relationship. Caring for dementia patients is difficult and requires a degree of perseverance that most caregivers are capable of learning if proper guidance and support is provided. Inexperienced caregivers, domineering caregivers, or caregivers who themselves are impaired by medical or psychiatric disturbances may exacerbate or cause a behavioral disturbance. Caregiver burden may be a problem both in community settings and in nursing homes. It is important for the clinician to assess the level of stress and burden on the caregiver as part of the evaluation of behavioral disturbances. Interventions to improve the patient-caregiver relationship and provide caregiver education and support are a vital part of treatment of behavioral disturbances in dementia. Providing resources to caregivers such as referral to support groups and respite services is often very helpful. (See the list of resources in the Appendix, p 466.)

After medical, environmental, and caregiving causes are excluded, it might be concluded that the behavioral problem is a manifestation of the dementia and may not be amenable to a pharmacologic intervention. Such disturbances that are closely linked to the dementia syndrome take on the form of a catastrophic reaction. A catastrophic reaction is an acute behavioral, physical, or verbal reaction to environmental stressors that result from an inability to make routine adjustments in daily life. The reaction might include anger, emotional lability, or aggression when the patient is confronted with a deficit, such as the inability to find a word, or confusion about where she is or what she is supposed to do. Catastrophic reactions are best treated by identifying and avoiding their precipitants, by providing structured routines and activities, and by recognizing early signs of the impending catastrophic reaction so that the patient can be distracted and supported before reacting.

If the disturbance is not related to an identifiable cause or environmental precipitant, it may be a consequence of the brain deterioration that occurs during the course of dementia. Disturbances with a more insidious onset or that are persistent are more likely to be symptoms of the underlying disease. Epidemiologic and clinical studies suggest that such disturbances fall into three groups: mood symptoms, psychosis, and specific behaviors. The overlap in the symptoms of these groups can make treatment choices difficult. One approach for the clinician is to decide whether the predominant symptom of a polysymptomatic disturbance is psychosis (delusions or hallucinations), mood symptoms (dysphoria, sadness, irritability, lability), aggression, or agitation, and then target treatment toward the prevailing feature.

Behavioral disturbances may occur in all types of dementias, including Alzheimer's type, vascular, and mixed. Frontotemporal dementia (Pick's disease) is a less common type of dementia often associated with prominent disinhibition, compulsive behaviors, and social impairment due to more advanced frontal lobe degeneration. In severe cases, a syndrome of hyperphagia, hyperactivity, and hypersexuality may occur that is related to bilateral temporal lobe atrophy. Another dementia associated with prominent psychiatric symptoms and behavioral disturbances is dementia with Lewy bodies (DLB). This form of dementia may be more common than previously thought. It is characterized by cognitive deterioration and parkinsonian features with prominent psychosis characterized by visual hallucinations. Patients with DLB often suffer from distressing hallucinations and a fluctuating clinical course. These patients are extremely sensitive to the extrapyramidal side effects of antipsychotic medications (such as muscle rigidity and tremor) and often cannot tolerate even low doses of atypical agents.

TREATMENT: BASIC APPROACH

The treatment of the psychiatric and behavioral disturbances in dementia is complex and may require several interventions applied as part of a comprehensive plan of care. Specialists should be consulted in refractory cases. In general, treatment begins with appropriate environmental and caregiver interventions. Nonpharmacologic interventions should always be used as a first-line treatment in the management of disruptive, aggressive, or agitated behavior. Table 31.1 provides a list of key behavioral interventions that might ameliorate behavioral symptoms in patients with dementia. The implementation of a daily routine and introduction of meaningful activities is vital. Patients with dementia may display a reduction in behavioral disturbances with the use of music, particularly during meals and bathing, and with light physical exercise or walking. Massage, pet therapy, white noise, videotapes of family, and cognitive stimulation programs may also be helpful. Educational materials are available for both

Table 31.1—Behavioral Interventions for Dementia Care

- Treat underlying medical precipitants
- Correct sensory deficits; replace poorly fitting hearing aids, eyeglasses, and dentures
- Remove offending medications, particularly anticholinergic agents
- Keep the environment comfortable, calm, and homelike with use of familiar possessions
- Provide regular daily activities and structure; refer patient to adult day care programs, if needed
- Monitor for new medical problems
- Attend to patient's sleep and eating patterns
- Install safety measures to prevent accidents
- Ensure that the caregiver has adequate respite
- Educate caregivers about practical aspects of dementia care and about behavioral disturbances
- Teach caregivers the skills of caregiving: communication skills, avoiding confrontational behavior management, techniques of ADL support, activities for dementia care
- Simplify bathing and dressing with the use of adaptive clothing and assistive devices if needed
- Provide access to experienced professionals and community resources
- Refer family and patient to local Alzheimer's Association
- Consult with caregiving professionals, such as geriatric case managers

NOTE: ADL = activity of daily living.

professional and non-professional caregivers that provide specific tips and suggestions to ease the challenge of providing personal care to agitated dementia patients. If the disturbances persist despite best efforts, pharmacologic interventions for specific target symptoms are often necessary. Their disorder-specific use, in conjunction with nonbiologic therapies, is discussed in the next section.

TREATMENTS FOR SPECIFIC DISTURBANCES

At the core of treatment is the identification of any possible underlying cause of the behavior change, with the recognition that multiple causes may be operating concurrently. First and foremost, managing pain, dehydration, hunger, and thirst is paramount. Consider the possibilities of positional discomforts or nausea secondary to medication effects, as these are common possible culprits. Environmental modifications can improve patient orientation. Good lighting, one-on-one attention, supportive care, and attention to personal needs and wants are also important aspects of treatment. If there is sleep-wake cycle disturbance, efforts should be made to stabilize the sleep cycle by maintaining a stable routine, using bright lights, or prescribing short-term use of medications (see the sleep disturbances section, below).

Mood Disturbances in Patients with Dementia

In dementia patients experiencing mood symptoms, procedures similar to those used with other behavior disturbances should be employed, that is, optimize the environment by reducing adverse stimuli and assess physical health comprehensively. Recreation programs and activity therapies have demonstrated positive results in improving mood in depressive symptoms in dementia. Criteria for the diagnosis of depression in Alzheimer's dementia have been proposed that note common features of irritability and social isolation or withdrawal. The waxing and waning course of mood symptoms in dementia is attributed to the cognitive loss and reduction in communication skills related to the dementia. Depression of 2 weeks' duration resulting in significant distress should likely receive a trial of an antidepressant medication. Similarly, sustained depressive features lasting more than 2 months following the initiation of behavioral interventions warrants treatment with antidepressant medications.

First-line agents are the selective serotonin-reuptake inhibitors, preferred for their favorable side-effect profiles. Studies of depression in patients with dementia have demonstrated the efficacy of sertraline and citalopram in comparison with placebo, but other studies using the same medications as well as paroxetine and fluoxetine have been inconclusive. Table 31.2 lists the antidepressants most commonly used to treat depressive symptoms in dementia.

The treatment of depression in dementia requires persistence. If a first agent has failed an adequate therapeutic dose for 8 to 12 weeks, an alternative agent should be tried. Venlafaxine, bupropion, mirtazapine, and the tricyclic agents desipramine and nortriptyline might be considered. Tricyclics should be avoided if a bundle branch block or other significant cardiac conduction disturbance is present. For patients who are partial responders to an antidepressant, augmentation strategies might be considered. The addition of a stimulant such as methylphenidate[OL] (2.5 to 10 mg per day) may be helpful in some cases, but there is some risk of increasing psychotic symptoms if the patient has a tendency to be suspicious or delusional. Also, the addition of stimulants such as methylphenidate to augment bupropion should be avoided, as bupropion already possesses stimulant effects. If the patient does not improve, the agents should be discontinued. If a patient continues to be significantly depressed after several antidepressant trials and is in danger because of serious weight loss or suicidal ideas, electroconvulsive therapy might be considered. This is the most efficacious and rapidly effective treatment for severe major depression and has a favorable safety profile even in mild dementia.

Manic-like Behavioral Syndromes in Dementia Patients

Occasionally mood syndromes may develop in dementia patients that are characterized by pressured speech, disinhibition, elevated mood, intrusiveness, hyperactivity, and reduced sleep. These syndromes therefore resemble manic episodes observed in the context of bipolar affective disorder in younger adults, although they are generally considered to be secondary to the dementing disorder. The important distinction in the dementia patient is the frequent co-occurrence with confusional states and a tendency to have more of a fluctuating mood, that is, the patient's mood may be irritable or hostile as opposed to euphoric. The appearance of hypersexual behaviors may be observed in this clinical scenario, although sexual disinhibition frequently occurs with dementia as a consequence of reduced frontal-executive functioning and may not necessarily be part of a manic syndrome. Treatment of manic-like states, emotional lability, disinhibition, or irritability typically begins with the use of mood-stabilizing agents such as divalproex sodium[OL] (see Table 31.3). The sustained-release preparation

---

[OL] Not approved by the U.S. Food and Drug Administration for this use.

Table 31.2—Drugs to Treat Depressive Features of Behavioral Disturbances in Dementia

Medication	Daily Dose	Uses	Precautions
Selective serotonin-reuptake inhibitors			
Citalopram	10–40 mg	Depression, anxiety[OL]	Gastrointestinal upset, nausea, insomnia
Escitalopram	5–20 mg	Depression, anxiety	
Fluoxetine	10–40 mg	Depression, anxiety	CNS stimulation
Paroxetine	10–40 mg	Depression, anxiety	Inhibits the cytochrome P-450 system
Sertraline	25–100 mg	Depression, anxiety	
Trazodone	25–150 mg	When sedation is desirable	Sedation, falls, hypotension
Serotonin norepinephrine-reuptake inhibitors			
Duloxetine	20–60 mg	Depression, diabetic neuropathy	Nausea, dry mouth, dizziness
Mirtazapine	7.5–30 mg	Useful for depression with insomnia	Sedation, hypotension
Venlafaxine	25–150 mg	Useful in severe depression	Hypertension may be a problem, insomnia
Tricyclic antidepressants			
Desipramine	10–100 mg	Depression, anxiety	Anticholinergic effects, hypotension, sedation, cardiac arrhythmias
Nortriptyline	10–75 mg	High efficacy for depression if side effects are tolerable; therapeutic range 50–150 ng/dL	Anticholinergic effects, hypotension, sedation, cardiac arrhythmias
Other			
Bupropion	75–225 mg	More activating, lack of cardiac effects	Irritability, insomnia

Table 31.3—Mood Stabilizers for Behavioral Disturbances in Dementia With Manic Features

Drug	Geriatric Dosage	Adverse Effects	Comments
Carbamazepine[OL]*	200–1000 mg/day (therapeutic level 4–12 µg/mL)	Nausea, fatigue, ataxia, blurred vision, hyponatremia	Poor tolerability in older adults; must monitor CBC, LFTs, electrolytes q 2 weeks for first 2 months, then q 3 months
Lithium[OL]*	150–1000 mg/day (therapeutic level 0.5–0.8 mEq/L)	Nausea, vomiting, tremor, confusion, leukocytosis	Poor tolerability in older adults; toxicity at low serum levels; monitor thyroid and renal function
Divalproex sodium[OL]*	250–2000 mg/day (therapeutic level 40–100 µg/mL)	Nausea, GI upset, ataxia, sedation	Requires monitoring of CBC, platelets, LFTs at baseline and q 6 months; better tolerated than other mood stabilizers in older patients

* Approved by the Food and Drug Administration for the treatment of bipolar disorder.

NOTE: CBC = complete blood cell count; GI = gastrointestinal; LFTs = liver function tests; q = every.

divalproex sodium is commonly recommended. In dementia patients, a typical starting dose of divalproex is 125 mg twice a day. The dose should be titrated upward slowly while the patient is monitored for sedation, ataxia, and falls. Blood levels in the range of 40 to 100 µg/dL have been shown to be effective, but individual variability in dose and response is great. Because of the potential adverse effects on the liver and thrombocytopenia, transaminase levels and a complete blood cell count (CBC) should be taken before therapy is initiated, rechecked with each dose increase, and repeated at least every 6 months while the patient remains on the drug. Alternatives to divalproex sodium are carbamazepine[OL], lamotrigine[OL], or lithium[OL]. Carbamazepine starting at 100 mg twice a day (with monitoring of liver enzymes and CBC) is an acceptable alternative for manic like states, mood lability, or irritability in dementia. Leukopenia is of concern with carbamazepine, and monitoring the CBC with every dose increase and at least every 3 months while the patient remains on the drug is needed. Lamotrigine has been used in the treatment of mania, but no geriatric trials have been conducted. Lithium is valuable as a mood stabilizer, but its use may be a problem in the elderly patient because of enhanced sensitivity to adverse effects. Elevated lithium levels may occur in the context of reduced renal function and dehydration, resulting in ataxia, tremor, gastrointestinal distress, and confusion.

[OL] Not approved by the U.S. Food and Drug Administration for this use.

Psychosis in Dementia: Delusions and Hallucinations

Delusions (paranoid or unfounded ideas) or hallucinations (false perceptions), whether occurring independently or in association with mood syndromes, typically require specific pharmacologic treatment if the patient is disturbed by these experiences, or if the experiences lead to disruptions in the patient's environment that cannot otherwise be controlled. Clinical criteria for the diagnosis of Alzheimer's dementia with psychosis specifies that the presence of delusions or hallucinations occur for at least 1 month, at least intermittently, and must cause distress for the patient. Antipsychotic drugs are listed in Table 31.4, along with dosing information. The atypical agents risperidone^OL, olanzapine^OL, quetiapine^OL, and aripiprazole^OL are being used more commonly than older agents such as haloperidol^OL. The older agents are more likely to cause extrapyramidal side effects, such as parkinsonism and tardive dyskinesia. Sedation, hypotension, and falls are common adverse effects among all antipsychotic agents. As these medications are more widely used, differences in side-effect profile are emerging. An increased risk of cerebrovascular events in patients with dementia has been identified with use of risperidone, olanzapine, and aripiprazole. The U.S. Food and Drug Administration (FDA) has required that warnings re-

garding diabetes mellitus, hyperglycemia, ketoacidosis, and hyperosmolar states be included as a risk of therapy with all of the atypical antipsychotic agents. Quetiapine is the most sedating of the atypical agents. Clozapine^OL, the first atypical agent introduced, is difficult to use because of the need for weekly CBC monitoring, adverse effects of sedation and orthostatic hypotension, and the risk of agranulocytosis. Clozapine is still helpful in a small group of patients with psychosis associated with Parkinson's dementia and those with DLB who are unable to tolerate the extrapyramidal adverse effects of other agents. It is clear that more information on side effects of all atypical agents will become available and should be considered by the clinician before prescribing them.

Although antipsychotic agents have demonstrated efficacy in large controlled trials in the treatment of dementia with psychosis and aggression, it is important to note that the overall positive effects have been relatively modest. Controlled studies of geriatric patients have had notorious difficulty with very high placebo responses. Although 45% to 55% of patients have been found to improve on antipsychotic medications, the response to placebo ranged from 30% to 50% across studies. Antipsychotic agents clearly play an important role in the treatment of delusions, hallucinations, and aggression in dementia, but they must be

Table 31.4—Antipsychotic Agents for the Treatment of Psychosis (Hallucinations and Delusions) in Dementia

Drug	Daily Dose	Adverse Effects	Comments	Formulations
Aripiprazole^OL	5–15 mg	Mild sedation, mild hypotension	Warning about increased cerebrovascular events in dementia, possible hyperglycemia	Tablet, liquid concentrate
Clozapine^OL	12.5–200 mg	Sedation, hypotension, anticholinergic effects, agranulocytosis	Weekly CBCs required, poorly tolerated by older adults, reserved for treatment of refractory cases, warning about hyperglycemia	Tablet, rapidly dissolving tablet
Olanzapine^OL	2.5–10 mg	Sedation, falls, gait disturbance	Warning about hyperglycemia and cerebrovascular events in patients with dementia	Tablet, rapidly dissolving tablet, IM injection
Quetiapine^OL	25–200 mg	Sedation, hypotension	Warning about hyperglycemia, ophthalmologic exam recommended every 6 months	Tablet
Risperidone^OL	0.5–2 mg	Sedation, hypotension, EPS with doses > 1 mg/day	Warning about cerebrovascular events in patients with dementia, hyperglycemia warning	Tablet, rapidly dissolving tablet, liquid concentrate, depot IM injection
Ziprasidone^OL	40–160 mg	Higher risk of QTc prolongation	Warning regarding increased QTc prolongation, possible hyperglycemia Little published information on use in older adults	Capsule, IM injection

NOTE: CBCs = complete blood cell counts; EPS = extrapyramidal symptoms; IM = intramuscular.

---

^OL Not approved by the U.S. Food and Drug Administration for this use.

part of a comprehensive treatment plan. The FDA has requested that the manufacturers of aripiprazole[OL], olanzapine[OL], quetiapine[OL], risperidone[OL], clozapine[OL], and ziprasidone[OL] add a boxed warning to their labeling describing an increased risk of mortality that has been observed in 17 placebo-controlled studies. In these studies, the rate of death for patients with dementia was approximately 1.6 to 1.7 times that of placebo. In most cases the cause of death appeared to be heart related or from infections (eg, pneumonia). More information on this warning is available at http://www.fda.gov/cder/drug/infopage/ antipsychotics/default.htm.

There is some evidence that cholinomimetic agents such as donepezil or galantamine may reduce the psychosis and behavioral disturbances of Alzheimer's disease. Studies comparing these agents with placebo in patients with mild to moderate Alzheimer's disease have suggested that they may reduce the rate of emergence of behavioral disturbances and psychosis. One area where cholinesterase inhibitors may be likely to improve psychosis is in the case of DLB; reduced visual hallucinations have been reported with cholinesterase inhibitors. Galantamine in dosages of 16 to 24 mg per day may be useful in the treatment of patients with DLB, who are uniquely sensitive to the extrapyramidal adverse effects of antipsychotic agents.

Disturbances of Sleep

Treatment of insomnia and sleep-wake cycle disturbance should begin with improvement of sleep hygiene (see Table 31.5). This consists of efforts to get the patient to go to sleep later every day, around 10:00 or 11:00 PM, while keeping the environment calm, comfortable, and conducive to sleep, into the next morning. If the sleep disturbance is associated with depression, suspiciousness, or delusions, those conditions should be treated.

For primary sleep disturbances when good sleep hygiene and increasing daytime activity level are not successful, trazodone[OL] (25 to 150 mg at bedtime) or mirtazapine[OL] (7.5 to 15 mg at bedtime) might be used. Benzodiazepines or antihistamines, such as diphenhydramine, should be avoided, since they carry a high risk for falls, hip fractures, disinhibition, and cognitive disturbance when prescribed for patients with dementia. (See also "Sleep Problems," p 229.)

Zolpidem[OL], zaleplon[OL], and eszopicione[OL] are short-acting nonbenzodiazepine sedative hypnotics that may be helpful for sleep disturbances in the elderly patient, although there have been no controlled trials for their use in sleep disturbances secondary to dementia. Zolpidem has been studied in elderly pa-

Table 31.5—Behavioral Management of Insomnia

- Establish a stable routine for going to bed and awakening
- Optimize sleep environment (attention to noise, light, temperature)
- Increase daytime activity and light exercise
- Reduce or eliminate caffeine, nicotine, alcohol
- Reduce evening fluid consumption to minimize nocturia
- Give activating medications early in the day if patient unable to eliminate
- Control nighttime pain
- Limit daytime napping to brief periods of 20 to 30 minutes
- Use relaxation, stress management, breathing techniques to promote natural sleep

tients without dementia and appears to be effective in improving sleep onset, although it does not improve sleep duration because of its short half-life. The recommended dose of zolpidem in the elderly person is 5 mg, as an increased risk of adverse effects appears to be dose related. Zaleplon has been less extensively studied in the older patient but appears to have similar properties.

Aggression and Hypersexuality

If hypersexuality occurs in association with another recognizable syndrome such as a mania-like state, treatment of the specific syndrome should be attempted. In men with dementia who are dangerously hypersexual or aggressive, a trial of an antiandrogen might be attempted to reduce the sexual drive. Patients may be tried on progesterone[OL] 5 mg orally once daily at first. The dose should be adjusted to suppress serum testosterone well below normal. If the patient responds well behaviorally, 10 mg of depot intramuscular progesterone may be given weekly to maintain a reduction of sexual drive. An alternative treatment to reduce sexual drive is leuprolide acetate[OL] (5 to 10 mg intramuscularly every month), also an antiandrogen. The use of antipsychotic medications is often adopted clinically, given the seriousness of hypersexual behaviors in institutionalized setting such as nursing homes; however, there are no controlled studies supporting this use. Presumably, the medication may enhance the cognitive focus of the individual's perceptions by reducing any psychotic thinking that may in some way be contributing to hypersexual behavior. Additional studies are needed for this problem.

Intermittent Aggression or Agitation

When disruptive behavior occurs intermittently or episodically, such as once per week or less, behavioral interventions focusing on identifying the antecedents of the behavior and avoiding the triggers are often

---

[OL] Not approved by the U.S. Food and Drug Administration for this use.

most useful. Behavior modification using positive rein-forcement of desirable behavior has been shown to be helpful, and it also helps encourage the caregiver to focus on times when behavior is not a problem. Reminiscence, validation therapy, aromatherapy, and environmental modifications of light, sound, and space may all help promote positive behavior. Distraction techniques, activity therapies, and exercise also show promise in reducing troublesome behaviors.

Physical restraint in any form should be avoided if at all possible. If restraining measures are necessary, careful supportive care should be provided to the patient. Over time, it is usually possible to reduce or eliminate the amount of restraint. (See also the section on quality issues in "Nursing-Home Care," p 114, and the section on restraints in the nursing home in "Legal and Ethical Issues," p 28.)

REFERENCES

- American Psychiatric Association. Practice guideline for the treatment of Alzheimer's disease and other dementias of later life. *Am J Psychiatry*. 1997; 154(5 Suppl):1–39.

- Ayalon L, Gum AM, Feliciano L, et al. Effectiveness of nonpharmacological interventions for the management of neuropsychiatric symptoms in patients with dementia: a systematic review. *Arch Intern Med*. 2006;166(20):2182–2188.

- Doody RS, Stevens JC, Beck C, et al. Practice parameter: management of dementia (an evidence-based review). Report of the quality standards subcommittee of the American Academy of Neurology. *Neurology*. 2001;56(9):1154–1166.

- Hoeffer B, Talerico KA, Rasin J, et al. Assisting cognitively impaired nursing home residents with bathing: effects of two bathing interventions on caregiving. *Gerontologist*. 2006;46(4):524–532.

- Tariot PN, Ryan JM, Porsteinsson AP, et al. Pharmacologic therapy for behavioral symptoms of Alzheimer's disease. *Clin Geriatri Med*. 2001;17(2):359–376.

- Weiner MF, Lipton AM, eds. *The Dementias Diagnosis Treatment and Research*. 3rd ed. Washington DC: American Psychiatric Press, Inc.; 2003.

CHAPTER 32—DELIRIUM

KEY POINTS

- Delirium is under-recognized and often inappropriately evaluated and managed. Approximately one third of patients aged 70 or older admitted to the general medical service experience delirium.

- The Confusion Assessment Method is the most clinically useful diagnostic tool.

- Most of the treatable causes of delirium lie outside the central nervous system, and these should be investigated first.

- The management of delirium requires an interdisciplinary effort by physicians, nurses, family members, and others involved in the care of the patient. A multifactorial approach is the most successful since many factors contribute to delirium.

Delirium has been described in the medical literature for more than two thousand years. Despite this, it remains under-recognized and often inappropriately evaluated and managed. Clinicians call delirium by many different names: up to 30 synonyms exist in the peer-reviewed literature, and far more in common medical parlance. *Acute confusional state* is the most common synonym, and the term still preferred today by many neurologists. Other synonyms for delirium range from the frequently used *acute mental status change*, *altered mental status*, *organic brain syndrome*, *reversible dementia*, and *toxic* or *metabolic encephalopathy* to the arcane *dysergastic reaction* and *subacute befuddlement*.

INCIDENCE AND PROGNOSIS

Delirium is common and associated with substantial morbidity. Approximately one third of patients aged 70 or older admitted to a general medical service experience delirium: one half of these are delirious on admission to the hospital; the other half develop delirium in the hospital. Among those admitted to intensive care units, the prevalence of delirium is much higher, and when rates for delirium are combined with those for stupor and coma, prevalence rates may exceed 75%. One third of older patients presenting to the emergency department are delirious. In postacute skilled nursing facilities, 16% of new admissions meet the full criteria for delirium, and an additional 49% have subsyndromal delirium. The prevalence of delirium among older patients discharged from the hospital into the community remains unknown.

Although delirium is traditionally viewed as a transient phenomenon, there is growing evidence that it may persist for weeks to months in a substantial portion of affected persons. A study of very old hospitalized medical and surgical patients found that approximately one third of those with incident delirium still met full criteria 3 and 6 months later. Subsequent studies performed in somewhat younger groups have found slightly lower but substantial persistence rates weeks to months after acute hospitalization. Risk factors for delirium persistence are starting to be defined—very elderly patients and those with preexisting cognitive impairment seem to be at highest risk for prolonged or permanent cognitive decline after the acute onset.

There is mounting evidence that delirium is strongly and independently associated with poor patient outcomes. Delirium has been associated with a tenfold increased risk of death in the hospital and three- to fivefold increased risk of nosocomial complications, prolonged hospital length of stay, and greater need for postacute nursing-home placement. Studies that have incorporated postdischarge follow-up have found that delirium is associated with poor functional recovery and increased risk of death up to 2 years after hospital discharge. Most of these associations persist after adjustment for factors such as patient age, preexisting dementia, and severity of illness. There is evidence that patients with persistent delirium have worse functional recovery than those whose delirium clears, suggesting that persistence of delirium may play an important role in poor long-term outcomes.

DIAGNOSIS AND DIFFERENTIAL DIAGNOSIS

Under-recognition of delirium is a major problem. The criteria of the 4th edition of the *Diagnostic and Statistical Manual of Mental Disorders* (*DSM-IV*), although precise, may be difficult to apply in clinical practice. More clinically useful is the Confusion Assessment Method (CAM), which was derived from *DSM-III-R* but is equally compatible with *DSM-IV*. (See Table 32.1 for a comparison of the *DSM-IV* and CAM criteria for delirium.) By judging the presence or absence of the four key CAM features shown in the

Table 32.1—A Comparison of the *DSM-IV* Diagnostic Criteria for Delirium and the Confusion Assessment Method

DSM-IV Criteria	Confusion Assessment Method
■ Disturbance of consciousness (ie, reduced clarity of awareness of the environment) with reduced ability to focus, sustain, or shift attention	1. Acute change in mental status and fluctuating course —Is there evidence of an acute change in cognition from the patient's baseline? —Does the abnormal behavior fluctuate during the day, ie, tend to come and go, or increase and decrease in severity?
■ A change in cognition (such as memory deficit, disorientation, language disturbance) or the development of a perceptual disturbance that is not better accounted for by a preexisting, established, or evolving dementia	2. Inattention —Does the patient have difficulty focusing attention, eg, being easily distractible, or having difficulty keeping track of what is being said?
■ The disturbance develops over a short period of time (usually hours to days) and tends to fluctuate during the course of the day	3. Disorganized thinking Is the patient's thinking disorganized or incoherent, eg, rambling or irrelevant conversation, unclear or illogical flow of ideas, or unpredictable switching from subject to subject?
■ There is evidence from the history, physical examination, or laboratory findings that the disturbance is caused by the direct physiologic consequences of a general medical condition or a drug, or both	4. Altered level of consciousness —Is the patient's mental status anything besides alert, ie, vigilant (hyperalert), lethargic (drowsy, easily aroused), stuporous (difficult to arouse), or comatose (unarousable)? **The diagnosis of delirium requires the presence of features 1 and 2 and either 3 or 4**

SOURCES: Data from (1) *Diagnostic and Statistical Manual of Mental Disorders.* 4th ed. Washington, DC: American Psychiatric Association; 1994 and (2) Inouye SK, van Dyck CH, Alessi CA, et al. Clarifying confusion: the Confusion Assessment Method: a new method for detection of delirium. *Ann Intern Med.* 1990;113(12):941–948.

table, the clinician can establish the diagnosis of delirium with better than 95% sensitivity and specificity. The CAM is a diagnostic algorithm, not a patient interview, and therefore the assessment done prior to its application is not specified. Although the CAM can be completed by using observations from routine care, recent evidence suggests that the use of a formal mental status evaluation is superior. In fact, one study examining nurses' application of the CAM using observations from routine care found a sensitivity of only 19% when compared with a formal mental status assessment by trained research staff. Factors associated with nonrecognition included hypoactive delirium, pre-existing cognitive impairment, advanced age, and visual impairment. A brief formal cognitive assessment such as the Mini–Mental State Examination, with supplemental attentional testing, is recommended prior to using the CAM. Table 32.2 shows some commonly used tests of attention. In the absence of a formal evaluation or when there is doubt, any older patient with acute change in mental status should be considered delirious, and evaluated and managed as described below.

Until recently, application of the CAM has required a conversant patient. The Confusion Assessment Method for the Intensive Care Unit (CAM-ICU) is a variant of the CAM that does not require verbal responses from the patient. Although it was designed for ventilated patients in the ICU, it can be used more generally for patients who are unable to speak. It uses the same four features as the CAM diagnostic algorithm but uses mental status testing that requires only yes-no answers that can be indicated by a nod or raised finger. Attention is tested using the Attention Screening Examination, in which patients are required to immediately recall simple pictures. Disorganized thinking is tested by answers to a series of simple yes-no

questions (eg, "Does 1 pound weigh more than 2 pounds?").

The differential diagnosis of delirium includes dementia, depression, and acute psychiatric syndromes. In many cases, it is not truly a "differential" diagnosis, since these syndromes can coexist and indeed are risk factors for one another. Instead, it is better thought of as a series of independent questions: Does this patient have delirium? . . . dementia? . . . depression? The most common diagnostic issue is whether a newly presenting confused patient has dementia, delirium, or both. To make this determination, the physician must know the patient's baseline status. In the absence of baseline data, information from family members, caregivers, or others who know the patient is essential. An acute change in mental status from baseline is not consistent with dementia and suggests delirium. In addition, a rapidly fluctuating course (over minutes to hours) and an abnormal level of consciousness are also highly suggestive of delirium. Depression may also be confused with hypoactive delirium. In one study, one third of psychiatric consultations for depression in the acute-care setting actually had hypoactive delirium. Finally, certain acute psychiatric syndromes, such as mania, can present similarly to hyperactive delirium. In the absence of known bipolar disease, it is best initially to evaluate and manage hyperactive patients as if they have delirium rather than attributing the presentation to psychiatric disease and missing a serious underlying medical disorder.

THE SPECTRUM OF DELIRIUM

The classic presentation of delirium is thought to be the wildly agitated patient. However, studies have demonstrated that agitated or hyperactive delirium represents only 25% of all cases. More common is

Table 32.2—Commonly Used Tests of Attention

Test	Patient Is Asked To:	Comments
Digit span	Repeat random sequence of numbers Repeat sequence of numbers in reverse order	Should be able to do at least 5 forward, 4 backward
Days, months	Recite the days of the week backward Recite the months of the year backward	Advantage: not much affected by poor memory, hearing, education, knowledge of English
Continuous performance task	Raise hand whenever he or she hears a certain letter or number in a list	Does not require a verbal response
Attention screening examination	Show 5 pictures; ask patient to remember them and to recall them out of a series of 10 pictures shown subsequently	Used in the CAM-ICU Does not require a verbal response
MMSE items	Subtract 7 from 100, then subtract 7 from each remainder ("serial sevens")	Requires ability to calculate
	Spell *world* backward	Requires knowledge of English

NOTE: CAM-ICU = Confusion Assessment Method for the Intensive Care Unit; MMSE = Folstein's Mini–Mental State Examination.

hypoactive or "quiet" delirium, or delirium with mixed features. Hypoactive delirium has no better prognosis than hyperactive delirium; it is recognized and appropriately treated less frequently. Special case-finding efforts are necessary to detect quiet delirium among high-risk elderly patients. If agitation is present, behavioral control measures may be necessary (see below), but such measures alone are not adequate treatment for delirium, and in some cases they may exacerbate or prolong the delirium.

Though we often speak of delirium as being either present or absent, it is important to recognize that the number and severity of symptoms vary widely. To more completely describe delirium, several severity scales have been validated and published: the Memorial Delirium Assessment Scale and the Delirium Rating Scale are among these. The Delirium Index is a severity measure based on the CAM and may be used in conjunction with it. When patients with delirium are stratified according to these scales, it is found that those with severe delirium have worse outcomes than those with mild delirium. Moreover, patients who do not fulfill all CAM or *DSM* criteria for delirium but who still demonstrate significant delirium symptoms have worse outcomes than patients with no symptoms of delirium. There is a gradient of worsening outcomes over the spectrum of delirium.

THE NEUROPATHOPHYSIOLOGY OF DELIRIUM

Research into the neuropathophysiology of delirium is in its infancy, but it suggests that different underlying mechanisms may pertain in different situations. Our understanding of the pathophysiology of delirium has not yet progressed to the point that it has an impact on the management of most delirious patients. One of the best-documented mechanisms for delirium is cholinergic deficiency. This is seen classically in overdoses of anticholinergic drugs such as atropine, which in severe cases can be reversed by the administration of physostigmine. In addition, many drugs not classified as anticholinergic (antihistamines, certain opioids, and antidepressants) have substantial anticholinergic activity and may also precipitate delirium. Delirium has been associated with increased serum anticholinergic activity measured by bioassay in both medical and surgical patients. Moreover, significant anticholinergic activity has been found in the serum of patients who were taking no drugs with anticholinergic properties, which suggests that there may be endogenous activity predisposing certain patients to the development of delirium.

A second potential mechanism for delirium is an alteration in the ratio of amino acids important in neurotransmitter production. Serotonin, a key central nervous system neurotransmitter, is dependent on the transport of tryptophan across the blood-brain barrier. Tryptophan competes with other large neutral amino acids, most notably phenylalanine, for transport into the central nervous system. Alterations in the tryptophan-to-phenylalanine ratio may result in serotonin excess or deficiency, which in turn may result in delirium. In fact, high levels of phenylalanine (common in postoperative or posttraumatic catabolic states) and low tryptophan-to-phenylalanine ratios have been associated with delirium in several medical and surgical cohorts.

Other mechanisms for delirium may be important in other settings. In patients with infections or cancer, delirium may be mediated through cytokines, particularly interleukin-2 and tumor necrosis factor. Other neurotransmitter systems, including γ-aminobutyric acid and dopamine, are also involved in some cases of delirium. The evidence for most of these mechanisms is based on cross-sectional comparisons of patients with and without delirium. Obtaining better longitudinal data, in which blood samples are examined at several time points in the same patient, is a crucial next step. In addition, more research is necessary to determine what mechanisms are most important in which patient populations, to begin to design targeted, pathophysiologically based preventive or treatment strategies.

RISK FACTORS

In the absence of a clear neuropathophysiologic basis for delirium, the cornerstone of its management focuses on the assessment and treatment of modifiable risk factors. Fortunately, research has identified several consistent risk factors for delirium. These risk factors classify into two groups: baseline factors that predispose patients to delirium, and acute factors that precipitate delirium. Among the predisposing factors, advanced age, preexisting dementia, preexisting functional impairment in activities of daily living, and high medical comorbidity are consistent risk factors. Male gender, sensory impairment (poor vision and hearing), and history of alcohol abuse have also been reported by some studies. Among acute precipitating factors, medications, especially those that are sedating or highly anticholinergic, uncontrolled pain, low hematocrit level, bed rest, and use of certain indwelling devices and restraints have been associated with the development of delirium. A useful model suggests that delirium is precipitated when the sum of predisposing and precipitating factors crosses a certain threshold. In such a model, the greater the predisposing factors, the fewer precipitating factors are required to initiate delirium. This would explain why older, frail persons develop delirium in the face of stressors that are much less severe than those that can cause delirium in younger, healthy persons. A mnemonic for reversible risk factors for delirium is presented in Table 32.3.

POSTOPERATIVE DELIRIUM

Delirium may be the most common complication after surgery in older persons. There is a 15% incidence after elective noncardiac surgery, and the incidence may exceed 50% after emergency procedures such as hip fracture repair. A prospectively validated clinical prediction rule for delirium after elective noncardiac surgery described seven risk factors that can be identified preoperatively: advanced age, cognitive impairment, physical functional impairment, history of alcohol abuse, markedly abnormal serum chemistries, intrathoracic surgery, and aortic aneurysm surgery. Patients with none of these risk factors had a 2% risk of delirium, those with one or two risk factors had a 10% risk, and those with three or more risk factors had a 50% risk.

In addition to baseline risk factors, postoperative management plays an important role in the development of delirium. Contrary to popular belief, the peak incidence of delirium is not immediately upon emergence from anesthesia, but on the second postoperative day. The stresses of surgery and anesthesia are not likely to be the sole precipitants of most cases of postoperative delirium.

Several studies have demonstrated that the route of intraoperative anesthesia, whether general, spinal, epidural, or other, has little impact on the risk of delirium. Postoperative medication management plays a much more important role. Postoperative use of benzodiazepines and certain opioids, especially meperidine, is strongly associated with the development of delirium. Although pain medications can cause delirium, adequate pain management is also important, because high levels of postoperative pain have also been associated with delirium. Strategies to provide adequate analgesia with minimal doses of opioids should be employed. These include the use of scheduled rather than as-needed dosing, patient-controlled or regional analgesia, and opioid-sparing analgesics such as acetaminophen or nonpharmacologic approaches, such as ice packs. Low postoperative hematocrit level (<30%) has also been associated with postoperative delirium. Appropriate transfusion of high-risk patients should be considered, especially after elective procedures for which autologous blood is available, though transfusions have not yet been shown to reduce delirium.

In recent years, several studies have documented the high incidence of cognitive dysfunction in patients who have undergone coronary artery bypass graft surgery (CABG). Although the exact nature and frequency of this dysfunction remains an area of active study, one large longitudinal study showed a 53% incidence of cognitive decline at hospital discharge, 36% at 6 weeks, and 24% at 6 months. Although post-CABG cognitive dysfunction is sometimes referred to as "pump head," studies have failed to find significant differences in cognitive outcomes of those undergoing on-pump as opposed to off-pump surgery, a finding that belies this name. None of the existing studies of cognitive outcomes after CABG have explicitly assessed for delirium, so the interplay between delirium and these more global measures of cognitive dysfunction remains unknown.

EVALUATION

All patients with newly diagnosed delirium require a careful history, physical examination, and targeted

Table 32.3—Mnemonic for Reversible Causes of Delirium

Drugs	Any new additions, increased doses, or interactions Consider over-the-counter drugs and alcohol Consider esp. high-risk drugs (see Table 32.5)
Electrolyte disturbances	Especially dehydration, sodium imbalance Thyroid abnormalities
Lack of drugs	Withdrawals from chronically used sedatives, including alcohol and sleeping pills Poorly controlled pain (lack of analgesia)
Infection	Especially urinary and respiratory tract infections
Reduced sensory input	Poor vision, poor hearing
Intracranial	Infection, hemorrhage, stroke, tumor Rare: consider only if new focal neurologic findings, suggestive history, or work-up otherwise negative
Urinary, fecal	Urinary retention: "cystocerebral syndrome" Fecal impaction
Myocardial, pulmonary	Myocardial infarction, arrhythmia, exacerbation of heart failure, exacerbation of chronic obstructive pulmonary disease, hypoxia

laboratory testing. Most of the treatable causes for delirium lie outside the central nervous system, and these should be investigated first. Moreover, multiple contributing factors are often present, so the work-up should not be terminated because a single "cause" is identified. Key steps in the evaluation and management of delirium are summarized in Table 32.4.

The history should focus on the time course of the changes in mental status and their association with other symptoms or events (eg, fever, shortness of breath, medication change). Because medications are the most common and treatable cause of delirium, a careful medication history, using the nursing administration sheets in the hospital or a "brown-bag" review in the outpatient setting, is imperative. In the outpatient setting, it is also important to review the patient's use of over-the-counter drugs and alcohol. The physical examination should include vital signs and oxygen saturation, a careful general medical examination, and a neurologic and mental status examination. The emphasis should be on identifying acute medical problems or exacerbations of chronic medical problems that might be contributing to delirium. Laboratory tests should be selected on the basis of history and examination findings. Most patients require at least a complete blood cell count, electrolytes, and kidney function tests. Urinalysis, tests for liver function, serum drug levels, and arterial blood gases, as well as chest radiograms, electrocardiogram, and appropriate cultures are helpful in selected situations. Cerebral imaging is often performed but is rarely helpful, except in cases of head trauma or new focal neurologic findings.

Table 32.4—Management of Delirium

Step	Key Issues	Proposed Treatment
1. Identify and treat reversible contributors	Medications	Reduce or eliminate offending medications, or substitute less psychoactive medications
	Infections	Treat common infections: urinary, respiratory, soft-tissue
	Fluid balance disorders	Assess and treat dehydration, heart failure, electrolyte disorders
	Impaired CNS oxygenation	Treat severe anemia (transfusion), hypoxia, hypotension
	Severe pain	Assess and treat; use local measures and scheduled pain regimens that minimize opioids Avoid meperidine
	Sensory deprivation	Use eyeglasses, hearing aid, portable amplifier
	Elimination problems	Assess and treat urinary retention and fecal impaction
2. Maintain behavioral control	Behavioral interventions	Teach hospital staff appropriate interaction with delirious patients Encourage family visitation
	Pharmacologic interventions	If necessary, use low-dose high-potency antipsychotics (see Table 32.6)
3. Anticipate and prevent or manage complications	Urinary incontinence	Implement scheduled toileting program
	Immobility and falls	Avoid physical restraints; mobilize with assistance; employ physical therapy
	Pressure ulcers	Mobilize Reposition immobilized patient frequently and monitor pressure points
	Sleep disturbance	Implement a nonpharmacologic sleep hygiene program, including a nighttime sleep protocol Avoid sedatives
	Feeding disorders	Assist with feeding; use aspiration precautions; provide nutritional supplementation as necessary
4. Restore function in delirious patients	Hospital environment	Reduce clutter and noise (esp. at night); provide adequate lighting; have familiar objects brought from home
	Cognitive reconditioning	Have staff reorient patient to time, place, person at least three times daily
	Ability to perform ADLs	As delirium clears, match performance to capacity
	Family education, support, and participation	Provide education about delirium, its causes, its reversibility, how to interact, and family's role in restoration of function
	Discharge	As delirium may persist, provide for increased ADLs support; follow mental status changes as "barometer" of recovery

NOTE: ADLs = activities of daily living; CNS = central nervous system.

In the absence of seizure activity or signs of meningitis, electroencephalograms and cerebrospinal fluid analysis rarely yield helpful results.

MANAGEMENT

Delirious hospitalized patients are particularly vulnerable to complications and poor outcomes and must be given special care. This requires an interdisciplinary effort by physicians, nurses, family members, and others involved in the care of the patient. A multifactorial approach is the most successful since many factors contribute to delirium; thus, multiple interventions, even if individually small, may yield marked clinical improvement (See Table 32.4). Failure to diagnose and manage delirium properly may result in costly and life-threatening complications and long-term loss of function.

Modifying the risk factors that contribute to delirium is critically important. Some factors, such as age and prior cognitive impairment, cannot be modified. However, even some predisposing factors, such as sensory impairment, may be modifiable through proper use of eyeglasses and hearing aids. Drugs are the most common reversible causes of delirium. Anticholinergics, H_2-blockers, benzodiazepines, opioids, and antipsychotic medications should be replaced with drugs that have no central effects. For example, H_2-blockers may be replaced by antacids or proton-pump inhibitors, and regular dosing of 1 g of acetaminophen three to four times daily may reduce or eliminate the need for opioids in many patients (see Table 32.5).

The delirious patient is susceptible to a wide range of iatrogenic complications, and careful surveillance is critical. Bowel and bladder function should be monitored closely, but urinary catheters, which can lead to urinary tract infection, are to be avoided unless absolutely required for monitoring fluids or treating urinary retention. Bowel stimulants and stool softeners can be used to prevent obstipation, particularly in those who are concomitantly using opioids. Complete bed rest should be avoided, as it may lead to increasing disability through disuse of muscles and the development of pressure ulcers and atelectasis in the lungs. Exercise and ambulation prevent the deconditioning often associated with hospitalization. Malnutrition can be avoided through the use of nutritional supplements and careful attention to intake of food and fluids. Some delirious patients may need assistance in feeding.

Managing behavioral problems while ensuring both the comfort and safety of the patient can be challenging. The patient should be placed in a room near the nursing station for close observation. Nonpharmacologic behavioral measures provide orientation and a feeling of safety. Orienting items such as clocks, calendars, and even a window view should be made available. Patients should be encouraged to wear their eyeglasses and hearing aids. Although physical restraint use has not been well studied in the hospital, evidence from the long-term-care setting suggests that such restraints probably do not decrease the rate of falls by confused ambulatory patients, and they may actually increase the risk of fall-related injury. Restraints, though objectionable, may be required because of violent behavior or to prevent the removal of important devices, such as endotracheal tubes, intra-arterial devices, and catheters. Even for persons with these devices, the calm reassurance provided by a sitter or family member may be much more effective than the use of physical restraints or drugs. Whenever restraints are used, the indicators for use should be frequently reassessed, and the restraints should be removed as soon as possible.

When medications are used as restraints to "save staff time," they extract a costly toll in accidents, adverse effects, and loss of mobility, and they should be avoided if possible. Pharmacological interventions may be necessary for symptoms such as delusions or hallucinations that are frightening to the patient when verbal comfort and reassurance are not successful (see Table 32.6). Some delirious patients display behavior that is dangerous to themselves or others and cannot be calmed by the provision of a sitter or family companionship. However, the mere presence of delirium is not an indication for pharmacologic intervention. Indications for such interventions should be clearly identified, documented, and constantly reassessed.

It is important to stress to family members that delirium is usually not a permanent condition, but rather that it improves over time. Unfortunately, the persistence of delirium is common. Thus, when counseling families, it is important to point out that many cognitive deficits associated with the delirium syndrome can continue, abating only weeks and even months following the illness. Advanced age (85 years or older), preexisting cognitive impairment, and severe illness are risk factors for slow recovery of cognitive function. Careful monitoring of mental status and provision of adequate functional supports during this period are necessary to give the patient the maximum chance of returning to his or her baseline level. Family members can play an important role in the hospital and postacute setting by providing appropriate orientation, support, and functional assistance. Hospitals are increasingly making provisions for family members to sleep overnight with relatives who are already delirious or at high risk for developing delirium. While symptoms of delirium may persist, acute exacerbation of cognitive dysfunction is not expected during the convalescent period and therefore likely heralds a new

Table 32.5—Drugs to Reduce or Eliminate in the Management of Delirium

Agent	Adverse Effects	Possible Substitutes	Comments
Alcohol	CNS sedation and withdrawal	If history of heavy intake, careful monitoring and benzodiazepines if withdrawal symptoms	Alcohol history is imperative
Anticholinergics (oxybutynin, benztropine)	Anticholinergic toxicity	A lower dose, behavioral measures	Rare at low doses
Anticonvulsants (esp. primidone, phenobarbital, phenytoin)	CNS sedation and withdrawal	Alternative agent or none	Toxic reactions can occur despite "therapeutic" drug levels
Antidepressants, esp. tertiary amine tricyclic agents (amitriptyline, imipramine, doxepin)	Anticholinergic toxicity	Secondary amine tricyclics (nortriptyline, desipramine) SSRIs or other agents	Secondary amines as good as tertiary for adjuvant treatment of chronic pain
Antihistamines (including diphenhydramine)	Anticholinergic toxicity	Nonpharmacologic protocol for sleep; pseudoephedrine for colds	Must take OTC medication history
Antiparkinsonian agents (levodopa-carbidopa, dopamine agonists, amantadine)	Dopaminergic toxicity	A lower dose; adjusted dosing schedule	Usually with end-stage disease and high doses
Antipsychotics, esp. low-potency anticholinergic agents and atypical agents (clozapine)	Anticholinergic toxicity; CNS sedation	No agents or, if necessary, low-dose high-potency agents	See note to Table 32.6 for warnings about atypical antipsychotics
Barbiturates	CNS sedation; severe withdrawal syndrome	Gradual discontinuation or benzodiazepine	In most cases, should no longer be prescribed; avoid inadvertent or abrupt discontinuation
Benzodiazepines, esp. long-acting (including diazepam, flurazepam, chlordiazepoxide)	CNS sedation	Nonpharmacologic sleep management; intermediate agents (lorazepam, temazepam)	Associated with delirium in medical and surgical patients
Benzodiazepines: ultra short-acting (including triazolam, alprazolam)	CNS sedation and withdrawal	Nonpharmacologic sleep management; intermediate agents (lorazepam, temazepam)	Associated with delirium in case reports and series
Chloral hydrate	CNS sedation	Nonpharmacologic sleep protocol	No better for delirium than benzodiazepines
H_2-blocking agents	Possible anticholinergic toxicity	A lower dosage; antacids or proton-pump inhibitors	Most common with high-dose intravenous infusions
Nonbenzodiazepine hypnotics (eg, zolpidem)	CNS sedation and withdrawal	Nonpharmacologic sleep protocol	Like other sedatives, can cause delirium
Opioid analgesics (esp. meperidine)	Anticholinergic toxicity, CNS sedation, fecal impaction	Local measures and nonpsychoactive pain medications around the clock; opioids only for breakthrough and severe pain	Higher risk in patients with renal insufficiency; must titrate risks from drugs versus risks from pain
Almost any medication if time course is appropriate			**Consider risks and benefits of all medications in the elderly patient**

NOTE: CNS = central nervous system; OTC = over-the-counter; SSRI = selective serotonin-reuptake inhibitor.

medical problem. Families should be counseled to seek prompt medical attention if patient's mental status acutely worsens.

PREVENTION

Finally, it should be stated that the most effective way to manage delirium is to prevent it from developing in the first place. A study demonstrated that a unit-based proactive multifactorial intervention can reduce the incidence of delirium among older hospitalized patients aged 70 or older by more than one third (adjusted odds ratio = 0.60, 95% confidence interval, 0.39 to 0.92). Six intervention components were used selectively on the basis of patient-specific risk factors determined at an admission assessment. These included interventions for cognitive impairment, sleep deprivation, immobility, visual impairment, hearing impair-

Table 32.6—Pharmacologic Therapy of Agitated Delirium

Agent	Mechanism of Action	Dosage	Benefits	Adverse Effects	Comments
Haloperidol[OL]	Antipsychotic	0.25–1.0 mg po or IV q 4 h prn agitation	Relatively nonsedating; few hemodynamic effects	EPS, esp. if > 3 mg per day	Usually, agent of choice*
Lorazepam[OL]	Sedative	0.25–1.0 mg po or IV tid prn agitation	Use in sedative and alcohol withdrawal, Parkinson's, Lewy body disease, and history of neuroleptic malignant syndrome	More paradoxical excitation, respiratory depression than haloperidol	Second-line agent, except in specific cases noted
Olanzapine[OL]	Antipsychotic	2.5–10 mg po qd	Fewer EPS than haloperidol	More sedating than haloperidol	Small case series only**
		dissolving tablet: 2.5–10 mg po qd			Oral formulations are less effective for acute management
		IV or IM: 2.5–10 mg qd			
Quetiapine[OL]	Antipsychotic	25–50 mg po bid	Fewer EPS than haloperidol	Hypotension	Small case series**
Risperidone[OL]	Antipsychotic	0.25–1.0 mg po q 4 h prn agitation	Similar to haloperidol	Might have slightly fewer EPS	Case series only**

NOTE: bid = twice a day; EPS = extrapyramidal symptoms; h = hour; IM = intramuscularly; IV = intravenously; prn = as needed; po = by mouth; q = each; qd = each day; tid = three times a day.

* In a randomized trial comparing haloperidol, chlorpromazine, and lorazepam in the treatment of agitated delirium in young patients with AIDS, all were found to be equally effective, but haloperidol had the fewest side effects or adverse sequelae.

** The U.S. Food and Drug Administration has attached warnings to the atypical antipsychotics because of the increased risk of stroke and mortality that as been found to be associated with their long-term use, primarily for agitation in dementia.

[OL] Not approved by the U.S. Food and Drug Administration for this use.

ment, and dehydration. Among these, the most creative and successful was a nonpharmacologic sleep protocol that involved trained volunteers offering patients warm milk, back rubs, and soothing music at bedtime; this intervention substantially reduced the use of sedative-hypnotic medication. Similar programs to prevent delirium should be developed and implemented in hospitals and other settings that care for acutely ill elderly patients. One example of such programs is the Hospital Elder Life Program (HELP), which is currently being disseminated to hospitals (see http://elderlife.med.yale.edu/public/public-main.php?pageid=01.00.00).

Although a unit-based intervention can be highly successful, it may be difficult to apply in all settings, especially in surgical patients. A randomized trial demonstrated that proactive geriatrics consultation can reduce the incidence of delirium in elderly patients undergoing hip fracture repair. Consultation began in most cases preoperatively and continued throughout the duration of hospitalization. Daily recommendations were based on a structured protocol that covered key elements in delirium prevention, such as limitation of

psychoactive medications; 77% adherence was achieved. The geriatrics consultation group achieved a reduction in the incidence of delirium (32% versus 50% usual care, $P < .05$) of similar magnitude to the unit-based protocol described above. Geriatrics consultation, if performed proactively and intensively, may be an important strategy for preventing delirium in high-risk surgical patients.

Even though multifactorial intervention is effective in preventing delirium, existing data suggest that it may be less effective in treating established delirium. The two studies cited above failed to show an effect on delirium once it developed. Moreover, a recent study randomized 227 patients with prevalent or incident delirium on a general medical unit to either geriatric specialist consultation and follow-up care by an intervention nurse, or usual care. No differences were found in the rate of improvement of delirium symptoms, functional recovery, or discharge to the community between the two groups. This study provides a sobering reminder of the need for more research on how to optimally manage the delirious patient and the development of novel approaches based on a better understanding of the pathophysiology of this common, morbid, and costly syndrome.

REFERENCES

- Bergmann MA, Murphy KM, Kiely DK, et al. A model for management of delirious postacute care patients. *J Am Geriatr Soc.* 2005;53(10):1817–1825.

- Inouye SK, Bogardus ST Jr, Charpentier PA, et al. A multicomponent intervention to prevent delirium in hospitalized older patients. *N Engl J Med.* 1999;340(9):669–676.

- Inouye SK, Foreman MD, Mion LC, et al. Nurses' recognition of delirium and its symptoms. *Arch Intern Med.* 2001;161(20):2467–2473.

- Kiely DK, Bergmann MA, Murphy KM, et al. Delirium among newly admitted post-acute facility patients: prevalence, symptoms, and severity. *J Gerontol A Biol Sci Med Sci.* 2003; 58(5): M441–M445.

- Trzepacz P, Breitbart W, Franklin J, et al. Practice guideline for the treatment of patients with delirium. Web site of the American Psychiatric Association; 1999. Available at http://www.psych.org/psych_pract/treatg/pg/pg_delirium.cfm (accessed October 2005).

CHAPTER 33—SLEEP PROBLEMS

KEY POINTS

- Studies show an association between sleep complaints and risk factors for sleep disturbance (eg, chronic illness, mood disturbance, less physical activity, and physical disability) but little association with older age, suggesting that these risk factors rather than aging itself account for insomnia in the majority of those studied.

- Notable age-related changes in sleep structure as measured by polysomnography include a decrease in stage 3 and stage 4 sleep (the deeper stages of sleep) with an increase or maintenance of stages 1 and 2 (the lighter stages of sleep).

- Insomnia is usually due to psychiatric, medical, or neurologic illness; excessive daytime sleepiness is usually due to a primary sleep disorder, such as sleep apnea.

- The appropriate treatment of sleep problems must be guided by knowledge of likely causes and potential contributing factors. Trials have shown that nonpharmacologic interventions can be quite effective in improving sleep in older adults.

EPIDEMIOLOGY

Several studies have documented a high prevalence of sleeping problems among older people. In one representative sample, the most common sleeping complaints among community-dwelling older people were found to be difficulty falling asleep (37% of the sample), nighttime awakening (29%), and early morning awakening (19%). Daytime sleepiness is also common, with 20% of noninstitutionalized Americans reporting that they are "usually sleepy in the daytime." As a result of such complaints, at least one half of community-dwelling older people use either over-the-counter or prescription sleeping medications.

Three large epidemiologic studies of older people found an association between sleep complaints and risk factors for sleep disturbance (eg, chronic illness, mood disturbance, less physical activity, and physical disability) but little association with older age, suggesting that these risk factors, rather than aging per se, account for insomnia in the majority of those studied. However, some primary sleep disorders, such as sleep apnea and periodic limb movements in sleep, increase in prevalence with age. Although some studies have shown an increased risk of sleep complaints in women, others have not. Studies have shown that self-reported sleeping difficulties are more common in older black Americans, particularly women and those with depression and chronic illness.

Unfortunately, late-life insomnia is commonly a chronic problem. A study of older people in Britain found that 36% of those with insomnia at baseline reported severely disrupted sleep 4 years later. Of those who reported the use of prescription hypnotics at baseline, 32% were still using these agents 4 years later. Another study of a volunteer sample of urban women aged 85 years and older found that all had health problems and sleeping difficulties, and the majority regularly used alcohol, an over-the-counter sleeping medication, or both, in an effort to improve their sleep. Previous research has suggested that insomnia is a predictor of death and nursing-home placement in older men, but not in older women.

CHANGES IN SLEEP WITH AGING

Older people have a decreased sleep efficiency (time asleep divided by time in bed), a stable or decreased total sleep time, and an increased sleep latency (time to fall asleep). Older people also report an earlier bedtime and earlier morning awakening, more arousals during the night, and more daytime napping. Notable age-related changes in sleep structure as measured by polysomnography include a decrease in stage 3 and stage 4 sleep (the deeper stages of sleep). Stages 1 and 2 (the lighter stages of sleep) increase or remain the same. The decline in deep sleep seems to begin in early adulthood and progresses throughout life. In persons over age 90 years, stages 3 and 4 may disappear completely. Other common findings include an earlier onset of rapid-eye-movement (REM) sleep in the night and decreased total REM sleep but no change or a decrease in percentage of REM sleep. Older people have more equal distribution of REM sleep throughout the night, whereas younger people have longer periods of REM sleep as the night progresses. Older persons also have a decrease in sleep spindles and K complexes on electroencephalogram during sleep.

The significance of these changes in sleep is unclear. Most experts believe that the decreased sleep in older people is due to a decreased *ability* to sleep, rather than a decreased *need* for sleep. However, some research has shown that after a period of sleep deprivation older people show less daytime sleepiness, less evidence of decline in performance measures, and a quicker recovery of normal sleep structure than younger people. Older people have more sleep disturbance with jet lag and shift work, which may reflect physiologic changes in circadian rhythm with age. In addition, it is not clear to what extent changes in sleep are due to changes of normal aging or to pathologic changes from other processes. In studies comparing good sleepers with poor sleepers, poor sleepers were found to take more medications, make more physician visits, and have poorer self-ratings of health. In addition, as noted above, chronologic age per se does not seem to correlate with higher prevalence of poor sleep.

EVALUATION OF SLEEP

To aid in screening older patients for sleep problems, several years ago the National Institutes of Health Consensus Statement on the Treatment of Sleep Disorders of Older People suggested that clinicians ask three simple questions:

- Is the person satisfied with his or her sleep?
- Does sleep or fatigue interfere with daytime activities?

- Does the bed partner or others complain of unusual behavior during sleep, such as snoring, interrupted breathing, or leg movements?

These, or similar screening questions, can be quite useful to identify sleep complaints in the older patient. Transient sleep problems (eg, those lasting less than 2 to 3 weeks) are usually situational; persistent sleep problems are likely to require more detailed evaluation.

The initial and subsequent office evaluations of a patient with persistent sleep complaints can be rather lengthy. To obtain a careful description of the sleep complaint, it may be helpful to have the patient keep a sleep log, recording each morning the time spent in bed, the estimated amount of sleep, the number of awakenings, the time of morning awakening, and any symptoms that occurred during the night. This should be supplemented by information from the bed partner, or others who may have observed unusual symptoms during the night. The focused physical examination depends on evidence from the history. For example, reports of painful joints should be followed by a careful examination of the affected areas. Reports of nocturia that disrupts sleep should be followed by evaluation for cardiac, renal, or prostatic disease, or diabetes mellitus. Careful mental status testing is also indicated. The findings of the history and physical examination should guide laboratory testing.

Polysomnography is indicated when the clinician suspects a primary sleep disorder, such as sleep apnea, periodic limb movement disorder, or violent or other unusual behaviors during sleep. Objective methods to measure sleep other than traditional polysomnography in a sleep laboratory have been developed and are being used more extensively in studies of sleep. Portable monitoring systems for use in the home have been developed and are used primarily to screen for sleep apnea. These systems generally measure pulse oximetry, heart rate, respiration, and nasal airflow. Although they are used extensively, research testing the validity of these systems is ongoing. Another methodology is a wrist-activity monitor, which estimates sleep versus wakefulness on the basis of the person's wrist activity. Some studies have demonstrated that the wrist monitor is sensitive enough to assess the efficacy of treatment for insomnia in older people. Observational measures for detecting sleep problems and sleep-related breathing disorders have been used for research in nursing-home residents.

COMMON SLEEP DISORDERS

Insomnia (ie, difficulty in initiating or maintaining sleep) is usually due to psychiatric, medical, or neurologic illness; excessive daytime sleepiness is usually due to a primary sleep disorder, such as sleep apnea. However, there is significant overlap among these symptoms. In one large study of patients of all ages referred to sleep disorders centers, insomnia was found to be most commonly due to psychiatric illness, psychophysiologic problems, drug or alcohol dependence, and restless legs syndrome; excessive daytime sleepiness was found to be most commonly due to sleep apnea, periodic limb movement disorder, or narcolepsy. However, patients referred to sleep centers are a select population, and the most common causes of excessive sleepiness in the community are probably chronic insufficient sleep (either voluntarily or because of work schedules), medical problems, or sleep-disruptive environmental conditions. Thus, the clinician should not exclude a primary sleep disorder in the patient presenting with insomnia and likewise should probably not refer every patient with daytime sleepiness to a sleep laboratory.

Psychiatric Disorders and Psychosocial Problems

Many studies report that psychiatric disorders are the cause of sleep problems in more than half of all patients presenting with insomnia. Depression is a particularly common cause. Early morning awakening is a common pattern, although increased sleep latency and more nighttime wakefulness are also seen. However, these changes may not be present or may be less marked in depressed persons who do not seek medical care. Conversely, sleep disturbance in older people who are not currently depressed may be an important predictor of future depression. In depressed older patients with sleep disturbance, treatment of depression may also improve the sleep abnormalities. Several studies using electroencephalography have found that antidepressant medications alter sleep architecture, suggesting that antidepressant drug efficacy may depend to some extent on regulation of sleep and changes in REM-sleep regulation. (See also "Depression and Other Mood Disorders," p 247.)

Bereavement can also affect sleep. Bereavement without major depression is not associated with significant changes in sleep measures, but people with bereavement and depression and those with major depression have identical sleep patterns. These sleep abnormalities improve with treatment of depression. Anxiety and stress can also be associated with sleeping difficulty, usually difficulty with initiating sleep or perhaps early awakening. Patients may have difficulty falling asleep because of excessive worrying at bedtime. (See also "Anxiety Disorders," p 258.) Research has found that older caregivers report more sleep complaints than do similarly aged noncaregivers. In one study, nearly 40% of older women who were family caregivers of adults with dementia reported using a sleeping medication for themselves in the past month. (See also the sections on caregiving in "Psychosocial Issues," p 16; "Community-Based Care," p 121; and "Elder Mistreatment," p 80.)

Drug and Alcohol Dependency

Drug and alcohol use account for 10% to 15% of cases of insomnia. Chronic use of sedatives may cause light, fragmented sleep. Many sleeping medications, when used chronically, lead to tolerance and the potential for increasing doses. When chronic hypnotic use is suddenly stopped, rebound insomnia may occur, and the person may start taking the medication again.

Alcohol abuse is often associated with lighter sleep of shorter duration. In addition, some persons try to treat their sleeping difficulties with alcohol. Older persons with poor sleep should be instructed to avoid nighttime alcohol because although alcohol causes an initial drowsiness, it can impair sleep later in the night. Finally, it is important to remember that sedatives and alcohol can worsen sleep apnea; the use of these respiratory depressants should be avoided in older persons with documented or suspected untreated sleep apnea. (See also "Substance Abuse," p 274.)

Medical Problems

Examples of treatable medical problems that may contribute to sleep difficulty in older people include pain from arthritis and other conditions, paresthesias, cough, dyspnea from cardiac or pulmonary illness, gastroesophageal reflux, and nighttime urination. In patients with sleeping difficulties who describe pain at night, assessment and management of the painful condition is the appropriate approach (see "Persistent Pain," p 131). Nighttime urination may be associated with sleep disorder, poorer quality of sleep, nighttime thirst, and increased fatigue in the daytime.

Sleep can be impaired by diuretics or stimulating agents (eg, caffeine, sympathomimetics, and bronchodilators) taken near bedtime. Some antidepressants, antiparkinson agents, and antihypertensives (eg, propranolol) can induce nightmares and impair sleep. Required medications that are sedating (eg, sedating antidepressants) should be given at bedtime if possible.

Sleep Apnea

Sleep apnea is a disorder of periodic reductions in ventilation during sleep. Various terms have been used for this syndrome (eg, *sleep-related breathing disorder*, *sleep-disordered breathing*), but *sleep apnea* remains the term used by most clinicians. Patients with obstructive sleep apnea usually present with excessive daytime sleepiness and are typically unaware of their frequent arousals at night that are associated with reductions in ventilation. Patients are often obese and may have morning headache, personality changes, poor memory, confusion, and irritability. A bed partner may report loud snoring, cessation of breathing, and choking sounds during sleep.

The reported prevalence of sleep apnea among older persons varies from 20% to 70%, depending on the population studied. The prevalence of sleep apnea increases with age. Sleep apnea is very common among patients referred to sleep centers for evaluation of daytime sleepiness, reportedly occurring in 70% of such patients. The most important predictor of obstructive sleep apnea is large body mass. Other reported predictors identified in community-dwelling elderly persons include falling asleep at inappropriate times, male gender, and napping. The classic sleep apnea patient is the obese, sleepy snorer with hypertension. Large neck circumference has also been reported as a marker for sleep apnea.

Alcoholism is an important risk factor for sleep apnea, and sleep-disordered breathing is a significant contributor to sleep disturbance in men over age 40 with a history of alcoholism. Finally, there appears to be an association between sleep apnea and dementia. One nursing-home study found that sleep apnea is associated with dementia, and the sleep disorder was found to be positively correlated with the severity of dementia. However, another study concluded that sleep-disordered breathing in Alzheimer's patients is mild and not associated with mental status or behavioral changes.

The importance of mild degrees of sleep-disordered breathing in elderly persons is unclear. One study found no association between mild or moderate sleep-disordered breathing and subjective sleep-wake disturbance. The long-term consequences of asymptomatic sleep-disordered breathing are also unclear.

Patients suspected of having sleep apnea should be referred to a sleep laboratory for evaluation and, if the diagnosis is documented, a trial of treatment. Home-based diagnostic systems are also available, but the validity of such systems (in comparison with polysomnography in a sleep laboratory) is not clear. There is conflicting evidence whether older patients tolerate the main treatment of obstructive sleep apnea, nasal continuous positive airway pressure (CPAP), as well as middle-aged patients. Careful efforts to use devices that improve comfort may improve adherence with CPAP. Unfortunately, there may be prejudice among clinicians against the use of nasal CPAP in older patients, perhaps because they assume that the treat-

ment will not be tolerated or successful in this population. Oral appliances are an alternative treatment in some patients. Several upper airway surgical approaches have also been used.

Periodic Limb Movements During Sleep and Restless Legs Syndrome

Periodic limb movements during sleep (PLMS) is a condition of debilitating, repetitive, stereotypic leg movements that occur in non-REM sleep. The leg movements occur every 20 to 40 seconds and can last hours or even much of the night, and each movement may be associated with an arousal. The occurrence of PLMS increases with age. One study found evidence of PLMS in over one third of community-dwelling older persons. Correlates of PLMS included dissatisfaction with sleep, sleeping alone, and reported kicking at night. Some authors have suggested that the high prevalence of PLMS with age is associated with delayed motor and sensory latencies noted on nerve conduction testing. PLMS may present as difficulty maintaining sleep or excessive daytime sleepiness. A bed partner may be aware of the leg movements, or these movements may remain occult until identified in a sleep laboratory. When PLMS is associated with sleep complaints that are not explained by another sleep disorder, this is called periodic limb movement disorder (PLMD). Polysomnography is required to establish a diagnosis of PLMD.

The restless legs syndrome is a condition of an uncontrollable urge to move one's legs at night. The symptoms occur while the person is awake, and symptoms can also involve the arms. The diagnosis is based on the patient's description of symptoms, and the patient's complaint is usually of nighttime leg discomfort or difficulty in initiating sleep. Polysomnography is not required to make this diagnosis. There may be a family history of the condition and, in some cases, an underlying medical disorder (eg, anemia, or renal or neurologic disease). The prevalence of restless legs syndrome also increases with age. Many patients with the condition also have PLMS. In older patients with PLMD or restless legs syndrome, dopaminergic agents are the initial agent of choice. An evening dose of a dopamine agonist (eg, pramipexole[OL] or ropinirole) are commonly used for patients with frequent (eg, nightly) symptoms. A nighttime dose of carbidopa-levodopa[OL] can be used for patients who need medication infrequently (ie, for as-needed use). Some patients may describe a shift of their symptoms to daytime hours with successful treatment of symptoms at night. There is some evidence that patients with restless legs syndrome and a low serum ferritin level may improve with iron-replacement therapy. Benzodiazepines, anticonvulsants, and narcotics have

---

[OL] Not approved by the U.S. Food and Drug Administration for this use.

also been used for restless leg syndrome but likely have more adverse effects in older people than the dopaminergic agents.

Disturbances in the Sleep-Wake Cycle

Disturbances in the sleep-wake cycle may be transient, as in jet lag, or associated with an obvious cause (eg, shift work). Some patients have persistent disturbance, with either a delayed sleep phase (fall asleep late and awaken late) or an advanced sleep phase (fall asleep early and awaken early). The advanced sleep phase is particularly common in older people. Some patients have persistent sleep-phase disturbance, in which circadian rhythms and sleeping period have become completely desynchronized (eg, persons who are always asleep during the day and awake at night), or sleep-wake cycles are irregular and sleep habits are very disjointed. It is unclear to what degree, if any, changes in sleep pattern in older people (such as increased daytime napping and disrupted nighttime sleep) are due to alterations in the circadian rhythm. Although results are mixed, several studies have shown age-related decreases in hormonal levels and evidence of earlier circadian rises in certain hormones, suggesting the existence of age-related alteration in circadian rhythm. Problems related to an advanced sleep phase may respond to appropriately timed exposure to bright light (see the section on nonpharmacologic interventions, p 235). Patients with a significant sleep-phase cycle disturbance should be referred to a sleep laboratory for evaluation. Dementia and delirium may also cause sleep-wake disturbance, frequent nighttime awakenings, nighttime wandering, and nighttime agitation.

REM Sleep Behavior Disorder

REM sleep behavior disorder is characterized by excessive motor activities during sleep and a pathologic absence of the normal muscle atonia during REM sleep. The presenting symptoms are usually vigorous sleep behaviors associated with vivid dreams. These behaviors may result in injury (to the patient or bed partner). The condition may be acute or chronic, and it is more common in older men. There may be a family predisposition. Transient REM sleep behavior disorder has been associated with toxic-metabolic abnormalities, primarily drug or alcohol withdrawal or intoxication. The chronic form of the disorder is usually idiopathic or associated with a neurologic abnormality (eg, drug intoxication, vascular disease, tumor, infection, neurodegeneration disorders such as Parkinson's disease, or trauma). Several psychiatric

medications have been associated with this disorder, including tricyclic antidepressants, monoamine oxidase inhibitors, fluoxetine, venlafaxine, cholinesterase inhibitors, and other agents. Polysomnography is recommended to establish the diagnosis. Removal of the offending agent is indicated for drug-induced REM sleep behavior disorder. Clonazepam [OL] is reported to be effective for the treatment of REM sleep behavior disorder, with little evidence of tolerance or abuse over long periods of treatment, but some patients may have adverse effects from this agent. There is some evidence for the use of melatonin in the treatment of REM sleep behavior disorder in patients with coexisting neurodegenerative disorders (eg, Parkinson's disease, dementia with Lewy bodies). Environmental safety interventions are also indicated, such as removing dangerous objects from the bedroom, putting cushions on the floor around the bed, protecting windows, and, in some cases, putting the mattress on the floor.

CHANGES IN SLEEP WITH DEMENTIA

Most studies of sleep in dementia have focused on Alzheimer's disease. Unfortunately, the baseline slowing of electroencephalographic activity often seen with dementia can cloud the distinction between sleep and wakefulness and between the various stages of non-REM sleep in the sleep laboratory. Older patients with dementia have more sleep disruption and arousals, lower sleep efficiency, a higher percentage of stage 1 sleep, and decreases in stage 3 and 4 sleep than do nondemented older people. Some authors have noted a decreased percentage of sleep spent in REM, but this has not been reported in all studies. Of interest, some studies suggest that older persons with dementia have less sleep disturbance than older depressed persons. Disturbances of the sleep-wake cycle are common with dementia, resulting in daytime sleep and nighttime wakefulness.

SLEEP DISTURBANCES IN THE HOSPITAL

Acute hospitalization is commonly cited as one of the stressors that can precipitate transient or short-term insomnia. This insomnia is likely multifactorial in origin and related to illness, medications, change from usual nighttime routines at home, and a sleep-disruptive hospital environment. For example, high noise levels have been documented in the acute hospital setting. Some nursing-based nonpharmacologic interventions to improve sleep have been tested. One small uncontrolled study described increased nighttime melatonin levels in hospitalized older patients treated with day-

---

OL Not approved by the U.S. Food and Drug Administration for this use.

time bright-light exposure. Another small study implemented "flexible medication times" that allowed inpatients to sleep longer in the morning, and their resulting in-hospital sleeping patterns were more similar to their at-home sleeping patterns. However, adherence with nonpharmacologic interventions may be difficult to achieve in the acute hospital. For example, one large clinical trial of nonpharmacologic interventions to prevent delirium in hospitalized older people reported only a 10% adherence rate for the sleep protocol portion of the intervention.

Sleeping medications are commonly prescribed in hospitalized older people. Benzodiazepine receptor agonists are very commonly used. Because of increased sensitivity in elderly patients, smaller doses may be effective as well as safer. Sedating antihistamines (eg, diphenhydramine) should not be used as a sleep aid in hospitalized older people because of possible complications related to anticholinergic adverse effects (eg, delirium, urinary retention, and constipation). In addition, it is important to keep in mind that sleep-related breathing disorders may be common in hospitalized adults, particularly among those with cardiac illness and stroke.

SLEEP IN THE NURSING HOME

Studies of sleep in nursing-home residents have demonstrated marked sleep disruptions and frequent nighttime arousals. In addition, sleep-related problems are a common reason for institutionalization. For example, up to 70% of caregivers report that nighttime difficulties played a significant role in their decision to institutionalize the older person, often because the sleep of the caregiver was being disrupted. Once in the nursing home, many residents nap on and off throughout the day and have frequent awakenings during the night. One study found that 65% of residents reported problems with their sleep and that the use of hypnotic medications was common, but no association was found between the use of sedative hypnotics and the presence, absence, or change in sleep complaints after 6 months of follow-up. Another study found the average duration of sleep episodes during the night in nursing-home residents to be only 20 minutes. Common conditions in nursing-home residents that may contribute to these sleep difficulties include multiple physical illnesses, the use of psychoactive medications, debility and inactivity, increased prevalence of sleep disorders, as well as environmental factors such as nighttime noise, light, and disruptive nursing care. The lack of exposure to bright light during the day may also be a factor.

MANAGEMENT OF SLEEP PROBLEMS

The appropriate treatment of sleep problems must be guided by knowledge of likely causes and potential contributing factors. It is not appropriate to start an older patient with persistent sleep complaints on a sedative hypnotic agent without a careful clinical assessment to identify the cause. Sedative hypnotics have a documented association with falls, hip fracture, and daytime carryover symptoms in older people. If the initial history and physical examination do not suggest a serious underlying cause for the sleep problem, a trial of improved sleep habits is usually the best first approach (see Table 33.1). If the patient takes daytime naps, it is important to determine whether these are needed rest periods or due to inactivity, boredom, or sedating medications. It is important to explain to the person that daytime naps will decrease nighttime sleep.

Short-term hypnotic therapy may be appropriate in conjunction with improved sleep habits in cases of transient, situational insomnia, particularly during bereavement, acute hospitalization, and other periods of temporary acute stress. The clinician should not withhold sedative hypnotic medication treatment in situations where it is clearly indicated. People generally do not feel well if they do not sleep well. However, in the older patient with chronic insomnia, sedative hypnotic

Table 33.1—Measures to Improve Sleep Hygiene

- Maintain a regular rising time.
- Maintain a regular bed time, but do not go to bed unless sleepy.
- Decrease or eliminate naps, unless necessary part of sleeping schedule.
- Exercise daily, but not immediately before bedtime.
- Do not use bed for reading or watching television.
- Relax mentally before going to sleep; do not use bedtime as worry time.
- If hungry, have a light snack (except with symptoms of gastroesophageal reflux or medical contraindications), but avoid heavy meals at bedtime.
- Limit or eliminate alcohol, caffeine, and nicotine, especially before bedtime.
- Wind down before bedtime, and maintain a routine period of preparation for bed (eg, washing up, going to the bathroom).
- Control the nighttime environment with comfortable cool temperature, quiet, and darkness.
- Try a familiar background noise (eg, a fan or other "white noise" machine).
- Wear comfortable bed clothing.
- If unable to fall asleep within 30 minutes, get out of bed and perform soothing activity such as listening to soft music or light reading (but avoid exposure to bright light).
- Get adequate exposure to bright light during the day.

agents should be used cautiously because of the complications associated with their long-term use (see the section on chronic hypnotic use, p 236). The chronic use of benzodiazepines can lead to dependence or cognitive impairment. It must be noted that there is increasing debate among sleep experts on the risks and benefits of long-term use of sleeping medications in adults of all ages. However, there is good evidence of increased risk of confusion, falls, and fracture with chronic sedative use by older people. Regardless, in chronic insomnia, it is imperative that the clinician exclude primary sleep disorders and review medications and other medical conditions that may be contributory.

Nonpharmacologic Interventions

Trials have shown that nonpharmacologic interventions can be quite effective in improving sleep in older people (see Table 33.2 for a summary of such interventions). A review of more than 12 studies of behavioral interventions in community-dwelling older people with insomnia concluded that these interventions produce reliable and durable therapeutic benefits, including improved sleep efficiency, sleep continuity, and satisfaction with sleep; treatment is also helpful in reducing chronic hypnotic use. Stimulus control and sleep restriction, which focus on poor sleep habits, seem to be especially helpful for older persons with insomnia. Cognitive and educational interventions are also important in changing inaccurate beliefs and attitudes about sleep. However, relaxation-based interventions seem less effective for older persons. One large randomized trial of insomniacs with a mean age of 65 years compared cognitive behavior therapy (stimulus control, sleep restriction, sleep hygiene, and cognitive therapy), pharmacotherapy (with temazepam), both cognitive behavioral therapy and pharmacotherapy, and placebo. All three active treatments were found to be effective in short-term follow-up in improving sleep, as indicated by sleep diaries and polysomnography. However, people reported more satisfaction with the cognitive behavioral therapy, and sleep improvements were found to be better sustained over time (up to 2 years) with behavioral treatment.

Several small studies have also tested the effectiveness of exposure to bright light (either natural sunlight or with commercially available light boxes) on the sleep of older persons with insomnia. Positive effects on sleep have been demonstrated with light exposure of various intensities for various durations and at various times during the day. Evening exposure seems to be particularly useful in the older person with an advanced sleep phase. Bathing before sleep has been demonstrated to enhance the quality of sleep in older people, perhaps related to changes in body temperature with bathing. Moderate-intensity exercise has also been shown to improve sleep in healthy, sedentary people aged 50 and older who reported moderate sleep complaints at baseline. However, strenuous exercise should not be performed immediately before bedtime.

Nonpharmacologic interventions have also been studied in institutional settings. A study of institutionalized demented residents with sleep and behavior problems found morning exposure to bright light to be associated with better nighttime sleep and less

Table 33.2—Examples of Nonpharmacologic Interventions to Improve Sleep

Intervention	Goal	Description
Stimulus control	To recondition maladaptive sleep-related behaviors	Patient is instructed to go to bed only when sleepy, not use the bed for eating or watching television, get out of bed if unable to fall asleep, return to bed only when sleepy, get up at the same time each morning, not take naps during the day.
Sleep restriction	To improve sleep efficiency (time asleep over time in bed) by causing sleep deprivation	Patient first collects a 2-week sleep diary to determine average total daily sleep time, then stays in bed only that duration plus 15 minutes, gets up at same time each morning, takes no naps in the daytime, gradually increases time allowed in bed as sleep efficiency improves.
Cognitive interventions	To change misunderstandings and false beliefs regarding sleep	Patient's dysfunctional beliefs and attitudes about sleep are identified; patient is educated to change these false beliefs and attitudes, including normal changes in sleep with increased age and changes that are pathologic.
Relaxation techniques	To recognize and relieve tension and anxiety	In progressive muscle relaxation, patient is taught to tense and relax each muscle group. In electromyographic biofeedback, the patient is given feedback regarding muscle tension and learns techniques to relieve it. Meditation or imagery techniques are taught to relieve racing thoughts or anxiety.
Bright light	To correct circadian rhythm causes of sleeping difficulty (ie, sleep-phase problems)	The patient is exposed to sunlight or a light box. Best evidence is from treatment of seasonal affective disorder (from 2500 lux for 2 hours/day to 10,000 lux for 30 minutes/day). For delayed sleep phase, 2 hours early morning light at 2500 lux. For advanced sleep phase, 2 hours evening light at 2500 lux. Shorter durations may be as effective. Routine eye examination is recommended before treatment; avoid light boxes with ultraviolet exposure.

daytime agitation. Another study of residents with dementia and behavioral problems found that a program of social interaction with nurses was effective in reducing behavioral problems and sleep-wake rhythm disorders in 30% of the residents. Another small trial of incontinent nursing-home residents demonstrated increased nighttime sleep and less agitation among those randomized to receive a combined daytime physical activity program plus nighttime intervention to decrease noise and light disruption. Another trial combined an enforced schedule of structured social and physical activity for 2 weeks in a small sample of assisted-living residents and found that treated residents had enhanced slow-wave sleep and improved performance in memory-oriented tasks.

Nonpharmacologic interventions may also be important in the acute hospital. A large study testing the feasibility of a nonpharmacologic sleep protocol for hospitalized older patients (consisting of a back rub, warm drink, and relaxation tapes) administered by nurses was successful in reducing sedative hypnotic drug use; the sleep protocol was found to have a stronger association than sedative-hypnotic drugs with improved quality of sleep.

Pharmacotherapy

Short-acting agents are recommended for patients with problems initiating sleep, and intermediate-acting agents are recommended for problems with sleep maintenance. Short-acting agents have lower associations with falls and hip fractures. However, agents with rapid elimination in general also produce the most pronounced rebound and withdrawal syndromes after discontinuation. Rebound insomnia after cessation of short-acting agents is dose dependent and can be reduced by tapering the dosage prior to discontinuing the drug. Triazolam is a short-acting benzodiazepine that is not listed in Table 33.3 because it has been associated with nocturnal amnesia and confusion and is generally not recommended for older persons.

Zolpidem, zaleplon, and eszopiclone are nonbenzodiazepine hypnotics. These agents are structurally unrelated to the benzodiazepines, but they share some of the pharmacologic properties of benzodiazepines and have been shown to interact with the central nervous system γ-aminobutyric acid (GABA) receptor complex at benzodiazepine (GABA-BZ) receptors. The selectivity of these newer agents to the GABA-BZ receptor may account for their decreased muscle-relaxant, anxiolytic, and anticonvulsant effects in comparison with benzodiazepines in some studies. Zolpidem is a nonbenzodiazepine imidazopyridine that has been studied in older persons with insomnia. In older patients, studies suggest that zolpidem does not produce rebound insomnia, agitation, or anxiety with cessation; does not seem to produce impaired daytime performance on cognitive and psychomotor performance tests; and may have a therapeutic effect that outlasts the period of drug treatment. Zaleplon is a nonbenzodiazepine hypnotic from the pyrazolopyrimidine class, which has also been studied for short-term use by older persons with insomnia. Because of their rapid onset of action, zolpidem and zaleplon should be taken only immediately before bedtime or after the patient has gone to bed and has been unable to fall asleep. Eszopiclone has been approved by the Food and Drug Administration for use in the United States. There is some evidence that it is effective in long-term management of insomnia. Guidelines recommend that zolpidem or zaleplon, like benzodiazepines, be used only for a short term (2 or 3 weeks) and that, if used longer, these agents be used no more than 2 or 3 nights per week. Concerns remain regarding the risks of confusion, falls, and fracture with chronic use of these medications in older people, and caution is warranted even with these newer agents.

Ramelteon, a melatonin receptor agonist, is the only prescription sleep medication not designated as a controlled substance. It is indicated specifically for patients who have difficulty falling asleep. It is contraindicated in patients with severe hepatic impairment. As with other hypnotics, ramelteon can possibly worsen depression in primarily depressed people. It should not be used with fluvoxamine and should be administered with caution with other CYP1A2, CYP3A4, and CYP29C inhibitors. Common adverse events include headache, somnolence, fatigue, dizziness, exacerbated insomnia, diarrhea, and arthralgias.

Low doses of sedating antidepressants such as trazodone[OL] or mirtazapine[OL] at bedtime may be used as a sleeping aid, particularly for patients with depression. These agents have been suggested for use as a nighttime adjuvant for sleep in depressed patients receiving another antidepressant at therapeutic doses during the daytime. Other indications may be patients with a history of psychoactive substance use problems, failure with other sleeping medications, suspected untreated sleep apnea (where further respiratory depression is a concern), and fibromyalgia (where there is some evidence for antidepressant medication treatment effect). However, the adverse effects of sedating antidepressants may limit their usefulness.

Chronic Hypnotic Use

European studies have reported the prevalence of regular (eg, daily) benzodiazepine use in older people to be at least 5%, with greater use among older women than among older men. There is strong epidemiologic evidence for increased morbidity and mortality with

---

[OL] Not approved by the U.S. Food and Drug Administration for this use.

Table 33.3—Prescription Medications Commonly Used for Insomnia in Older People

Class, Drug	Starting Dose	Usual Dose	Half-Life (hours)	Comments
Intermediate-acting benzodiazepines				
Temazepam	7.5 mg	7.5–30 mg	8.8	Psychomotor impairment, increases risk of falls
Short-acting nonbenzodiazepines				
Eszopiclone	1 mg	1–2 mg	6	Reportedly effective for long-term use in selected individuals; may be associated with unpleasant taste, headache; avoid administration with high-fat meal.
Zaleplon (a pyrazolopyrimidine)	5 mg	5–10 mg	1 (reported unchanged in elderly persons)	Reportedly little daytime carryover, tolerance, or rebound insomnia
Zolpidem (an imidazopyridine)	5 mg	5–10 mg	1.5–4.5 (3 in elderly persons, 10 in hepatic cirrhosis)	Reportedly little daytime carryover, tolerance, or rebound insomnia
Sedating antidepressants				
Mirtazapine[OL]	15 mg	5–45 mg	31–39 in older adults; 13–34 in younger adults; mean = 21	Increased appetite, weight gain, headache, dizziness, daytime carryover; used for insomnia with depression
Trazodone[OL]	25–50 mg	25–150 mg	Reportedly 6 ± 2; prolonged in elderly and obese persons	Moderate orthostatic effects; reportedly effective for insomnia with depression; administration after food minimizes sedation and postural hypotension
Melatonin receptor agonist				
Ramelteon	8 mg	8 mg	1–2.6	Slight decrease in sleep latency; mild adverse events

[OL] Not approved by the U.S. Food and Drug Administration for this use.

chronic use of prescription sleeping pills; however, much of this evidence predates the availability of newer, nonbenzodiazepine hypnotics. It has been reported that the nightly use of prescription sleeping pills is associated with an increased mortality that is similar to the mortality hazard of smoking one to two packs of cigarettes per day. In addition, after tolerance to hypnotics develops, long-term use of these agents may actually make sleep worse. In data reported from a longitudinal study of older people in Germany, those who took sleeping medications had a higher rate of sleep-related complaints than those who did not take a medication for sleep. Additional research is needed to help clarify the consequences of long-term use of the newer, nonbenzodiazepine hypnotics in older people.

Several studies have shown that the bulk of prescription sleeping medication use is occurring among chronic users, and not those with transient sleeping difficulties. A cross-sectional study in Spain found that 88% of prescription hypnotic users reported daily use of the drug, and 72% of people reported use for more than 3 months. Long-term use was two to three times more common in older people than in middle-aged respondents. Likewise, studies in Canada and France have shown that sleep-promoting medications were prescribed for a year or longer in more than two thirds of people who were

taking these medications. Studies in the United States have also demonstrated more benzodiazepine use by older persons and by women, with chronic use being more common in older people. The association between long-acting benzodiazepines and falls in older people has been known for some time. A prospective, population-based Finnish study found this association to be particularly true in older people with physical disability, but not in independent older people.

It is important for the clinician to help older chronic hypnotic users to reduce or eliminate their use of these agents. This can be difficult to achieve, but telling patients that their age predisposes them to developing the side effect so forgetfulness and falls can help. In addition, other methods to help older chronic hypnotic users reduce or eliminate their use of these agents have been reported. One small controlled trial in older women found that decreasing the hypnotic dose by one half for 2 weeks, followed by full withdrawal (perhaps with the use of a substitute pill to maintain the ritual of nightly pill taking) was effective (over short-term follow-up) in eliminating hypnotic use without adverse effects on nighttime sleep, depressive symptoms, or daytime sleepiness. Another small controlled trial involving tapering benzodiazepine use to complete withdrawal over as many as 6 weeks found better success in those persons randomized to receive a nightly dose of 2 mg of controlled-release melatonin rather than placebo. At follow-up 6 months later, nearly 80% of persons who successfully discontinued benzodiazepines continued to report good sleep quality.

Nonprescription Sleeping Agents

Nearly half of older people report using nonprescription sleeping products. The most commonly used products are sedating antihistamines, acetaminophen, alcohol, and melatonin. Sedating antihistamines (eg, diphenhydramine) are common ingredients in over-the-counter sleeping agents as well as in combination analgesic–sleeping agents that are marketed for nighttime use. Diphenhydramine has potent anticholinergic effects, and tolerance to its sedating effects develops after several weeks, so it is generally not recommended for older people. Patients with mild discomfort and sleeping difficulties may have adequate relief with a simple pain reliever (eg, acetaminophen) at bedtime and thus avoid risking the adverse effects of the combination agent. Although alcohol causes some initial drowsiness, it can interfere with sleep later in the night and may actually worsen sleeping difficulties. Evidence is mixed regarding the effectiveness of melatonin as a treatment for insomnia. Because of these mixed results and the lack of regulative control in the currently available melatonin products, it is difficult for the clinician to recommend use of these products. The exception may be chronic hypnotic users, for whom there is some evidence for success in withdrawal of the hypnotic with concomitant use of melatonin.

Valerian is an herbal product with mild sedative action that has been marketed for insomnia. The mechanism of action of valerian is uncertain, and it contains several potentially active compounds. Given this information, its use is not recommended.

REFERENCES

■ Alessi CA, Martin JL, Webber AP, et al. Randomized, controlled trial of a nonpharmacological intervention to improve abnormal sleep/wake patterns in nursing home residents. *J Am Geriatr Soc.* 2005;53(5):803–810.

■ Cole CS, Richards KC. Sleep in persons with dementia: Increasing quality of life by managing sleep disorders. *J Gerontol Nurs.* 2006; 32(3):48–53; quiz 54–55.

■ Kripke DF. Chronic hypnotic use: deadly risks, doubtful benefit. *Sleep Med Rev.* 2000;4(1):5–20.

■ Lee CY, Low LP, Twinn S. Understanding the sleep needs of older hospitalized patients: a review of the literature. *Contemp Nurse.* 2005;20(2):212–220.

■ Mauk KL. Promoting sound sleep habits in older adults. *Nursing.* 2005;35(2):22–25.

■ Moul DE, Hall M, Pilkonis PA, et al. Self-report measures of insomnia in adults: rationales, choices, and needs. *Sleep Med Rev.* 2004;8(3):177–198.

■ Nagel CL, Markie MB, Richards KC, et al. Sleep promotion in hospitalized elders. *Medsurg Nurs.* 2003;12(5): 279–289; quiz 290.

CHAPTER 34—PRESSURE ULCERS

KEY POINTS

■ A pressure ulcer is defined as damage caused to skin and underlying soft tissue by unrelieved pressure when the tissue is compressed between a bony prominence and external surface over a prolonged period of time.

■ Three main factors are believed to play a role in pressure-ulcer formation: pressure, friction, and shear forces. Intrinsic and extrinsic factors determine the tolerance of soft tissue to the adverse effects of pressure.

■ Risk assessment and preventive strategies are required to decrease the incidence of pressure ulcers.

■ The stage of an ulcer determines the appropriate treatment plan.

Pressure ulcers are a serious and common problem for older persons, affecting approximately 1 million adults in the United States. As the population ages, pressure ulcers will continue to be a major health care problem. The surgeon general's Healthy People 2010 document has identified pressure ulcers as a national health issue for long-term care, and the Centers for Medicare and Medicaid Services (CMS) has designated pressure ulcers as one of the three primary markers of quality of care in the long-term-care setting. The prevention and healing of pressure ulcers requires the cooperation and skills of the entire multidisciplinary health care team.

EPIDEMIOLOGY

A pressure ulcer is defined as damage caused to skin and underlying soft tissue by unrelieved pressure when the tissue is compressed between a bony prominence and external surface over a prolonged period of time. Because pressure is the major physiologic factor that leads to soft-tissue destruction, the term *pressure ulcer* is most widely used and preferred over *decubitus ulcer* or *bedsore*.

The causes of pressure ulcers are still not fully understood. Most research into the causes of pressure ulcers has been done in animal models. Three main factors are believed to play a role in pressure-ulcer formation: pressure, friction, and shear forces. It appears that the amount of pressure, friction, or shear force needed to create a pressure ulcer depends on the quality of tissue, the blood flow, and the amount of pressure applied. Hence, for patients with poor-quality tissue (ie, tissue with inadequate blood perfusion), it may take less sustained pressure over a shorter period of time to develop a pressure ulcer. Conversely, patients with good-quality tissue may be able to sustain higher loads of pressure over a longer period of time before an ulcer develops. Ulcers caused by shearing forces tend to develop deep in the fascia, whereas ulcers caused by friction tend to be quite superficial, starting in the epidermal and dermal layers. With aging, local blood supply to the skin decreases, epithelial layers flatten and thin, subcutaneous fat decreases, and collagen fibers lose elasticity. These changes in aging skin and the resultant lowered tolerance to hypoxia may predispose the older person to pressure-ulcer development.

The incidence and prevalence of pressure ulcers vary greatly, depending on the setting. In the hospital, incidence rates have ranged from 0.4% to 38%. Higher rates are noted in intensive care units, where patients are less mobile and have severe systemic illnesses. The Fourth National Pressure Ulcer Prevalence Survey found an annual hospital prevalence rate of 10.1%. In the long-term-care setting, incidence and prevalence rates have ranged from 3% to 30%. Less is known about pressure ulcers in home care, but studies have reported incidence rates of 4% to 17% and prevalence rates of 5% to 15%.

The incidence of pressure ulcers not only differs by health care setting but also by stage of ulceration. The stage I pressure ulcer (persistent erythema) occurs most commonly, accounting for 47% of all pressure ulcers. The stage II pressure ulcers (partial thickness loss involving only the epidermal and dermal layers) are second, at 33%. Stage III (full-thickness skin loss involving subcutaneous tissue) and stage IV (full thickness involving muscle or bone or supporting structures) pressure ulcers make up the remaining 20%. Several studies have noted that the incidence rates of pressure ulcers among black Americans and white Americans may differ; blacks tend to have a greater incidence of stage III and stage IV pressure ulcers than whites have. Whether this can be attributed to structural skin changes or socioeconomic factors is unknown

because of the paucity of pressure-ulcer research among patients in U.S. minority groups.

RISK FACTORS AND RISK-ASSESSMENT SCALES

The literature abounds with lists of risk factors associated with pressure-ulcer development. However, any disease process that renders an elderly person immobile for an extended period of time will increase the risk for pressure-ulcer development. There are intrinsic and extrinsic factors that determine the tolerance of soft tissue to the adverse effects of pressure. Intrinsic risk factors are physiologic factors or disease states that increase the risk for pressure-ulcer development, for example, age, poor nutritional status, and decreased arteriolar blood pressure. Extrinsic factors are external factors that damage the skin, for example, friction and shear, moisture, and urinary or fecal incontinence or both. Variables that appear to be predictors of pressure-ulcer development include age of 70 years or older, impaired mobility, current smoking history, low body mass index, altered mental status (eg, confusion), urinary and fecal incontinence, malnutrition, restraints, malignancy, diabetes mellitus, stroke, pneumonia, heart failure, fever, sepsis, hypotension, kidney failure, dry and scaly skin, history of pressure ulcers, anemia, lymphopenia, and hypoalbuminemia. Some physiologic risk factors (eg, diabetes mellitus, cerebral vascular accident) have been associated with microcirculatory impairment, thus leading to neural and endothelial compromise and increasing the risk of ulceration.

Because of the myriad of risk factors associated with pressure-ulcer development, various scales have been developed to quantify a person's risk by identifying the presence of factors in several categories. The Braden Scale (http://www.bradenscale.com/bradenscale.htm) and the Norton Scale (http://www.woundcarehelpline.com/NortonScale.pdf) are probably the most widely used tools for identifying elderly patients who are at risk for developing pressure ulcers and have been validated. Both tools are recommended by the Agency for Healthcare Research and Quality (AHRQ). The Braden Scale has a sensitivity of 83% to 100% and a specificity of 64% to 77%; the Norton Scale has a sensitivity of 73% to 92% and a specificity of 61% to 94%.

The AHRQ guidelines for preventing pressure ulcers recommend that bed- and chairbound patients or those with impaired ability to be repositioned should be assessed upon admission to the hospital or the nursing home for additional factors that increase the risk for developing pressure ulcers. Pressure-ulcer risk should also be reassessed at periodic intervals and when there is a change in level of activity or mobility. Studies have demonstrated that the incorporation of systematic risk-assessment tools has significantly reduced the incidence of pressure ulcers. To date, the Braden Scale is the only tool to be validated in nonwhite populations. It is important to note that the use of risk-assessment tools will not guarantee that all elderly persons at risk for pressure ulcers will be identified.

PREVENTION

The AHRQ sponsored the development of recommendations for the prevention of pressure ulcers in adults. These clinical practice guidelines (*Pressure Ulcers in Adults: Prediction and Prevention*, published in May 1992) provide an excellent approach to evidenced-based pressure-ulcer prevention (available at http://www.guideline.gov/summary/summary.aspx?doc_id=2601&nbr=1827&string=pressure+ulcers).

Skin Care

There is limited evidence on the role of skin care in pressure-ulcer prevention. Most recommendations are based on expert opinions. After identification of the older person at risk for pressure ulcers, the goal of skin care is to maintain and improve tissue tolerance to pressure in order to prevent injury.

All older persons at risk should have a systematic skin inspection at least once a day, with emphasis on the bony prominences. The skin should be cleansed with warm water and a mild cleansing agent to minimize irritation and dryness of the skin. Every effort should be made to minimize environmental factors leading to skin drying, such as low humidity (less than 40%) and exposure to cold. Decreased skin hydration has been found to result in decreased pliability, and severely dry skin has been noted to damage the stratum corneum. Dry skin should be managed with moisturizers.

Massaging over bony prominences should be avoided. Previously, it was believed that massaging the bony prominences promoted circulation. However, postmortem biopsies found degenerated tissue in those areas exposed to massage but no degenerated tissue on those areas that were not massaged. All efforts should be made to avoid exposing the skin to perspiration, wound drainage, or urine and fecal matter resulting from incontinence. When disposable briefs are used to manage incontinence, the patient must be checked and changed frequently, since perineal dermatitis can develop quickly. The use of disposable underpads to control excessive moisture and perspiration may help wick moisture away from skin. The use of moisturizers and moisture barriers should also be considered to protect the skin.

Nutrition

An association has been observed between pressure-ulcer development and malnutrition; several studies have identified malnutrition as a risk factor for pressure-ulcer formation. Ensuring an adequate diet to prevent malnutrition that is compatible with an individual's ability to eat and goals of care is a reasonable strategy to reduce the risk of ulcer formation.

Mechanical Loading

Minimizing friction and shear is also important. This can be accomplished through proper repositioning, transferring, and turning techniques. The use of lubricants (eg, cornstarch and creams), protective films (eg, transparent film dressings and skin sealants), protective dressings (eg, hydrocolloids), and protective padding may be used to reduce the possibility of friction and shear. Older persons who are at risk for developing pressure ulcers should be repositioned at least every 2 hours. Bed-positioning devices such as pillows or foam wedges should be used to keep bony prominences from direct contact with one another. The head of the bed should be at the lowest degree of elevation consistent with medical conditions. The use of lifting devices, such as trapezes or bed linen, to move the person in bed will also decrease the potential for friction and shear forces. The heel is quite vulnerable to pressure-ulcer development; studies suggest that approximately 20% of all pressure-ulcer development occurs at the heels. This may be attributed to the limited amount of soft tissue over the heel. Specific clinical interventions to prevent heel pressure ulcers have been developed (see Table 34.1).

Patients seated in a chair should be assessed for good postural alignment, distribution of weight, and balance. They should be taught or reminded to shift

Table 34.1—Prevention of Heel Pressure Ulcers

- Assess the heels of patients at high risk for pressure ulcers every day.
- Use moisturizer on the heels twice a day; do not massage.
- Apply transparent film dressings to the heels of older persons prone to friction problems (eg, stroke patients).
- Apply hydrocolloid dressing (either single or extra-thick) to the heels of older persons with reactive hyperemia (pre-stage I).
- Have older persons wear socks to help prevent friction; remove at bedtime.
- Have older persons in wheelchairs wear properly fitting padded sneakers or shoes.
- Place pillow vertically under the person's legs (without hyperextending them) to support heels off the bed surface.
- Turn the person every 2 hours, repositioning heels.

weight every 15 minutes. The use of doughnuts as seating cushions is contraindicated because they increase pressure over the area of contact and may actually cause pressure ulcers.

Mobility

Maintaining or improving mobility is also extremely important. It is one of the most effective ways to decrease pressure on bony prominences. For bedbound patients there are benefits of both active and passive range-of-motion exercises. Those patients not confined to bed should be encouraged to move from bed to chair to standing to ambulating to minimize the risk of developing pressure ulcers.

Support Surfaces

Any elderly person identified as being at risk for developing pressure ulcers should be placed on a pressure-reducing device. Two types exist: static (foam, static air, gel or water, or a combination) and dynamic (alternating air, low air loss, or air fluidized). Most static devices are less expensive than dynamic surfaces. Table 34.2 provides details about the various types of support surfaces that can guide selection for particular situations. Most experts would agree that for pressure-ulcer prevention, the use of static devices is appropriate. Two conditions warrant consideration of a dynamic surface:

- bottoming-out occurs (the static surface is compressed to less than 1 inch), or
- the patient is at high risk for pressure ulcers and reactive hyperemia is noted on a bony prominence despite the use of a static support surface.

Although effective at reducing pressure, dynamic airflow beds have several potential adverse effects,

including dehydration, sensory deprivation, loss of muscle strength, and difficulty with mobilization.

MANAGEMENT

The AHRQ developed evidence-based guidelines on the management of pressure ulcers. This guideline, *Treatment of Pressure Ulcers*, published in December 1994, reviews the foundation for providing evidence-based pressure-ulcer management (available at http://www.guideline.gov/summary/summary.aspx?doc_id=810).

Assessment

A pressure ulcer will not heal unless underlying causes are identified and effective interventions are implemented. When a pressure ulcer has developed, a systematic evaluation is necessary. Table 34.3 presents an approach to assessment and documentation when a pressure ulcer develops.

There is no universal agreement on a single system for classifying pressure ulcers. Most experts do agree that the stage of an ulcer determines the appropriate treatment plan. It should be noted that staging alone does not determine the seriousness of the ulcer. Most systems use four stages to classify ulceration. Table 34.4 describes one staging system. When eschar, a thick brown or black devitalized tissue, is covering the ulcer, the ulcer cannot be accurately staged.

The challenge for most staging systems occurs in the definition of the stage I pressure ulcer. There is more variability in attempts to classify the first stage of ulcer development than in any other stage. Most systems define the stage I pressure ulcer as nonblanchable erythema of intact skin; both the AHRQ prediction and prevention guidelines and the Minimum Data Set (required by CMS for all patients in long-term-care facilities) refer to stage I pressure ulcer in these terms. However, it is difficult (at best) to blanch the skin of persons with darkly pigmented skin. To address this

Table 34.2—Support Surfaces for Persons at Risk for Pressure Ulcers

Type	Examples	Support Area	Low Moisture Retention	Reduced Heat Accumulation	Shear Reduction	Pressure Reduction	Cost per Day
Static surfaces	Foam	Yes	No	No	No	Yes	Low
	Standard mattress	No	No	No	No	No	Low
	Static flotation—air or water	Yes	No	No	Yes	Yes	Low
Dynamic surfaces	Air fluidized	Yes	Yes	Yes	Yes	Yes	High
	Low-air-loss	Yes	Yes	Yes	?	Yes	High
	Alternating air	Yes	No	No	Yes	Yes	Moderate

SOURCE: Adapted from Bergstrom N, Bennett MA, Carlson CE, et al. *Treatment of Pressure Ulcers. Clinical Practice Guideline No. 15.* Rockville, MD: US Department of Health and Human Services, Public Health Service, Agency for Health Care Policy and Research. December 1994:38. AHCPR Pub. No. 95-0652.

Table 34.3—A Systematic Approach to the Management of Pressure Ulcers

Evaluate and Document:	Consider These Strategies:
Location	Examine high-risk sites.
	Develop targeted pressure-relieving strategies (eg, positioning and repositioning, padding, seat cushions, and heel elevation).
	Limit shearing forces by special attention to positioning when the head of bed is elevated.
	Lift rather than slide the patient.
	Cleanse and dry regularly if wetted frequently.
Stage	Differentiate between minor stage I lesions (nonblanchable erythema related to extravasation of red blood cells into the interstitium) and deep tissue injuries that can progress to full-thickness lesions.
	Discuss with caregivers and families the possibility of significant pressure-ulcer development when deep tissue injury is identified.
Area	Record diameter for circular lesions.
	Record lengths of largest perpendiculars for irregular lesions.
Depth	Measure depth from plane of skin.
	Probe and measure extent of undermining or depth of sinus tracts.
Drainage	Estimate amount.
	Identify degree of odor and purulence.
	Monitor hematocrit if more than minor blood loss with dressing changes occurs.
	Monitor serum albumin if volume of ulcer drainage is large.
Necrosis	Consider simple blunt debridement of small amounts of necrotic tissue.
	Involve general or plastic surgeons for extensive debridement.
	Monitor damage to healthy tissue whenever using blunt, enzymatic, or wet-to-dry dressings for debridement.
	Monitor use of pressure dressings (which can cause necrosis) after blunt debridement.
Granulation	Identify granulation as an indication that wound healing is occurring.
	Look for regression when other infections (eg, urinary tract infection or pneumonia) occur.
	Develop strategies to protect and enhance growth of granulation tissue (eg, nourishment, vitamins, and minerals; use of dressings to ensure moist wound surfaces).
	Avoid damage with dressing changes.
Cellulitis	Differentiate from a thin rim of erythema surrounding most healing wounds.
	Look for tender, warmth, redness, particularly if there is progression.
	Consider treatment with systemic antibiotics active against gram-positive cocci.

SOURCE: Bennett RG. Pressure ulcers. In: Cobbs EL, Duthie EH Jr, Murphy JB. *Geriatrics Review Syllabus: A Core Curriculum in Geriatric Medicine,* 4th ed. Dubuque, IA: Kendall Hunt Publishing Company for the American Geriatrics Society; 1996:155.

Table 34.4—Staging System for Pressure Ulcers

Stage I	Persistent nonblanchable erythema of intact skin.*
Stage II	Partial-thickness skin loss involving epidermis or dermis, or both. The ulcer is superficial and presents clinically as an abrasion, blister, or shallow crater.
Stage III	Full-thickness skin loss involving damage or necrosis of subcutaneous tissue that may extend down to, but not through, underlying fascia.
Stage IV	Full-thickness skin loss with extensive destruction, tissue necrosis, or damage to muscle, bone, or supporting structures (eg, tendon or joint capsule). Undermining and sinus tracts may also be associated with stage IV pressure ulcers.

* The National Pressure Ulcer Advisory Panel further expands this definition as follows: A Stage I pressure ulcer is an observable pressure-related alteration of intact skin whose indicators as compared with the adjacent or opposite area on the body may include changes in one or more of the following: skin temperature (warmth or coolness), tissue consistency (firm or boggy feel), and/or sensation (pain, itching). The ulcer appears as a defined area of persistent redness in lightly pigmented skin, whereas in darker skin tones, the ulcer may appear with persistent red, blue, or purple hues.

SOURCE: Adapted from definitions by the Agency for Health Care Policy and Research. See Bergstrom N, Bennett MA, Carlson CE, et al. *Treatment of Pressure Ulcers. Clinical Practice Guideline No. 15.* Rockville, MD: US Department of Health and Human Services, Public Health Service, Agency for Health Care Policy and Research. December 1994:47–49. AHCPR Pub. No. 95-0652.

concern, the National Pressure Ulcer Advisory Panel (NPUAP) revised its definition of a stage I pressure ulcer to encompass the skin alterations that might be seen in stage I pressure ulcers regardless of skin pigmentation. This system defines a stage I ulcer as an observable pressure-related alteration of intact skin whose indicators, as compared with an adjacent or opposite area on the body, may include changes in one or more of the following: skin temperature (warmth or coolness), tissue consistency (firm or boggy feel), or sensation (pain, itching). The NPUAP definition further states that the pressure ulcer appears as a defined area of persistent redness in lightly pigmented skin, whereas in darker skin tones, the pressure ulcer may appear with persistent erythema, or blue or purple hues. Although this definition is cumbersome, it is the only definition that includes patients with darkly pigmented skin.

Treatment

Debridement

Debridement is necessary when there is necrotic, devitalized tissue within the wound. Such tissue supports the growth of pathologic organisms and prevents healing. There are four major types of debridement methods: mechanical, enzymatic, autolytic, and sharp (Table 34.5) used in the United States. It should be noted that biosurgery (maggot or larva therapy), which is used widely in Europe, is another potential debridement option. The debridement method should be selected on the basis of the patient's health condition, the ulcer presentation, the presence or absence of infection, and the patient's ability to tolerate the procedure.

Dressings

Numerous dressings are used in the healing of pressure ulcers. The use of gauze wet-to-dry has been discouraged by experts; it is actually a debriding technique that can damage the tissue matrix and prolong healing. Many experts advocate the use of hydrocolloid dressings. These dressings, when compared with gauze, have been found to significantly speed the healing process. This is most likely because hydrocolloids require fewer dressing changes (inflicting less trauma), block bacteria from penetrating the wound bed, and maintain a moist wound environment (facilitating increases in the growth factors needed in the healing process). Moreover, studies have demonstrated that the use of hydrocolloids, when compared with the use of gauze, decreases direct and indirect institutional costs. It is essential to select an appropriate dressing, not on the basis of the stage of the pressure ulcer, but rather on the amount of wound exudate. Table 34.6 identifies some of the most common dressings and the indications for their use.

Surgical Repair

The use of surgical repair of a pressure ulcer remains a viable option for stage III and stage IV pressure ulcers. However, because many stage III and stage IV pressure ulcers eventually heal over a long period of time with the use of modern wound-healing principles and the rate of recurrence of surgically closed pressure ulcers is high, the practitioner must carefully weigh the benefits of the surgery. When the surgical option is exercised, the most common type of surgical repairs are direct closure, skin grafting, skin flaps, musculocutaneous flaps, and free flaps.

Table 34.5—Methods of Debridement

Type	Description	Advantages, Disadvantages
Mechanical	Use of physical forces to remove devitalized tissues; methods include wet-to-dry irrigation (using 19-gauge needle with 35-cc syringe), hydrotherapy, and dextranomer	May remove both devitalized and vitalized tissues; may cause pain
Surgical, Sharp	Use of scalpel, scissors, and forceps to remove the devitalized tissue; laser debridement is also under this category	Quick, effective if performed by skilled professional; should be used when infection is suspected; pain management is needed
Enzymatic	Use of topical debriding agent to dissolve the devitalized tissue (chemical force)	Appropriate when there are no signs or symptoms of local infection; some may damage surrounding skin
Autolytic	Use of synthetic dressings to allow the devitalized tissue to self-digest from the enzymes found in the ulcer fluids (natural force)	Recommended when the older person cannot tolerate other forms of debridement and when infection is not suspected; may take a long time to be effective
Biosurgery	Use of larvae to digest devitalized tissue	Quick, effective; good option when older person cannot tolerate surgical debridement

SOURCE: Data from Bergstrom N, Bennett MA, Carlson CE, et al. *Treatment of Pressure Ulcers. Clinical Practice Guideline No. 15.* Rockville, MD: US Department of Health and Human Services, Public Health Service, Agency for Health Care Policy and Research. December 1994:47–49. AHCPR Pub. No. 95-0652.

Table 34.6—Common Dressings for Treating Pressure Ulcers

Dressing	Indications	Contraindications	Example	Comments
Transparent film	Stage I, II Protection from friction Superficial scrape	Draining ulcers Suspected skin infection or fungus	Bioclusive Tegaderm Op-site	Apply skin prep to intact skin to protect from adhesive
Foam island	Stage II, III Low to moderate exudate Can apply as window to secure transparent film	Excessive exudate Dry, crusted wound	Allevyn Lyofoam	
Hydrocolloids	Stage II, III Low to moderate drainage Good peri-wound skin integrity Autolytic debridement of necrotic tissue	Poor skin integrity Infected ulcers Wound needs packing	DuoDERM Extra thin film DuoDERM Tegasorb RepliCare Comfeel Nu-derm	Left in place 3–5 days Can apply as window to secure transparent film Can apply over alginate to control drainage Must control maceration Apply skin prep to intact skin to protect from adhesive
Alginate	Stage III, IV Excessive drainage	Dry or minimally draining wound Superficial wounds with maceration	Sorbsan Kaltostat Algosteril AlgiDERM	Apply dressing within wound borders Requires secondary dressing Must use skin prep Must control for maceration
Hydrogel (amorphous gels)	Stage II, III, IV	Macerated areas Wounds with excess exudate	IntraSite gel SoloSite gel Restore gel	Needs to be combined with gauze dressing Stays moist longer than saline gauze Changed 1–2 times/day Used as alternative to saline gauze for packing deep wounds with tunnels, undermining Reduces adherence of gauze to wound Must control for maceration
(gel sheet)	Stage II	Macerated areas Wounds with moderate to heavy exudate	Vigilon Restore Impregnated Gauze	Needs to be held in place with topper dressing
Gauze packing (moistened with saline)	Stage III, IV Wounds with depth, especially those with tunnels, undermining		square 2 × 2s, 4 × 4s Fluffed Kerlix Plain NuGauze	Must be remoistened often to maintain moist wound environment
Silver dressings (silver with alginates, gels, charcoal)	Malodorous wounds High level of exudates Wound highly suspicious for critical bacterial load Peri-wound with signs of inflammation Slow-healing wound	Systemic infection Cellulitis Signs of systemic side effects, esp. erythema multiforme Fungal proliferation Sensitivity of skin to sun Interstitial nephritis Leukopenia Skin necrosis Concurrent use with proteolytic enzymes	Silvercel Silvadene Aquacel Ag Acticoat	

SOURCE: Copyright © 2006 by Rita Frantz. Reprinted from Reuben DB, Herr K, Pacala JT, et al. *Geriatrics At Your Fingertips. 2006.* 8th ed. New York: American Geriatrics Society; 2006:187. Reprinted with permission.

Diet and Nutritional Supplements

If a patient with a pressure ulcer is malnourished, the importance of diet and dietary supplements is controversial. The AHRQ treatment guideline rates the strength of the evidence as "C," the weakest rating, for nutritional support that achieves approximately 30 to 35 calories per kg per day and 1.25 to 1.50 g of protein per kg per day. Evidence to support the use of supplemental vitamins and minerals is equally weak.

New or Unproven Therapies

Throughout the years a number of treatments have been advocated for the healing of pressure ulcers without sufficient data to support their various claims. Data on the therapeutic efficacy of hyperbaric oxygen, low-energy laser irradiation, and therapeutic ultrasound have not been established. However, areas of great promise include the use of recombinant platelet-derived growth factors to stimulate healing and skin equivalents that may prove to heal stage III and stage IV pressure ulcers. Preliminary data on the uses of electrical stimulation, vacuum-assisted closures, and warm-up therapy, which increases the basal temperature of the ulcer to promote healing, are promising.

Monitoring Healing

Monitoring the healing of pressure ulcers can pose a challenge to the practitioner. The accurate measurements of a pressure ulcer can inform the practitioner about the effectiveness of ulcer treatment. However, the use of traditional measurements (rulers and tracing paper) produces highly variable results among raters. In the past 8 years, two instruments to measure healing of pressure ulcers with some level of validity and reliability have been developed. The Pressure Sore Status Tool and the Pressure Ulcer Scale for Healing (http://www.npuap.org/push3-0.html) are excellent tools for monitoring pressure-ulcer healing. The use of high-frequency portable ultrasound to measure wound healing has been introduced. The use of this technology, which can capture three-dimensional measurements, has been shown to be quite beneficial in objectively monitoring healing. Moreover, because ultrasound is "color blind," it can detect stage I pressure ulcers in darkly pigmented skin.

There has been considerable debate regarding the use of reverse staging of pressure ulcers to monitor healing. Staging of pressure ulcers is appropriate only for defining the maximum anatomic depth of tissue damage. Since pressure ulcers heal to a progressively more shallow depth, they do not replace lost muscle, subcutaneous fat, or dermis before they re-epithelialize. Instead, pressure ulcers are filled with granulation (scar) tissue composed primarily of endothelial cells, fibroblasts, collagen, and extracellular matrix. A stage IV pressure ulcer cannot become a stage III, stage II, and then stage I; reverse staging does not accurately characterize what is physiologically occurring as the pressure ulcer heals. When a stage IV pressure ulcer has healed, it should be classified as a healed stage IV pressure ulcer, not a stage 0. The progress of healing can be documented only by describing ulcer characteristics or measuring wound characteristics with a validated tool.

Ulcer care should be evaluated for healing progress on a weekly basis. There are no standard healing rates for pressure ulcers. Review of the literature suggests that a majority of stage I pressure ulcers heal within 1 day to 1 week; stage II, within 5 days to 3 months; stage III, within 1 month to 6 months; and stage IV, within 6 months to 1 year. Clearly, some full-thickness pressure ulcers may never heal, depending on comorbidity; however, no clear guidelines exist to determine when a pressure ulcer can be truly defined as recalcitrant or what characteristics must be present to predict that an ulcer will never heal.

Control of Infections

All pressure ulcers become colonized with both aerobic and anaerobic bacteria, and superficial swab cultures of the wounds have not been shown to be helpful in determining which organism may be causing the infection. Therefore, routine swab cultures are not recommended. However, there is some evidence to suggest that quantitative tissue swab cultures can be used to determine the wound bioburden. Wound cleansing and dressing changes are two of the most important methods for minimizing the amount of bacterial colonization. Increasing the frequency of wound cleansing and dressing changes is an important first step when purulent or foul-smelling drainage is observed on the ulcer. When ulcers are not healing or have persistent exudate after 2 weeks of optimal cleansing and dressing changes, it is reasonable to consider the use of antimicrobials.

The use of topical antimicrobials has been shown to decrease the bioburden in pressure ulcers. The use of antimicrobials such as silver sulfadiazine and mupirocin ointment can be applied up to three times a day for 1 to 2 weeks, with careful monitoring for allergic reactions. Because prolonged use of these antimicrobials may result in resistant organisms, they should not be used indefinitely. In the past several years, the uses of silver-impregnated dressings to decrease the bioburden has become quite popular. Although the exact mechanism of how silver kills the infection remains unknown, it is hypothesized that it stops the enzyme that feeds the proliferation of bacteria, viruses, and fungi. These dressings (Aquacel Ag, Acticoat, Actisorb, and Arglaes) control bacterial load and ideally control odor caused by the bacteria. The dressing selected determines how the silver is delivered, the length of treatment, the amount of exudate absorption, the incidence of maceration, the ease of dressing removal, and the pain intensity at dressing changes. It is important to select a dressing that meets the needs of the patient and the staff.

Because most topical antibiotics do not penetrate the wound bed, they are not effective for control of infections. When ulcers fail to heal despite the treatments described above, it is reasonable to consider the possibility of cellulitis or osteomyelitis. Biopsy of the ulcer for quantitative bacterial cultures or of the underlying bone can be used to establish these diagnoses. Cellulitis, osteomyelitis, bacteremia, and sepsis are all indications for the use of systemic antibiotics.

The use of topical antiseptics (eg, povidone iodine, iodophor, sodium hypochlorite, hydrogen peroxide, and acetic acid) is not recommended because of their tissue toxicity. There is some new literature suggesting that diluted povidone iodine (<5%) is not cytotoxic to healthy granulation tissue.

COMPLICATIONS FROM PRESSURE ULCERS

The development of pressure ulcers can lead to several complications. Probably the most serious complication is sepsis. When a pressure ulcer is present and there is aerobic or anaerobic bacteremia, or both, the pressure ulcer is most often the primary source of the infection. Additional complications of pressure ulcers include localized infection, cellulitis, and osteomyelitis. Quite often, a nonhealing pressure ulcer may indicate underlying osteomyelitis. Mortality can also be associated with pressure-ulcer development. Several studies have noted the association of pressure-ulcer development and mortality in both the hospital and nursing-home settings. In fact, the mortality rate has been noted to be as high as 60% for those older persons who develop a pressure ulcer within 1 year of hospital discharge. Thus, careful assessment of a pressure ulcer is essential. Finally, other complications of pressure ulcers include pain and depression. Both pain and depression have been associated with decreased wound healing.

REFERENCES

■ Allman RM, Goode PS, Patrick MM, et al. Pressure ulcer risk factors among hospitalized patients with activity limitation. *JAMA* 1995;273(11):865–870.

■ Berlowitz DR, Bezerra HQ, Brandeis GH, et al. Are we improving the quality of nursing home care: the case of pressure ulcers. *J Am Geriatr Soc.* 2000;48(1):59–62.

■ Lyder CH, Preston J, Grady JN, et al. Quality of care for hospitalized Medicare patients at risk for pressure ulcers. *Arch Intern Med.* 2001;161(12):1549–1554.

■ Lyder CH, Shannon R, Empleo-Frazier O, et al. A comprehensive program to prevent pressure ulcers in long-term care: exploring costs and outcomes. *Ostomy Wound Manage.* 2002;48(4):52–62.

■ Stotts NA, Rodeheaver GT, Thomas DR, et al. An instrument to measure healing in pressure ulcers: development and validation of the Pressure Ulcer Scale for Healing (PUSH). *J Gerontol A Biol Sci Med Sci.* 2001;56(12):M795–M799.

PSYCHIATRY

CHAPTER 35—DEPRESSION AND OTHER MOOD DISORDERS

KEY POINTS

- Symptoms of depression below the threshold for a diagnosis of major depression are common in late life and may incur disability, therefore warranting an intervention.

- Selective serotonin-reuptake inhibitors (SSRIs) such as sertraline and citalopram are most commonly used as first-line agents for older adults with depression.

- Treatment of depression may require up to 12 weeks before a response to medication is noted; trials of more than one antidepressant may be required before a satisfactory response is achieved.

- The side-effect profile and propensity to interact with other medications are key factors to consider in selecting an antidepressant for an older patient.

EPIDEMIOLOGY

Prevalence studies of community residents demonstrate surprisingly low rates of depressive disorders among those aged 65 years and older. Only 1% to 2% of women and fewer than 1% of men interviewed with standardized instruments meet diagnostic criteria for major depression. Both current and lifetime prevalence rates for older persons are lower than those for middle-aged persons; furthermore, these relatively low rates persist after accounting for possible premature death and institutionalization, both of which may be associated with depression. Similarly, the incidence of first-episode major depression decreases after age 65. Data demonstrating that older persons are less likely to recognize depression and to endorse depressed mood offer one explanation for the lower prevalence and incidence of depressive syndromes among older community residents.

However, the prevalence of depressive symptoms that do not meet the threshold for a clinical diagnosis is substantial in seniors, with most studies reporting rates in the range of 15%. These subsyndromal states are not inconsequential. "Minor" or subsyndromal depression has been associated with increased use of health services, excess disability, and poor health outcomes, including higher mortality rates.

The prevalence rates of both major and subsyndromal depression are related to the setting in which older persons are seen and methods used to identify cases. Thus, major depression has been identified in 6% to 10% of older persons in primary care clinics and 12% to 20% of nursing-home residents. More varied rates of 11% up to 45% have been reported among elderly patients requiring inpatient medical care. The reported prevalence rates of minor depression in outpatient medical settings have been varied as well, with rates from 8% to over 40% reported. Studies that count symptoms due to physical illness toward a diagnosis of depression may inflate prevalence rates among medical patients because of symptom overlap. In the psychiatric clinic setting, major depression is the most common disorder seen among elderly patients and accounts for more than 40% of outpatient caseloads and inpatient psychiatry admissions.

CLINICAL PRESENTATION AND DIAGNOSIS

The Geriatric Syndrome of Late-Life Depression

Symptoms used to diagnose major depression are listed in Table 35.1, which summarizes the criteria for major depression from the fourth edition of the *Diagnostic and Statistical Manual of Mental Disorders* (*DSM-IV*). Although aging does not markedly affect the overall phenomenology of major depression, some differences between younger and older depressed patients have been reported. Older patients are more preoccupied with somatic symptoms and less frequently report depressed mood and guilty preoccupations. Among patients who do not acknowledge sustained feelings of sadness, the demonstration of the second core symptom, a persistent loss of pleasure and interest in previously enjoyable activities (*anhedonia*), is necessary for a diagnosis of major depression. Thus, one need not exhibit depressed mood to meet criteria for major depressive disorder. The core symptoms are particularly important to detect in primary care settings and have been found to identify most medically ill patients who also meet full diagnostic criteria. Furthermore, these core symptoms are less likely to overlap with those of a medical illness.

The diagnosis of major depression in older persons is complicated by the overlap among symptoms of major depression with those of physical illness. Patients

Table 35.1—*DSM-IV* Diagnostic Criteria for Major Depression

Depressed mood*

Loss of interest or pleasure*

Appetite change or weight loss

Insomnia or hypersomnia

Psychomotor agitation or retardation

Loss of energy

Feelings of worthlessness or guilt

Difficulties with concentration or decision making

Recurrent thoughts of death or suicide

* "Gateway" (or "core") symptoms, at least one of which must be present for a diagnosis of major depression.

NOTE: The diagnosis requires that the patient have at least one gateway or core symptom and that five or more symptoms have occurred nearly every day for most of the day for at least 2 weeks. Also, the symptoms must be causing significant distress or impaired functioning and must not be due to a direct physiologic cause.

SOURCE: Data from the American Psychiatric Association. *Diagnostic and Statistical Manual of Mental Disorders*. 4th ed. Washington, DC: American Psychiatric Association; 1994.

with serious medical illness may be preoccupied with thoughts about death or feel worthless because of concomitant disability. The *DSM-IV* criteria require that the depressive symptoms are not a direct effect of a general medical condition or medication used to treat it, but this distinction based on cause may be difficult to make reliably. Alternative diagnostic criteria have been suggested for medical patients, including an inclusive approach that counts all symptoms regardless of cause. Inclusive approaches result in the highest prevalence rates. Furthermore, a depressed person's thoughts of death and worthlessness appear to differ from those of a patient with a serious medical illness. In depression, these thoughts are not based on a realistic assessment of prognosis or overall self-worth. The perspective of depressed patients is influenced by the feelings of sadness or guilt that accompany the disordered mood. The alternative diagnosis of mood disorder due to a general medical condition should be used for patients with depression that appears to result directly from a specific medical condition (eg, hypothyroidism).

The recognition of psychotic depression has particular relevance to primary care clinicians. Patients with psychotic depression have sustained irrational beliefs (delusions) in association with their depression, and these beliefs not infrequently focus on physical or medical preoccupations, such as the belief that one's bowels are "blocked with cancer." Psychotic depression may be suspected when the irrational belief focuses on somatic symptoms or around fears of a serious physical condition such as cancer when there is no medical source identified to support the belief.

Screening for mood symptoms is an important part of a comprehensive assessment of all older patients regardless of socioeconomic or ethnic status, although cultural variation may influence how emotional states are expressed. Since the diagnosis of depression hinges on a qualitative change from a patient's normal mood state, it is essential to obtain information from involved family members or caregivers to determine whether a clinically meaningful syndrome has developed. Recent large-scale studies of mental health in the elderly age group (eg, the Primary Care Research in Substance Abuse and Mental Health for the Elderly, PRISM-E) have shown that among older persons with depression, there is a preponderance of women and ethnic minorities. This suggests that a higher degree of vigilance for mood disorders is warranted in these groups.

Bipolar Disorder

A diagnosis of mania requires a distinct period of persistently elevated mood lasting for 1 or more weeks and three additional symptoms that may include inflated self-esteem or grandiosity, hypersexuality, increased activity, decreased need for sleep, pressured speech, racing thoughts or flight of ideas, and distractibility. Grandiose or paranoid delusions may be present. Although the criteria for diagnosing bipolar disorder in younger and older patients are identical, some differences in phenomenology have been noted. Elderly patients with bipolar disorder are more likely to have a mixture of depression and marked irritability. Pressured speech that tends to go off on tangents is common, although the severity of thinking disturbance is less pronounced than in young adults and flight of ideas is less common. Hypersexuality and grandiosity may be present but are less prominent, as well. Manic-like syndromes in late life are also distinguished by a greater likelihood of confusion, often a reflection of an underlying cognitive disturbance, such as an incipient dementia.

DIFFERENTIAL DIAGNOSIS

Approximately 30% to 50% of patients with late-life depression are experiencing a recurrence of episodes that began in early adulthood. Despite the associations between late-onset depression and chronic medical illness, disability, and psychosocial stresses, most episodes develop without an identifiable precipitant. Because late-onset depression is less likely than typical recurrent depression to be familial, a positive family history is less useful for establishing a diagnosis.

Differentiation From Medical Illness

Medical disorders that may imitate depression are particularly important to consider in elderly patients because of the increased vulnerability of this population to physical illnesses. Hyperthyroidism merits special consideration, because older hyperthyroid patients may present with apathy and diminished energy that mimics depression. Although apathy may be commonly associated with the core depressive symptom of anhedonia, apathy may also occur in persons who retain a reactive capacity for experiencing pleasure. The distinction of apathy from true depression becomes particularly important among patients with Parkinson's disease, carcinoma of the pancreas, and dementia, because depressive syndromes that occur commonly in these disorders are responsive to antidepressant medications.

Depression Associated With Structural Brain Disease

Major depression may be a prodrome of dementia such as Alzheimer's disease or may develop after the onset of cognitive decline. Differentiation may be confounded because depression is commonly accompanied by symptoms of impaired concentration, indecisiveness, and lack of motivation that are also associated with dementia. An older person with depression may both report memory loss and poor concentration and be unable to perform simple cognitive tests without having dementia. Differentiation from dementia requires evidence that the cognitive impairment, developed concurrently with the onset of depression, reverses with improvement in mood. Conversely, patients with true dementia may have symptoms that imitate depression. These include loss of interest, apathy, psychomotor retardation, and disrupted sleep. A diagnosis of major depression requires the presence of at least one core symptom and the persistence of symptoms for at least 2 weeks; approximately 20% of patients with early Alzheimer's disease meet these criteria.

Studies have described a syndrome of "vascular" depression that is associated commonly with anhedonia, executive dysfunction, and the absence of guilty preoccupations. The syndrome is thought to result from prefrontal and subcortical lesions due to microinfarcts. These patients tend to have a late age of onset, risk factors for vascular disease, prefrontal or subcortical white matter hyperintensities on T2 weighted magnetic resonance imaging, and evidence of non-amnestic neuropsychologic deficits in tasks requiring initiation, persistence, and self-monitoring. Execution of tasks requiring planning and shifting between cognitive sets is impaired. Depressed patients with such defects in executive function may experience a remission of disturbed mood in response to standard pharmacotherapies but remain substantially disabled because of the cognitive dysfunction.

Bereavement

Bereavement is common among older persons. Feelings of sadness, disturbed sleep, and diminished appetite are common among bereaved persons but generally resolve within a few months. Up to 14% of bereaved adults develop a major depression within 2 years of the loss, which occurs with a lower frequency among bereaved elderly persons. Bereavement that has evolved into a major depression is characterized by morbid preoccupations with guilt or suicidal ideas beyond transient thoughts of joining the deceased that would be expected in association with the loss. Also, bereavement is not associated with sustained functional impairment, so a marked decline in self-care may be a sign of a depressive syndrome.

COURSE

Major depression is often a recurrent disorder in both younger and older adults. Evidence from observational studies in which treatment was not provided systematically indicate that up to one third of patients run a chronic course, and another third have partial recovery with residual disability. Patients who suffer their first episode in later life take longer to recover. Depressed elderly persons also use health services, including outpatient visits, specialist consultations, and laboratory assessments, more than nondepressed elderly persons do.

Comorbid medical illness is associated with more refractory mood symptoms, and medical morbidity and mortality are themselves increased in patients who have suffered a depressive episode. The relationship between depression and increased mortality rates from cardiovascular causes is particularly striking. Depressed patients have an increased risk of cardiovascular mortality generally, and the development of depression in patients following a myocardial infarction, heart failure, or cardiac bypass surgery increases mortality from cardiovascular events.

Old age is associated with an increased risk for suicide. Persons aged 65 and over represent less than 13% of the population but account for 25% of suicides. The likelihood that an attempt will be fatal approximates 25%, a rate far greater than in young adults. "Psychologic autopsy" studies that use interviews with relatives and physicians to reconstruct a suicide victim's premorbid mental state have demonstrated that as many as 75% of older adults who commit suicide were suffering from depression. The vast majority had seen a primary care physician within the previous month. In addition to depression, risk factors for late-life suicide include a comorbid physical illness, living alone, male gender, and alcoholism. Older men and women commit suicide violently; firearms and hanging are the methods most commonly employed.

TREATMENT

Overview

The course of treatment for major depression can be conceptualized as follows: acute treatment to reverse the current episode, continuation treatment to prevent relapse, and maintenance treatment to prevent recurrence. Continuation treatment to stabilize the recovery involves ongoing antidepressant therapy for an additional 6 months. Maintenance treatment (3 years or longer) is provided to patients with a history of recurrent depression. The duration of maintenance therapy should be based on the frequency and severity of previous episodes. Recurrent episodes complicated by suicidal ideas or attempts warrant lifelong treatment. Psychotherapy, antidepressants, and electroconvulsive therapy (ECT) are empirically proven treatments for depression in older persons.

Initiatives have been developed to increase the likelihood that patients with major depression treated in primary care settings will receive antidepressant treatment that is adequate in dose and duration. The increased attention to this problem results from findings that most elderly patients prefer being treated for depression by their primary care physicians. Studies have shown that the majority of patients who are prescribed antidepressants by their primary care physicians do not obtain refills of their initial prescription. Educational programs and the use of depression nurse specialists have been developed to increase recognition and treatment intensity.

Psychotherapy

Table 35.2 lists the variety and characteristics of psychotherapies advocated for older adults. Research demonstrating the efficacy of psychotherapy for major depression in older adults has included cognitive-behavioral therapy, interpersonal psychotherapy, and problem-solving therapy. Problem-solving therapy involves working with the patient to identify practical life difficulties that are causing distress and providing guidance to help the patient identify solutions. The treatment is delivered generally in six to eight meetings spaced 1 to 2 weeks apart. Cognitive and interpersonal psychotherapy are also time-limited but less highly structured. Psychotherapy for minor depression has been promising, with efficacy demonstrated particularly in persons who have suffered a loss. Also, caregivers of older persons may develop minor or major depressive syndromes that benefit from psychotherapy. Psychotherapy may be combined with an antidepressant, and the combination has been associated with a longer period of remission following recovery from the acute episode. Psychotherapy combined with antidepressant medication is recommended for all patients with severe or suicidal depression.

Table 35.2—Psychotherapy for the Geriatric Syndrome of Late-Life Depression

Therapy	Distinguishing Characteristics
Cognitive-behavioral	Directive, symptom focused Techniques practiced outside of therapy Counters negativistic misperceptions and mistaken pessimistic beliefs
Interpersonal	Exploratory but not open ended Focused on interpersonal conflict, role change, role deficits
Short-term psychodynamic	Problem focused Transference not examined
Life review, reminiscence	Recall of personal history to master one's present and future
Problem solving	Brief, focused on patient-defined solutions Accepts that some problems cannot be changed May be useful to counter executive deficits
Supportive	Meant to maintain present level of function or symptom control
Dementia caregiver counseling	Focused on the caregiver role and activities Combines elements of cognitive-behavioral, problem-solving, and interpersonal therapy
Bereavement therapy	Restructuring (not restoration) the experience of the lost loved one through review of both positive and negative aspects of the relationship
Behavioral	Educational, pragmatic Directed at reducing negative and increasing positive experiences
Dialectical-behavioral therapy	Focused on reduction of counterproductive behaviors Emphasis on acceptance of affect and the inevitability of conflict

Choice of Antidepressants: First Considerations

Psychotherapy if not effective alone should be combined with pharmacotherapy for depression. The choice of agent depends on the patient's comorbid medical conditions, the side-effect profile of the antidepressant, and the individual patient's sensitivity to these effects. Potential interactions with other medications also should be considered. Prominent complaints of sleep disturbance, anxiety, or psychomotor retardation will direct the practitioner toward agents that are, respectively, more sedative or more activating. And because the SSRIs are now the mainstay of antidepressant prescribing, a hierarchy of choices is available in published protocols designed for either primary care or older patient practices. Sertraline and citalopram are often preferred because adverse effects and drug interactions may be less likely than with some other SSRIs, such as fluoxetine and paroxetine.

A number of researchers have explored various strategies to optimally manage depressive syndromes in older persons, recognizing that a systematic approach is often helpful. One such treatment strategy, developed by Steffans and colleagues at Duke University, is called the Duke Somatic Treatment Algorithm for Geriatric Depression. The graded approach in this algorithm begins with a 6- to 12-week trial of the SSRI sertraline for the older depressed patient who has not previously been treated. The only stipulation at this point is that the patient's illness not be severe enough to warrant an intervention such as ECT (eg, an imminent risk of suicide, life-threatening food refusal, psychosis). For an initial SSRI trial, it is recommended that the dose be gradually titrated upward at weekly intervals for the first 3 weeks, as tolerated. If the SSRI is not well tolerated, the clinician may proceed to the venlafaxine trial described below. For patients who have had a previous successful response to an antidepressant, that particular agent would be the medication of choice.

If, after 6 to 12 weeks, a satisfactory response is not evident, then a trial of sustained-release venlafaxine is recommended at a dosage of 150 mg daily for 6 to 12 weeks. If the symptoms do not remit with venlafaxine, other options may be considered at this point, such as augmentation with another medication. For example, if there is a partial response to the SSRI but with residual low energy and low interest, then the SSRI may be augmented with sustained-release bupropion for an additional 6 weeks. Other options in the context of incomplete response may include augmenting with lithium carbonate or switching to a tricyclic antidepressant or monoamine oxidase inhibitor (MAOI). However, at this juncture it might be helpful to obtain consultation from a psychiatrist or other mental health professional.

Selective Serotonin-Reuptake Inhibitors

SSRIs and tricyclic antidepressants are comparably effective for treating mild to moderate major depression, but SSRIs are often better tolerated. Table 35.3 provides a detailed summary of dosing, formulations, precautions, and advantages of the individual SSRIs. Controversy continues about whether the most severe melancholic form of depression that generally requires treatment in a psychiatric hospital responds better to a tricyclic antidepressant. Melancholic patients typically suffer from marked appetite and weight loss, diurnal mood variation that is worse in the morning, early morning awakening, and either retardation of motor movement or agitation.

Although the SSRIs are generally free of severe side effects, a small proportion of elderly patients develop hyponatremia that is due to the syndrome of inappropriate antidiuretic hormone secretion during SSRI treatment, particularly at higher doses. In rare cases, patients are unable to tolerate SSRIs because of induced anxiety, sleep disturbance, or agitation. This reaction appears to be more common in older persons and may in some cases be related to the inhibition of the metabolism of other medications, discussed later in this section. Beginning at lower doses may reduce the incidence of anxiety with activating SSRIs such as fluoxetine and may decrease the gastrointestinal adverse effects of nausea or diarrhea that occur with SSRIs. Sexual side effects occur commonly with all SSRIs, and many patients may not wish to continue SSRI treatment because of them, so inquiring about sexual function is an important part of follow-up care. Although SSRIs have been associated with mild weight loss initially, long-term use with many of these medications has been associated with weight gain. Pseudoparkinsonism and other movement disorders may occur, particularly if these medications are used in combination with other drugs that block dopamine (eg, metoclopramide).

SSRIs inhibit various P-450 hepatic cytochrome isoenzymes that metabolize most medications. Fluoxetine and paroxetine are potent inhibitors of the P-450 2D6 isoenzyme responsible for the metabolism of most psychiatric medications, as well as dextromethorphan, codeine, tricyclic antidepressants, and metoprolol. Sertraline is a weak inhibitor of both the 2D6 and 3A4 isoenzymes. Inhibition of 2D6 can decrease the analgesic effects of codeine (and related compounds) and tramadol by preventing their conversion to their active metabolites, morphine and O-desmethyltramadol. Fluoxetine's active metabolite, norfluoxetine, also inhibits the 3A4 isozymes. The SSRI fluvoxamine inhibits the 3A4, 2D6, and 1A2 systems. Because P-450 1A2 is required to metabolize theophylline, olanzapine, and phenacetin, concurrent

Table 35.3—Selective Serotonin-Reuptake Inhibitors for Older Adults

Generic (Trade) Name	Initial Dosage	Final Dosage	Sedative Potential	Precautions	Advantages
Citalopram (Celexa)	10 mg am	20–40 mg am	Low	Side effects include nausea, tremor, dizziness, sweating, agitation	Few drug interactions, well tolerated
Escitalopram (Lexapro)	10 mg am	10–20 mg am	Low	Nausea, tremor, dizziness, sweating, agitation	May have fewer side effects than citalopram, well tolerated
Fluoxetine (Prozac)	10 mg am	20–40 mg am	Low	Nausea, tremor, dizziness, sweating, agitation, prolonged half-life, insomnia, drug interactions	Liquid preparation available
Paroxetine (Paxil)	10 mg hs	20–40 mg hs	Low	Nausea, tremor, dizziness, sweating, agitation, drug interactions, anticholinergic effects	Mild sedative effect
Sertraline (Zoloft)	25 mg am	100–200 mg am	Low	Nausea, tremor, dizziness, sweating, agitation	Few drug interactions, well tolerated

NOTE: am = *ante meridiem* or before noon; hs = *hora somni* or at bedtime.

use of fluvoxamine may result in markedly increased concentrations of these medications. Given its potential for multiple interactions, the use of fluvoxamine in older patients is best limited unless monitored very closely.

SSRIs may increase the anticoagulant effects of medications such as warfarin, potentially through cytochrome isoenzyme inhibition or the inhibition of platelet activity. Careful monitoring of prothrombin times or another suitable index of blood clotting is indicated following the introduction of an SSRI to patients being treated with warfarin.

SSRIs have been considered particularly safe for older persons because these antidepressants do not cause orthostatic hypotension, arrhythmias, or marked sedation. However, evidence indicates that nursing-home residents treated with SSRIs are at increased risk for falling and suffering hip fractures. It is not clear whether these findings are due to patient selection in that patients considered at greatest risk for falling may be treated with SSRIs preferentially. Alternatively, SSRIs may contribute to falls by causing a subtle balance disturbance or pseudoparkinsonism in vulnerable patients. Or depression itself may be a risk factor.

With the introduction of serotonergic reuptake inhibitors, reports emerged of a serotonergic withdrawal syndrome following discontinuation lasting 2 to 3 weeks and characterized by lightheadedness, insomnia, agitation, nausea, headache, and sensory disturbances. Mood disturbance may also occur. The shorter-acting SSRIs (sertraline, paroxetine) appear to induce this syndrome, but venlafaxine and other SSRIs have also been implicated. Therefore, these agents should be tapered rather than stopped abruptly.

Tricyclic Antidepressants

The tricyclic antidepressants nortriptyline and desipramine are the most appropriate for use in older persons. Table 35.4 provides a detailed summary of dosing, formulations, precautions, and advantages of these agents. They are effective in the most severe forms of depression but are associated with anticholinergic side effects that may be problems in older patients. For nortriptyline, therapeutic response is associated with blood levels between 50 and 150 ng/mL and for desipramine, levels above 120 ng/mL. Over 60% of patients with nonpsychotic major depression or with depression that is not associated with dementia respond within 6 weeks to levels in these ranges. Although 5% of the population requires lower dosing because of the absence of the enzyme required to metabolize secondary amine tricyclics, most patients achieve target concentrations at dosages of 50 to 75 mg per day of nortriptyline and 100 to 150 mg per day of desipramine.

The potential for side effects that are due to the anticholinergic and sedative properties of tricyclics limits their use in older patients. These medications are particularly inappropriate for patients who are sensitive to constipation or vulnerable to orthostatic hypotension and for men with benign prostatic hyperplasia. Also, tricyclic antidepressants have a quinidine-like effect that delays ventricular conduction. Among patients with a pretreatment first-degree heart block, 10% may develop a second-degree block during treatment. Patients with bundle branch block or prolonged QT_c interval are at risk for developing a ventricular arrhythmia.

Table 35.4—Tricyclic Antidepressants for Older Adults

Generic (Trade) Name	Initial Dosage	Final Dosage	Sedative Potential	Precautions	Advantages
Desipramine (Norpramin)	10–25 mg hs	25–150 mg hs	Low	May be fatal in overdose May exacerbate glaucoma, anticholinergic effects	Therapeutic plasma level 115–200 ng/mL May have stimulant properties
Nortriptyline (Pamelor, Aventyl)	10–25 mg hs	25–100 mg hs	Moderate	Lower final dose May be fatal in overdose May exacerbate glaucoma, anticholinergic effects	Therapeutic window for plasma levels of 50–150 ng/mL

NOTE: hs = *hora somni* or at bedtime.

Other Antidepressants

Table 35.5 provides a detailed summary of dosing, formulations, precautions, and advantages of other antidepressants, including a stimulant. Bupropion is generally safe, free of sexual side effects, and well tolerated when used at recommended doses. Bupropion has been associated with a 0.4% risk of seizures, which is much higher when recommended doses are exceeded, and is contraindicated in persons with a seizure disorder. Bupropion appears to act by increasing the activity of dopamine and norepinephrine and therefore has stimulant-like qualities. Because of the activating property of bupropion, dosing of the short-acting form in the morning and mid-afternoon may help to avoid insomnia. Long-acting bupropion has a smaller seizure risk and is less likely to cause insomnia. Dosages are increased gradually by the use of a twice-a-day regimen to achieve target dosages of 150 to 300 mg per day of the short-acting form. The dosage range of sustained-release bupropion is 150 to 300 mg per day given as a single daily dose.

Venlafaxine acts as an SSRI at lower doses while also inhibiting the reuptake of norepinephrine at the high end of the therapeutic range of 75 to 225 mg per day. Venlafaxine is effective for both generalized anxiety and major depression and may treat both effectively at dosages of 75 to 150 mg per day. A dose-response relationship for severe depression has been demonstrated, and patients with melancholia may require dosages of 225 mg per day or greater. Initial dosing should use gradual increases to minimize the early side effect of nausea. The noradrenergic properties of higher doses may explain the association between doses of 225 mg and higher with hypertension. Patients requiring doses at the high end of the therapeutic range should have blood-pressure monitoring. This side effect does not occur in patients with hypertension controlled by a β-blocker. Venlafaxine should also be discontinued several days prior to ECT to avoid hypertension during ECT. Venlafaxine, like other SSRIs, has been associated with decreased sexual functioning. Venlafaxine should be discontinued by gradual tapering to avoid the risk of flu-like discontinuation symptoms.

Duloxetine is an antidepressant medication that has been approved for the treatment of both depression and neuropathic pain secondary to diabetes mellitus. Duloxetine is a serotonin- and nore-pinephrine-reuptake inhibitor, and its pharmacodynamic characteristics are generally like those of venlafaxine, although it is structurally unique. Because of its effects of increasing neural sphincter activity and bladder capacity, it has also been approved for the treatment of urinary incontinence and has been shown to reduce stress incontinence in women. These features may make duloxetine advantageous for the older patient.

Mirtazapine is a norepinephrine, 5-HT$_2$, and 5-HT$_3$ antagonist. The total daily dose is 15 to 45 mg. Mirtazapine is given as a single bedtime dose to capitalize on its sedative properties and is available in rapidly dissolving form for patients who have difficulty swallowing pills. Mirtazapine is also associated with increased appetite and weight gain. This side-effect profile has contributed to the use of mirtazapine before bedtime in nursing-home residents with depression and dementia who demonstrate nighttime agitation and weight loss. Mirtazapine is also free of sexual side effects.

The MAOIs are effective antidepressants that have been in use for nearly half a century. Orthostatic hypotension is a common adverse effect of MAOIs and in older patients may increase the risk of falling. Concomitant ingestion of a food product rich in tyramine (eg, cheese) or of pseudoephedrine or pressor amines can cause a life-threatening hypertensive crisis. The use of MAOIs with an SSRI or meperidine can cause a fatal serotonin syndrome associated with delirium and hyperthermia. Selegiline has just been approved as the first transdermal patch (Ensam) for depression. It is available in 6, 9, and 12 mg; at the lowest dose, no dietary restrictions are needed.

Although methylphenidate and other stimulants have been used for decades to treat major depression, controlled data demonstrating their efficacy are limited. However, these agents may have a role in reversing the apathy and lack of energy seen in some patients with

Table 35.5—Other Antidepressants, Including Stimulants, for Older Adults

Generic (Trade) Name	Initial Dosage	Final Dosage	Sedative Potential	Precautions	Advantages
Other Antidepressants					
Bupropion (Wellbutrin SR)	SR: 75 mg qd	SR: 150–300 mg qd	Low	Dopaminergic, noradrenergic, agitation, insomnia, seizures Dose should be divided	May help apathetic depression Sustained-release form available
Duloxetine (Cymbalta)	20 mg	30–60 mg	Low	Drug interactions (CYP 1A2, 2D6 substrate)	Equally SSRI and SNRI, narrow dose range FDA approved for neuropathic pain
Hypericum perforatum, or St. John's wort	300 mg bid	900 mg tid	Low	Use standardized, freeze-dried extract, 0.3% hypericin Drug interactions with other antidepressants	Low side-effect profile, OTC
Mirtazapine (Remeron, Sol-tabs)	7.5 mg hs	15–45 mg hs	Moderate	Prolonged half-life, renal clearance Dry mouth, weight gain Serotonergic and noradrenergic	Sedative effects may improve sleep
Trazodone (Desyrel)	25–50 mg hs	100–200 mg hs	High	Very sedative	For sleep disturbance
Venlafaxine (Effexor, Effexor XR)	37.5 mg bid XR: 75 mg qd	75–225 mg qd	Low	Headache, nausea, vomiting Hypertension, withdrawal syndrome	Fewer drug interactions Extended-release preparation available, may be more effective than SSRIs
Stimulants					
Methylphenidate (Ritalin)	5 mg am	20 mg bid	Low	Side effects include anorexia, insomnia Daytime use only	Quick results For frail and apathetic patients
Modafinil (Provigil)	200 mg am	400 mg am	Low	Little used in elderly patients	Once-daily dosing, reverses daytime sedation sometimes observed with SSRIs

NOTE: am = *ante meridiem* or before noon; bid = *bis in die* or twice a day; FDA = U.S. Food and Drug Administration; hs = *hora somni* or at bedtime; OTC = over-the-counter; qd = *quaque die* or every day; SR = sustained release; SNRI = serotonin-norepinephrine reuptake inhibitor; SSRI = selective serotonin-reuptake inhibitor; TCA = tricyclic antidepressant; tid = *ter in die* or three times a day; XR = extended release.

dementia or disabling medical conditions. Benzodiazepines may be useful temporary adjuncts to treat anxiety and sleep disturbance associated with a major depression, but older persons are particularly sensitive to the adverse effects of these medications on cognition and gait stability.

Management of Partial Response and Nonresponse: Optimize, Switch, or Augment

Approximately 50% of patients with major depression demonstrate a robust response to treatment within 6 weeks. An additional 15% to 25% who have begun to improve achieve remission if treatment is continued for an additional 4 to 6 weeks. Some published studies using SSRIs have reported 6-week response rates of 40% that increase to more than 60% when treatment extends to 12 weeks. However, noticeable improvement within the first 2 weeks of treatment predicts

the likelihood of successful recovery with the initial medication. The admonition to "start low, go slow" in treating the older patient is too often interpreted as "start low, stay low," which can lead to mistaken classification of the patient as a nonresponder. A less than 30% reduction in symptom severity by the sixth week of treatment at the indicated dose defines nonresponse. A 50% reduction in symptom severity indicates partial response. In either case the dose should be "optimized" by increasing to the upper limit of the final recommended dose range, depending on patient tolerance. Patients with a genuine nonresponse should be switched from an SSRI to a non-SSRI. Patients experiencing a partial response to an SSRI may receive augmentation (combination) therapy with a non-SSRI.

The options of switching to an antidepressant from another class or consulting a psychiatrist are more appropriate than initiating unfamiliar combination treatments.

Electroconvulsive Therapy for Psychotic Depression

Psychotic depression is often resistant to standard antidepressant regimens. Aggressive pharmacotherapy is required, with best results obtained in young adults when high doses of antidepressants and antipsychotic medications are combined. However, the effectiveness of combination treatment for older patients with psychotic depression remains uncertain. Available evidence suggests that most elderly patients who have depression with pronounced psychotic features either cannot tolerate adequate doses of conventional medications or do not respond to them. Therefore, ECT has become the standard treatment for late-life psychotic depression.

MANAGEMENT OF BIPOLAR DISORDER

Most persons with bipolar disorder have a history of episodes in early adulthood and often receive chronic treatment with an anti-manic medication. Occasionally this regimen may need adjustment if a new episode of mania emerges. Evidence to support an array of medications for mania has increased substantially in the past decade (see Table 35.6). In addition to lithium and established mood stabilizers for mania, newer antipsychotic and anticonvulsant medications are used in managing manic symptoms, although controlled trials in elderly patients are lacking.

Lithium Carbonate

Lithium carbonate is highly effective for the acute and maintenance treatment of classical manic episodes. It is important to recognize that much lower plasma levels are recommended for older patients than for younger patients. For example, plasma ranges of 0.8 to 1.2 mEq/L are used when treating acute mania in younger adults, and levels of 0.6 to 0.8 mEq/L are used for mania prophylaxis. The use of lithium for treating elderly patients is complicated by the 30% decrease in renal functioning that accompanies normal aging and the increased sensitivity of older persons to neurologic side effects from this medication, particularly if structural brain disease is present.

The decreased renal clearance of lithium in the older patient is addressed simply by reducing the total daily dose. Furthermore, lower concentrations may be adequate in older adults; some patients respond acutely to levels in the range of 0.6 to 0.8 mEq/L or less. Levels of 0.4 to 0.6 mEq/L may provide effective prophylaxis. Also, older persons develop neurologic

side effects at concentrations that are well tolerated in young adults. A fine resting tremor, diarrhea, myoclonus, an intention tremor, or pseudo-parkinsonism may develop with levels in the standard therapeutic range. Sensitivity to these effects and to increased confusion is increased among patients with dementia and when lithium is coadministered with an antipsychotic medication. Clinicians are advised to balance the therapeutic effects of a concentration at the low end of the usual target range against side effects that develop in a particular patient. Consideration should be given to a time lag of 1 to 2 weeks that may occur between achieving a steady-state dose and either therapeutic efficacy or the development of neurologic side effects.

Drugs that inhibit lithium excretion may raise concentrations by up to 50% and result in toxicity if the lithium dose is not decreased. Many of the nonsteroidal anti-inflammatory agents, including ibuprofen, have this effect. Thiazide and potassium-sparing diuretics, angiotensin-converting enzyme inhibitors, and angiotensin-receptor blockers raise lithium levels as well. The effect of furosemide is less clear, but lithium levels should be checked a few days after this diuretic is added in an older patient receiving lithium. Both dehydration and salt depletion are known to raise lithium levels. With adequate monitoring, bipolar patients who have benefited from lithium need not be deprived of this medication because of advanced age.

Anticonvulsants

Valproic acid (valproate, divalproex) has been approved for the treatment of bipolar disorder and is comparable in efficacy to lithium. Target concentrations of 50 to 100 µg/mL used when treating seizure disorders appear to be appropriate. Divalproex has been used effectively to treat agitation in patients with dementia and may be particularly useful for the treatment of behavioral disturbance associated with mood lability. However, upward titration in the frail elderly person must be carried out carefully because dementia patients may be particularly vulnerable to developing excessive sedation during valproic acid treatment. As with other anticonvulsants used to treat mania, valproic acid is associated with allergic skin rashes in 5% to 10% of patients. Decreased platelet counts occur at higher doses, and platelet functioning may be diminished. Patients with hepatic disease may develop liver toxicity during valproic acid treatment. Patients with low albumin concentrations will also have a higher proportion of free drug in their blood and are at greater risk for toxicity.

Carbamazepine[OL] is another antiepileptic medication that has been used to treat mania. Leukopenia and

---

[OL] Not approved by the U.S. Food and Drug Administration for this use.

Table 35.6—Agents Used to Stabilize Mania and Manic-Like Symptoms

Generic (Trade) Name	Initial Dosage	Final Dosage	Sedative Potential	Precautions	Advantages
Anticonvulsants					
Divalproex sodium (Depakote, Depakote ER)	250 mg bid; ER: 500 mg hs	1000 mg bid; ER: 1000 mg hs	Moderate	Delayed onset of action, drug interactions GI upset, tremor, weight gain, edema, thrombocytopenia Inhibits hepatic enzymes; increases other drug levels Hepatoxicity, pancreatitis	Better tolerated than carbamazepine Therapeutic level 50–100 µg/mL
Carbamazepine (Tegretol, Epitol)	100 mg bid	400 mg bid	Moderate	Delayed onset of action, drug interactions Dizziness, unsteady gait, rare agranulocytosis Enhances cytochrome P-450 activity and decreases other drug levels Not FDA approved for bipolar disorder	Therapeutic level 4–12 µg/mL Available as a liquid
Antipsychotics					
Olanzapine (Zyprexa, Zyprexa Zydis [oral dissolving])	2.5 mg qd	5–15 mg qd	Moderate	Anticholinergic as dose increases Cost Weight gain, hyperglycemia	FDA approved for acute mania and maintenance monotherapy for bipolar I disorder but not for bipolar depression
Quetiapine (Seroquel)	25 mg bid	100 mg bid	More than moderate	Slit-lamp examination for cataracts	Sedative, not anticholinergic, fewer EPS, less TD FDA approved for mania
Risperidone (Risperdal, Risperdal Consta [injectable])	0.25 mg qd Inj: 25 mg q 2 weeks	6 mg qd Inj: 50 mg q 2 weeks	Moderate	EPS likely at doses above 2 mg, high potency, cost, reports of stroke	Available in liquid form FDA approved for acute mania
Benzodiazepine					
Clonazepam (Klonopin)	0.5 mg bid	5 mg bid	Moderate	Long half-life Fall risk limits use in elderly patients May exacerbate confusion in dementia Not FDA approved for bipolar disorder	Calming, sedation
Lithium					
Lithium carbonate (Eskalith, Eskalith CR)	300 mg qd; CR: 450 mg qd	300 mg tid; CR: 450 mg bid	Low	Renal clearance is sole route of elimination Toxicity may appear below therapeutic range Nausea, vomiting are signs of toxicity Risk of hypothyroidism with long-term use Drug interactions	Patient preference, otherwise, none Therapeutic level 0.4–1.0 mEq/mL

NOTE: bid = *bis in die* or twice a day; CBC = complete blood cell count; CR = controlled release; EPS = extrapyramidal symptoms; ER = extended release; FDA = U.S. Food and Drug Administration; GI = gastrointestinal; hs = *hora somni* or at bedtime; q = *quaque* or every; qd = *quaque die* or every day; TD = tardive dyskinesia; tid = *ter in die* or three times a day.

thrombocytopenia occurs in 5% to 10% of patients within the first 2 weeks of treatment. However, life-threatening agranulocytosis and aplastic anemia occur rarely.

Lamotrigine is a newer anticonvulsant that has been approved for the treatment of depression in the context of bipolar affective disorder, although trials specifically in elderly patients are not available. Titration should be conducted very carefully in patients who may also be taking hepatic cytochrome isoenzyme-inducing drugs or valproic acid. In the absence of these, titration begins at 25 mg per day for 2 weeks, then 50 mg per day for 2 weeks, then 100 mg per day for 1 week, then 200 mg per day for usual maintenance. As with most of the anticonvulsants, for patients with moderate liver dysfunction the doses should be reduced by approximately 50%, and with more severe dysfunction the doses should be reduced by approximately 75%.

For patients in whom ECT is anticipated, anticonvulsants agents should be tapered and discontinued if at all possible because of the likelihood of interfering with an adequate seizure duration during the course of treatments.

Antipsychotics

Most antipsychotic medications are observed clinically to exert some anti-manic effects; however, olanzapine has been approved for the acute treatment of mania. Concerns about olanzapine-associated metabolic syndrome need to be considered. Mania in late life may be associated with confusion and cognitive dysfunction; the anticholinergic effects of olanzapine may exacerbate these symptoms. Risperidone and quetiapine are also approved for the acute treatment of mania.

Electroconvulsive Therapy

ECT is highly effective for the treatment of major depression and mania, with response rates exceeding 70% in older adults. ECT is the first-line treatment for patients at serious risk for suicide or life-threatening poor intake due to a major depression. Patients with delusional depression may demonstrate paranoia about their food or caregivers, precluding pharmacologic treatment because of the unreliable oral intake. Also, delusional depression is less responsive to standard medication regimens. Therefore, ECT is generally the first-line treatment for these patients and is associated with response rates that approximate 80%.

The cognitive side effects of ECT are the principal factor limiting its acceptance. Anterograde amnesia or the inability to learn new information may be pronounced initially, particularly during bilateral ECT, but it improves rapidly following completion of treatment. Retrograde amnesia is more persistent, and the recall of events that immediately preceded ECT may be lost permanently. Although patients may complain that ECT has had a long-term effect on their memory, longitudinal studies have failed to demonstrate lasting cognitive effects; furthermore, improved memory, perhaps owing to recovery from depression, has been reported. There are few absolute medical contraindications other than the presence of increased intracranial pressure or unstable angina. Patients with coronary artery disease or cerebral vascular disease may be administered ECT safely by the use of appropriate pharmacologic management of the autonomic responses that may occur during treatment. Nevertheless, a recent myocardial infarction or cerebral vascular event and unstable coronary artery disease increase the risk of complications. Right unilateral treatment produces fewer cognitive side effects than bilateral treatment but is less effective unless doses markedly exceeding a patient's seizure threshold are used.

The selection of ECT over aggressive pharmacotherapy is generally made by weighing the risk of waiting for a medication to work against the burden of hospital treatment, any medical conditions that may complicate general anesthesia, and patient biases against this treatment. After a course of ECT, patients should be continued on pharmacotherapy following recovery. Patients who did not respond to intensive antidepressant treatment before receiving ECT have lower acute response rates and are more likely to relapse subsequently, even when antidepressant continuation treatment with a new medication is provided. Although maintenance ECT is sometimes used to prevent relapse, the burden that maintenance ECT places on patients and their families may limit its usefulness for the long-term management of late-life major depression.

REFERENCES

- Alexopoulos GS, Meyers BS, Young RC, et al. Executive dysfunction and long-term outcomes of geriatric depression. *Arch Gen Psychiatry*. 2000;57(3):285–290.

- Denihan A, Kirby M, Bruce I, et al. Three-year prognosis of depression in the community-dwelling elderly. *Br J Psychiatry*. 2000;176(5):453–457.

- Fava M, Rush AJ, Trivedi MH, et al. Background and rationale for the Sequenced Treatment Alternatives to Relieve Depression (STAR*D) study. *Psychiatr Clin N Am*. 2003;26(2):457–494.

- Kennedy GJ, Marcus P. Use of antidepressants in older patients with co-morbid medical conditions: guidance from studies of depression in somatic illness. *Drugs Aging.* 2005;22(4):273–287.

- Mulsant BH, Alexopoulos GS, Reyolds CF 3rd, et al. Pharmacologic treatment of depression in older primary care patients: the PROSPECT algorithm. *Int J Geriatr Psychiatry.* 2001;16(6):585–592.

- Steffens DC, McQuoid DR, Krishnan KR. The Duke Somatic Treatment Algorithm for Geriatric Depression (STAGED) approach. *Psychopharmacol Bull.* 2002; 36(2):58–68.

CHAPTER 36—ANXIETY DISORDERS

KEY POINTS

- Late-life anxiety is often a comorbid condition with other problems such as cognitive decline and depression.
- Comorbid medical problems that commonly lead to anxiety include cardiovascular and pulmonary disorders.
- Selective serotonin-reuptake inhibitor medications such as sertraline are often used as first-line treatment for anxiety in late life.
- Nonpharmacologic therapies such as relaxation training may be helpful, particularly for generalized anxiety and anxiety secondary to medical conditions.

Older adults suffer from the entire range of anxiety disorders. The clinician treating older persons therefore needs to be familiar with the hallmarks and available treatments for each type of anxiety disorder. Since the published literature on anxiety in elderly patients is relatively sparse, some of the characterizations and treatment strategies described here are based on research carried out in younger populations. They have been modified to take into account the physiologic and psychologic differences between older and younger adults.

Familiarity with the various diagnostic criteria, along with the skill to conduct a thorough psychologic assessment, is crucial in determining the most appropriate treatment for anxiety. Clinicians need to be aware of difficulties in proper assessment of geriatric anxiety; these include medical comorbidity, the difficulty of differentiating anxiety from depression, falsely high scores on anxiety rating scales resulting from overemphasis of cardiac and respiratory problems, and the tendency of older patients to resist psychiatric evaluation.

Anxiety assessment begins with a clinical interview to determine the course and nature of symptoms, along with the nature of the patient's mental status and external support. Supplemental rating scales, which aid in comparing a patient's level of difficulties with that of others and assessing difficulties over time, along with laboratory investigations, can result in an accurate clinical picture and the ability to formulate an effective management plan. Even though discrete anxiety disorders such as panic disorders are less prevalent among older than among younger adults, anxiety as a symptom is a common problem. The ability to recognize and effectively treat anxiety in older persons is important, given the debilitating effects that an unhealthy level of anxiety can have in this vulnerable population.

CLASSES OF ANXIETY DISORDERS

The types of anxiety disorders as currently defined in the fourth edition of the *Diagnostic and Statistical Manual of Mental Disorders* (*DSM-IV*) are listed in Table 36.1.

Panic Disorder

Panic attacks are acute, discrete episodes of intense anxiety that result as a reaction to some perceived threat (eg, emotional, environmental). The term *panic attack* is used when a person experiences an intense and acute reaction to an internal or external cue; it lasts between a few minutes and a half hour. The physiologic symptoms may include trembling, accelerated heart rate, sweating, shortness of breath, chest pain, dizziness, nausea, and the sense that one is somehow detached from the surroundings. For example, a person might have a fear of being trapped on an elevator and report feeling dizzy and nauseated when entering one. Another might report high levels of acute anxiety at the mere sight of elevator doors. A clinically significant degree of panic symptoms exists if a review of the patient's history reveals that recurrent and unpredictable panic attacks have occurred for at least 1 month and time is being spent in worried anticipation of possible reccurrence. Diagnostically, one needs also to consider whether agoraphobia related to

Table 36.1—Types of Anxiety Disorders Defined in *DSM-IV*

Panic disorder without agoraphobia

Panic disorder with agoraphobia

Agoraphobia without history of panic disorder

Specific phobias

       Animal type

       Natural environment type

       Blood-injection-injury type

       Situational type

       Other type

Social phobia

Obsessive-compulsive disorder

Posttraumatic stress disorder

Acute stress disorder

Generalized anxiety disorder

Anxiety disorder due to a general medical condition

Substance-induced anxiety disorder

Anxiety disorder not otherwise specified

SOURCE: Data from *Diagnostic and Statistical Manual of Mental Disorders.* 4th ed. Washington, DC: American Psychiatric Association; 1994.

the panic attacks is present. In such cases, agoraphobia involves the persistent fear of situations that result in a panic attack, as when a patient reports remaining at home in order to avoid an attack. Common examples of feared situations include being caught in a crowd or trapped in traffic. Comparison of young and older adults with panic disorder indicates that age of onset can affect the clinical presentation. Patients with late-onset panic disorder (at or after age 55) report fewer panic symptoms and less avoidance, and they score lower on somatization measures than do those with early-onset panic disorder. Also, earlier-onset panic more commonly persists into old age.

Phobic Disorders

Phobias include several distinct disorders, categorized as specific phobia and social phobia. A specific phobia involves a distinct trigger, such as a specific person, animal, place, object, event, or situation that results in symptoms of anxiety. Commonly, the patient's anxiety level increases instantly when the feared trigger is encountered. Interestingly, he or she is able to identify this fear as unrealistic and unsupported, even though the cognitive and physiologic responses persist. Specific phobias often involve a great amount of anticipatory anxiety (thoughts of just the possibility of encountering the feared stimulus), and avoidance behaviors are likely to be reported. The consequence of such a clinical profile is that the person experiences a variety of personal difficulties as a result of the anxiety. These behaviors interfere with work and daily routines, and they decrease the person's opportunities to experience pleasurable situations (for fear that a trigger might be present). They may also contribute to secondary symptoms, such as frustration, hopelessness, and a sense that one lacks control in one's life. The level of anxiety or fear usually varies as a function of both the degree of proximity to the phobic stimuli and the degree to which escape is limited. Examples of common phobias include fear of specific animals, closed spaces, flying, or heights. Frequently, specific phobias occur with panic disorder, with or without agoraphobia. Among elderly persons, especially in urban settings, fear of crime seems to be particularly prevalent. Phobic disorders tend to be chronic and persist into old age. However, fear of falling is a specific phobia that is increasingly recognized to have an onset in later life.

Persons with social phobia suffer from fears that they will behave in a manner that is inept or embarrassing. Commonly, the fear is that of trembling, blushing, or sweating profusely in social situations. Other common feared situations involve giving public speeches, going on dates, or simply socializing with others at a function or party. Again, as with specific phobias, social phobia is often accompanied by a significant degree of anticipatory anxiety or avoidance, or both. Though systematic studies of this disorder in elderly persons are lacking, epidemiologic data indicate that this disorder is chronic and persistent in old age. Common manifestations in old age include the inability to eat food in the presence of strangers, and, especially in men, being unable to urinate in public lavatories.

Obsessive-Compulsive Disorder

Obsessive-compulsive disorder involves persistent thoughts (obsessions) and behaviors (compulsions) that are performed in an effort to decrease the anxiety experienced as a result of the thoughts. Obsessions are thoughts or ideas that come to a person's mind, commonly while completing a specific task or during a particular type of situation. For example, a person may wash his hands repeatedly, for hours at a time, after shaking a stranger's hand; the unwanted thought is that he may have exposed himself to a serious disease. The act of washing in this example is the compulsion. Obsessive-compulsive disorder is chronic and often disabling. Depression and other symptoms of anxiety may also be comorbid in an older population. A new occurrence of obsessive-compulsive disorder in late life is unlikely. More commonly, symptoms of obsessions occur along with a depressive syndrome or early dementia. For example, obsessions about paying bills on time may occur in the context of difficulty in estimating time and planning.

Posttraumatic Stress Disorder

The distinctive feature of posttraumatic stress disorder is that the person has experienced, either as a witness or a victim, a traumatic event to which he or she has reacted with feelings of fear and helplessness. Examples of such events include those that involve actual or threatened death or serious injury, other threats to one's integrity, witnessing an event that involves death or serious injury of another, or even hearing about death or serious injury to a family member or close associate. Commonly observed symptoms include the re-experiencing of the traumatic event, avoidance (both cognitively and behaviorally) of stimuli associated with the event, psychologic numbing, and increased physiologic arousal. Symptoms of hyperarousal include difficulty falling or staying asleep, hypervigilance, and exaggerated startle response. Disorders often found to occur with posttraumatic stress disorder include depression, panic disorder, and substance-use disorders. Symptoms must be present for at least 1 month and cause clinically significant distress or impairment in social, occupational, or other important areas of functioning. In the short term, that is, between 2 days and 1 month after the traumatic event, a diagnosis of acute stress disorder is given; thereafter, one must consider a diagnosis of posttraumatic stress disorder.

Generalized Anxiety Disorder

The distinctive symptoms of generalized anxiety disorder include feeling easily tired and experiencing other physical symptoms, such as muscle tension, having trouble sleeping through the night, difficulty concentrating on a task, and feeling irritable or on edge. These symptoms need to have occurred for at least 6 months and must be accompanied by the sense that one cannot control the feelings of anxiety. In addition, these feelings of intense worry must be a result of more than one stressor. For example, intense worry over financial matters or a medical illness alone, even with all the associated symptoms, in and of itself does not qualify a person for a diagnosis of generalized anxiety disorder. Because many elderly patients with this disorder also present with features of depression, the clinician may try to distinguish between the two diagnoses. Commonly the overlap is sufficiently extensive to preclude this distinction, as described below.

COMORBIDITY

Mixed Anxiety and Depression

Mixed anxiety and depression is a presentation that is included in the *DSM-IV* "Criteria for Further Study."

The essential features of this proposed disorder are dysphoric mood for at least 1 month that is composed of at least four anxious or depressive symptoms, such as irritability, worry, sleep disturbance, anticipating the worst, concentration or memory difficulties, and hopelessness. Clinicians working with elderly persons have long observed the significant overlap in symptoms of anxiety and depression. In fact, it is quite common to see individuals with a combination of anxiety and depression, although one or both disorders might be present only at subsyndromal levels.

Anxiety and Agitation in Dementia

Patients with dementia, whether living at home or in a long-term-care institution, commonly display behaviors described as agitation. Agitation takes the form of verbal or motor activity that is either appropriate behavior but repeated frequently or inappropriate behavior that suggests lack of judgment. As many as 85% of dementia patients eventually develop disruptive, agitated behavior. Early identification of triggers, including environmental stimuli, medication side effects, and uncommunicated internal needs, can result in effective treatment and relief for already overburdened caregivers. See "Dementia" (p 204) and "Behavioral Problems in Dementia" (p 213) for details on diagnosing and managing disruptive, agitated behavior.

Anxiety and Medical Disorders

It is common to encounter patients with comorbid anxiety and medical disorders. This could be due to longstanding anxiety disorder that coincidentally occurs alongside a medical illness, or there could be interplay between the two. There are conditions exacerbated by anxiety, such as the common cold or influenza, and also those that are precipitated by high levels of anxiety, such as angina pectoris or myocardial infarction. Other medical illnesses that commonly accompany an anxiety disorder include cardiovascular illnesses, pulmonary disorders, drug side effects (eg, thyroid hormone replacements, antipsychotics, caffeine, theophylline, selective serotonin-reuptake inhibitors [SSRIs]) or interactions, and hyperthyroidism. Given the complicated clinical picture that results when anxiety and medical disorders coexist, a thorough assessment, including a clinical history, is imperative before treatment begins.

PHARMACOLOGIC MANAGEMENT

Behavioral interventions should be initiated and combined with pharmacologic treatment when behavioral interventions alone are not effective. Numerous compounds have been used over the years as anxiolytics: alcohol, barbiturates, antihistamines, benzodiazepines, antipsychotic medications, and β-blockers. Although empirical studies of the use of anxiolytics in treating elderly persons are lacking, the efficacy of these medications is inferred from clinical practice with younger patients, and their use is modified by age-appropriate dosing. A brief description of the various classes of compounds currently favored as anxiolytics follows. Table 36.2 summarizes the treatment strategies for anxiety disorders in late life.

Antidepressants

Antidepressants are efficacious in the treatment of panic disorder, obsessive-compulsive disorder, generalized anxiety disorder, and posttraumatic stress disorder in younger patients. Given their relatively favorable side-effect profile, the SSRIs or serotonin–norepinephrine reuptake inhibitors (eg, venlafaxine) should now be considered the drugs of choice for these disorders. Further, SSRIs should also be considered treatments of choice for treating mixed anxiety and depression. Compounds such as venlafaxine should be considered as alternatives for those patients who do not respond to SSRIs or who develop adverse effects. Case reports, open-label trials, and, more recently, controlled trials of serotonergic antidepressants like trazodone and SSRIs have also suggested a modest degree of efficacy in the management of anxiety and agitation in dementia, particularly when patients are not psychotic and comorbid depression is a strong possibility. (See also "Behavioral Problems in Dementia," p 213.)

Benzodiazepines

Over the past several decades benzodiazepines have been the most commonly prescribed anxiolytics for both young and older patients, but their use is now discouraged. When needed because symptoms are severe, benzodiazepines with a short half-life, such as lorazepam and oxazepam, are preferable in treating elderly patients because they are metabolized by direct conjugation, a process relatively unaffected by aging. However, it is preferable to limit the use of even short-acting benzodiazepines to less than 6 months because long-term use is fraught with multiple complications, such as motor incoordination and falls, cognitive impairment, depression, and the potential for abuse and dependence.

Buspirone, Antihistamines, and Atypical Antipsychotics

Several studies have suggested that buspirone, an anxiolytic medication with some serotonin-agonist properties, is efficacious in the treatment of patients

Table 36.2—Treatment Strategies for Anxiety Disorders in Late Life

Disorder	First-Line Treatments	Second-Line Treatments
Panic disorder with or without agoraphobia	SSRIs,* SNRIs,* CBT	Newer antidepressants, benzodiazepines**
Social phobia		
Generalized	SSRIs* or phenelzine[OL] plus CBT	Benzodiazepines**
Specific	β-blockers plus CBT	Buspirone
Simple (specific) phobia	CBT or benzodiazepines**	β-blockers
Obsessive-compulsive disorder	SSRIs* plus CBT	Clomipramine, combination pharmacotherapy
Posttraumatic stress disorder	SSRIs* or SNRIs*	CBT, newer antidepressants
Generalized anxiety disorder	SNRIs,* SSRIs,* CBT	TCAs, benzodiazepines,** newer antidepressants
Anxiety and medical disorders	Identify and treat underlying cause, use SSRIs* or SNRIs* in primary anxiety disorder	Benzodiazepines**
Mixed anxiety depression	SSRIs* or SNRIs*	Buspirone, benzodiazepines,** CBT
Anxiety and agitation in dementia	Atypical antipsychotics[OL] or trazodone[OL]	Benzodiazepines,** anticonvulsants

* Not all SSRIs and SNRIs are approved for anxiety disorders or all types of anxiety disorders. For example, the SSRI escitalopram is not approved for anxiety, nor is the SNRI duloxetine.

** Preferably, benzodiazepines with a short half-life and no active metabolites (eg, lorazepam).

NOTE: CBT = cognitive-behavioral therapy; SNRIs = serotonin–norepinephrine reuptake inhibitors (eg, venlafaxine); SSRIs = selective serotonin-reuptake inhibitors (eg, sertraline); TCAs = tricyclic antidepressants.

[OL] Not approved by the U.S. Food and Drug Administration for this use.

with generalized anxiety disorder, although clinical experience is less positive. Buspirone appears to be a safer choice than benzodiazepines for patients taking several other medications or needing to be treated for longer periods of time. One drawback of buspirone is the amount of time required to see a clinical response (approximately 4 weeks). This suggests that con-comitant use of a short-acting benzodiazepine in the initial stage of treatment would be useful for some patients. Buspirone may also be efficacious in reducing symptoms of anxiety and agitation in patients with dementia. Antihistamines such as hydroxyzine and diphenhydramine[OL] are sometimes used to manage mild anxiety, but there are few data that demonstrate efficacy and the anticholinergic properties of these agents can cause serious problems. Finally, atypical antipsychotics, such as risperidone[OL], olanzapine[OL], and quetiapine[OL], are increasingly being used to man-age anxiety and agitation associated with dementia, particularly when an underlying psychosis may be present.

BEHAVIORAL INTERVENTIONS

Although pharmacotherapy is commonly the first-line treatment for late-life anxiety disorders, behavioral interventions are often adequate, either alone or as adjuncts to medication. Techniques generally fall into three categories. Relaxation training uses music, visual imagery, aromatherapy, or instruction in relaxation techniques. Cognitive restructuring helps the patient identify triggers and stimuli that maintain anxiety and helps him or her to slowly gain more control over the effect of such stimuli and develop a range of coping strategies and tools. Finally, exposure, with response prevention, has been shown to be particularly effective

[OL] Not approved by the U.S. Food and Drug Administration for this use.

with both panic disorder and obsessive-compulsive disorder. Treatment of the elderly person typically includes a combination of these behavioral approaches. Their success depends on the appropriateness of the patient for psychotherapy; the patient's support system, intellectual functioning, and motivation level; the de-gree of coordination of care with medical professionals; and the nature of the disorder. Consultation with a mental health professional can assist in determining the appropriateness of a referral.

REFERENCES

■ De Beurs E, Beekman AT, Deeg DJ, et al. Predictors of change in anxiety symptoms of older persons: results from the Longitudinal Aging Study Amsterdam. *Psychol Med.* 2000;30(3):515–527.

■ Demertzis KH, Craske MG. Anxiety in primary care. *Curr Psychiatry Rep.* 2006;8(4):291–297.

■ Kogan JN, Edelstein BA, McKee DR. Assessment of anxiety in older adults. *J Anxiety Disord.* 2000; 14(2):109–132.

■ Montorio I, Wetherell JL, Nuevo R. Beliefs about worry in community-dwelling older adults. *Depress Anxiety.* 2006;23(8):466–473.

■ Mostofsky DI, Barlow DH, eds. *The Management of Stress and Anxiety in Medical Disorders.* Needham Heights, MA: Allyn & Bacon; 2000.

■ Ostir GV, Goodwin JS. Anxiety in persons 75 and older: findings from a tri-ethnic population. *Ethn Dis.* 2006;16(1):22–27.

■ Sheikh JI. Anxiety in older adults: assessment and manage-ment of three common presentations. *Geriatrics.* 2003;58(5):44–45.

CHAPTER 37—PSYCHOTIC DISORDERS

KEY POINTS

■ Hallucinations are perceptions without stimuli that may occur in any sensory modalities (ie, visual, tactile, auditory, olfactory, gustatory). In late life, multimodal hallucinations are common.

■ Delusions are abnormal beliefs that in late life are often paranoid or persecutory, such as a belief that one's safety is in jeopardy or belongings are being stolen.

■ Psychosis occurring for the first time in late life is often due to dementia or neurologic conditions such as dementia or stroke, as opposed to a primary psychotic disorder, such as schizophrenia.

■ Dementia with Lewy bodies is associated with characteristically vivid visual hallucinations, often consisting of people or animals.

■ When psychotic symptoms arise in the context of depression, the symptoms are often "mood congruent"; examples are delusions that one is penniless or that one is already dead.

Psychotic symptoms are defined as either *hallucinations*, that is, perceptions without stimuli, or *delusions*, that is, fixed, false, idiosyncratic ideas. Hallucinations are abnormal perceptions that can be in any of the five sensory modalities (auditory, visual, tactile, olfactory, gustatory). Delusions are unfounded ideas that can be suspicious (paranoid), grandiose, somatic, self-blaming, or hopeless. This chapter focuses on conditions in which psychotic symptoms are prominent and central to making the diagnosis. It only briefly discusses other disorders, such as dementia, delirium, and the mood disorders, in which psychotic symptoms can occur but whose defining features are in the cognitive or mood realms and which are discussed elsewhere. (See "Dementia," p 204; "Delirium," p 220; "Depression and Other Mood Disorders," p 247.)

Hallucinations and delusions occur in a variety of disorders. The evaluation of a person with hallucinations and delusions (Figure 37.1) should first evaluate for underlying sources such as delirium, dementia,

stroke, or Parkinson's disease. An acute onset of altered level of consciousness or inability to sustain attention suggests delirium. Next, a primary mood disorder should be considered. Only after other causes are excluded should the diagnosis of a schizophrenia-like state be made. It should be noted that delirium, most often superimposed on an underlying dementia, is the most common cause of new-onset psychosis in late life.

SCHIZOPHRENIA AND SCHIZOPHRENIA-LIKE SYNDROMES

Schizophrenia is defined as a chronic psychiatric disorder characterized by positive symptoms (eg, hallucinations, delusions, and thought disorder) and negative symptoms (eg, social dilapidation and apathy). Mood disorder and cognitive disorder should be excluded. In men, schizophrenia has a modal onset at age 18; onset after age 45 years is uncommon. In women, on the other hand, modal age of onset is 28, and 20% to 30% of cases begin after age 45. Ten percent to 15% of

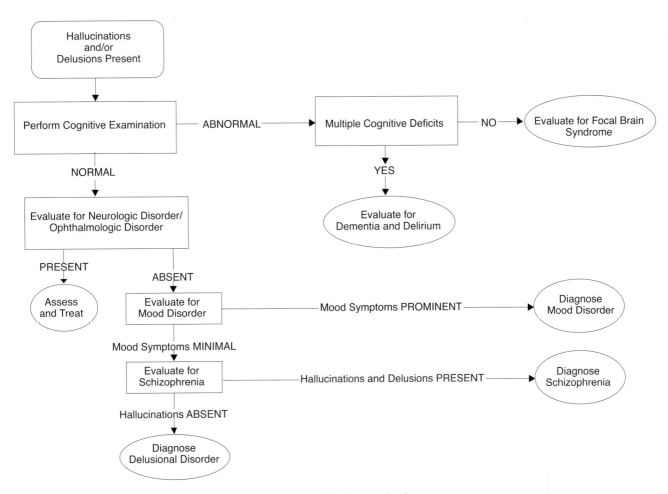

Figure 37.1—Evaluating the patient with hallucinations or delusions, or both.

cases of schizophrenia first come to clinical attention after patients have reached 59 years of age.

In older persons, schizophrenia-like conditions are characterized by onset after age 44, prominent persecutory (paranoid) delusions, and multimodal hallucinations. For example, patients commonly complain that items are being stolen or report that they are being persecuted unjustly. Hallucinations often manifest in complaints, for example, that a neighbor is persistently banging on walls or the roof, that someone is pumping gas under the door, or that electrical sensations are being sent through the walls of the person's home and into his or her body. A schizophrenia-like psychosis can be diagnosed only when cognitive disorder, mood disorder, or other explanatory medical conditions such as delirium or focal brain pathology have been excluded (Figure 37.1).

The schizophrenia-like psychoses of late life differ from schizophrenia beginning in early life in two ways. First, thought disorder, a sign described as speech in which a series of thoughts are not connected to one another in a logical fashion, is much less common in elderly patients, comprising only 5% of cases. In early-onset schizophrenia, thought disorder is present in approximately 50% of cases. It is important to note that thought disorder in schizophrenia occurs in the absence of an impaired sensorium (ie, delirium). When illogical speech occurs in late life, a delirium or dementia should be excluded. A second significant difference is the rarity of social deterioration and dilapidation among elderly patients. Thus, personality is often intact in late-onset cases. However, there is a dearth of long-term follow-up studies, so it is unknown whether social deterioration and personality changes occur after many years of symptoms.

Epidemiology and Clinical Characteristics

Late-onset schizophrenia is more common among women. The population-based incidence of late-onset schizophrenia is unknown, but the lifetime prevalence of schizophrenia is 1% among both men and women.

Late-onset schizophrenia-like psychoses affect predominantly women, with the female:male ratio ranging from 5:1 to 10:1. It has been speculated that later onset is due to decreasing natural estrogen levels, but there is little evidence to support this hypothesis. Many persons with late-onset schizophrenia-like psychosis have been able to hold responsible jobs and work efficiently, but premorbid isolation and "schizoid" (socially isolated personality) traits are common. Studies report greater degrees of brain white matter hyperintensities on magnetic resonance imaging scans in late-onset schizophrenia, a finding that suggests that brain vascular disease is a risk factor. However, this finding has not been adequately replicated, and other causes of white matter hyperintensities are plausible.

One condition that may be confused with late-onset schizophrenia is frontotemporal dementia (formerly referred to as Pick's disease), as it may involve features of socially inappropriate and odd behaviors as well as premorbidly odd or "schizoid" personality features. (See "Dementia," p 204.)

Treatment and Management

Nonpharmacologic

Because suspiciousness and paranoid delusions are commonly the most prominent symptoms, the physician's first task in treating late-onset psychosis is often to establish a trusting therapeutic relationship with the patient. On occasion, the suspicious ideas are plausible (eg, the claim that the patient is being financially abused by a relative), but usually the delusions are bizarre and implausible. It is rarely effective to confront the patient with the unreality or implausibility of his or her ideas. The patient is more likely to respond positively if the physician empathizes with the distress that the symptoms cause ("I can see how upset you are by all of this"). If patients ask whether the physician "believes" them, a response such as, "I don't hear anything like that, but I appreciate the fact that you do" is both honest and empathic. The symptoms are usually frightening and distressing to the patients and can lead to unusual behaviors. For example, patients who develop concerns that their food is being poisoned may exhibit unusual eating habits or food avoidance. Furthermore, suspiciousness can isolate the patient from friends and family. Therefore, encouraging patients to maintain important relationships and seeking their permission to discuss the source of symptoms with close family members or friends may help these patients maintain important, supportive relationships.

Pharmacologic

Clinical experience and descriptive case series suggest that antipsychotic drugs are as effective in late-onset schizophrenia as in early-onset cases. Most specialist physicians recommend the newer atypical antipsychotic drugs because they are less likely to cause tardive dyskinesia, a side effect for which older age is a predisposing factor. Doses should be increased at semi-weekly or weekly intervals, as needed. While doses are being titrated, patients should be monitored for the emergence of extrapyramidal side effects (parkinsonian tremor, rigidity, dystonia) and other movement disorders. These should be treated by lowering dosage and switching to an alternative antipsychotic if necessary. Polypharmacy should be avoided by reducing or switching antipsychotic medication rather than adding a medication for extrapyramidal symptoms. The more common side effects with quetiapine are sedation and orthostatic hypotension; with risperidone, extrapyramidal symptoms; and with olanzapine, weight gain and sedation (Table 37.1).

No studies are available to guide the length of treatment. Clinical experience suggests that patients who respond to antipsychotic medications should be continued on the minimal effective dose for at least 6 months. For patients who relapse on treatment or when the dosage is lowered, maintenance over a longer term (at least 1 to 2 years) is recommended. Patients should be monitored for the emergence of tardive dyskinesia, a syndrome characterized by repetitive involuntary movements of the oral and limb musculature. If tardive dyskinesia develops, the dosage of the antipsychotic agent should be lowered, if possible. Depending on the duration of exposure, tardive dyskinesia may worsen or appear when the antipsychotic is discontinued or the dose is lowered, or when switching from one antipsychotic to another. At the time antipsychotic drugs are initiated or as soon as symptoms improve enough so that the patient can understand the risk, he or she should be informed of the risk of tardive dyskinesia and the possibility that it can be irreversible.

PSYCHOTIC SYMPTOMS IN DELIRIUM

Hallucinations, particularly visual hallucinations, can be a symptom of delirium, even when it is mild. The onset of delirium is usually acute, and there is often an identifiable metabolic or infectious cause. The mental status examination reveals multiple cognitive impairments and a diminished level of consciousness. (See "Delirium," p 220.)

PSYCHOTIC SYMPTOMS IN MOOD DISORDER

Delusions can be seen in major depression and in the manic phase of bipolar disorder. These delusions are described as "mood congruent." That is, in patients with depression, the delusional content usually reflects self-deprecation, self-blame, hopelessness, or the conviction of ill health. A patient may complain that she has no blood or that her intestines are not working, for example; another patient may believe that he has caused a terrible wrong and deserves to be punished (a self-blaming delusion). Some patients become convinced that they are dying and that nothing can be done to help them when there is no physiologic evidence to support their concerns. Other common depressive delusions are the conviction that one has no insurance, no clothing, or no money when this is not true (delusion of poverty). Delusions congruent with mania are grandiose. Examples include the person's belief that that he or she is infallible, can do impossible physical or intellectual activities, has skills and abilities that no other human being has, or is a special personage such as Jesus Christ. (See "Depression and Other Mood Disorders," p 247.)

PSYCHOTIC SYMPTOMS IN DEMENTIA

Patients with dementia experience both hallucinations and delusions. These are usually less complex than the delusions seen in schizophrenia or mood disorder. Common delusions in dementia are the belief that one's belongings have been stolen or moved, or the conviction that one is being persecuted. Delusions that one's spouse is unfaithful (delusions of infidelity) are also common. (See "Dementia," p 204.)

Management of psychosis in dementia is particularly challenging, as the use of antipsychotic medication warrants careful consideration of risks and side effects.

Table 37.1—Commonly Used Antipsychotic Medications: Dosing and Side Effects

Agent	Starting Daily Dose (*mg*)	Maximum Daily Dose (*mg*)	Side Effects*		
			EPS**	Drowsiness	Weight Gain
Clozapine	12.5	75	1	3	3
Haloperidol	0.5–1	8	3	2	1
Olanzapine	2.5	10	1	2	3
Quetiapine	25	200	1	3	2
Risperidone	0.5–1	4	2	1	2

* Key: 1 = uncommon to 3 = common.

** EPS = extrapyramidal side effects: rigidity, parkinsonian tremor, dystonia, akathisia.

There has been recent attention to potential side effects of the newer antipsychotic medications in the class of atypical antipsychotics when used in patients with dementia. This group includes aripiprazole, olanzapine, risperidone, clozapine, quetiapine, and ziprasidone. One concern involves the risk of cerebrovascular adverse events (eg, stroke, transient ischemic attack) with risperidone, when such events were observed in clinical trials of risperidone in elderly patients with dementia-related psychosis. It is important to note that these clinical trials included patients with vascular dementia. The mechanism for the risk of cerebrovascular events has not yet been clarified. The observation of increased cerebrovascular events resulted in the addition of a warning to the product information. A class warning regarding atypical antipsychotics has already been applied concerning the risk of hyperglycemia in both younger and older patients with schizophrenia. The U.S. Food and Drug Administration has asked all manufacturers of atypical antipsychotic drugs to include a warning on the increased risk of developing hyperglycemia and diabetes. The mechanism for these adverse effects is unclear, although the fact that weight gain occurs with most of these medications may account for the increased rate of hyperglycemia.

ISOLATED SUSPICIOUSNESS

Suspiciousness can be viewed as a personality trait, that is, an aspect of all human beings that varies among people in its degree of prominence. One epidemiologic study has found that suspiciousness becomes more common in older Americans and affects 4% of those aged 65 and over. It is distinguished from psychotic disorders by the understandable nature of the ideas (for example, excessive worry about safety) and the absence of other psychotic symptoms.

SYNDROMES OF ISOLATED HALLUCINATIONS

Charles Bonnet Syndrome

Between 10% and 13% of patients with significant visual impairment (bilateral acuity worse than 20/60) experience visual hallucinations. These can take the form of shapes such as diamonds or rectangles but more commonly consist of complex hallucinations such as small children, multiple animals, or a vivid scene such as one would see in a movie. This condition, first

OL Not approved by the U.S. Food and Drug Administration for this use.

described more than 200 years ago, goes by the eponym *Charles Bonnet syndrome*. The criteria for this syndrome are as follows:

- visual hallucinations,
- partially or fully intact insight (the patient is aware that the perceptions cannot be real but still reports that they appear absolutely real and vivid),
- visual impairment, and
- lack of evidence of brain disease or other psychiatric disorder.

It has been suggested that this syndrome is a concomitant of the phantom limb syndrome caused by retinal lesions. However, visual hallucinations have also been reported in persons with field defects due to cortical lesions of the visual pathways.

The best treatment of the Charles Bonnet syndrome is information and support. Patients should be told that the hallucinations are a sign of eye disease, not mental illness. An occasional patient has partial insight or loses insight and becomes very distressed by this symptom. When this distress is significant or leads to dangerous behavior, a cautious trial of low doses of an atypical antipsychotic medication is occasionally beneficial.

Organic Hallucinosis

Patients with Parkinson's disease, stroke, and other brain disorders occasionally experience delusions and hallucinations without prominent cognitive impairment or other evidence of psychiatric disorder. Delirium due to a superimposed condition should be excluded. In patients with Parkinson's disease, the symptoms may be secondary to prescribed dopaminergic agent, but some patients experience visual hallucinations prior to the onset of any pharmacotherapy. Education and support should be offered to all patients with these symptoms. If the patients experience significant emotional distress or the symptoms lead to dangerous or upsetting behavior, cautious use of an antipsychotic medication is appropriate. For patients with Parkinson's disease and hallucinations, quetiapine^OL 12.5 to 75 mg or olanzapine^OL 2.5 to 5 mg daily may be beneficial. Some patients require clozapine^OL 12.5 to 75 mg daily. However, clozapine requires a complete blood cell count once a week for 6 months and then biweekly thereafter because of the risk of granulocytopenia.

Dementia associated with Lewy bodies is increasingly recognized as an important cause of hallucinations in late life. The clinical scenario typically involves cognitive decline accompanied by motor features of parkinsonism. However, prominent visual hallucinations are a key part of the diagnosis. These hallucinations are often vivid and troubling. (See "Dementia," p 204.)

Dementia associated with Lewy bodies presents a challenge similar to that of psychosis in Parkinson's disease because the drugs in the class approved to treat psychosis, the antipsychotics, have been shown to worsen the parkinsonian symptoms. No trial data are available to guide drug choice, but there are case reports of significant improvement through the use of cholinesterase inhibitors[OL]. If an antipsychotic medication must be used, then the treatment strategies outlined above are appropriate if there is careful attention to the risk of extrapyramidal side effects. Nonpharmacologic treatments include redirection, reassurance, and explanation.

REFERENCES

- Kertesz A, Munoz DG. Frontotemporal dementia. *Med Clin North Am.* 2002;86(3):501–518.

- Marsh L, Berk A. Neuropsychiatric aspects of Parkinson's disease: recent advances. *Curr Psychiatry Rep.* 2003;5(1):68–76.

- Marsh L. Neuropsychiatric aspects of Parkinson's disease. *Psychosomatics.* 2000; 41(1):15–23.

- Mittal D, Davis CE, Depp C, et al. Correlates of health related quality of well being in older patients with schizophrenia. *J. Nerv Ment Dis.* 2006;194(5):335–340.

- McKeith IG, Burn DJ, Ballard CG, et al. Dementia with Lewy bodies. *Semin Clin Neuropsychiatry.* 2003;8(1):46–57.

CHAPTER 38—PERSONALITY AND SOMATOFORM DISORDERS

KEY POINTS

- Personality disorders persist into late life and pose complex challenges to clinicians across various medical and psychiatric settings.

- Personality disorders may be more difficult to detect in late life because of age-associated changes in symptoms, comorbid psychopathology, and lack of age-adjusted diagnostic instruments.

- The goal of treatment of personality disorders in late life is not to cure the disorder, but to decrease the frequency and intensity of symptoms. To this end, both psychotherapeutic and psychopharmacologic strategies are needed.

- Somatoform disorders represent the presence of physical symptoms without established underlying pathology and with strongly associated psychologic factors. Undifferentiated somatoform disorder and hypochondriasis are likely the most common forms seen in late life.

- Treatment of somatoform disorders must attend to the affected individual's distress and belief in the veracity of his or her symptoms. The prognosis may be guarded, but repeated reassuring clinical visits help to build a therapeutic relationship.

[OL] Not approved by the U.S. Food and Drug Administration for this use.

PERSONALITY DISORDERS

Personality disorders are defined in the fourth edition of the *Diagnostic and Statistical Manual of Mental Disorders, Text Revision (DSM-IV-TR)* by the presence of chronic and pervasive patterns of inflexible and maladaptive inner experiences and behaviors. These patterns lead to significant disruptions in several spheres of function, including cognitive perception and interpretation, affective expression, interpersonal relations, and impulse control. People with personality disorders are often distinguished by repeated episodes of disruptive or noxious behaviors, and as a result they often receive pejorative labels, depending on their form. Descriptive terms often applied to those with personality disorders include "difficult," "dramatic," and "overbearing," to name just a few. The developmental roots of personality disorders are believed to lie in childhood and adolescence, but their features can present clinically at any age. These features represent the influence of both genetic and environmental factors.

The *DSM-IV-TR* describes ten personality disorders, grouped into three broad clusters that are based on common phenomenology. Depressive and passive-aggressive personality disorders are two additional categories, but they are considered provisional since they appear to lack the empirical support of the other ten diagnoses. Brief definitions and late-life features of all twelve personality disorders are provided in Table 38.1. Mixed diagnoses and those that do not

Table 38.1—Features of Personality Disorders

Cluster, Disorder	General Features*	Features Specific to Geriatric Patients
Cluster A: Odd or Eccentric Behaviors		
Paranoid	Pervasive suspiciousness of the motives of others, which often leads to irritability and hostility	Episodes of paranoid psychosis, agitation, and assaultivenes
Schizoid	Disinterest in social relationships, coupled with isolative and sometimes odd behaviors	Poor, strained, or absent relationships with caregivers
Schizotypal	Characteristic appearance, behaviors, and beliefs that are strange, unusual, or inappropriate	Beliefs that may become delusional and that may lead to conflicts with others; relationships with caregivers that may be strained or absent
Cluster B: Dramatic, Emotional, or Erratic Behaviors		
Antisocial	Poor regard for social norms and laws; lack of conscience and empathy for others; frequent reckless and criminal behaviors	Frequent remission of antisocial behaviors with less aggression and impulsivity
Borderline	Impaired control of emotional expression and impulses associated with unstable interpersonal relations, poor self-identity, and self-injurious behaviors	Persistent emotional lability and unstable relationships, but less self-injurious and impulsive behaviors
Histrionic	Excessive emotionality and attention-seeking behaviors, sometimes appearing overly seductive or provocative	Behaviors that may become excessively disinhibited and disorganized, appearing manic
Narcissistic	Pervasive sense of entitlement, grandiosity, and arrogance, coupled with lack of empathy	May present as hostile, rageful, paranoid, or depressed
Cluster C: Anxious or Fearful Behaviors		
Avoidant	Excessive sensitivity to rejection and social scrutiny; social demeanor that may be timid and inhibited	Social contacts that may be extremely limited, providing for inadequate support
Dependent	Excessive dependence on others to help make decisions and provide support	Commonly, comorbid depression; clinical appearance often with demanding or clinging behaviors if dependency needs not met
Obsessive-Compulsive	Pervasive preoccupation with orderliness and cleanliness; a perfectionistic, rigid, and controlling approach that may become more inflexible and indecisive under stress	Obsessive-compulsive traits that may become exaggerated in efforts to maintain control over somatic and environmental changes
Provisional Personality Disorders		
Passive-Aggressive	Pervasive pattern of passive resistance to demands and authority, such as through procrastination; attitudes toward others and responsibilities that are often critical and resentful	No clear changes in late life
Depressive	Outlook on life that is pervasively gloomy and pessimistic; excessively guilt prone with poor self-esteem	Commonly seen with comorbid depression in late life

* Descriptions of the clusters and of the disorders in each cluster are based on the *Diagnostic and Statistical Manual of Mental Disorders. 4th ed. Text Revision,* Washington, DC: American Psychiatric Association; 2000. The provisional disorders are described in the *DSM-IV–TR* appendix.

fit into any existing category are labeled "personality disorder, not otherwise specified" (NOS).

Many older persons with personality disorders can easily become overwhelmed by age-associated losses and stresses, largely because they lack appropriate coping skills and the personal, social, or financial resources to buffer their losses. In particular, admission to a hospital or long-term-care setting poses a unique stress on all persons with personality disorders in late life. The loss of a familiar environment, personal items, privacy, and the control over one's schedule can lead to a sense of disorganization and displacement. Conflict in an institutional setting begins when patients with personality disorders try to cope with the stresses from their new environment by exaggerating their maladaptive behaviors. An obsessive-compulsive person may attempt to maintain a sense of control by demanding rigid adherence to schedules and rules of hygiene. Dependent persons may feel helpless and panicked without enough attention to their needs, and they respond with clinging behaviors and excessive questions or requests for assistance. Paranoid, antisocial, and borderline patients may refuse to cooperate with treatment plans or institutional rules.

Epidemiology

Prevalence rates of late-life personality disorders in the community range from 5% to 10%, which is a slightly lower range than the 10% to 18% prevalence estimates for persons of all ages in the community. Prevalence rates in inpatient settings and with comorbid depression are much higher, ranging from 10% to over 50%, depending on the method of diagnosis. The most common personality disorders in late life are dependent, obsessive-compulsive, paranoid, and NOS. Although most research has demonstrated fewer diagnoses in older age groups, it is unclear whether this represents an actual difference in prevalence or merely reflects the fact that it is more difficult to make a diagnosis in late life. Some researchers have suggested that prevalence rates may be influenced by increased mortality among those with personality traits that are associated with higher rates of reckless, impulsive, and self-injurious behaviors. Other research exploring the neural substrates of emotion has demonstrated an attenuation of emotional reactivity in late life across a number of physiologic and behavioral parameters. These findings may partially explain the reduction in prevalence of the more impulsive and emotionally reactive personality features, such as those associated with borderline personality disorder.

Diagnostic Challenges

Establishing a diagnosis of personality disorder in the older patient can be especially challenging because it requires a detailed, longitudinal psychiatric and psychosocial history. Elderly patients and their informants are not always able to provide sufficient history, especially when it may span 50 years or more. The history may be distorted by recall bias (the tendency to present more socially desirable traits) or memory impairment. Furthermore, schizotypal and paranoid persons may be reluctant to engage in clinical interviews and share personal history, and antisocial and narcissistic persons who lack insight into their problems may refuse to divulge relevant experiences. Records often do not provide sufficient information to determine prior personality dynamics. Remote diagnoses from previous decades cannot be easily correlated with current ones because the diagnostic criteria for personality disorders have changed significantly in the past 50 years. As a result of all of these limitations, clinicians often are reluctant to make a diagnosis or to make judgments that are based on insufficient information.

A further diagnostic challenge for clinicians is the need to isolate lifelong personality characteristics from a multitude of comorbid problems. Acute and chronic episodes of major depression, psychosis, and other major psychiatric disorders can distort personality features considerably. Even the current diagnostic nomenclature might serve to handicap late-life diagnosis since it is not age adjusted, and many criteria fail to apply in late life. A final barrier to diagnosis may be present if the clinician erroneously considers all older patients to have disruptive personality features as a normal function of age.

Differential Diagnosis

In clinical settings, it is important to remember that not every older person with prominent or troubling personality features has a personality disorder. Those who demonstrate rigid and maladaptive personality traits but without the pervasiveness or severity as represented by *DSM-IV-TR* criteria are better described as suffering from personality dysfunction or an adjustment disorder. An adjustment disorder might best characterize previously healthy and well-adjusted persons who demonstrate acute changes in personality as a result of severe stresses. For example, physical pain and disability can lead to dependent or avoidant behaviors that resemble those seen in personality disorders, but without the pervasive pattern and degree of maladaptiveness. There is also considerable overlap between symptoms of major psychiatric disorders and those of personality disorders, and without longitudinal history it can be difficult to distinguish between them. For example, the odd thinking and unusual perceptual experiences seen in psychotic disorders may resemble behaviors seen in schizotypal personality disorder. The emotional lability of bipolar states can mimic behaviors of borderline and histrionic diagnoses, and depressive symptoms from dysthymic and depressive disorders can be almost indistinguishable from depressive personality traits. Diagnosis of a personality disorder becomes more certain when seemingly acute behaviors emerge as enduring and pervasive personality traits. This process depends on the opportunity to observe a person over time and in multiple settings or situations.

Personality disorders as described in *DSM-IV-TR* must also be differentiated from the diagnosis of personality change due to a specific medical condition. When personality change is a direct result of brain damage, it has classically been described within the context of an "organic" personality disorder, although this term is no longer used in *DSM* nomenclature. Most often, personality changes with an "organic" source involve impairments in executive functioning, consisting of poor impulse control, poor planning, and greater vulnerability to irritability or agitation. Along these lines, Alzheimer's disease and other dementias are often associated with personality changes, including apathy, egocentricity, and impulsivity. Frontal lobe injury may result in a disinhibited impulsive syndrome, or conversely, an apathetic, avolitional syndrome may result. Frontotemporal dementia has been associated with distinct personality changes characterized by odd social interactions and compulsive behaviors such as hoarding. (See "Dementia," p 204.) Temporal lobe epilepsy has been associated with personality change, including emotional deepening, verbosity, hypergraphia, hypersexuality, and preoccupation with religious, moral, and cosmic issues.

Long-Term Course

Personality disorders may follow one of four possible courses: they persist unchanged, evolve into a different form or major psychiatric disorder (eg, depression), improve, or remit. Few disorders have actually been studied over time, and rarely into late life. Several studies have suggested that personality disorders may enter a period of relative quiescence in middle age, with fewer and less intense symptoms and increased adaptation. However, this period may precede their reemergence in late life. Other researchers have proposed that personality disorders characterized by emotional and behavioral lability, including antisocial, borderline, histrionic, narcissistic, and dependent, tend to improve over time, although patients remain vulnerable to depression. Personality disorders characterized by an overcontrol of affect and impulses, including paranoid, schizoid, schizotypal, and obsessive-compulsive personality disorders, are thought to either remain stable or to worsen in late life.

Only antisocial and borderline personality disorders have been looked at longitudinally, and both have shown symptom improvement and even remittance into middle and later life for a significant percentage of patients. At the same time, there can be persistent psychopathology that is not recognized within the context of existing antisocial or borderline diagnostic criteria. In other words, longstanding personality dynamics may manifest in new behaviors. For example, those with antisocial personality disorders demonstrate less aggressiveness, violence, and criminal acts as they age, but they still have antisocial tendencies expressed through substance abuse, disregard for safety, and noncompliance with institutional rules. Elderly borderline patients display less impulsivity, self-mutilation, and risk-taking, but more age-appropriate symptoms, such as the use of multiple medications and nonadherence with treatment.

Treatment

The treatment of personality disorders in late life is complicated and often has limited success. Given the chronic and pervasive nature of personality disorders, the overall goal of treatment in late life is not to cure the disorder, but to decrease the frequency and intensity of disruptive behaviors. The first step should always be to clarify the diagnosis and then to identify recent stressors that may account for the current presentation. The resultant formulation will guide the selection of realistic target symptoms and therapeutic approaches and will allow a treatment team to anticipate future stressors. Treatment of personality disorders in late life uses the same basic approaches as with younger patients, but clinicians must incorporate a much broader understanding of the impact of age-related stressors and comorbid disorders. All forms of psychotherapy have been used to treat personality disorders in older adults, ranging from intensive and long-term insight-oriented approaches to equally intensive but more focused cognitive-behavioral models. In late life, however, there may be more limitations on time and intensity of therapy, and as a result treatment must focus more on short-term, cognitive-behavioral, and pharmacologic approaches. Studies in adults generally find that comorbid personality disorders complicate the treatment of psychiatric illness, but that with consistent treatment, the prognosis is often favorable. The prognosis in late life is more guarded, especially for persons with comorbid major depression. One study of elderly persons with major depression found that those with a concomitant personality disorder were less likely to benefit from psychotherapy.

In outpatient settings, clinicians have limited control over a patient's environment and must therefore rely on one-to-one interventions if the patient is willing to cooperate with treatment. With some patients, it may be necessary to convey a basic formulation of their behaviors, along with suggested approaches, to caregivers and affiliated health care professionals, such as internists, social workers, and visiting nurses. This communication is important when patients are vulnerable to self-harm or likely to cause significant disruptions in other settings when they are not understood and approached in a therapeutic manner. Table 38.2 suggests therapeutic approaches that clinicians can employ with various personality disorders.

The interdisciplinary team meeting provides the best forum to discuss disruptive persons and to coordinate a consistent treatment plan.

Disruptive behaviors can sometimes be traced to particular activities or staff interactions, which can be adapted as part of an overall treatment strategy. Sometimes, disengagement from patients will reduce the intensity of disruptive interactions. In other situations, the continuity of staffing and of daily schedules is critical. In all situations, a treatment plan should be well documented and conveyed to the patient, as well as all involved staff and caregivers. All plans must provide appropriate limits to ensure the safety of patients and staff. A written contract, signed by all

Table 38.2—Therapeutic Strategies for Personality Disorders in Late Life

Cluster A—Paranoid, Schizoid, Schizotypal Personality Disorders

- Always assess for and treat comorbid psychosis.

- Do not force social interactions, but offer support and problem-solving assistance in a professional and consistent manner.

- Do not challenge paranoid ideation; instead, solicit and empathize with emotional responses to the inner turmoil and fear of paranoid states.

Cluster B—Antisocial, Borderline, Histrionic, and Narcissistic Personality Disorders

- Assess for and treat underlying mood lability, depression, anxiety, and substance abuse.

- Adopt a consistent, structured, and predictable approach with strict boundaries to contain disruptive behaviors.

- Adopt a team approach with all involved clinicians to devise a common plan; avoid staff splits between "supporters" and "detractors" of the patient.

- Use behavioral contracts and authority figures when necessary to address recurrent disruptive behaviors.

- Do not personalize belligerent behaviors directed toward staff members; instead, provide opportunities for staff to ventilate frustration and negative thoughts and emotions with professional colleagues.

Cluster C—Avoidant, Dependent, and Obsessive-Compulsive Personality Disorders

- Assess for and treat underlying anxiety, panic, and depression.

- Provide regularly scheduled clinical contacts rather than on an as-needed basis.

- When possible, provide case managers to solicit the needs of avoidant patients and to provide extra reassurance and attention to the needs of dependent and obsessive-compulsive patients.

Depressive and Passive-Aggressive Personality Disorders

- Differentiate between the depressive and negative attitudes and the actual symptoms of major depression. Provide appropriate and adequate antidepressant treatment.

- Avoid becoming too pessimistic or burnt-out with attempts at providing care; shift focus to a supportive and nonjudgmental therapeutic relationship, with minimal expectations as to outcome.

- Encourage individual psychotherapy to identify underlying emotions and to redirect negative attitudes toward more constructive activities.

parties, may be needed with nonadherent persons in order to eliminate ambiguity. Although it is important to involve family members in the treatment plan, clinicians must recognize that patients with personality disorders often have conflictual relationships with them. Attention should also be given to individual staff members who must work with difficult patients. They need opportunities to vent feelings of anxiety and frustration, and to feel acknowledged and supported by administrative and clinical staff.

There have been no studies looking specifically at pharmacologic strategies for personality disorders in late life, so clinicians must instead extrapolate from guidelines used for younger persons. Psychotropic medications can be targeted at a particular personality disorder, specific symptoms or symptom clusters, or comorbid depression, anxiety, or psychosis. The goal is not to cure the disorder, but to reduce the frequency and intensity of targeted symptoms. Antidepressant medication may be helpful for the target symptoms of depression and anxiety found in most personality disorders. Mood stabilizers (eg, lithium carbonate[OL] and divalproex sodium[OL]) and antipsychotic medica-

tions have been found to reduce mood lability and impulsivity in borderline patients, and they may be useful with similar symptoms in antisocial personality disorder. Antianxiety agents are commonly used for transient agitation seen in borderline, antisocial, narcissistic, and paranoid disorders, and they may reduce social anxiety and panic in avoidant and dependent patients. Antidepressants are used commonly to treat obsessive-compulsive personality symptoms, although efficacy has not been established for the treatment of these symptoms as opposed to obsessive-compulsive disorder. Antipsychotic agents can treat the transient psychosis, agitation, and impulsivity seen in dramatic cluster and paranoid disorders, as well as the borderline psychosis and paranoia seen in odd cluster disorders.

For personality disorders, psychotropic medications are best used as adjuncts to psychotherapy. In older persons, multiple medications should be avoided in general, and particularly when there is a history of nonadherence, confusion, or impulsivity. Attention must be given to potential interactions with multiple other medications used to treat medical disorders. It is important to obtain and document informed consent (or consent of family members or guardians) for the use of psychotropics when there is a history of

---

[OL] Not approved by the U.S. Food and Drug Administration for this use.

dementia, recent delirium, paranoia, or conflictual doctor-patient relationships.

Finally, clinicians must recognize that in some cases it is best not to prescribe a psychotropic medication. Such cases include older persons with personality disorders and comorbid substance abuse, chronic non-adherence, or a history of or potential for abusive or self-injurious use of medications. Antisocial and borderline persons often demonstrate such behaviors. Dependent patients may insist upon medications as a means of fostering dependency on the clinician, and obsessive-compulsive patients may perpetuate a maladaptive relationship with the clinician through detailed and controlling discussions of medication management. In each example, medication management is corrupted by dysfunctional interpersonal behaviors that lie at the heart of personality disorders.

SOMATOFORM DISORDERS

Somatoform disorders encompass a heterogeneous group of seven diagnoses that have in common the presence of physical symptoms or complaints without objective organic causes, and that are strongly associated with psychologic factors. Clinical characteristics of each diagnosis are summarized in Table 38.3. These disorders are especially relevant to geriatric care because affected older persons are seen in all health care settings, and they tend to overutilize medical services. Somatoform disorders in late life have not been well studied, and existing research has usually focused on select diagnoses, such as hypochondriasis, in limited or biased samples. Research also has looked at somatic symptom reporting rather than at specific diagnoses. Prevalence rates in middle and late life have been found to be less than 1%, except for one study, which found a prevalence rate of more than 36% for somatization disorder in women over 55 years old seen in health care clinics. The presence of these disorders has not been found to be strongly associated with age, although there is weak evidence for a slight increase in hypochondriasis with age. Increased somatic preoccupation and symptoms are, however, associated with depression in late life, and older age of onset for depression may be most predictive. In addition to depression, increased somatic preoccupation is associated with the presence of the personality trait of neuroticism, in which a person displays a tendency to experience more negative emotions. Somatoform disorders are found more commonly in women and in lower socioeconomic groups. Late onset of a somatoform disorder may suggest associated neurologic illness.

Table 38.3—Clinical Characteristics of Somatoform Disorders*

Somatization Disorder

Multiple physical complaints in excess of what would be expected, given history and examination, prior to the age of 30 and lasting several years; complaints not fully explained by medical work-up; must include four different sites of pain, two gastrointestinal symptoms, one sexual symptom, one pseudoneurologic symptom (not pain).

Undifferentiated Somatoform Disorder

One or more physical complaints, lasting at least 6 months, that cannot be fully explained by appropriate medical work-up and that result in considerable social, occupational, or functional impairment.

Conversion Disorder

One or more motor or sensory deficits that cannot be fully explained by appropriate medical work-up and that appear to be causally related to psychologic factors.

Pain Disorder

Pain is the major focus of clinical presentation, and psychologic factors are believed to be playing a critical role in the onset, severity, exacerbation, and maintenance of the pain.

Hypochondriasis

A preoccupation with fears of having a serious illness, based on misinterpretation of bodily symptoms and resistant to appropriate medical evaluation and reassurance.

Body Dysmorphic Disorder

Preoccupation with an imagined defect in appearance. If there is an actual physical defect, this preoccupation greatly exceeds what would be expected.

Somatoform Disorder, Not Otherwise Specified

The presence of somatoform symptoms that do not meet the criteria for other categories.

* Descriptions of the clusters and of the disorders in each cluster are based on the *Diagnostic and Statistical Manual of Mental Disorders. 4th ed. Text Revision*, Washington, DC: American Psychiatric Association; 2000.

Clinical Characteristics and Causes

It is important to recognize that somatoform disorders do not represent intentional, conscious attempts by older patients to present factitious physical symptoms. Somatoform symptoms are experienced by the affected person as real physical pain and discomfort, usually without insight into associated psychologic factors. Somatoform disorders do not represent delusional thinking as found in psychotic states (although body dysmorphic disorder can be associated with beliefs of delusional quality), and they are different from psychosomatic disorders, which are characterized by actual disease states with presumed psychologic triggers. Rather, somatoform disorders represent a complex interaction between mind and brain in which an affected person is unknowingly expressing psychologic stress or conflict through the body. It is not surprising, then, that depression and anxiety are associated with increased somatic expressions. In late life, somatoform disorders, in particular hypochondriasis, may be a way for a person to express anxiety and attempt to cope with accumulating fears and losses. These may include fears of abandonment by family and caregivers, loss of beauty and strength, financial setbacks, loss of independence, loss of social role (eg, through retirement, loss of spouse, occupational disability), and loneliness. The psychologic distress and anxiety over such losses may be less threatening and more controllable when shifted to somatic complaints or symptoms. In turn, the adoption of a sick role might be reinforced by increased social contacts and support.

The causes of somatoform disorders are usually multifactorial, and often they are rooted in early developmental experiences and personality traits. Psychodynamic approaches suggest that these disorders result from unconscious conflict in which intolerable impulses or affects are expressed through more tolerable somatic symptoms or complaints. One reason for this may be the presence of alexithymia, in which a person is unable to identify and express emotional states, so that the body becomes the available mode of expression.

Although psychodynamic explanations can apply across the life span, these conflicts often begin early in life, perhaps accounting for the relatively young age of onset for most somatoform disorders. In late life, psychologic conflict that results in significant depression and anxiety are for the most part the same conflicts that can lead to somatization. In addition, the presence of so many comorbid medical problems and the use of multiple medications may provide readily available somatic symptoms around which psychologic conflict can center. In long-term care, older persons are faced with many overwhelming losses, and their own bodies often serve as the last bastion of control. Somatic preoccupation thus serves as a means of coping with stress, even though it is maladaptive and can result in excessive and unnecessary disability.

Treatment

Persons with somatoform disorder do not usually present as such; by their definition they present to clinicians with what appear to be legitimate somatic complaints with an unknown physical cause. It is only after repeated but fruitless work-ups, multiple and persistent complaints and requests, and sometimes angry and inappropriate reactions to treatment that clinicians begin to suspect a somatoform disorder. In some cases the manner of presentation and symptom complex is more immediately suggestive of a particular somatoform disorder. In any event, it is important for the clinician to remember that from the perspective of the patient, the symptoms and complaints are quite real and disturbing. It is never wise to challenge the patient or to suggest that the symptoms are "all in your mind," even after work-up has made it obvious that psychologic factors are involved. The typical response to such advice is for the patient to seek additional opinions and medical tests, which in turn can perpetuate a cycle of somatization that never addresses the underlying issues.

Instead, the clinician should attempt to foster an ongoing, supportive, consistent, and professional relationship with the affected person. Such a relationship will serve to provide reassurance as well as to protect the patient from excessive and unnecessary medical visits and procedures. The clinician should focus on responding to individual complaints, perhaps with periodic but regularly scheduled appointments, and to set limits on work-up and treatment in a firm but empathetic manner. This can be difficult to do when patients become demanding and attempt to consume excessive clinic time, but the clinician must endeavor to remain professional and not to personalize the situation or to feel that he or she is failing the patient. Overall, the role of the clinician is to focus on symptom reduction and rehabilitation, and not to attempt to force the patient to have insight into the potential psychologic nature of his or her symptoms. It would be hazardous to prematurely diagnose a somatoform disorder when there might actually be an underlying medical problem that has eluded diagnosis. For example, disorders such as multiple sclerosis, systemic lupus erythematosus, and acute intermittent porphyria commonly have complex presentations that elude initial diagnostic work-up. Moreover, many somatoform disorders coexist with actual disease states; for example, many persons with pseudoseizures also have an actual seizure disorder. At the same time, it is important for the clinician to set limits on what he or she can offer, and to make appropriate referrals to specialists and mental health clinicians.

The mental health clinician will play a more active role in addressing the somatoform disorder. Unfortunately, no particular treatment for any somatoform disorder has been found to have good efficacy, and most disorders tend to be lifelong. As a result, the goal of treatment is not to cure, but to control symptoms. The clinician first forms a therapeutic alliance based on empathetic listening and acknowledgment of physical discomfort, without trivializing the somatic complaints. Sometimes an offer to review all available medical records can be a tangible way of conveying one's seriousness to the patient. Underlying anxiety and depression must be identified and treated with psychotherapy and, when necessary, antidepressant or antianxiety medications, or both. Cognitive-behavioral therapy focuses on identifying distorted thought patterns and anxious triggers, and replacing them with more realistic and adaptive strategies. A mental health professional may assist in determining whether cognitive-behavioral therapy may be of benefit. In many cases, however, the supportive nature of regular visits to a primary care provider may be sufficient to meet the needs of persons with somatoform disorders as well as other personality disorders.

REFERENCES

■ Agronin ME. Somatoform disorders. In: Blazer DG, Steffens DC, Busse EW, eds. *Textbook of Geriatric Psychiatry*. 3rd ed. Washington, DC: American Psychiatric Press; 2004:295–302.

■ Rabinowitz T, Hirdes JP, Desjardins I. Somatoform disorders. In: Agronin ME, Maletta GJ, eds. *Principles and Practice of Geriatric Psychiatry*. Philadelphia: Lippincott Williams & Wilkins; 2006:489–504.

■ Sheehan B, Lall R, Bass C. Does somatization influence quality of life among older primary care patients? *Int J Geriatr Psychiatry*. 2005;20(10):967–972.

■ Zweig RA, Agronin ME. Personality disorders. In: Agronin ME, Maletta GJ, eds. *Principles and Practice of Geriatric Psychiatry*. Philadelphia: Lippincott Williams & Wilkins; 2006:449–470.

CHAPTER 39—SUBSTANCE ABUSE

KEY POINTS

■ Alcohol and other substance-abuse problems may not be detected when screening questions are omitted during routine medical visits.

■ Alcohol use may be an unrecognized cause of falls, cognitive decline, and medical problems (eg, anemia, elevated liver function tests, thrombocytopenia).

■ A diagnosis of alcohol withdrawal should be considered in older adults who develop delirium with hospitalization or facility placement.

■ Cognitive impairment from chronic alcoholism in older adults may improve with sustained abstinence.

The abuse and misuse of alcohol, psychoactive medications, illicit drugs, and nicotine have become significant public health concerns for the growing population of elderly people. This concern is highlighted by the growth in the literature demonstrating that substance abuse and dependence among older people is common. Moreover, elderly adults are particularly vulnerable to the cognitive and physical effects of these substances.

Clinicians and researchers therefore may need to change their thinking about the risks of use in this segment of the population. Typically, substance-use problems are thought to occur only in people who use substances in high quantities and at regular intervals. Among elderly adults, however, negative health consequences have been demonstrated at consumption levels previously thought of as light to moderate, and certainly not in the amounts usually associated with a diagnosis of substance dependence. A growing number of effective treatments for these problems lead not only to reduced substance use but also to improved general health. Taken together, both the risks and the emergence of new treatments underscore the need to identify problems and provide appropriate treatment for older adults suffering from the effects of substance misuse.

DEFINITIONS OF SUBSTANCE ABUSE

Establishing valid criteria for determining which older adults would benefit from reducing or eliminating their substance use is the first step in successful intervention. *Substance dependence* has been defined by the medical community as any use that imparts significant disability and warrants treatment. Many older adults are not recognized as having problems that are related to their substance use, partly because the diagnostic criteria are difficult to interpret and to apply consistently to older adults. For instance, many older people drink at home by themselves; thus, they are less likely than younger drinkers to be arrested, to get into arguments, or to have difficulties in employment. Moreover, because many of the diseases caused or affected by substance misuse (eg, hypertension, stroke, and peptic ulcer disease) are common disorders in late life, the clinician may overlook the effects of substance use on the older patient who presents with these disorders. The literature indicates that older problem drinkers are identified less often by clinicians and are less often referred for treatment than are their younger counterparts.

Because of the difficulties in assessing older adults for substance dependence, many experts have advocated screening to identify people who are at risk for problem behaviors or who have at-risk or problem use. *At-risk use* is defined as any use of a substance at a quantity or frequency greater than a recommended level. The level of use is often determined empirically based on association with significant disability. For instance, the recommended upper limit of alcohol consumption for elderly adults has been established as no more than seven standard drinks per week with no more than two episodes of binge drinking (four or more drinks in a day) during a period of 3 months. *Problem substance use* is defined as the consumption of any amount of an abusable substance that results in at least one problem related to this use. For example, the use of benzodiazepines by a patient who has an unsteady gait would be considered problem use.

On the other end of the spectrum, *abstinence* refers to drinking no alcohol in the previous year. If an older patient is abstinent, it is useful to ascertain why alcohol is not used. Some individuals are abstinent because of a previous history of alcohol problems. For this reason, it is particularly important to obtain a history of both current and past use. Some are abstinent because of recent illness; others have lifelong patterns of low-risk use or abstinence. Patients who have a previous history of alcohol problems may require preventive monitoring to determine if any new stresses could exacerbate an old pattern. In addition, a previous history of at-risk drinking or alcohol dependence increases the risk of developing other mental health problems in late life, such as depressive disorders or cognitive problems, and may limit treatment response because of brain damage.

Low-risk or moderate use of alcohol is that which falls within the recommended guidelines for consump-

tion and is not associated with problems. Older adults in this category not only consume amounts that fall within recommended drinking guidelines but are also able to set reasonable limits on alcohol consumption, ie, they do not drink when driving a motor vehicle or boat, or when using contraindicated medications. It is important to note, however, that a change in physical health or change in prescription medications may mean that even low-risk use can become a problem.

The most practical method for identifying people who could benefit from intervention is to determine the quantity and frequency of their use of abusable substances. This method has advantages over formal diagnostic interviews because of its brevity, easily interpretable results, and absence of stigmatizing language, such as "addiction," "alcoholism," "alcoholic" or "alcohol dependence." For more on screening, see identifying substance-use disorders (p 278).

MAGNITUDE OF THE PROBLEM

Drug Use

Little is known about the epidemiology of substance-use disorders among elderly adults other than alcoholism. The general belief is that older drug addicts are only younger addicts who have grown old, and that few older adults initiate drug use in their later years. The Epidemiologic Catchment Area study provides perhaps the only community study of the prevalence of drug abuse and dependence among elderly adults. Using the Diagnostic Interview Schedule to determine prevalence rates for psychiatric diagnoses as defined by the third edition of the *Diagnostic and Statistical Manual of Mental Disorders* (*DSM-III*), the study found the lifetime prevalence rates of drug abuse and dependence to be 0.12% for elderly men and 0.06% for elderly women. The lifetime history of illicit drug use was found to be 2.88% for men and 0.66% for women. No active cases were reported in either gender. In contrast, a more recent study of an elder-specific drug program in a veteran population found that one quarter had either a primary drug problem or concurrent drug and alcohol problems. This study may be a reflection of the growing number of elderly adults who used drugs during a time of expanded drug experimentation in the United States in the 1960s. Recent increases in hepatitis C among patients aged 60 and over may reflect both a history of intravenous drug use as well as increased risk of nosocomial infection with advanced age. Other studies to determine the prevalence and incidence of substance-use disorders involving nicotine, caffeine, benzodiazepines, marijuana, and opiates (in later life) are needed.

Medication Use

Perhaps a unique problem with the elderly age group is the misuse or inappropriate use of prescription and over-the-counter medications. This problem includes the misuse of substances such as sedatives, hypnotics, narcotic and non-narcotic analgesics, diet aids, decongestants, and a wide variety of over-the-counter medications. Community surveys have found that 60% of elderly people are taking an analgesic, 22% are taking a central nervous system medication, and 11% are taking a benzodiazepine. Many medications used by elderly people have the potential for inducing tolerance, withdrawal syndromes, and harmful medical consequences, such as cognitive changes, falls, and kidney or liver disease. There is a growing body of literature demonstrating a concerning increase in morbidity and mortality associated with the misuse of prescription and nonprescription medications, even though this is not considered as a disorder in *DSM-IV*.

Medication use by all elderly patients needs to be monitored carefully; it is important to avoid prescribing potentially hazardous combinations of drugs, medications with a high risk of adverse effects, and ineffective or unnecessary medications. (See "Pharmacotherapy," p 66.) A practical approach to monitoring psychoactive medications is to reevaluate the older patient's use every 3 to 6 months. Only those patients with specific target symptoms and a documented response to the treatment should continue on maintenance treatment. Patients without a response or partial response to the treatment should be reevaluated for appropriate diagnosis and further care. In such cases, consultation with a geriatric mental health professional could be advantageous. (See also "Depression and Other Mood Disorders," p 247; "Anxiety Disorders," p 258; "Psychotic Disorders," p 262; and "Personality and Somatoform Disorders," p 267.)

Alcohol Use

Community-based epidemiologic studies define the extent and nature of alcohol use in the older population by reporting percentages of abstainers, heavy drinkers, and daily drinkers. Abstention from alcohol ranges from 31% to 58%, and daily drinking ranges from 10% to 22% in samples of older patients. "Heavy" drinking, defined as a minimum of 12 to 21 drinks per week, is present in 3% to 9% of the older population; alcohol abuse, as defined clinically, is present in approximately 2% to 4%.

Longitudinally designed community studies give valuable insight regarding the natural course of drinking patterns in elderly age groups. In studies that examined longitudinal alcohol use the incidence of heavy drinking was 0.2% to 4% of older adults per year. It is also important to keep in mind that most of the literature on drinking indicates that although elderly people are likely to decrease the quantity of alcohol consumed on a given day, the frequency of use or pattern of use changes very little over time.

Cultural and Demographic Factors

Numerous studies have shown that the prevalence of alcohol use and alcohol-related problems among older adults is much higher for men than for women. Among younger adults, however, the ratio of men to women drinkers has changed over the past several decades, with the result that more women present for treatment. These changes are likely to continue to be reflected in the next generation of older women. Similar patterns by gender are seen with illicit drug use, except that benzodiazepines are much more commonly used by older women than by older men.

Conclusions are less clear from the few studies addressing differences among various ethnic groups. Depending on the study, older black Americans and older Hispanic Americans have been found to consume amounts of alcohol similar to or lower than the amounts consumed by older white Americans. The Epidemiologic Catchment Area data demonstrated nonsignificant differences in the 1-year diagnosis of alcohol abuse and dependence among black Americans (2.93% among men, 0.60% among women), white Americans (2.85% among men and 0.47% among women), and Hispanic Americans (6.57% among men and 0.0% among women). More relevant risk factors than race or ethnicity for alcohol consumption among elderly people are increased leisure time and higher disposable income.

Clinical Settings

Elderly people constitute the majority of admissions to acute-care facilities and are frequent users of outpatient medical services, including primary care. The prevalence rates for alcohol problems among hospital populations are substantially higher than for community dwellers. High prevalence rates for problems related to drinking are also becoming more common in retirement communities. Data from a survey of a Veterans Affairs nursing home has demonstrated that 35% of the patients interviewed had a lifetime diagnosis of alcohol abuse. A significant number of patients seen in outpatient clinics also have been found to have an active alcohol-use disorder. The high prevalence of alcohol-related problems in both hospital and outpatient populations underscores the need for thorough screening of older patients in medical settings.

Risks and Benefits of Substance Use

Benefits of Alcohol Consumption

Moderate alcohol consumption among otherwise healthy older adults has been promoted as having significant beneficial effects, especially with regard to cardiovascular disease and mortality. The findings from the cardiovascular literature have led to a host of articles in the popular press espousing the benefits of alcohol use.

Alcohol in moderate amounts may promote relaxation and reduce social anxiety. However, even though there are benefits of moderate drinking, the practice of recommending drinking to people who currently do not drink is not advocated. Many older adults do not drink because of past problems with drinking, family problems with drinking, the expense related to drinking, and the adverse effects of intoxication. There is no evidence to support a therapeutic effect of alcohol for heart disease or any other condition in people who previously did not drink.

Excess Physical Disability

Substance abuse has clear and profound effects on the health and well-being of elderly people in all spheres of life. Older people are prone to the toxic effects of substances on many different organ systems. The social and economic impact is also tremendous. Substance abuse has adverse effects on self-esteem, coping skills, and interpersonal relationships, which may be compounded by losses that are common in the late stages of life. Elderly adults are particularly prone to these toxic effects because of both the physiologic changes associated with aging and the changes associated with other illnesses common in late life.

Levels of alcohol consumption above seven drinks per week, so called at-risk drinking, have been associated with a number of health problems, including an increased risk of stroke caused by bleeding, impaired driving skills, and an increased rate of injuries, such as falls and fractures. The risk of breast cancer in women who consume three to nine drinks per week has been shown to be increased by approximately 50% over that of women who drink fewer than three drinks per week. Of particular importance to older persons are the potential harmful interactions between alcohol and both prescribed and over-the-counter medications, especially psychoactive medications such as benzodiazepines and antidepressants. Alcohol is also known to interfere with the metabolism of many medications, including digoxin and warfarin.

Older adults who consume more than an average of four drinks per day or whose drinking has led to a diagnosis of alcohol dependence are at greatest risk of excess physical disability and physical illness that are related to the drinking. The most common problems associated with alcohol dependence are alcoholic liver disease, chronic obstructive pulmonary disease, peptic ulcer disease, and psoriasis. Moreover, unexplained multisystem disease should alert the clinician to probe more closely for alcohol use. With smoking, the risks are much clearer, including increased rates of pulmonary disease, especially cancer. Medications such as benzodiazepines are also associated with excess physical disability, with increased rates of falls, and driving-related impairment. Research is beginning to demonstrate that the disability associated with these problems is also reversible with reductions in substance use.

Mental Health Problems

Substance use can be a significant factor in the course and prognosis of nearly all mental health problems of late life. Alcohol, benzodiazepine, opioid, and cigarette use have all been demonstrated to be related etiologically to mood disturbances, but they also complicate the treatment of concurrent mood disorders. People with both alcoholism and depression have a more complicated clinical course of depression with an increased risk of suicide and more social dysfunction than nondepressed people with alcoholism. Overall, elderly people with alcohol abuse or dependence are nearly three times more likely to have a lifetime diagnosis of another mental disorder. Alcoholism has been implicated in mood disorders, suicide, dementia, anxiety disorders, and sleep disturbances.

As might be expected, patients with alcohol-related dementia who become abstinent do not show a progression in cognitive impairment comparable to that of people with Alzheimer's disease. The complex role of alcoholism in the development of Alzheimer's disease is not fully understood, but certainly alcoholism is known to lead to a syndrome of dementia independently. Interesting new hypotheses implicate glutamatergic toxicity, but overall, the mechanisms are not well understood. The criteria for alcohol-related dementia are as follows:

- clinically evident dementia at least 60 days after last alcohol exposure;
- a history of significant use for at least 5 years, ie, at least 35 drinks per week for men and 28 per week for women;
- the occurrence of this period of significant use within 3 years of the onset of cognitive deficits.

Clinical features supporting the diagnosis include end-organ damage (eg, liver disease), cognitive stabilization or improvement after abstinence, and evidence of cerebellar atrophy in brain imaging. Further research is greatly needed to understand the potential benefits of long-term abstinence in this condition. Similarly, those with comorbid depression and alcohol use are likely to have better depression outcomes if abstinence is achieved. Moderate alcohol use has also been demonstrated to have negative effects on the treatment of late-life depression, further underscoring the need for reducing moderate use in the context of chronic health problems in older adults.

IDENTIFYING SUBSTANCE-USE DISORDERS

Although clinical examination remains the most valuable tool for identifying substance-use problems, screening instruments help increase the sensitivity and efficiency of the diagnosis of various disorders. Several instruments have been developed for identifying alcohol-use disorders, including self-administered questionnaires and laboratory studies. Self-administered questionnaires provide the busy clinician with a rapid, sensitive, and inexpensive method of screening for alcohol problems. Two questionnaires—the Michigan Alcoholism Screening Test (MAST) and the CAGE (see Table 39.1)—have been developed with these principles in mind. Both of these instruments have high sensitivity and specificity for identifying alcohol-use disorders in young and middle-aged people. The geriatric version of the MAST (MAST-G), which asks questions relevant to an aging cohort, is 95% sensitive and 78% specific for identifying alcohol problems in older people. Other widely used questionnaires include the Alcohol Use Disorders Identification Test (AUDIT) and the Drinking Problems Index.

Biologic markers of substance use can be useful in managing patients with known substance-use disorders, but they have proved less valuable in detecting illness. These markers include γ-glutamyl transferase, which has a low sensitivity and a moderate specificity for diagnosing an alcohol-use disorder; mean corpuscular volume, which has a low sensitivity but a high specificity; and carbohydrate-deficient transferrin, which has a low sensitivity and low specificity. Further research on

these markers is needed, but clinically any combination of macrocytic anemia, thrombocytopenia, and elevated γ-glutamyl transferase should flag the need for further screening. Urine drug screens are an effective method of screening for or identifying illicit drug use as well as prescription drug use.

TREATMENT

Older adults with a substance-use problem often present with a variety of treatment needs. It is therefore important to have an array of services available for older adults that can be tailored to these individual needs and to have the flexibility to adapt to changing needs over time. The most important aspect of treating an older adult who is misusing a substance is to engage the patient in the intervention. Older adults engaged in treatment have shown very robust improvement, especially in comparison with younger cohorts. The spectrum of interventions for alcohol abuse in older adults range from prevention and education for persons who are abstinent or low-risk drinkers, to minimal advice or brief structured interventions for at-risk or problem drinkers, and formalized alcoholism treatment for drinkers who meet criteria for abuse or dependence. The array of formal treatment options available includes psychotherapy, education, rehabilitative and residential care, and psychopharmacologic agents. An example of the necessity to tailor care is the contrast between the at-risk drinker or benzodiazepine user and the severely dependent patient. It is unlikely that the at-risk user will need the intensity of services required for the severely dependent patient. Indeed, requiring the at-risk drinker to accept a set of rigorous services may be more detrimental than helpful.

Dependency on medications such as benzodiazepines is managed by placing the patient on a 24-hour equivalent of the dosage of the drug on which the patient is dependent, tapering the dosage by 10% every three half-lives, and by providing supportive counseling via groups, psychosocial support, and 12-step programs. Symptoms of withdrawal from narcotics can be controlled when necessary with oral clonidine. Assuring that the patient enters a long-term treatment program increases the likelihood of long-term success.

Because of the high prevalence of smoking-related diseases in the older population, smoking cessation is especially important and should be given the same emphasis as the treatment of other chronic diseases, such as diabetes and hypertension. For smoking cessation, it is important to prepare the patient for quitting by discussing management strategies before quitting, setting a quit date, and implementing a monitoring

Table 39.1—The CAGE Questionnaire

C	Have you ever tried to Cut down on your drinking?
A	Have you ever gotten Annoyed at someone for criticizing your drinking?
G	Do you ever feel Guilty about your drinking?
E	Have you ever had an Eye-opener to steady your nerves or get rid of a hangover?

A positive answer to one or more questions suggests problem drinking

plan for maintaining success. The rate of success in older adults has been found to parallel that in younger populations.

Detoxification and Stabilization

The assessment of any substance abuser starts with a thorough history, physical, and laboratory examination. Included in the initial assessment is an assessment of the patient's potential to suffer acute withdrawal. Severe withdrawal such as that from alcohol use can be life threatening and warrants careful attention. Patients with severe symptoms of dependency or withdrawal potential and patients with significant medical or psychiatric comorbidity may require inpatient hospitalization for acute stabilization before implementing an outpatient management strategy. Detoxification is achieved by placing the patient on the minimal amount of drug that suppresses withdrawal symptoms and then decreasing the dosage by 10% every three half-lives. In general, longer acting formulations of the drug being abused are preferred to shorter acting formulations, but many clinicians find that prescribing the specific drug that a patient was abusing makes the process more acceptable to the patient and minimizes the time needed to determine the initial dose.

For the patient hospitalized for an elective surgery or condition unrelated to the substance problem, it is extremely important to be vigilant for any evidence of withdrawal. Unrecognized alcohol withdrawal can result in serious morbidity and mortality for the elderly patient. Early symptoms include tachycardia, diaphoresis, tremulousness, and hypertension. These symptoms may progress to overt delirium, psychosis, and seizures.

Outpatient Management

Traditionally, outpatient substance-abuse treatment has been reserved for specialized clinics focused on substance abuse. It is becoming increasingly apparent that this model is inadequate in addressing the broader public health demand, and there is a need to involve a variety of clinicians and clinical settings to deliver substance-abuse treatment. This is particularly important for older adults, who frequently seek medical services but rarely seek specialized addiction services. The traditional addiction clinic is focused on supportive group psychotherapy and encouragement to attend regular self-help group meetings such as Alcoholics Anonymous, Alcoholics Victorious, Rational Recovery, or Narcotics Anonymous. For older adults, peer-specific group activities are considered superior to mixed-age group activities. Outpatient rehabilitation, in addition to focusing on active addiction issues, usually

needs to address issues of time management. Abstinence reduces the time spent in maintaining the substance-use disorder. The management of this time, which is often the greater part of a patient's day, is critical to the prognosis of treatment. Clinicians should be wary of focusing on abstinence as the only positive outcome of treatment and should commend patients for making progress in cutting down on use as well as for stopping. This may be particularly relevant for misuse of medications such as benzodiazepines, because eliminating the use may be more difficult. For benzodiazepines, the risks of adverse events such as falls are greater with higher doses and medications with a longer half-life such as diazepam or clonazepam. Therefore, using medications with a half-life of 6 to 12 hours reduces the risks for that patient. If benzodiazepines seem to be indicated for an anxiety condition and treatment is initiated for the first time, the long-acting preparations are best avoided in favor of shorter-acting agents that do not have active metabolites (eg, lorazepam). However, for patients already receiving long-acting benzodiazepines (eg, 50 mg or more per day of diazepam), the risk of withdrawal complications is increased, and therefore the dose should be reduced very gradually. If the daily dose is greater than the equivalent of 100 mg of diazepam, then the patient should be hospitalized to initiate withdrawal. Ultimately, a transition to shorter-acting agents is ideal, but this should be initiated very carefully and should involve an equivalent dose initially before any reductions are considered. The use of resources such as day programs and senior centers can be beneficial, especially for cognitively impaired patients. Social services such as financial support are often needed to stabilize the patient in early recovery. Supervised living arrangements, such as halfway houses, group homes, nursing homes, and residing with relatives, should also be considered.

Brief Interventions

Low-intensity, brief interventions have been suggested as cost-effective and practical techniques that can be used as an initial approach to at-risk and problem drinkers in primary care settings. Studies of brief intervention have been conducted in a wide range of health care settings, from hospitals and primary health care locations to mental health clinics. Two trials of brief alcohol intervention with older adults have been reported. Both studies were randomized trials of brief intervention to reduce hazardous drinking by older adults, and both used advice protocols in primary care settings. These studies have shown that older adults can be engaged in brief intervention protocols, that the protocols are acceptable in this population, and that drinking is substantially reduced among at-risk drinkers receiving the interventions compared with a control group.

Pharmacotherapy

The use of medications to support abstinence may be of benefit, but it is not well studied. Small-scale studies have demonstrated that naltrexone is well tolerated and efficacious in older patients. Studies are currently under way using various antidepressants, including the selective serotonin-reuptake inhibitors. Some of the general principles used in treating younger patients should be applied to older drinkers as well. For example, benzodiazepines are important in the treatment of alcohol detoxification, but they have no clinical place in maintaining long-term abstinence because of their abuse potential and the potential for fostering further abuse of alcohol or benzodiazepines. Disulfiram may benefit some well-motivated patients, but cardiac and hepatic disease limits its use by the older adult who abuses alcohol. The use of methadone maintenance has proven efficacy in opioid dependence. Older patients can be initiated and maintained on methadone, following the same principles of use as in younger patients. Comorbid medical and psychiatric disorders must be identified and properly treated, and they may necessitate the need for referral to, or consultation with, a psychiatrist with expertise in these areas. Buprenorphine and buprenorphine with naloxone are approved for outpatient treatment of opioid dependence. However, given the complexity of the treatment of this condition, systematic training, practice, monitoring, regulation, and evaluation are necessary in a multidisciplinary treatment setting to optimize outcomes. Guidelines for developing treatment programs using buprenorphine are available on the Web site of the Substance Abuse and Mental Health Services Administration (see http://buprenorphine.samhsa.gov/index.html).

Establishing abstinence from nicotine follows the same principles as that from other addicting substances. Initially, pharmacologic substitution with either nicotine gum or patch is followed by a gradual decrease in dosage. Several trials demonstrated that antidepressant medications improve rates of continued abstinence, but only bupropion has been approved for this purpose by the U.S. Food and Drug Administration. As with other abstinence regimens, psychotherapy plus pharmacotherapy is better than pharmacotherapy alone. See also "Respiratory Diseases and Disorders" (p 300).

REFERENCES

- Andrews JO, Heath J, Graham-Garcia J. Management of tobacco dependence in older adults: using evidence-based strategies. *J Gerontol Nurs*. 2004;30(12):13–24.

- Blow FC, Brower KJ, Schulenberg JE, et al. The Michigan Alcoholism Screening Test–Geriatric Version (MAST-G). *Alcohol Clin Exp Res*. 1992;16:372.

- Korper SP, Council CL, eds. *Substance Use by Older Adults: Estimates of Future Impact on the Treatment System* (DHHS Publication No. SMA 03-3763, Analytic Series A-21). Rockville, MD: Substance Abuse and Mental Health Services Administration, Office of Applied Studies; 2002.

- Moore AA, and the American Geriatrics Society Clinical Practice Committee. Clinical guidelines for alcohol use disorders in older adults. Updated November 2003. Available at: http://www.americangeriatrics.org./products/positionpapers/alcohol.shtml (accessed October 2005).

- Stevenson JS. Alcohol use, misuse, abuse, and dependence in later adulthood. *Annu Rev Nurs Res*. 2005;23:245–280.

CHAPTER 40—MENTAL RETARDATION

KEY POINTS

- Difficulties with behavioral problems and impairment in adaptive skills are a major problem among adults with mental retardation.

- Poor communication skills often lead to under-recognition of medical problems, which may precipitate behavioral problems.

- Menopausal symptoms should be considered when women with mental retardation exhibit behavioral changes in later life.

- Dementia of the Alzheimer's type occurs almost invariably among persons with Down syndrome, but dementia is not a necessary outcome among persons with other types of mental retardation.

Mental retardation continues to be a widely used term to describe the condition of subaverage intellectual function in the presence of deficits in adaptive behavior. Critics have attacked this definition for a variety of reasons. These include reliance on intelligence tests to demonstrate intellectual difficulties, which has been criticized because of difficulties in determining cut-off values for normality, the questionable cultural fairness of the tests, and the questionable relevance of the tests for performance in real-life situations. Similar controversies regarding the imprecision of definition and measurement of adaptive behavior remain unresolved. However, the key concept of a central, biologically based deficit in intellectual function appears to be valid; persons with mental retardation have a condition in which nearly every cognitive process that has been studied is deficient. For mild mental retardation, the same genetic and environmental influences appear to operate that determine individual differences throughout the normal range of variation in general cognitive ability. Importantly, the heritability of general cognitive ability is substantial, probably around 50%; the effects of shared environmental influences in families become negligible after adolescence, and genetic influence increases from infancy to adulthood. Persons with severe degrees of mental retardation are more likely to have structural defects of the brain or metabolic or chromosomal derangements. The challenge for the future is to determine how these biologic abnormalities interact with the aging process.

PREVALENCE

The number of aging persons with mental retardation is increasing, probably because of increased longevity. Life expectancy in mental retardation has increased from 20 years in the 1930s to 60 years in 1980. For those with Down syndrome, life expectancy has increased by about 30 years. The prevalence of mental retardation and developmental disability (cerebral palsy, autism, epilepsy) is generally assumed to be around 1%. Thus, estimates are that in the United States there are 525,000 persons aged 60 and over with these conditions, and the numbers are expected to double by 2030.

PSYCHIATRIC AND MENTAL DISORDERS IN AGING ADULTS WITH MENTAL RETARDATION

The prevalence of psychiatric disorders among adults with mental retardation is about five times that of age-matched control groups. Depending on the exact population studied and the type of diagnoses included, rates range from 10% to 40%.

Dementia

Adults with Down syndrome have an increased risk for the early onset of Alzheimer's disease, with nearly 100% developing the neuropathology by age 40. Although not all develop symptoms in their 40s, approximately 40% aged 50 and over have symptoms of dementia, with 50% developing seizures as a result of the degenerative changes. Approximately 75% of persons with Down syndrome in their 60s have symptoms of dementia (compared with a prevalence in the general population of 5% at age 65). Symptoms also include loss of adaptive skills and increased maladaptive behavior; the dementia is often associated with depression, indifference, and social inappropriateness. The average age at death for persons with Down syndrome and Alzheimer's disease is approximately 50. One study has demonstrated that in women with Down syndrome, an early age of menopause is associated with earlier dementia symptoms. Menopause may be an important factor among women with mental retardation who experience a behavioral or cognitive change in late life.

The incidence of dementia in persons with mental retardation who do not have Down syndrome is the same as in the general population; however, these persons also have a higher prevalence of the neuropathology of Alzheimer's disease: 54% for ages 50 to 65, 76% for ages 66 to 75, 87% for ages >75.

Other Major Mental Disorders

For persons with mental retardation, the lifetime prevalence of other major mental illnesses appears to be similar to or slightly higher than that of the general population. In those aged 65 and over, approximately 70% may reach criteria for a psychiatric diagnosis, often with higher rates than for a younger age group. Autistic traits are common, occurring in up to approximately half of adults with learning disability or mental retardation. These traits are more common in those with severe or profound degrees of mental retardation and in younger individuals; they are typically associated with behavioral difficulties.

Adaptive Behavioral Difficulties

Difficulties that adults with mental retardation have with adaptive behavior may be severe, and difficulties may occur with increasing frequency in later life as a consequence of cognitive decline and increasingly impaired mobility. For example, surveys concerning adults with mental retardation have revealed that 25% have no useful speech and 10% have no receptive comprehension. Half do not have basic self-care skills, half have a physical disability, and half have a mobility impairment; 10% are totally dependent. Support services for these people are usually deficient.

Behavioral Disorders

As many as 50% to 60% of adults with mental retardation have a maladaptive behavior (such as withdrawal, self-injury, stereotypy) that is severe or that occurs frequently, and follow-up studies show that these behaviors may persist for years. The proportion decreases with age, except in Down syndrome, in which the proportion is higher and the incidence of behavioral problems increases with the degree of mental retardation. Aggression occurs with similar frequency in all age groups. About half of the persons with behavioral disorders have had an experience in the preceding 12 months that may have precipitated the disorder, such as a change in environment or loss of a familiar companion.

DIAGNOSIS AND TREATMENT

The diagnosis of a mental disorder in the older adult with mental retardation is based on the same principles of history and examination that apply in the general population. However, presentations of mental illness may be different in these patients. Typically, verbal skills are poor, and reports of mood or mental experiences are difficult to obtain. Often, mental disorders present as behavioral changes, for example, social withdrawal, apathy, and vegetative changes occurring in depressed persons, or agitation, sleeplessness, or aggression in those experiencing delusions or hallucinations. It is more difficult for persons with limited coping skills to adjust to changes in living or work situations, and inquiries should be made about whether such changes have occurred.

It is important to identify the cause of the person's mental retardation. Careful physical, laboratory, and neurologic investigation (electroencephalography and neuroimaging) may establish a cause in 40%. Different conditions are associated with different problems (see Table 40.1). Elderly persons with mental retardation who have not been previously evaluated should be referred to a specialist for assessment if asymmetric neurologic signs are present, if there is a history of cognitive or neurologic deterioration, or if behavioral symptoms cannot be reversed. Medical disorders commonly present as psychiatric or behavioral disorders, and they occur in persons with mental retardation twice as commonly as in the average psychiatric population.

Maladaptive behaviors, such as aggression, are common in persons with mental retardation and may not indicate a mental disorder. An impulsive response to a stressor may reflect only suboptimal judgment in a particular situation. An appropriate treatment in such

Table 40.1—Disorders That Are Associated With Specific Types of Mental Retardation in the Older Adult

Type of Retardation	Associated Disorders
Down syndrome	Hypothyroidism, Alzheimer's disease
Fragile X syndrome	Autistic behaviors, gaze avoidance, attentional difficulty
Frontal lobe damage	Apathy, irritability, distractibility, perseveration, impulsivity
Prader-Willi syndrome	Hyperphagia, obesity, ritualistic behaviors, aggression
Temporal lobe lesions	Gastaut-Geschwind syndrome (an interictal syndrome with hypergraphia, irritability, elation, paranoia) Kluver-Bucy syndrome (hypersexuality, hyperorality, visual agnosia, diminished aggression, anxiety)

cases would be instructional or behavioral; the preferred behavior programs are ones that reward good behavior. A disorder of impulse control, however, may also produce aggressive responses; diagnosis of such a disorder requires a pattern of impulsivity that is disproportionate to the degree of intellectual impairment. With an impulse-control disorder, aggression may be preceded by a period of increasing tension and arousal, occur explosively and out of proportion to the stressor, and seem to have a driven, sustained nature. Appropriate treatment would consist of instructional and behavioral methods, but also with pharmacologic interventions to reduce impulsivity (eg, selective serotonin-reuptake inhibitors[OL]) or arousal (eg, β-blockers[OL]). Pharmacologic treatment of aggression is similar to that in the general population and includes the use of mood stabilizers[OL], selective serotonin-reuptake inhibitors[OL], β-blockers[OL], and antipsychotic medications[OL].

The diagnosis of dementia among persons with mental retardation is made according to the same criteria as in the general population. These criteria include the presence of cognitive and adaptive deterioration; demonstration of deficits on examination (preferably with longitudinal follow-up showing progression of deficits); and exclusion of other possible causes of deterioration, such as medical or environmental factors, or other mental disorders, such as depression or delirium. Standardized scales are available that help structure the interview and history and produce a score that indicates the likelihood that dementia is present and its severity. The Washington University Clinical Dementia Rating Scale that is widely used with the general population can also be used in many individuals with mental retardation. Neuroimaging studies may be helpful in establishing the diagnosis and in differentiating Alzheimer's disease from vascular dementia; longitudinal and volumetric studies may help differentiate normal aging from dementia. There are insufficient

[OL] Not approved by the U.S. Food and Drug Administration for this use.

studies to demonstrate the efficacy of standard treatments (such as donepezil) in persons with mental retardation.

MEDICAL DISORDERS

Adults with mental retardation have more medical problems than do age-matched persons (approximately five medical conditions per person; those with more severe mental retardation have more problems). Approximately two thirds of those in a community setting have chronic conditions or major physical disability. It is estimated that 50% of these medical conditions go undetected. Prompt detection and treatment is associated with better survival. Visual or hearing impairments are more common in persons with mental retardation; they increase with age and affect approximately 25%.

Persons with Down syndrome and others with mental retardation have similar age-specific mortality until ages 30 to 34, after which there is an exponential increase in mortality with age for those with Down syndrome, probably because of the onset of dementia. Life expectancy decreases with increasing severity of mental retardation, and with other morbidity such as inability to ambulate, lack of feeding skills, and incontinence. Life expectancy for adults with mental retardation is lower than for the general population and is about 65 years. The commonest causes of death are cardiovascular and respiratory disorders, cancer, and dementia (particularly in Down syndrome).

SOCIAL CONDITIONS

At least 80% of adults with mental retardation live at home and are cared for by aging family members; 20% live in residential programs. It is estimated that about 40% of eligible persons may not be served by the formal service system. This situation often leads to a crisis when the parent is no longer able to provide adequate care or is unable to manage a behavioral problem. It is estimated that about half of developmentally disabled adults with a behavior problem need a different living arrangement. Typically, more than half of the families have not made plans for the future care of adult relatives with mental retardation; those in day programs or workshops do not typically have pensions or Social Security benefits to allow retirement. Not surprisingly, the degree of mental retardation, physical health, and functional skills of the aging person correlate with the degree of parental stress and burden, although maternal and family characteristics such as education and income are more correlated with overall life satisfaction and maternal well-being.

REFERENCES

■ Bosch JJ. Health maintenance throughout the life span for individuals with Down syndrome. *J Am Acad Nurse Pract.* 2003;15(1):5–17.

■ Melville CA, Finlayson J, Cooper S, et al. Enhancing primary health care services for adults with intellectual disabilities. *J Intellect Dis Res.* 2005;49(Part 3):190–198.

■ Powrie E. Primary health care provision for adults with a learning disability. *J Adv Nurs.* 2003;42(4):413–423.

■ Ryan R, Sunada K. Medical evaluation of persons with mental retardation referred for psychiatric assessment. *Gen Hosp Psychiatry.* 1997;19(4):274–280.

■ Sutherland G, Couch MA, Iacono T. Health issues for adults with developmental disability. *Res Dev Disabil.* 2002;23(6):422–445.

DISEASES AND DISORDERS

CHAPTER 41—DERMATOLOGIC DISEASES AND DISORDERS

KEY POINTS

- Seborrheic dermatitis and rosacea are chronic conditions that can be suppressed, but not entirely eliminated.

- Neurodermatitis, or lichen simplex chronicus, occurs most commonly in the age group over 60 years old.

- Stasis dermatitis is most commonly caused by incompetency of venous valves and is best treated by control of venous hypertension.

- Most lower extremity chronic ulcers are caused by venous insufficiency.

- The risk of metastasis from squamous cell carcinoma increases with the size of the lesion, depth of invasion, lack of differentiation, and location of the lesion.

Skin disease increases with aging and sun exposure. Dermatologic care of the older patient requires an awareness of cutaneous changes of aging and the effects of cumulative ultraviolet (UV) radiation exposure, as well as knowledge of the common tumors, inflammatory diseases, and infections seen in older persons.

AGING AND PHOTOAGING

Skin is composed of the epidermis, dermis, basement membrane zone (the area between the epidermis and dermis that serves to hold the two together), and the subcutaneous fat. In normal young skin the epidermis interdigitates with the dermis. Over time these interdigitations are flattened, with decreased contact between the epidermis and dermis. This results in decreased nutrient transfer and increased skin fragility. There is also a change with age in the barrier function because fewer lipids are present in the top layer of the skin, leading to dryness and roughness. The turnover of epidermal cells is slower and may account for the decrease in the rate of wound healing. In aging skin, there is a decrease in the number of immune antigen-presenting cells, such as Langerhans cells, which may have consequences for cutaneous immune surveillance. Changes in the dermis, such as decreased ground substance, correlate with wrinkling and atrophy of the skin in the older person. A decrease in the amount of collagen and elastin is associated with striking changes in fiber orientation, notably a fragmented and more haphazard architecture.

Changes in hair in the older person include graying of hairs that is due to changes in follicular melanocytes, and a decrease in scalp hair density secondary to shortening of anagen (the growth phase of the hair cycle) duration and an increase in the proportion of hairs in telogen (the resting phase).

Photoaging refers to the effects of UV exposure on skin. The depth of penetration of UV light depends on the wavelength, and shorter wavelengths are more biologically active. Ultraviolet B (UVB; 290 to 320 nm) radiation causes most of the acute and chronic damage. Ultraviolet A (UVA; 320 to 400 nm) also plays an important role because it makes up more of the sunlight that reaches the earth's surface and has greater depth of penetration. Mechanisms by which UV light causes changes in the skin probably include DNA injury or decreased DNA repair or both, oxidative damage, lysosomal damage, and altered collagen structure.

Photodamaged skin appears wrinkled, coarse, or rough, and it has mottled pigmentation (due to solar lentigos, seborrheic keratoses, and ephelides or freckles), hypopigmentation, and telangiectasias. Cutaneous malignancies are also more common in photodamaged skin. Prevention of photodamage involves the use of broad-spectrum sunscreens—sunscreens that protect against both UVB and UVA radiation—as well as the avoidance of direct sunlight and use of protective clothing along with hats and sunglasses. Although there are claims that various topical agents decrease photodamage, only topical tretinoin has been shown to increase the thickness of the superficial skin layers, reduce pigmentary changes and roughness, and increase collagen synthesis.

Surgical therapies are used to treat photodamage through controlled partial injury to the skin. These include chemical peeling agents, dermabrasion, and laser resurfacing. All rely on the destruction of surface populations of keratinocytes, followed by repopulation with keratinocytes deep from within the sun-protected follicular structures. Controlled trials to evaluate the effectiveness of these expensive modalities are rare and inconclusive.

SEBORRHEIC DERMATITIS

Seborrheic dermatitis is a common chronic dermatitis that is characterized by symmetric erythema and greasy-looking scales in areas rich in sebaceous glands, such as the hairline (scalp), forehead, nasolabial fold, and the retroauricular and midline chest areas. Dandruff may be an early precursor of this condition. The prevalence of seborrheic dermatitis is higher in persons infected with human immunodeficiency virus (HIV) and those with Parkinson's disease. At all ages, seborrheic dermatitis is more common in males than females.

Although the cause of seborrheic dermatitis is unclear, it is thought that the normal yeast flora (*Malassezia furfur*) play some role in inducing inflammation of the skin, which leads to increased epidermal proliferation and desquamation. The name is misleading, and patients affected with seborrheic dermatitis do not have more seborrhea than the normal population. On the face, it can involve only the eyebrows, glabella, and nasolabial folds, or it can cause a mild blepharitis with red eyelid margins. It should be stressed to patients that seborrheic dermatitis can be suppressed but not cured. It is often treated with medicated shampoos that act against yeast, including selenium sulfide, ketoconazole, and various tar shampoos. Acute forms can also be treated with mild topical corticosteroids such as hydrocortisone 1% to 2%. Once the dermatitis is under control, patients can use the medicated shampoos for maintenance.

ROSACEA

Rosacea (Figure 41.1) is a common condition in fair-skinned persons and affects young to middle-aged as well as elderly persons. The cause of rosacea remains elusive; recurrent facial flushing resulting from a variety of stimuli is a common symptom. The flushing is often induced by sunlight exposure, alcohol, hot beverages, and drugs that cause vasodilatation. Medications such as oral niacin (for hyperlipidemia) and topical steroids can often induce or worsen rosacea. Rosacea has several variants, each of which requires a different approach to treatment. Usually the central convex areas of the face are affected (nose, forehead, cheeks, and chin) with erythema and telangiectasias. More advanced cases show follicular and nonfollicular papules and pustules. Recurrent flushing and edema cause thickening of the skin; in the most severe cases a rhinophyma may develop. Rosacea can also involve the eye, causing irritation and burning that may present as conjunctival injection, blepharitis, episcleritis, chalazion, or hordeolum. Often, rosacea and seborrheic dermatitis coexist.

The treatment of rosacea is based on the clinical picture. It is important for patients to understand that it is a chronic condition with frequent flares. They should be educated on avoiding skin irritants or strong soaps and cleansers, and instructed to reduce sun exposure and regularly apply sunscreens. Oral antibiotics such as tetracylines (doxycycline, minocycline) and erythromycin are used to treat the moderate to severe papular-pustular rosacea. Topical agents such as azelaic acid cream, erythromycin, clindamycin, and metronidazole can be

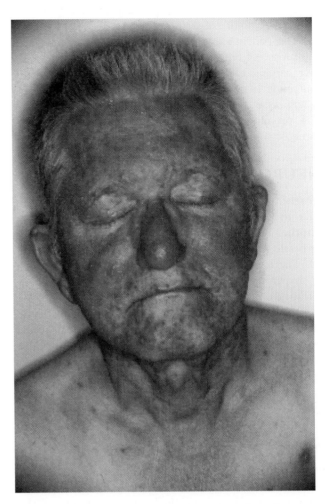

Figure 41.1—Rosacea. Diffuse erythema and erythematous papules and papulopustules are seen on the cheeks, forehead, and chin. The nose shows thickening of the skin and changes consistent with an early rhinophyma.

used for mild rosacea or as maintenance once the oral antibiotics have been tapered. Severe or refractory rosacea can be treated with oral isotretinoin. Lasers, such as the potassium-titanyl-phosphate (KTP) laser, intense pulsed light and the pulsed dye laser, can be used to reduce the redness and improve cosmetic appearance. Rhinophyma occurs less commonly and can be treated with surgical excision or CO_2 laser ablation.

XEROSIS

Dryness of the skin, often a concern for the older patient, is due to the reduction in water content and barrier function of the aging epidermis. It is exacerbated by environmental factors, such as decreased humidity from cold weather or central heating, irritation by hot water, and too frequent washing with harsh soaps and cleansers. Skin findings are often more pronounced on the legs. Depending on the severity of the dryness, xerosis can present as rough, itchy skin or as scales that give the skin a dry, cracked appearance known as *eczema craquelé* (Figure 41.2).

The patient's awareness of exacerbating factors and regular use of tepid showers and emollients immediately after bathing can be quite helpful. Moisturizing agents containing lactic acid or α-hydroxy acids can reduce the roughness and scaliness. When irritation or inflammation is a prominent finding, episodic use of mild topical corticosteroids for a short time provides relief.

NEURODERMATITIS

Neurodermatitis is a nonspecific term that is used to refer to chronic, pruritic conditions of unclear cause. Another term commonly used is *lichen simplex chronicus.* It is most common in adults over the age of 60. The lesions show signs of chronic scratching, such as hyperpigmentation and lichenification (leathery thickness) along with redness and scaling. Scratching these lesions often leads to pleasure and a vicious cycle of skin changes that then induce more pruritus. Treatment consists of potent topical corticosteroids, often under occlusion, emollients, as well as behavior modification. Other causes of pruritus such as irritant or allergic contact dermatitis, drug allergy, or xerosis must be excluded.

STASIS DERMATITIS

Stasis dermatitis can be an early sign of chronic venous insufficiency of the lower extremities. Chronic venous hypertension, caused mostly by incompetency of the venous valves, is the initial trigger for stasis dermatitis. Venous hypertension slows down the flow of blood in the microvasculature, damages the permeability barrier of the small vessels, and allows for the passage of fluid

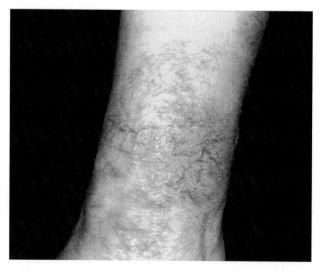

Figure 41.2—Eczema craquelé. Dry, erythematous, fissured, and cracked skin is seen on the lower legs of this patient.

and plasma proteins into the tissue, leading to the edema and extravasation of erythrocytes. These processes lead to decreased oxygen diffusion and metabolic exchange and to activation and attraction of inflammatory cells and mediators to the site. Stasis dermatitis typically occurs in the medial supramalleolar areas. It is often associated with intense pruritus. Initially, pitting edema to the ankle is noted, which is often worse at night. Over time, these events lead to the progressive induration and adherence of the skin and subcutaneous tissues. Venous ulcers can develop spontaneously or secondary to trauma, arising most often in the supramalleolar areas.

The goal of therapy is to control the venous hypertension with the regular use of compression bandages or stockings and exercising the calf muscles to improve venous return. Topical treatment includes the judicious use of corticosteroids and emollients. Sensitization to ingredients in topical medications and emollients, including topical antibiotics, is commonly encountered but frequently overlooked. Patch testing to exclude contact sensitization to these agents should be considered before use.

VENOUS AND ARTERIAL ULCERS

An ulcer is a wound with loss of epidermal and dermal layers, in contrast to an erosion, which is loss of the epidermal layer only. Chronic leg wounds are defined as open wounds that fail to heal within a period of 6 weeks. Venous disease causes 72% of leg ulcers, 22% have a mixed arterial and venous etiology, and only 6% are due to pure arterial disease. (See Table 41.1.)

To achieve healing of arterial ulcers, changes in life style such as increasing exercise, following a diet low in cholesterol, ceasing smoking, losing weight, and achieving better diabetic control should be encouraged. Oral systemic agents that have hematologic effects such as pentoxifylline[OL] or cilostazol[OL] or antiplatelet medications such as aspirin[OL] and clopidogrel[OL] can be used, although their effectiveness has not been proven to decrease the risk of thrombotic events or accelerate the healing of existing ulcers. Occlusive dressings can be used to help the wound heal; the type of dressing used depends on the ulcer type and amount of drainage. Debridement of necrotic and fibrinous debris is key to the healing process and can be achieved by mechanical or chemical methods. Vascular bypass surgery or angioplasty may be necessary to provide revascularization. Other surgical measures such as pinch grafts, split thickness skin grafts, or allografts can be used to cover a wound. Tissue-engineered skin such as Apligraf (composed of an epidermal layer of keratinocytes derived from human

---

[OL] Not approved by the U.S. Food and Drug Administration for this use.

Table 41.1—The Characteristics of Venous and Arterial Ulcers

	Venous Disease	Arterial Disease
Signs and symptoms	Limb heaviness, aching and swelling that is associated with standing and is worse at end of day	Claudication (pain in leg with walking), poor peripheral pulses, sluggish capillary refill
Risk factors	Age, obesity, history of deep-vein thrombosis or phlebitis	Age > 40, cigarette smoking, diabetes mellitus, hyperlipidemia, hypertension, male gender, sedentary life style
Location of ulcers	Along the course of the long saphenous vein, between the lower medial calf to just below the medial malleolus	Over bony prominences

neonatal foreskin and a dermal layer containing bovine type I collagen and with cultured human fibroblasts) has been shown to shorten healing time.

PRESSURE ULCERS

See "Pressure Ulcers" (p 238).

INTERTRIGO

Intertrigo (Figure 41.3) is more common in older persons because of the increased skin folds secondary to decreased dermal elasticity; environmental factors such as decreased mobility, moisture, friction, and poor hygiene also contribute. Diabetic and obese patients are more prone to develop intertrigo.

Commonly involved areas, such as the inframammary abdominal folds, groin, and axillae, will appear erythematous, macerated, moist, and mildly malodorous. Often there is secondary candidal or mixed bacterial colonization. Frequent airing, keeping involved areas dry, and using topical antifungal powders and creams, such as 2% miconazole powder or nystatin cream, constitute the treatment. Occasionally, a very mild topical corticosteroid such as 1% to 2% hydrocortisone is needed for a short period to reduce inflammation and irritation. (See also the section, p 298, on candidiasis.)

BULLOUS PEMPHIGOID

Most cases of bullous pemphigoid (Figure 41.4) occur in patients in their 60s and 70s. This is a chronic autoimmune blistering disorder characterized by large tense blisters on normal or erythematous skin. The blisters heal without scar formation. They are usually filled with clear fluid but on occasion may be hemorrhagic and can be found anywhere on the body. Mucous membranes are involved in up to a third of patients and show erosions or blisters on the mucosa. In some cases there is intense pruritus, and instead of blisters, one may find urticarial lesions. Systemic medications such as diuretics, analgesics, antibiotics, and

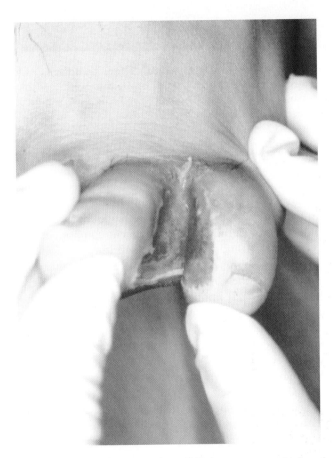

Figure 41.3—Intertrigo and candidiasis are commonly found in the web space between the 4th and 5th toes. Moist erythema, maceration, and superficial erosion is apparent.

angiotensin-converting enzyme inhibitors can lead to the development of bullous pemphigoid.

The antibodies directed against bullous pemphigoid are antigens in the hemidesmosomes (proteinaceous plaques that help the epidermis adhere to the basement membrane). The cause of antibody formation is still unclear. It is thought that the antibodies bind to the bullous pemphigoid antigen, which then activates the complement cascade. The activated complement components then attract leukocytes and cause degranulation of mast cells, and proteases from these cells cause separation of the epidermis from the basement membrane.

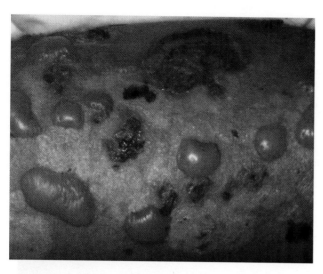

Figure 41.4—Bullous pemphigoid. Tense, fluid-filled, and hemorrhagic bullae on an erythematous base were seen on the trunk and extremities. Some of the bullae have ruptured and left a scab with crusting.

Diagnosis is clinical and confirmed by biopsy and immunofluorescence studies. On histopathology, one sees that the blister occurs below the epidermis. Direct immunofluorescence reveals immunoreactants in a linear pattern at the basement membrane between the epidermis and dermis. The complement component C3 is detected in almost all patients, and immunoglobulin G is found in most patients. One can also measure antibodies to the basement membrane antigens in sera through indirect immunofluorescence; however, the antibody titer does not correlate with disease activity.

Though it may last for months to years, bullous pemphigoid is often a self-limited disease. Treatment depends on severity. When the lesions are localized, they may be treated with topical corticosteroids. More extensive disease can be treated with oral corticosteroids, especially for control of acute flares. Because of the adverse effects of corticosteroids, particularly in older persons, other immunosuppressive, steroid-sparing agents, such as azathioprine or cyclophosphamide, are usually added as steroids are tapered. Combination therapy with tetracylines and niacinamide has been shown to be effective.

PRURITUS

Pruritus, a very common skin complaint, is associated with many cutaneous and systemic conditions. In older persons pruritus at times can be very severe, compromising quality of life. Although xerosis is the most common cause of pruritus in the older patient, it is important to perform a complete history and examination to exclude skin conditions such as scabies, allergic, irritant or atopic dermatitis, or bullous pemphigoid.

Systemic diseases such as renal disease, cholestasis or chronic liver disease, thyroid disease, anemia, occult malignancies, or drug side effects must also be considered. Generalized pruritus can also be associated with generalized anxiety disorder, depression, and even psychosis, including delusions of parasitosis.

Treatment depends on the underlying cause; symptomatic relief can often be achieved with topical corticosteroids, emollients, or menthol in calamine preparations. Oral antihistamines should be used with caution in older persons. For severe, refractory cases, UVB phototherapy has been used.

PSORIASIS

Psoriasis (Figure 41.5) affects 2% of the population and has bimodal incidences: one in the mid-20s and the other at about 50 to 60 years of age. There is a genetic predisposition, with multigene mode of inheritance, and environmental factors also play a role in triggering the disease.

The skin findings in psoriasis are rather characteristic: well-demarcated erythematous papules and plaques with overlying silvery scale. Extensor surfaces, areas prone to trauma, scalp, and nails are commonly involved. Various forms of psoriasis exist:

- inverse pattern, where lesions occur in skin folds, such as the neck, axillae, and genital area;
- guttate, where small 1-cm papules appear over the upper trunk and proximal extremities, usually after an infection;
- pustular, which is acute with generalized eruption of 2- to 3-mm sterile pustules and fever;
- palmoplantar; and
- erythrodermic psoriasis, in which the patient has generalized erythema.

Various factors may trigger psoriasis. Physical trauma (known as Koebner's phenomenon), infections, stress, medications (oral corticosteroids, lithium, β-blockers, angiotensin-converting enzyme inhibitors, as well as nonsteroidal anti-inflammatory drugs) have been shown to initiate or exacerbate psoriasis. Five percent to 30% of patients with psoriasis also suffer from psoriatic arthritis, which is characterized by pain, swelling, and stiffness in the small joints. Some patients may also suffer from spondylitis or sacroiliitis.

Several treatment options are available for patients with psoriasis, but each method must be evaluated in terms of risks and benefits for the older patient. Topical treatments such as corticosteroids, vitamin D derivatives (calcipotriene), topical retinoids (tazarotene), salicylic acid, or tar compounds may be sufficient to treat and control mild plaque psoriasis. Some of these treatments

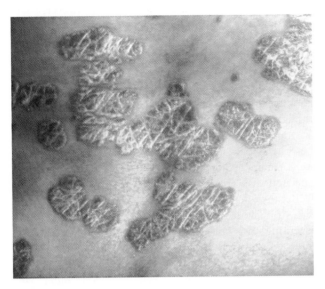

Figure 41.5—Psoriasis. Characteristic well-demarcated beefy red plaques with overlying silvery-white scales are evident on the back of this patient.

may be irritating or messy to apply. Long-term use of topical corticosteroids is limited by the cutaneous atrophy and decreased potency (tachyphylaxis) that occur over time. Patients who do not improve with topical treatments may be candidates for systemic treatment, such as phototherapy or immunosuppressive agents. UV therapy, including PUVA (psoralen with UVA light) and UVB therapies, can be adjunctive treatment along with topical agents; several treatments per week may be required. Patients with longstanding psoriasis who receive phototherapy must be carefully examined for skin cancer. Agents such as cyclosporine and methotrexate are quite effective in treating psoriasis. However, each of these medications has significant side effects that require careful monitoring through laboratory tests and physical examinations. In addition to drug interactions, systemic illnesses such as poor kidney function, hypertension, and lung disease may limit the use of these medications. As the pathophysiology of psoriasis is elucidated, newer and more effective therapies that target specific cytokines and T-lymphocyte surface molecules and that inhibit signaling are showing promise. One such drug, etanercept, a TNF antagonist, has been approved for the treatment of moderate to severe chronic plaque psoriasis.

ONYCHOMYCOSIS

See "Diseases and Disorders of the Foot" (p 416).

HERPES ZOSTER

More than two thirds of reported cases of herpes zoster (Figure 41.6) occur in persons aged 50 years and older. The incidence of herpes zoster is 20 to 100

times higher in immunosuppressed patients than in other groups, and the severity and likelihood of recurrence is also higher. Patients with herpes zoster are contagious to those who lack immunity, but less so than patients with varicella. Patients with uncomplicated dermatomal zoster spread infection by means of direct contact with their lesions, whereas patients with disseminated zoster may also transmit infection in aerosol and thus need respiratory isolation.

The pathogenesis of zoster is due to the passage of the varicella zoster virus (VZV) from skin and mucosal surfaces into sensory nerves and then into sensory ganglia, where latent infection is established. Although reactivation is associated with several immunosuppressive conditions, such as HIV infection, malignancy, or the use of immunosuppressive drugs or corticosteroids, the most important is the senescence of the cellular immune response to VZV with increasing age. (See Table 44.1, p 305.) These settings lead to reactivation of the virus, with the neuronal necrosis and inflammation that account for the severe neuralgia. The infection spreads down the sensory nerve and is released around the sensory nerve endings in the skin, producing the characteristic lesions: a cluster of vesicles on an erythematous base in a dermatomal pattern that is unilateral and does not cross the midline. Patients often complain of symptoms of pain, burning, paresthesias, tenderness, pruritus, or hyperesthesia several days before the rash appears. The vesicles turn into pustules and eventually crust over in 7 to 10 days.

Ten percent to 15% of cases of herpes zoster involve the ophthalmic branch of the trigeminal nerve. Involvement of the nasociliary branch, which presents as vesicles on the tip of the nose (known as Hutchinson's sign), requires careful ophthalmic exami-

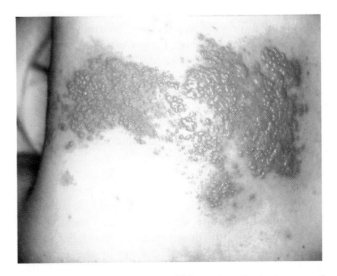

Figure 41.6—Herpes zoster. This patient had clusters of vesicles and pustules on an erythematous base involving a thoracic dermatome.

nation to monitor for complications, such as neurotrophic keratitis and ulceration, scleritis, or uveitis. Involvement of the facial or auditory nerves that presents as herpes zoster of the external ear or tympanic membrane leads to facial palsy with or without tinnitus, vertigo, and deafness. This is known as Ramsay Hunt syndrome. Another complication is secondary bacterial infection. Pain is a chief complaint of patients with zoster; it can precede, be concomitant with, or persist after the rash. Pain that persists or appears after the rash has healed or at 30 days after onset of rash is called *post-herpetic neuralgia*. Age is the most significant risk factor, and post-herpetic neuralgia occurs in 70% of zoster patients aged 70 and older. It is often difficult to treat.

Although the symptoms of herpes zoster can be confused with a variety of conditions causing localized pain (eg, pleurisy, myocardial infarction, renal colic, cholecystitis, and glaucoma), the lesions and their distribution make the diagnosis rather easy. However, it is very difficult, if not impossible in some situations, to differentiate herpes simplex from zoster. In both infections, a Tzanck smear from the base of vesicle (stained with either hematoxylin-eosin, Giemsa, or Papanicolaou) shows multinucleated giant cells and epithelial cells containing intranuclear inclusion bodies. A smear from the base of the vesicle can be sent for direct fluorescent antibody staining. This test can differentiate between herpes simplex virus and the VZV. Definitive diagnosis is made by viral culture; however, isolation of the virus can be difficult.

If the patient's immunity is intact, herpes zoster is usually self-limited. Treatment in all patients should be initiated early, within 72 hours of the onset of rash. Acyclovir is effective, and in patients aged 50 years and older it is dosed at 800 mg five times a day for 7 to 10 days; the dosage should be adjusted if renal function is decreased. Valacyclovir or famciclovir are prodrugs of acyclovir that provide greater oral bioavailability and allow less frequent dosing. Early treatment halts progression of disease, increases the rate of clearance of virus from vesicles, decreases the incidence of visceral and cutaneous dissemination, decreases the ocular complications when the eye is involved, and in some cases it may decrease pain and the incidence of post-herpetic neuralgia. Wet compresses and topical antibiotics such as bacitracin or mupirocin can treat secondary bacterial infection.

There is no definitive treatment for post-herpetic neuralgia. Narcotics, nonsteroidal anti-inflammatory drugs, epidural injection of local anesthetics, glucocorticoids, low-dose tricyclic antidepressants, capsaicin, and acupuncture are some of the therapies that are mentioned in literature. Debate over the efficacy of corticosteroids given with antiviral therapy has been fueled by two large randomized controlled trials that reached opposite conclusions. However, risks do not appear to be significantly increased with the use of corticosteroids for zoster, especially when used with antiviral therapy, and the steroids may decrease the acute neuropathic pain and reduce pain medication requirements. Pregabalin and gabapentin are non-narcotic analgesics labeled for use in post-herpetic neuralgia. Capsaicin, an extract of hot chili peppers that depletes substance P, is the only compound labeled for use in post-herpetic neuralgia. Unfortunately, many patients cannot tolerate the burning associated with this topical medication.

Because definitive treatment for post-herpetic neuralgia is lacking, efforts have been directed toward preventing this debilitating complication of herpes zoster. Zostavax (zoster vaccine live) received FDA approval in 2006 for use in the prevention of herpes zoster in individuals 60 years old and older. In placebo-controlled studies, Zostavax significantly reduced the risk of developing herpes zoster. Its effectiveness is believed to be related to the documented "boost" it gives to the cellular response to VZV. Its benefit with regard to prevention of post-herpetic neuralgia is directly related to its effect on the prevention of herpes zoster.

CANDIDIASIS

Factors that contribute to intertrigo also predispose a person to candidiasis. (See the section, p 287, on intertrigo.) Involved areas appear clinically similar to intertrigo, but there may be peripheral satellite pustules. Candida pustules can also occur on the backs of bedridden patients and on other areas prone to moisture and occlusion. Oral thrush may also develop in patients on corticosteroid inhalers, antibiotics, or immunosuppressive medications or with concomitant systemic illnesses, such as diabetes mellitus. To confirm the diagnosis, a KOH preparation of scrapings of the involved site is performed. The presence of spores and pseudohyphae is consistent with candidiasis.

Treatment resembles that of intertrigo: keeping the moist areas dry, improving hygiene, and treating with topical or oral treatment with anticandidal agents such as nystatin or ketoconazole.

SCABIES

Scabies refers to infestation with the human mite *Sarcoptes scabiei*. It is spread by person-to-person contact and is common in institutionalized older persons. Epidemics are described in long-term-care facilities, and eradication can be difficult. The adult female mite becomes fertilized on skin and burrows into the top superficial layer, where she lays eggs. The clinical manifestations occur days to weeks later when the patient develops hypersensitivity reaction to the mite saliva and excretions. Therefore, it is often difficult to pinpoint the initial infested patient, and spreading of mites may have occurred before diagnosis.

Infested patients complain of severe pruritus, especially of the hands, axillae, genitalia, and peri-umbilical region. Clinically one finds erythematous papules and occasionally nodules along with linear burrows (crooked, raised lines). The patient may have scratched to the point of causing bleeding or weeping eczematous lesions. Scabies should be suspected in anyone who complains of pruritus or displays signs of excoriation. Diagnosis is confirmed by performing a scraping on a suspected lesion and finding mite excreta, eggs, or, rarely, the mite itself, under the microscope.

Treatment of scabies is often initiated when there is strong clinical suspicion of infestation. Treatment involves eradicating the mite, decreasing the pruritus, and treating any contacts. Topical permethrin 5% is most commonly used. It is applied from the neck to the toes and rinsed off after 8 to 12 hours. This treatment should be repeated in 1 week to prevent development of resistance. Persons who may have been exposed should also be treated. Topical corticosteroids may help to reduce pruritus, but it is important to reassure patients that the itching may persist for weeks or months. Cleaning the bedding, clothes, and towels (bath, linen) with hot water is sufficient to eradicate the mite from the surroundings.

There have been reports in the literature of treating scabies effectively with an oral dose of an antihelminthic agent called ivermectin (250 to 400 µg per kg) that is repeated in a week. However, there are no long-term studies, and it is not yet approved for this use by the U.S. Food and Drug Administration.

LOUSE INFESTATIONS

Lice can infest the body (pediculosis corporis), scalp (pediculosis capitis), or pubic hair (pediculosis pubis). With pediculosis corporis or capitis, lice are spread from person to person through physical contact or fomites. Pediculosis pubis is usually spread by sexual contact. In all cases, patients complain of pruritus of the involved areas, and there can be secondary infection. In cases of pediculosis corporis, the lice feed on the body but live on clothing, where they lay eggs, often near the seams. In cases of pediculosis capitis, the lice lay eggs on the proximal part of the hair shaft. The eggs (or nits) are visible as white specks cemented to the hair at an oblique angle. Patients with pediculosis pubis also have nits on the pubic hair and commonly have more organisms.

Treatment involves eradicating the lice and larvae, treating close contacts, and treating the secondary infection. Pyrethrin or its derivatives (permethrin) are ovicidal and can be used as single 10-minute topical

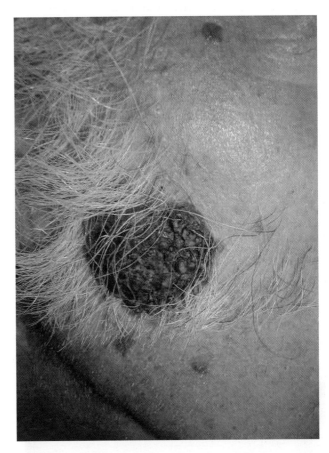

Figure 41.7—Seborrheic keratoses. These lesions present as waxy, warty stuck-on papules in a variety of colors.

treatment for patients and those who have been exposed. Combs, brushes, hats, clothing, bedding, and towels (bath, linen) must be washed with hot water.

BENIGN GROWTHS

Seborrheic Keratoses

Seborrheic keratoses (Figure 41.7) are very common benign growths that present as tan to gray or black waxy or warty papules and plaques. They commonly occur on the trunk and extremities but can be found anywhere on the body. Occasionally some lesions may be darkly pigmented, and differentiation from a melanoma may be difficult without a biopsy. These growths are irksome to patients and can be removed with cryosurgery or shave excision if necessary.

Cherry Angiomas

Cherry angiomas are the most common acquired cutaneous vascular proliferations. They usually appear in persons in their 20s and increase in number over time. Clinically they appear as round to oval, bright red, dome-shaped papules ranging in size from less than 1 mm to several millimeters. Cherry angiomas are benign but can bleed when traumatized. Removal of these lesions can be achieved with excision, electrodessication, or laser ablation.

Actinic Keratoses

Actinic keratoses (also known as *solar keratoses*) are lesions caused by chronic UV radiation (Figure 41.8) that occur in fair-skinned persons. They are considered premalignant growths, precursors of squamous cell carcinoma. It is unclear how many progress to squamous cell carcinoma; reports vary from 0.24% to 20%. They appear as poorly circumscribed, occasionally scaly, erythematous macules and papules on sun-exposed areas, such as the face, ears, and dorsum of hands and arms. Some may have an overlying thick, hard growth known as a *cutaneous horn*. Lesions on the lips are called *actinic cheilitis*.

Actinic keratoses are most often treated to prevent progression to squamous cell carcinoma but also to decrease discomfort. They respond to a variety of treatments, such as cryotherapy with liquid nitrogen,

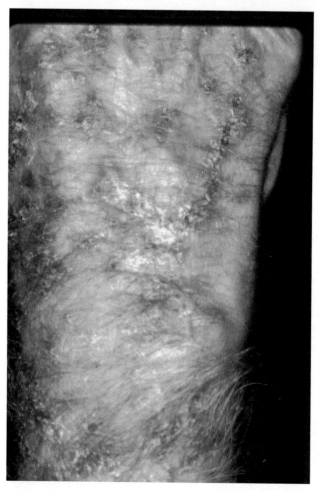

Figure 41.8—Actinic keratoses are rough, scaly, red-brown macules on sun-exposed skin and are premalignant.

topical agents such as chemical acids, 5-fluorouracil, immunomodulators such as imiquimod [OL], or excision. Although treating the lesions with liquid nitrogen for 10 to 15 seconds is very effective, it can be somewhat uncomfortable and can cause pigmentary changes. When there are several lesions in an area, treatment that the patient can perform at home, such as topical 5-fluorouracil or imiquimod, is helpful because it can also treat subclinical lesions. However, patients must be monitored and warned about the bright erythema and discomfort that can occur with these treatments.

SQUAMOUS CELL CARCINOMA

Squamous cell carcinoma is the second most common form of skin cancer. It affects patients in mid- to late life and occurs most commonly on chronically sun-exposed areas. Squamous cell carcinomas cause local tissue destruction if not treated and have a low risk (but greater risk than basal cell carcinomas) to metastasize. The risk of metastases and recurrence increases with the size of the tumor (greater than 2 cm), poor differentiation, and increased depth of invasion. Squamous cell carcinoma also tends to behave more aggressively when it occurs on sites such as the lip and ear. These tumors present as chronic erythematous papules, plaques, or nodules with scaling, crusting, or ulceration. They also have a propensity to occur in longstanding nonhealing wounds and in burn and radiation scars.

Treatment consists of surgical excision. In cosmetically important areas or with aggressive tumors, Mohs micrographic surgery is performed. In patients who are poor surgical candidates or who have multiple comorbidities, destruction with cryotherapy or local radiation has been used.

BASAL CELL CARCINOMA

Basal cell carcinoma is the most common cancer in the United States. As with other cutaneous malignancies, fair-skinned persons with chronic sun exposure are at risk. It presents in three major clinical patterns:

- nodular—this is the most common variant and appears as a waxy, translucent papule with overlying telangiectasias;
- morpheaform—this has a scar-like appearance and can look atrophic;
- superficial—this appears as an erythematous macule or papule with fine scale or superficial erosion.

Some basal cell carcinomas appear as superficial ulcers with characteristic rolled borders (Figure 41.9).

OL Not approved by the U.S. Food and Drug Administration for this use.

Others may be pigmented and confused for melanoma, especially in darker skinned individuals.

Treatment of basal cell carcinoma is surgical excision. Some basal cell carcinomas, particularly those located in cosmetically important areas, those that are nodular or morpheaform, and those that are recurrent should be excised by use of Mohs micrographic surgery to ensure adequate excision and tissue sparing. Like squamous cell carcinomas, basal cell carcinomas occurring in poor surgical candidates can also be treated with ablative methods, such as cryosurgery, radiation, and curettage with electrodessication.

MELANOMA

The incidence of melanoma continues to increase, and it affects all adult age groups. The risk factors for melanoma include very fair skin type, family history, dysplastic or numerous nevi, and sunlight exposure, particularly intermittent blistering sunburns in childhood. Melanomas are usually asymptomatic; thus, regular skin examinations and early recognition are key for favorable prognosis.

A new pigmented skin lesion or a change in the color, size, surface, or borders of a preexisting mole should be suspected for melanoma and biopsied. A useful mnemonic is ABCD: **A**symmetry, **B**orders, **C**olor, **D**iameter. There are four clinical types:

- lentigo maligna—the type seen most commonly on atrophic, sun-damaged skin of an elderly patient; this appears as an irregularly shaped tan or brown macule that has been enlarging slowly;

- superficial spreading—this type can occur anywhere and presents often as an irregularly shaped macule, papule, or plaque with great variation in color (Figure 41.10);

- nodular—a papule or nodule, often black or gray, that has been growing rapidly;

- acral lentiginous—this type is found on the palms, soles, or nail beds (Figure 41.11); it is found in all skin types and presents as a dark brown or black patch; its incidence is highest in persons aged 65 or older.

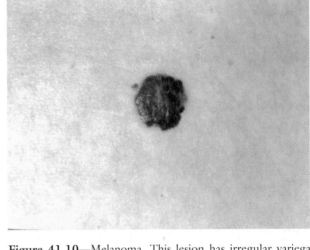

Figure 41.10—Melanoma. This lesion has irregular variegation in pigment (shades of brown and blue-black) as well as irregular borders, suggesting melanoma.

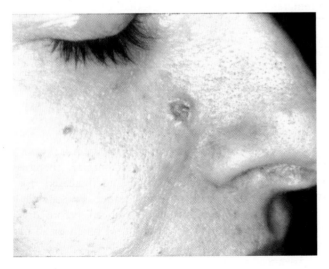

Figure 41.9—Basal cell carcinoma, ulcerated. This is also a pearly, fleshy papule but is ulcerated in the center and has a characteristic rolled border.

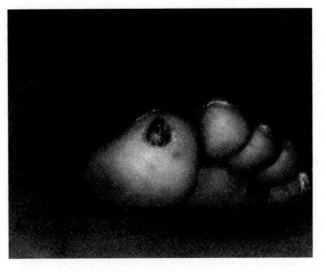

Figure 41.11—Acral lentiginous melanoma. This type of melanoma presents as a dark macular growth with irregular borders on volar surfaces of palms and soles (as in this case), and nails.

The treatment of melanoma consists of surgical excision and, depending on depth, may also involve sentinel node mapping and biopsy, lymph node dissection, or adjuvant therapy.

REFERENCES

- Chosidow O. Scabies and pediculosis. *Lancet.* 2000; 355(9206):819–826.

- Gnann JW Jr, Whitley RJ. Clinical Practice. Herpes zoster. *N Engl J Med* 2002;347(5):340–346.

- Martin ES, Elewski BE. Cutaneous fungal infections in the elderly. *Clin Geriatr Med.* 2002;18(1):59–75.

- McCarberg B. Managing the comorbidities of postherpetic neuralgia. *J Am Acad Nurse Pract.* 2003;15(12 Suppl):16–21; quiz 22–24.

- Sieggreen MY, Kline RA. Arterial insufficiency and ulceration: diagnosis and treatment options. *Adv Skin Would Care.* 2004;17(5 Pt 1):242–251; quiz 252–253.

- Valencia IC, Falabella A, Kirsner RS, et al. Chronic venous insufficiency and venous leg ulceration. *J Am Acad Dermatol.* 2001;44(3):401–421.

- Yosipovitch G, Tang MB. Practical management of psoriasis in the elderly: epidemiology, clinical aspects, quality of life, patient education and treatment options. *Drugs Aging.* 2002;19(11):847–863.

CHAPTER 42—ORAL DISEASES AND DISORDERS

KEY POINTS

- Since teeth become less sensitive with age, it is not uncommon to observe profound yet asymptomatic untreated dental disease in older persons, which justifies a need for regular dental evaluation every 6 to 12 months.

- Periodontitis caused by plaque formation within the gingival sulcus may lead to loss of alveolar bone height, decreased support around the tooth, malposition, loosening, and eventual loss of the tooth.

- Dentures usually aid in speech and restore diminished facial contours, but improved ability to masticate is unpredictable and enhanced oral intake is a less likely outcome.

- Oral cancer screening is critical to early detection and treatment of asymptomatic early-stage oral cancer, translating into improved outcomes and better survival rates.

The oral cavity is responsible for initiating food intake, producing speech, and protecting the alimentary tract and upper airway. Dysfunction and disease in the mouth can profoundly affect overall health and social functioning and may be particularly important for elderly patients who are frail or nutritionally at risk. Findings prevalent in older patients (eg, decay, missing teeth, periodontal disease, and salivary hypofunction) do not represent normal aging, and patients with such findings should be urged to seek preventive and therapeutic care.

THE AGING OF THE TEETH

Most age-related changes in teeth are subtle (see Table 42.1) but become significant in the presence of environmental factors or disease. For a combination of reasons, the teeth of an older person are typically less sensitive or wholly insensitive to temperature changes and, importantly, to the sensations that commonly herald dental disease in younger adults. It is not uncommon to observe profound yet asymptomatic untreated dental disease in an older person's mouth.

DENTAL DECAY

Dental *caries*, or decay, is a bacterially derived demineralization and cavitation that can attack teeth throughout the life span. *Recurrent caries* refers to decay at the interface between a dental restoration (such as a filling or crown) and the tooth. (See Figure 42.1 for the anatomy of the tooth.) Older persons have more restored teeth (and usually the restorations are older and more extensive) and thus are more likely to have recurrent caries. The teeth of older persons may feature more caries of the root surfaces than are typically observed in younger persons because prior periodontal disease exposes the root surface, thereby predisposing it to demineralization and increased risk for caries. Both recurrent and root caries are generally asymptomatic and may become advanced before discovery, often resulting in destruction of much or all of the tooth.

Advanced caries commonly results in necrosis of the remaining pulp, which usually leads to acute or chronic dental abscess. Even if such infections do not

Table 42.1—The Clinical Significance of Selected Age-Related Changes in Oral Tissues

Tissue Affected	Nature of Change	Clinical Significance
Tooth dentin	Increased thickness	Diminished pulp space
	Diminished permeability resulting from sclerosis of dentinal tubules	Diminished sensitivity of dentin; diminished susceptibility to effects of bacterial metabolites; increased tooth brittleness
Dental pulp	Diminished volume	Diminished reparative capacity; diminished sensitivity and alteration in nature of sensitivity
	Shift in proportion of nervous, vascular, and connective tissues	Diminished reparative capacity; diminished sensitivity and alteration in nature of sensitivity
Salivary glands	Fatty replacement of acini	Possibly less physiologic reserve

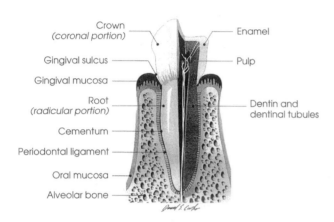

Figure 42.1—Dental and periodontal anatomy.

Labels: Crown (coronal portion) — Enamel; Gingival sulcus — Pulp; Gingival mucosa; Root (radicular portion) — Dentin and dentinal tubules; Cementum; Periodontal ligament; Oral mucosa; Alveolar bone

cause pain, they should not be ignored, since severe metastatic infections of dental and oral origin have been reported in virtually every organ system. In particular, α-hemolytic (viridans) streptococci of the oral cavity have long been implicated in close to one third of the cases of bacterial endocarditis reported annually in the United States, and bacteria associated with dental abscesses (eg, *Staphylococcus aureus)* have been cultured from the aspirates of infected hip arthroplasties.

The risk factors for dental caries are the same at any age, but many of the risk factors increase in prevalence as people age. A primary risk factor is poor oral hygiene, which often occurs in an older person when visual acuity, manual dexterity, or upper extremity flexibility is impaired, or when salivary flow is diminished. Another risk factor is frequent ingestion of sticky foods with a high content of sucrose, such as cake, candy, and cookies. Other risk factors include infrequent dental visits because of financial, access, or educational barriers; the presence of permanent or removable artificial teeth (more common with increasing age); and limited lifetime exposure to fluoride, widely used in the United States only in the past four decades. White elderly Americans display a higher incidence of root caries than either black

elderly Americans or Hispanic elderly Americans, but they are more likely to have received dental treatment for the lesions. Recurrent caries are also more common in white elderly Americans because of the greater likelihood that they have received prior dental treatment.

The prevention of caries involves daily oral hygiene with fluoride toothpaste, limitation of sugar intake, and regular dental examinations. The treatment of dental caries includes topical high-potency fluoride for remineralization, removal of demineralized tooth structure ("drilling"), and replacement of removed tooth structure with fillings or crowns. When caries involves the dental pulp, root canal treatment becomes necessary. This in turn usually requires reinforcement of the remaining tooth structure with a crown ("cap").

DISEASES OF THE PERIODONTIUM

The investing tissues of the teeth, termed the *periodontium,* consist of the gingiva, the alveolar bone, and a collagenous sleeve (termed the *periodontal ligament)* located between the tooth root and the surrounding bone. Periodontal disease occurs when microorganic colonies *(plaque)* form on the teeth near the gingiva and between the gingiva and the root surface within the gingival sulcus. The most common form of periodontal disease is gingivitis, in which the inflammatory reaction to plaque is limited to the gingiva. Gingivitis develops more rapidly in healthy older adults than in younger ones, but in both groups the changes—including gingival edema and light bleeding on brushing—are rapidly reversible following removal of plaque. If the inflammatory process extends to the periodontal ligament and alveolar bone, the process is termed *periodontitis.* In periodontitis there is destruction of the hard and soft tissues of the periodontium. In most adults periodontitis is a process marked by long periods of disease quiescence punctuated by bursts of localized destructive inflammation. The prevalence of active periodontitis is 20% to 40% of dentate adults. By their 50s, more than 90% of

Americans with teeth show 2 mm or more of lost alveolar bone height, the primary marker of prior periodontal disease activity. In advanced cases of periodontitis, the decreased support around a tooth leads to its malposition, loosening, and eventual loss.

Epidemiologic data support the concept that those who reach advanced age without significant periodontal bone loss will not likely experience a worsening of the disease in senescence. In contrast, other adults who have experienced a more rapid rate of bone loss commonly will have lost teeth in their 40s and 50s. In addition to age, risk factors for periodontitis include smoking and poor oral hygiene. Black and Hispanic Americans have a significantly higher prevalence of advanced periodontitis than do white Americans. Preventing gingivitis and periodontitis is largely a matter of oral hygiene and regular dental examinations and cleanings. Managing periodontal disease involves debriding the roots below the gingiva, which may require surgical access. Topical antibiotics (chlorhexidine, tetracycline) and systemic antibiotics (minocycline, metronidazole) are increasingly used as adjuncts to other periodontal therapy.

Periodontitis has been long reported to be worse in patients with poorly controlled diabetes mellitus. Investigations also support the contention that periodontitis, as an active infection, impairs diabetic control. Periodontal disease may be rapidly destructive in a patient whose immune system is impaired by disease or immunosuppression therapy. Epidemiologic data also correlate osteoporosis and tooth loss due to periodontitis. Periodontal disease and the pathogens responsible for it have been linked epidemiologically and immunologically with peripheral vascular disease, cerebrovascular disease, and pneumonia. Similar correlations have been reported for coronary heart disease, although one report disputes this. There is also epidemiologic association between gram-negative pneumonia, gram-negative periodontal pathogens, salivary hypofunction, and impaired swallowing function.

The prevention and control of periodontal disease revolve around daily oral care: tooth brushing and flossing to remove bacterial plaque on the teeth, particularly within the gingival sulcus. Regular dental evaluation, every 6 to 12 months, is important to ensure that the periodontium is healthy or to provide early intervention if it is not.

TOOTHLESSNESS

Advanced age was once considered synonymous with the need for false teeth, but that stereotype is fading. In the early 1960s more than 70% of adult Americans aged 75 or over were edentulous. By the 1990s fewer than 40% of this group were edentulous, most likely because of a rising tendency for exposure to some level of preventive and restorative dental care in childhood or early adulthood.

Nevertheless, removal of one or more teeth in an older adult may be necessitated by various combinations of physiologic and behavioral factors. The leading cause is inability or unwillingness to access and pay for restorative dental treatment in the face of a symptomatic dental disease, usually stemming from dental caries. A second common cause is loosening of teeth as a consequence of periodontal disease, to the point that mastication becomes painful or ineffective, or both. The third common cause is removal of otherwise healthy teeth that, because of the absence or loss of other teeth for the preceding or other reasons, would hinder the fabrication or function of a dental prosthesis.

Nearly 50% of Americans aged 85 and over have no natural teeth, and there are unique problems associated with the edentulous state. Functionally, the teeth aid in mastication and enunciation. Aesthetically, the teeth support the lips and cheeks and keep the nose and chin at a fixed distance apart. When a person has lost all teeth and there are no prosthetic replacements, the facial appearance is dramatically changed because of the lack of tissue support and diminished vertical height in the lower half of the face. Chewing ability is severely compromised, yet the impact on nutritional intake is difficult to characterize. One longitudinal study employing diet diaries demonstrated a correlation between loss of teeth and increased carbohydrate intake, decreased protein intake, and diminished intake of selected micronutrients.

As a modality of compensation for loss of all of the teeth, removable dentures can aid in speech and restore diminished facial contours, but they are less predictably successful in restoring the ability to masticate. Edentulous persons with dentures are generally capable of eating a wider range of foods than edentulous persons without dentures. Yet dentures restore, on average, only about 15% of the chewing ability of the natural dentition. The range of foods regularly eaten by denture wearers is significantly restricted in comparison with the dietary range of persons with natural teeth. Denture wearers also have to chew more times before they swallow food, and they swallow their food in larger particles. Older patients and their physicians who hope that dentures will restore oral intake in cases of malnutrition or unexplained weight loss are usually disappointed, whereas those who hope for a more socially acceptable appearance, clearer speech, and modest improvement in chewing comfort and range of dietary choices are more likely to be satisfied.

Dentures often are a considerable source of discomfort, dysfunction, and embarrassment for older people. This is because the alveolar processes that originally held the natural teeth continually remodel and diminish in volume once the natural teeth are gone. For most patients, dentures require frequent professional adjustment and periodic replacement. Alveolar ridge resorption is most severe in the oldest patients who have had the longest time without natural teeth; this effect is more pronounced in those with osteoporosis.

For health of the oral mucosa, dentures should be kept clean by removing them and cleaning them after meals, and soaking them in a commercial disinfectant several times each week. Dentures should remain out of the mouth for several hours each day; most people choose to leave their dentures out during sleep. Fractured or broken dentures, as well as denture looseness or soreness, should be brought to a dentist's attention without delay. However, since neither dental services nor dentures are currently covered by Medicare and fewer than 10% of older Americans have private dental insurance, many elderly people continue to use inadequate or even damaging dentures.

SALIVARY FUNCTION IN AGING

Saliva is critical for protecting the tissues of the oral cavity and maintaining their function in speech, mastication, swallowing, and taste perception. Saliva buffers the intraoral pH, contains a wide spectrum of antimicrobial factors, remineralizes and lubricates the oral surfaces, and keeps the taste pores patent. In the absence of disease, the major salivary glands undergo regressive histologic changes with age. Yet data from the Baltimore Longitudinal Study on Aging and the Veterans Affairs Dental Longitudinal Study have demonstrated that with healthy aging, flow from the parotid glands under both resting and stimulated conditions remains essentially unchanged. Both groups of investigators have reported that flow from the submandibular glands undergoes no change with age; other centers have reported a measurable but clinically minor decrease. It has been suggested that the major salivary glands show "organ reserve" in which the capacity of youthful glands exceeds ordinary demands, but that with age-related changes, functional reserves dwindle. By extreme old age, healthy glands function adequately under normal conditions but are more susceptible to factors that impede function, such as dehydration or drug-induced hypofunction.

Complaints of dry mouth are very common among older people. The leading causes are the commonly prescribed drugs that have this adverse effect. Commonly implicated are drugs with anticholinergic effects, including tricyclic antidepressants, opioids, antihistamines, and anti-arrhythmic agents. Separate studies have found that 72% of institutionalized elderly patients received at least one (and some as many as five) potentially xerostomic medications daily and that 55%

of more than 4000 rural community-dwelling elderly persons took at least one potentially xerostomic medication daily. Dry mouth may also be due to local disease, such as salivary gland tumors and blocked ducts, or to systemic disease. Sjögren's syndrome affects approximately 3 million Americans—predominantly women—aged 50 or over. Depression has been reported to diminish saliva flow, as have poorly controlled diabetes mellitus and hypothyroidism.

Dry mouth is also an adverse effect of therapeutic irradiation of the head and neck. In the total dose range administered for oral and oropharyngeal squamous cell carcinoma, salivary flow is commonly obliterated as a consequence of short-term direct effects on the glands and long-term fibrosis of their vascular supply. As a result, patients who have undergone radiation of the head may experience rapidly destructive dental caries and painful oral mucositis, which may affect nutritional status.

Treatment of the older person with dry mouth requires attention to both diagnosis and prevention. Diminished oral secretions increase the risk for serious oral disease. A history of irradiation of the head and neck as well as systemic causes should be excluded. Medications that reduce salivary flow should be decreased, discontinued, or substituted for, if possible. Patients who have had irradiation should be considered for a 3-month course of oral pilocarpine (5 to 10 mg three times a day), which may restore some salivary function. Saliva substitutes and oral lubricants, available without prescription and used as needed, can provide transient relief but have none of the protective properties of saliva. Patients should be counseled on the greatly elevated risk for oral disease and educated on the need to limit sugar in their diet and optimize their daily oral hygiene practices.

ORAL MUCOSAL PROBLEMS

Squamous cell carcinoma accounts for 96% of oral and oropharyngeal malignancies. Of the 28,000 new cases of oral cancer reported in the United States annually, more than 95% occur in people aged 40 or over; age is the primary risk factor identified in epidemiologic analyses. The 5-year survival rate for white Americans is approximately 55% and for black Americans, 34%. Carcinoma of the lip, tongue, and floor of mouth represents more than 65% of all oropharyngeal cases. Lip cancer affects men eight times more frequently than women; most other sites affect men at a ratio slightly below 2:1. Oral cancer is strongly linked with the use of tobacco, particularly cigarettes. Lip cancer has a strong correlation with pipe and cigar smoking. Ethanol is a potent cofactor that enhances the effects of tobacco. Other potential risk factors—dentures, poor oral care, oral viral disease, oral lichen planus, candidosis—have been suggested, but none has shown the unambiguous associations of age, smoking, and alcohol use.

Oral malignancy appears clinically as painless red, white, or mixed red and white areas of the oral mucosa that may be ulcerated or indurated. Red and mixed lesions (termed *erythroplakia*) (Figure 42.2) display cellular atypia in as many as 93% of cases and should be biopsied immediately. White lesions (*leukoplakia*) (Figure 42.3) are malignant or premalignant less than 10% of the time and merit close monitoring; biopsy is indicated if a lesion does not disappear in 14 days or is increasing in size. Clinicians also have less invasive diagnostic tools available for determining whether a white or red lesion in the mouth merits biopsy, such as scraping (exfoliative cytology) and in situ staining. Early identification markedly improves outcome: 5-year survival without nodal involvement in white Americans is 80% and in black Americans is 69%, but survival rates decline with nodal involvement (41% and 30%, respectively) and with distant metastases (18% and 12%). A thorough oral cancer screening, which can be completed in less than 2 minutes, consists of a head and neck nodal assessment followed by inspection of the oral cavity using gauze to retract the tongue and tongue blades to enhance visualization of the cheeks, lips, and vestibules. Although oral cancer screening is easy to learn, straightforward to perform, requires minimal instrumentation, and causes no discomfort to the patient, few elderly smokers receive oral evaluations as part of the routine physical examination.

The treatment of localized oral squamous cell carcinoma is generally surgical, although large but localized tumors can be managed with radioactive implants. More extensive disease necessitates surgery followed by beam irradiation. Concern over the deleterious adverse effects of irradiation (described in the preceding section) has led to the development of techniques that seek to limit destruction of healthy tissues surrounding a tumor. Radiation alone has been used to shrink inoperable tumors. Newer protocols combine surgery and chemotherapy with the goal of a cure.

Candidiasis presents as diffuse erythema, cracking at the corners of the mouth, curd-like white patches, or erythema in denture areas; it can result in taste dysfunction, burning, itching, and pain. Older patients are particularly susceptible to candidiasis because of denture use, salivary hypofunction, the prevalence of diabetes mellitus, and the use of antibiotics for pulmonary and urologic diseases. Patients who use inhaled corticosteroids also are at higher risk and should be instructed to rinse out their mouth after using the inhaler. Management of candidiasis involves, first, excluding any immunopathic cause for the disease, fol-

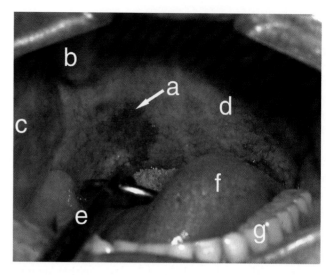

Figure 42.2—Erythroplakia in a 72-year-old man with a history of cigar smoking and alcohol abuse. Lesion confirmed by biopsy to be invasive squamous cell carcinoma, poorly differentiated.

Key: a = erythroplakia; b = right posterior maxillary alveolar ridge; c = inner aspect of right cheek; d = soft palate; e = tongue retractor; f = tongue dorsum; g = mandibular denture.

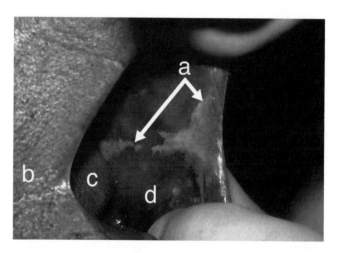

Figure 42.3—Leukoplakia in a 66-year-old man with a history of smoking. Lesion confirmed by biopsy to be carcinoma in situ.

Key: a = leukoplakia; b = right lip commissure; c = tongue; d = inner aspect of left cheek.

lowed by administration of topical or systemic antifungal agents and optimal oral and denture hygiene.

Burning mouth syndrome is a chronic oral-facial pain disorder usually without other clinical signs. It typically affects women aged 50 or over, with a particularly high attack rate in Asian Americans and Native Americans. The pain most commonly affects the lips, tongue, and palate. Multiple causes have been suggested, including xerostomia, denture use, candidiasis, nutritional deficiencies, and psychiatric disorders. Treatment is empirical.

CHEMOSENSORY PERCEPTION

Olfactory function declines with age. A decreased ability to identify odors and to rank their intensities affects both elderly men (to the greater extent) and women. Several drugs have been implicated in smell dysfunction, as has Alzheimer's disease, among other disorders common among older persons. Impaired olfaction in older persons has been anecdotally implicated as a risk factor for eating spoiled food or failing to notice gas leaks or domestic fires.

Taste perception changes with aging. The subjective perception of saltiness and sweetness shows blunting with advancing age. This change potentially has clinical significance, possibly playing a role in a person's tendency to oversalt foods or crave sweets.

Complaints of taste and smell dysfunction are common among older persons. Often the complaint derives from medication use, but other causes are possible (see Table 42.2 and Table 42.3). Some drugs

Table 42.2—Drugs That Interfere With Gustation (Taste) and Olfaction (Smell)

Gustation*		
Acyclovir	Enalapril	Pentoxifylline
Allopurinol	Ethacrynic acid	Phenytoin
Amiloride	Ethambutol	Procainamide
Amitriptyline	Fenoprofen	Prochlorperazine
Amphotericin B	Gemfibrozil	Promethazine
Ampicillin	Hydrochlorothiazide	Propafenone
Baclofen	Imipramine	Propranolol
Buspirone	Labetalol	Ritonavir
Captopril	Levamisole	Saquinavir
Chlorpheniramine	Lomefloxacin	Sulfamethoxazole
Desipramine	Mexiletine	Sulindac
Doxepin	Nabumetone	Terfenadine
Dexamethasone	Nelfinavir	Tetracyclines
Diclofenac	Ofloxacin	Trifluoperazine
Dicyclomine	Nifedipine	Zidovudine
Diltiazem	Pentamidine	

Olfaction**		
Amitriptyline	Enalapril	Pentamidine
Amphetamine	Flunisolide	Pirbuterol
Beclomethasone dipropionate	Flurbiprofen	Propafenone
	Hydromorphone	Tocainide
Cocaine	Levamisole	Zalcitabine
Codeine	Morphine	
Dexamethasone		

* Gustation: source lists more than 250 agents reported to disturb the sense of taste. Agents listed above are limited to those for which taste disturbance was objectively determined through threshold or intensity scaling or both, employing one or more standardized solutions.

** Olfaction: source lists more than 40 agents reported to disturb the olfactory sense. Agents listed above are limited to those for which olfactory disturbance was determined objectively through experiment or clinical trial.

SOURCE: Data from Schiffman SS, Zervakis J. Taste and smell perception in the elderly: effect of medications and disease. *Adv Food Nutr Res.* 2002; 44:247–346.

Table 42.3—Nonpharmacologic Causes of Taste and Smell Dysfunction in Elderly Persons

Gustatory dysfunction
  Oral causes
    Burning mouth syndrome
    Candidiasis
    Laceration
    Malignancy
    Salivary hypofunction
    Therapeutic irradiation of head
    Thermal or chemical burn
  Other causes
    Alzheimer's disease, other neurodegenerative disorders
    Central nervous system tumor
    Endocrinopathies (eg, diabetes mellitus, Cushing's syndrome, adrenocortical insufficiency, hypothyroidism)
    Head trauma
    Nutritional deficiencies (vitamin B_{12}, zinc)
    Psychiatric disorder
    Stroke
Olfactory dysfunction
  Upper aerodigestive and respiratory causes
    Dental infection
    Periodontal disease
    Poor oral hygiene, including poor denture hygiene
    Sinusitis
    Tobacco smoking or use of nasal snuff
    Tumor of airway or sinus
    Upper respiratory infection (bacterial or viral)
  Other causes
    Alzheimer's disease, other neurodegenerative disorders
    Central nervous system tumor
    Exposure to volatile or particulate toxins
    Head trauma
    Nutritional deficiencies (niacin, zinc)
    Psychiatric disorder
    Stroke

may have no primary effect on taste but cause diminished saliva flow and lead to impaired taste perception. One's sense of "taste" may actually be more accurately termed "flavor"—that is, the full range of sensations that accompany eating, including temperature, texture, sound, and smell in addition to the perception of sweet, salt, sour, and bitter. Flavor perception is prone to impairment in the older person because of changes in olfaction and oral stereognosis, salivary hypofunction, and the presence of dentures, which present physical and thermal barriers. Flavor-enhancement strategies have been shown to have positive effects on both food preference and caloric intake among frail elderly patients.

REFERENCES

■ Bailey R, Gueldner S, Ledikwe J, et al. The oral health of older adults: an interdisciplinary mandate. *J Gerontol Nurs.* 2005;31(7):11–17.

■ Gil-Montoya JA, de mello AL, Cardenas CB, et al. Oral health protocol for the dependent institutionalized elderly. *Geriatr Nurs.* 2006;27(2):95–102.

- Lamster IB. Oral health care services for older adults: a looming crisis. *Am J Public Health.* 2004;94(5):699–702.

- Schiffman SS, Zervakis J. Taste and smell perception in the elderly: effect of medications and disease. *Adv Food Nutr Res.* 2002;44:247–346.

- Sciubba JJ. Oral cancer: the importance of early diagnosis and treatment. *Am J Clin Dermatol.* 2001:2(4):239–251.

- Shay K. Infectious complications of dental and periodontal diseases in the elderly population. *Clin Infect Dis.* 2002;34(9):1215–1223.

CHAPTER 43—RESPIRATORY DISEASES AND DISORDERS

KEY POINTS

- With age, there is a decline in forced vital capacity, forced expiratory volume in 1 second, and Pao$_2$, while the A-a gradient increases.

- Five percent to 10% of people aged 65 years and over meet criteria for asthma.

- Smoking cessation may slow the decline in lung function at any age.

- Descriptive studies show that older people recover pulmonary physiology at the same rate as their younger cohorts, but in some disease states they may require a longer time to be liberated from the ventilator.

- Most patients with chronic obstructive pulmonary disease derive little or no benefit from routine inhaled corticosteroids, but a brief course of systemic corticosteroids may reduce the duration of an acute exacerbation of the disease.

AGE-RELATED PULMONARY ALTERATIONS

Studies of age-specific alterations in pulmonary function are limited by common and important comorbidities experienced by older adults, including smoking-related diseases, occupational and industrial exposures, and other significant organ dysfunction such as heart failure or deconditioning. These limitations notwithstanding, decrements in various aspects of pulmonary function occur with aging.

Because of alterations in connective tissue, the size of the airways is reduced and the alveolar sacs become shallow. Chest wall compliance is reduced as a consequence of kyphoscoliosis, calcification of the costal cartilage, and arthritic changes in the costovertebral joints. Sarcopenia results in intercostal muscle atrophy and a reduction in diaphragmatic strength by 25%. These processes result in a decline of forced vital capacity and forced expiratory volume in 1 second of

25 to 30 mL per year in nonsmokers and approximately double that (60 to 70 mL per year) in smokers aged 65 years and over. The normal A-a gradient increases with age and can be approximated by the following formula: (Age / 4) + 4. The Pao$_2$ decreases with age and can be approximated by the following equation: Pao$_2$ = 110 − (0.4 × age).

COMMON RESPIRATORY SYMPTOMS AND COMPLAINTS

A common misperception is that older adults tend to overestimate or exaggerate respiratory symptoms; however, the opposite is more often true. For example, many older adultss and their physicians tend to underestimate the importance of dyspnea, which may go undiagnosed until advanced disease is evident. This is partly due to the fact that dyspnea is blamed on deconditioning and age. Older adults will often adjust their activity level to compensate for insidiously shrinking lung function and disabling dyspnea. Such changes in life style often go unnoticed by family, the patient's physician, and even the patient. Pulmonary or cardiac disorders, or both, may underlie such modifications in life style, and testing (eg, pulmonary function tests or chest radiography) may reveal major abnormalities such as asthma, emphysema, or pulmonary fibrosis. Another complicating feature of symptom recognition in older adults is that older adults often have more than one explanation for their problems. A patient may have overlapping symptoms of dyspnea, cough, and wheezing because of a combination of diseases such as asthma or emphysema, obstructive sleep apnea, heart failure, and gastroesophageal reflux.

Dyspnea

Dyspnea becomes prominent in end-stage lung diseases such as chronic obstructive pulmonary disease (COPD) and idiopathic pulmonary fibrosis. Importantly, the level of dyspnea is the best predictor of quality of life, yet it does not correlate with either oxygenation or pulmonary function tests. A thorough history and physical examination can help tailor both testing and empirical treatment choices. For example, in an older patient presenting with dyspnea and associated nocturnal cough, common diseases such as asthma, emphysema, allergic rhinitis with postnasal drip, and gastroesophageal reflux disease would be considered first. Minimal testing (eg, pulmonary function tests only) followed by an empiric trial directed toward the most likely cause would be a reasonable approach. In the same patient, the presence of significant weight loss or constitutional symptoms (fever, night sweats) could suggest other diseases, such as malignancy or tuberculosis. At times, the particular language the patient choses to describe the dyspnea can be revealing, such as "heavy" for cardiac dysfunction or deconditioning or "tight" for angina or asthma. The common causes of dyspnea in older patients to consider include COPD, cardiac disease, asthma, interstitial lung disease, and deconditioning.

Chronic Cough

Fortunately, most patients can be reassured that chronic cough, although particularly annoying, usually has a benign cause. By far, the most common causes of chronic cough are postnasal drip, asthma, and gastroesophageal reflux. These three diagnoses account for over 90% of the causes identified in most series, and a reasonable approach to the treatment of chronic cough, then, is empiric treatment for these conditions. Not infrequently, a combination of these conditions may contribute, so treatment for multiple causes may be warranted when single therapies are ineffective. Less common yet important differential diagnostic considerations of cough in older patients include drug effects (eg, angiotensin-converting enzyme inhibitors), heart failure, laryngeal dysfunction, *Bordetella pertussis* infection, chronic cough after viral upper respiratory tract infection or secondary bacterial infections, recurrent aspiration, or respiratory tract abnormalities such as bronchiectasis or airway tumors.

Wheezing

Although asthma is a common cause of wheezing in all age groups, it is not the most common cause, particularly if the wheezing is not associated with cough or dyspnea. Postnasal drip is another common cause to consider; also, the rates of heart failure rise in older age groups, and associated pulmonary edema may present as "cardiac asthma." Finally, airway hyperresponsive-ness from chronic bronchitis is not uncommon in older patients with a history of wheezing and sputum and tobacco use.

MAJOR PULMONARY DISEASES IN OLDER PATIENTS

Asthma

After childhood, the prevalence of asthma has a second peak after the age of 65; 5% to 10% of older adults meet criteria for obstruction and bronchial hyper-reactivity. The rate of death from asthma has increased most significantly in those aged 65 and over, accounting for up to 45% of all deaths caused by asthma. This is likely due to reduced awareness of bronchial constriction on the part of the patient (with delays in seeking medical attention), as well as under-recognition and undertreatment on the part of clinicians. Therapy of asthma in older and younger people differs in several ways. Paramount to the care of the elderly asthmatic patient is adequate instruction in the proper use of peak expiratory flow monitoring (because of the older person's decreased perception of bronchoconstriction) and in the correct activation of the metered-dose inhaler. Neurologic, muscular, and arthritic diseases in older people can lead to suboptimal timing and discoordination in using the inhaler device. The clinician should observe the patient actually using the inhaler. Inhaled corticosteroids (or other controller drugs such as leukotriene receptor antagonists) represent the mainstay of therapy in both older and younger people. The lowest effective dosage should be used, and counsel given regarding rinsing of the oropharynx to avoid thrush. In older people, theophylline is fraught with adverse effects and drug interactions, and it should be considered a third-line drug to be used only as a once-daily medication in the evening for severe asthma or COPD, targeting a serum level of 10 to 12 mg/dL if tolerated. Oral corticosteroids are discussed in the next section on COPD. Although controversy persists as to whether the response to relievers such as β-agonists varies with age, these drugs remain a mainstay of as-needed reliever medication. The potential for adverse effects of β-agonists—for example, hypokalemia or possible QT prolongation in cardiac patients on digoxin or other medications— warrants adequate controller use by asthmatic patients to minimize overreliance on the β-agonist. The use of long-acting β-agonists is controversial and should be considered with caution and only in those patients who are reliably able to manage medications. (See Table 43.1 for commonly used medications taken with metered-dose inhalers.)

Table 43.1—Commonly Used Inhaled Medications, With Packaging Colors

Class of Drug	Generic Name	Trade Name	Color (Body/Cap)
β-Agonists	Albuterol	Proventil	Yellow/orange
		Ventolin	Light blue/dark blue
	Formoterol*	Foradil	White/light blue
	Levalbuterol	Xopenex HFA	
	Pirbuterol	Maxair	Blue/white
	Salmeterol	Serevent	Teal/light teal
Corticosteroids	Beclomethasone	Beclovent	White/brown
		Vanceril	Pink/dark pink
		QVAR	Mauve/gray
	Budesonide	Pulmicort	White/brown
	Flunisolide	AeroBid	Gray/purple or green
	Fluticasone	Flovent	Orange/light orange
	Mometasone	Asmanex	
	Triamcinolone	Azmacort	White/white
Combination β-agonist and corticosteroid	Fluticasone propionate and salmeterol	Advair	Purple/light purple
Others	Cromolyn	Intal	White/blue
	Ipratropium	Atrovent	Silver/green
	Tiotropium*	Spiriva	Gray/green
	Nedocromil	Tilade	White/white
	Albuterol-ipratropium	Combivent	Silver/orange

NOTE: Generics may differ.

* Powder for oral inhalation.

Chronic Obstructive Pulmonary Disease

COPD affects approximately 15 million people in the United States and is the fourth most common cause of death after heart disease, cancer, and stroke. The prevalence and mortality rate from COPD is increasing, especially in older adults. Episodes of acute respiratory failure that require mechanical ventilation are associated with mortality rates ranging from 11% to 46%. The National Lung Health Education Program Executive Committee has noted that the morbidity and mortality from COPD accounts for more than $15 billion per year in U.S. medical care expenditures. Hospitalization continues to represent the largest component of cost for COPD patients.

The diagnosis of airflow limitation is challenging in that no single item or combination of items from the history and clinical examination excludes airflow limitation. The finding most strongly associated with a decreased likelihood of airflow limitation is a history of never having smoked cigarettes (especially in patients without a history of wheezing and without wheezing on examination). Wheezing noted on physical examination is the most potent predictor of airflow limitation,

and patients with obstructive airflow limitation are 36 times more likely to have wheezing than are patients without this problem. Other findings associated with an increased likelihood of airflow limitation include a barrel-shaped chest, hyperresonance on percussion, and a forced expiratory time of greater than 9 seconds measured during the clinical bedside examination.

Smoking cessation at any age has been shown to slow the decline in lung function, and aggressive cessation efforts are appropriate even in the oldest-old patient. The basic elements of the approach are the "Five A's" from the Agency for Health Care Policy and Research:

- **A**sk patients about use of tobacco at every office visit.
- **A**ssess readiness to quit.
- **A**dvise patients to quit.
- **A**ssist patients in the quit attempt with aids such as a local cessation program and pharmacologic agents such as bupropion or nicotine replacement.
- **A**rrange both a quit date and a follow-up visit or contact to discuss the quit attempt.

The chief components of daily drug therapy in emphysema consist of a β-agonist, ipratropium bromide or tiotropium, or both drugs in combination. For more severe disease, the use of long-acting β-agonists such as salmeterol along with a combined albuterol and ipratropium bromide metered-dose inhaler can achieve improved adherence and long-term control by reducing the number of inhalers by one (ie, the patient will have only the long-acting inhaler and the combination short-acting inhaler rather than three inhalers). Inhaled corticosteroids have been tested in several multicenter randomized controlled trials in COPD with negative results overall; however, there appears to be a benefit in subgroup analyses of patients with "asthmatic COPD" as defined by spirometry testing with documented bronchodilator responsiveness. A landmark investigation documented that the use of systemic corticosteroids (intravenous followed by oral) reduces the duration and recurrence of acute exacerbations of COPD for up to 6 months. Importantly, there is no benefit to a course of steroids longer than 14 days. For the few patients (5% to 10%) who do benefit or who require prolonged use of corticosteroids, the risks should be considered, discussed, and documented in the patient's medical record. These risks include peptic ulcer disease, hypertension, cataracts, diabetes mellitus, osteoporosis, psychosis, seizures, poor wound healing, infections, and aseptic necrosis of the hip. Appropriate preventive measures should also be taken in these circumstances of prolonged use, such as using the lowest possible dosage of corticosteroids and using supplemental vitamin D, calcium, and perhaps a bisphosphonate for those at risk of osteoporosis. Other possible beneficial interventions in older emphysema patients include pulmonary rehabilitation via exercise training and respiratory therapy and education. Both major depression and anxiety have been shown to be present in up to 40% of COPD patients, and their treatment must be considered. In fact, unprovoked anxiety attacks often result in patients' seeking help in emergency departments, being admitted to the hospital, and being treated with potentially avoidable courses of oral corticosteroids when the anxiety is not diagnosed and treated.

Obstructive Sleep Apnea

Sleep-related breathing disorders are very common in older people, and obstructive sleep apnea is the most common type of sleep-related breathing disorder. Obstructive sleep apnea has been associated with cerebrovascular accidents, myocardial infarctions, and a threefold increase in mortality. Most patients with obstructive sleep apnea remain undiagnosed and there-

fore without treatment of this life-threatening, yet potentially correctable disease. Treatment options include addressing upper-airway obstruction via weight loss, avoiding alcohol and sedatives, sleeping on one's side or upright, correcting of metabolic disorders such as hypothyroidism, and providing continuous positive airway pressure (CPAP) via a nasal mask. To increase adherence with the use of CPAP, it may be combined with "nasal pillows" to increase comfort and "ramping technique" to provide a delayed rise in the applied pressure after the patient has fallen asleep. Treatment issues are generally the same regardless of age, and the major consideration for the clinician is a high index of suspicion and clinical recognition of this disease.

Idiopathic Pulmonary Fibrosis

Restricting lung disease has more than 100 causes; however, the history, examination, serologic testing, and biopsy often leave the patient with the diagnosis of idiopathic pulmonary fibrosis. This disease is increasing in prevalence with the aging of our population. Rarely is it an inherited disorder. Pulmonary fibrosis is extremely frustrating for all involved because of its relentless progression. The median survival is 3 to 5 years. The presentation is normally one of insidious dyspnea (often unrecognized because of a decrease in the activity level on the part of the patient) and cough. Clubbing is often a prominent finding on physical examination in pulmonary fibrosis, as opposed to emphysema, which rarely causes clubbing (prompting a search for another disease such as occult lung cancer). Oral corticosteroids (0.5 mg/kg/day) for 3 to 6 months is the most common initial therapy, yet only 10% to 20% of patients respond and adverse effects are often prominent. Early referral to a subspecialist is warranted if the patient wishes to consider further therapeutic measures so that steroid-sparing agents such as azathioprine[OL] or enrollment in a randomized controlled trial of newer pharmacologic agents (eg, interleukin-10 or interferon gamma) can be considered.

Pulmonary Thromboembolism

The incidence of pulmonary thromboembolism triples between the ages of 65 and 90 years and has a reported 10% recurrence rate within 1 year. Age above 70 years has been independently associated with missed antemortem diagnosis. Importantly, 10% to 20% of patients with documented pulmonary embolism have an entirely normal blood gas profile (ie, normal Pao_2 and normal A-a gradient for age). Age-specific risk factors for pulmonary thromboembolism include hypercoagulability due to increases in fibrinogen, activated protein-C resis-

[OL] Not approved by the U.S. Food and Drug Administration for this use.

tance due to factor-V Leiden gene mutation, malignancy, stasis (decreased mobility due to stroke, heart failure, or arthritis), or vessel injury (due to trauma or varicosities). The diagnostic evaluation is not different for younger and older patients. Anticoagulants are central to therapy and generally guided by the same principles in younger and older patients. Because of lessened cardiopulmonary reserve in older patients, achieving therapeutic levels of heparinization quickly may be even more important to avoid major adverse hemodynamic or oxygenation defects. The trend toward increased use of outpatient low-molecular-weight heparin preparations, while achieving anticoagulation with warfarin, is supported by large, well-designed randomized controlled trials. Heparinization and adequate warfarin therapy should overlap for approximately 1 to 3 days, with an INR target of 2 to 3. Warfarin interacts with many drugs that are commonly used in the older age group (for lists of drugs that increase or decrease INR with warfarin, see the section on anticoagulation in the Appendix, p 453). Studies have inconsistently shown that age itself is a risk factor for bleeding risk with use of warfarin. Duration of therapy for at least 6 months has been shown to be superior to 3 months, and the shorter duration should be used only for those patients with either a specific risk factor that is now removed or for those in whom the risk of prolonged anticoagulant therapy clearly outweighs that of completing 6 months of therapy. Indeed, patients with multiple ongoing risk factors for pulmonary thromboembolic disease should be considered for anticoagulation therapy for up to 2 years or longer. Recurrent pulmonary thromboembolism is usually treated with lifelong anticoagulation.

Pneumonia

See "Infectious Diseases" (p 304).

Lung Cancer

See "Oncology" (p 442).

REFERENCES

- Barua P, O'Mahony MS. Overcoming gaps in the management of asthma in older patients: new insights. *Drugs Aging.* 2005;22(12):1029–1059.

- Bosson JL, Pouchain D, Bergmann JF; for the ETAPE Study Group. A prospective observational study of a cohort of outpatients with an acute medical event and reduced mobility: incidence of symptomatic thromboembolism and description of thromboprophylaxis practices. *J Intern Med.* 2006;260(2):168–176.

- Kwon NH, Oh MJ, Min TH, et al. Causes and clinical featurs of subacute cough. *Chest.* 2006;129(5):1142–1147.

CHAPTER 44—INFECTIOUS DISEASES

KEY POINTS

- Immune function and host resistance is compromised in elderly persons not only as a consequence of age-related declines in immunity (immune senescence) but more importantly because of comorbid disease.

- Because of the older person's altered febrile response to infection, a redefinition of fever should be considered in the frail older patient (temperature >2°F over baseline or oral temperature >99°F).

- The application of minimum criteria for initiating antibiotic therapy for residents of long-term-care facilities is likely to reduce inappropriate antibiotic use without jeopardizing patient safety.

- Careful selection of first-line therapy is warranted in older patients with pneumonia because of the associated high mortality rates and because the causes of pneumonia differ in younger and older patients.

- The response to aggressive, highly active antiretroviral therapy is similar in younger and older adults with human immunodeficiency virus (HIV) infection.

Infection is the major cause of mortality in 40% of those aged 65 years and older, and it contributes to death in many others. Infection is also a significant cause of morbidity in older adults, often exacerbating underlying illness or leading to hospitalization. Four of the top twenty diagnosis-related groups paid by Medicare are infection-related diagnoses (pneumonia, number 2; urinary tract infections, number 14; septicemia, number 15; and other respiratory infections, number 17). Further, because of their increased susceptibility to infection, older adults often herald the arrival of new infections or the return of annual epidemics. Associations of infection and inflammation with age-related chronic diseases suggest that infectious diseases may play an even larger role in the morbidity and mortality of the elderly population than previously realized. This chapter explores the biologic, cultural, and societal factors that influence susceptibility to infection, the presentation of disease, and the management of infections in elderly patients.

PREDISPOSITION TO INFECTION

Fundamental alterations in the immune response occur with aging in large measure because of comorbidities but also because of age-related declines in immunity, a phenomenon known as *immune senescence* (Table 44.1). The main features of immune senescence are depressed T-cell responses and T-cell–macrophage interactions (clinically reflected as delayed-type hypersensitivity responses), but deficits of innate immunity are increasingly being recognized, particularly in frail elderly patients.

Although age itself influences immune function, comorbidities have the greatest impact on innate im-

mune function and nonspecific host-resistance factors; for example, skin integrity and cough or gag reflexes are local defense mechanisms that are often impaired. Perhaps the best example is chronic obstructive pulmonary disease, in which impaired mucociliary clearance and alveolar macrophage dysfunction are likely to be factors that increase the risk of lower respiratory tract infection. Comorbid diseases also indirectly complicate infections in elderly persons. For example, community-acquired pneumonia in otherwise healthy patients under age 50 is typically treated on an outpatient basis and rarely causes mortality; however, in elderly patients with community-acquired pneumonia and multiple comorbid conditions, the greatly increased risk of morbidity and mortality often necessitates hospitalization. Furthermore, cognitive impairment and other barriers to adherence may increase the difficulty of treating elderly patients, increasing complications and costs.

A major influence on immune function in the older person is nutritional status. Protein and calorie undernutrition is present in 30% to 60% of persons

Table 44.1—Changes in Immune Function Associated With Aging

	Change With Age		
	Direction	Degree	Comment
Innate immunity			
Skin, mucous membranes	decrease	+++	Skin thins and dries with aging
Complement		—	Most changes are due to comorbidity
Polymorphonuclear neutrophils			Most changes are due to comorbidity
Adherence, chemotaxis		—	
Ingestion		—	
Intracellular killing	decrease	+	Most changes are due to comorbidity
Adaptive immunity			
Thymic hormones	decrease	+++	
Lymphocyte subsets			
T cells		+++	Shift from naive to memory subtypes
Natural killer cells	decrease	++	Number increases, but function declines
Lymphocyte functions			
Proliferative responses	decrease	++	
Cytokine production, secretion			
IL-2, IL-2 receptor	decrease	+++	
IL-4, IL-6, IL-10	increase	++	
IFN-γ	increase	+	
PGE$_2$	increase	++	
Delayed-type hypersensitivity	decrease	++	
Autoimmunity	increase	++	Autoantibodies common, but of unclear significance

NOTE: — = no age-related changes; + = mild; ++ = moderate; +++ = marked; IL = interleukin; IFN = interferon; PGE$_2$ = prostaglandin E$_2$.

aged 65 years or older on admission to the hospital. In the outpatient arena, 11% of older adults suffer from undernutrition, 90% of which is due to reversible underlying conditions (depression, poorly controlled diabetes mellitus, medication side effects). Delayed wound healing, increased risk of nosocomial infection, extended lengths of hospital stay, and increased mortality are all associated with malnutrition. Even mildly undernourished older adults (those with a serum albumin of 3.0 to 3.5 g/dL) have evidence of immune compromise, poor vaccination responses, and diminished cytokine responses to specific challenges. Nutritional interventions may boost immune function in some older adults, but this remains controversial. Some studies suggest a clinical benefit, particularly in those with subclinical nutritional deficiencies, whereas others do not. Differences in study design, population enrolled, duration of follow-up, and definitions of infection (self-reported versus physician diagnosed) may account for many of these differences. (See "Malnutrition," p 161.)

Institutionalization places elderly persons at greatly increased risk for epidemic disease such as influenza. Widespread antibiotic use also increases their risk for acquiring diseases caused by more resistant organisms. Methicillin-resistant *Staphylococcus aureus*, vancomycin-resistant enterococci, and multiply resistant gram-negative rods are more common causes of infection in institutionalized elderly persons. Resistance is fostered in the nursing home by debilitated hosts, close proximity of residents, and difficulties in implementing infection-control measures in long-term care, as well as by high levels of antibiotic use.

DIAGNOSIS AND MANAGEMENT OF INFECTIONS

Presentation

It has long been recognized that older adults may present without typical signs and symptoms, even in the face of very significant infection. Fever, the most readily recognized feature of infection, may be absent in 30% to 50% of frail older adults with serious infections, even pneumonia or endocarditis. The cause of impaired febrile responses in older adults is incompletely understood, but diverse mechanisms of thermoregulation are involved, including blunted thermogenesis by brown adipose tissue.

Because of the altered febrile response to infection, many authors have suggested a redefinition of *fever* in older adults. Given the sensitivity, specificity, and positive and negative predictive values, fever in elderly nursing-home residents can be redefined appropriately as a body temperature >2°F (1.1°C) over baseline (if a baseline is available) or, perhaps more practically, an oral temperature >99°F (37.2°C) or a rectal temperature >99.5°F (37.5°C) on repeated measures. This definition of fever has a sensitivity of 82.5% in nursing-home residents, and the specificity remains high at 89.9% (Table 44.2). Although these data were generated in a trial of frail older veteran men in a nursing home, it would seem reasonable to apply the same definitions to frail older adults of either gender in the community. However, the performance characteristics of this definition of fever in otherwise healthy older adults has not been validated.

The absence of fever is only one atypical presentation of infectious disease in the elderly person. For example, infective endocarditis may be heralded by a nonspecific decline in baseline functional status, such as confusion or falling. Subsequent anorexia and decreased oral intake may follow, and exacerbation of an underlying illness (eg, atrial fibrillation) may become the predominant feature. Cognitive impairment further contributes to the atypical presentation of infections in older adults. Many cognitively impaired older patients are unable to communicate symptoms accurately, and clinicians must be ready to pursue objective assessments such as laboratory and radiologic evaluations at a lower threshold, unless advance directives indicate otherwise.

Antibiotic Management

Drug distribution, metabolism, excretion, and interactions may be altered with age. Aging in the absence of

Table 44.2—Defining Fever in Frail, Older Residents of Long-Term-Care Facilities

Definition	Sensitivity	Specificity	(+) Likelihood Ratio	(−) Likelihood Ratio
T > 101°F (38.3°C)	40.0%	99.7%	133	0.6
T > 100°F (37.7°C)	70.0%	98.3%	41	0.3
T > 99°F (37.2°C)	82.5%	89.9%	8	0.2

NOTE: (+) Likelihood ratio = sensitivity / (1 − specificity); (−) Likelihood ratio = (1 − sensitivity) / specificity; T = temperature.

SOURCE: Data from Castle SC, Yeh M, Toledo S, et al. Lowering the temperature criterion improves detection of infections in nursing home residents. *Aging Immunol Infect Dis.* 1993;4(2):67–76.

any comorbid disease is associated with a reduction in renal function, and reductions in antibiotic dose may be required in the elderly patient. (See "Pharmacotherapy" p 72.) Furthermore, antibiotic interactions occur with many medications commonly prescribed for elderly persons. Digoxin, warfarin, oral hypoglycemic agents, theophylline, antacids, lipid-lowering agents, antihypertensive medications, and H_2-receptor antagonists all have significant interactions with commonly prescribed antibiotics. Drug concentrations can increase (eg, enhanced digoxin toxicity associated with macrolides, tetracyclines, and trimethoprim) or decrease (eg, reduced absorption of some fluoroquinolones with antacids) with concomitant drug administration. Atrophic gastritis, a common problem in older adults, and H_2 blockers or proton-pump inhibitors can reduce the absorption of some antibiotics, such as ketoconazole or itraconazole. Finally, adherence to prescribed regimens may be limited as a consequence of poor cognitive function, impaired hearing or vision, use of multiple medications, and financial constraints.

The choice and timing of antibiotics may also be important in the treatment of older infected adults. In sepsis, a preponderance of data suggests that initially broad coverage is warranted, since outcomes (mortality, length of stay in intensive care) are improved when the offending organism is covered by the initial antibiotic regimen. In older adults with pneumonia, data suggest that delaying initiation of therapy for 4 or more hours after admission to the hospital is associated with an increased risk of mortality. However, these and similar data in other infectious syndromes and the atypical presentation of

infection noted above often leads to early initiation of antimicrobials in older adults, particularly in long-term care. However, in long-term care, up to 75% of antibiotic use may be inappropriate. The use of strict, minimum criteria for initiation of antimicrobials in long-term care is most likely to reduce inappropriate antibiotic use without jeopardizing patient safety (Table 44.3).

INFECTIOUS SYNDROMES

Bacteremia and Sepsis

Bacteremia is a common cause of hospitalization for older patients. Older patients with bacteremia are less likely than their younger counterparts to have chills or sweating, and fever is commonly absent. Gastrointestinal and genitourinary sources of bacteremia are more common; thus, the causative bacteria are more likely to be gram-negative rods.

Bacteremia carries a poor prognosis in older adults. For example, nosocomial gram-negative bacteremia carries a mortality rate of 5% to 35% for young adults, but of 37% to 50% in older adults. Major contributing factors include coexisting diseases that reduce physiologic reserve and the more common use of invasive devices (eg, intravenous or urinary catheters) that make eradication of organisms difficult.

The management of bacteremia and sepsis in older and younger patients is similar. Rapid administration of appropriate antibiotics aimed at the most likely sources is essential. The use of activated protein C as adjunctive therapy in septic older adults had raised concern

Table 44.3—Suggested Minimum Criteria for Initiation of Antibiotic Therapy in the Long-Term-Care Setting

Condition	Minimum Criteria
Urinary tract infection, without catheter	Fever AND one of the following: new or worsening urgency, frequency, suprapubic pain, gross hematuria, CVA tenderness, incontinence
Urinary tract infection, with catheter	Fever OR one of the following: new CVA tenderness, rigors, or new-onset delirium
Skin and soft-tissue infection	Fever OR one of the following: redness, tenderness, warmth, new or increasing swelling of affected site
Respiratory infection	■ Fever > 102°F (38.9°C) AND one of the following: RR > 25, productive cough ■ Fever > 100°F < 102°F AND one of the following: RR > 25, pulse > 100, rigors, new-onset delirium ■ Afebrile with COPD AND new or increased cough with purulent sputum ■ Afebrile without COPD AND new or increased cough AND either RR > 25 or new-onset delirium
Fever without source of infection	■ At least one of the following: new-onset delirium, rigors ■ If these are not present, evaluate without initiating antibiotics ■ Antibiotics probably should not be instituted as a diagnostic test, but if initiated as such, discontinue in 3–5 days if no improvement and evaluation negative

NOTE: COPD = chronic obstructive pulmonary disease; CVA = costovertebral angle; RR = respiratory rate.

SOURCE: Data from Loeb M, Bentley DW, Bradley S, et al. Development of minimum criteria for the initiation of antibiotics in residents of long-term-care facilities: results of a consensus conference. *Infect Control Hosp Epidemiol.* 2001;22:120–124.

about increased bleeding. However, a recent analysis of patients aged 75 and over enrolled in a randomized trial of activated protein C in sepsis demonstrated preservation of the survival benefit in older adults despite a slightly increased risk of serious bleeding.

Pneumonia

Patients aged 65 years and older account for more than 50% of all pneumonia cases, and annual hospitalization rates for pneumonia range from 12 per 1000 among community-dwelling adults aged 75 and older to 32 per 1000 among nursing-home residents. In fact, the cumulative 2-year risk of pneumonia for long-term-care residents is approximately 30%. Pneumonia mortality in older adults is three to five times that of young adults, but the rate is profoundly influenced by comorbidity. Comorbidity is the strongest independent predictor of mortality in community-acquired pneumonia in older adults, with a relative risk of 4.1 (in the article that determined this relative risk, comorbidity was defined as cancer, collagen vascular disease, or advanced liver disease). Other independent risk factors include age of 85 years and older, debility (decreased motor function), serum creatinine >1.5 mg/dL, and the presence of hypothermia ($<36.1°F$), hypotension (<90 mm Hg systolic), or tachycardia (>110 beats per minute) on admission. Long-term follow-up data also suggest that community-acquired pneumonia in older adults indicates a higher risk of subsequent all-cause mortality over the next 12 years as a consequence of both recurrent pneumonia (relative risk 2.1 [1.3 to 3.4]) but also cardiovascular disease (relative risk 1.4 [1.0 to 1.9]).

The causes of pneumonia in younger and elderly adults differ. In elderly patients, *Streptococcus pneumoniae* is still the predominant organism, but gram-negative bacilli (eg, *Haemophilus influenzae, Moraxella catarrhalis, Klebsiella* spp.) are much more common than in younger adults, particularly in patients with chronic obstructive pulmonary disease or who reside in long-term-care facilities. *S. aureus* and respiratory viruses are also common causes of community-acquired pneumonia in nursing-home residents (Figure 44.1).

Pneumonia therapy has changed significantly in the past few years because of the emergence of resistant bacteria, particularly drug-resistant *S. pneumoniae*, leading many practitioners to rely heavily on fluoroquinolones, even for routine community-acquired pneumonia. This practice, however, has led to increased rates of fluoroquinolone resistance in several areas of the world, and some fluoroquinolones can have significant adverse effects, including dizziness and cardiac conduction abnormalities (QT prolongation),

that may limit their use in certain older adults. The current Infectious Diseases Society of America treatment guidelines for community-acquired pneumonia suggest the following as first-line therapy in adults over the age of 60 with or without comorbidity: a β-lactam and β-lactamase combination or advanced-generation cephalosporin (ceftriaxone or cefotaxime) with or without a macrolide. Alternatively, one of the newer fluoroquinolones with enhanced activity against *S. pneumoniae* (levofloxacin, moxifloxacin) may be used. Given the resistance already emerging to fluoroquinolones, it is prudent to use these drugs only in situations with highest risk for drug-resistant *S. pneumoniae* or other resistant organisms. In the outpatient setting, this is limited to residents of long-term-care facilities or patients with marked chronic obstructive pulmonary disease (FEV_1 $<30\%$ predicted). In the inpatient setting, the sicker the patient (ie, the closer to needing intensive care), the stronger the justification for use of a fluoroquinolone. This is true because the margin for error is small, fluoroquinolones are currently the most effective therapy for drug-resistant *S. pneumoniae*, they are effective against most gram-negative bacilli, and they can be used to treat atypical organisms such as *Legionella* spp. that are more likely in the intensive-care setting.

Nursing-home acquired pneumonia (NHAP) or hospital acquired pneumonia (HAP) in older adults requires more broad initial therapy than community-acquired pneumonia because of the broader spectrum of organisms causing infection (see Figure 44.1). In the nursing-home setting, polymicrobial infection, often due to aspiration, and *S. aureus* are much more common than in the community setting. In the hospital setting, gram-negative bacilli predominate, but *S. aureus* is more common as well and is more likely to affect specific antibiotic choices because of resistance. Outcomes data suggest that response to therapy is greater when the initial antibiotic regimen covers the offending agent. Thus, initial regimens should be broadly inclusive, followed by step-down therapy to more narrow coverage if the causative agent is identified. Importantly, if patients are known to be colonized with methicillin-resistant *S. aureus* (MRSA), initial regimens should include vancomycin or linezolid until MRSA is excluded as the cause. Further, data suggest that patients with clinically improving HAP not caused by nonfermenting gram-negative bacilli (eg, *Pseudomonas, Stenotrophomonas*) can be treated with shorter courses of antibiotics, 7 or 8 days, rather than the 2 weeks commonly employed in the past. Shorter courses (8 days versus 15 days) of antibiotics are associated with equivalent efficacy and less antibiotic resistance.

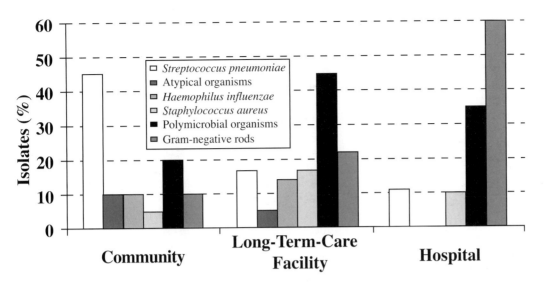

Figure 44.1—Causes of pneumonia by domiciliary setting. A specific cause for pneumonia is isolated only 30% to 50% of the time. Isolates here were pooled from several studies and were microbiologically confirmed. When a specific causative agent is identified, the predominant organisms vary by domiciliary setting, as indicated. Atypical organisms include *Mycoplasma pneumoniae*, *Chlamydia pneumoniae*, viruses, and, rarely, *Legionella* spp.

The prevention of pneumonia in older adults is a complex issue, and a multipronged approach is most likely to be effective. Immunization of at-risk persons is far and away the most well-studied measure (see "Prevention," p 63). In addition to vaccines, smoking cessation and aggressive treatment of comorbidities (eg, minimizing aspiration risk in post-stroke patients, limited use of sedative hypnotics) may reduce the risk of infection. Finally, system changes with attention to infection control (isolation, cohorting, skin testing for tuberculosis with purified protein derivative [PPD], and immunization policies) may be particularly effective in the nursing home.

Influenza

Influenza results in approximately 40,000 deaths annually in the United States, and nearly all of these deaths occur in the older adult population. The clinical syndrome of influenza is easily recognized by most clinicians, particularly in the setting of local activity or outbreak settings frequently seen in the nursing home. Annual influenza vaccine is 60% to 80% efficacious in older adults for preventing severe disease, hospitalization, and death. Therefore, annual immunization is recommended for all adults over the age 50, and for anyone of any age who wishes to reduce the risk of serious influenza.

According to current CDC recommendations, amantadine and rimantadine should not be used because of resistance. In contrast, neuraminidase inhibitors (zanamivir and oseltamivir) are effective against both influenza A and B; they inhibit the virus by interference with an essential enzyme, neuraminidase, that cleaves sialic acid to expose host cell receptors for the virus. Oseltamivir, a capsule, is preferred over zanamivir in older adults because zanamivir must be inhaled, and it is difficult for many older adults to properly use the product. Treatment of influenza is effective if initiated in the first 48 hours, but it is most effective if initiated within 24 hours of symptom onset. Neuraminidase inhibitors, oseltamivir and zanamivir, can be used for the treatment and prevention of influenza. The safety of these compounds is based on evidence from only one or two randomized controlled trials and systematic reviews. These findings suggest that neuraminidase inhibitors have a reasonable adverse event profile if being used to treat or protect patients against a life-threatening disease.

Urinary Tract Infection

Urinary tract infection (UTI) is among the most common of clinical illnesses in older adults, with an incidence of 10.9 per 100 person years in men and 14 per 100 person years in women age 65 and older. As in young adults, gram-negative bacilli (eg, *Escherichia coli*, *Enterobacter* spp., *Klebsiella* spp., *Proteus* spp.) are most common, but there is an increase in more resistant isolates, such as *Pseudomonas aeruginosa*, and in gram-positive organisms, including enterococci, coagulase-negative staphylococci, and *Streptococcus agalactiae* (group B strep). In patients with indwelling catheters, the microbes listed still predominate, but it is also common to encounter additional organisms, including enterococci, *S. aureus,* and fungi, particularly *Candida* spp. The organisms colonizing urinary catheters commonly develop biofilms and are difficult to clear with the same urinary catheter in place.

Asymptomatic Bacteriuria

Up to 15% of women in the community and 40% of women in nursing homes will have asymptomatic bacteriuria; the incidence in men is approximately half that in women. Rates are even higher with the use of condom catheters (87%) or Foley catheters (nearly 100%). Numerous studies have suggested that there is no clinical benefit from the treatment of asymptomatic bacteriuria and that treatment is associated with significant adverse effects, expense, and the potential for selection of resistant organisms. Thus, no treatment is recommended. The clinical difficulty faced almost daily by clinicians is deciding what is symptomatic. The presentation of infection can be quite subtle in older adults, and a change in functional status often prompts the collection of a urine specimen even in the absence of fever, dysuria, or other typical clinical features. However, since no controlled trial has ever shown a decreased incidence of urosepsis or mortality with antibiotic treatment of asymptomatic bacteriuria, a period of observation rather than a therapeutic trial would seem most prudent when symptoms are not clearly related to bacteriuria.

Urinary Tract Infection in Women

In contrast to asymptomatic bacteriuria, symptomatic UTI does require therapy. Therapy is based on the location of infection (upper versus lower tract disease) and likely causative agent. Lower tract UTI (cystitis), characterized by dysuria, frequency, and urgency (note: not fever, which generally indicates upper tract disease), is often treated in young women for 1 to 3 days, and recent data suggest 3 days of therapy is sufficient for uncomplicated cystitis in older women. Randomized trials in older women indicate that fluoroquinolones are more efficacious than trimethoprim-sulfamethoxazole (TMP-SMX), likely because of *E. coli* TMP-SMX resistance rates of 10% to 20% in most areas of the country. Other reasonable choices in some settings include amoxicillin (particularly for enterococcal infection) and first-generation cephalosporins in the patient with multiple antibiotic intolerances. Culture is not required unless first-line therapy fails.

Upper UTI (pyelonephritis), characterized by fever, chills, nausea, and flank pain and commonly accompanied by lower tract symptoms, requires more prolonged therapy, 7 to 21 days. Because of the excellent bioavailability of many antibiotics, particularly the fluoroquinolones, intravenous therapy is not essential if the patient can tolerate oral medications. A study comparing fluoroquinolones with TMP-SMX for upper tract UTI in younger women (aged 18 to 58) suggests that fluoroquinolones are more effective (microbiologic cure rate 99% versus 89% for TMP-SMX; clinical cure rates 96% versus 83%, respectively) because of the presence of TMP-SMX–resistant organisms. This is likely to be true in older adults as well. Intravenous administration of antibiotics remains the standard of care for patients with suspected urosepsis, those with upper tract disease due to relatively resistant bacteria such as enterococci, or those unable to tolerate oral medications. Culture and sensitivity data are more useful in guiding antimicrobial therapy in upper tract UTIs than in lower tract disease and should be obtained in most cases.

Prophylactic antibiotics intended to prevent frequently recurrent UTIs in older women are not recommended because of the high incidence of the development of resistant organisms. Several measures may decrease the frequency of recurrence, including intravaginal or systemic estrogen replacement that changes the vaginal flora, thus reducing the risk of UTI, or perhaps ingestion of at least 300 mL of cranberry juice each day, though data in support of these measures remain preliminary.

Urinary Tract Infection in Men

Prostatic disease (primarily hyperplasia) or functional disability, such as autonomic neuropathy from diabetes mellitus with incomplete bladder emptying, account for the majority of both lower and upper UTIs in elderly men. Thus, short-course therapy for UTIs in elderly men is inappropriate and should be avoided. A minimum of 14 days of therapy should be provided, and if prostatic involvement is suspected (ie, acute or chronic prostatitis), at least 6 weeks of therapy is usually required. The causative organisms and treatment choices are similar to those outlined above for elderly women. Fluoroquinolones and TMP-SMX are most widely used when prostatic involvement is suspected and culture data confirms the organism's susceptibility because, of the available agents, these two penetrate the prostate the best. Because treatment for all UTIs in men is generally longer than in women and the prostate is a common reservoir for recurrent UTIs, culture and sensitivity data should guide therapy for virtually all UTIs in men.

Tuberculosis

Worldwide, approximately 1.7 billion persons are infected with *Mycobacterium tuberculosis* (MTB), 16 million in the United States. Adults aged 65 and older account for one fourth of all active tuberculosis cases in the United States. The vast majority of active MTB in older adults occurs in community-dwelling elderly persons, but the rate of infection in long-term-care residents is much higher: skin-test studies show prevalence rates of skin-test reactivity in the range of 30% to 50%. This high prevalence is due to MTB exposure in the early 1900s, when it was estimated that 80% of all persons were infected with MTB by the age of 30. Most active cases of tuberculosis in older adults are, therefore, due to reactivation disease, but primary infection may account for 10% to 20% of cases and is of particular concern in nursing-home outbreaks.

As with most other infections, tuberculosis may not present in classic fashion (cough, sputum, fever, night sweats, weight loss) in the elderly patient. Often fatigue, anorexia, decreased functional status, or low-grade fever are the presenting manifestations. Most tuberculous disease in elderly persons occurs with lung involvement (75%), and pneumonic processes in older adults, particularly those that develop in a postacute manner, should raise a high index of suspicion for MTB. Older adults are more likely than their younger counterparts to have extrapulmonary disease. Other sites include miliary (disseminated) disease, tuberculous meningitis or osteomyelitis, and urogenital disease, but virtually any body structure can be involved, and that organ system can account for the major presenting symptom.

A diagnosis of active disease usually requires isolation of the organism from sputum, urine, or other clinical specimen. Current techniques have improved the speed of diagnosis, particularly for identifying the species of *Mycobacterium* after isolation. This is now typically accomplished within 24 hours of obtaining a positive culture by use of DNA probes. Direct polymerase chain reaction of clinical specimens or other rapid diagnostic techniques are not available or reliable in most local laboratories, but such tests can be obtained in research settings. They are most likely to be helpful for establishing a diagnosis from cerebrospinal or pleural fluid, which yields positive cultures in only 10% to 15% of cases.

The most confusing area of MTB diagnostics for most practitioners is the interpretation of the results of PPD skin tests. In all populations, induration of ≥15 mm 48 to 72 hours after placement of a 5-tuberculin-unit PPD indicates a positive test. Induration ≥10 mm is considered a positive test in nursing-home residents, recent converters (previous PPD <5 mm), immigrants from countries with high endemicity of MTB, underserved populations in the United States (homeless persons, black Americans, Hispanic Americans, and Native Americans), and per-

sons with specific risk factors (gastrectomy, >10% below ideal body weight, chronic kidney failure, diabetes mellitus, or immune suppression, including that caused by corticosteroids or malignancy). In patients infected with human immunodeficiency virus (HIV), those with a history of close contact with persons with active MTB, and those with chest radiographs consistent with MTB, ≥5 mm induration is considered a positive PPD test. Anergy panel testing in conjunction with PPD testing is of little value and is not recommended.

Long-term-care facilities should employ a two-step procedure for PPD testing during the initial evaluation of residents. Two-step testing requires retesting of patients with <10 mm induration within 2 weeks. If the second skin test results in ≥10 mm of induration or the increase in the size of the induration from the first to the second skin test is ≥6mm, the patient is considered PPD positive.

The treatment of active MTB in the elderly person is similar to that in young adults. Four-drug therapy (usually isoniazid [INH], rifampin, pyrazinamide, and ethambutol or streptomycin) is recommended as initial therapy, with tapering to one of several two- or three-drug regimens once susceptibility testing is available. The most common regimen is INH, rifampin, and pyrazinamide for 2 months, followed by INH and rifampin for an additional 4 months.

Prophylaxis with 9 months of INH for asymptomatic persons with a positive PPD should be provided *regardless of age* in adults who are recent converters (defined in persons >35 years of age with a PPD that has gone from <10 mm to ≥15 mm within 2 years), or regardless of duration of PPD positivity if one is afflicted with any of the specific risk factors highlighted above. Patients with a positive PPD of unknown duration, particularly those over the age of 35 years, should receive INH prophylaxis with close monitoring for symptoms and signs of peripheral neuropathy (due to INH and preventable by coadministration of pyridoxine) and hepatitis (due to INH, rifampin, or pyrazinamide). Shorter course therapy with 2 months of rifampin and pyrazinamide is effective but has a much higher incidence of hepatotoxicity than INH and thus should be used only in very specific circumstances.

Infective Endocarditis

Since the early part of the 20th century, infective endocarditis (IE) has undergone a transformation, from a disease of young adults primarily due to rheumatic or congenital valve anomalies to one of older adults associated with degenerative valvular disorders and prosthetic valves. Native-valve endocarditis is typically caused by viridans streptococci, *S. aureus*, and occasional infections are due to HACEK organisms (a group of typically nonfermenting gram-negative rods that primarily inhabit the oral cavity and include the genera *Haemophilus, Actinobacillus, Cardiobacterium, Eikenella,* and *Kingella*). Gastrointestinal and genitourinary organisms, such as enterococci and gram-negative rods, are more common in native-valve IE in older adults, and coagulase-negative staphylococci are a common cause of prosthetic-valve endocarditis, particularly in the first 60 days following placement of a prosthetic valve.

The diagnosis of endocarditis is often difficult in the elderly patient. Fever and leukocytosis are less common in elderly than in younger patients, occurring in only 55% and 25%, respectively, versus 80% and 60%, respectively. Blood culture positivity rates do not vary by age; however, degenerative, calcific valvular lesions and prosthetic valves lower the sensitivity of transthoracic echocardiography (TTE) to 45% in older patients (sensitivity is 75% in younger patients). Transesophageal echocardiography (TEE) improves the diagnostic yield for IE, but the absence of positive findings on TEE never excludes IE. TEE is of particular value in resolving the clinical problem of *S. aureus* bacteremia. Positive findings on TEE support prolonged antibiotic administration (4 to 6 weeks) versus short-course (2-week) therapy. On the other hand, TEE is invasive and expensive. Interestingly, age does not appear to play a major role in mortality risk, with a 2-year survival of 75% for IE in all age groups unless major comorbidities are also present.

Antibiotic treatment of IE is directed at the identified pathogen or the most likely causes, if blood cultures are negative. Therapy is administered intravenously for 2 to 6 weeks. Surgical therapy should be considered for severe valvular dysfunction, recurrent emboli, marked heart failure, myocardial abscess formation, fungal endocarditis, or the failure of appropriate antibiotics to sterilize blood cultures.

Prophylaxis is available for bacterial endocarditis in at-risk patients undergoing dental, upper respiratory tract, gastrointestinal, or genitourinary procedures. Recommendations for endocarditis prophylaxis have been published and are widely available (eg, the American Heart Association, see http://www.amhrt.org).

Prosthetic Device Infections

Permanent implantable prosthetic devices are common in the elderly age group. Prosthetic joints, cardiac pacemakers, artificial heart valves, intraocular lens implants, vascular grafts, penile prostheses, and a variety of other devices are more often placed in older than in younger adults. A discussion of all prosthetic device infections is beyond the scope of this chapter, but several general concepts can be summarized.

Prosthetic device infections are usually separated into early versus late infection because the causative agents differ significantly. Early prosthetic device infection (PDI), most commonly defined as occurring less than 60 days after device implantation, is primarily due to contamination at the time of implantation or events associated with the acute hospitalization (such as occult bacteremias due to intravenous catheters). Thus, coagulase-negative staphylococci predominate, and *S. aureus* and diphtheroids are common as well; gram-negative bacilli and fungi are relatively rare causes of early PDI. Late PDI is usually caused by organisms that commonly cause transient bacteremia (in the elderly person this is most often skin, respiratory, gastrointestinal, or genitourinary organisms). Staphylococci, including coagulase-negative staphylococci, play a major role in PDIs in both the early and late periods, though their relative importance is greater early. Thus, empiric staphylococcal therapy should be provided in either early or late PDI if a specific causative agent is not identified.

In general, hardware removal is required to clear PDIs. However, early antibiotic intervention, in some instances combined with aggressive surgical drainage, may be successful. Small studies in prosthetic joint infection suggest that initial debridement and culture and a brief course (2 weeks) of intravenous antibiotics followed by combination oral therapy with fluoroquinolones and rifampin for 3 to 6 months may obviate the need for device removal. Until more definitive data are available, it is prudent to restrict this approach to patients with a short duration of symptoms (<3 weeks), those who are likely to have difficulty tolerating another surgical procedure, or those in whom return to full functional status is not a realistic goal because of comorbidities. In those older adults in whom full functionality is the goal, the best chance for cure is a two-stage procedure in which the device is removed and antibiotics are given for an extended period (6 to 8 weeks), followed by delayed reimplantation. For life-saving devices such as mechanical valves or implantable defibrillators, this is not an option. Infected prosthetic devices are usually surrounded by microbial biofilms, such as microbe-derived glycocalyx. Biofilms reduce antibiotic penetration and greatly increase the bactericidal concentrations of antibiotic without changing the inhibitory concentrations (ie, the amount of drug necessary to inhibit the organism does not change, but it takes tremendously increased concentrations to kill the organism). Furthermore, many conditions associated with infected prostheses are also accompanied by poor blood flow to the area. Thus, it is preferable to use bactericidal antibiotics, often in combination with a second agent that penetrates biofilms and poorly perfused areas (eg, rifampin for staphylococci).

The use of prophylactic antibiotics in situations other than prosthetic heart valves remains a point of contention. Antimicrobial prophylaxis is indicated for dental, gastrointestinal, and genitourinary procedures for patients with prosthetic valves and is probably reasonable for vascular grafts, particularly within the first few months after placement, but no randomized controlled trial has ever clearly shown benefit. The need for prophylaxis for patients with prosthetic joints, intraocular lens implants, cerebrospinal fluid shunts, breast implants, or less common prostheses is even less clear. However, a joint statement by the American Dental Association and American Academy of Orthopaedic Surgeons (AAOS) recommends very limited use of antibiotic prophylaxis in specific patients undergoing dental procedures with a higher bacteremic risk (eg, dental extraction) and who are also at high risk for hematologic seeding (eg, first 2 years after prosthetic joint replacement, immunocompromised or immunosuppressed, or previous prosthetic joint infection). For more information, see the advisory statement posted on the AAOS Web site (http://www.aaos.org/wordhtml/papers/advistmt/1014.htm).

Bone and Joint Infections

Native bone and joint infections in the absence of prostheses occur in older adults. Septic arthritis is more likely to occur in joints with underlying pathology (rheumatoid changes, gout, osteoarthritis), and early arthrocentesis is indicated in any mono- or oligo-articular syndrome to exclude infection. *S. aureus* is the most likely pathogen; only rarely are infections due to gram-negative bacilli and streptococci. Aggressive antibiotic therapy combined with serial arthrocentesis may be as effective as open surgical drainage in uncomplicated septic arthritis, and it preserves better functionality in the joint. Surgical drainage is required for patients failing this more conservative strategy.

Osteomyelitis in older adults can be due to hematogenous seeding from a bacteremia or contiguous spread from an adjacent focus. *S. aureus* is the predominant organism, but gastrointestinal and genitourinary flora are again more common in older adults, which emphasizes the advantage of a specific microbiologic diagnosis to guide therapy. Infections of pressure ulcers and diabetic foot infections are very common, particularly in institutionalized older adults, and they commonly require surgical consultation combined with aggressive antimicrobial therapy aimed at mixed aerobic and anaerobic bacteria.

HIV Infection and AIDS

HIV infection in elderly adults was initially limited to those who had received blood transfusions for surgical procedures. However, increasing numbers of older Americans with HIV have acquired their infection via sexual activity. Older adults constitute approximately 10% of all new diagnoses of acquired immunodeficiency syndrome (AIDS) in the United States, but this group suffers from a lack of HIV awareness among their clinicians. Nonspecific symptoms such as forgetfulness, anorexia, weight loss, and recurrent pneumonia are often dismissed as age-related, and HIV testing can be delayed. Untreated HIV infection in the elderly person tends to pursue a more rapid downhill course, perhaps because of impaired T-cell replacement mechanisms with advanced age and the impact of additional comorbidities. However, if older adults are treated with aggressive highly active antiretroviral therapy (HAART), the response is similar to that seen in young adults. In fact, older adults often adhere better to complicated HAART regimens than young adults. Treatment regimens and opportunistic infection prophylaxis with the HAART combination are similar to those used in younger persons. Indications that HIV therapies may accelerate atherosclerosis and glucose intolerance suggest that an aggressive approach to cardiovascular prevention in older HIV-infected adults is warranted and may lead to specific recommendations in older adults if associations of metabolic changes with specific HIV therapies become clearer.

HIV prevention is rarely discussed in the geriatric community but is important if the trend of increasing sexual acquisition of HIV in older adults is to be reversed. Most older women do not believe that they are at risk for HIV infection, yet heterosexual activity is the primary mode of infection in this group. The concept of HIV-risky behavior is not pervasive in the geriatric community because HIV was not a problem during their adolescence or young adulthood. Elderly persons must be included in educational programs aimed at ensuring safe sexual practices and increasing awareness of the benefits of testing and effective HIV therapy.

Additional Common Infectious Syndromes

Advancing age is the major risk factor for reactivated varicella-zoster virus, herpes zoster or "shingles"; the most disabling complication, post-herpetic neuralgia, is common in elderly persons. (See "Dermatologic Diseases and Disorders," p 290, for diagnosis and treatment.) There is now compelling evidence from the Shingle Prevention Study that the zoster vaccine significantly reduces the incidence of and morbidity associated with varicella zoster virus. Although not yet covered by third-party payers, the vaccine is available for use.

Facial nerve palsy (Bell's palsy) is common in older adults and associated with at least three infectious causes: herpes simplex virus, varicella zoster virus, and *Borrelia burgdorferi* (which causes Lyme disease). There are no strong data, at present, to suggest benefit of antiviral therapy for facial nerve palsies due to herpes simplex virus, but trials are under way. If facial nerve palsy occurs as part of an episode of varicella zoster virus, treatment is indicated (see "Dermatologic Diseases and Disorders," p 289). If Lyme disease is suspected on a clinical basis, the patient should receive oral amoxicillin, 500 mg four times a day for 14 days; or doxycycline, 100 mg twice a day for 14 days; or intravenous ceftriaxone, 2 g per day for 14 days.

Gastrointestinal infections are common among elderly persons. Diverticulitis, appendicitis, cholecystitis, intra-abdominal abscess, and ischemic bowel can present diagnostic dilemmas in the absence of fever or elevated white blood cell counts. A high index of suspicion is necessary in older adults. Computed tomography or labeled white cell studies are most likely to be of value in establishing the diagnosis of intra-abdominal infection, and ultrasound is an easy, readily available tool to assist in diagnosing cholecystitis, appendicitis, or abscess. Ischemic bowel often requires angiography.

Infectious diarrhea is also common in elderly persons. Older patients with achlorhydria are at particular risk because a lower bacterial inoculum is necessary to cause disease. Decreased intestinal motility associated with specific medications and advanced age may further increase susceptibility to infection. Epidemics occurring in the long-term-care setting are commonly due to *E. coli*, viruses, salmonellae, or *Shigella* spp. Frequent use of antimicrobials in older adults also increases the risk for *Clostridium difficile* colitis. Moreover, there is increased evidence of resistant strains of *Clostridium difficile* creating challenges to management of these individuals. Probiotic therapy is often recommended, although there is not yet sufficient support to indicate routine administration of probiotics for all patients.

FEVER OF UNKNOWN ORIGIN

Fever of unknown origin (FUO) is currently defined as temperature greater than 38.3°C (101°F) that lasts for at least 3 weeks and is undiagnosed after 1 week of medical evaluation. Several studies have examined this syndrome in elderly patients and demonstrated interesting differences between older and younger adults. The cause of FUO can be determined in more than 90% of cases in elderly persons, and one third have treatable infections, such as intra-abdominal abscess, bacterial endocarditis, tuberculosis, perinephric abscess, or occult osteomyelitis, with an incidence of infection similar to that in younger patients. In contrast, collagen vascular diseases are more common causes of FUO in elderly than in younger patients. These are primarily due to giant cell arteritis, polymyalgia rheumatica, and polyarteritis nodosa, but rarely due to Wegener's granulomatosis. In several published series, 28% of all FUOs in elderly persons were due to collagen vascular diseases (Table 44.4). Neoplastic disease accounts for another 20%, but, with rare exceptions, fever due to cancer is primarily confined to hematologic malignancies (eg, lymphoma and leukemia), and not solid tumors. Drugs are another cause of FUO in elderly persons. Rare causes in this age group include deep-vein thrombosis with or without recurrent pulmonary emboli and hyperthyroidism.

A diagnostic approach to FUO in older adults is presented in Table 44.5.

Table 44.4—Fever of Unknown Origin in Older Adults

Causes	Approximate % of Cases
Infections	35
Intra-abdominal abscess	12
Infective endocarditis	10
Other	7
Tuberculosis	6
Collagen vascular disorders	28
Giant cell arteritis, polymyalgia rheumatica	19
Polyarteritis nodosa	6
Other	3
Malignancy	19
Lymphoma	10
Carcinoma	9
Others (pulmonary emboli, drug fever)	9
No diagnosis	5–10

SOURCE: Data pooled from multiple studies: Esposito AL, Gleckman RA. Fever of unknown origin in the elderly. *J Am Geriatr Soc.* 1978;26(11):498; Knockaert DC, Vanneste LJ, Bobbaers HJ. Fever of unknown origin in elderly patients. *J Am Geriatr Soc.* 1993;41(11):1187–1192.

Table 44.5—Evaluation of Fever of Unknown Origin in Older Adults

1. Confirm fever; conduct thorough history (include travel, MTB exposure, drugs, constitutional symptoms, symptoms of giant cell arteritis) and physical examination. Discontinue nonessential medications.

2. Initial laboratory evaluation: CBC with differential, liver enzymes, ESR, blood cultures × 3, PPD skin testing, TSH, antinuclear antibody, consider antineutrophilic cytoplasmic-antibody or HIV-antibody testing in specific cases.

3. a) Chest or abdomen or pelvic CT scan—if no obvious source; *or*

   b) Temporal artery biopsy—if symptoms or signs consistent with giant cell arteritis or polymyalgia rheumatica and increased ESR; *or*

   c) Site-directed work-up on basis of symptoms or laboratory abnormalities, or both.

4. If 3a is performed and no source is found, then 3b, and vice versa.

5. a) BM biopsy—yield best if hemogram abnormal—send for H&E, special stains, cultures, *or*

   b) Liver biopsy—very poor yield unless abnormal liver enzymes or hepatomegaly.

6. Indium-111 labeled white blood cell or gallium-67 scan—nuclear scans can effectively exclude infectious cause of FUO if negative.

7. Laparoscopy or exploratory laparotomy.

8. Empiric trial—typically reserved for antituberculosis therapy in rapidly declining host or high suspicion for tuberculosis (ie, prior [+] PPD).

NOTE: BM = bone marrow; CBC = complete blood cell count; CT = computed tomography; ESR = erythrocyte sedimentation rate; FUO = fever of unknown origin; HIV = human immunodeficiency virus; H&E = hematoxylin and eosin stain; MTB = *Mycobacterium tuberculosis*; PPD = (tuberculin) purified protein derivative; TSH = thyroid stimulating hormone.

REFERENCES

- American Thoracic Society and Infectious Diseases Society of America. Guidelines for the management of adults with hospital-acquired, ventilator-associated, and health-care associated pneumonia. *Am J Respir Crit Care Med.* 2005;171(4):388–416.

- Boyce JM, Havill NL, Maria B. Frequency and possible infection control implications of gastrointestinal colonization with methicillin-resistant Staphylococcus aureus. *J Clin Microbiol.* 2005;43(12):5992–5995.

- Lawrence SJ, Korzenik JR, Mundy LM. Probiotics for recurrent Clostridium difficile disease. *J Med Microbiol.* 2005;54(Pt 9):905–906.

- Millan-Rodriguez F, Palou J, Bujons-Tur A, et al. Acute bacterial prostatitis: two different sub-categories according to a previous manipulation of the lower urinary tract. *World J Urol.* 2006;24(1):45–50.

- Oxman MN, Levin MJ, Johnson GR, et al. A vaccine to prevent herpes zoster and postherpetic neuralgia in older adults. *N Engl J Med.* 2005;352(22):2271–2284.

- Woolery WA, Franco FR. Fever of unknown origin: keys to determining the etiology in older patients. *Geriatrics.* 2004;59(10):41–45.

- Zimmerli W, Trampuz A, Ochsner PE. Prosthetic-joint infections. *N Engl J Med.* 2004;351(16):1645–1654.

CHAPTER 45—CARDIOVASCULAR DISEASES AND DISORDERS

KEY POINTS

- Coronary artery disease is the most common cause of death in people aged 65 years and older. Autopsy studies show that 70% of people older than 70 have the disease.

- Double-blind, randomized controlled studies have demonstrated that the absolute reduction in cardiovascular mortality and morbidity in elderly adults with dyslipidemia treated with statins is greater than for people younger than 65 years.

- Heart failure is the most common cause of hospitalization and rehospitalization in people aged 65 years and older. The prevalence and incidence increase with age.

- Atrial fibrillation is the most common type of arrhythmia in adults and is more common as patients age. Evidence-based recommendations for the management of newly detected atrial fibrillation now exist.

- Older adults with peripheral vascular disease are at increased risk of all-cause mortality, cardiovascular mortality, and mortality from coronary artery disease.

AGE-RELATED CARDIOVASCULAR CHANGES

See Table 45.1.

ISCHEMIC HEART DISEASE

Epidemiology

Coronary artery disease (CAD) is the most common cause of death in people aged 65 years and older. Autopsy studies show that 70% of people older than 70 years have CAD with $\geq$50% atherosclerotic obstruction of one or more coronary arteries. More than 30% of people aged 65 years and older have clinical manifestations of CAD. In one study the prevalence of CAD among 1802 community-dwelling older adults (mean age = 80 years) was 33% for the white Americans, 35% for the black Americans, 35% for the Hispanic Americans, and 38% for the Asian Americans. Eighty percent of deaths from CAD occur in people aged 65 years and older; 60% of people hospitalized with acute myocardial infarction (MI) are aged 65 years and older. The prevalence of CAD and the incidence of new

Table 45.1—Age-Related Changes That Affect Heart Action and Circulation

Structure or Function	Change With Age
Myocytes	Progressive loss of cells; hypertrophy
Left-ventricular stiffness	Increased
Left-ventricular compliance	Decreased
Left-ventricular wall thickness	Increased
Left-ventricular diastolic filling	Decreased, with increased contribution to filling resulting from left atrial systole
Left-ventricular relaxation	Decreased
Maximal heart rate	Progressive decrease
Maximal cardiac output	Progressive decrease
Maximal Vo_2	Progressive decrease
Systemic vascular resistance	Increased
Vasodilator response to exercise	Decreased
Ability to secrete sodium	Decreased

coronary events are similar among men and women aged 75 years and older, but they are higher among men who are younger than 75. Eighty-three percent of MIs in women occur after menopause. Women are less likely than men to survive the initial MI.

CAD may be diagnosed in older adults if there is coronary angiographic evidence of significant CAD, a documented MI, a typical history of angina pectoris, or clinical findings of myocardial ischemia. The incidence of sudden cardiac death as the initial manifestation of CAD increases with age.

Risk Factors

It is important to address modifiable risk factors for CAD in older persons. Cessation of cigarette smoking, treatment of hyperlipidemia, treatment of hypertension, ingestion of a diet low in saturated fat and cholesterol, maintenance of ideal body weight, and regular physical activity will lead to a reduction of CAD and new coronary events. Whether decreasing elevated plasma homocysteine levels by increasing folate supplements will reduce the incidence of new coronary events is not yet known.

If hypertension is present, lower blood pressure to <140/90 mm Hg. If CAD is present and the serum low-density lipoprotein (LDL) cholesterol is >125 mg/dL despite use of the American Heart Association (AHA) Step II diet, lipid-lowering drug therapy, preferably statin drug therapy, is recommended. The National Cholesterol Education Program Adult Treatment Panel (ATP) III guidelines have been updated and now recommend that physicians set an LDL goal of <70 mg/dL for very high-risk patients, on the basis of studies such as the Heart Protection Study. Very high-risk people are those with diabetes mellitus and cardiovascular disease, acute coronary syndrome, or multiple severe or poorly controlled risk factors. In high-risk people, the recommended LDL goal is <100 mg/dL. High-risk people are those with cardiovascular disease, diabetes mellitus, or a 10-year risk of CAD of >20%. If a second lipid-lowering drug is needed in addition to a statin drug to achieve this, preferably the cholesterol absorption inhibitor ezetimibe or a bile acid resin such as colesevelam can be used.

The LDL goals for moderate and low-risk individuals currently remain the same: that is, <130 mg/dL in older adults with two or more risk factors and a 10-year risk for CAD of 10% to 20%; <160 mg/dL for older adults with one or no risk factors.

It may be beneficial to treat hypertriglyceridemia in patients who also have hypercholesterolemia or hypoalphalipoproteinemia, or both. Possible indications for treatment of isolated hypertriglyceridemia include overt CAD, a strong family history of CAD, and multiple coexisting cardiac risk factors. Consider treating with gemfibrozil or nicotinic acid. People with CAD and a low serum high-density lipoprotein (HDL) cholesterol in the presence of a normal serum LDL cholesterol should be treated with gemfibrozil. These recommendations may need to be modified in the presence of comorbid conditions.

Presentation

In older adults, myocardial ischemia caused by CAD is more commonly manifested by dyspnea on exertion than by chest pain typical of angina pectoris. The dyspnea is caused by a transient increase in left ventricular (LV) end-diastolic pressure caused by ischemia superimposed on reduced ventricular compliance. Angina pectoris in older adults may cause pain in the back and shoulders or a burning epigastric pain. A substernal location of anginal pain is less commonly observed in older adults. The pain of angina pectoris in older persons may be described as less severe and of shorter duration. Myocardial ischemia may cause clinical heart failure. Acute pulmonary edema in older adults unassociated with acute MI may be a clinical manifestation of unstable angina pectoris resulting from extensive CAD.

In studies of older adults with clinically recognized acute MI, the prevalence of presenting symptoms ranged from 19% to 66% for chest pain, 20% to 59% for dyspnea, 15% to 33% for neurologic symptoms, and 0% to 19% for gastrointestinal symptoms. Other symptoms associated with acute MI in older adults include sudden death, peripheral gangrene, increased claudica-

tion, palpitations, kidney failure, weakness, pulmonary embolism, restlessness, and sweating. Older adults with acute MI are more likely than younger people to die from the MI and to have pulmonary edema, heart failure (HF), LV systolic dysfunction, cardiogenic shock, conduction disturbances requiring insertion of a pacemaker, atrial fibrillation (AF) or atrial flutter, and rupture of the LV free wall, septum, or papillary muscle.

Diagnostic Testing

For terms on interpreting screening and diagnostic tests, see the Appendix, p 464.

Coronary angiography is the gold standard for detecting CAD and determining its severity. Resting electrocardiography (ECG) may be used to diagnose MI or ischemia, whether silent or symptomatic, in older adults. The diagnosis of CAD by treadmill exercise-induced ischemic ST-segment depression ≥1.0 mm in older adults has a sensitivity of 84% and a specificity of 70%. The diagnosis of CAD by upright bicycle exercise–induced ischemic ST-segment depression ≥1.0 mm in older adults has a sensitivity of 62% and a specificity of 93%. Older adults with the following are more likely to have multivessel CAD and a higher incidence of new coronary events:

- exercise-induced hypotension,
- an inadequate blood-pressure response to exercise,
- marked ischemic ST-segment depression (≥2.0 mm),
- ischemic ST-segment depression in both anterior and inferior leads,
- poor exercise duration (<6 minutes using a standard Bruce treadmill protocol),
- ischemic ST-segment depression occurring within 6 minutes of exercise, and
- persistence of ST-segment depression past 8 minutes in the recovery period.

Older adults with CAD and complex ventricular arrhythmias or silent myocardial ischemia detected by 24-hour ambulatory ECG monitoring have a higher incidence of new coronary events.

Exercise stress testing using thallium perfusion scintigraphy or radionuclide ventriculography may be useful in the diagnosis and prognosis of CAD in older adults, especially for those in whom ST-segment changes cannot be reliably interpreted because of left bundle branch block, LV hypertrophy, or treatment with digitalis. In older adults unable to perform exercise stress testing because of musculoskeletal disorders or pulmonary disease, intravenous dipyridamole-thallium imaging may be used for the diagnosis and prognosis of CAD. The diagnosis of CAD by intravenous dipyridamole-thallium imaging in people aged 70 years or older has a sensitivity of 86% and a specificity of 75%.

Echocardiography may be useful for detecting regional LV wall motion abnormalities, acute myocardial ischemia, and complications due to acute MI, LV aneurysm, cardiac thrombi, left main CAD, LV hypertrophy, and associated valvular heart disease; it is also useful for evaluating LV systolic and diastolic function and cardiac chamber size in older adults with CAD. Echocardiographic LV hypertrophy and abnormal LV ejection fraction are also associated with an increased incidence of new coronary events in older adults with CAD.

Stress echocardiography using exercise or dobutamine or adenosine is useful in diagnosing CAD and determining the prognosis in older adults. Exercise echocardiography has a sensitivity of 85% and a specificity of 77% in diagnosing CAD in older adults. In persons aged ≥70 years, dobutamine stress echocardiography has a sensitivity of 87%, a specificity of 84%, and an accuracy of 86%. In people aged ≥70 years, adenosine stress echocardiography has a sensitivity of 66%, a specificity of 90%, and an accuracy of 73%.

The American College of Cardiology (ACC)/American Heart Association (AHA) guidelines do not recommend electron-beam computed tomography for diagnosing obstructive CAD because of its low specificity. These guidelines also state that the published data do not answer the question of whether the electron-beam computed tomography score is additive to the Framingham score for defining CAD risk in asymptomatic persons.

Management

The management decisions described below are based on data from randomized controlled trials that included highly variable percentages of older adults. Few trials included older adults with serious comorbidities or frailty.

Stable Angina Pectoris

The physician needs to identify and correct reversible factors that can aggravate angina pectoris and myocardial ischemia, for example anemia, infection, obesity, hyperthyroidism, uncontrolled hypertension, arrhythmias such as AF with a rapid ventricular rate, and severe valvular aortic stenosis. Smoking should be stopped. Treatment of hypertension and hyperlipidemia can be initiated. An exercise program will improve exercise tolerance. Aspirin 160 to 325 mg daily de-

creases the incidence of MI, stroke, and vascular death. Patients intolerant to aspirin can be treated with clopidogrel 75 mg daily to reduce the incidence of MI, stroke, and vascular death.

β-Blockers are effective antianginal agents and are the drug of choice to prevent myocardial ischemia. They reduce MI, sudden coronary death, and mortality, and they should be given to all people with CAD without contraindications to β-blockers.

Nitrates relieve and prevent angina pectoris. Nitroglycerin administered as a sublingual tablet 0.3 to 0.6 mg or as a sublingual spray 0.4 mg is the drug most commonly used to relieve an acute anginal attack. Long-acting nitrates help prevent recurrent episodes of angina. A 12- to 14-hour nitrate-free interval every 24 hours is necessary to avoid nitrate tolerance. If anginal symptoms persist despite treatment with nitrates and β-blockers, a nondihydropyridine calcium channel blocker such as verapamil or diltiazem should be used in people with normal LV ejection fraction, and amlodipine or felodipine should be used in people with HF or abnormal LV ejection fraction.

If people with stable angina have persistent angina interfering with their quality of life despite therapy with nitrates, β-blockers, and calcium channel blockers, consider coronary revascularization by coronary artery bypass graft (CABG) surgery or by percutaneous transluminal coronary angioplasty (PTCA).

Unstable Angina Pectoris and Non-Q-Wave Myocardial Infarction

People with unstable angina or non-Q-wave MI are generally admitted to a coronary care unit after treatment has begun in the emergency department. Reversible factors are then identified and corrected. Continuous nasal oxygen should be administered at 1 to 2 liters per minute to patients with cyanosis, respiratory distress, HF, or high risk factors. Aspirin 75 to 325 mg should be given at admission and daily indefinitely. The first dose of aspirin is chewed. A loading dose of 300 mg of clopidogrel should be given at admission and continued in a dosage of 75 mg daily for 9 months. The combination of aspirin plus clopidogrel reduces the incidence of cardiovascular death, nonfatal MI, or stroke by 20% in comparison with aspirin plus placebo. In patients in whom PTCA is performed, the combination of aspirin plus clopidogrel has been shown to reduce the incidence of cardiovascular death, nonfatal MI, or urgent target-vessel revascularization within 30 days of PTCA by 30% in comparison with aspirin plus placebo.

Subcutaneous enoxaparin or dalteparin (low-molecular-weight heparins) can be used instead of unfractionated heparin for the acute phase of management of people with non-Q-wave MI or unstable angina pectoris. Platelet glycoprotein IIb/IIIa receptor blockade with administration of abciximab is used for 12 to 24 hours in patients in whom PTCA is planned within the next 24 hours. Tirofiban or eptifibatide can be administered to patients with continuing myocardial ischemia, an elevated cardiospecific troponin I or T, or with other high-risk features in whom an invasive management is not planned.

People whose anginal symptoms are not fully relieved with three sublingual nitroglycerin tablets should be treated with continuous intravenous nitroglycerin for at least 24 hours. When the patient is angina free for 24 hours, he or she can be switched to an oral or transdermal preparation of long-acting nitrates. β-Blockers, unless contraindicated, should be given in the emergency department, intravenously initially and then orally and continued indefinitely. Oral angiotensin-converting enzyme (ACE) inhibitors are another important element in the pharmacologic armamentarium, especially if diabetes mellitus, hypertension, HF, or abnormal LV ejection fraction is present, unless there are contraindications to its use. If the serum LDL cholesterol is ≥100 mg/dL 24 to 96 hours after hospitalization, a statin is indicated for long-term use.

Table 45.2 shows the ACC/AHA Class I indications for an early invasive strategy in the treatment of patients with unstable angina pectoris or non-Q-wave MI. Table 45.3 shows the ACC/AHA guidelines for coronary revascularization in the treatment of patients with unstable angina pectoris or non-Q-wave MI.

Acute Myocardial Infarction

Aspirin should be administered in a dosage of 160 mg to 325 mg daily as soon as acute MI is suspected and continued indefinitely. The first dose of aspirin should be chewed. Clopidogrel 75 mg daily may be used in people unable to tolerate aspirin. Intravenous metoprolol or atenolol (the two β-blockers approved by the Food and Drug Administration for intravenous use in acute MI) should be administered at admission to older adults with acute MI without contraindications to β-blockers. Early intravenous blockade is followed by oral β-blocker therapy continued indefinitely to reduce the incidence of recurrent MI and mortality.

In the absence of contraindications, older adults with ischemic symptoms of at least 30 minutes' duration occurring within 6 to 12 hours of clinical presentation and with at least 1 to 2 mm of ST-segment elevation in two or more ECG leads or the presence of left bundle branch block are potential candidates for reperfusion therapy with either thrombolytic therapy or PTCA. Primary PTCA is the therapy of choice because it is associated with improved survival compared with

Table 45.2—AAC/AHA Class I Indications for Early Invasive Treatment of Patients With Unstable Angina or Non-Q-Wave Myocardial Infarction Without Serious Comorbidity

- Recurrent angina or myocardial ischemia at rest or with low-level activities despite intensive anti-ischemic therapy
- Increased cardiospecific troponin T or I
- New or presumably new ST-segment depression
- Recurrent angina or myocardial ischemia with heart failure symptoms, an S_3 gallop, pulmonary edema, worsening rales, or new or worsening mitral regurgitation murmur
- High-risk findings on noninvasive stress testing
- Abnormal LV systolic function (LV ejection fraction < 40%)
- Hemodynamic instability
- Sustained ventricular tachycardia
- Percutaneous coronary intervention within 6 months
- Prior CABG surgery

NOTE: AAC = American College of Cardiology; AHA = American Heart Association; CABG = coronary artery bypass graft; LV = left ventricular.

SOURCE: Data from Braunwald E, Antman EM, Beasley JW, et al. ACC/AHA 2002 guideline update for the management of patients with unstable angina and non-ST-segment elevation myocardial infarction—summary article: a report of the American College of Cardiology/American Heart Association Task Force on Practice Guidelines (Committee on the Management of Patients With Unstable Angina). *J Am Coll Cardiol.* 2002;40(7):1366–1374.

Table 45.3—ACC/AHA Guidelines for Coronary Revascularization in the Treatment of Patients With Unstable Angina or Non-Q-Wave Myocardial Infarction

- CABG surgery is recommended for patients with left main CAD, three-vessel CAD, or two-vessel CAD with significant proximal left anterior descending CAD and either an LV ejection fraction < 50% or treated diabetes mellitus.
- PTCA or CABG surgery is recommended for patients with one-vessel CAD or two-vessel CAD without significant proximal left anterior descending CAD but with a large area of viable myocardium and high-risk criteria on noninvasive testing.
- PTCA is recommended for patients with multivessel CAD with a suitable coronary anatomy and with normal LV function and without diabetes mellitus.

NOTE: AAC = American College of Cardiology; AHA = American Heart Association; CABG = coronary artery bypass graft; CAD = coronary artery disease; LV = left ventricular; PTCA = percutaneous transluminal coronary angioplasty.

SOURCE: Data from Braunwald E, Antman EM, Beasley JW, et al. ACC/AHA guidelines for the management of patients with unstable angina and non-ST-segment elevation myocardial infarction: a report of the American College of Cardiology/American Heart Association Task Force on Practice Guidelines (Committee on the Management of Patients with Unstable Angina). *J Am Coll Cardiol.* 2000;36(3):970–1062.

thrombolytic therapy. There are also data which suggest that thrombolytic therapy increases mortality in patients older than 75 years of age with acute MI.

Intravenous heparin is recommended in patients with acute MI undergoing PTCA or CABG surgery and in people with acute MI at high risk of systemic embolization, for example, people with a large or anterior MI, AF, history of pulmonary or systemic embolus, or known LV thrombus. If intravenous heparin is not given, subcutaneous heparin is administered to reduce the incidence of deep-vein thrombosis.

Nitrates may be used for the treatment of chest pain and HF in older adults with acute MI. To reduce mortality, severe HF, or severe LV systolic dysfunction, ACE inhibitors should be used to treat people with acute MI who are hemodynamically stable (systolic blood pressure ≥100 mm Hg) with HF, or who have a large anterior MI, or an LV ejection fraction ≤40%. Calcium channel blockers are not recommended in the treatment of acute MI. Older adults taking calcium channel blockers before the onset of their acute MI should be switched to β-blockers at the time of their acute MI.

Prophylactic use of antiarrhythmic drugs other than β-blockers does not improve clinical outcome in people with acute MI. The use of lidocaine during MI is limited to the treatment of life-threatening ventricular arrhythmias. Supraventricular tachyarrhythmias may be treated with β-blockers or direct-current cardioversion.

Treatment After Myocardial Infarction

Every attempt to control coronary risk factors must be made after MI. Aspirin 160 to 325 mg daily should be administered indefinitely. Long-term oral anticoagulant therapy is necessary as secondary prevention of MI in people unable to tolerate daily aspirin or clopidogrel, people with persistent AF, and people with LV thrombus.

People without contraindications to β-blockers should receive them indefinitely after MI. Avoid β-blockers with intrinsic sympathomimetic activity. High-risk subgroups of people with a history of MI (eg, all older adults and people with HF, asymptomatic abnormal LV ejection fraction, complex ventricular arrhythmias, peripheral arterial disease, or diabetes mellitus) are most likely to benefit from the use of β-blockers.

ACE inhibitors are recommended for use indefinitely in older adults after MI unless there are specific contraindications to their use. Calcium channel blockers are not to be used after MI unless there is persistent angina pectoris despite the use of β-blockers and nitrates. On the basis of data from the Heart Estrogen-Progestin Replacement study, hormonal therapy is contraindicated in the treatment of postmenopausal women after MI.

β-Blockers are the only antiarrhythmic drugs that reduce mortality after MI. To reduce mortality in older adults with life-threatening ventricular tachycardia or ventricular fibrillation after MI, an automatic implantable cardioverter-defibrillator is indicated.

Risk Stratification After Myocardial Infarction

Clinical factors, including age and coronary risk factors, can be used to classify people as high or low risk after MI (see Table 45.4). Exercise stress tests using thallium perfusion scintigraphy or radionuclide ventriculography and stress echocardiography using exercise or dobutamine or adenosine are useful for classifying people as high or low risk after MI.

After MI, older adults with spontaneous episodes of myocardial ischemia or episodes of myocardial ischemia provoked by minimal exertion, before treatment of a mechanical complication of MI (eg, acute mitral valve regurgitation, postinfarction septal deficit, left ventricular free wall rupture, or ventricular aneurysm), or with persistent hemodynamic instability can be referred for coronary angiography and consideration of coronary revascularization.

Coronary Revascularization After Myocardial Infarction

The benefits of revascularization in older adults after MI are prolongation of life and relief of unacceptable symptoms that persist despite optimal medical management.

Table 45.4—Factors Predicting a High Risk of New Coronary Events in Older Persons With a History of Myocardial Infarction

Findings on Echocardiogram
- Abnormal LV ejection fraction detected by echocardiography or radionuclide ventriculography
- Echocardiographic LV hypertrophy

Findings on ECG
- Abnormal signal-averaged ECG
- Complex ventricular arrhythmias or silent myocardial ischemia detected by a 24-hour ambulatory ECG
- Ischemic ST-segment depression on a resting ECG

Findings on Exercise Tolerance Testing
- Exercise-induced hypotension
- Exercise-induced ischemic ST-segment depression in both anterior and inferior leads
- Exercise-induced marked ischemic ST-segment depression (≥ 2 mm)
- Inadequate blood-pressure response to exercise
- Ischemic ST-segment depression occurring within 6 minutes of exercise
- Persistence of exercise-induced ST-segment depression past 8 minutes in the recovery period
- Poor exercise duration (< 6 minutes using a standard Bruce treadmill protocol)

NOTE: ECG = electrocardiogram; LV = left ventricular.

CABG surgery can improve survival in patients with significant left main CAD; in patients with significant three-vessel CAD, especially if decreased LV ejection fraction and myocardial ischemia are present; in patients with significant two-vessel CAD, proximal left anterior descending CAD, and decreased LV ejection fraction; in diabetic patients with multivessel CAD; and in patients with clinical evidence of HF during ischemic episodes with ischemic but viable myocardium.

PTCA with stenting is preferred in severely symptomatic patients with significant one-vessel or two-vessel CAD and a normal LV ejection fraction, in patients with multiple medical problems including prior MI, in patients at increased risk of developing stroke because of cerebrovascular disease or diffuse aortic disease, in patients at increased risk of developing postoperative cognitive dysfunction, and in patients who are frail. See Table 45.3.

DYSLIPIDEMIA

Double-blind, randomized controlled studies have demonstrated that the absolute reduction in cardiovascular mortality and morbidity in older adults with dyslipidemia treated with statins is greater than for people younger than 65 years of age. In older adults with prior MI and a serum LDL cholesterol of ≥125 mg/dL, statins have been demonstrated to reduce new coronary events in people aged 60 to 100 years and new stroke in people aged 60 to 90 years. Older adults in whom the serum LDL cholesterol was reduced to <90 mg/dL had the greatest reduction in new coronary events and in stroke. In the Cardiovascular Health Study, at 7.3-year follow-up of 1250 women and 664

men aged 65 to 80 years with hypercholesterolemia and free of cardiovascular disease, statins were found to significantly reduce all-cause mortality by 44% and cardiovascular events by 56%.

See Table 45.5 and Table 45.6 for treatment indications and drug regimens.

HEART FAILURE

Epidemiology and Etiology

HF is the most common cause of hospitalization and rehospitalization in people aged 65 years and older. The prevalence and incidence of HF increase with age. CAD, hypertension, valvular heart disease, and cardiomyopathies are the most common causes of HF in older adults.

Not only do older adults experience an age-related decrease in LV diastolic relaxation and early LV diastolic filling (see Table 45.1), they are more likely to have LV diastolic dysfunction because they have an increased prevalence of hypertension, myocardial ischemia due to CAD, LV hypertrophy due to hypertension, valvular aortic stenosis, hypertrophic cardiomyopathy, and other cardiac disorders. In older adults, the increased stiffness of the LV and prolonged LV relaxation time impair LV early diastolic filling and cause higher LV end-diastolic pressures at rest and during exercise.

In HF associated with LV diastolic dysfunction with normal LV systolic function, the LV ejection fraction is ≥50%. The prevalence of a normal LV ejection fraction associated with HF increases with age and is higher in older women than in older men.

Table 45.5—Treatment Indications for Dyslipidemia

Risk Category	Conditions	LDL-Cholesterol Goal	Initiate Nonpharmacologic Management	Consider Drug Therapy
Low	0–1 risk factor*	< 160 mg/dL	≥ 160 mg/dL	≥ 190 mg/dL; optional: 160–189 mg/dL
Moderate	2+ risk factors; 10-year CAD risk < 10%†	< 130 mg/dL	≥ 130 mg/dL	≥ 160 mg/dL
Moderately high	2+ risk factors; 10-year CAD risk 10%–20%†	< 130 mg/dL	≥ 130 mg/dL	≥ 130 mg/dL; optional: 100–129 mg/dL
High	CVD‡, DM, or 10-year CAD risk > 20%†	< 100 mg/dL	≥ 100 mg/dL	≥ 100 mg/dL
Very high	DM + CVD‡; acute coronary syndrome; multiple severe or poorly controlled risk factors	< 70 mg/dL	≥ 100 mg/dL	≥ 100 mg/dL; optional: 70–99 mg/dL

NOTE: CAD = coronary artery disease; CVD = cardiovascular disease; DM = diabetes mellitus; HDL = high-density lipoprotein; LDL = low-density lipoprotein.

* Risk factors are cigarette smoking, hypertension, HDL < 40 mg/dL, family history of premature CAD, male age ≥ 45 years, female age ≥ 55 years.

† Calculation of 10-year risk of CAD is available at http://www.nhlbi.nih.gov/guidelines/cholesterol/ (accessed October 2005).

‡ CVD is signified by CAD, angina, peripheral artery disease, transient ischemic attack, stroke, abdominal aortic aneurysm, or 10-year CAD risk > 20%.

SOURCE: Reuben DB, Herr KA, Pacala JT, et al. *Geriatrics At Your Fingertips: 2006*, 8th ed. New York: American Geriatrics Society; 2006:30. Reprinted with permission.

Table 45.6—Drug Regimens for Dyslipidemia

Condition	Drug	Dosage	Formulations
Elevated LDL, normal TG	Statin (HMG-CoA reductase inhibitor*):		
	Atorvastatin	10–80 mg qd	T: 10, 20, 40, 80
	Fluvastatin	20–80 mg qd in PM, max 80 mg	C: 20, 40; T: ER 80
	Lovastatin	10–40 mg qd in PM (max dose 80 mg); extended release max dose 60 mg)	T: 10, 20, 40
	Pravastatin	10–40 mg qd	T: 10, 20, 40, 80
	Rosuvastatin	10–40 mg qd	T: 5, 10, 20, 40
	Simvastatin	5–80 mg qd in PM	T: 5, 10, 20, 40, 80
Elevated TG (> 500 mg/dL)	Fenofibrate	54–160 mg qd	T: 54, 160
	Gemfibrozil	300–600 mg po bid	T: 600
	Omega-3-acid ethyl esters	4 g/d in single or divided doses	C: 1 g
Combined elevated LDL, low HDL, elevated TG	Fenofibrate, gemfibrozil, or HMG-CoA if TG < 300 mg/dL	as above	as above
Alternative for any of above	Niacin†	100 mg tid to start; increase to 500–1000 mg tid; ER 150 mg qhs to start, increase to 2000 mg qhs as needed	T: 25, 50, 100, 250, 500, ER 150, 250, 500, 750, 1000; C: TR 125, 250, 400, 500
Elevated LDL or combined with inadequate response to one agent	Lovastatin/niacin combination*†	20 mg/500 mg qhs to start; increase to 40 mg/2000 mg as needed	T: 20/500, 20/750, 20/1000
	Colesevelam	Monotherapy: 1850 mg po bid; combination therapy: 2500–3750 mg/d in single or divided doses	T: 625
	Ezetimibe	10 mg qd	T: 10
	Ezetimibe/simvastatin* combination	1 tab qd	T: 10/10, 10/20, 10/40, 10/80

NOTE: bid = twice a day; C = capsule; d = day; ER = extended release; HDL = high-density lipoprotein; LDL = low-density lipoprotein; max = maximum; po = by mouth; qd = once a day; qhs = each bedtime; T = tablet; TG = triglycerides; tid = three times a day.

*Measure transaminases at baseline and at 3 months, then periodically. Watch for statin-induced myopathy, usually presenting as diffuse, symmetric myalgias. If myopathy is suspected (higher risk at higher statin doses or in combination with fenofibrate, gemfibrozil, or niacin), measure creatinine phosphokinase and transaminases; creatinine phosphokinase levels above 10 times the upper limit of normal indicate serious myopathy or rhabdomyolysis. Even if creatinine phosphokinase and transaminases are normal, myalgias still may be due to statin; if this is the case, myalgias should disappear within 1 week of discontinuing statin.

† Monitor for flushing, pruritus, nausea, gastritis, ulcer. Dosage increases should be spaced 1 month apart. Aspirin 325 mg po 30 minutes before first niacin dose of the day is quite effective in preventing adverse events.

SOURCE: Reuben DB, Herr KA, Pacala JT, et al. *Geriatrics At Your Fingertips: 2006*, 8th ed. New York: American Geriatrics Society; 2006: pp 30–31. Reprinted with permission.

During exercise, people with normal LV systolic function but abnormal LV diastolic function are unable to normally increase stroke volume, even in the presence of increased LV filling pressure. Myocardial hypertrophy, ischemia, or fibrosis causes slow or incomplete LV filling at normal left atrial pressures. Left atrial pressure rises to increase LV filling, resulting in pulmonary and systemic venous congestion. The development of AF (the prevalence of which increases with age) may also cause a decrease in cardiac output and the development of pulmonary and systemic venous congestion, because of the loss of left atrial contribution to LV late diastolic filling and reduced diastolic filling time due to a rapid ventricular rate.

In HF associated with LV systolic dysfunction, the LV ejection fraction is <50%. The amount of myocardial fiber shortening is reduced, the stroke volume is decreased, the LV is dilated, and the patient is symptomatic.

LV ejection fraction must be measured in all people with HF, preferably by echocardiography (because of the additional information provided, eg, the presence and severity of valvular heart disease, LV thrombus), to determine appropriate therapy for HF.

Presentation

Increased pulmonary capillary wedge pressure causes pulmonary congestion, resulting in dyspnea. Dyspnea may progress from exertional dyspnea to orthopnea, to paroxysmal nocturnal dyspnea, to dyspnea at rest, and to the development of acute pulmonary edema. Pulmonary congestion may cause coughing and wheezing. Decreased cardiac output may cause weakness, a feeling of heaviness in the limbs, nocturia, oliguria, confusion, insomnia, headache, anxiety, memory impairment, bad dreams or nightmares, and, rarely, psychotic manifestations. Congestive hepatomegaly may cause epigastric or right upper quadrant heaviness or a dull ache, a sense of fullness after eating, anorexia, nausea, and vomiting.

LV failure with transudation of fluid into the alveoli causes moist rales, which are heard over the lung bases posteriorly. Congestion of bronchial mucosa causes rhonchi and wheezes. During acute pulmonary edema, coarse, bubbling rales and wheezes are heard over the lung fields. Signs of pleural effusion may occur with left or right ventricular failure. Systemic venous hypertension causes distention of the jugular veins.

Right ventricular failure may cause an enlarged, tender liver and ascites. Compression of the liver causes the hepatojugular reflux sign. Pressure applied to the middle of the abdomen can cause the abdominal jugular reflux sign. A pulsating liver indicates tricuspid regurgitation. Right ventricular failure causes edema that first develops in the dependent parts of the body. Severe right ventricular failure will cause anasarca.

An LV third heart sound (best heard at the apex) and jugular venous distention are the most sensitive and specific physical findings in HF. Most people with HF have cardiomegaly. However, HF may develop in people with acute MI or other conditions before the heart has had a chance to enlarge. Heart murmurs due to valvular heart disease may become faint or absent because of a low cardiac output. Physical examination cannot distinguish between HF associated with abnormal and HF associated with normal LV ejection fraction.

Chest radiographs should be obtained for all people with suspected HF and will show pulmonary vascular congestion in those with LV failure. When the pulmonary capillary pressure reaches 20 to 25 mm Hg, interstitial pulmonary edema is present. When the pulmonary capillary pressure exceeds 25 mm Hg, alveolar edema and pleural effusion occur.

Management

Precipitating causes of HF, such as excess sodium ingestion, myocardial ischemia, infection, anemia, fever, hypoxia, tachyarrhythmias, bradyarrhythmias, hyperthyroidism, hypothyroidism, and obesity must be identified and treated. Sodium intake should be decreased to 1.6 g (4 g of sodium chloride) daily. Drugs known to precipitate or aggravate HF, such as nonsteroidal anti-inflammatory drugs, calcium channel blockers, and most antiarrhythmic drugs, should be withdrawn.

It is important to identify the underlying causes of HF and treat when possible. People with myocardial ischemia due to severely stenotic coronary arteries without contraindications to coronary revascularization who have exercise-limiting angina, frequent episodes of angina occurring at rest, or recurrent episodes of acute pulmonary edema despite optimal medical management can be referred for coronary angiography with CABG surgery or PTCA. Surgical correction of valvular lesions and surgical excision of a dyskinetic LV aneurysm is a potential intervention for some people with HF.

Anticoagulants should be given if there is prior systemic or pulmonary embolism, AF, or cardiac thrombi detected by echocardiography. People with HF who have complete atrioventricular block or severe bradycardia are candidates for a transvenous pacemaker implanted into the right ventricle.

People with HF who are dyspneic at rest or at a low work level may benefit from a formal cardiac rehabilitation program. Disease management strategies, either self-or nurse-directed, have been shown to be effective at reducing rehospitalization rates among older adults with HF. Frequent weighing, careful attention to symptoms, and adjustment of diuretic dosing are components of HF disease management.

Angiotensin-Converting Enzyme Inhibitors

ACE inhibitors improve symptoms, quality of life, and exercise tolerance, and they decrease mortality and hospitalization for HF in people who have HF associated with abnormal LV ejection fraction. In a review of 32 randomized trials of ACE inhibitors in people with HF and abnormal LV ejection fraction revealed that the ACE inhibitors significantly reduced total mortality by 23% and mortality or hospitalization for HF by 35%. ACE inhibitors should be administered to all people with HF and abnormal LV ejection fraction unless there are specific contraindications to their use.

ACE inhibitors also improve symptoms, exercise tolerance, and LV systolic and diastolic function in people with HF and normal LV ejection fraction. ACE inhibitors are indicated for people with HF and normal LV ejection fraction if HF persists despite diuretic and β-blocker therapy. In one study, people with HF and normal LV ejection fraction treated with ACE inhibitors for 6 months had a 63% significant reduction in mortality if the LV ejection fraction was 40% to 49% and a 39% insignificant reduction in mortality if the LV ejection fraction was ≥50%. In this study, ACE inhibitors significantly improved quality-of-life scores in patients with LV ejection fractions of 40% to 49% and ≥50%.

Asymptomatic hypotension with a systolic blood pressure between 80 and 90 mm Hg and a serum creatinine level that increases but is <2.5 mg/dL are side effects of ACE inhibitors that should not necessarily cause cessation of this drug, but require a decreased dose of diuretic if the jugular venous pressure is normal and a possible decreased dose of ACE inhibitor. Contraindications to the use of ACE inhibitors are symptomatic hypotension, progressive azotemia, angioneurotic edema, hyperkalemia, intolerable cough, and rash.

Angiotensin II Type 1 Receptor Antagonists

Studies have found that older patients with HF and abnormal LV ejection fraction treated with losartan have fewer adverse effects, such as cough, rash, or altered taste sensation, than do patients treated with captopril. In the second Evaluation of Losartan in the Elderly study, patients with HF and abnormal LV ejection fraction treated with losartan or with captopril were found to have a similar mortality and hospitalization for HF. In this study mortality in people receiving captopril who were also receiving β-blockers was significantly reduced. Older adults with HF should be treated with an angiotensin II type 1 receptor antagonist if they are unable to tolerate ACE inhibitors because of cough, rash, altered taste sensation, or angioneurotic edema. Treatment with a β-blocker plus an ACE inhibitor plus an angiotensin II type 1 receptor blocker is not recommended because the Valsartan Heart Failure Trial showed that administration of these three drugs together significantly increases mortality.

β-Blockers

Chronic administration of β-blockers after MI reduces mortality, sudden cardiac death, and recurrent MI, especially in older adults. These benefits are more marked in people with a history of HF. One study showed that after 6 to 12 months of therapy, carvedilol caused a 65% significant reduction in mortality in patients with HF and abnormal LV ejection fraction treated with diuretics, ACE inhibitors, and digoxin. At 1-year follow-up of those with New York Heart Association class II, III, or IV HF and abnormal LV ejection fraction who were treated with diuretics, ACE inhibitors, and optional digoxin, metoprolol CR/XL was shown to cause a 34% significant reduction in mortality. Older adults with HF and abnormal LV ejection fraction should be treated with diuretics, ACE inhibitors, and β-blockers.

β-Blockers are beneficial in the treatment of HF associated with normal LV ejection fraction by:

- reducing the ventricular rate to <90 beats per minute, thereby increasing LV diastolic filling time and causing an increase in LV end-diastolic volume;
- decreasing myocardial ischemia;
- reducing elevated blood pressure;
- decreasing LV mass; and
- improving LV relaxation.

The increase in ventricular rate that occurs with exercise can also be prevented with modest doses of β-blockers, especially in older adults.

β-Blockers have also been demonstrated at 32-month follow-up of elderly patients with New York Association class II or III HF and a normal LV ejection fraction treated with diuretics and ACE inhibitors to significantly reduce mortality by 35%.

β-Blockers along with loop diuretics should be used to treat older adults with HF and normal LV ejection fraction.

Diuretics

Diuretics are used in the treatment of HF associated with abnormal or normal LV ejection fraction. Mild HF may be treated with a thiazide diuretic. However, the thiazide diuretic is ineffective if the glomerular filtration rate is <30 mL per minute. Older adults with moderate or severe HF should be treated with a loop diuretic such as furosemide. People with severe HF or concomitant renal insufficiency may need metolazone in addition to the loop diuretic. The minimum effective dose of diuretic should be given. Older adults with HF associated with abnormal LV ejection fraction tolerate higher doses of diuretics than do older adults with normal LV ejection fraction. Older adults with HF and normal LV ejection fraction need high LV filling pressures to maintain an adequate stroke volume and cardiac output, and they cannot tolerate intravascular depletion.

Aldosterone Antagonists

One study showed that among people with severe HF and abnormal LV ejection fraction who were treated with diuretics, ACE inhibitors, and digoxin, those randomized to spironolactone 25 mg daily had a 30% significant decrease in mortality and a 35% significant reduction in hospitalization for HF at 2-year follow-up. However, only 10% of patients were treated with β-blockers. In the Eplerenone Post-Acute Myocardial Infarction Heart Failure Efficacy and Survival Study, 86% of patients were treated with ACE inhibitors or angiotensin II type 1 receptor blockers and 75% with β-blockers. In comparison with placebo, eplerenone significantly reduced mortality by 15%. The ACC/AHA guidelines recommend (with a Class IIa indication) the use of an aldosterone antagonist in patients with systolic HF and class IV symptoms despite diuretics, ACE inhibitors, β-blockers, and digoxin, preserved kidney function, and normal serum potassium.

Digoxin

Digoxin may be used in the treatment of older adults with HF and supraventricular tachyarrhythmias such as AF. In the Digitalis Investigator Group trial, digoxin in comparison with placebo significantly increased mortality by 23% in women with HF and an abnormal LV ejection fraction. In this study, in men with HF and an abnormal LV ejection fraction, digoxin significantly reduced mortality by 6% if the serum digoxin level was 0.5 to 0.8 ng/mL, insignificantly increased mortality by 3% if the serum digoxin level was 0.9 to 1.1 ng/mL, and significantly increased mortality by 12% if the serum digoxin level was ≥1.2 ng/mL. On the basis of these data, digoxin can be administered to men with HF and an abnormal LV ejection fraction if they have persistent HF despite diuretics, ACE inhibitors, and β-blockers. However, the serum digoxin level must be maintained between 0.5 to 0.8 ng/mL.

Digoxin should not be used for treating people with HF in sinus rhythm associated with a normal LV ejection fraction. By increasing contractility through an increased intracellular calcium concentration, digoxin may increase LV stiffness in these people, increasing LV filling pressure and aggravating HF with normal LV ejection fraction. In the Digitalis Investigator Group trial, digoxin insignificantly increased all-cause hospitalization by 4% in patients with HF and a normal LV ejection fraction.

Isosorbide Dinitrate Plus Hydralazine

The combination of oral isosorbide dinitrate and hydralazine may be beneficial in the treatment of HF and abnormal or normal LV ejection fraction. Isosorbide dinitrate plus hydralazine is indicated if:

- HF with abnormal ejection fraction persists despite treatment with diuretics, ACE inhibitors, β-blockers, and digoxin, or

- HF with normal LV ejection fraction persists despite treatment with diuretics, β-blockers, and ACE inhibitors.

The ACC/AHA guidelines recommend with a Class IIa indication the use of isosorbide dinitrate plus hydralazine in patients with HF who cannot be given an ACE inhibitor or angiotensin II type 1 receptor blocker because of hypotension or renal insufficiency.

BIDIL is a combination of isosorbide dinitrate and hydralazine approved for HF in African-Americans.

Calcium Channel Blockers

Calcium channel blockers such as nifedipine, diltiazem, and verapamil exacerbate HF in patients with HF and abnormal LV ejection fraction. Studies show that diltiazem significantly increases mortality in patients with pulmonary congestion and abnormal LV ejection fraction after MI and that the vasoselective calcium channel blockers amlodipine and felodipine do not significantly affect survival in patients with HF and abnormal LV ejection fraction. In these studies, a significantly higher incidence of pulmonary edema and peripheral edema was observed in patients treated with amlodipine than in those treated with placebo, and a significantly higher incidence of peripheral edema was observed in patients treated with felodipine than in those treated with placebo. Therefore, calcium channel blockers are not indicated in older adults with HF and abnormal LV ejection fraction. However, calcium channel blockers may be given to people with HF and normal LV ejection fraction if they have persistent HF despite the use of diuretics and are unable to tolerate β-blockers, ACE inhibitors, and isosorbide dinitrate plus hydralazine. Felodipine is the only calcium channel blocker labeled for the treatment of heart failure by the Food and Drug Administration.

Self-Management

The number-one cause of recidivism in HF patients is volume and sodium retention. Patients must be instructed to adhere to a low-sodium diet. They need to weigh themselves daily and call the primary care clinician immediately if they gain more than 2 pounds in 1 day. Over-the-counter drugs to avoid that can exacerbate sodium and fluid retention include sodium-based antacids, high-dose aspirin, nonsteroidal anti-inflammatory drugs, ginseng (germanium), ginkgo, echinacea, and decongestants. Black licorice has the same effect.

VALVULAR HEART DISEASE

Valvular Aortic Stenosis

Valvular aortic stenosis (AS) in older adults is usually due to stiffening, scarring, and calcification of the valve leaflets.

Angina pectoris, syncope or near syncope, and HF are the three classic manifestations of severe AS. Doppler echocardiography is used to diagnose AS and determine the severity.

Older adults with AS have an increased incidence of new coronary events; those with symptomatic severe AS have a poor prognosis. However, those with asymptomatic severe AS are at low risk of death and can be followed until symptoms develop.

The American Heart Association guidelines for the use of prophylactic antibiotics to prevent bacterial endocarditis are available at http://www.amhrt.org. Older adults with HF, exertional syncope, or angina associated with moderate or severe AS can be considered for aortic valve replacement. People with asymptomatic AS should report the development of symptoms possibly related to AS immediately to their physicians. Nitrates should be used with caution in people with AS and angina to prevent orthostatic hypotension and syncope; vasodilators should be avoided. Diuretics should be prescribed cautiously in people with AS and HF to prevent a decrease in cardiac output and hypotension.

If LV systolic dysfunction in people with severe AS is associated with critical narrowing of the aortic valve rather than with myocardial fibrosis, it often improves after successful aortic valve replacement. Balloon aortic valvuloplasty is a potential intervention for older adults with symptomatic severe AS who are not candidates for aortic valve surgery and possibly for people with severe LV dysfunction as a bridge to subsequent aortic valve surgery.

Aortic Regurgitation

Acute aortic regurgitation (AR) in older adults may be due to infective endocarditis, rheumatic fever, aortic dissection, trauma after prosthetic valve surgery, or rupture of the sinus of Valsalva. It causes sudden severe HF. Chronic AR in older adults may be caused by aortic valve leaflet disease (secondary to any cause of AS, infective endocarditis, rheumatic fever, congenital heart disease, rheumatoid arthritis, ankylosing spondylitis, after prosthetic valve surgery, or myxomatous degeneration of the valve) or by aortic root disease.

The prevalence of AR increases with age; in one study it was found to be 31% among 554 older men and 28% among 1243 older women. The AR murmur is typically a high-pitched blowing diastolic murmur that begins immediately after the aortic second sound. The diastolic murmur is best heard along the left sternal border in the third and fourth intercostal spaces when AR is due to valvular disease and is best heard along the right sternal border when AR is due to dilatation of the ascending aorta. The severity of AR correlates with the duration of the diastolic murmur, not with the intensity of the murmur. Doppler echocardiography is used to diagnose the presence and severity of AR.

People with acute AR develop symptoms as a consequence of the sudden onset of HF. People with acute AR should have immediate aortic valve replacement because death may occur within hours to days. People with chronic AR may be asymptomatic for many years. The prognosis of older adults with HF and severe AR is poor.

Prophylactic antibiotics should be used to prevent bacterial endocarditis in older adults with chronic AR, according to American Heart Association guidelines (available at http://www.amhrt.org). Older adults with asymptomatic chronic severe AR should be treated with ACE inhibitors to reduce the LV volume overload. Echocardiographic evaluation of LV end-systolic dimension should be performed yearly if the measurement is <50 mm, but every 3 to 6 months if the measurement is 50 to 54 mm. Aortic valve replacement should be considered if the LV end-systolic dimension exceeds 55 mm, even in the absence of cardiac symptoms. Aortic valve replacement should also be considered when the LV ejection fraction approaches 50% before the decompensated state.

Mitral Regurgitation

In one study, mitral regurgitation (MR) was present in 32% of 554 older men and in 33% of 1243 older women. The most common cause of MR in older adults is mitral annular calcium deposition. Other disorders causing MR in older adults include CAD, mitral valve prolapse, and rheumatic heart disease. Symptoms associated with severe MR are primarily those of HF, especially dyspnea. The heart murmur associated with MR is heard as an apical holosystolic murmur, late systolic murmur, or early systolic murmur beginning with the first heart sound but ending in mid-systole. The presence of an LV third heart sound suggests that the MR is severe. Doppler echocardiography is used to diagnose the presence and monitor the severity of MR.

In MR, the LV ejection fraction should be >55% to 60% and the LV end-systolic dimension <45 mm. Mitral valve surgery should be considered in older adults with New York Heart Association class III or IV symptoms caused by MR or in older adults with severe MR and an LV ejection fraction <50% or an LV end-systolic dimension above 45 to 50 mm.

Mitral Stenosis

The most common cause of mitral stenosis (MS) in older adults is mitral annular calcium. The prevalence of MS in older adults is low. Older adults with MS have a low-pitched mid-diastolic murmur heard at the point of maximal apical impulse with or without presystolic accentuation. Doppler echocardiography is used to diagnose the presence and severity of MS.

Long-term oral warfarin therapy to reduce thromboembolic events must be considered for all older adults with MS, especially those with AF. Mitral valvular surgery or valvuloplasty may be indicated if the patient has recurrent embolization on anticoagulants. A β-blocker will slow the ventricular rate if AF is present. Diuretics will control congestive symptoms.

In the absence of clot, MR, and severe subvalvular involvement, the therapy of choice for symptomatic MS is balloon valvuloplasty. However, many older adults with symptomatic MS have poor valve morphology for valvuloplasty (heavy calcification) and require mitral valve replacement. Older persons with MS and a critical valve area of 1.0 cm^2 need interventional therapy. Mitral valve replacement is usually necessary because stenotic mitral valves in older adults are commonly calcified and severely deformed, with associated significant MR, and successful open mitral commissurotomy is not possible.

ARRHYTHMIAS

Ventricular Arrhythmias

The presence of three or more consecutive ventricular premature complexes on an ECG is diagnosed as ventricular tachycardia (VT). VT is considered sustained if it lasts ≥30 seconds and nonsustained if its lasts <30 seconds. Complex ventricular arrhythmias (VAs) include VT or paired, multiform, or frequent (≥30 per hour on a 24-hour ambulatory ECG or ≥6 per minute on a 1-minute rhythm strip of an ECG) ventricular premature complexes. Researchers using a 24-hour ambulatory ECG to detect VAs in older adults found a prevalence of 10% for nonsustained VT (N = 554) and a rate of 55% for complex VAs (N = 843).

Nonsustained VT and complex VA are not associated with an increased incidence of new coronary events in older adults with no clinical evidence of heart disease, and asymptomatic people should not be treated with antiarrhythmic drugs. Simple VA (ie, VAs that are not paired, multiform, or frequent) in older adults with heart disease should also not be treated with antiarrhythmic drugs. Nonsustained VT and complex VA are associated with an increased incidence of new coronary events in older adults with heart disease, especially in those with abnormal LV ejection fraction, LV hypertrophy, or silent myocardial ischemia.

Available data show that older adults with nonsustained VT or complex VA and heart disease should be treated with β-blockers if there are no contraindications. Older adults should not be treated with any of the class I antiarrhythmic drugs (ie, encainide, flecainide, lorcainide, moricizine,

propafenone, quinidine, procainamide, disopyramide, mexiletine, phenytoin, or tocainide), calcium channel blockers, d-sotalol, or d,l-sotalol. Amiodarone was found to not reduce mortality in people with VT or complex VA associated with prior MI or HF, and it had a high incidence of toxicity.

Analysis of data from the Cardiac Arrhythmia Suppression Trial showed that β-blockers are an independent factor for decreasing arrhythmic death or cardiac arrest by 40%, for reducing all-cause mortality by 33%, and for decreasing occurrence of new or worsened HF by 32%. However, the automatic implantable cardioverter-defibrillator (AICD) is the most effective treatment for reducing mortality in older adults with life-threatening VT or ventricular fibrillation. Table 45.7 lists the ACC/AHA indications for an AICD.

Atrial Fibrillation

AF is the most common type of arrhythmia in adults. It is more common as patients age; the prevalence is 1% among those younger than 60 years and increases to more than 8% in those older than 80 years. Data, when adjusted for age, indicate that more men are affected than women. Cardiac conditions associated with the development of AF are hypertension, rheumatic mitral valve disease, CAD, and HF. Noncardiac causes include hyperthyroidism, hypoxic pulmonary

Table 45.7—ACC/AHA Indications for an Automatic Implantable Cardioverter-Defibrillator

- Cardiac arrest due to VF or VT not due to a transient or reversible cause*

- Spontaneous sustained VT in association with structural heart disease*

- Syncope of undetermined origin with clinically relevant, hemodynamically significant sustained VT or VF induced at electrophysiologic study when drug therapy is ineffective, not tolerated, or not preferred*

- Nonsustained VT in patients with coronary disease, prior MI, LV dysfunction, and inducible VF or sustained VT at electrophysiologic study not suppressible by a class I antiarrhythmic drug*

- Spontaneous sustained VT in patients without structural heart disease not amenable to other therapy*

- An LV ejection fraction ≤ 30% at least 1 month post-MI and 3 months post–coronary artery surgery**

NOTE: AAC = American College of Cardiology; AHA = American Heart Association; LV = left ventricular; MI = myocardial infarction; VF = ventricular fibrillation; VT = ventricular tachycardia.

* Class I indication.

** Class IIa indication.

SOURCE: Data from Gregoratos G, Abrams J, Epstein AE, et al. ACC/AHA/NASPE 2002 guideline update for implantation of cardiac pacemakers and antiarrhythmia devices: summary article: a report of the American College of Cardiology/American Heart Association Task Force on Practice Guidelines (ACC/AHA/NASPE Committee to Update the 1998 Pacemaker Guidelines). *Circulation.* 2002;106(16):2145–2161.

conditions, surgery, and alcohol intoxication. Patients with AF may have symptoms of hemodynamic compromise, such as irregular palpitations and lightheadedness, or more vague symptoms, such as malaise, but they may be asymptomatic. Patients with AF are at increased risk of thromboembolic disease.

The management of AF includes treatment of the underlying disease (such as pneumonia, hyperthyroidism, or pulmonary embolus) when possible and treatment of precipitating factors. Immediate direct-current cardioversion should be performed in patients with paroxysmal AF with a very rapid ventricular rate associated with acute MI, chest pain caused by myocardial ischemia, hypotension, severe HF, or syncope. Intravenous β-blockers, verapamil, or diltiazem may be used to slow immediately a very rapid ventricular rate associated with AF.

Amiodarone may be used in patients with symptomatic life-threatening AF refractory to other drug therapy. Radiofrequency catheter modification of atrioventricular conduction or complete atrioventricular block produced by radiofrequency catheter ablation followed by permanent pacemaker implantation can be performed in patients with symptomatic AF in whom a rapid ventricular rate cannot be slowed by drug therapy.

Paroxysmal AF associated with the tachycardia-bradycardia syndrome is indication for treatment with a permanent pacemaker, in combination with drugs used to slow a rapid ventricular rate in AF. A permanent pacemaker should also be considered in people with AF who develop cerebral symptoms such as dizziness or syncope associated with ventricular pauses >3 seconds that are not drug induced, as documented by a 24-hour ambulatory ECG.

BRADYARRHYTHMIAS

Numerous drugs can cause bradyarrhythmias and conduction disturbances. Hyperkalemia, hypokalemia, hypothyroidism, and hypoxia can also depress cardiac impulse formation and conduction. Drugs and endocrine and metabolic disorders causing reversible cardiac impulse formation and conduction abnormalities must be considered before a decision to implant a permanent pacemaker can be made.

A 12-lead ECG with a 1-minute strip may diagnose bradyarrhythmias caused by a sick sinus syndrome, atrioventricular block, right and left bundle branch block, bifascicular block, and trifascicular block. ECG manifestations of sick sinus syndrome include severe sinus bradycardia, sinus pause or arrest, sinus exit block, sinus node reentrant rhythm, AF or atrial flutter with a slow ventricular rate that is not drug induced, failure of restoration of sinus rhythm after cardioversion for tachyarrhythmias, a pause longer than

3 seconds after carotid sinus massage, and a tachycardia-bradycardia syndrome. The tachycardia-bradycardia syndrome is characterized by paroxysmal AF, atrial flutter, or supraventricular tachycardia followed by periods of sinus bradycardia, sinus arrest, or sinoatrial block.

Dyspnea, weakness, fatigue, falls, angina pectoris, HF, episodic pulmonary edema, dizziness, faintness, slurred speech, personality changes, paresis, and convulsions in older adults may be caused by bradyarrhythmias. Death may result from prolonged ventricular asystole. Older adults with symptoms that may be due to bradyarrhythmias should have a 12-lead ECG with a 1-minute rhythm strip. Because ECG abnormalities may be intermittent, a 24-hour ambulatory ECG may need to be performed.

In some older adults without clinical evidence of heart disease and recurrent episodes of unexplained syncope, a patient-activated memory loop event recorder may be used to capture the ECG tracings preceding and during syncope. Those with unexplained syncope and heart disease should undergo an electrophysiologic study.

Table 45.8 shows ACC/AHA class I indications for permanent pacemaker implantation in patients with bradyarrhythmias. Telephone telemetry can be used to evaluate the pacemaker battery and determine that the pacemaker functions appropriately. However, the pacemaker cannot be reprogrammed over the telephone and this is best performed in an office where expertise and equipment are available.

Single-chamber pacemakers should be checked by telephone telemetry twice in the first month after implantation, every 3 months from month 2 to 48 after implantation, every 2 months from month 49 to 72 after implantation, and monthly thereafter. Dual chamber pacemakers should be checked by telemetry twice in the first month after implantation, monthly from month 2 to 6 after implantation, every 2 months from month 7 to 36 after implantation, and monthly thereafter.

PERIPHERAL ARTERIAL DISEASE

Aneurysms and Dissections

Aneurysms and dissections are primarily disorders of older adults. Aneurysms are most commonly found in the abdominal aorta, thoracic aorta, popliteal arteries, and iliac arteries, and they are usually atherosclerotic. Symptomatic aneurysms are medical emergencies that require immediate surgery. Asymptomatic aneurysms should be followed for rate of growth. Older adults with an abdominal aortic aneurysm >5 cm are potential candidates for surgical repair. Elective surgical

Table 45.8—ACC/AHA Class I Indications for Permanent Pacemaker Implantation in Patients With Bradyarrhythmias

- Third-degree and advanced second-degree AV block associated with:

  —bradycardia with symptoms

  —necessity for drugs that result in symptomatic bradycardia

  —documented period of asystole ≥ 3 seconds or any escape rate < 40 beats per minute in awake, symptom-free patient

  —after catheter ablation of the AV junction

  —postoperative AV block not expected to resolve

  —neuromuscular diseases with AV block

- Chronic bifascicular and trifascicular block with:

  —intermittent third-degree AV block

  —type II second-degree AV block

  —alternating bundle branch block

- AV block after acute myocardial infarction with:

  —persistent second-degree AV block in the His-Purkinje system with bilateral bundle branch block or third-degree AV block within or below the His-Purkinje system

  —transient advanced (second- or third-degree) infranodal AV block and associated bundle branch block

  —persistent and symptomatic second- or third-degree AV block

- Sinus node dysfunction with documented symptomatic bradycardia or with symptomatic chronotropic incompetence

NOTE: AAC = American College of Cardiology; AHA = American Heart Association; AV = atrioventricular.

SOURCE: Data from Gregoratos G, Abrams J, Epstein AE, et al. ACC/AHA/NASPE 2002 guideline update for implantation of cardiac pacemakers and antiarrhythmia devices: summary article: a report of the American College of Cardiology/American Heart Association Task Force on Practice Guidelines (ACC/AHA/NASPE Committee to Update the 1998 Pacemaker Guidelines). *Circulation*. 2002;106(16):2145–2161.

repair of a descending thoracic aortic aneurysm or a thoracoabdominal aortic aneurysm in older adults should be considered if the aneurysm is ≥5 cm in maximal diameter. All older adults considered for elective surgical repair must be evaluated for coexistent CAD. The treatment of abdominal aortic aneurysms with endovascular stent-graft prostheses has been demonstrated to be efficacious as an alternative to major open abdominal surgery. Endovascular techniques are especially useful in older adults with multiple comorbidities.

The pain associated with thoracic aortic dissection is severe and often tearing. Stroke, paraplegia, syncope, pulse loss with or without ischemic pain, and HF resulting from severe AR secondary to the dissection may occur. Diagnosis is best made by transesophageal echocardiography, magnetic resonance imaging, or computed tomography. Surgical intervention is the treatment of choice for acute proximal dissection and for complicated acute distal dissection (ie, complicated by rupture, expansion, saccular aneurysm formation,

vital organ or limb ischemia, or continued pain). Endostenting, a new procedure for treating aneurysm, is under investigation. Medical treatment with afterload reduction and β-blockers is the treatment of choice for uncomplicated distal dissection, for stable, isolated arch dissection, and for uncomplicated dissection presenting 2 weeks or later after onset.

Occlusive Peripheral Vascular Disease

The prevalence of occlusive peripheral vascular disease (PVD) increases with age. Significant independent risk factors for symptomatic PVD in older men and women are age, cigarette smoking, hypertension, diabetes mellitus, and serum LDL cholesterol and serum HDL cholesterol (inverse association). People with diabetes mellitus commonly have more distal and diffuse atherosclerosis.

Atherosclerotic vascular disorders, especially CAD, may coexist with PVD. If CAD is present, the prevalence of severe CAD is higher in older adults with PVD than in older adults without PVD. Older adults with PVD are at increased risk for all-cause mortality, cardiovascular mortality, and mortality from CAD.

Atherosclerotic vascular disease affecting the lower extremities may cause asymptomatic arterial insufficiency or symptomatic disease presenting as intermittent claudication or pain at rest, ulceration, and gangrene. Because the superficial femoral and popliteal vessels are most commonly affected by the atherosclerotic process, the pain of intermittent claudication is most often localized to the calf. Atherosclerotic narrowing of the distal aorta and its bifurcation to the two iliac arteries may cause pain in the buttocks or thighs, as well as the legs. People with rest pain are at increased risk of developing ulcers and infection.

Only one half of older adults with documented PVD are symptomatic. Older adults with PVD may not walk far or fast enough to induce muscle ischemic symptoms because of comorbidities such as arthritis or pulmonary disease, may have atypical symptoms unrecognized as intermittent claudication, or may have sufficient collateral arterial channels to tolerate their arterial obstruction.

The diagnosis of PVD is usually made by a thorough history and physical examination. People with asymptomatic arterial insufficiency are identified by a low ankle-brachial index (ABI), which is determined by dividing the systolic blood pressure measured at the ankle by that obtained in the brachial artery. Lower extremity arterial disease is defined as an ABI <0.9. An ABI of <0.90 is 95% sensitive and 99% specific for the diagnosis of PVD. The lower the ABI, the more severe the restriction of arterial blood flow and the more serious the ischemia. An ABI <0.4 is indicative of severe disease that would require intervention to promote wound healing. With ABIs below 0.25 to 0.40, rest pain and tissue loss are often found. Patients with calcified arteries from diabetes mellitus or kidney failure occasionally have relatively noncompressible arteries leading to falsely elevated ABI values in the normal range.

Doppler flow velocity measurements may be useful in grading the severity of vascular obstructions, predicting the healing of ischemic ulcers, and studying diabetic patients with noncompressible arteries. Ultrasonic duplex scanning with color provides detailed information about the arterial system and should be performed when the patient is scheduled for balloon angioplasty or direct arterial surgery; it is also useful in follow-up studies of these patients.

Medical therapy of PVD includes cessation of cigarette smoking and treatment of other risk factors. Exercise therapy is the most effective medical treatment for intermittent claudication. In the Scandinavian Simvastatin Survival Study, simvastatin, in comparison with placebo, was found to reduce the risk of new or worsening intermittent claudication by 38%. Statins have been demonstrated to reduce the incidence of new coronary events in older adults with PVD and a serum LDL cholesterol $\geq$125 mg/dL with and without CAD. Compared with placebo, simvastatin has also been shown to significantly increase the treadmill exercise time until the onset of intermittent claudication by 24% at 6 months and by 42% at 1 year after treatment in older adults with PVD, a serum LDL cholesterol $\geq$125 mg/dL, and a mean ABI of 0.63.

Aspirin therapy delays the progression of PVD and reduces the incidence of stroke, MI, or vascular death. The Clopidogrel versus Aspirin in Patients at Risk for Ischaemic Events trial compared aspirin 325 mg daily with clopidogrel 75 mg daily; clopidogrel significantly reduced the annual incidence rate of stroke, MI, or vascular death by 24% in patients with significant PVD. Therefore, clopidogrel 75 mg daily is preferable to aspirin in the treatment of PVD. Vasodilators should be avoided. The use of pentoxifylline has generally been disappointing. Cilostazol has been demonstrated in numerous studies to increase exercise capacity in people with intermittent claudication and has been shown to be superior to pentoxifylline. However, cilostazol is a phosphodiesterase inhibitor and is contraindicated if HF is present.

People with PVD must wear properly fitted shoes. Careless nail clipping or injury from walking barefoot must be avoided. Feet should be washed daily and the skin kept moist with topical emollients to prevent cracks and fissures, which may be portals for bacterial infection. Fungal infection of the feet must be treated. Socks should be wool or another thick fabric, and padding or shoe inserts may be used to prevent pressure ulcers. When a wound of the foot develops, specialized foot gear, including casts, boots, and ankle foot orthoses, are helpful in taking weight off the affected area.

Indications for percutaneous transluminal angioplasty with intravascular stenting or lower extremity bypass surgery include:

- incapacitating claudication interfering with work or quality of life;
- limb salvage in people with life-threatening ischemia, as indicated by one or more of the following: pain at rest, nonhealing ulcer, infection, or gangrene;
- vasculogenic impotence.

VENOUS DISORDERS

Chronic deep venous insufficiency usually results from prior deep-vein thrombosis (DVT). Symptoms of chronic deep venous insufficiency include edema of the lower extremities, which resolves after nighttime recumbency. Chronic edema with pigmentation of the leg may develop. Compression treatment is the mainstay of therapy. Venous insufficiency predisposes patients to stasis ulcer formation. Venous ulcers develop in the lower aspect of the tibial region, typically above the medial malleolus. Treatment of venous stasis ulcers include different methods of ulcer debridement using gels, proteolytic enzymes, and mechanical debridement. Venous ulcers that do not respond to these therapies may be treated with surgical intervention. Adjunctive procedures include skin grafting of the ulcers using autogenous or tissue-engineered skin with or without venous surgery.

People with chronic deep venous insufficiency are at increased risk of developing DVT, a potentially life-threatening disorder. The gold standard diagnostic test for DVT of the lower extremity is ascending phlebography. Other diagnostic tests include impedance plethysmography and venous Doppler duplex ultrasonography.

See also the Appendix (p 453) for more on anticoagulation.

Superficial venous insufficiency with development of varicose veins may be caused by primary valvular degeneration of veins or by chronic deep venous insufficiency. The most common symptom is aching leg pain, most often exacerbated by standing. Ulcers rarely develop unless deep venous insufficiency is present. Stasis dermatitis may also be seen. Superficial phlebitis develops in severe cases as a result of localized clotting of the vessels. Treatment consists of limb elevation, elastic supportive stockings, and exercise to increase muscle tone. Anticoagulation is not indicated in the absence of deep venous disease.

REFERENCES

- Aronow WS. Hypercholesterolemia: the evidence supports use of statins. *Geriatrics.* 2003;58(8):18–20,26–28,31–32.

- Aronow WS. Epidemiology, pathophysiology, prognosis, and treatment of systolic and diastolic heart failure in elderly patients. *Heart Disease.* 2003;5(4):279–294.

- Aronow WS. Management of peripheral arterial disease of the lower extremities in elderly patients. *J Gerontol A Biol Sci Med Sci.* 2004;59(2):M172–M177.

- Braunwald E, Antman EM, Beasley JW, et al. ACC/AHA 2002 guideline update for the management of patients with unstable angina and non-ST-segment elevation myocardial infarction—summary article: a report of the American College of Cardiology/American Heart Association Task Force on Practice Guidelines (Committee on the Management of Patients With Unstable Angina). *J Am Coll Cardiol.* 2002;40(7):1366–1374.

- Gregoratos G, Abrams J, Epstein AE, et al. ACC/AHA/NASPE 2002 guideline update for implantation of cardiac pacemakers and antiarrhythmia devices: summary article: a report of the American College of Cardiology/American Heart Association Task Force on Practice Guidelines (ACC/AHA/NASPE Committee to Update the 1998 Pacemaker Guidelines). *Circulation.* 2002;106(16):2145–2161.

- Grundy SM, Cleeman JI, Merz CN, et al. Implications of recent clinical trials for the National Cholesterol Education Program Adult Treatment Panel III Guidelines. *Circulation.* 2004;110(2):227–239.

CHAPTER 46—HYPERTENSION

KEY POINTS

- Treating hypertension is beneficial in older adults, as it leads to reductions in heart attack, stroke, heart failure, and overall mortality.

- Thiazide-type diuretics are more effective in preventing cardiovascular disease than other agents and are the preferred first-line therapy in most older adults.

- α-Receptor antagonist agents may increase morbidity and should not be used for first-line therapy. β-Blockers should not be used as first-line therapy in most older adults. Both α-receptor antagonists and β-blockers may be useful in specific patients, depending on comorbid conditions.

- Caution is needed in treating older adults with antihypertensives. Monitoring for falls, orthostatic hypertension, and other adverse drug events is essential. "Start low and go slow."

EPIDEMIOLOGY AND PHYSIOLOGY

Blood pressure, particularly systolic pressure, increases with increasing age. The risk associated with hypertension does not decline with age, and the criteria that define hypertension, outlined in the Seventh Report of the Joint National Committee on Prevention, Detection, Evaluation, and Treatment of High Blood Pressure (JNC 7; see references at end of chapter and Table 46.1), are not age adjusted. Epidemiologic studies, including the National Health and Nutrition Examination surveys, suggest that the prevalence of hypertension in persons aged 65 years and older is between 50% and 70%; the prevalence is highest among older black Americans. In contrast to younger hypertensive populations, among whom men predominate, in the older hypertensive population the prevalence rate is higher for women, particularly for those above the age of 75 years. Over the past 50 years the use of antihypertensive medications has increased, and the prevalence rates of elevated blood pressure, left ventricular hypertrophy, and cardiovascular and stroke mortality have all declined. However, these trends have been delayed among the older population, and blood pressure remains poorly controlled in many older patients despite treatment for hypertension.

Table 46.1—Classification of Blood-Pressure Levels

Category	Systolic (mm Hg)		Diastolic (mm Hg)
Normal	< 120	and	< 80
Prehypertension	120–139	or	80–89
Hypertension			
Stage 1	140–159	or	90–99
Stage 2	≥ 160	or	≥ 100

NOTE: Diagnoses should be based on the average of two or more readings taken at each of two or more visits after an initial screening.

SOURCE: Data from *JNC 7 Express: the seventh report of the Joint National Committee on Prevention, Detection, Evaluation, and Treatment of High Blood Pressure.* Bethesda, MD: National High Blood Pressure Education Program, National Heart, Lung, and Blood Institute, National Institutes of Health, US Department of Health and Human Services; May 2003:3 (Table 1).

Many of the physiologic changes that occur with aging contribute to the increase in blood pressure, but life-style factors such as obesity and physical inactivity and the presence of comorbid diseases are also important contributors. Several physiologic changes combine to increase peripheral vascular resistance, the physiologic hallmark of hypertension in older persons. Several mechanisms contribute to the age-associated increase in arterial vascular stiffness. Arterial stiffness, or reduced vascular compliance, provides the best explanation for the relatively greater increase in systolic pressure and the increase in pulse pressure (the difference between systolic and diastolic pressure) observed with aging. Decreased sensitivity of the baroreflex, perhaps related to decreased arterial distensibility, contributes to an increase in blood-pressure variability and sympathetic nervous system activity. The dynamic regulation of vascular tone is affected by impairments in vasodilator systems (eg, production of nitric oxide by vascular endothelial cells and vasodilatation mediated by β-adrenergic receptors) and heightened vasoconstriction mediated by α-adrenergic receptors. Alterations in kidney function as well as in neurohumoral systems that are involved in sodium balance combine to increase the proportion of older hypertensive persons whose blood pressure increases with increased sodium intake. Approximately two thirds of older hypertensive persons have sodium-sensitive hypertension.

The regulation of blood-pressure homeostasis may be impaired in older hypertensive persons, making older people with elevated systolic blood pressure more likely to develop both orthostatic and postprandial hypotension. Maintaining normal blood pressure and cerebrovascular and coronary perfusion in the face of hypotensive stimuli related to postural challenge, meals, or medications requires the integrated coordination of multiple compensatory mechanisms. The age-associated decline in baroreflex sensitivity and alterations in sympathetic nervous system function impair the dynamic regulation of blood pressure. Because of the blunted sensitivity of the baroreflex, a greater reduction in blood pressure occurs before the increase in heart rate and other compensatory mechanisms are activated. Other pathophysiologic changes that impair blood-pressure regulation include arterial and cardiac stiffness and a decrease in early diastolic filling.

CLINICAL EVALUATION

Accurate measurement of blood pressure is the most critical aspect of the diagnosis of hypertension in the older patient. Because variability in blood pressure increases with age, the diagnosis of hypertension should be made by using the average of several blood-pressure readings taken on each of three visits.

Ambulatory blood-pressure monitoring may be necessary for patients with extreme blood-pressure variability or possible "white-coat" hypertension. Clinicians should be aware of an auscultatory gap, which can lead to underestimation of the true systolic blood pressure and can indicate arterial stiffness. Determining the systolic blood pressure by palpation avoids this problem.

Once a diagnosis of hypertension has been made, the remainder of the clinical evaluation centers on excluding secondary forms of hypertension (using an approach similar to that used in younger patient populations), identifying target organ damage, and determining cardiovascular risk factors and the presence of comorbid conditions. Although most older patients have essential hypertension, secondary forms of hypertension should be suspected in the presence of malignant hypertension, a sudden increase in diastolic blood pressure, worsening level of control, or poorly controlled blood pressure on a regimen of three antihypertensive medications. Renovascular disease is the most common secondary form of hypertension among older patients. Treatment decisions should take into account cardiovascular disease, target-organ damage (eg, left ventricular hypertrophy), diabetes mellitus, and other comorbid diseases. Finally, the patient's smoking history, dietary intake of sodium and fat, alcohol intake, and the level of usual physical activity should be determined to allow the clinician to individualize advice about life-style modifications to help control blood pressure as well as reduce overall cardiovascular disease risk factors.

TREATMENT

The overwhelming consensus derived from the results of several randomized placebo-controlled clinical trials is that treatment of hypertension in older persons is safe and effective. Meta-analyses of more than forty randomized clinical trials of antihypertensive therapy have provided compelling evidence that treatment is effective in reducing cardiovascular (eg, chronic heart failure) and cerebrovascular (eg, stroke) morbidity and mortality. A meta-analysis of outcome trials in systolic hypertension among older patients demonstrated that treatment was associated with significant reductions in overall mortality, cardiovascular events, and stroke. The treatment effect was largest in men, in those aged 70 years and over, and in those who had greater pulse pressures. Of note, few participants in randomized controlled trials of hypertension treatment were over 80 years old and almost none were over 85 years. As the treatment effect is delayed about 5 years, consideration needs to be given to initiating or continuing antihypertensive medication in very elderly persons.

As with other chronic conditions in older patients, it is important to balance the recognized beneficial effects of antihypertensive therapy with the potential impact on the patient's functional status and quality of life (eg, with the development of orthostatic hypotension). A treatment approach using modalities least likely to produce adverse effects and targeting a reduction in systolic blood pressure to 135 to 140 mm Hg and diastolic blood pressure to 85 to 90 mm Hg should be developed. For individuals with type 2 diabetes, a systolic blood pressure goal of less than 130 mm Hg is recommended. For persons with markedly elevated systolic blood pressure, an intermediate target, such as 160 mm Hg, may be an appropriate initial goal in the absence of target-organ damage. The focus of treatment should be on the systolic blood pressure and pulse pressure, since among older hypertensive persons, they are stronger predictors than the diastolic blood pressure of adverse outcomes. The systolic blood pressure alone correctly classifies the blood-pressure stage of more than 99% of older hypertensive patients. In addition, analysis of data from the Systolic Hypertension in the Elderly Program study demonstrates a significant relationship between pulse pressure and the risk for stroke and overall mortality that is independent of the level of mean arterial pressure.

Life-Style Modification

Nonpharmacologic therapy may be effective for older persons with stage 1 hypertension (140 to 159 mm Hg systolic or 90 to 99 mm Hg diastolic blood pressure) and is an important adjunct to drug treatment because of synergistic effects with antihypertensive drugs and the benefits realized through the reduction in other cardiovascular risk factors (see Table 46.2). Life-style modifications that target the typical characteristics of the older hypertensive person—overweight, sedentary, and salt-sensitive—are likely to be effective. The randomized Trial of Nonpharmacologic Interventions in Elderly study, which evaluated the effects of dietary sodium restriction and weight loss in elderly patients, demonstrated that relatively modest reductions in dietary sodium intake (40 mmol per day) and in body weight (4 kg) are accompanied by a 30% decrease in the need to reinitiate pharmacologic treatment. A meta-analysis of randomized trials assessing the effects of dietary sodium restriction demonstrated a significant reduction in systolic (a mean decrease of 3.7 mm Hg for each decrease of 100 mmol per day in sodium intake) but not in diastolic blood pressure. This differential reduction in systolic pressure is particularly well suited for the older hypertensive patient. Persons with stage 1 hypertension who do not have diabetes

mellitus should complete a 6-month trial of nonpharmacologic therapy before adding an antihypertensive medication if the target blood pressure is not achieved. (See also "Physical Activity," p 51; "Malnutrition," p 161.)

Pharmacologic Treatment

The general approach to pharmacologic management of the older hypertensive patient is presented in the JNC 7. General principles regarding drug selection are reviewed here and summarized in Table 46.3. Drug selection may be affected by whether the patient has simple hypertension or hypertension complicated by any of several comorbid conditions (eg, diabetes mellitus, coronary artery disease or history of myocardial infarction, heart failure, prostatism) that may influence the choice of drug. Racial and ethnic background likely has an effect on an individual's response to antihypertensive drug therapy; the blood-pressure reduction resulting from monotherapy with angiotensin-converting enzyme (ACE) inhibitors or angiotensin receptor blockers is somewhat attenuated among blacks. Given the available evidence to date, for those with simple, uncomplicated hypertension, the initial antihypertensive drug choice is a low-dose thiazide-type diuretic. A majority of patients will not

Table 46.2—Nonpharmacologic Therapy for Stage 1 Hypertension

- Weight reduction
- Aerobic and strength-training exercise programs
- Smoking cessation
- Moderation of alcohol intake
- Dietary changes to decrease sodium, saturated fat, and cholesterol while maintaining adequate intake of potassium, magnesium, and calcium

Table 46.3—General Treatment Recommendations for Stage 1, Simple Hypertension

- Begin with a nonpharmacologic approach (see Table 46.2).
- Use a low dose diuretic as the first choice for initial pharmacologic therapy.
- Base alternative drug selection or combination therapies on individual patient characteristics.
- When initiating drug therapy, begin at half of the usual dose, increase dose slowly, and continue nonpharmacologic therapies.
- Focus treatment goal on systolic blood-pressure reduction to 135 to 140 mm Hg.
- Avoid excessive reduction in diastolic blood pressure (below 70 mm Hg).
- Do not use aggressive therapy whenever adverse effects (eg, postural hypotension) cannot be avoided.

reach their systolic blood pressure goal on a single drug; JNC 7 recommends considering starting patients on two drugs if the initial blood pressure is more than 20 mm Hg above the target level. In this circumstance, partly in light of the results from the Second Australian National Blood Pressure Study, adding an ACE inhibitor to a low-dose thiazide-type diuretic is a combination that is reasonable to consider. Beyond these general recommendations for initial therapy, there is no universally accepted approach to choosing alternative agents or combination therapies; these decisions should be made on an individual basis that considers the advantages and disadvantages of the drug together with the patient's comorbidities. Finally, centrally acting agents (eg, clonidine, methyldopa) and those more likely to produce orthostatic hypotension should be avoided in most older patients.

Diuretics

Therapy with low-dose thiazide-type diuretics (eg, hydrochlorothiazide ≤25 mg daily, or the equivalent) has demonstrated significant benefits in mortality, stroke, and coronary events in randomized clinical trials in older hypertensive patients. The two thiazide-type diuretics in common usage—the benzothiadiazine hydrochlorothiazide and the benzene sulfonamide chlorthalidone—differ markedly in their chemical structure, potency, and pharmacokinetics. The effectiveness of both drugs has been demonstrated in clinical trials, although many recent trials, such as the Antihypertensive and Lipid-Lowering Treatment to Prevent Heart Attack Trial (ALLHAT), have used chlorthalidone. Although the direct comparability of these two diuretics has not been rigorously examined, the available evidence suggests that their blood-pressure lowering and other effects are comparable. These beneficial effects, combined with their relative safety, favorable adverse-effect profile (their adverse metabolic effects—hypokalemia, hyperuricemia, and glucose intolerance—are attenuated at lower doses), once-daily dosing, and low cost have led to the recommendation that diuretics are preferred for initial therapy. Another advantage is that diuretic therapy leads to a disproportionate reduction in systolic relative to diastolic blood pressure, and it is better than other agents at achieving a reduction in systolic blood pressure. Thiazide diuretics are also well suited for use in combination therapies because of synergistic effects with other antihypertensive drug classes. The importance of maintaining a normal potassium level during therapy with thiazide-type diuretics deserves emphasis. Adequate potassium replacement during diuretic-based treatment has been shown to prevent the risk of arrhythmias as well as decrease the impairment in glucose tolerance.

Angiotensin-Converting Enzyme Inhibitors

ACE inhibitors have been demonstrated to be effective in lowering blood pressure in older hypertensive patients. Given the results from the Second Australian National Blood Pressure randomized controlled trial, there is support for using ACE inhibitors as initial monotherapy for simple hypertension in older hypertensive patients, especially in men. Drugs in this class are generally well tolerated (with the exception of cough during ACE inhibitor therapy), and they do not adversely affect the central nervous system or metabolic profile. There are compelling benefits from using ACE inhibitors in those patients with coexisting diabetes mellitus (particularly when there is microalbuminuria), as well as in those with left ventricular systolic dysfunction.

Angiotensin-Receptor Blockers

There have been no randomized controlled trials that have compared outcomes from treatment with angiotensin receptor blockers (ARBs) with diuretics among older hypertensive patients. The recently completed ALLHAT study did not include an ARB arm. Results from a network meta-analysis suggest that diuretic therapy is superior to ARBs for most outcomes. In the absence of data from randomized controlled trials to support their benefit with respect to cardiovascular events and mortality, therapy with an ARB generally should not be considered as initial monotherapy for simple hypertension. ARB therapy may be considered in patients with underlying diabetes, heart failure, or chronic kidney disease, especially if they are not able to tolerate ACE inhibitor therapy.

Calcium Channel Antagonists

Therapy with calcium channel antagonists (CCAs), in particular, long-acting agents in the dihydropyridine (nifedipine-like) class, has been shown in the Systolic Hypertension in Europe and China trials to lead to significant reduction in stroke risk in older hypertensive patients. The pathophysiologic (reduction in peripheral vascular resistance) and adverse-effect (absence of central or metabolic effects) profiles of the CCA class are other factors that support their use in this patient population. Although these agents are not recommended as first-step therapy, they may be considered as second-line drugs, generally in combination with a thiazide-type diuretic. Because of age-related changes in their pharmacokinetics, lower doses of CCAs should be used. Short-acting CCAs should not be used to treat hypertension.

β-Receptor Antagonists

β-Receptor antagonists are recommended in the JNC 7 report as another option for second-line drug therapy. β-Receptor antagonists should not be considered as first-line monotherapy for simple hypertension in older patients. Analysis of evidence from randomized controlled trials has questioned the efficacy of β-blockers in older hypertensive persons. Results from these studies suggest that therapy with a β-receptor antagonist is less effective than therapy with low-dose thiazide diuretics with respect to blood-pressure reduction and in the prevention of cardiovascular events, stroke, and death. In addition, β-blockers are more likely to be discontinued because of adverse effects. Because of their effectiveness in the management of symptomatic coronary artery disease, in secondary prevention following myocardial infarction, and in certain heart failure settings, β-receptor antagonists should be considered for older patients whose hypertension is complicated by these comorbid conditions.

α-Receptor Antagonists

Although the reduction in peripheral vascular resistance that occurs with therapy using an α-receptor antagonist is particularly appropriate for the pathophysiologic profile of geriatric hypertension, and although these agents are effective in blood-pressure reduction, the development of postural hypotension has limited the widespread use of this class of antihypertensive for treating elderly patients. The treatment arm that included persons randomized to therapy with the α-receptor antagonist doxazosin in the ALLHAT study was stopped early because of a higher rate of cardiovascular end points, including a twofold greater likelihood of being hospitalized for heart failure. α-Receptor antagonist therapy, usually in combination with another drug, might be considered for treating older hypertensive men with prostatism since these drugs have been shown to be efficacious in improving obstructive urinary symptoms.

The J-Curve Hypothesis

Although it is clear that an increase in blood pressure above normal (>130/85 mm Hg) is positively and linearly associated with morbidity and mortality, concerns have been expressed that reduction of blood pressure below a given threshold level may be linked to adverse outcomes. Some studies have shown an increase in mortality with blood-pressure reduction below a certain threshold, creating a J-shaped curve of mortality. The significance of these concerns remains controversial. Many of the studies that have suggested a J-curve relationship have been confounded by

comorbid illnesses among those with the lowest blood pressures. However, the results from several longitudinal studies have identified an increased risk for stroke and overall mortality in persons in the lowest systolic and, particularly, diastolic blood-pressure levels. Until additional prospective data are available to provide guidance in this therapeutic dilemma, it is prudent to use caution in lowering blood pressure in older persons with hypertension much below 140/90 mm Hg. Excessive reductions in blood pressure (eg, diastolic levels below 70 mm Hg) and treatment-induced postural hypotension should be avoided.

Follow-Up Visits

The frequency of follow-up visits should reflect the patient's degree of blood-pressure elevation at presentation, with closer follow-up indicated for those with more severe hypertension (ie, a systolic blood pressure greater than 180 mm Hg). With the exception of hypertensive emergencies (discussed below), attempts to reduce the patient's blood pressure to target levels too rapidly are unnecessary and likely deleterious. For most patients, an interval of 1 to 2 months is appropriate between visits to determine the need for dose adjustment.

Given the age-related changes in systems that regulate blood pressure and impaired blood-pressure homeostasis, overtreatment of hypertension may result in situational (postural or postprandial) hypotension. At all follow-up visits, it is imperative to determine the supine and standing blood pressure (Table 46.4). It is good practice to adjust antihypertensive drug doses to achieve the target (seated) blood pressure only after determining whether postural hypotension is present.

The patient's adherence to the current antihypertensive medication regimen should be assessed before an increased dosage is recommended or an alternative medication is considered. For some patients, additional information derived from blood-pressure measurements taken at home or another nonclinical setting may be important; home blood-pressure monitoring may also aid in promoting a

---

Table 46.4—Hypertension Management: Follow-Up Visits

- Assess adherence to therapy.
- Monitor for adverse effects, especially postural hypotension.
- Measure supine and upright blood pressure.
- Encourage self-monitoring of blood pressure.
- Reinforce life-style modifications (eg, diet, exercise).
- Adjust dose cautiously.
- Evaluate for refractory hypertension.

patient's adherence to therapy. Patient education regarding the significant benefits to be gained from adequate blood-pressure control is of particular importance, since hypertension is usually asymptomatic. The interdisciplinary geriatric team is well suited to promote this approach (eg, nurses to provide feedback on the degree of blood-pressure control, dietitians to review dietary information and adherence, pharmacists to promote adherence to the medical regimen, and social workers to review and, where possible, alleviate the financial burden associated with the cost of medical therapy). This evaluation should include a careful review of the patient's other medications to identify those (eg, nonsteroidal anti-inflammatory drugs and corticosteroids) that may worsen blood-pressure control.

When a patient's blood pressure has not been successfully reduced to the target level, cautiously increasing the dose, adding another agent (particularly a thiazide diuretic, if the patient is not already receiving this drug), or switching to another class of medication should be considered. Patients also should be counseled to continue their life-style modifications. It may take many months to achieve the target blood-pressure goal. When this goal is not attained despite adherence to a three-drug regimen, an evaluation for refractory hypertension (especially renovascular disease) should be considered. Once a patient has achieved appropriate stable blood-pressure control for more than a year, step-down treatment may be considered; a cautious downward dosage adjustment may be attempted, with close blood-pressure monitoring. Patients who have been successful at achieving weight loss or other nonpharmacologic interventions are most likely to be successfully weaned from antihypertensive medications.

SPECIAL CONSIDERATIONS

Hypertensive Emergencies and Urgencies

Elevated blood pressure per se in the absence of signs or symptoms of target-organ damage does not constitute a hypertensive emergency or urgency. Rapidly and too aggressively reducing blood pressure in a patient with incidentally discovered elevated blood pressure is potentially harmful and may produce complications, such as coronary or cerebral hypoperfusion syndromes.

Examples of true hypertensive emergencies in older patients include hypertensive encephalopathy, acute heart failure with pulmonary edema, dissecting aortic aneurysm, and unstable angina. These situations present with symptoms and signs of vascular compromise of the affected organs. The management of these emergencies requires an acute hospital setting, with the parenteral administration of an antihypertensive agent and continuous blood-pressure monitoring to achieve an immediate reduction in blood pressure, although not initially to a normal target level. Blood pressure should not be lowered emergently more than 25% within the first 2 hours, with a goal of achieving 160/100 mm Hg gradually over the first 6 hours of therapy.

Hypertensive urgencies, situations in which blood pressure should be lowered within 24 hours to prevent the risk of target-organ damage, are more common than true emergencies. The majority may be managed with oral administration of antihypertensive medications to achieve a gradual blood-pressure reduction.

Hypertension in the Long-Term-Care Setting

Approximately one third to two thirds of residents in long-term-care facilities have hypertension. Special considerations are warranted in the care of residents with respect to making the correct diagnosis and defining the goals of therapy and its effects on quality of life. Blood-pressure measurements in long-term-care settings may not be accurate. Inaccuracies result from measurement errors and from the temporal variability in blood pressure, particularly in relation to meals. Blood pressure appears to be highest in the morning before breakfast. Postprandial hypotension is common among long-term-care residents, affecting about one third of this population. The presence of postprandial hypotension has been associated with otherwise unexplained syncope, and it has been found to be a significant independent risk factor for falls, syncope, stroke, and overall mortality.

There are several factors to consider in the management of hypertension in this setting. First, the advanced average age of persons in long-term care raises controversy surrounding the question whether the benefits of antihypertensive therapy extend to the very old (ie, those aged 80 years and older). If the beneficial effects of treatment are less evident, the potential adverse effects and risks of therapy should be weighed more heavily in defining the goals of therapy. Even an intervention as seemingly innocuous as a sodium-restricted diet needs to be evaluated in the context of the high prevalence of protein-energy malnutrition among nursing-home residents. Second, the average resident in long-term care takes seven medications, and most have three or more comorbid conditions. The addition of an antihypertensive medication increases the possibility of an adverse drug event in this frail, at-risk group. Third, several studies have identified the use of antihypertensive medications, particularly vasodilators, as a risk factor for falls in this high-risk population, who experience an average of two falls each year. It is therefore important to assess both postural and postprandial blood pressure in this population. Randomized controlled trials that could provide clear risk-benefit evidence to support an approach to antihypertensive management in the long-term-care population have not yet been conducted. The available data suggest that diuretic therapy is effective in controlling systolic blood-pressure elevations and that blood-pressure reduction with diuretics lowers the prevalence of postural hypotension.

REFERENCES

- Chobanian AV, Bakris GL, Black HR, et al. The Seventh Report of the Joint National Committee on Prevention, Detection, Evaluation, and Treatment of High Blood Pressure; The JNC 7 Report. *JAMA*. 2003;289(19):2560–2572. Available at http://www.nhlbi.nih.gov/guidelines/hypertension (accessed October 2005).

- Domanski MJ, Davis BR, Pfeffer MA, et al. Isolated systolic hypertension: prognostic information provided by pulse pressure. *Hypertension*. 1999;34(3):375–380.

- Psaty BM, Lumley T, Furberg CD, et al. Health outcomes associated with various antihypertensive therapies used as first-line agents: a network meta-analysis. *JAMA*. 2003;289(19):2534–2544.

- The ALLHAT Collaborative Research Group. Major outcomes in high-risk hypertensive patients randomized to angiotensin-converting enzyme inhibitor or calcium channel blocker vs. diuretic. *JAMA*. 2002;288(23):2981–2997.

- Vasan RS, Beiser A, Seshadri S, et al. Residual lifetime risk for developing hypertension in middle-aged women and men. *JAMA*. 2002;287(8):1003–1010.

- Wing LM, Reid CM, Ryan P, et al. A comparison of outcomes with angiotensin-converting–enzyme inhibitors and diuretics for hypertension in the elderly. *N Engl J Med*. 2003;348(7):583–592.

CHAPTER 47—ENDOCRINE AND METABOLIC DISORDERS

KEY POINTS

- Older adults with severe hypothyroidism should undergo testing to exclude concomitant adrenal insufficiency before receiving thyroid hormone replacement.

- Vitamin-D deficiency not only contributes to osteoporosis but has been associated with muscle weakness and falls.

- Malignant causes of hypercalcemia include squamous cell cancers, breast cancer, lymphoma, and myeloma.

- There is little evidence of long-term benefit from supplementation with growth hormone, testosterone, or estrogen in older adults.

Impaired homeostatic regulation, a hallmark of aging, occurs in many endocrine systems but may become manifest only during stress. For example, fasting blood glucose levels change little with normal aging, increasing 1 to 2 mg per dL per decade of life. In contrast, glucose levels after a glucose challenge increase much more in healthy older persons than in young adults. In some cases, a loss of function in one aspect of endocrine function may result in a compensatory change in endocrine regulation and associated alterations in catabolism that maintain homeostasis. For example, the reduction in testicular testosterone production that occurs in many older men may be partially compensated for by an increase in pituitary luteinizing hormone secretion and a decrease in testosterone metabolism. In other instances, compensatory changes or alterations in hormone catabolism do not fully offset age-related impairment in endocrine functions, as illustrated by the age-related decline in basal serum aldosterone levels. In this case, a decline in aldosterone clearance fails to offset the decrease in aldosterone secretion.

As with diseases in other organ systems, endocrine disorders in older adults often present with nonspecific, muted, or atypical symptoms and signs. Some of these presentations are well-defined syndromes that are seen almost exclusively in older adults, such as apathetic thyrotoxicosis or hyperosmolar nonketotic state in patients with diabetes mellitus. However, more commonly, endocrine disorders present with subtle, nonspecific symptoms, such as cognitive impairment, or an absence of any complaints. Indeed, the diagnosis of endocrinopathies such as hyperparathyroidism, diabetes mellitus, hypothyroidism, and hyperthyroidism in older adults is commonly established as a result of abnormalities found on routine laboratory screening.

Laboratory evaluation of older adults for endocrine disorders may be complicated by coexisting medical illnesses and medications. For example, the presence of serious acute nonthyroidal illness may lead to the mistaken impression of a thyroid disorder because of the reduction in free thyroxine (T_4) levels and sometimes increased or decreased thyrotropin (TSH) levels in sick but euthyroid older patients. Furthermore, ranges of normal laboratory values for endocrine testing are commonly established in younger adults, and even age-adjusted norms for laboratory tests may be confounded by the inclusion of older adults who are ill. Therefore, normal ranges for healthy older people are not available for most laboratory tests.

THYROID DISORDERS

With aging, a reduction in T_4 secretion is balanced by a decrease in T_4 clearance, resulting in unchanged circulating T_4 levels. Triiodothyronine (T_3) levels are unchanged until extreme old age, when they decrease slightly. However, T_3 levels are commonly reduced in the setting of nonthyroidal illness because of decreased T_4-to-T_3 conversion. TSH levels are unchanged or minimally changed in healthy older people.

Nonspecific, atypical, or asymptomatic presentations of thyroid disease are common in older adults. In the outpatient setting, laboratory testing in the stable outpatient is the most reliable way to identify hypothyroidism or hyperthyroidism in older adults who are not acutely ill. Given a 1.4% prevalence of thyroid disease in ambulatory women aged 50 and over, some clinicians recommend routine screening with a highly sensitive TSH test, although treatment may not affect outcomes. In addition, the prevalence of hypothyroidism or hyperthyroidism is sufficiently high to warrant TSH testing in all older adults with a recent decline in clinical, cognitive, or functional status, or upon admission to the nursing home. However, the results of thyroid function testing may be confusing in euthyroid patients with significant concurrent illnesses, as discussed below.

Hypothyroidism

Most prevalence estimates of hypothyroidism in older adults range from 0.5% to 5% for overt disease, and from 5% to 10% for subclinical hypothyroidism, depending on the population studied. As in younger people, most cases of hypothyroidism in older people are due to chronic autoimmune thyroiditis.

Symptoms of hypothyroidism are often atypical in older adults. Some clinical features of hypothyroidism (eg, dry skin, decreased skin turgor, slowed mentation, weakness, constipation, anemia, hyponatremia, arthritis, paresthesias, gait disturbances, elevated myocardial band of creatine phosphokinase) may misleadingly suggest other diseases. Furthermore, these symptoms usually have an insidious onset and a slow rate of progression. As a result, the diagnosis of hypothyroidism is recognized on clinical examination in only 10% to 20% of cases in older adults, and laboratory screening is necessary to detect most cases of hypothyroidism in this population. In addition, older patients with mild hypothyroidism who develop serious nonthyroidal illness may rapidly become severely hypothyroid, and older adults are more susceptible to myxedema coma in this setting. Demented older people with hypothyroidism rarely recover normal cognitive function with thyroid replacement, but cognition, functional status, and mood may improve with treatment of the hypothyroidism.

Subclinical hypothyroidism, with elevated serum TSH and normal free T_4 levels, occurs in up to 15% of people aged 65 and over, and is more common in women. Subclinical hypothyroidism is associated with impaired left ventricular diastolic and systolic function, and is an important risk factor for atherosclerosis and myocardial infarction in older women. An approach to the management of subclinical hypothyroidism is outlined in Figure 47.1. The presence of elevated thyroid peroxidase antibody titers portends the eventual development of thyroid failure and overt hypothyroidism, and it is appropriate to initiate T_4 replacement therapy in these patients. In addition, T_4 replacement is indicated in older adults with progressively increasing TSH levels or a TSH level persistently above 10 mIU/L.

By itself, an increased TSH level is usually due to primary hypothyroidism, but TSH levels may be transiently elevated during recovery from acute illnesses. Therefore, the diagnosis of hypothyroidism should be confirmed with the combination of an elevated TSH level and a decreased free T_4 or free T_4 index, or by the demonstration of a persistently increased TSH level, or both. Other potentially confusing scenarios in the diagnosis of hypothyroidism include the *low T_4 syndrome*, seen in euthyroid patients with severe nonthyroidal illnesses and presenting with a decreased free T_4 index without an increase in TSH levels. Free T_4 levels are usually normal in the low T_4 syndrome, with elevated levels of reverse T_3. Thyroid hormone supplementation has not been shown to be beneficial in these patients. A normal (or low) TSH together with a low free T_4 level may also suggest *secondary hypothyroidism*, which is differentiated from the low T_4 syndrome by the presence of hypopituitarism (deficiencies in other pituitary hormones) and decreased reverse T_3 levels. Rarely, older people with primary hypothyroidism may also present with inappropriately normal TSH levels resulting from suppression of TSH by fasting, acute illnesses, and medications such as dopamine, phenytoin, or glucocorticoids.

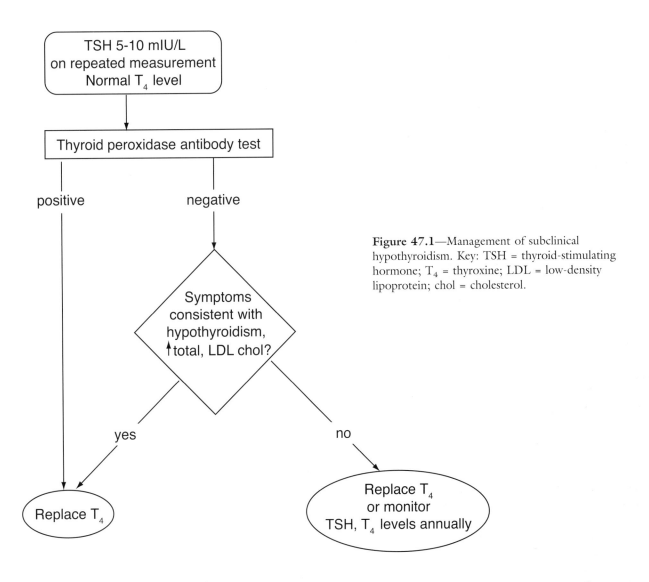

Figure 47.1—Management of subclinical hypothyroidism. Key: TSH = thyroid-stimulating hormone; T_4 = thyroxine; LDL = low-density lipoprotein; chol = cholesterol.

T_4 replacement is usually initiated at a low dosage (eg, 25 µg per day) in older adults, increasing the dose every few weeks until TSH levels normalize. However, in patients with cardiac disease, it is prudent to begin replacement therapy at even lower dosages (eg, 12.5 µg per day). In these patients, thyroid replacement should not be withheld for fear of exacerbating cardiac disease; instead, the goal is to reduce or eliminate symptoms of hypothyroidism without causing intolerable exacerbation of cardiac symptoms, such as angina. Older adults who are severely hypothyroid at presentation should receive larger initial T_4 replacement doses of 50 to 100 µg, or as high as 400 µg intravenously for those with myxedema stupor or coma, even if there is preexisting heart disease. Such patients should also receive testing to exclude concomitant adrenal insufficiency as well as stress doses of glucocorticoids before receiving T_4 to avoid precipitating an adrenal crisis with T_4 replacement.

Thyroid hormone requirements decrease with aging because of a reduction in clearance rate, and T_4 replacement doses are as much as a third lower in older than in younger adults. The average T_4 replacement dosage in older adults is approximately 110 µg per day. Overreplacement of thyroid hormone should be avoided, because osteopenia related to increased bone turnover and exacerbation of heart disease may occur. With correction of the hypothyroid state, the clearance rate of medications such as anticonvulsants, digoxin, and opiate analgesic agents may be affected, necessitating dosage adjustments. T_4 supplementation may have beneficial effects on some parameters of cognitive and cardiac function in some older adults with subclinical hypothyroidism, although randomized trials of such treatment have yielded mixed results. Finally, elevations in total and low-density lipoprotein cholesterol levels in hypothyroid patients may resolve with restoration of the euthyroid state, even in those with subclinical hypothyroidism, suggesting that T_4 replacement may reduce the risk of atherosclerotic vascular disease in older adults with good long-term survival prospects.

Hyperthyroidism

Hyperthyroidism develops in 0.5% to 2.3% of older people, and 15% to 25% of all cases of thyrotoxicosis occur in adults aged 60 and over. In the United States, most cases in older adults are due to Graves' disease, but toxic multinodular goiter and autonomously functioning adenomas are more common in older than in young adults, especially in populations with low iodine intake.

Hyperthyroidism often presents with vague, atypical, or nonspecific symptoms in frail older patients. Many findings that are common in younger adults (eg, tremor, heat intolerance, tachycardia, ophthalmopathy, increased perspiration, goiter, brisk reflexes) are less common or absent in older persons, whereas other manifestations, such as atrial fibrillation, heart failure, constipation, anorexia, muscle atrophy, and weakness, are more common in older adults. Older persons may present with *apathetic thyrotoxicosis*, a well-known clinical presentation of hyperthyroidism that is rarely seen in younger persons, in which the usual hyperkinetic presentation is replaced by depression, inactivity, lethargy, or withdrawn behavior, often in association with symptoms such as weight loss, muscle weakness, or cardiac symptoms. A low TSH level is associated with a threefold higher risk of developing atrial fibrillation within 10 years, and hyperthyroidism is present in 13% to 30% of older people with atrial fibrillation. Hyperthyroidism is a cause of secondary osteoporosis and should be considered in the evaluation of patients presenting with decreased bone mass.

A highly sensitive TSH test is adequate as an initial test for hyperthyroidism in relatively healthy older patients, but the diagnosis should be confirmed with a free T_4 test. Figure 47.2 illustrates the approach to diagnosing the cause of a low TSH level. Most asymptomatic older adults with low serum TSH levels are clinically euthyroid and have normal T_4 and T_3 levels, with normal TSH on repeat testing 4 to 6 weeks later. T_3 *thyrotoxicosis*, with elevated T_3 but normal T_4 levels, occurs in a minority of hyperthyroid patients, but it is more common with aging, especially in patients with toxic adenomas or toxic multinodular goiter. However, in contrast to young adults, many older persons with hyperthyroidism do not have increased T_4 or T_3 levels, probably because of decreased conversion of T_4 to T_3 associated with aging and nonthyroidal illness. Diagnostic confusion may occasionally occur in euthyroid patients with conditions or medications causing elevated T_4 levels (*high T_4 syndrome*). The high T_4 syndrome may occur with drugs or illnesses that decrease T_4-to-T_3 conversion (high-dose glucocorticoids or β-blocking agents, acute fasting) or that increase circulating levels of thyroid-binding globulin (estrogens, clofibrate, hepatitis).

Subclinical hyperthyroidism is present in less than 2% of older people and is associated with adverse cardiovascular events such as atrial fibrillation, increased left ventricular mass, and impaired ventricular relaxation; osteoporosis; neuropsychiatric problems including dementia; and excess cardiovascular and all-cause mortality. Accordingly, treatment for this condition may be justifiable, but there is a lack of data from randomized controlled trials to support this approach.

Thyroid scanning and measurement of radioactive iodine uptake may be useful in confirming hyperthyroidism and defining the cause (Figure 47.2). Radioactive iodine therapy is the treatment of choice for most older people with hyperthyroidism. Higher or repeated doses are often necessary for patients with toxic multinodular goiter. Antithyroid drugs such as methimazole or propylthiouracil are given before radioactive iodine, to control symptoms and to avoid a worsening of thyrotoxicosis due to transient release of thyroid hormone after radioactive iodine. β-Blocking agents are helpful to manage symptoms such as tachycardia, tremor, and anxiety, but patients should be monitored for changes in cardiopulmonary function. Following radioactive iodine therapy, patients should be followed with serial TSH levels for the eventual development of hypothyroidism, or persistent or recurrent hyperthyroidism. With resolution of hyperthyroidism, the clearance rate of other drugs may decrease, necessitating dosage adjustments to avoid excessive drug levels.

Nodular Thyroid Disease and Thyroid Cancer

The incidence of multinodular goiter increases with aging, and approximately 90% of women aged 70 years and over, and 60% of men aged 80 years and over have thyroid nodules. Most of these are nonpalpable. Multinodular goiters often have autonomously functioning areas, so that administration of exogenous thyroid hormone to suppress these goiters may cause iatrogenic hyperthyroidism. Older persons with multinodular goiter may develop iodine-induced thyrotoxicosis after receiving radiocontrast or amiodarone.

Solitary thyroid nodules are more likely to be malignant in people over 60 years of age, especially men. The incidence of differentiated thyroid cancers is similar in older and younger adults, whereas anaplastic

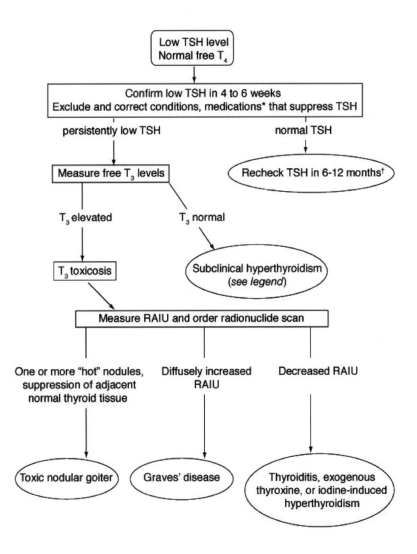

Figure 47.2.—Diagnostic algorithm for a low TSH level.
Key: TSH = thyroid-stimulating hormone; T_4 = thyroxine; T_3 = triiodothyronine; RAIU = radioactive iodine uptake.
* Glucocorticoids, dopamine agonists, and phenytoin.
† If TSH is again normal, discontinue monitoring.
NOTE: The management of subclinical hyperthyroidism is controversial. If subclinical hyperthyroidism is diagnosed, the patient should be assessed for clinical findings consistent with thyrotoxicosis, such as atrial fibrillation, osteoporosis, and neuropsychiatric symptoms. If these findings are present, the clinician may wish to consider further evaluation as suggested for T_3 toxicosis. Otherwise, it is reasonable to recheck TSH, free T_4, and free T_3 and monitor clinically for manifestations of thyrotoxicosis every 6 months.

thyroid carcinomas occur almost exclusively in older adults. However, even well-differentiated papillary and follicular carcinomas are more aggressive and are associated with increased mortality in older persons. Accordingly, a new solitary nodule or an enlargement of an existing nodule warrants a careful evaluation, including a fine-needle aspiration. An approach to the management of a solitary thyroid nodule is outlined in Figure 47.3. Levothyroxine suppressive therapy is indicated to reduce the risk of cancer recurrence and mortality for some patients with thyroid cancer (eg,

those at highest risk), but adverse effects on the heart and osteoporosis may occur with long-term thyroid suppression. β-Blocking agents and bone antiresorptive agents may be useful to minimize these untoward effects.

DISORDERS OF PARATHYROID AND CALCIUM METABOLISM

Important changes occur with aging in several systems that regulate calcium homeostasis, ultimately leading to

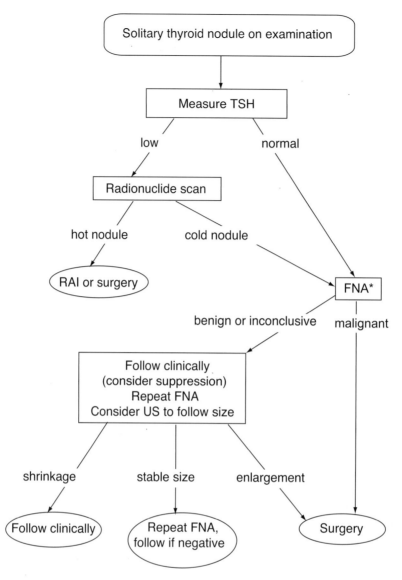

Figure 47.3—Management of a solitary thyroid nodule. This evaluation should be performed in consultation with an endocrinologist.

Key: TSH = thyroid-stimulating hormone; RAI = radioactive iodine; FNA = fine needle aspiration biopsy; US = ultrasound.
* Repeat FNA if inadequate specimen.

a reduction in bone mass and in some cases osteoporosis in older people (Table 47.1). The net effect of these changes is to increase circulating levels of parathyroid hormone (PTH), which increases 30% between 30 and 80 years of age. Serum calcium levels remain normal as a result of the increase in PTH, but the balance between bone resorption and bone formation is altered in favor of resorption, resulting in a decrease in bone mass and an increased risk of osteoporosis with aging.

Vitamin-D Deficiency

Dietary calcium intake is inadequate in most older people. However, as a consequence of factors men-

tioned in Table 47.1, older people are less able than younger adults to compensate by increasing their intestinal absorption of ingested calcium. In addition, vitamin-D deficiency is common in older adults, especially in hospitalized patients, nursing-home residents, and homebound community-dwelling people. Increased bone turnover and bone loss, especially of cortical bone, is a major consequence of secondary hyperparathyroidism in vitamin D-deficient older adults. Furthermore, vitamin-D deficiency is associated with muscle weakness and may contribute to fall risk in some patients.

Adequate dietary calcium and vitamin-D supplementation may reverse age-related hyperparathyroidism, increase bone mineral density, and reduce falls and

Table 47.1—Age-Related Alterations in Calcium Homeostasis

Factors leading to decreased 1,25(OH)$_2$D levels

    Decreased renal 1α-hydroxylase activity, leading to decreased renal parathyroid hormone responsiveness

    Decreased vitamin-D synthesis by the skin

    Decreased sunlight exposure (housebound and institutionalized elderly persons)

Factors leading to decreased intestinal absorption of dietary calcium

    Inadequate dietary calcium and vitamin-D intake

    Decreased intestinal responsiveness to 1,25(OH)$_2$D

    Decreased gastric acid secretion

    Lactase deficiency (avoidance of dairy products)

Factors leading to age-related increase in serum parathyroid hormone levels

    Slight decrease in serum calcium levels

    Decreased renal clearance of parathyroid hormone

    Decreased 1,25(OH)$_2$D levels

NOTE: 1,25(OH)$_2$D = 1,25 dihydroxyvitamin D.

osteoporotic fracture rates, although the effectiveness of vitamin D alone in preventing osteoporotic fractures is unclear. For many older people, an elemental calcium intake of at least 1000 to 1500 mg per day is desirable, together with at least 600–800 IU of vitamin D per day. High-dose supplementation may cause vitamin-D intoxication with hypercalcemia, hypercalciuria, impairment of kidney function, and bone loss. A few patients who are unable to take daily oral supplements may benefit from 100,000 IU of oral or parenteral vitamin D every 6 months with minimal risk of hypercalcemia. (See also the section on prevention and treatment of osteoporosis in "Osteoporosis and Osteomalacia," p 198.)

Hypercalcemia

Primary hyperparathyroidism and malignancy are the most common causes of hypercalcemia in older adults. The annual incidence of primary hyperparathyroidism is approximately 1 per 1000, and the disease is threefold more prevalent in women than in men. Most patients with primary hyperparathyroidism are asymptomatic, and the diagnosis is made after an incidental finding of hypercalcemia. When the disease is symptomatic, older persons are more likely than younger adults to present with neuropsychiatric symptoms such as depression and cognitive impairment, neuromuscular symptoms such as proximal muscle weakness, or osteoporosis. Typical laboratory findings in primary hyperparathyroidism and other common causes of hypercalcemia are described in Table 47.2. The diagnosis of primary hyperparathyroidism is confirmed with an elevated or high normal PTH level by the use of an assay for intact PTH, in the presence of hypercalcemia.

Surgery is the treatment of choice for primary hyperparathyroidism with total serum calcium levels more than 1 mg/dL above the normal range, 24-hour urine calcium levels above 400 mg, creatinine clearance reduced by more than 30% in comparison with normal persons of the same age, markedly decreased bone density (T score below −2.5 at any site on bone densitometry), or nephrolithiasis. Patients with serum calcium levels less than 1 mg/dL above the normal range who are asymptomatic and managed conservatively should avoid thiazide diuretics, dehydration, and immobilization. Baseline assessment in these patients should include blood pressure, serum calcium and creatinine, creatinine clearance, 24-hour urine calcium, abdominal radiography, and bone densitometry. Follow-up assessments should include blood pressure and serum calcium every 6 months, and serum creatinine and bone densitometry can be considered periodically. In addition, these patients should be followed clinically for the development of nephrolithiasis, minimal trauma fractures, and neuropsychiatric or neuromuscular symptoms. Medical management options for hyperparathyroidism also include β-blocking agents, oral phosphate in patients with low serum phosphate levels and good kidney function, and possibly bisphosphonates or raloxifene.

Table 47.2—Typical Laboratory Results in the Differential Diagnosis of Hypercalcemia

Laboratory Test	Primary Hyperparathyroidism	Humoral Hypercalcemia of Malignancy	Local Osteolytic Hypercalcemia
Serum calcium	↑	↑ or ↑↑	↑ or ↑↑
Serum phosphate	↓ or low-normal	↓	↑
Urine calcium	↑	↑	↑
Parathyroid hormone	↑	↓↓	↓↓
Parathyroid hormone-related peptide	0	↑	0

NOTE: The diagnosis of malignancy-related hypercalcemia is normally straightforward, and extensive diagnostic testing is rarely required. ↑ = increased; ↓ = decreased; ↑↑ = markedly increased; ↓↓ = markedly decreased; 0 = undetectable.

In hospitalized patients, the most common cause of hypercalcemia is a malignancy that produces PTH-related peptide, with hypercalcemia resulting primarily from increased net bone resorption. The presence of an underlying cancer is usually evident on examination and routine diagnostic testing. Squamous cell cancers of the lung or head and neck are common causes of hypercalcemia due to PTH-related peptide production. Other common malignancies associated with hypercalcemia include breast cancer, lymphoma, and myeloma, although the mechanism of the hypercalcemia is different for many of these cancers. Acute treatment for hypercalcemia includes volume replacement with intravenous saline, followed by diuresis with a loop diuretic when rehydration is complete. A parenteral bisphosphonate such as pamidronate should be given, along with treatment of the underlying malignancy, if possible. In addition to their usefulness in the treatment of hypercalcemia, bisphosphonates may decrease bone pain and the risk of pathologic fractures in patients with osteolytic bone metastases from a variety of cancers.

Paget's Disease of Bone

Paget's disease is characterized by localized areas of increased bone remodeling, resulting in a change in bone architecture and an increased tendency to deformity and fracture. Its prevalence increases with aging, affecting 2% to 5% of people aged 50 years and over. Paget's disease is usually asymptomatic and is often diagnosed as an incidental finding on radiographs or during evaluation for an unexplained elevation in serum alkaline phosphatase. The most commonly affected sites are the pelvis, spine, femur, tibia, and skull. When Paget's disease is symptomatic, pain is the most common presenting symptom, either localized to the affected bones or resulting from secondary osteoarthritic changes, often in the hips, knees, and vertebrae. When bone deformities occur, the long bones of the lower extremities are usually affected, often with a bowing of the involved extremity. Skull involvement may result in compression of the eighth cranial nerve and sensorineural hearing loss. The most devastating complication of Paget's disease is malignant transformation of the affected bone, especially osteosarcoma. Treatment is not usually necessary for asymptomatic disease, unless there is concern for hearing loss from skull involvement, nerve root or spinal cord compression from vertebral involvement, or hip fracture from femoral neck involvement. Bisphosphonates suppress the accelerated bone turnover and bone remodeling that is characteristic of this disease, and they are the treatment of choice. During treatment, patients should be monitored clinically for changes in bone pain, joint function, and neurologic

status, and with biochemical indices of bone formation (eg, serum osteocalcin or bone-specific alkaline phosphatase) or resorption (eg, urinary N-telopeptide), or both.

HORMONAL REGULATION OF WATER AND ELECTROLYTE BALANCE

Unlike young adults, older persons are predisposed to both volume depletion and free water excess. This impairment in regulation of volume status and osmolality is multifactorial, reflecting decreased total body water content as well as alterations in antidiuretic hormone (ADH) secretion, osmoreceptor and baroreceptor systems, urine-concentrating capability, renal hormone responsiveness, and thirst sensation. ADH secretion tends to be excessive in older people, with normal to elevated basal ADH levels, increased ADH responses to osmoreceptor stimuli such as hypertonic saline infusion, and decreased ethanol-induced inhibition of ADH secretion. This state of relative ADH excess with aging, together with the common occurrence of renal insufficiency, heart failure, hypothyroidism, and diuretic use, predisposes older adults to hyponatremia by impairing free water clearance. (Medications causing syndrome of inappropriate antidiuretic hormone or SIADH include the selective serotonin-reuptake inhibitors, sulfonylureas, carbamazepine, oxcarbazepine, and tricyclic antidepressants.)

Under other circumstances, older people are at increased risk of volume depletion. With aging, basal aldosterone secretion declines disproportionately to the decrease in clearance, with a net reduction in circulating aldosterone levels of about 30% by the age of 80 years. At the same time, atrial natriuretic hormone secretion (and renal responsiveness to this hormone) increases with aging. Atrial natriuretic hormone inhibits aldosterone production and causes natriuresis and diuresis through its effects on the kidneys. Taken together, these changes predispose older people to volume depletion by decreasing the ability of the kidneys to conserve sodium under conditions of fluid deprivation. Baroreceptor ADH responses to hypotension and hypovolemia are decreased in older people, placing them at additional risk of dehydration. Moreover, renal responsiveness to ADH is decreased with aging, resulting in a decreased ability of the kidneys to maximally concentrate urine. Finally, even healthy older adults have decreased thirst sensation and may not be aware that they are becoming dehydrated. Demented and immobile older people are at the highest risk for severe dehydration.

In addition to predisposing to volume depletion, age-related hyporeninemic hypoaldosteronism also increases the risk of hyperkalemia, especially in patients with diabetes mellitus or renal insufficiency. The addition of angiotensin-converting enzyme inhibitors, nonsteroidal anti-inflammatory drugs, β-blocking agents, and diuretics with aldosterone-antagonist properties may lead to potentially lethal hyperkalemia in some of these patients.

DISORDERS OF THE ADRENAL CORTEX

Basal serum cortisol levels do not change with aging, because decreased cortisol secretion is balanced by a decrease in clearance. Adrenocorticotropic hormone (ACTH) stimulation of cortisol production is unchanged, and cortisol and ACTH responses to stress and secretagogues are unimpaired with aging. Clinically, acute cortisol responses to stress may be higher and more prolonged in older than in younger adults. Accordingly, unless it is emergent, adrenal function testing should be deferred at least 48 hours after major stressors, such as surgery or trauma. In older patients with a normal ACTH stimulation test in whom adrenal insufficiency is suspected, endocrinology consultation is recommended to assist with further testing.

Hypoadrenocorticoidism

Chronic glucocorticoid therapy is also the most common cause of adrenal failure in older adults, because of chronic suppression of adrenal function. Recovery of adrenal axis function is variable and may take several months to occur. Autoimmune-mediated adrenal failure is less common in older than in younger adults, but tuberculosis, adrenal metastases, and adrenal hemorrhage in anticoagulated patients are more common causes of adrenal insufficiency in older persons. Older patients with chronic adrenal insufficiency may present with nonspecific symptoms such as anorexia, weight loss, or impaired functional status, and hyperkalemia may not be present initially. Accordingly, a high index of suspicion is required to make the diagnosis. When adrenocortical insufficiency is suspected, the ACTH stimulation test should be performed and therapy initiated, although the best test to exclude secondary adrenal insufficiency (decreased pituitary ACTH secretion) is controversial. In older people who are stopping chronic glucocorticoid therapy, the replacement regimen should be tapered gradually, and stress dose coverage should be given for major surgery and other acute physiologic stresses until adrenocortical function has normalized.

Hyperadrenocorticoidism

Exogenous glucocorticoids are the most common cause of Cushing's syndrome in older adults, often causing adverse effects, including psychiatric and cognitive symptoms, osteoporosis, myopathy, and glucose intolerance. For patients beginning long-term glucocorticoid therapy, baseline and follow-up bone densitometry measurements are indicated, and calcium, vitamin D, and antiresorptive treatments such as bisphosphonates should be initiated as appropriate. Management of subclinical glucocorticoid hypersecretion is discussed in the following section.

Adrenal Neoplasms

In autopsy studies, the prevalence of clinically inapparent adrenal masses (*adrenal incidentalomas*) ranges from less than 1% of people younger than 30 years of age to 7% of persons older than 70 years of age. Most adrenal incidentalomas are benign adrenocortical adenomas, although pheochromocytomas and adrenocortical carcinomas also occur.

The goals of assessment are to determine whether the tumor is functional (hormone-secreting) (Table 47.3), and whether it is benign or malignant. Screening for *subclinical glucocorticoid hypersecretion* is controversial. Many adrenocortical adenomas have a degree of functional autonomy, and some patients may develop hypertension, insulin resistance, and other metabolic derangements. However, it is unclear whether subclinical glucocorticoid hypersecretion is associated with long-term morbidity, or whether adrenalectomy or medical management of metabolic

Table 47.3—Screening Tests for Hormone Hypersecretion in Patients With Adrenal Incidentalomas

Diagnosis	Test	Indications
Functional adrenocortical adenoma	24-hour urine free cortisol 1 mg overnight dexamethasone suppression test	Cushing's syndrome manifestations Before major surgery
Pheochromocytoma	24-hour urine metanephrines and catecholamines Plasma metanephrines	Patients with incidentaloma
Primary aldosteronism	Serum potassium Ratio of morning plasma aldosterone concentration to plasma renin activity	Hypertension

derangements improves outcomes. Moreover, screening all older adults with adrenal incidentalomas for glucocorticoid hypersecretion would yield a high proportion of false-positive results. Accordingly, it may be prudent to limit testing to patients with a symptom complex suggesting Cushing's syndrome and patients scheduled for major surgery who are at risk for postoperative adrenal crisis.

The assessment of malignancy risk in adrenal incidentaloma patients is based on lesion size, its imaging characteristics, and its rate of growth. The prevalence of adrenal cortical carcinoma in these patients increases from 2% of lesions smaller than 4 cm to 25% of lesions larger than 6 cm. Surgical excision is generally recommended for adrenal masses larger than 6 cm, and for imaging findings including rapid growth rate that suggest the mass is not an adenoma. However, the individual's treatment preferences and clinical condition must be taken into account before recommending treatment.

Adrenal Androgens

In contrast to cortisol, circulating levels of the principal adrenal androgen, dehydroepiandrosterone (DHEA), decline progressively with aging and in octogenarians are only 10% to 20% of young adult levels. Low DHEA levels are associated with poor health, whereas DHEA levels are positively correlated with some measures of longevity and functional status. Given these associations, there has been interest in the potential therapeutic effects of DHEA administration in older adults.

Most studies involving physiologic to mildly supraphysiologic DHEA supplementation in middle-aged and older persons have not found beneficial effects on body composition, although bone mineral density was found to increase modestly in postmenopausal women after 1 year of DHEA. DHEA improved mood and subjective well-being in patients with primary adrenal insufficiency and mid-life dysthymia, but improvements in mood and well-being were not consistently observed in healthy middle-aged and older persons. DHEA decreased circulating high-density lipoprotein cholesterol levels in older women, suggesting potential long-term atherogenic effects. Furthermore, DHEA is metabolized to estrogens and to androgens, including testosterone and dihydrotestosterone, and its effects on the risk of breast cancer in women and prostate cancer in men are unknown. Finally, higher doses of DHEA may cause androgenization in some women and gynecomastia in men. Thus, the safety and efficacy of DHEA supplementation in older adults have not been established, and its use is inappropriate outside of clinical studies.

TESTOSTERONE

Despite former controversy, there is now general agreement that total and free testosterone levels and testosterone secretion are lower in healthy older men than in younger men. Many healthy older men exhibit moderate primary testicular failure, with decreased sperm production, testosterone levels, and testosterone secretory responses to gonadotropin administration. In addition, many of these men have inappropriately normal (ie, not increased) gonadotropin levels in the presence of low testosterone levels, suggesting secondary (hypothalamic or pituitary) testicular failure. Overt testicular failure is common in chronically ill and debilitated older men, manifested by total testosterone levels well below the normal range and symptoms suggesting androgen deficiency, including decreased libido and potency, gynecomastia, and hot flushes. Testosterone replacement therapy is generally warranted in these patients, as in hypogonadal young men. However, it is more common to encounter older men with low-normal or mildly decreased serum testosterone levels and nonspecific manifestations, such as decreased libido, weakness, decreased muscle mass, osteopenia, and memory loss. In most cases, these manifestations have multiple causes, but it has been hypothesized that declining testosterone levels with aging contribute to their development, and that testosterone supplementation may help to prevent or treat these disorders.

Men with suspected hypogonadism should be evaluated with a serum free or bioavailable (non–sex hormone–binding globulin-bound) testosterone level, either measured by equilibrium dialysis or calculated from measurements of total testosterone and sex hormone–binding globulin. Concentrations of sex hormone–binding globulin, the main circulating binding protein for testosterone, increase with age. Therefore, the age-related decline in serum free or bioavailable testosterone is greater than that of total testosterone, and total testosterone measurements do not accurately reflect the decrease in biologically active testosterone with aging. Direct radioimmunoassays using "analog" kits for free testosterone are widely used but are not recommended because they may underestimate androgen deficiency in older men and overestimate androgen deficiency in men with low sex hormone–binding globulin (eg, moderately obese men). Luteinizing hormone and follicle-stimulating hormone levels should be obtained. In addition, a review (and if possible, discontinuation) of medications that may suppress gonadotropins (eg, glucocorticoids and central nervous system–active drugs) and a prolactin level are indicated if gonadotropins are low-normal or low in the presence of low testosterone levels. High prolactin levels inhibit gonadotropin secretion and could be due to either a pituitary adenoma or hypothalamic disorder. Further studies may be warranted in such patients, including magnetic resonance imaging of the pituitary fossa and assessment of other pituitary functions (eg, cortisol response to ACTH and T_4). Baseline bone densitometry measurements should be obtained in men with decreased testosterone levels to exclude osteoporosis.

Data from controlled studies of testosterone supplementation of up to 3 years' duration in older men with low-normal or mildly decreased serum testosterone levels are summarized in Table 47.4. However, it is unknown whether these potential benefits and risks are clinically important, or whether the benefits outweigh the risks. Bearing these uncertainties in mind, a trial of testosterone supplementation may be appropriate in older men with serum total testosterone levels below 3.0 ng/mL and clinical features suggesting hypogonadism (eg, osteoporosis, muscle wasting or weakness, mild anemia of unclear cause, loss of libido), although the U.S. Food and Drug Administration has not labeled the use of testosterone for this indication. Notably, bisphosphonates have clearly demonstrated efficacy in treating older men with osteoporosis. Androgen replacement therapy is inappropriate in asymptomatic older men with low-normal total testosterone levels who do not have clinical manifestations consistent with androgen deficiency. Men should be monitored closely for adverse androgenic effects of treatment, including erythrocytosis and potential exacerbation of prostatic disease. However, there is no direct evidence that testosterone therapy increases the risk of prostate cancer or symptomatic benign prostatic hyperplasia. (See also "Disorders of Sexual Function," p 382.)

ESTROGEN REPLACEMENT THERAPY

Many of the symptoms and signs of hormone deficiency mimic those classically associated with aging. The fact that many hormones also decline with aging has led to an enthusiasm for attempting to reverse unwanted changes associated with aging by the use of hormonal replacement. Based on very compelling epidemiologic data, replacement of estrogen, with or without progesterone, was once standard care for postmenopausal women, but this practice has fallen out of favor in the past several years given new data from randomized clinical trials. Estrogen replacement therapy (ERT) now is largely limited to treatment of menopausal symptoms (See the section on treatment of

Table 47.4—Potential Short-Term Benefits and Risks of Testosterone Supplementation in Older Men With Low-Normal or Mildly Decreased Testosterone Levels

Study End Point	Effect of Testosterone
Lean body mass	Increased
Fat mass	Decreased
Bone mineral density	Variable
Strength	Variable Improved strength and performance of some functional tasks in some studies
Sexual function	Variable Activation in sexual behavior and increased libido (most consistent findings)
Mood	Variable Mood, subjective well-being improved (in some studies)
Cognitive	Some cognitive domains improved Worsened effect of practice on verbal fluency
Lipid profile	Decreased total, LDL cholesterol HDL cholesterol unchanged
Coronary heart disease	In men with established disease, improved ECG evidence of exercise-induced coronary ischemia (in most studies) Variable effect on angina pectoris
Prostate	PSA increased slightly in many patients No effect on voiding symptoms, prostate examination
Hematocrit	Increased 2.5% to 5% versus baseline Erythrocytosis developed in 6% to 25% of subjects
Long-term clinical outcomes	Unknown

NOTE: This table summarizes results of placebo-controlled studies. LDL = low-density lipoprotein; HDL = high-density lipoprotein; ECG = electrocardiographic; PSA = prostate-specific antigen.

menopausal symptoms in "Gynecologic Diseases and Disorders," p 377).

Three meta-analyses of observational studies have demonstrated an association of ERT use in women with a reduction in heart disease by half. Current use of estrogen is the factor most strongly associated with reducing risk, and prolonged use is the second most important factor. Preliminary studies suggest that the effects are similar when progesterone is added. However, a few long-term prospective studies are now available, and further studies are being completed to determine if the cardiovascular benefit of ERT is present, as suggested by epidemiologic studies. A randomized controlled trial of estrogen with progesterone replacement in women with established coronary disease did not find that estrogen improves cardiac outcome. In fact, the estrogen treatment group demonstrated increased mortality in the first year on therapy, with improved survival in years 2 through 5, leading to no net benefit. Another trial of women with coronary artery disease found no benefit from estrogen for angiographic changes of atherosclerosis.

The Women's Health Initiative (WHI) is a set of clinical trails to test primary prevention of coronary artery disease with estrogen and estrogen-progesterone combinations. In the WHI, the estrogen-progesterone arm was discontinued early because of the increased risk of coronary disease, breast cancer, stroke, and deep-vein thrombosis in this group. Aspirin and lipid-lowering agents were not found to have an effect on the outcomes. The estrogen-alone arm of the study was discontinued early (February 2004 rather than March 2005) because the hormone increased the risk of stroke and did not reduce the risk of coronary heart disease.

Some observational studies also suggested that estrogen may have a role in preventing dementia. Studies of estrogen in women with mild dementia demonstrate improved memory, orientation, and calculation skills, but these studies are small and limited by selection bias. A placebo-controlled trial of estrogen replacement given for 1 year to 120 women with early to moderate Alzheimer's dementia found no improvement in affective or cognitive outcomes. In the WHI, more women in the estrogen-progesterone arm of the trial had clinically important declines in their Mini–Mental State Examination scores. Similarly, in the estrogen-alone arm of the cognitive substudy, 76 women taking estrogen developed mild cognitive impairment, compared with 58 women receiving placebo (hazard ration [HR], 1.34; 95% confidence interval [CI], 0.95 to 1.89), and when this was combined with the estrogen-plus-progestin trial, the HR was 1.25 (95% CI, 0.97 to 1.60), not clear evidence of harm. Conjugated equine estrogen (CEE) alone did not protect against dementia, as 47 participants were diagnosed with probable dementia, 28 assigned to CEE, and 19 to placebo (HR, 1.49; 95% CI, 0.83 to 2.66). When the estrogen-alone trial was combined with the estrogen-plus-progestin trial, per the original WHI mental status protocol, the overall HR for probable dementia was 1/76 (95% CI, 1.19 to 2.60; $P = .005$).

The risks of breast cancer, endometrial cancer, and deep-vein thrombosis associated with the use of estrogen have been well established. Meta-analyses suggest that women who used estrogen for 5 years or less have no increased risk of breast cancer, but that treatment for 15 years or more is associated with a 30% increased risk. Information about estrogen-progesterone combinations, with various derivatives and dosing schedules, are incomplete; it is therefore not possible to conclude that any particular formulation may lessen these risks compared to other formulations. Unopposed estrogen increases the risk for endometrial cancer by 2% to 8%, and the risk increases with increasing duration of use. Risk may be decreased with lower doses than in standard use. Progesterone reduces or negates the risk of endometrial cancer associated with estrogen. Finally, data demonstrate a two- to fourfold increase in risk of thromboembolic disease with the use of estrogen. (See also the section on estrogen replacement therapy for osteoporosis prevention in "Osteoporosis and Osteomalacia," p 201.)

GROWTH HORMONE

Growth hormone secretion declines with aging, and by 70 to 80 years of age, about half of adults have no significant growth hormone secretion over 24 hours. A corresponding decline occurs in levels of insulin-like growth factor 1, which mediates most of the effects of growth hormone; it falls to levels comparable to those in growth hormone–deficient children in 40% of adults aged 70 to 80 years.

Adults with growth hormone deficiency due to hypothalamic-pituitary disease exhibit decreased muscle strength, lean body mass, and bone density; increased abdominal obesity; unfavorable lipid profiles; and an increased risk of cardiovascular disease. All improve with growth hormone replacement. Older adults without hypothalamic-pituitary disease have many of the same conditions, which leads to the hypothesis that growth hormone supplementation may have a beneficial effect on these clinically important age-related disorders.

Randomized controlled trials of growth hormone supplementation in older adults have reported increased lean body mass and bone density and decreased fat mass. However, growth hormone was not found to augment improvements in muscle strength achieved with exercise alone, and no improvements in functional status were demonstrated. Furthermore, significant adverse effects were common, including carpal tunnel syndrome, arthralgias, edema, and gynecomastia. The long-term efficacy and safety of growth hormone administration in older people are unknown. Short-term growth hormone supplementation may improve nitrogen balance in older persons with severe illness and catabolic states. However, growth hormone is very expensive, and at present it is not recommended for clinical use in older people who do not have established hypothalamic-pituitary disease.

MELATONIN

Melatonin, a hormone secreted by the pineal gland, is thought to be involved in the regulation of circadian and seasonal biorhythms. Melatonin secretion is inhibited by exposure to light, resulting in a marked circadian variation in circulating melatonin levels, and its sedative effects suggest a role in sleep induction. Most studies show that plasma melatonin levels decline throughout life after early childhood, but the physiologic significance of this decline in melatonin secretion is unclear. Numerous claims have been made in the lay press regarding the "anti-aging" benefits of melatonin supplementation for various conditions, including insomnia, immune deficiency, cancer, and the aging process itself. Although melatonin may have sleep-inducing properties in older people with insomnia, the long-term risks and benefits of melatonin supplementation have not been established for insomnia or any other indication.

REFERENCES

■ Bilezikian JP, Potts JT Jr, Fuleihan Gel-H, et al. Summary statement from a workshop on asymptomatic primary hyperparathyroidism: a perspective for the 21st century. *J Clin Endocrinol Metab*. 2002;87(12):5353–5361.

■ Giannoulis MG, Sonksen PH, Umpleby M, et al. The effects of growth hormone and/or testosterone in healthy elderly men: a randomized controlled trial. *J Clin Endocrinol Metab*. 2006;91(2):477–484.

■ Grady D, Wenger NK, Herrington D, et al. Postmenopausal hormone therapy increases risk for venous thromboembolic disease. *Ann Intern Med*. 2000;132(9):689–696.

■ Gruenewald DA, Matsumoto AM. Aging of the endocrine system. In: Hazzard WR, Blass JP, Halter JB, et al., eds. *Principles of Geriatric Medicine and Gerontology*. 5th ed. New York: McGraw-Hill; 2004:819–835.

■ Grumbach MM, Biller BM, Braunstein GD, et al. Management of the clinically inapparent adrenal mass ("incidentaloma"). *Ann Intern Med*. 2003;138(5):424–429.

■ Rossouw JE, Anderson GL, Prentice RL, et al. Writing Group for the Women's Health Initiative Investigators. Risks and benefits of estrogen plus progestin in healthy postmenopausal women: principal results from the Women's Health Initiative randomized controlled trial. *JAMA*. 2002;288(3):321–333.

CHAPTER 48—DIABETES MELLITUS

KEY POINTS

■ Diabetes mellitus, one of the most common chronic ailments in older adults, results in decreased life expectancy, excess complications and comorbidities, and a higher risk of geriatric conditions (polypharmacy, urinary incontinence, falls, cognitive impairment, depression, chronic pain), functional impairment, and disability.

■ Both diabetes and impaired glucose tolerance are important to identify and address by changes in life style.

■ Because of the great heterogeneity in the older population, treatment goals for older diabetic patients must be carefully individualized.

■ Though the target blood pressure is debated, attempts to lower blood pressure, as tolerated, are important for older hypertensive diabetic patients.

■ Diabetes self-management is an essential part of diabetes care, and annual self-management training is a covered benefit under Medicare Part B.

Diabetes mellitus is a group of metabolic diseases characterized by hyperglycemia due to abnormalities in insulin secretion, insulin action, or both. It is one of the most common chronic diseases affecting older persons. Estimates of the prevalence among persons aged 65 years and over range between 15% and 20%. Because the general population is aging and rates of obesity are increasing among middle-aged adults, people aged 65 and older will constitute the majority of diabetic persons in the United States and in other developed countries in the coming decades. In the United States, people aged 65 and older now account for more than 40% of all people with diabetes.

The age-adjusted prevalence of diabetes mellitus is higher among black Americans and Hispanic Americans than white Americans. Further, black Americans have been found to suffer from complications of diabetes at disproportionately higher rates than white Americans. Research is only starting to decipher the effects of race on diabetes development and outcomes.

Because diabetes may be asymptomatic for many years, it is estimated that up to one third of older adults with diabetes mellitus are unaware of their condition. Despite the early asymptomatic period, diabetes mellitus is a serious condition associated with significant morbidity and a shortened survival. Older persons with diabetes can expect a 10-year reduction in life expectancy and a mortality rate nearly twice that of persons without this disease. In addition, older adults disproportionately experience the clinical complications and comorbidities associated with diabetes. These complications include atherosclerosis, neuropathies, loss of vision, and renal insufficiency. The rates of myocardial infarction, stroke, and kidney failure are increased approximately twofold, and the risk of blindness is increased approximately 40% in older persons with diabetes. Most patients aged 65 and older who require dialysis have diabetes.

Research data are accumulating about important clinical consequences of diabetes that are common in older adults and that have serious consequences on health status and quality of life. When diabetes is poorly controlled in older patients, hyperglycemia alone can be the cause of insidious decline characterized by fatigue, weight loss, muscle weakness, and decline in function. Older adults with diabetes are at higher risk than those without diabetes for geriatric syndromes, including incontinence, falls, frailty, cognitive impairment, and depressive symptoms. They also have a higher prevalence of functional impairment and disability than older adults without diabetes. Mobility disability is about 2 to 3 times more likely, and disability in activities of daily living is about 1.5 times more likely, in older adults with diabetes than in those without.

PATHOPHYSIOLOGY OF DIABETES IN OLDER ADULTS

The American Diabetes Association classifies diabetes mellitus affecting older adults into three types. Type 1 is the result of an absolute deficiency in insulin secretion due to autoimmune destruction of the β cells of the pancreas. Type 2 is most commonly due to tissue resistance to insulin action and relative insulin deficiency. A third category is reserved for other specific types of diabetes: injuries to the exocrine pancreas; endocrinopathies characterized by excesses of hormones, such as growth hormone, cortisol, glucagon, and epinephrine, which antagonize insulin action; drug- or chemical-induced diabetes; and infections leading to the destruction of the β cells of the pancreas.

In about 90% of cases, older adults with diabetes have the type 2 form of the disease. Most older adults with type 2 diabetes have had years of glucose intolerance, insulin resistance, and the metabolic syndrome. This "pre-diabetes" syndrome is also associated with increased risk for atherosclerotic disease, as well as development of type 2 diabetes.

The prevalence of both type 2 diabetes and glucose intolerance increases with age. The reasons for the increased prevalence of glucose intolerance and type 2 diabetes among older persons are not fully known; there appears to be an interaction among several factors, including genetics, life style, and aging influences. Obesity and decreased physical activity, common among older persons, contribute to impairments in insulin action. Glucose intolerance has also been shown to be related to age-associated decline in pancreatic β-cell function and to reductions with aging of the insulin-signaling mechanisms that limit the mobilization of glucose transporters needed for insulin-mediated glucose uptake and metabolism in muscle and fat. Changes in body composition that occur with aging, such as increased visceral fat leading to insulin resistance, may also contribute to alterations in carbohydrate metabolism in aging. Decreased levels of physical activity that may occur in some older adults may exacerbate age-related changes in body composition and increased carbohydrate intolerance. An altered inflammatory environment with aging may also contribute to the higher rates of diabetes in older adults.

In addition to intrinsic physiologic mechanisms, external factors may contribute to glucose intolerance and type 2 diabetes. Some medications commonly used by older adults—diuretics, estrogen, sympathomimetics, glucocorticoids, niacin, and olanzapine—alter carbohydrate metabolism and increase glucose levels. Intercurrent illnesses, such as infections, myocardial infarction, and stroke, as well as other physiologic stresses can lead to worsened hyperglycemia. The heterogeneity in the severity of hyperglycemia among older patients with type 2 diabetes is related to the varying contributions of each of these factors in each individual.

The pathophysiology of the complications of diabetes is similar in younger and older persons. Prolonged hyperglycemia leads to glycosylation of proteins; the accumulation of these abnormal proteins can cause tissue damage. Also, metabolic products of the aldose-reductase system, such as sorbitol, accumulate in the presence of hyperglycemia. These products can impair cellular energy metabolism and contribute to cell injury and death.

Physiologic changes that occur with diabetes and its complications may interact with physiologic changes associated with aging to further decrease physiologic reserve. Type 2 diabetes and obesity are associated with inflammatory dysregulation, which may also be associated with aging and lead to clinical sequelae such as sarcopenia. Aging is associated with decreased physiologic reserve in multiple organ systems (renal, cardiovascular, central nervous system), which may interact with end-organ damage due to diabetes, resulting in increased vulnerability to physiologic stressors.

DIAGNOSIS AND EVALUATION

The current American Diabetes Association diagnostic criteria for diabetes mellitus do not include any adjustments that are based on age. Three ways to establish the diagnosis of diabetes mellitus are possible, and each must be confirmed, on a subsequent day, by any one of the three methods:

- Symptoms of polyuria, polydipsia, and unexplained weight loss plus a casual plasma glucose concentration of ≥200 mg/dL (11.1 mmol/L). *Casual* is defined as any time of day without regard to time since last meal.

- A plasma glucose concentration after an 8-hour fast of ≥126 mg/dL (7.0 mmol/L).

- A plasma glucose concentration of ≥200 mg/dL (11.1 mmol/L) measured 2 hours after ingestion of 75 g of glucose in 300 mL of water administered after an overnight fast.

In clinical practice, the presence of two fasting glucose levels of ≥126 mg/dL is the most common method of diagnosis. Older adults with fasting blood glucoses from 110 to 125 mg/dL are defined as having impaired fasting glucose (IFG), a condition associated with increased risk for diabetes development. Some older adults have isolated postchallenge hyperglycemia (IPH) but do not have high fasting blood glucoses; many of these people would be diagnosed as type 2 diabetes by oral glucose tolerance testing criteria. IPH does appear to confer increased risk for atherosclerotic complications, but not as much as diagnosed type 2 diabetes.

Several recent diabetes prevention trials demonstrated that in people with glucose intolerance, progression to type 2 diabetes can be prevented by medications and life-style changes. Life-style changes were found to be slightly more efficacious in older than in younger adults and superior to medications in the older group. These results demonstrate the importance of preventive measures and life-style changes in older adults who are at risk for developing type 2 diabetes.

MANAGEMENT

Clinical Evaluation

Older patients with diabetes require a comprehensive evaluation, which in the primary care setting may be done over several patient visits. For patients with significant functional impairments and comorbidities, including those with psychosocial problems and caregiver requirements, a formal, comprehensive geriatric assessment may be needed. Regardless of how the comprehensive evaluation of an older adult with diabetes mellitus is handled, four issues deserve special attention.

First, the history and physical examination must include evaluation of risk factors for atherosclerotic disease and the presence of all comorbid diseases. Diabetes is a well-established risk factor for atherosclerotic cardiovascular disease, so other risk factors such as smoking, family history, hypertension, and hyperlipidemia should also be explored. Diabetes is also associated with multiple vascular complications that may be subclinical or clinical. The presence of coronary artery disease, peripheral vascular disease, neuropathy, foot problems, and medical eye disease must be determined. In many cases, subspecialty consultation (as for retinopathy) and laboratory testing will be indicated. In addition, older adults with diabetes are also likely to have prevalent chronic diseases that are not necessarily associated with their diabetes, such as osteoarthritis.

Second, a thorough drug history is important. As previously stated, certain medications can contribute to hyperglycemia. More often, older patients may be on multiple medications for multiple comorbidities and may experience adverse drug effects or trouble with medication management or finances.

Third, an assessment of functional status is important in order to help determine whether the patient is able to independently manage his or her diabetes, or whether caregiver input is also needed. Functional assessment will also assist the clinician and the patient in setting diabetes management targets.

Fourth, older patients should be screened for the use of multiple medications, depression, cognitive impairment, urinary incontinence, injurious falls, and pain. Multiple observational studies have shown that these geriatric conditions are more common in older people with diabetes than without. Finally, each patient's needs for diabetes education and self-management support, and whether to involve a caregiver, should be assessed.

General Principles of Diabetes Management

The clinician develops goals for diabetes management and individualized clinical targets with each older adult with diabetes, involving the caregiver when appropriate. The goals of diabetes management in older adults include

- control of hyperglycemia and its symptoms,
- evaluation and treatment of associated risks for atherosclerotic and microvascular disease,
- evaluation and treatment of diabetes complications,
- support for diabetes self-management and education, and
- maintenance or improvement of general health status.

Although these goals are similar for older and younger people with diabetes, the management of older patients is complicated by the medical and functional heterogeneity of this group. In fact, this heterogeneity is a key consideration for clinicians in developing individualized diabetes management interventions and clinical targets for older diabetes patients. Some may have developed diabetes in middle age and have developed multiple related comorbidities. Functional heterogeneity is found among older diabetics. Some may be recently diagnosed but may have had undiagnosed diabetes for years and have complications at diagnosis. Others may have just converted from impaired glucose tolerance to diabetes and may have few complications or comorbidities, or may be disabled and frail, with advanced cognitive impairment, multiple comorbidities and complications, or significant limitations in functioning. Still others may be healthy and active with minimal comorbidities and excellent function. Many older diabetes patients are in between, with mild or early functional limitations, several related comorbidities, and multiple risks for worsening morbidity.

Another consideration in treating older diabetic patients is life expectancy and the time needed for clinical benefit from a specific intervention. Clinical trials have demonstrated that approximately 8 years are needed before the benefits of glycemic control are reflected in a reduction in microvascular complications such as diabetic retinopathy or kidney disease, but that only 2 to 3 years are required to see benefits from better control of blood pressure and lipids. It is important to remember that the median remaining life

expectancy for a 70-year-old woman is 14 years, which is plenty of time for the development of diabetes complications. Therefore, for a person in her or his early 70s who is newly diagnosed or highly functional, diabetes management is no different from that of younger people. However, management must be designed to fit the clinical status of older adults who are significantly functionally impaired or have multiple comorbidities. In all cases, patient preferences and quality of life must be considered.

Solid evidence supports the effectiveness of several components of diabetes care, including control of lipids and blood pressure, control of hyperglycemia, aspirin use, smoking cessation, appropriate eye and foot care, prevention of nephropathy, and diabetes education and self-management support for medication adherence, blood-glucose self-management, appropriate nutrition, weight loss if indicated, and increased physical activity. However, very few of the data supporting these interventions were obtained from research studies of older people. It is likely that many management guidelines can be generalized to many older adults with diabetes, particularly those who are healthy and functional. These older adults should have the same opportunity as younger adults for intensive diabetes management, reduction of the risks associated with diabetes, and treatment of comorbid conditions that can lead to worse disease and poorer health status in the future. However, intensive diabetes management of all diabetes-associated conditions may not be feasible for some older patients, and clinicians may have to prioritize the reduction of some risks over others. For some older patients, particularly those with severe comorbidities and disabilities, aggressive management is not likely to provide benefit and may even result in harm, such as hypoglycemia with aggressive glycemic control or hypotension with aggressive blood-pressure control.

Therefore, it is important to establish individual diabetes management goals and clinical targets with patients, to re-evaluate the clinical, functional and social status of the patient if these goals and targets are not being met, and to determine if caregiver support or specialty input is needed (Table 48.1).

The California Healthcare Foundation and the American Geriatrics Society collaborated to develop guidelines for improving the care of the older person with diabetes mellitus. Many of the specific management interventions outlined below are adapted from this guideline.

Prevention and Management of Atherosclerotic Complications

Older adults with diabetes are at high risk for atherosclerosis and its complications. In fact, virtually all older adults with diabetes have either clinical or preclinical atherosclerotic disease. Therefore, interventions that reduce the risk of atherosclerotic diseases are extremely important (Table 48.2). Smoking cessation counseling and pharmacologic intervention should be offered to any older diabetic person who smokes. Daily aspirin therapy should be offered to older adults with diabetes if there is not a contraindication to aspirin. Available evidence suggests that dosages from 81 to 325 mg per day are appropriate.

There is strong evidence from a number of randomized controlled trials that the management of hypertension in older adults reduces cardiovascular events and mortality; some of these studies included substantial numbers of older people with diabetes. The best target blood pressure for older diabetic patients is not clear, but in the majority of patients the target blood pressure should be 140/80. Observational studies suggest that lowering blood pressure to less than 130/80 may provide increased benefit. Because some older adults may not be able to tolerate aggressive blood-pressure lowering, hypertension should be treated gradually to avoid complications. Patient preference and medication side effects should be considered. (See also "Hypertension," p 331.)

Evidence for medication choice in older patients with diabetes suggests that most classes chosen (diuretics, angiotensin-converting enzyme inhibitors, β-blockers, and calcium channel blockers) have comparable effectiveness in reducing cardiovascular disease and mortality. Evidence suggests that angiotensin-converting enzyme inhibitors and angiotensin II receptor blockers have cardiovascular and renal benefit for persons with diabetes.

Evidence supports the use of lipid-lowering therapy and therapy to increase high-density lipoprotein (HDL) in older adults with diabetes; randomized controlled trials and meta-analysis have confirmed the benefit of the statin drugs. The use of fibrates in the setting of low HDL may also be of benefit. Therefore, lipid abnormalities should be corrected in the older adult with diabetes, as long as this is reasonable after considering the individual's overall health status. Evidence suggests that the target low-density lipoprotein (LDL) level is 100 mg/dL. Dietary modification can be tried for 6 months if the LDL level is 100 to 129 mg/dL. If the LDL level is 130 mg/dL or higher, pharmacologic therapy is needed in addition to life-style modifications in diet and activity level. Older persons are always at risk for adverse drug effects, so when an older person with diabetes is prescribed a statin or niacin, or when the dose is increased, an alanine aminotransferase level should be measured within 12 weeks of the dose initiation or change. Also, some people may develop muscle inflammation with the statins, so symptoms of

Table 48.1—Key Elements of Care for Older Persons with Diabetes Mellitus

- Individualized care and education
- Prevention and management of cardiovascular risk factors
- Glycemic control; prevention and management of microvascular complications
- Screening for and treatment of geriatric syndromes

Table 48.2—Preventing and Managing Cardiovascular Risk Factors in Older Diabetic Patients

Counsel the patient regarding:

- Maintenance of appropriate weight
- Increasing physical activity
- Discontinuing smoking
- Limiting fat and carbohydrate intake

Consider drug therapy to:

- Treat hypertension
- Prevent myocardial infarction (ie, aspirin)
- Treat dyslipidemia

muscle pain and weakness in the presence of statin therapy must be evaluated. If a fibrate has been started or increased, liver enzymes should be evaluated annually.

Prevention and Management of Microvascular Complications

Microvascular complications of diabetes are major problems among older adults with diabetes and may be important contributors to disability. Diabetic retinopathy may result in decreased vision in older people with diabetes. It is important to remember that other medical eye diseases, such as glaucoma and cataracts, are also very common in older diabetic persons. Any older person with new-onset diabetes should have a screening dilated-eye examination by an eye-care specialist. If there is evidence of retinopathy, other medical eye disease, eye symptoms, or high risk (poorly controlled hyperglycemia or blood pressure), a dilated-eye examination should be done every year. If there is no eye disease or high risk, eye examinations can be performed every other year.

Serious foot problems and amputations are more common among older people with diabetes, so these patients should have a careful foot examination each visit. This also provides an excellent opportunity for teaching and reinforcement of foot care with the patient and caregivers. To screen for kidney disease, a test for the presence of microalbuminuria should be performed at diagnosis and annually if no abnormalities are detected. (See also "Kidney Diseases and Disorders," the section on kidney disease and the vascular system, p 371.) Finally, given a higher mortality rate among diabetic patients who develop pneumonia, pneumococcal vaccination is strongly recommended.

Management of Hyperglycemia

There are many options for drug therapy in older persons with type 2 diabetes and no clearly preferred algorithm. Regimens can consist of any of the classes of drugs shown in Table 48.3 and Table 48.4, used alone or in combination. It is important to adjust the regimen over the course of the illness as goals change, the disease progresses, or complications develop. Sulfonylurea preparations have a long record of safety and effectiveness. However, hypoglycemia is a serious adverse event, and long-acting sulfonylureas such as chlorpropamide and glyburide should be avoided in older patients. In addition, these drugs must be used cautiously in patients with significant renal and hepatic insufficiency, since the liver is the primary site of metabolism and they are excreted by the kidneys. α-Glucosidase inhibitors impair the breakdown of carbohydrates in the gut and limit absorption. The residual carbohydrates in the intestinal lumen are responsible for diarrhea in about 25% of patients who use this drug. The biguanide preparations also have gastrointestinal side effects and can cause lactic acidosis in patients with renal insufficiency. Metformin is contraindicated for older men with a serum creatinine level of 1.5 mg/dL or higher, or for older women with a serum creatinine level of 1.4 mg/dL or higher. If an older patient receives metformin, the serum creatinine should be measured at least annually and with any increase in dose. For those aged 80 or older or those suspected to have reduced muscle mass, a timed urine collection for creatinine clearance should be obtained. The thiazolidinediones are generally well tolerated, but there is a risk of idiosyncratic hepatic toxicity. Finally, insulin can be used effectively in patients with type 2 diabetes. It is often possible to achieve good glycemic control with one or two injections a day of an intermediate-acting insulin preparation. The greatest risk of insulin therapy is hypoglycemia, and some evidence suggests that frail older adults are at higher risk for serious hypoglycemia than are healthier, more functional older adults. Therefore, it is important that the older adult's ability to self-administer insulin is assessed carefully. The management plan for an older adult with diabetes who has severe or frequent hypoglycemia should be evaluated. The patient may require referral to subspecialty diabetes care, or more frequent contact with the health care team. Psychosocial reasons for hypoglycemia must be investigated and treated, such as an inability to understand self-management that is due to cognitive problems, inadequate diabetes knowledge, difficulty in implementing therapy that is due to disability, or lack of caregiver support.

EDUCATION AND SELF-MANAGEMENT SUPPORT

Because diabetes is a disease for which the patient and caregivers have the primary responsibility for management and ultimate control, it is imperative that the patient understands the mechanisms of the metabolic derangements and their management and becomes fully involved in diabetes self-management. Therefore, diabetes education about diabetes and particularly diabetes self-management is a key part of effective care.

Often, this can be accomplished in the primary care setting. However, for patients who have complex clinical conditions, referral to a diabetes educator for one-on-one counseling or group classes, a comprehensive diabetes disease management program, or specialty physician care may improve control. It is important to note that annual diabetes self-management training is a covered benefit under Medicare Part B. Diabetes mellitus education programs may be particularly important in older adults with diabetes who are members of minority groups, particularly black Americans or Hispanic Americans, in whom diabetes is more prevalent than in white Americans. It is critically important to recognize when caregiver involvement in diabetes self-management activities is required. The caregiver must be highly involved and educated about diabetes and its self-management when the patient is cognitively impaired, is significantly disabled or frail, or has limited proficiency in English.

Diabetes self-management and support must cover several important areas. It is important that the older patient, and caregiver if appropriate, be educated about hypo- and hyperglycemia, including precipitating factors, prevention, symptoms, monitoring, treatment, and when to notify the physician. Although hypoglycemia is unusual in older adults when they are treated with sulfonylurea or insulin, older adults with diabetes are still at higher risk than middle-aged adults with diabetes. When appropriate, the patients and caregiver should be taught blood-glucose self-monitoring, and their technique should be reassessed and reinforced periodically.

Diet and physical activity remain important components of the initial and ongoing management of patients with diabetes. The term "meal planning" has replaced the term "diet" in the management of diabetes. There is no special "diabetic diet"—people with diabetes have the same nutritional needs as anyone else. Meal planning should focus on strategies that improve glycemic control as well as lipids and blood pressure. An individualized meal plan of regular, well-balanced meals consisting of healthy foods in the right amounts, with the goal of keeping weight under

Table 48.3—Non-insulin Agents for Treating Diabetes Mellitus

Drug	Dosage	Formulations	Comments (Metabolism)
Oral Agents			
2nd-Generation Sulfonylureas			Increase insulin secretion; lower HbA_{1c} by 1.0%–2.0%
Glimepiride (Amaryl)	4–8 mg once, begin 1–2 mg	T: 1, 2, 4	Numerous drug interactions, long-acting (L, K)
Glipizide (generic or Glucotrol)	2.5–40 mg once or divided	T: 5, 10	Short-acting (L, K)
(Glucotrol XL)	5–20 mg once	T: ER 2.5, 5, 10	Long-acting (L, K)
Glyburide (generic or Diaβeta, Micronase)	1.25–20 mg once or divided	T: 1.25, 2.5, 5	Long-acting, risk of hypoglycemia (L, K)
Micronized glyburide (Glynase)	1.5–12 mg once	T: 1.5, 3, 4.5, 6	(L, K)
α-Glucosidase Inhibitors			Delay glucose absorption; lower HbA_{1c} by 0.5%–1.0%
Acarbose (Precose)	50–100 mg tid, just before meals; start with 25 mg	T: 25, 50, 100	GI adverse effects common, avoid if Cr > 2 mg/dL, monitor liver enzymes (gut, K)
Miglitol (Glyset)	25–100 mg tid, with 1st bite of meal; start with 25 mg qd	T: 25, 50, 100	Same as acarbose but no need to monitor liver enzymes (L, K)
Biguanides			Decrease hepatic glucose production; lower HbA_{1c} by 1.0%–2.0%
Metformin (Glucophage)	500–2550 mg divided	T: 500, 850, 1000	Avoid in patients > 80 yr, Cr > 1.5 in men, Cr > 1.4 in women, HF, COPD, elevated liver enzymes; hold before contrast radiologic studies; may cause weight loss (K)
(Glucophage XR)	1500–2000 mg qd	T: ER 500	Same as above
Meglitinides			Increase insulin secretion; lower HbA_{1c} by 1.0%–2.0%
Nateglinide (Starlix)	60–120 mg tid	T: 60, 120	Give 30 min before meals
Repaglinide (Prandin)	0.5 mg bid–qid if HbA_{1c} < 8% or previously untreated	T: 0.5, 1, 2	Give 30 min before meals; adjust dose at wkly intervals; potential for drug interactions, caution in hepatic, renal insufficiency (L)
	1–2 mg bid–qid if HbA_{1c} ≥ 8% or previously treated		
Thiazolidinediones			Insulin resistance reducers; lower HbA_{1c} by 0.5%–1.0%; risk of HF; avoid if NYHA Class III or IV cardiac status; D/C if any decline in cardiac status
Pioglitazone (Actos)	15 or 30 mg qd; max 45 mg/d as monotherapy, 30 mg/d in combination therapy	T: 15, 30, 45	Check liver enzymes at start, q 2 mo during 1st yr, then periodically; avoid if clinical evidence of liver disease or if serum ALT levels > 2.5 upper limit of normal (L, K)
Rosiglitazone (Avandia)	4 mg qd–bid	T: 2, 4, 8	Check liver enzymes at start, q 2 mo during 1st yr, then periodically; avoid if clinical evidence of liver disease or if serum ALT levels > 2.5 upper limit of normal (L, K)
Glipizide and metformin (METAGLIP)	2.5/250 once; 20/2000 in 2 divided doses	T: 2.5/250, 2.5/500, 5/500	Avoid in patients > 80 yr, Cr > 1.5 in men, Cr > 1.4 in women; see individual drugs (L, K)
Glyburide and metformin (Glucovance)	1.25/250 mg initially if previously untreated; 2.5/500 mg or 5/500 mg bid with meals; max 20/2000/d	T: 1.25/250, 2.5/500, 5/500	Starting dose should not exceed the total daily dose of either drug; see also individual drugs

(table continued on next page)

Table 48.3—Non-insulin Agents for Treating Diabetes Mellitus (continued)

Drug	Dosage	Formulations	Comments (Metabolism)
Combinations			
Rosiglitazone and glimepiride (Avandaryl)	Previously on rosiglitazone alone: initially 4/1, may increase glimepiride component in 1- to 2- mg increments every 1–2 weeks; maximum 8/4 per day	4/1, 4/2, 4/4	Do not start with active liver disease; monitor liver function tests; avoid in HF
Pioglitazone and metformin (Actoplus Met)	Previously on metformin alone: initially 15/500 or 15/850 once or twice daily Previously on pioglitazone alone: initially 15/500 twice daily or 15/850 once daily	15/500, 15/850	Confirm normal renal function before starting and monitor, especially in patients older than 80 years; avoid in hepatic disease; caution with HF
Rosiglitazone and metformin (Avandamet)	4/1000–8/2000 in 2 divided doses	T: 1/500, 2/500, 4/500, 2/1000, 4/1000	Avoid in patients > 80 yr, Cr > 1.5 in men, Cr > 1.4 in women; see individual drugs (L, K)
DPP-4 Inhibitor			
Sitagliptan (Januvia)	100 mg daily	T: 25, 50, 100	Decrease dosage to 25–50 mg daily in renal impairment
Injectable Agents			
Exenatide (Byetta)	5–10 µg SC bid	1.2-, 2.4-mL prefilled syringes	Incretin mimetic; lowers HbA$_{1c}$ by 0.4%–0.9%; nausea and hypoglycemia common; less weight gain than insulin; avoid if CrCl < 30 mL/min (K)
Pramlintide (Symlin)*	60 µg SC immediately before meals	0.6 mg/mL in 5-mL vial	Amylin analogue; lowers HbA$_{1c}$ by 0.4%–0.7%; nausea and hypoglycemia common; reduce pre-meal dose of short-acting insulin by 50% (K)

NOTE: ALT = alanine aminotransferase; bid = twice a day; Cr = creatinine; CrCl = creatinine clearance; d = day; D/C = discontinue; ER = extended release; GI = gastrointestinal; HF = heart failure; K = renal elimination; L = hepatic elimination; max = maximum; min = minute(s); qd = each day; qid = four times a day; SC = subcutaneously; T = tablet; tid = three times a day; wkly = weekly; yr = year(s).

*Although patients up to 78 years were enrolled in the pramlintide clinical trials, the manufacturer states that no consistent age-related differences in pramlintide activity were identified. Hypoglycemia can be severe; hence, pramlintide should be prescribed only for patients who are able to recognize and respond to the signs and symptoms of hypoglycemia and for whom close monitoring and supervision are available.

SOURCE: Reuben DB, Herr KA, Pacala JT, et al. *Geriatrics At Your Fingertips: 2006*, 8th ed. New York: American Geriatrics Society; 2006:Table 35. Reprinted with permission.

Table 48.4—Insulin Preparations

Preparations	Onset	Peak	Duration
Insulin glulisine (Apidra)	20 min	0.5–1.5 h	3–4 h
Insulin lispro (Humalog)	15 min	0.5–1.5 h	6–8 h
Insulin (eg, Humulin, Novolin)*			
Regular	0.5–1 h	2–3 h	8–12 h
NPH	1–1.5 h	4–12 h	24 h
Insulin aspart (NovoLog)	30 min	1–3 h	3–5 h
Insulin detemir (Levemir)	3–4 h	6–8 h	6–24 h
Long-acting (Ultralente)	4–8 h	16–18 h	> 36 h
Insulin glargine (Lantus)**	1–2 h	—	24 h
Insulin inhaled (Exubera)† (1 mg inhaled = approximately 3 IU regular insulin SC)	10–20 min	2 h	6 h
Insulin, zinc (Lente)	1–2.5 h	8–12 h	18–24 h
Isophane insulin & regular insulin inj. (Novolin 70/30)	30 min	2–12 h	24 h

NOTE: h = hour(s); inj = injectable; min = minute(s); NPH = neutral protamine Hagedorn (insulin).

* Also available as mixtures of NPH and regular in 50:50 proportions.

** To convert from NPH dosing, give same number of units once a day. For patients taking NPH twice a day, decrease the total daily units by 20% and titrate on basis of response. Starting dose in insulin-naive patients is 10 U once daily at bedtime.

† Pulmonary spirometry before beginning, at 6 months, and annually thereafter. If decline in FEV$_1$ is ≥20%, monitor more frequently and consider discontinuing. Not recommended in patients with underlying lung disease (eg, asthma, COPD). Absorption 20% lower in mild asthma, 2 times higher in COPD. Cough is common. Do not use in patients who smoke or have quit smoking in the last 6 months; if patient begins smoking, discontinue immediately because of increased risk of hypoglycemia.

SOURCE: Reuben DB, Herr KA, Pacala JT, et al. *Geriatrics At Your Fingertips: 2007-2008*, 9th ed. New York: American Geriatrics Society; 2007:Table 36. Reprinted with permission.

control, is key to diabetes management. Physical activity programs should also be individualized based on functional status and presence of diabetic complications. The patient should be assessed regularly for level of physical activity, and the benefits of exercise and available resources for becoming more active should be reinforced.

When a new medication is prescribed, the older adult with diabetes and the caregiver should receive education about the purpose of the drug, how to take it, the common side effects, and important adverse reactions. Reassessment and reinforcement of this education should be done periodically as needed. Finally, every older adult with diabetes and all caregivers should receive education about risk factors for foot ulcers and amputation and appropriate foot care measures to reduce this risk. Physical ability to provide foot care should be evaluated, with periodic reassessment and reinforcement.

For patient education to be an effective tool in diabetes management, it must take into account the level of adjustment to the disease. In addition, it is critical that the patient and caregiver understand not only "what" needs to be done but "why" it needs to

be done. Self-efficacy strengthening and coping skills training should also be addressed. Support groups, such as those available through the American Diabetes Association, can be extremely helpful for the older patient and caregivers.

REFERENCES

■ American Diabetes Association: Clinical Practice Recommendations 2005. *Diabetes Care.* 2004;28(Suppl 1):S1–S79.

■ Brown AF, Mangione CM, Saliba D, et al.; California Health Care Foundation/American Geriatrics Society Panel on Improving Care for Elders with Diabetes. Guidelines for improving the care of the older person with diabetes mellitus. *J Am Geriatr Soc.* 2003;51(5 Suppl Guidelines):S265–S280.

■ Feil D, Weinreb J, Sultzer D. Psychiatric disorders and psychotrophic medication use in elderly persons with diabetes. *Ann Long Term Care.* 2006.14(7):39–48.

■ Hainer TA. Managing older adults with diabetes. *J Am Acad Nurse Pract.* 2006;18(7):309–317.

CHAPTER 49—GASTROINTESTINAL DISEASES AND DISORDERS

KEY POINTS

■ Though physiologic changes of aging may affect gastrointestinal function, most gastrointestinal symptoms and signs are due to pathologic conditions.

■ Drugs used to treat many of the illnesses affecting older persons can cause gastrointestinal symptoms and disorders.

■ Colon cancer is a common and often preventable cause of death.

The structure and function of the gastrointestinal tract are affected both by physiologic changes of aging and by the effects of accumulating disorders involving many body systems. In association with advancing age, there can be changes in connective tissue that limit the elasticity of the gut and alterations in the nerves and muscles that impair motility. Accumulating disorders and diseases are often associated with increased use of medications by older persons, many of which have direct effects on intestinal mucosa and motility. Some disease states, like atherosclerosis and diabetes mellitus, can adversely influence gastrointestinal function and

lead to symptoms and complications. Gastrointestinal problems may quickly compromise the older person's ability to maintain adequate nutrition and lead to fatigue and weight loss.

ESOPHAGUS

Dysphagia

Dysphagia implies either the inability to initiate a swallow or a sensation that solids or liquids do not pass easily from the mouth into the stomach; it is a common problem among older adults. Dysphagia in a patient with dyspepsia requires immediate evaluation and therapy. Patients with oropharyngeal dysphagia complain of foods getting stuck shortly after they swallow, inability to initiate a swallow, impaired ability to transfer food from the mouth to the esophagus, nasal regurgitation, and coughing. Cerebrovascular accidents, Parkinson's disease and other neuromuscular disorders, Zenker's diverticulum, oropharyngeal tumors, and prominent cervical osteophytes are the most common causes of oropharyngeal dysphagia in elderly persons. In particular, hesitancy in swallowing and defects in swallowing related to tremor of the tongue occur in patients with Parkinson's disease. In contrast, patients with esophageal dysphagia usually point to the sternum when asked to localize the site. Dysphagia for both solids and liquids from the onset usually implies a motility disorder of the esophagus. In contrast, dysphagia for solids which progresses later to involve liquids suggests mechanical obstruction. Progressive dysphagia results from either cancer or peptic stricture, whereas intermittent dysphagia is most often related to a lower esophageal ring or esophageal dysmotility, such as achalasia or diffuse esophageal spasm. It is particularly important to obtain a detailed review of medications, because anticholinergics, antihistamines, and certain antihypertensive agents can reduce salivary flow. Slurred speech may indicate weakness or incoordination of muscles involved in articulation and swallowing. Dysarthria and nasal regurgitation of food suggest weakness of the soft palate or pharyngeal constrictors. Food regurgitation, halitosis, a sensation of fullness in the neck, or a history of pneumonia accompanying dysphagia may be the result of a pharyngoesophageal (or Zenker's) diverticulum, which may be associated with a poorly relaxing or hypertensive upper esophageal sphincter. Painful swallowing (odynophagia) typically results from infection or malignancy.

Endoscopy is the best first test to evaluate dysphagia; it allows biopsies and therapeutic interventions, such as dilation. However, lower esophageal rings or extrinsic esophageal compression can be overlooked during endoscopy. In such cases, radiologic evaluation with a 13-mm barium tablet or a solid bolus with barium, such as a marshmallow or bread, may identify the level and nature of obstruction. If results of these tests are normal, an esophageal motility study should be performed. For patients with oropharyngeal dysphagia, videofluoroscopy allows detailed analysis of swallowing mechanics, identifies whether aspiration is present, and evaluates the effects of different barium consistencies. Naso-pharyngo-laryngoscopy is a bedside procedure that evaluates the oropharynx, vallecula, and piriform sinuses, as well as the larynx and perilaryngeal regions, for pooled secretions or retained food; its utility is uncertain.

The treatment of dysphagia depends on its underlying cause. Esophageal cancer requires resection, chemotherapy, or radiation therapy. For patients who are poor surgical candidates, palliative endoscopic techniques, such as endoscopic mucosal resection for early esophageal cancer, photodynamic therapy for high-grade dysplasia in Barrett's esophagus, and stent placement in obstructing esophageal cancer, may be considered. Following stroke or head or neck surgery,

or in degenerative neurologic diseases, swallowing rehabilitation and dietary modifications to facilitate oral intake are required. In some cases, feeding with a cup, straw, or spoon may improve swallowing. Endoscopic dilation is performed in patients with esophageal webs or strictures. Cricopharyngeal myotomy may benefit patients who have inadequate pharyngeal contraction, pharyngoesophageal diverticulum, or lack coordination between the pharynx and the upper esophageal sphincter. Endoscopic incision of the septum between the pharyngoesophageal (Zenker's) diverticulum and the esophagus with a flexible endoscope and needle-knife may also be performed. Botulinum toxin [OL] injection to the cricopharyngeus muscle is an alternative to surgery for patients with cricopharyngeal achalasia. (See also "Eating and Feeding Problems," p 167.)

Gastroesophageal Reflux Disease

Gastroesophageal reflux disease (GERD) is defined as chronic symptoms or mucosal damage produced by the abnormal reflux of gastric contents into the esophagus. Highly specific symptoms for GERD include heartburn, regurgitation, or both, which occur often after meals and are aggravated by recumbency and relieved by antacids. Among persons aged 65 and over, symptoms of heartburn or acid regurgitation occur at least weekly in 20% of the population and at least monthly in 59%, rates similar to those observed in younger adults.

In more than 80% of patients, GERD is caused by transient inappropriate lower esophageal sphincter relaxations that lead to acid reflux into the esophagus. Some patients may have reduced lower esophageal sphincter tone, which permits reflux when intra-abdominal pressure rises. Sliding hiatal hernia occurs in about 30% of patients aged 50 years or over and may contribute to acid reflux and regurgitation. Poor esophageal peristalsis leads to delayed clearance of the refluxate and increased acid exposure time. In patients receiving anticholinergic drugs, reduced salivary secretion decreases the buffering capacity of the esophagus against refluxed acid and may aggravate mucosal injury.

Patients with uncomplicated heartburn or regurgitation should be treated empirically with acid-suppressing drugs. If such therapy is unsuccessful, or if there are symptoms suggesting complicated disease, an upper endoscopy should be performed. Individuals, particularly white men, who have longstanding symptoms or who require continuous therapy for reflux need endoscopic screening for Barrett's esophagus. The frequency and severity of reflux symptoms are poorly predictive of the presence of Barrett's esophagus, particularly in patients aged 65 or over.

[OL] Not approved by the U.S. Food and Drug Administration for this use.

The presence of anemia, dysphagia, gastrointestinal bleeding, recurrent vomiting, and weight loss suggests complicated GERD. Patients with these signs and symptoms should be considered for endoscopy. This is the procedure of choice to evaluate mucosal integrity and confirm the diagnosis of dysplasia or cancer in cases of Barrett's esophagus. However, many patients with reflux symptoms do not have esophagitis. In such cases, 24-hour ambulatory esophageal pH testing helps to confirm the diagnosis. This noninvasive test is also useful for patients with noncardiac chest pain or reflux-associated pulmonary and upper respiratory symptoms or to monitor the esophageal acid exposure in patients with refractory symptoms. Esophageal manometry is used to document the presence of effective esophageal peristalsis in patients in whom antireflux surgery is being considered and to exclude underlying esophageal motility disorder, such as achalasia, as the cause of the patients' symptoms.

Proton-pump inhibitors are the treatment of choice for patients with GERD, but they are expensive. One of them, omeprazole, is now available over the counter. The use of these drugs heals esophagitis in 85% of cases and eradicates heartburn and regurgitation in 80%. In comparison, H_2 antagonists ameliorate symptoms and heal esophagitis in only 60% of cases. For the dysphagic elderly patient, various formulations of proton-pump inhibitors, such as orally disintegrating tablets, are available. Regardless, therapy should be maintained for at least 8 weeks. After acute medical therapy alleviates symptoms, the patient should be given a trial off medication. Endoscopy, esophageal motility, and ambulatory 24-hour pH monitoring should be performed if the most potent medical therapy still results in a poor response.

Recurrence of symptoms is common after therapy is stopped, and lifelong therapy is commonly needed. Intermittent therapy with an H_2 antagonist or proton-pump inhibitor may be successful in some patients with mild to moderate symptoms without severe esophagitis. Depending upon the initial therapy rendered, the medical regimen is adjusted in a step-up or step-down fashion to the most cost-effective regimen. The need for maintenance medical therapy is determined by the rapidity of recurrence. Among patients whose symptoms recur less than 3 months after stopping therapy, their disease may best be managed with continuous drug therapy. Patients whose symptoms recur 3 months or more after stopping treatment may be adequately managed with intermittent use of drugs. The induction of hypergastrinemia and gastric carcinoid tumors in rats treated with omeprazole has raised safety concerns about the long-term safety of proton-pump inhibitors. However, although patients treated with omeprazole for up to 5 years have shown gastritis and gastric atrophy, no

neoplastic changes have been seen. Since gastric acidity normally protects against ingested pathogens, another concern with gastric acid inhibition is an increased risk of enteric infections. In a similar fashion, acid-suppressive therapy also allows pathogen colonization of the upper gastrointestinal tract with an increased risk of community-acquired pneumonia.

Older patients with large hiatal hernia, with persistent regurgitation despite proton-pump inhibitor therapy, or who do not wish to take proton-pump inhibitors over the long term, should be considered for antireflux surgery. This can be performed laparoscopically, with success rates of more than 90%. Endoscopic anti-reflux procedures may also be used to treat reflux symptoms in selected patients who are not controlled by anti-secretory drugs.

Drug-Induced Esophageal Injury

Decreased esophageal peristaltic clearance, which is common among older persons, may be associated with pill retention. Esophageal injury may then occur as a result of prolonged contact of the caustic contents of the medication with the esophageal mucosa. The site of injury is commonly at the level of the aortic arch, of an enlarged left atrium, or of the esophagogastric junction. Because salivation and swallowing are markedly reduced during sleep, pill intake immediately before lying down and without adequate fluid bolus favors pill retention and injury. Taking medications with at least 8 fluid ounces of water helps dissolve tablets or capsules and may also reduce the risk of injury or gastrointestinal complaints. Patients with medication-induced esophageal injury present with sudden odynophagia to a degree that even swallowing saliva is difficult. A classic example is the elderly patient in a nursing home given a number of medications with a small amount of water while recumbent before sleep.

Tetracyclines, particularly doxycycline, are the most common antibiotics that induce esophagitis. Aspirin and all of the nonsteroidal anti-inflammatory drugs (NSAIDs) can also damage the esophagus. Other offenders include potassium chloride, quinidine, iron, and alendronate, an agent increasingly used for the treatment of osteoporosis in older adults. Because of this, alendronate should be used cautiously in patients with esophageal dysfunction and taken with at least 8 ounces of water to minimize the risk of the tablet's getting stuck in the esophagus and causing damage. In addition, patients should stand or sit upright for at least 30 minutes and should not eat during this interval. Etidronate, another bisphosphonate used to treat postmenopausal osteoporosis and Paget's disease, has not been associated with esophageal injury.

Upper endoscopy, the most sensitive diagnostic tool, may reveal a discrete ulcer of variable size with normal surrounding mucosa. These lesions typically heal spontaneously within a few days, and it is unclear whether therapy is needed. Suspension of sucralfate[OL] provides a protective coat on the esophageal mucosa and promotes healing. (Sucralfate is approved only for treating duodenal ulcers, so its use for treating stomach or esophageal ulcers would be off label.) Strictures may be noted in users of NSAIDs. Endoscopic dilation may be needed if a stricture is found. If possible, discontinue potentially caustic oral medications or substitute with a liquid preparation.

Esophageal Cancer: Endoscopic Palliation

Esophageal cancer is commonly diagnosed at an advanced, incurable stage in older patients who are not candidates for tumor resection. These patients are plagued by symptoms of esophageal obstruction or fistula formation, dysphagia, aspiration, and weight loss. In such instances, endoscopic palliation can be achieved with either laser therapy or a single stent placement. Laser therapy with neodymium-yttrium-aluminum-garnet (Nd:YAG) laser fulgurates the malignant obstructing tissue and restores luminal patency in more than 90% of cases, with a 5% risk of perforation. Relief may last for up to several months; treatments may be repeated. Photodynamic therapy uses a photosensitizing agent in combination with endoscopic laser exposure. It is more effective than Nd:YAG laser for palliation and has fewer complications, but it may cause skin photosensitivity.

Stenting with self-expanding metal stents is preferable therapy for patients with a malignant stricture or an esophago-bronchial fistula, as it relieves dysphagia and aspiration in up to 95% of patients and has a low complication rate. The disadvantages of stents include their high cost, tumor ingrowth, and stent migration.

STOMACH

Dyspepsia

Dyspepsia implies chronic or recurrent pain or discomfort in the upper abdomen. The major causes of dyspepsia are gastric or duodenal ulcer, gastroesophageal reflux, and gastric cancer. Because symptom pattern is inadequate for accurate diagnosis, endoscopy is the test of choice. Endoscopy is normal in up to 60% of patients, who are then classified as having functional dyspepsia. It is unclear whether *Helicobacter pylori* gastritis causes symptoms of dyspepsia.

Because the incidence of gastric cancer increases with age, upper endoscopy should be considered in older patients presenting with new onset of dyspepsia. Treatment is then targeted at the underlying diagnosis. For patients with ulcer and documented *H. pylori* infection, a trial of anti-*H. pylori* therapy should heal the ulcer and abolish the ulcer diathesis. For the majority of patients with functional (or nonulcer) dyspepsia, reassurance and a course of antisecretory therapy using either H_2-receptor antagonists or proton-pump inhibitors is recommended.

Treatment of *H. pylori* may lead to or possibly exacerbate reflux esophagitis. One possibility is that ammonia production by *H. pylori* buffers acid. Alternatively, reversal of *H. pylori*–induced gastritis (and associated hypochlorhydria) may increase gastric acid secretion and precipitate previously asymptomatic reflux. Despite this association, eradication of *H. pylori* should not be avoided solely to prevent the development or exacerbation of reflux esophagitis.

NSAID-Induced Gastric Complications

The risk of ulcers and their complications is three times greater in NSAID users than in nonusers. For those aged 60 or over, the relative risk increases even more, to fivefold. Older patients, particularly women, are two to four times more likely than younger patients to be hospitalized with peptic ulcer disease. The presence of *H. pylori* infection may have a synergistic effect on NSAID-induced ulcer disease. Elderly patients with NSAID-induced ulcers tend to present with anemia, bleeding, or perforation without the warning symptoms of dyspepsia or abdominal pain. In addition, elderly NSAID users commonly require emergency surgery for serious complications and have higher rebleeding rates, greater transfusion requirements, longer hospital stays, and higher mortality rates than do younger patients. When NSAIDs are used in older patients, the concomitant use of misoprostol or a proton-pump inhibitor may reduce the risk of gastric bleeding. Risk factors for upper gastrointestinal complications of NSAIDs use are shown in Table 49.1. COX-2 inhibitor therapy with celecoxib may be substituted for selected patients at risk for gastric complications from conventional NSAIDs, but a careful evaluation of underlying cardiovascular risk and risk-to-benefit assessment is mandatory.

Peptic Ulcer Disease

In the United States, *H. pylori* infection is responsible for about 80% of duodenal ulcers and approximately 60% of gastric ulcers. The majority of older patients with ulcers complain of dyspepsia, although bleeding,

---

[OL] Not approved by the U.S. Food and Drug Administration for this use.

Table 49.1—Risk Factors for Upper Gastrointestinal Adverse Events in Patients Treated With Nonsteroidal Anti-Inflammatory Drugs

Age 65 years and older

Comorbid medical conditions

Use of oral glucocorticoids

History of peptic ulcer disease

History of upper gastrointestinal bleeding

Use of anticoagulants

SOURCE: Data from American College of Rheumatology Subcommittee on Osteoarthritis Guidelines: recommendations for the medical management of osteoarthritis of the hip and knee, 2000 update. *Arthritis Rheum.* 2000;(43):1905–1915.

anemia, and acute abdominal pain may also occur. Typically, the diagnosis of peptic ulcer is made by upper gastrointestinal radiography or endoscopy. Endoscopy is more sensitive and specific than double-contrast barium study (92% versus 54% and 100% versus 91%, respectively). It is important to differentiate benign gastric ulcers from gastric cancer by obtaining multiple endoscopic biopsies.

The goal in evaluating an older patient with upper gastrointestinal symptoms is to quickly establish a definitive diagnosis, avoiding costly and risky diagnostic procedures. Drugs that may cause dyspepsia, especially NSAIDs, should be eliminated when possible. If early satiety, weight loss, occult gastrointestinal bleeding, or otherwise unexplained anemia is present, an endoscopy should be performed to exclude malignancy.

Among patients with dyspepsia who test positive for *H. pylori*, antibiotic therapy may be beneficial for up to 30% of those with underlying peptic ulcer, but those with nonulcer (functional) dyspepsia will have a variable response. *H. pylori* testing should not be performed in asymptomatic people.

Biliary Disease

Gallstones primarily form in the gallbladder and may obstruct the cystic or common bile duct, causing biliary pain, cholecystitis, and cholangitis. When stones obstruct the ampulla, pancreatitis may occur. Biliary pain is acute, severe upper abdominal pain, usually in the epigastrium or right upper quadrant, and it may last for more than 1 hour. The pain may radiate to the back or scapula and is often associated with restlessness, nausea, or vomiting. Episodes are typically separated by several weeks. Postprandial epigastric fullness, fatty food intolerance, and regurgitation are nonspecific symptoms and are not related to gallstones. If biliary disease is suspected in older patients, ultrasonography should be the initial imaging modality. Computed abdominal tomography scanning may be used if common bile duct stones or ductal obstruction are sus-

pected. Magnetic resonance cholangiography (MRC) and endoscopic ultrasonography are two new, very accurate imaging modalities to detect common bile duct pathology, including gallstones. However, for patients with obstructive jaundice, cholangitis, or suspected biliary pancreatitis where the probability of common bile duct stones is high, therapeutic endoscopic retrograde cholangiopancreatography (ERCP) is preferred.

Isolated alkaline phosphatase elevation without jaundice may be a presenting manifestation of biliary obstruction in older patients and should always be evaluated. If cholelithiasis is detected in patients with biliary pain, laparoscopic cholecystectomy is the procedure of choice. However, this procedure is not indicated in patients with gallstones without biliary pain or complications. The incidental finding of gallstones in a patient with dyspepsia may lead to an unnecessary cholecystectomy and a poor long-term outcome. In the rare older patient who is unable to undergo surgery, treatment with ursodeoxycholic acid or lithotripsy, or both, may be attempted. In patients with common bile duct obstruction due to gallstones, endoscopic sphincterotomy and bile ductal drainage is adequate in preventing recurrent cholangitis, and the gallbladder may be left *in situ*. In any older patient with gallstones, the possibility of gallbladder cancer should be entertained. In older patients presenting with biliary pain who have had a cholecystectomy, a retained common bile duct stone should be suspected and evaluated by ERCP, MRC, or endoscopic ultrasonography. In patients with abnormal liver function tests, right upper quadrant pain, and an increased common bile duct diameter, biliary manometry should also be considered. If sphincter of Oddi dysfunction is confirmed, endoscopic sphincterotomy should be performed. For patients with malignant jaundice, treatments are mostly palliative, with either surgery or percutaneous or endoscopic stenting. Such drainage improves quality of life, decreases pruritus, and improves the nutritional state of the patient, but it does not improve survival.

COLON

Constipation

Chronic constipation affects about 30% of adults aged 65 years or older, more commonly women. Although it commonly occurs as a side effect of drugs, it may be a manifestation of metabolic or neurologic disease. Regardless, colonic obstruction must always be excluded. Constipation has been defined as a stool frequency of less than three per week. However, some individuals may complain of straining at defecation or a sense of incomplete defecation despite a daily bowel evacuation. A more objective diagnosis of constipation is based upon colonic transit times.

Patients with irritable bowel syndrome often complain of constipation, which alternates with periods of diarrhea or normal bowel evacuation. Such patients have normal colonic transit times. Lumbosacral spinal disease may lead to colonic hypomotility and dilatation, decreased rectal tone and sensation, and impaired defecation. Older patients with Parkinson's disease may have constipation worsened by physical inactivity or medication use. In middle-aged and older women, the pelvic floor muscles that contribute to the external sphincter of the rectum may acquire laxity that contributes to problems with fecal incontinence.

Most patients with prolonged colonic transit have colonic inertia, defined as the delayed passage of radiopaque markers through the proximal colon. Outlet delay is a form of idiopathic constipation in which markers move normally through the colon but stagnate in the rectum. This is typically seen in older female patients with fecal impaction and megarectum, and in women with pelvic floor dyssynergia who demonstrate abnormal responses of the pelvic floor muscles during defecation. Older patients with megacolon or megarectum have chronic fecal retention, increased rectal compliance and elasticity, and blunted rectal sensation, all leading to fecal impaction and soiling.

Defecography is a technique in which thick barium simulating stool is introduced into the rectum and evacuation is monitored by fluoroscopy while the patient sits on a commode. Assessment of the anorectal structure and function is then made at rest and during barium expulsion. Anorectal manometry evaluates rectal sensation and compliance, reflex relaxation of the internal anal sphincter, and the competence of the anal sphincters.

For most patients with constipation and normal colonic transit time, fluids, dietary fiber, and bulk laxatives, such as psyllium seed or calcium polycarbophil, are effective in increasing the frequency and softening the consistency of stool with a minimum of adverse effects. Patients who respond poorly or who do not tolerate fiber may require laxatives. Chronic use of stimulant laxatives such as bisacodyl and senna may lead to hypokalemia, protein-losing enteropathy, and impairment of bowel motility. Stool softeners such as docusate sodium have few side effects but are less effective than laxatives. Constipation among patients with dementia is common, especially if psychotropic medications are being used. Because the patient cannot be relied upon to describe symptoms, a proactive approach is needed.

Management of slow-transit constipation requires daily osmotic laxatives, such as sorbitol, lactulose, or a polyethylene glycol solution. A new laxative approved for idiopathic chronic constipation, lubiprostone, is a chloride channel activator that increases intestinal water secretion. Because of this mechanism, it may also be effective in slow-transit constipation. Severe intractable colonic inertia with megacolon may require subtotal colectomy and ileorectostomy. Pelvic floor dysfunction requires biofeedback, relaxation exercises, and the use of suppositories.

Patients with fecal impaction should first have their colon evacuated with enemas or polyethylene glycol electrolyte solution until cleansing is complete. Recurrence of fecal impaction is then prevented with a fiber-restricted diet together with cleansing enemas twice weekly or daily oral intake of 12 to 16 fluid ounces of polyethylene glycol solution.

Fecal Incontinence

Fecal incontinence, defined as the recurrent uncontrolled passage of fecal material for at least 1 month, is a disturbing disability because it affects quality of life and may lead to social isolation. Fecal incontinence may be minor, with inadvertent passage of flatus or soiling of underwear with liquid stool, or it may be major, with involuntary leakage of feces. Fecal incontinence affects 2% to 7% of adults, mostly older persons in poor general health.

Fecal continence depends on many factors, such as physical and mental function, stool consistency, colonic transit, rectal compliance, internal and external anal sphincter function, as well as anorectal sensation and reflexes. Normal defecation is a complex sequential process that starts with the entry of stool into the rectum that leads to reflex relaxation of the internal anal sphincter. If defecation is desired, the anorectal angle is voluntarily straightened, and abdominal pressure is increased by straining. This results in descent of the pelvic floor, contraction of the rectum, and inhibition of the external anal sphincter, which causes evacuation of the rectal contents.

Decreased anal sphincter tone can result from trauma (eg, anal surgery) or neurologic disorders (eg, spinal cord injury or a secondary effect of diabetes mellitus). Vaginal delivery associated with anal sphincter tears or trauma to the pudendal nerve may result in fecal incontinence immediately or after many years. Decreased rectal compliance resulting from ulcerative or radiation proctitis leads to increased fecal frequency and urgency. Impaction is a common cause of fecal incontinence in elderly persons because it inhibits the internal anal sphincter tone, permitting leakage of liquid stool. Idiopathic fecal incontinence caused by denervation of the pelvic floor musculature occurs most commonly in middle-aged and elderly women.

The history and physical examination often provide clues to the cause of fecal incontinence. A flexible sigmoidoscopy may be considered in order to exclude inflammation or tumor. The next step is anorectal manometry, which measures resting anal sphincter tone, the squeeze pressure, the rectoanal inhibitory reflex, rectal sensation, and rectal compliance. Abnormalities of the anal sphincters, the rectal wall, and the puborectalis muscle can be further evaluated by the use of endorectal ultrasound. Typically, a defect in the internal anal sphincter is associated with low resting sphincter pressure, whereas defects in the external sphincter are associated with lower anal squeeze pressure.

Medical therapy is aimed at reducing stool frequency and improving stool consistency. The former is achieved with antidiarrheal drugs, such as loperamide; the latter, by supplementing the diet with a bulking agent, such as methylcellulose. Older patients with incontinence related to cognitive impairment or physical debility may benefit from a regular defecation program. Biofeedback therapy is a painless noninvasive method of retraining the pelvic floor and the abdominal wall musculature and is recommended for patients with fecal incontinence associated with structurally intact sphincter. Surgery may involve sphincter repair or implantation of an artificial sphincter. Colostomy may be needed for patients with intractable symptoms in whom other treatments have failed. A synthetic sphincter device, consisting of an inflatable cuff that maintains continence, is a valve that allows the cuff to deflate for defecation. Radiofrequency energy delivery to the anal sphincters (Secca procedure) may also improve continence in selected patients.

Diverticular Disease

The prevalence of diverticular disease is age dependent, increasing to 30% by age 60 and to 65% by age 85. Although most patients remain asymptomatic, 20% develop diverticulitis, and 10% may develop diverticular bleeding. Therefore, the mere presence of diverticulosis does not require specific therapy. A diet high in fiber appears to be associated with a reduced risk of the development of diverticular disease and may reduce the risk of subsequent complications.

Uncomplicated diverticulosis is often an incidental finding on screening sigmoidoscopy, colonoscopy, or barium enema. Some patients may complain of nonspecific abdominal cramping, bloating, flatulence, and irregular bowel habits. Diverticular bleeding is usually painless and self-limited, and it rarely coexists with acute diverticulitis. Diverticulitis usually presents with left lower quadrant pain, although nausea, vomiting, constipation, diarrhea, and dysuria or frequency may occur. The physical examination usually reveals left lower quadrant tenderness, a tender mass, and abdominal distention. Generalized tenderness suggests perfora-

tion and peritonitis. Low-grade fever and leukocytosis are common, but their absence in older patients does not exclude the diagnosis. Urinalysis may reveal sterile pyuria induced by adjacent colonic inflammation; the presence of mixed colonic flora on urine culture suggests a colovesical fistula. Other complications that can occur include perforation, obstruction, and abscess formation.

Computed tomographic (CT) scanning is the optimal imaging method in acute diverticulitis. CT features of acute diverticulitis include increased density of soft tissue within pericolic fat and colonic diverticula, bowel wall thickening, soft-tissue masses (phlegmon), and pericolic fluid collections (abscess formation). CT can also identify peritonitis, obstruction, and fistula to the bladder, vagina, and abdominal wall. However, in approximately 10% of patients, diverticulitis cannot be distinguished from colon cancer, since both may show focal thickening of the bowel wall. In such cases, upon resolution of the acute inflammation, a colonoscopy is indicated. In older persons, CT-guided percutaneous drainage of localized abscesses may obviate emergent surgery and permit single-stage elective surgical resection.

The majority of patients (85%) with simple diverticulitis respond to medical therapy. In contrast, all patients with complicated diverticulitis require surgery. Indications for emergency surgery are free perforation with peritonitis, obstruction, clinical deterioration or failure to improve with conservative management, and an abscess that cannot be drained percutaneously. Indications for elective surgical intervention are recurrent or intractable symptoms, persistent mass, obstruction, and fistula or abscess formation.

Mild diverticulitis with left lower quadrant pain, low-grade fever, and minimal physical findings is often treated on an outpatient basis, with clear liquids and oral antibiotics, such as ciprofloxacin 500 mg twice a day or metronidazole 500 mg three times a day, or both. Hospitalization is needed only if the patient fails to improve. Once the episode resolves, solid food is reintroduced and the colon is evaluated, preferably by colonoscopy. For patients with moderate to severe symptoms, treatment with bowel rest, fluids, and intravenous antibiotics is initiated, with the aim to avoid urgent surgery. Antibiotics should be active against gram-negative rods and anaerobes. Possible regimens include cefoxitin, piperacillin-tazobactam, or gentamicin plus clindamycin. If there is no improvement, the diagnosis is incorrect or an abscess, peritonitis, fistula, or obstruction is present. Older immunosuppressed patients with multiple underlying medical conditions may present with minimal symptoms or signs even with frank peritonitis, and the diagnosis is commonly delayed. In such cases, early surgical intervention should be considered. Diffuse peritonitis requires fluid resuscitation, broad-spectrum antibiotics, and emergency laparotomy. Colonic resective surgery removes the septic focus, corrects the obstruction or fistula formation, and restores bowel continuity. In most elective cases, resection and primary anastomosis are possible, if the disease is well localized or has significantly resolved.

After successful medical therapy of the first episode of diverticulitis, one third of patients will remain asymptomatic, another third will have episodic abdominal cramps (painful diverticulosis), and the remaining will proceed to a second attack of diverticulitis. Therefore, elective surgery is not necessary for all patients with diverticulitis who respond to medical therapy. If surgery is performed, progression of diverticulosis in the remaining colon occurs in only 15%, and the need for further surgery is reduced to less than 10%.

Irritable Bowel Syndrome

Irritable bowel syndrome (IBS) is a functional gastrointestinal disorder with remissions and exacerbations, characterized by abdominal pain (A), bloating (B), and either constipation (C) or diarrhea (D), or both. IBS results from altered bowel motility, visceral hypersensitivity, and enhanced perception by the brain of many visceral stimuli. A common mediator for all these abnormalities is serotonin, and serotonin-receptor agonists and antagonists are used in the management of IBS. Although psychosocial factors are commonly involved in IBS, they are not known to have a causative role.

Since the clinical symptoms characteristic of irritable bowel syndrome are not specific, it is important to be mindful of features that are not consistent with IBS. These include weight loss, first onset of symptoms after age 50, nocturnal diarrhea, family history of cancer or inflammatory bowel disease, rectal bleeding or obstruction, and laboratory abnormalities, such as anemia, leukocytosis, abnormal chemistries, positive fecal cultures, or the presence of parasites in the stool. In the older patient the diagnosis should be made only after other conditions (ie, ischemia, diverticulosis, colon cancer, or inflammatory bowel disease) have been carefully excluded. An appropriate work-up of an older person with symptoms consistent with IBS should include a colonoscopy to exclude structural abnormalities of the colon. A CT scan of the abdomen and a small bowel series may also be useful. If the history, physical examination, and laboratory or imaging studies are negative, the diagnosis of IBS can then be made and subcategorized as IBS with constipation (IBS-C) or diarrhea (IBS-D) or IBS with alternating constipation and diarrhea.

Depending on the IBS subtype, treatment includes reassurance, antispasmodics, antidiarrheals, fiber supplements, and serotonin-receptor agents (eg, alosetron). Although quite effective, the latter drugs may precipitate intestinal ischemia and should be used with caution, particularly in the elderly patient. Try to establish a definitive diagnosis of IBS, avoid repetitive investigations, and clarify that although IBS is not life threatening, it can certainly negatively impact quality of life. As part of chronic disease management, it is also important that clinicians listen actively to patients' symptoms, validate their feelings, provide empathy, set realistic shared goals, negotiate treatment strategies instead of issuing directives, help patients take responsibility for treatment decisions, establish limits on the duration and frequency of visits and phone calls, and maintain a continuing relationship.

Occult Gastrointestinal Bleeding

Older patients are commonly noted to have a positive stool test for occult blood or are diagnosed with unexplained iron-deficiency anemia. Although colorectal cancer is a leading concern in such patients, many other causes, such as esophagitis, peptic ulcers, esophageal and gastric malignancies, intestinal or colonic angiodysplasia, benign colon polyps, inflammatory bowel disease, or hemorrhoids may be the cause. A positive fecal occult blood test should not be attributed to esophageal varices or colonic diverticula, because it is rare for such lesions to bleed in an occult fashion. The presence of fecal occult blood should not be attributed to aspirin or warfarin use or alcohol ingestion.

Detection of occult blood in the stool has a low sensitivity and a high rate of false-positive results, leading to more invasive and expensive tests. Despite these limitations, annual screening is currently recommended and has been associated with up to a 33% reduction in mortality from colorectal cancer. Because of the high prevalence of colorectal cancer and adenomatous polyps in older adults with a positive fecal occult blood test, colonoscopy is performed and, if negative, is followed by an upper endoscopy. If symptoms of upper gastrointestinal disease are present, there is a high likelihood for a positive endoscopy. However, in older patients at risk for colon cancer, the presence of a proximal lesion should not preclude evaluation of the colon. Patients with normal upper and lower tract may require evaluation for a small bowel source. The most common cause for bleeding from the small bowel is angiodysplasia, followed by tumors or ulcers that are commonly caused by NSAIDs. Unrecognized gluten-sensitive enteropathy can result in iron-deficiency anemia, since iron is absorbed in the proximal small bowel.

In one prospective study that evaluated patients with iron-deficiency anemia with colonoscopy, endoscopy, and, if these tests were negative, radiographic examination of the small intestine, a source of bleeding was identified in 62%. A lesion was seen on colonoscopy in 25%, on upper endoscopy in 36%, and on both in 1% of patients. Peptic ulcer disease was the primary abnormality in the upper gastrointestinal tract, but cancer was detected on colonoscopy in 11% of patients. Even after endoscopic examination of both the upper and lower parts of the gastrointestinal tract, the source of bleeding remains unidentified in approximately 10% of older patients presenting with iron-deficiency anemia and occult gastrointestinal bleeding. In such cases, video capsule endoscopy has a high diagnostic yield and is simple and noninvasive.

Colonic Angiodysplasia

The terms *angiodysplasia*, *arteriovenous malformation*, and *vascular ectasia* have been used interchangeably. Angiodysplasias occur most often in the cecum and ascending colon, where they may cause bleeding, particularly in patients aged 60 or over. However, angiodysplasias occur throughout the gastrointestinal tract and may be multiple or coexist in several different regions of the gastrointestinal tract. They may be asymptomatic or cause occult or clinically overt gastrointestinal bleeding.

Angiodysplasias are dilated, thin-walled vessels in the mucosa and submucosa that are lined by endothelium or by smooth muscle. Although they are mostly tortuous veins, arteriovenous communications or enlarged arteries may be present, leading to brisk bleeding. The pathogenesis of angiodysplasias is not well understood. They may result from local ischemia associated with cardiac, vascular, or pulmonary disease. Researchers have detected increased expression of angiogenic factors, basic fibroblast growth factor and vascular endothelial growth factor, in segments of colon with angiodysplasia.

Angiodysplasias are usually diagnosed during colonoscopy, appearing as 5- to 10-mm cherry-red, ectatic blood vessels radiating from a central vascular core. Angiodysplasias can also be diagnosed by angiography. If they are serendipitously detected during routine endoscopy or colonoscopy, angiodysplasias should not be treated. However, an actively bleeding angiodysplasia should be treated. Whether angiodysplasias were the cause of bleeding in patients who have stopped bleeding and, in particular, in patients who are found to have both angiodysplasias and diverticula is a more difficult problem. In such cases, bleeding from angiodysplasias is almost always from the cecum or ascending colon.

Many endoscopic ablation techniques have been used in the treatment of angiodysplasias. Although acute bleeding can be successfully controlled with these approaches, rebleeding is common. Angiography may localize the site of active bleeding and allows embolization or infusion of vasopressin. Surgical resection is definitive for lesions that have been clearly identified as the source of bleeding. However, recurrent bleeding may occur from other proximal or distal lesions in more than 30% of cases. Hormonal therapy with estrogen (with or without progesterone) has also been used in women, but its benefit should be weighed against the potential risks of thromboembolic disease, estrogen-dependent tumors, or uterine bleeding.

Colonic Ischemia

Ischemic colitis is typically encountered in patients aged 65 years and older who have atherosclerosis or atrial fibrillation or who have had surgical bypass or vascular grafting procedures. The main symptoms at presentation are abdominal pain and lower gastrointestinal bleeding. Colonoscopy reveals segmental edema, hemorrhages, gray-black pseudomembrane formation, and focal ulcers, mostly in the region of the splenic flexure and typically sparing the rectum. Treatment is mostly supportive, but even with treatment colonic strictures may ensue. The development of peritoneal signs calls for surgical intervention with colonic resection of the involved segment.

Clostridium difficile Infection and Pseudomembranous Colitis

C. difficile infection is becoming increasingly recognized among hospitalized patients and as the source of epidemics in hospitals and long-term-care facilities for elderly persons. The infection is often precipitated by the use of antibiotics, such as cephalosporins, penicillins, or clindamycin. Clinically it presents with watery diarrhea, crampy abdominal pain, fever, abdominal tenderness and distention, and an elevated white blood cell count. Serious complications, such as ileus with dehydration and electrolyte abnormalities, toxic megacolon, perforation, and death, may occur. *C. difficile* infection should be considered when acute abdominal distention occurs in older hospitalized adults without diarrhea but with associated severe leukocytosis; it carries high mortality. *C. difficile* infection can be recognized endoscopically by the appearance of diffuse or segmental pseudomembranes coating an edematous mucosa, but the diagnosis is often made by the detection of *C. difficile* cytotoxins in the stool either by cytotoxin tissue culture assay, latex agglutination, or enzyme-linked immunoassays. Metronidazole

250 mg orally every 6 hours is effective in 85% of cases, and it may be given intravenously in severe cases of ileus or megacolon. Vancomycin (125 mg every 6 hours) is also highly effective but only if given orally. Antibiotic treatment for *C. difficile* colitis should be for 10 to 14 days to reduce the risk of relapse. Relapses may occur in up to 20% of cases and require repeat treatment with metronidazole, vancomycin, or a combination of vancomycin and rifampin. In order to prevent the disease in predisposed individuals and to avoid relapses, restitution of the colonic flora with lactobacilli or *Saccharomyces boulardii* has been used.

Acute Colonic Pseudo-Obstruction

Acute colonic pseudo-obstruction is manifested by acute massive dilation of the colon without evidence of mechanical obstruction. In the older adult, it is often related to neurologic disease, such as Parkinson's or cerebrovascular disease, trauma, recent orthopedic surgery, or use of narcotics. Infections, particularly *C. difficile*, and colonic ischemia need to be excluded. Urgent colonoscopy not only can assist with the diagnosis but allows placement of a decompression colonic tube. Parenteral fluids and supportive measures, discontinuation of narcotics, and the use of neostigmine intravenously often lead to rapid resolution.

Colonic Polyps and Colon Cancer

Polyps are usually asymptomatic, but they may bleed or predispose the patient to cancer. Colonic polyps are usually classified as neoplastic (adenomas) or non-neoplastic (hyperplastic). Approximately 40% of the U.S. population aged 50 or over have one or more adenomas. Detection and removal of adenomas significantly decreases the morbidity and mortality associated with colorectal cancer. Old age and male gender are major risk factors. First-degree relatives of patients with adenomas are also at increased risk for colorectal cancer and should undergo screening. Adenomas are most often detected by colon cancer screening tests, primarily sigmoidoscopy. Because adenomas do not typically bleed, the fecal occult blood test is an insensitive screening method. Older age, villous histology, and size are independent risk factors for malignancy within an adenoma. The risk of colon cancer also increases with the number of high-risk adenomas that are present.

Colorectal cancer is the third leading cause of cancer in the United States and the second leading cause of cancer death. The risk of colorectal cancer increases dramatically with age, with more than 90% of cases occurring in people over age 50. Women are more likely than men to harbor right-sided colonic adenomas. The risk of colorectal cancer in patients with rectal bleeding is age related and may reach to 25% in patients aged 80 and over. Up to 40% of colorectal cancer arises proximal to the splenic flexure, and less than 10% is within the reach of the digital rectal examination. Since it is impossible to identify the source of bleeding by clinical criteria, a colonoscopy should be performed in all cases of hematochezia, occult gastrointestinal bleeding, iron-deficiency anemia, or even melena after a negative upper endoscopy. Other symptoms, such as abdominal pain, altered bowel habits, or pencil-thin stools are less predictive of colorectal cancer but do require thorough investigation, starting with a colonoscopy. Typically, right-sided cancers present with iron-deficiency anemia and occult gastrointestinal bleeding, whereas left-sided cancers lead to obstructive symptoms, changes in bowel habits, and overt hematochezia.

Colonoscopy with endoscopic polypectomy is the ideal examination for the detection and removal of adenomatous polyps. Large adenomas that cannot be safely or completely resected endoscopically should generally be removed by segmental colectomy. If a polyp is detected by barium enema, colonoscopy is recommended to establish the histology, remove the polyp, and search for other lesions. If a single polyp is detected by sigmoidoscopy, it should be biopsied. If the polyp is hyperplastic, colonoscopy is not required. If the polyp is adenomatous, full colonoscopy is warranted.

A 3-year interval for surveillance colonoscopy is safe and cost-effective for most patients with adenomas. If only a small tubular adenoma is found, the interval may be extended to 5 years; in contrast, after removal of a large villous adenoma, a 1-year follow-up is recommended. After a negative screening or surveillance colonoscopy, an examination interval of 5 years appears to be safe. Patients with colorectal cancer should also have regular colonoscopic surveillance for adenomas starting 1 year after surgery, since these patients have adenoma or cancer recurrence rates of 25% to 30% at 3 years. Because the greatest impact of colorectal cancer on life expectancy occurs between the ages of 70 and 80 years and the protective effect of colonoscopy on colorectal cancer mortality is approximately 10 years, the optimal and most cost-effective age for one-time colonoscopic screening is 60 to 65 years of age.

Colonoscopic screening for cancer and subsequent surveillance lose their cost-effectiveness after the age of 80 years. Screening for colorectal cancer should also cease when the risk of screening outweighs any potential benefits, in patients with less than 10 years' estimated survival, or when tests are unlikely to prolong patient survival. In patients with known history ofpolyps, discontinuation of surveillance should be considered in those aged over 75 years in whom a follow-up examination is normal or shows only small tubular adenomas.

REFERENCES

■ De Lillo AR, Rose S. Functional bowel disorders in the geriatric patient: constipation, fecal impaction, and fecal incontinence. *Am J Gastroenterol.* 2000; 95(4):901–905.

■ Gostout CJ. Gastrointestinal bleeding in the elderly patient. *Am J Gastroenterol.* 2000; 95(3):590–595.

■ Miller KM, Waye JD. Approach to colon polyps in the elderly. *Am J Gastroenterol.* 2000;95(5):1147–1151.

■ Richter JE. Gastroesophageal reflux disease in the older patient: presentation, treatment and complications. *Am J Gastroenterol.* 2000;95(2):368–373.

■ Tendler DA. Acute intestinal ischemia and infarction. *Semin Gastrointest Dis.* 2003; 14(2):66–76.

CHAPTER 50—KIDNEY DISEASES AND DISORDERS

KEY POINTS

■ The older kidney is capable of maintaining homeostasis of body fluids and electrolytes under most circumstances.

■ Therapies directed at controlling blood pressure and minimizing proteinuria are key in patients with chronic kidney disease.

■ Adjusting medication dosages appropriately and avoiding nephrotoxic medications are important aspects of the management of patients with chronic kidney disease.

■ Early referral to a nephrologist is useful for optimal planning of kidney replacement therapy.

Kidney function declines after age 40 years at a mean rate of approximately 1% per year, accelerating some in the later years. This observation was first reported in cross-sectional studies and confirmed in a population of normal aging persons followed over time. However, although two thirds of individuals followed for up to 20 years in the Baltimore Longitudinal Study developed a decline in glomerular filtration rate (GFR) with aging, one third had no decline, indicating that a decline in kidney function with age is not inevitable.

Although there is loss of glomerular mass with aging, the loss of tubular mass is proportional, so that glomerular-tubular balance is usually maintained. Despite significant anatomic and functional changes, the older kidney is capable of maintaining homeostasis of body fluids and electrolytes under most circumstances. However, under environmental and disease-related stresses, such as volume changes or alterations in acid-base status, the older kidney is slower to respond to correct the abnormality.

FLUID AND ELECTROLYTE DISTURBANCES

Hyponatremia and Hypernatremia

Surveys of older adults in both acute and long-term-care facilities show a high prevalence of hyponatremia (serum sodium concentration <132 mmol/L). By definition, these patients have an excess of water relative to solute. Clinically, older adults with hyponatremia can be separated into those with decreased extracellular fluid (ECF) volume (eg, gastrointestinal losses, adrenal and renal salt-losing conditions), increased ECF volume (eg, heart failure), or normal ECF volume (eg, syndrome of inappropriate antidiuretic hormone, or SIADH). The last is the most common. Regardless of cause, nonosmotic (baroreceptor) stimulation of arginine vasopressin (AVP) release is a major factor in the development of hyponatremia. Older adults appear to have an increased osmoreceptor sensitivity, as evidenced by the greater increase in serum AVP in response to any given increase in serum osmolality. Postoperative and diuretic-induced hyponatremia are much more common in older than in younger patients.

Hyponatremia does not usually produce symptoms until the serum sodium concentration falls below 125 mmol/L. At about this level, central nervous symptoms begin to appear, including somnolence, cognitive impairment, seizures, and ultimately coma, secondary to brain edema. Although therapy is not different for older adults, it is important to proceed slowly and to monitor regularly the older patient's response to avoid the development of cardiovascular or neurologic symptoms, or both.

Hypertonic dehydration (serum sodium >148 mmol/L) is common in older adults, especially among acutely hospitalized and nursing-home patients. It also is largely avoidable. A number of factors may contribute to this condition. Body water is decreased as a proportion of total body weight because of the relative increase in fat content of normal older adults. Although AVP release from the posterior pituitary is normal (or even supernormal) in response to hypertonicity in older adults, the ability to concentrate the urine in response to AVP is decreased. Probably most important is the blunted or even absent thirst response to hypertonicity seen in normal older adults. This thirst response is even more impaired in patients with cerebral disease, such as stroke. Therefore, in hot weather and in the absence of air conditioning, it is important to make certain that older adults increase their consumption of fluids. An inability to obtain water because of functional or cognitive barriers may further limit the older adult's ability to adequately replenish lost body fluids. It is helpful to instruct older adults to drink a specific amount of water each day. For institutionalized older adults, particularly those with decreased mobility or impaired cognition, placing a specific amount of fluid within easy reach and assuring that it is gone by the end of the day is helpful. In addition, on very hot days, it may be wise to hold or decrease the dosage of diuretics in some patients. Symptoms of hypernatremia (obtundation, lethargy, coma) are predominantly neurologic, presumably because of shrinkage of the brain cells. As intravascular volume is preserved at the expense of cell water, changes in blood pressure, pulse rate, and skin turgor may not be evident early on.

Hypokalemia and Hyperkalemia

The list of potential causes of hypokalemia in older adults is long. A low serum potassium measurement usually represents total body potassium depletion. This may be secondary to gastrointestinal losses, as occurs with vomiting, diarrhea, nasogastric suction, or fistula drainage. Vomiting results in a metabolic alkalosis that shifts potassium into cells and increases urinary potassium losses. Another commonly overlooked cause of hypokalemia is excessive use of purgatives and enemas.

Total body depletion of potassium may also develop secondary to renal losses. In older adults this is commonly secondary to diuretic usage and may be completely avoided with supplemental potassium. Although the liquid form of potassium supplement has an unpleasant taste, it is generally absorbed better than potassium tablets and is not associated with the same risk of gastric ulceration. Potassium wasting may also result from excessive adrenal hormone production or a primary underlying kidney disease. Primary and sec-

ondary aldosteronism (the latter from renal artery stenosis or volume contraction resulting from diuretic usage in patients with heart, liver, or kidney disease) may be a contributing factor. Hypomagnesemia-induced hypokalemia with ongoing renal potassium wasting is also seen with diuretic usage.

Potassium deficiency affects the cardiovascular system, neurologic system, muscles, and kidneys. The major side effects affecting the cardiovascular system are hypokalemia-induced ventricular arrhythmias. Muscle symptoms include weakness, easy fatigability, cramping, myalgias, and muscle tenderness secondary to rhabdomyolysis. Effects on the kidneys result in polyuria and development of a metabolic alkalosis with paradoxical aciduria (low urine pH).

Because an alkalosis (chloride depletion) usually accompanies hypokalemia and is responsible for a shift of potassium intracellularly, replacement therapy should be with potassium chloride. The exception is the patient with renal tubular acidosis, in which case the alkaline salts of potassium should be given. Azotemia and age are the two significant risk factors for life-threatening hyperkalemia in patients receiving potassium-supplementation. The latter may be related to the lower levels of aldosterone seen in elder patients under any given set of conditions (low-salt versus high-salt diet, supine versus upright posture).

Most episodes of hyperkalemia are seen in patients with chronic kidney disease (CKD). However, significant hyperkalemia is uncommon until the azotemia becomes life threatening or another factor contributes, such as an increased endogenous or ingested potassium load, severe acidosis, administration of a diuretic to block sodium potassium exchange (triamterene, spironolactone), a deficiency of endogenous aldosterone or mineralocorticoid, or, importantly, administration of drugs, such as nonsteroidal anti-inflammatory drugs (NSAIDs) or angiotensin-converting enzyme (ACE) inhibitors. Older patients with an interstitial nephritis, especially patients with diabetes, develop a failure of the renin-aldosterone system with a hyperkalemia and mild metabolic acidosis, often referred to as *type IV renal tubular acidosis*.

CLINICAL PRESENTATIONS OF KIDNEY DISEASES

In general, the presentation of kidney disease in older and younger adults is not significantly different. Recognizing a decline in kidney function is important for early diagnosis of treatable causes of renal insufficiency. If no treatment is available, then interventions to retard disease progression should be started whenever possible. As detailed below, national guidelines have been developed to guide care in pre–end-stage renal disease (ESRD). Equally important, the impact of kidney function on other aspects of a person's health care needs to be considered. For example, the dosage of medications that are excreted by the kidney may need adjustment to prevent toxic drug levels. In addition, some medications may adversely affect kidney function or complicate kidney disease. Patients with CKD may also have alterations in feelings of well-being and changes in functional status that must be addressed.

The medical history and physical examination may be very helpful in determining the cause of renal insufficiency. The clinical symptoms and signs are variable but often are related to the underlying disease. Nephrotic syndrome may present with edema and hypertension. Kidney stones may present with flank pain, hematuria, nausea, and vomiting. These same symptoms are also seen with acute renal artery embolization. Renal artery stenosis may be silent or present with multiple episodes of pulmonary edema. The symptoms commonly reported as a direct result of CKD (eg, fatigue, nausea, cognitive difficulties) are generally not experienced until the creatinine clearance (CrCl) is less than 20 mL/min. However, complications of CKD, including anemia, metabolic acidosis, and alterations in calcium-phosphate metabolism, may develop as the GFR falls below 60 mL/min.

The first hint of kidney disease may be seen on a screening urinalysis with asymptomatic abnormalities (hematuria, proteinuria, pyuria, casts). It may also present with an asymptomatic elevated serum concentration of nitrogen or creatinine. It is important to remember that muscle mass decreases with age. Therefore, a normal serum creatinine may represent a decline in kidney function. For example, a serum creatinine of 1.0 mg/dL in an 80-year-old person weighing 65 kg corresponds to an estimated CrCl of 54 mL/min. It also is helpful to look for changes in serum creatinine over time. A change in serum creatinine from a steady-state concentration of 0.7 mg/dL to 1.4 mg/dL indicates that the kidney function has decreased by 50% and signals the need for further evaluation.

In summary, hematuria, proteinuria, abnormal urinary sediment, or a decreased CrCl in an older adult indicates the need to more fully evaluate kidney function. Although it is not clear that age alone is a risk factor for CKD, the comorbidity associated with the aging process, including vascular disease, diabetes mellitus, and cardiac disease, places older adults at increased risk of a renal insult.

Hematuria

Whether macroscopic or microscopic (>3 to 5 red blood cells per high-power field), hematuria in older adults deserves evaluation. A microscopic examination of the urine may suggest the source of the hematuria. Dysmorphic red blood cells (normal biconcave shape is distorted) or red cell casts in freshly voided urine suggest a glomerular source. Associated proteinuria or an elevated serum creatinine concentration also suggests kidney parenchymal disease. Biconcave red blood cells suggest a disease of the collecting system. Systemic coagulation defects should also be considered. In addition to a microscopic urine evaluation, the work-up of isolated hematuria should include a urine culture, imaging (kidney ultrasound or intravenous pyelography) to exclude a renal parenchymal mass, and if these are nondiagnostic, a urologic consultation for cystoscopy. In addition, a platelet count, prothrombin time, and partial thromboplastin time should be obtained to exclude a coagulopathy. In approximately 80% of older adults, the source of hematuria is the bladder, prostate, or urethra. Malignancies, most often bladder but also hypernephroma and prostate, account for one third of the cases of hematuria. Less than 10% of the hematuria is glomerular in origin (in the absence of proteinuria). It is important to remember that hematuria in patients on warfarin is not normal and suggests underlying pathology. Hematuria with proteinuria in a patient with diabetic nephropathy also needs evaluation to exclude underlying malignancy. When hematuria is noted on dipstick examination of the urine and no red blood cells are seen on the microscopic examination, the clinician needs to consider the presence of myoglobin.

Proteinuria

Normal protein excretion in older and younger adults does not differ significantly. Significant proteinuria is defined as greater than 150 mg per 24 hours. The urine dipstick is a good screening method for the detection of proteinuria, but it detects only albumin; light chains, which would be present in a patient with multiple myeloma, and low-molecular-weight protein (tubular protein) need to be detected by the use of a sulfa salicylic acid test. This test may be easily performed in the outpatient clinical setting.

When urinary proteins are primarily albumin and higher-molecular-weight proteins, the pathology is likely glomerular. Three grams of protein in a 24-hour urine sample is used to distinguish nephrotic from non-nephrotic proteinuria. The evaluation of proteinuria should begin with a careful examination of fresh urinary sediment (cells, casts), because this can provide helpful clues as to the mechanism of the proteinuria.

The urine dipstick method for detection of proteinuria is relatively insensitive, requiring urinary albumin concentrations of nearly 30 mg/dL. This means that a person with a urine output of 1 liter per day must be excreting nearly 300 mg of albumin per day before proteinuria can be detected. Micro-albuminuria, defined as a urinary albumin excretion of more than 30 mg per day (less than that detectable with the dipstick method), is an early indicator of progressing renal injury. This has become important because antihypertensive therapy, specifically ACE inhibitors, are being used to lower glomerular capillary pressures. This therapy reduces the proteinuria, which itself may be nephrotoxic, and retards the further development of renal damage, not only in diabetic but in nondiabetic kidney disease. Quantification of the severity of microalbuminuria does not require a 24-hour urine sample, as accurate enough estimates can be obtained with a timed early morning sample or simultaneous measurement of urinary creatinine concentration, or both.

Chronic Kidney Disease

The most useful measure of kidney function is an estimate of the GFR, because reductions in other functions (eg, tubular functions, concentrating ability, acid excretion) tend to parallel decline in GFR. The CrCl is the most reproducible measure of GFR available for clinical decision making. In older patients, creatinine production falls at nearly the same rate as the renal clearance of creatinine and, as noted previously, a normal serum creatinine may actually reflect a decline in kidney function. This pattern of change is important to recognize when the older patient is using drugs cleared primarily by the kidney. The relationship between serum creatinine and GFR has prompted a number of investigators to suggest that confounding variables could be corrected, so they have developed formulas to estimate CrCl as a measure of GFR. The most widely used formula is that of Cockcroft and Gault:

$$CrCl = \frac{(140 - age) \times weight}{72 \times serum\ creatinine}$$

Weight in kg; serum creatinine in mg/100 mL; 85% less in women.

This formula was developed and validated on highly selected samples of older adults that did not include many very old individuals. Only moderate correlations have subsequently been found between calculated and actual CrCls, especially in older populations.

Currently, no available method of estimating GFR from easily obtainable variables, such as age, sex, weight, and serum creatinine, is very accurate, and no method will be available until we have an easy method

for estimating muscle mass. In older adults, the lower limit of a normal GFR is not well defined. Nevertheless, in clinical practice, the use of an estimated GFR from the Cockcroft and Gault formula will provide a prompt and reasonable guide for clinical decision making in most situations. Cystatin C is an alternative measure of kidney function that may have prognostic importance among elderly adults who do not meet standard criteria for CKD (estimated GFR ≥60mL/min per 1.73m^2). Cystatin C seems to identify a "preclinical" state of kidney dysfunction that is not detected with serum creatinine or estimated GFR. Finally, it is important to recognize that certain commonly prescribed drugs (trimethoprim-sulfamethoxazole, cimetidine, and cefoxitin) compete with creatinine for tubular secretion, causing an increase in serum creatinine concentration without changing GFR. (See also the section on elimination in "Pharmacotherapy," p 68.)

IMAGING TECHNIQUES AND KIDNEY BIOPSY

Many imaging techniques are available to evaluate the genitourinary system. Ultrasonography is noninvasive and safe, and it can provide many diagnostic clues, showing kidney size, hydronephrosis of the collecting system, and solid and cystic parenchymal renal masses. An intravenous pyelogram shows more detail of the collecting system, including sites of obstruction and other pathology, such as papillary necrosis. However, it is best to avoid intravenous contrast in older adults with diabetes mellitus, CKD, hypertension, and, most notably, multiple myeloma, given the increased risk of contrast media-induced acute renal failure (ARF), especially if the person is dehydrated. If intravenous contrast absolutely must be used, the patient should be well hydrated before and for at least 24 hours after the procedure. Although the studies are controversial, use of N-acetylcysteine before procedures with contrast dye in high-risk patients is done in most clinical centers. Computed tomography scans, magnetic resonance imaging, isotopic renography, and angiography are additional techniques available to further evaluate selected kidney disorders.

For patients with suspected primary glomerular disease or unexplained kidney failure, a kidney biopsy may be indicated after all other available means for establishing a diagnosis have been exhausted. Kidney biopsy should be avoided because of age alone. At least half of all primary glomerular lesions responsible for the nephrotic syndrome are potentially treatable (eg, membranous glomerulopathy, minimal-change disease, vasculitis), and trials of immunosuppressive or corticosteroid therapies, or both, are warranted. However, when a condition unresponsive to these agents is diagnosed, such as primary amyloidosis, it is important not to subject older adults to the potentially serious side effects of these medications. In one study, more than 200 kidney biopsy samples in adults aged 60 and over with ARF were reviewed to evaluate whether the biopsy was useful in predicting organ and patient survival. The authors found that in more than 90% of the biopsies, a diagnosis of ARF was made; in many of these cases, a treatment was available; and in 30% of the cases, the diagnosis on biopsy did not match the clinical diagnosis. In summary, when a cause for ARF is unclear based on clinical and laboratory evaluation, a kidney biopsy is warranted. The exception would be the older adult who is unable to tolerate the indicated treatment for ARF because of comorbidity. It is important to work with the nephrologist and make certain that the patient is clinically stable for the procedure. This includes optimumally controlling blood-pressure and holding medications that might increase the risk of bleeding, (eg, aspirin).

DISEASES OF THE KIDNEY AND VASCULAR SYSTEM

A retrospective analysis examining the reason for kidney biopsy in 1368 older adults showed that the three most common reasons for referral were nephrotic syndrome (31%), acute renal insufficiency (26%), and chronic renal insufficiency (25%).

The incidence of nephrotic syndrome is at least as common in older adults as it is in younger people. The most common cause in older adults is membranous nephropathy (35%), followed by minimal-change disease (16%) and primary amyloidosis (12%). The incidence of membranous nephropathy, crescentic glomerulonephritis (GN), and amyloidosis is higher in older adults; the incidence of proliferative GN and immunoglobulin A nephropathy is lower; and the incidence of minimal-change disease is comparable to that for young adults but much lower than the rate seen in children. Diabetic nephropathy is probably the most common cause of nephrotic syndrome in older adults. The diagnosis is usually made based on a long (15- to 20-year) history of diabetes mellitus and the finding of diabetic retinopathy, and a biopsy is not necessary. Glomerulopathies resulting from systemic disease are more common in older adults because of the increased incidence of underlying diseases, such as amyloidosis (dysproteinemias), collagen vascular diseases (vasculitis), and neoplastic disease.

Membranous nephropathy (MN) is the most common form of primary kidney disease in older adults and is twice as common in older than in younger people. In a cohort of 155 patients over age 60 years followed for 20 years, older patients were more likely to be hypertensive, have worse kidney function, and experi-ence more thrombotic complications than younger patients. Possible causes of MN include medications (eg, NSAIDs, penicillamine), malignancies, and hepatitis B infection. One review reported that 11% of patients with MN had an underlying malignancy. In most patients the malignancy is clinically evident when MN is diagnosed, and probably only 1% to 2% of patients have an occult malignancy. Screening older adults with MN for malignancy should probably include a complete history and physical examination, chest radiograph, fecal occult blood tests, and colonoscopy. Older patients do seem more susceptible to the extra-renal complications of the nephrotic syndrome and its treatment, most notably, cardiovascular, thrombotic, and infectious events. The primary care physician is likely the first person called when acute symptoms develop, so it is essential that he or she be aware of these potential complications.

Minimal-change nephropathy presents similarly in young and old patients, but older people are more likely to have nonselective proteinuria, microscopic hematuria, hypertension, and renal insufficiency.

Most older adults with diabetic nephropathy have type 2 (non-insulin-dependent) diabetes. Control of blood pressure is important in slowing the rate of deterioration of kidney function. The use of ACE inhibitors or angiotensin-II receptor blockers, even in normotensive diabetic patients, promotes efferent arteriolar vasodilatation and decreases glomerular capillary pressure, which also slows the rate of deterioration of kidney function. Current recommendations are that in most patients with hypertension and CKD, an ACE inhibitor alone or in combination with an angiotensin-II receptor blocker should be used.

After diabetes, the next most common group of systemic diseases associated with kidney disease in older adults is the dysglobulinemias. These include amyloidosis, multiple myeloma, fibrillary GN, essential mixed cryoglobulinemia, and macroglobulinemia.

Acute Renal Insufficiency or Failure

ARF is at least as common in older as in younger adults. Controversy remains as to whether the prognosis is poorer in older adults, but there are no reasons to deny treatment for ARF, using any of the available techniques, on the basis of age. In older adults, azotemia and other consequences of ARF may induce acute behavioral changes that are usually reversible, and treatment should not be stopped on the assumption that the patient's mental status is irreversible. The primary physician is in a unique position to have an impact on both prevention and early detection of acute renal insufficiency. With a comprehensive medical history, physical examination, laboratory values, and urinalysis, it is usually possible to determine whether the cause of acute renal insufficiency is pre-renal, intra-renal, or post-renal. In general, a normal urinalysis suggests the cause is either pre-renal or post-renal.

Two clinical situations must be considered. The first is the development of acute renal insufficiency in the hospitalized or institutionalized patient being treated for a non-nephrologic illness. In this setting, intravascular volume depletion and acute tubular necrosis (ATN) are the major contributors—both of which may often be avoided with appropriate measures. The diagnosis is usually made based on the history, physical examination, and laboratory data, so that a kidney biopsy is not necessary. ARF has been reported in up to 8% of acutely hospitalized older adults aged 60 years and older. Although the studies vary, in general, ATN accounts for approximately 40% to 50% of the cases of ARF, and intravascular volume depletion for most of the remaining cases.

The second clinical situation to consider is whether acute renal insufficiency results from a primary kidney disease or is secondary to a systemic disease (such as diabetes mellitus, hypertensive or atherosclerotic vascular disease, or collagen vascular disease). Post-renal obstruction should always be excluded, because it is usually amenable to treatment.

Pre-Renal Acute Renal Insufficiency

Pre-renal ARF occurs when poor perfusion is causing the failure of kidney function. This type of ARF is of special importance in older adults. With acute hypotension, the decrease in kidney perfusion stimulates sympathetic activity and release of vasoconstrictor substances that further reduce GFR, contributing to ARF. Once the hemodynamic disturbances are corrected, the patient usually, but not always, recovers from the ARF. Loss of fluids (intravascular volume depletion), internal redistribution, decreased cardiac output, sepsis, and certain drugs (diuretics, ACE inhibitors) are responsible for the vast majority of cases of pre-renal ARF. In several series, intravascular volume depletion alone accounted for more than half of the cases of pre-renal ARF in older adults. The slow response to sodium retention, the decreased ability to concentrate urine, and most importantly, the impaired thirst regulation, all characteristics of the older patient, contribute to this high incidence.

The use of drugs that alter intrarenal hemodynamics is a growing cause of pre-renal ARF in older adults. The rapid development of pre-renal ARF in a patient recently started on an ACE inhibitor should make the clinician think about bilateral renal arterial stenosis. However, in one series, two thirds of the ACE inhibitor-related cases of ARF occurred in patients without renal arterial stenosis. Other factors that alter intrarenal hemodynamics include cardiac failure, concomitant use of NSAIDs (which inhibit prostaglandin production, an important regulator of kidney blood flow and GFR), diabetes mellitus, and volume depletion from any cause. (See the section on kidney diseases associated with NSAID use, p 374.)

It is important to distinguish between pre-renal ARF and ATN, which can develop in more severe cases. In patients who are oliguric, a urinary osmolality >500 mOsm/kg, a urinary sodium concentration <20 mEq/L, a urine-to-plasma creatinine ratio >40, or a fractional excretion of sodium <1% suggests pre-renal ARF. Generally, with pre-renal ARF the ratio of blood urea nitrogen to serum creatinine is >20. These urinary indices are not always reliable in differentiating pre-renal ARF from other forms of ARF. Probably the most reliable indicator of the pre-renal state is the response to treatment with volume (salt and water) repletion, but, again, older patients may have a delayed response to volume expansion.

Acute Tubular Necrosis

ATN can be either ischemic or nephrotoxic in origin. The causes of ischemic ATN are basically the same as those described in the preceding section as causes of pre-renal ARF, only more severe. In addition, surgical interventions, most notably cardiac surgery and repair of aortic aneurysms, as well as sepsis, account for most of the remaining cases in older adults. Hypotension during and after surgery, postoperative fluid loss, and arrhythmias may be important contributors. Measures to decrease the risk of ATN in the postoperative patient include careful attention to nutritional issues, avoidance of hypotension, prevention and treatment of postoperative infection, appropriate medication dosing, and hydration. (See also "Perioperative Care," p 92.)

Most of the antibiotics effective in treating serious infections have been associated with nephrotoxic ATN. Age is a well-known risk factor for the development of aminoglycoside nephrotoxicity. Preexisting kidney disease and volume depletion may contribute to medication accumulation, leading to ATN. When it is necessary to use an aminoglycoside antibiotic in an older adult, monitoring blood levels is essential.

Older adults also are at increased risk of developing radiocontrast-induced ARF. Although the non-ionic contrast dye has been reported in the literature to be less toxic to the kidneys, in practice, the risk of an acute renal insult is likely not significantly reduced. As mentioned earlier, it is best to avoid the use of intravenous contrast dye in any patient with preexisting impaired of kidney function, multiple myeloma, vascular disease, intravascular volume depletion, or diabetes. Hydration before and after procedures using contrast agents has been reported to be effective in reducing the incidence and severity of ARF in high-risk patients.

Clearly, when ARF develops, it needs to be managed promptly—but perhaps one of the most important roles of the clinician is preventing hospital-acquired ARF. With daily attention to changes in fluid intake, urine production, weight, and orthostatic blood-pressure measurements, the development of intravascular volume contraction in many older adults can be identified before significant symptoms develop. Another common cause of intravascular volume depletion is the order for "nothing by mouth" written in anticipation of a procedure, or the order for enemas written as a bowel preparation. When a procedure is delayed and maintenance intravenous fluids are not given, symptomatic intravascular volume depletion may develop in the frail older adult, with all the associated risks, including falls. (See also "Perioperative Care," p 92.)

Although the older kidney is able to defend against changes in volume, the response to correction is delayed. Avoiding the simultaneous use of multiple medications that may interact also is of benefit. For example, in the treatment of heart failure, the combination of a diuretic and an ACE inhibitor together with an NSAID can lead to development of renal insufficiency unless the patient is carefully monitored. When an older hospitalized patient is being treated by several clinicians, it may be prudent to write orders for "no NSAIDs" when appropriate.

Other Intrarenal Causes of Acute Renal Failure

In one review of 259 kidney biopsies done for ARF on adults aged 60 and older (remembering that when the cause of ARF has been established by the history, physical examination, and laboratory data, a kidney biopsy is not done), the following diagnoses were made: pauci-immune crescentic GN (with or without arteritis) in 31% of the biopsy samples, acute interstitial nephritis (AIN) in 19%, ATN with nephrotic syndrome in 8%, atheroemboli in 7%, ATN alone in 7%, light chain cast nephropathy in 6%, postinfectious GN in 5.5%, antiglomerular membrane antibody nephritis in 4%, and immunoglobulin A nephropathy or Henoch-Schönlein syndrome in 4%.

Acute GN in older adults often presents with circulatory congestion that suggests heart failure, in contrast to the hypertension and edema seen in younger patients. This observation, together with low urinary sodium concentrations and high ratios of blood urea nitrogen to serum creatinine that suggest pre-renal ARF, results in the misdiagnosis of acute GN as heart failure.

Acute or subacute GN may be an immunologic consequence of a systemic disease, for example, lupus erythematosus, vasculitis, Wegener's granulomatosis, mixed cryoglobulinemia, or a primary kidney disease of unknown cause, for example, crescentic GN with or without glomerular immune deposits. Other forms of proliferative GN include mesangioproliferative GN (including immunoglobulin A nephropathy), focal proliferative GN, crescentic GN (including antiglomerular basement membrane disease), and vasculitis. It is important to remember that acute postinfectious GN remains a common entity.

AIN is caused by a variety of agents and probably has no special implications for older adults except for the higher prevalence of NSAID-induced AIN, discussed below, and the fact that older adults tend to be on multiple medications.

Renal vascular causes of ARF are discussed below. Rhabdomyolysis with ARF is seen in the setting of acute immobilization, infectious diseases, stroke, hyperosmolar states, hyponatremia, hypernatremia, and after falls associated with muscle trauma.

Obstructive Nephropathy

Urinary obstruction is one of the most common causes of ARF in older adults. It is an important diagnosis to make because it is usually reversible. Prostatic hypertrophy or carcinoma is the most common cause, but other causes include retroperitoneal or pelvic neoplasia, such as lymphoma and carcinoma of the bladder, cervix, uterus, ovaries, or rectum. Another cause of post-renal obstruction may be a blocked indwelling Foley catheter.

Laboratory findings with obstructive ARF tend to be nonspecific, with high urinary sodiums and decreased osmolalities and a nondiagnostic urinalysis. The ratio of blood urea nitrogen to serum creatinine is usually increased. Ultrasonography is safe and readily available, and it has become the initial evaluation of choice in most settings. In most cases, obstruction can be diagnosed based on a dilated collecting system or large distended bladder.

Renal Vascular Disease

Nearly half of both normotensive and hypertensive people aged 60 and over with evidence of atherosclerotic aortoiliac or peripheral vascular disease, or both, show some obstruction (>50% narrowing) of the renal artery. In most of these patients, the obstruction goes unrecognized and is not clinically important. However, in some individuals, severe hypertension or progressive kidney disease, or both, may develop. Correction of stenosis may reverse these consequences. Therefore, any patient with suspected severe renal artery stenosis should have a diagnostic evaluation. If a significant stenosis is found, the patient should be referred for evaluation for either percutaneous transluminal renal angioplasty or surgical revascularization of the renal artery. Clues suggesting hemodynamically significant renal artery stenosis include the new onset of severe hypertension, significant worsening of preexistent hypertension, failure to control hypertension on previously effective medications, repeated episodes of pulmonary edema, and renal insufficiency in the absence of urinary abnormalities or other known cause. The last may be most dramatic in patients started on ACE inhibitors. A vascular bruit may be heard in the mid-abdomen or flank.

Occlusive arterial disease can cause either acute or chronic kidney failure with or without changes in the urinalysis and urinary sediment. Renal arterial embolization or thrombosis may be seen in patients with acute myocardial infarction, chronic atrial fibrillation, and subacute bacterial endocarditis. Symptoms vary from a slowly progressive, clinically silent event to severe acute flank pain and tenderness, hematuria, hypertension, fever, nausea, and vomiting. Serum lactic dehydrogenase concentrations increase dramatically after 1 to 2 days and remain elevated for a week or more.

Renal cholesterol embolization may be seen after vascular manipulation (ie, aortic surgery or angiography) or in association with anticoagulation or thrombolytics. Although less common, cholesterol emboli may also develop spontaneously. The usual course is a progressive kidney disease and worsening hypertension, but it can be acute with a vasculitic picture, including oliguria or anuria, fever, eosinophilia, eosinophiluria, hypocomplementemia, and embolization to other organs, including the extremities (digital infarctions). Hints to this diagnosis include livedo reticularis and cholesterol emboli on a dilated funduscopic examination (which should be performed on every patient when this diagnosis is suspected). The urinalysis is usually unremarkable, although hematuria and mild proteinuria may be seen. If the diagnosis remains unclear or other diagnoses exist as valid possibilities (radiocontrast nephropathy, endocarditis with left-sided emboli, vasculitis, thrombotic emboli), a definitive diagnosis may be made on visualization of cholesterol crystals on a biopsy of the skin or kidney.

Kidney Diseases Associated With NSAID Use

NSAIDs are widely taken by older adults because of their effectiveness in relieving pain in a variety of common chronic musculoskeletal disorders. Older adults are more predisposed than younger ones to the adverse effects of NSAIDs on the kidneys because of the age-associated decline in kidney function, the increased prevalence of such comorbid conditions as heart failure, hypertension, cirrhosis, and CKD, and the high use of concomitant drugs that affect kidney function (eg, diuretics, antihypertensives). It should be possible to use these drugs safely in older adults and maintain a low risk-to-benefit ratio, because those who are at risk of NSAID-induced kidney disease can be identified and monitored.

As mentioned above, NSAIDs can alter intrarenal hemodynamics and decrease GFR. NSAIDs can induce a variety of acute and chronic renal lesions. AIN can follow the use of nearly all NSAIDs. The typical clinical picture includes the nephrotic syndrome with acute renal insufficiency in a patient who has been on NSAIDs for months. An increase in eosinophils in blood or urine, or both, with NSAID-induced AIN is not nearly as common as in AIN caused by penicillin or other agents. The kidney abnormalities usually improve after the medication is discontinued, with or without corticosteroid therapy, but chronic renal insufficiency and even ESRD may occur. The AIN results primarily from a delayed hypersensitivity response to NSAIDs, and the nephrotic syndrome results from changes in glomerular permeability mediated by prostaglandins and other hormones. Less commonly, nephrotic syndrome may occur without AIN; rarely, an immune complex glomerulopathy is observed. Patients taking NSAIDs for months or years can develop papillary necrosis, chronic interstitial nephritis, and even ESRD. Case-control studies show that patients at increased risk are older men with chronic heart disease and kidney hypoperfusion. Impaired medullary circulation and direct toxicity due to a drug metabolite appear to play a critical role in inducing interstitial fibrosis, which can be facilitated by a sustained production of some growth factors and cytokines. The newer COX-2 inhibitors may also injure to the kidneys.

Chronic Kidney Failure

An examination of kidney biopsy results in older adults with chronic kidney failure showed that the most common histologic findings are hypertensive nephrosclerosis, focal segmental glomerulosclerosis, interstitial nephritis, and amyloidosis. Again, in patients with chronic kidney failure in which a cause is clear from the history and physical examination (eg, diabetes mellitus), no biopsy would be necessary.

Several points are made with regard to chronic renal insufficiency in older adults: First, although chronic elevation of serum creatinine represents a loss of kidney function that likely will not be recovered, defining the underlying pathology can help to prevent further loss of function. Second, the degree of kidney failure may be much greater than indicated by the serum creatinine, so that cognitive difficulties may develop at lower-than-expected serum creatinine levels. Third, although this area needs considerable research, some data suggest that erythropoietin serum levels do not change with age. Data also suggest that anemia secondary to erythropoietin deficiency may develop with more mild cases of renal insufficiency than previously thought. Preventing a further decline in kidney function or the development of "acute or chronic" kidney failure is critical. This requires careful attention to medication dosing, measurement of serum blood levels of medications when available, and avoidance of medications known to accumulate in renal insufficiency, including magnesium-containing compounds and meperidine. In addition, older adults with renal insufficiency are even less able than healthy older adults to defend against physiologic stress, including a free water load, salt challenge, or acidosis; this should be considered during acute illness. Lastly, as detailed below, early referral to a nephrologist and pre-ESRD care are very important.

Early Referral to a Nephrologist and Pre-ESRD Care

Early referral of older adults with evidence of kidney disease to a nephrologist is important. In general, when the serum creatinine is ≥1.5 mg/dL, patients should be referred for a nephrology consultation. A national effort is being made to improve pre-ESRD care, with national guidelines established by the Kidney Disease Outcomes Quality Initiative (KDOQI). The goal of the nephrology consultation is to determine the type of kidney disease, to define any associated comorbid conditions, and to assess the severity of renal dysfunction and any associated risk factors. A plan should be developed to address specific therapies for CKD and associated complications, maximize GFR, treat comorbid conditions, prevent cardiac disease, and when indicated, begin planning for replacement therapy. In addition, data suggest that beginning dialysis early in older adults may improve clinical outcomes and patient survival; early referral contributes to this positive outcome.

With regard to blood-pressure control, in patients with CKD the goal blood pressure is less than 130/80 mm Hg. High blood pressure is both a cause and consequence of CKD. Poorly controlled blood pressure may accelerate a decline in kidney function and exacerbate underlying cardiovascular disease. Whenever tolerated, an ACE inhibitor or angiotensin receptor blocker (ARB) should be used together with a diuretic. Attention to life-style change, including weight control, smoking, and an adherence to a low-salt diet, is also very important.

A normocytic, normochromic anemia is associated with CKD and is usually secondary to either decreased production of erythropoietin (EPO) or possibly inhibitors of erythropoiesis. However, before this diagnosis is made other common causes of anemia need to be excluded. Peripheral blood smear, screening for fecal occult blood, serum B_{12}, and iron studies should be done in all patients. If folate deficiency is suspected, a red blood cell folate should be measured. After other causes for anemia are excluded, a patient may be considered for EPO therapy. The goal hematocrit/hemoglobin is 33–36/11–12 to reduce the risk of heart disease, cognitive dysfunction, higher hospitalization rates, and increased mortality.

Individuals with CKD (GFR <60 mL/min) are at risk of alterations in calcium-phosphate metabolism that place them at risk of underling bone disease. The histologic types of bone disease vary in different clinical settings. Several therapies are available, but again, need to be individualized, depending on bone histology and clinical setting. All patients should have a serum phosphate, calcium, and parathyroid hormone measurement done before being referred to a nephrologist.

Individuals with CKD are also at risk of metabolic acidosis and loss of bone mineral. The national guidelines include recommendations that the serum CO_2 be greater than 22 mEq/L to protect against bone loss.

Dialysis and Transplantation

A 1999 report from the U.S. Renal Data System indicates that in 1997 more than half of all patients on chronic dialysis were aged 65 years or older. Diabetes mellitus, hypertension, GN, and obstructive nephropathy are the most common causes of ESRD in this group. The number of older adults started on dialysis has increased for two reasons. First, there is increased referral and acceptance of older adults, especially those with serious comorbid conditions. Second, the increased survival rates of other competing diseases, such as coronary artery disease or diabetes, increase the chances that a person will survive to develop ESRD.

The results of studies looking at life satisfaction and functional status in older adults on dialysis have varied. One prospective cohort study found that life satisfaction of older adults on dialysis and those in the control group did not differ significantly at 3 years. For some older adults living alone or in isolation, time spent on dialysis was a time to interact both with their "neighbors" on dialysis and with nursing staff; in a sense, this becomes their social life. It is also clear that rehabilitation (occupational and physical therapy) is important in slowing the loss of function in the dialysis patient. The choice of hemodialysis or peritoneal dialysis (chronic ambulatory peritoneal dialysis) depends on the patient's wishes and overall condition, the physician's expertise, and available resources. Neither method offers any advantage in survival rates when patients with similar risk factors are compared.

An alternative therapy for ESRD in older adults is kidney transplantation. The results have improved because of better patient selection, improved perioperative care, and the use of safer, more effective immunosuppression. Despite improved survival, kidney transplantation in persons aged 65 years and over remains uncommon and controversial, largely because of a reluctance to allocate a scarce resource (the donor kidney) to an older adult with a limited life expectancy. Because older adults have a senescent immune system, they may require less aggressive immunotherapy.

One report comparing older adults with a kidney transplant with those on dialysis (matched by age, underlying diagnosis leading to ESRD, and number of comorbid conditions) showed that after adjusting for known prognostic factors, the transplant patients had a much better (twofold) survival probability than did the patients on dialysis. The 5-year survival rates were 81% for transplant patients and 51% for dialysis patients. In addition, a study comparing graft survival in patients aged 18 to 59 with that in patients 60 years and older found that in the absence of risk factors (pretransplant history of nonskin cancer, vascular disease, or being an active smoker), the survival rates were similar. These findings have important implications for future management of ESRD patients aged 60 years and older.

REFERENCES

■ Fried LF, Lee JS, Shlipak M, et al. Chronic kidney disease and functional limitation in older people: health, aging and body composition study. *J Am Geriatr Soc.* 2006;54(5):750–756.

■ Levey AS, Coresh J, Balk E, et al. National Kidney Foundation practice guidelines for chronic kidney disease: evaluation, classification and stratification. *Ann Intern Med.* 2003;139(2):137–147.

■ Loos C, Briancon S, Frimat L, et al. Effect of end-stage renal disease on the quality of life of older adults. *J Am Geriatr Soc.* 2003;51(2):229–233.

■ Luckey AE, Parsa CJ. Fluid and electrolytes the elderly. *Arch Surg.* 2003;138(10):1055–1060.

■ Shlipak MG, Katz R, Sarnak MJ, et al. Cystatin C and prognosis for cardiovascular and kidney outcomes in elderly persons without chronic kidney disease. *Ann Intern Med.* 2006;145(4):237–246.

CHAPTER 51—GYNECOLOGIC DISEASES AND DISORDERS

KEY POINTS

■ Many older women do not spontaneously discuss gynecologic problems, yet many of these problems are treatable.

■ Symptomatic urogenital atrophy is common in postmenopausal women and is readily reversed with the administration of local estrogen.

■ Half of all cases of invasive cancer of the vulva occur in women over the age of 70 years.

■ Pessaries may improve comfort and bladder function in some older women with pelvic organ prolapse.

Most older women do not seek regular gynecologic care. This may be in part because they are reticent about discussing personal gynecologic problems. Important and treatable disorders consequently go undiagnosed until they become severely disabling. For example, although urinary incontinence affects 16 million adults in the United States, the average time between onset and reporting to a physician is 8.5 years; gynecologic problems such as genital prolapse and atrophic vaginitis often exacerbate urinary incontinence. Full gynecologic examination should be a routine part of a complete history and physical examination for all older women who are amenable to screening.

HISTORY AND PHYSICAL EXAMINATION

The latest American College of Obstetrics and Gynecology recommendations for primary care of women aged 65 and older include inquiring about not only routine gynecologic issues but also about involuntary loss of urine or feces, sexual behavior patterns and potential exposure to sexually transmitted diseases, and use of alternative medical treatments.

Nongynecologic medical problems that can have significant gynecologic effects should be noted in the history. For example, breast cancer therapy typically leads to severe urogenital atrophy, obesity can result in hyperestrogenic states due to peripheral conversion of androgens to estrogen, and osteoporotic lordosis causes increased intra-abdominal pressure and resultant predisposition to genital prolapse. Previous obstetrical events may cause pelvic floor neuromuscular damage and eventual development of urinary incontinence and genital prolapse.

If a woman is on hormone replacement, the regimen should be reviewed annually to assure adherence, need for continued therapy, and absence of abnormal side effects. If the uterus is present, estrogen must be combined with a progestin in order to prevent the development of endometrial hyperplasia (see the section on hormone replacement therapy in "Endocrine and Metabolic Disorders," p 347). The history should also include inquiry about abdominal distention (sign of ovarian cancer) and abnormal vaginal discharge or bleeding (signs of endometrial, cervical, or vaginal cancer).

The pelvic examination also presents an opportunity to discuss sexual function with the patient. Although the lack of available, sexually capable men may limit an elderly woman's sexual activities, many older women are interested in maintaining sexual relationships. Issues related to sexual activity such as atrophy-related dyspareunia, postcoital bleeding, and sexually transmitted diseases should be addressed. Many women require reassurance that enjoyable sexual activity is possible and normal at their age. Also, women who maintain regular sexual activity are less likely to have significant vaginal atrophy.

Most ambulatory elderly women can assume the lithotomy position. Because the vaginal introitus may be small and stenotic, smaller speculums may be needed. The dorsal position, in stirrups for a pelvic examination, requires flexion and external rotation of the hips. Patients with osteoarthritis who find the lithotomy position uncomfortable or impossible to assume will need to use an alternative position. The left lateral decubitus position is one alternative. The patient lies on her left side, with knees flexed. The upper hip (right) is flexed to a greater degree and the right leg is elevated, exposing the perineum. An adequate speculum and bimanual examination can usually be done in this position. To examine a bedbound patient, position an inverted bedpan under the sacrum to elevate the pelvis. Water-based lubricants facilitate the examination and can be used if a Pap smear will be performed.

In performing the pelvic examination of an older woman, the examiner should:

- examine the vulva for abnormal pigmentation, erythema, or raised lesions;

- look for signs of urogenital atrophy, including urethral caruncle, vaginal dryness, pale vaginal mucosa, loss of rugae, and reduced vaginal caliber and depth;

- have the patient perform Valsalva's maneuver to evaluate for pelvic organ prolapse and urinary incontinence;

- carefully palpate for pelvic masses or ovarian enlargement on bimanual examination;

- perform a Pap smear if indicated (see the section on cervical cancer in "Prevention," p 62).

The presence of significant vaginal mucosal atrophic changes may lead to inadequate or abnormal Pap smear interpretation. In this situation, the Pap smear should be repeated after 2 to 3 months of local estrogen therapy. Bimanual examinations and perineal inspection performed annually may detect vulvar, vaginal, or ovarian pathology. A rectal examination could also be performed at the same time in order to identify masses, detect occult bleeding, and evaluate the anal sphincter.

Ovaries become smaller with aging, and any palpable adnexal tissue should prompt consideration of malignancy. Although uterine fibroids are common, any increase in uterus size should be investigated. An ovarian or uterine mass could be evaluated by abdominal or pelvic ultrasound (using a vaginal probe) to determine location and character. Sonography, however, cannot definitively establish the nature (benign or malignant) of the mass, so further evaluation with laparoscopy ultimately depends on clinical judgment.

TREATMENT OF MENOPAUSAL SYMPTOMS

Estrogen is labeled by the U.S. Food and Drug Administration (FDA) for the treatment of menopausal symptoms and urogenital dryness and for the prevention of osteoporosis, but estrogen replacement therapy (ERT) has historically been used by clinicians for other reasons as well. The common short- and long-term uses, common prescribing practices, and risks of ERT are reviewed herein.

Menopause on average occurs at age 51 in the United States. With a life expectancy of 78 years, the average woman is postmenopausal one third of her life. Despite some controversy about the risks and benefits of ERT, many women and their physicians choose to treat or prevent the sequelae of estrogen deficiency in menopause, although the popularity of this therapy is waning in response to findings of the Women's Health Initiative (WHI) trial.

Vasomotor symptoms or hot flushes are the most common symptom of the climacteric, occurring in up to 80% of perimenopausal women. Symptoms persist beyond 5 years in 25% of women and are lifelong in a small minority. Although the cause of the vasomotor response remains unknown, vasomotor symptoms are usually relieved within the first cycle of estrogen treatment. Low-dose therapy can be initiated and estrogen doses titrated until symptoms improve. When estrogen is contraindicated or not acceptable, selective serotonin-reuptake inhibitors or progestins are considered the second most effective therapies. Clonidine[OL], methyldopa[OL], or herbal remedies such as yams and black cohosh have also been tried with little evidence to support their use.

See also the section on hormone replacement therapy in "Endocrine and Metabolic Disorders" (p 347) and the section on ERT and osteoporosis prevention in "Osteoporosis and Osteomalacia" (p 201).

TREATMENT OF UROGENITAL SYMPTOMS

Estrogen deficiency causes atrophy of both the vaginal and urethral mucosa. Both have a high density of estrogen receptors. Although randomized trials are few and have yielded variable results, a Cochrane Database Review suggests that estrogen may improve urge incontinence more than placebo.

See also "Disorders of Sexual Function" (p 382) and "Urinary Incontinence" (p 171).

UROGENITAL ATROPHY

The lower genital tract is exquisitely sensitive to estrogen. Urogenital atrophy occurs in all postmenopausal women. Proliferation and maturation of the vaginal epithelium depends on adequate estrogen stimulation. With reduction of estrogen production, genital blood flow decreases, leading to further decline in delivery of estrogen to those tissues. This reduction in microvascularity leads to vaginal dryness, mucosal pallor, decreased rugation, mucosal thinning, inflammation with discharge, and, ultimately, decreased vaginal caliber and depth. With progressive atrophy, the vaginal Pap smear–maturation index shows atrophic changes with a decrease in mucosal superficial cells and an increase in intermediate and basal cells. Many women experience dyspareunia, burning, and even vaginal bleeding in some cases (Figure 51.1).

These changes are somewhat readily reversed with the administration of local estrogen. The intravaginal use of estrogen cream, one half an applicator (1 to 2 g) as infrequently as two nights per week, allows topical estrogen therapy with minimal (if any) absorption, endometrial proliferation, or other systemic ef-

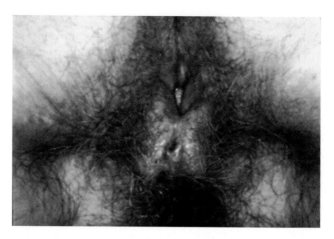

Figure 51.1—Severe vulvovaginal atrophy, including labial fusion secondary to lichen sclerosus.

fects. The available prescription estrogen creams appear to be therapeutically equivalent. The estrogen ring may be used for 3 months per ring, and vaginal tablets are available for use twice a week. Estrogen cream is also an excellent lubricant for use during intercourse or for pessary insertion. (See also "Disorders of Sexual Function," p 382.)

VULVOVAGINAL INFECTION AND INFLAMMATION

Postmenopausal women are susceptible to a broad range of vulvovaginal infections. Candidal infection, common in diabetic and obese patients who are plagued with moisture and irritation, can be treated with oral, intravaginal, and topical antifungal agents. Patients should be questioned about their ability to insert a vaginal applicator before beginning therapy. Topical corticosteroids can be used to hasten relief of symptoms. Combination therapy may be necessary, as older women commonly present with more chronic, untreated candidal infections that spread from the vulva to the inguinal areas. Other vaginal infections common in reproductive age women such as trichomonas and *Gardnerella* vaginosis are less common in elderly women, likely because of the higher vaginal pH. A wet preparation revealing sheets of inflammatory cells without bacterial forms may represent advanced atrophy rather than an infectious cause. Local estrogen cream in the case of a symptomatic woman with atrophic vaginitis is effective.

DISORDERS OF THE VULVA

With aging, the skin of the vulva loses elasticity, and the underlying fat and connective tissues undergo degeneration, with loss of collagen and thinning of the epithelial layer. Consequently, postmenopausal women not on estrogen are predisposed to a variety of dermatologic disorders and symptoms. The assessment of vulvar complaints must include direct examination. Any pigmented lesion or lesions that do not respond to topical corticosteroid or estrogen treatment *must* be promptly biopsied.

Vulvar skin irritation occurs from a variety of agents and causes burning, itching, and edema. Hygienic products used for urinary or fecal incontinence may lead to chemical dermatitis, as does urine itself. Treatment of incontinence is important to solving this problem. Vulvar burning or pain is rarely due to estrogen deficiency, and this complaint should be investigated rather than treated with ever-increasing doses of estrogen. Vulvar excoriation can result from scratching of an inflamed vulva. Local corticosteroids such as hydrocortisone 1% ointment applied daily, sitz baths, or use of a bidet can help alleviate vulvar irritation. Any chronically irritated area should be biopsied to exclude a malignancy.

Vulvar dystrophy is a somewhat outdated term used to describe both benign and malignant vulvar squamous changes. The preferred terminology set out by the International Society for the Study of Vulvovaginal Disease outlines three classes of non-neoplastic vulvar lesions. These are lichen sclerosus, squamous cell hyperplasia, and other dermatoses. A separate classification is used for biopsy-proven dysplastic lesions. These vulvar intraepithelial neoplasias (VIN) are graded on the basis of the level of atypia (dysplasia).

Nonneoplastic Vulvar Lesions

Lichen sclerosus causes over one third of all vulvar dystrophies and may extend beyond the vulva to the perirectal areas. It is rarely precancerous. There is epithelial thinning with edema and fibrosis of the dermis. It can progress to shrinkage and adherence of the labia minora with reduction in introital caliber. Lesions are typically shiny, white or pink, and parchment-like. Lesions may be asymptomatic or may cause itching, vaginal soreness, and dyspareunia. Diagnosis is confirmed on biopsy of the involved vulvar areas. Recommended treatment involves daily application of a rather potent topical corticosteroid, clobetasol propionate 0.05%. Treatment should be continued for at least 3 months. Testosterone had been the mainstay of therapy but has been shown to be significantly less effective than clobetasol. Further measures include wearing cotton underwear and avoiding irritant soaps. Topical emollient agents including lanolin can be helpful, but petroleum jelly should be avoided.

Squamous hyperplasia appears as thickened, hyperplastic, elevated white keratinized lesions that can be difficult to distinguish clinically from VIN or condylomata. However, it is benign. Biopsy should precede treatment. Topical mid-potency corticosteroids such as triamcinolone 0.1% twice daily for a few weeks (or longer with thick lesions) resolves the lesions; intermittent therapy may be necessary.

Other vulvar lesions include lichen simplex chronicus, which presents with vulvar pruritus, and lichen planus, which presents as erosive, ulcerative lesions that can result in significant vulvar scarring. Mid-potency corticosteroids applied topically or intravaginally are recommended. In lichen planus involving the vagina, local estrogen cream should also be used.

Vulvar Neoplasia

All suspicious, unusual, or symptomatic vulvar lesions should be biopsied. VIN lesions are not usually precancerous. VIN is most often seen in postmenopausal women, but the incidence of VIN does not increase with age. Over half of cases are asymptomatic. When symptoms are present, the most common is pruritus. The clinical appearance is the same as squamous hyperplasia or may be simply pigmentation. Lesions are often multifocal.

Invasive cancer of the vulva is an age-related malignancy; half of all cases occur after age 70. The vast majority are squamous cell carcinomas. Malignant melanoma, sarcoma, basal cell, carcinoma, and adenocarcinoma account for under 20% of cases. Treatment involves surgery (radical vulvectomy), occasionally accompanied by radiation.

DISORDERS OF PELVIC FLOOR SUPPORT

Child bearing and activities that increase intra-abdominal pressure cause progressive weakening of the connective tissue and muscular supports of the genital organs and can lead to genital prolapse. Conditions such as constipation, chronic coughing, and heavy lifting commonly increase intra-abdominal pressure. Common symptoms of prolapse include pelvic pressure, lower back pain, urinary or fecal incontinence, difficulty with rectal emptying, or a palpable mass. Traditional classification of vaginal prolapse differentiated protrusion of the posterior vaginal wall (enterocele or rectocele), descent of the anterior vaginal wall (cystocele), and prolapse of the vaginal apex. These conditions are demonstrated by having the patient bear down or cough while in the dorsal lithotomy position, but the full extent of prolapse is better appreciated with a standing Valsalva's maneuver.

Vaginal prolapse represents a pelvic organ hernia through the vaginal hiatus.

The 1995 American College of Obstetrics and Gynecology classification of pelvic organ prolapse is outlined in Table 51.1. The International Continence Society and the American Urogynecologic Association adopted a new, rather complex prolapse classification system that is based on measurement of the distance between vaginal anatomic sites and the hymeneal ring. The purpose of this classification, which is used by specialty societies, is to more objectively and reproducibly describe a patient's degree of prolapse.

Mild prolapse (1st or 2nd degree; see Table 51.1) can be retarded with adequate estrogenization and Kegel's exercises to strengthen the pelvic floor musculature (see the Appendix, p 500, for exercise instructions for the patient). Genital prolapse does not always lead to bladder dysfunction and should not be assumed to be the cause of incontinence (see "Urinary Incontinence," p 171). Correcting the prolapse will in some cases cause or exacerbate incontinence. On the other hand, large cystoceles or rectoceles may produce urinary retention, and reduction of the cystocele may restore normal bladder function.

Pessaries

Pessaries are commonly employed in an effort to delay or avoid surgery. Their use in older women may be indicated to provide comfort and restore bladder function when comorbid illness makes surgery undesirable. Such women may elect long-term pessary use under medical supervision. Available pessaries are made from rubber, plastic, or silicone. A variety of shapes and sizes are available: doughnuts, rings, cubes, inflatable balls, and foldable models. Pessary care requirements often influence the selection of a device and the amount of follow-up required.

The choice of pessary is influenced by the degree of prolapse, presence of incontinence, type of accompanying tissue relaxation, and ease of care. Patients with prolapse and no incontinence require only space-occupying types. Those with stress incontinence benefit from a foldable type, which restores bladder neck support. Ring pessaries are easier to insert and remove and may be preferred by older women.

Pessary selection often proceeds by trial and error; the optimal pessary fits snugly but comfortably and allows voiding and defecating without difficulty. After pessary selection and insertion, clinical follow-up within a few days is essential to ascertain satisfactory usage. After initial fitting and recheck, pessaries should be removed and cleaned, and the vaginal walls inspected. Pessary care requirements often influence the selection of a device and the amount of follow-up required for individual patients. If an older woman's mobility or manual dexterity permit, she should be

Table 51.1—Classification of Pelvic Organ Prolapse

Class	Description
1st degree	Extension to the mid-vagina
2nd degree	Approaching the hymenal ring
3rd degree	At the hymenal ring
4th degree	Beyond the hymenal ring

SOURCE: Data from American College of Obstetricians and Gynecologists. *Pelvic Organ Prolapse*. Washington, DC: American College of Obstetricians and Gynecologists. Technical Bulletin No. 214; 1995.

advised to remove the pessary twice a week, wash it with soap and water, and reinsert it with a water-soluble lubricant; she should use 1 g vaginal estrogen cream twice a week as well. Patients who cannot provide this level of self-care should be assisted at periodic office visits or by a visiting nurse. All patients with pessaries should be instructed to report any unusual discharge, bleeding, or discomfort, and any changes in bladder or bowel function, and all should have a pelvic examination once or twice a year. If discomfort is present or the device becomes uncomfortable, a different size or type should be tried. Pessaries do not work as well with marked vaginal outlet relaxation. If a pessary is left in place for long periods without monitoring, fibrous tissue may form around the pessary, and removal under anesthesia may be necessary.

Surgery for Prolapse

Surgical treatment of vaginal prolapse can be classified as either reconstructive or obliterative. Reconstructive procedures are designed to restore normal anatomy, whereas obliterative procedures result in closure of the vaginal canal. Vaginal reconstructive procedures include sacrospinous fixation (for apical prolapse), anterior repairs (for a cystocele), and posterior repairs (for a rectocele). These can safely be done under regional anesthesia, which minimizes anesthetic risks. Abdominal reconstructive procedures include sacrocolpopexy (for apical prolapse) and paravaginal repairs (for a cystocele). They typically require general anesthesia. Urinary incontinence procedures can be done either vaginally or abdominally at the time of the prolapse surgery. (See also "Urinary Incontinence," p 171.)

Obliterative procedures are restricted to elderly women who are not, and will not be, sexually active. In a LeFort colpocleisis, the anterior and posterior vaginal walls are sutured together, obliterating the vaginal canal. The simplicity and safety are very attractive for the oldest-old women, as the procedure can be done under local anesthesia in the outpatient setting. Anti-incontinence procedures can be done at the same time, as well. Limitation of physical activities and intra-abdominal pressure increase for 6 to 12 weeks postoperatively, the performance of pelvic floor exercises, and use of vaginal estrogen cream are key in optimizing the success rate of surgical therapy. The impact on quality of life of prolapse surgery for the patient can be quite remarkable, as a large, exteriorized prolapse can markedly limit a woman's ability to perform physical and social activities.

Age, in itself, is not a contraindication to surgery for genital prolapse. When a proven protocol for perioperative care, including preoperative medical clearance, regional anesthesia, infection prophylaxis, and deep-vein thrombosis prophylaxis, is followed, vaginal surgery offers a safe alternative to pessary use for elderly women with symptomatic genital prolapse. (See also "Perioperative Care," p 92.)

POSTMENOPAUSAL VAGINAL BLEEDING

Postmenopausal bleeding (defined as bleeding after 1 year of amenorrhea) occurs in a significant number of older women. The challenge is not only to exclude gynecologic malignancies but also to alleviate the symptoms and eliminate the cause of benign conditions. Causes of bleeding can be grouped according to anatomic areas and endocrine dysfunction (Table 51.2). Not all complaints of postmenopausal bleeding are related to the reproductive organs but may be confused by the patients as originating from these areas. Proper evaluation involves complete physical examination and directed diagnostic studies. Endometrial hyperplasia and cancer can be evaluated with endometrial biopsy or by measuring the endometrial thickness on vaginal probe ultrasound. Though neither ultrasound nor biopsy is 100% specific, an endometrial thickness of less than 5 mm on ultrasound essentially excludes hyperplasia and malignancy. Dilation and curettage is reserved for cases where tissue cannot otherwise be adequately sampled or when bleeding persists. The use of direct visualization (hysteroscopy) during the procedure is the most accurate method for tissue sampling. New techniques for destruction of the endometrial lining (ablation) by heat, cold, or excision may be helpful in women whose bleeding is proven to be due to nonmalignant conditions.

Exogenous hormone replacement is a common cause of postmenopausal bleeding. Women on continuous combined estrogen-progesterone replacement who continue to have bleeding after 1 year must be evaluated. Some specialists recommend biopsy if bleeding persists beyond 6 months. Women on cyclic hormone therapy who bleed at an unexpected time during the cycle should also be evaluated. (See also the section on hormone replacement therapy in "Endocrine and Metabolic Disorders," p 347.)

Table 51.2—Causes of Postmenopausal Vaginal Bleeding

Cervical
  Carcinoma
  Cervicitis
  Polyp

Endocrinologic
  Exogenous hormones
  Perimenopausal ovarian function

Ovarian
  Functioning ovarian tumor

Uterine
  Endometrial atrophy
  Hyperplasia
  Neoplasia
  Polyp
  Submucosal leiomyoma

Vaginal
  Atrophy
  Inflammation
  Tumor
  Ulceration

Vulvar
  Carcinoma
  Laceration or ulceration
  Urethral caruncle

Other
  Coagulation disorder
  Rectal lesion
  Urinary tract infection

CLIMACTERIC SYNDROMES

See the section on estrogen replacement therapy in "Endocrine and Metabolic Disorders" (p 347).

REFERENCES

■ Adams E, Thomson A, Maher C, et al. Mechanical devices for pelvic organ prolapse in women. *Cochrane Database Syst Rev.* 2004(2):CD004010.

■ Bash KL. Review of vaginal pessaries. *Obstet Gynecol Surv.* 2000;55(7):455–460.

■ Fernando RJ, Thakar R, Sultan AH, et al. Effect of vaginal pessaries on symptoms associated with pelvic organ prolapse. *Obstet Gynecol.* 2006;108(1):93–99.

■ Lachance JA, Everett EN, Greer B, et al. The effect of age on clinical/pathologic features, surgical morbidity, and outcome in patients with endometrial cancer. *Gynecol Oncol.* 2006;101(3):470–475.

■ Rivkin ME Nonneoplastic epithelial disorders of the vulva www.emedicine.com/med/topic3294.htm. *WebMD.* September 3, 2006.

CHAPTER 52—DISORDERS OF SEXUAL FUNCTION

KEY POINTS

- Normal age-associated changes in sexuality lead to declines in sexual function; however, sexual dysfunction should not be viewed as part of healthy aging.

- Physiologic changes in sexual response occur in both men and women. It is important to distinguish between normal age-associated changes and pathologic conditions that may be related to medications or medical disorders.

- Many older women have sexual dysfunction but may not report it to their primary care practitioners unless asked.

- Multiple options are available for the treatment of erectile dysfunction.

- Sexuality is an important part of quality of life for older adults; treatment of sexual dysfunction in older adults may lead to improvements in quality of life.

Our understanding of sexual function and dysfunction in older men has increased significantly in recent years. However, there is less scientific information on the sexuality of older women, possibly because of the difficulty of measuring the female sexual response and the exclusion of older adults from research. For example, the National Health and Social Life Survey, a study of adult sexual behavior, sampled adults only up to age 59.

FEMALE SEXUALITY

Age-Associated Changes

Many factors play an important role in the sexual response of older women, including changes that occur with menopause, cultural expectations, relationship problems, previous sexual experiences, chronic illnesses, and depression. American women live about 29 years after menopause and outlive their spouses an average of 8 years. Although the frequency of intercourse decreases with aging, sexuality remains important for older women. One study found that among Swedish women aged 61 years, 59% were sexually active, but 43% experienced vaginal dryness and 10%, vaginal burning. In a study of British women aged 55 to 85, only 24% were found to be sexually active; 62% did not have a sexual partner. Lack of sexual activity among women with partners was found to be due to lack of

the woman's interest in intercourse (43%), lack of the man's interest (24%), or the man's illness or erectile dysfunction (29%).

The female sexual response cycle changes with aging. During the excitement phase, the clitoris may require longer direct stimulation, and genital engorgement is decreased. Vaginal lubrication is reduced, although with increased foreplay and gentle stimulation lubrication is usually adequate for intercourse. During the plateau phase, there is less expansion and vasocongestion of the vagina. During orgasm, fewer and weaker contractions occur, although older women can still achieve multiple orgasms. Occasionally during orgasm, the older woman experiences spastic and painful contractions of the uterine musculature. During the resolution phase, vasocongestion is lost more rapidly. Most of these changes are thought to be due to a decline in serum estrogen concentration after menopause, but a vasculogenic component may contribute to postmenopausal sexual dysfunction.

Female Sexual Dysfunction

For the most part, menopause is accompanied by decreased sexual function, with decreased sexual interest, responsiveness, and coital frequency. In addition, there is an increase in urogenital symptoms, often not discussed with the physician. For example, a study of older British women found that 16% reported urinary urgency, dysuria, or frequency, 9% urinary incontinence, 11% vaginal itching, 8% vaginal dryness, and 2% painful intercourse. Among the women affected by vaginal dryness or painful intercourse, 33% did not seek professional advice and 36% resorted to over-the-counter medication (ie, lubricating jelly).

Dyspareunia, defined as pain with intercourse, can be due to organic or psychologic factors, or a combination of the two. For example, a woman may experience an episode of dyspareunia because of postmenopausal vaginal atrophy. With each subsequent sexual encounter she anticipates pain, causing inadequate arousal with decreased lubrication. Because of this cycle, the woman continues to experience dyspareunia, even after the vaginal atrophy has been treated. The most common organic cause of dyspareunia is atrophic vaginitis due to estrogen deficiency. Other causes include localized vaginal infections, cystitis, Bartholin cyst, retroverted uterus, pelvic tumors, excessive penile thrusting, or improper angle of penile entry.

Estrogen replacement can improve vaginal lubrication and sense of well-being, but it has little effect on libido. Libido is thought to be dependent on testosterone (even in women), rather than estrogen. The ovaries and adrenals are the main sources of androgens in women. Many investigators believe that there is a "female androgen deficiency syndrome," with impaired sexual function, loss of energy, depression, and serum total testosterone concentrations in the lower end of normal for women (<15 ng/dL), but there is no clear-cut definition. The effects of female androgen deficiency were originally identified in women treated for advanced breast cancer with oophorectomy and adrenalectomy. When deprived of androgens, these women reported loss of libido. In a double blind, randomized controlled trial, surgically menopausal women on estrogen replacement were randomized to placebo or testosterone patches that deliver 150 or 300 μg of testosterone daily. After 12 weeks, only the women randomized to the higher dose reported improvements in frequency of sexual activity, pleasure, orgasm, sexual fantasies, masturbation, and positive well-being. This dose increased mean serum free testosterone into the upper normal range for healthy younger women. In naturally postmenopausal women, some, but not all, studies have shown that the addition of testosterone[OL] to estrogen replacement therapy improves sexual function. (Testosterone has not been approved by the U.S. Food and Drug Administration [FDA] for the treatment of sexual dysfunction in women.)

Older women commonly have multiple medical ailments, some of which affect sexuality. However, there are limited scientific studies of the effect of chronic diseases and medications on the sexuality of older women. Women with diabetes mellitus report decreased libido and lubrication, and longer time to reach orgasm. Rheumatic diseases affect sexuality via functional disability. After mastectomy for breast cancer, 20% to 40% of women experience sexual dysfunction, possibly because of disruption of body image, marital and family problems, spousal reaction, adjuvant therapy, or the psychologic impact of a breast cancer diagnosis. Several drugs can adversely affect sexual function, including antihistamines, antihypertensives, antidepressants, antipsychotics, antiestrogens, central nervous system stimulants, narcotics, alcohol, and anticholinergic drugs.

Psychosocial factors have an important role in sexual dysfunction. Women commonly marry men older than themselves and live longer than men. Consequently, heterosexual older women are likely to spend the last years of their lives alone. Even when a partner is available, he might have erectile dysfunction. Finally, lack of privacy may be a problem when the older couple lives with their children or in a nursing home.

[OL] Not approved by the U.S. Food and Drug Administration for this use.

Evaluation and Treatment

The history is the most important part of the evaluation of sexual function, and careful questioning can detect problems that the woman might not otherwise volunteer. First, it is important to attempt to provide a comfortable atmosphere. Clinicians should ask about dyspareunia, lack of vaginal lubrication, and previous negative experiences, like rape, child abuse, or domestic violence. Medications should be carefully reviewed. A woman with dyspareunia should undergo a pelvic examination to exclude organic causes.

Dyspareunia due to atrophic vaginitis and decreased lubrication responds well to topical or systemic estrogen therapy. However, it is important to explain to the patient that complete restoration of vaginal tissue function may take up to 2 years. A vaginal estradiol ring delivers low-dose estrogen locally with lower systemic absorption and risks of systemic side effect than do vaginal estrogen creams. The ring is inserted into the upper third of the vaginal vault and replaced every 3 months. If the patient is not a candidate for or does not want to use estrogen, water-soluble vaginal lubricants (eg, Replens, Astroglide, K-Y jelly) are beneficial. Importantly, local stimulation through regular intercourse helps maintain a healthy vaginal mucosa. Longer foreplay allows more time for vaginal lubrication, just as older men often need longer and more direct stimulation to achieve an adequate erection.

Decreased libido may respond to testosterone, but no androgen preparation is approved by the FDA for female sexual desire disorders. Testosterone for women is available only in combination with estrogens and is FDA approved for moderate to severe vasomotor symptoms that are not improved with estrogens alone. Therapy is usually initiated with oral esterified estrogen 0.625 mg and methyltestosterone 1.25 mg. If symptoms do not improve, the dose can be doubled to esterified estrogen 1.25 mg and methyltestosterone 2.5 mg. Pharmacokinetic studies identifying appropriate replacement doses are lacking. The masculinizing side effects of testosterone, such as increased facial hair, are infrequent, dose dependent, and, for the most part, reversible upon discontinuation. Hepatic toxicity has been noted only in female-to-male transsexuals receiving very high doses of oral methyltestosterone. Oral methyltestosterone should not be used in women with liver disease and uncontrolled hyperlipidemia, as it may decrease high-density lipoproteins. In a 9-week study of postmenopausal women, esterified estrogens (1.25 mg a day) were found to decrease low-density lipoproteins and increase high-density lipoproteins, while the same dose of estrogens plus oral methyltestosterone (2.5 mg a day) decreased high-density lipoproteins. Lipid profile and liver function should be checked at baseline and every 6 months during therapy. Further studies of the best dosage, delivery system, long-term efficacy, and safety of testosterone are needed.

Randomized trials of sildenafil for female sexual dysfunction yielded conflicting results. The manufacturer has therefore decided not to apply for a license to use sildenafil in women.

Finally, the older woman should receive education about male sexual aging in addition to female sexual aging. Otherwise, she might mistakenly attribute her partner's diminished erection and need for more genital stimulation to her own inability to arouse her partner. Other psychologic issues, including depression, history of sexual abuse, and relationship problems, should be addressed and treated with antidepressants, psychotherapy, and marital therapy, as necessary. Table 52.1 summarizes treatments for female sexual dysfunction.

MALE SEXUALITY

Age-Associated Changes

As men age, their sexuality changes. The frequency of sexual intercourse and the prevalence of engaging in any sexual activity decrease. Young men report having intercourse three to four times per week, whereas only 7% of men aged 60 to 69 years and 2% of those aged 70 years and older report the same frequency. Fifty percent to 80% of men 60 to 70 years old engage in any sexual activity, a prevalence rate that declines to 15% to 25% among those aged 80 years and older. However, sexual interest often persists despite decreased activity. The man's level of sexual activity, interest, and enjoyment in younger years often determines his sexual behavior with aging. Factors contributing to a man's decreased sexual activity include poor health, social issues, partner availability, decreased libido, and erectile dysfunction.

Aging is associated not only with changes in sexual behavior but also with changes in the stages of sexual response. During the excitement phase, there is a delay in erection, decreased tensing of the scrotal sac, and loss of testicular elevation. The duration of the plateau stage is prolonged, and pre-ejaculatory secretion is decreased. Orgasm is diminished in duration and intensity, with decreased quantity and force of seminal emission. During the resolution phase, there is rapid detumescence and testicular descent. The refractory period between erections is also prolonged. However, erectile dysfunction is not a part of healthy aging.

Erectile Dysfunction

Erectile dysfunction is the inability to achieve or maintain an erection adequate for sexual intercourse. The prevalence of erectile dysfunction increases with age; by age 70 years, 67% of men have erectile dysfunction. This high prevalence is important; in a study comparing affected and unaffected men, men with sexual dysfunction reported impaired quality of life. The causes of sexual dysfunction in men are summarized in Table 52.2.

The most common cause of erectile dysfunction in older men is vascular disease. Risk for vascular erectile dysfunction increases with traditional vascular risk factors such as diabetes mellitus, hypertension, hyperlipidemia, and smoking. In fact, erectile dysfunction is a predictor of future major atherosclerotic vascular disease (ie, myocardial infarction and stroke).

Obstruction from atherosclerotic arterial occlusive disease likely impedes the intracavernosal blood flow and pressure needed to achieve a rigid erection. In

Table 52.1—Treatment Options for Sexual Dysfunction in Older Women

Symptom	Possible Cause	Therapy
Decreased desire	Postmenopausal status	Estrogen ± testosterone[OL]
	Chronic illness	Treatment of underlying illness
	Depression	Antidepressant medication
	Relationship problems	Marital therapy
	Drugs	Review of drugs ingested
Decreased lubrication	Postmenopausal status	Longer foreplay, regular intercourse, lubricants, estrogen
	Anticholinergic drugs	Review of medications, including over-the-counter drugs
Delayed or absent orgasm	Postmenopausal status	Estrogen ± testosterone[OL]
	Psychological problems	Sex therapy, antidepressant medication[OL]
Pain with intercourse	Organic cause	Treatment of underlying physical condition
	Vaginal dryness, atrophy	Longer foreplay, regular intercourse, lubricants, estrogen
	Vaginismus (involuntary vaginal contractions)	Sex therapy

[OL] Not approved by the U.S. Food and Drug Administration for this use.

Table 52.2—Causes of Sexual Dysfunction in Older Men

Causes (in order of prevalence)	Characteristics
Vascular disease	Gradual onset Vascular risk factors: diabetes mellitus, hypertension, hyperlipidemia, tobacco use
Neurologic disease, eg, spinal cord injury, autonomic dysfunction, surgical procedures	Gradual onset Neurologic risk factors: diabetes mellitus, history of pelvic injury, surgery, or irradiation, spinal injury or surgery, Parkinson's disease, multiple sclerosis, or alcoholism Loss of bulbocavernosus reflex
Medications, eg, anticholinergics, antihypertensives, cimetidine, antidepressants	Sudden onset Lack of sleep-associated erections or lack of erections with masturbation Temporal association with a new medication
Psychogenic, eg, relationship conflicts, performance anxiety, childhood sexual abuse, fear of sexually transmitted diseases, "widower's syndrome"	Sudden onset Sleep-associated erections or erections with masturbation are preserved
Hypogonadism	Gradual onset Decreased libido more than erectile dysfunction Small testes, gynecomastia Low serum testosterone concentration
Endocrine, eg, hypothyroidism, hyperthyroidism, hyperprolactinemia	Rare, < 5% of cases of erectile dysfunction

addition, atherosclerotic disease may cause ischemia of trabecular smooth muscle and result in fibrotic changes leading to failure of venous closure mechanisms. Venous leakage leading to vascular erectile dysfunction may also result from Peyronie's disease, arteriovenous fistula, or trauma-induced communication between the glans and the corpora. In anxious men who have excessive adrenergic-constrictor tone and in men with injured parasympathetic dilator nerves, erectile dysfunction can occur from insufficient relaxation of trabecular smooth muscle.

The second most common cause of erectile dysfunction in older men is neurologic disease. Disorders that affect the parasympathetic sacral spinal cord or the peripheral efferent autonomic fibers to the penis impair penile smooth muscle relaxation and prevent the vasodilation necessary for erection. In patients with spinal cord injury, the extent of erectile dysfunction largely depends on the completeness and the level of the spinal injury; those who have complete lesions or injury to the sacral spinal cord are more likely to have loss of erectile function. Common health problems such as diabetes mellitus, stroke, and Parkinson's disease can cause autonomic dysfunction that results in erectile failure. Finally, surgical procedures such as radical prostatectomy, cystoprostatectomy, and proctocolectomy commonly disrupt the autonomic nerve supply to the penis, resulting in postoperative erectile dysfunction.

Numerous commonly used medications have been associated with erectile dysfunction for which the mechanism, for the most part, is unknown. Those medications with anticholinergic effects, such as antide-pressants, antipsychotics, and antihistamines, may cause erectile dysfunction by blocking parasympathetic-mediated penile artery vasodilatation and trabecular smooth muscle relaxation. Almost all antihypertensive agents have been associated with erectile dysfunction; of these, β-blockers, clonidine, and thiazide diuretics have higher incidence rates. One mechanism may be the lowering of blood pressure below the critical threshold needed to maintain sufficient blood flow for penile erection, especially in those men who already have penile arterial disease. Over-the-counter medications such as cimetidine and ranitidine may also cause erectile dysfunction. Cimetidine, an H_2-receptor antagonist, acts as an antiandrogen and increases prolactin secretion and thus has been associated with loss of libido and erectile failure. Ranitidine can also increase prolactin secretion, although less commonly than does cimetidine.

The prevalence of psychogenic erectile dysfunction correlates inversely with age. Psychogenic erectile dysfunction may occur via increased sympathetic stimuli to the sacral cord, inhibiting the parasympathetic dilator nerves and thus inhibiting erection. Common causes of psychogenic erectile dysfunction include relationship conflicts, performance anxiety, childhood sexual abuse, and fear of sexually transmitted diseases. Older men may have "widower's syndrome," in which the man involved in a new relationship feels guilt as a defense against subconscious unfaithfulness to his deceased spouse.

The role of androgens in erection is unclear. Hypogonadal men show smaller and slower developing erections in response to fantasy, which is improved with androgen replacement. However, even men with castrate levels of testosterone can attain erections in response to direct penile stimulation. It may be that erection to certain types of sexual stimuli (ie, direct penile stimulation) are androgen independent, whereas response to fantasy may be androgen sensitive. Overall, testosterone appears to play a minor role in erectile function and a larger role in libido. In addition, hypogonadal patients respond better to phosphodiesterase inhibitors after testosterone replacement therapy.

Hyperthyroidism, hypothyroidism, and hyperprolactinemia have been associated with erectile dysfunction. However, less than 5% of erectile dysfunction is caused by endocrine abnormalities. Thus, endocrine evaluation of men with erectile dysfunction but intact libido is of limited value.

Evaluation of Erectile Dysfunction

The initial step in evaluation is to obtain a sexual, medical, and psychosocial history. Sexual history should clarify whether the problem consists of inadequate erections, decrease in libido, or orgasmic failure. The onset and duration of erectile dysfunction, the presence or absence of sleep-associated erections, and associated decline in libido may lead the clinician to the likely cause.

Sudden onset suggests psychogenic or drug-induced erectile dysfunction. A psychogenic cause is likely if there is sudden onset but sleep-associated erections or if erections with masturbation or another partner are intact. However, if the sudden onset is accompanied by lack of sleep-associated erections and lack of erection with masturbation, temporal association with new medication should be sought. A gradual onset of erectile dysfunction associated with loss of libido suggests hypogonadism.

Medical history is directed at discerning those factors likely to be contributing to erectile dysfunction. Vascular risk factors include diabetes mellitus, hypertension, coronary artery disease, peripheral arterial disease, hyperlipidemia, and smoking. Neurogenic risk factors include diabetes mellitus, history of pelvic injury or surgery, spinal injury or surgery, Parkinson's disease, multiple sclerosis, and alcoholism. An extensive medication review, including over-the-counter medications, is also essential. Finally, the psychosocial history should assess the patient's relationship with the sexual partner, the partner's health and attitude toward sex, economic or social stresses, living situation, alcohol use, and affective disorders.

On physical examination, signs of vascular or neurologic diseases must be sought. Peripheral pulses should be palpated. Signs of autonomic neuropathy and loss of the bulbocavernosus reflex suggest neurologic dysfunction. The genital examination includes palpating the penis for Peyronie's plaques and assessing for testicular atrophy. A femoral bruit and diminished (or absent) pedal pulses suggests arterial insufficiency. An absent bulbocavernosus reflex in a patient with diabetes mellitus suggests penile neuropathy. A loss of secondary sexual characteristics, small testes, and gynecomastia suggest hypogonadism.

Appropriate laboratory evaluation are those that target relevant comorbid conditions such as diabetes mellitus and vascular disease or that evaluate neurologic disorders if suggested by the physical examination. Consider the measurement of total testosterone in the setting of other symptoms of androgen deficiency. (See "Endocrine and Metabolic Disorders," p 337.)

An office-based diagnostic tool that can help direct the treatment of erectile dysfunction is intracavernous injection of a vasoactive drug, such as papaverine or alprostadil (formerly prostaglandin E_1, or PGE_1). An initial test dose of 15 to 30 mg of papaverine is used if the history and examination suggest a neurogenic cause. A 30-gauge needle and 1-cc syringe are typically used for the injection. Hold the glans of the penis with one hand and clean the injection site with an alcohol swab. Then, holding the needle parallel to the floor, insert the needle into the side of the penis to avoid the urethra. Inject the vasoactive agent over 30 to 60 seconds. After withdrawing the needle, apply pressure to the injection site for 1 minute to prevent bruising. An erectile response will occur within 15 minutes and may last up to 40 minutes. A poor response suggests arteriogenic or venogenic erectile dysfunction, inadequate dose of vasoactive agent, or anxiety with excessive adrenergic tone. A second trial injection at the next office visit with a higher dose (30 to 60 mg papaverine) or alprostadil (5 to 20 μg) may be used.

An at-home therapeutic trial of a phosphodiesterase inhibitor (sildenafil or vardenafil) is easier than the in-office diagnostic penile injection of a vasodilator. The initial dose should be low (sildenafil 25 to 50 mg or vardenafil 5 to 10 mg) in men suspected of having neurogenic erectile dysfunction. A poor response suggests vasculogenic erectile dysfunction. Further therapeutic trial with sildenafil 100 mg or vardenafil 20 mg may prove to be effective. An at-home therapeutic trial using tadalafil (5 to 10 mg) can be considered, but the long half-life complicates matters if an adverse reaction occurs with the first dose.

More extensive diagnostic tools are available but not commonly used. Nocturnal penile tumescence testing is of little value, except to confirm a psychogenic cause. The penile brachial pressure index may be helpful in assessing arteriogenic erectile dysfunction. This index measures the loss of systolic pressure between the arm and the penis. When measured before and after exercise, it can be used to assess for a pelvic steal syndrome, which is the loss of erection associated with initiation of active pelvic thrusting, presumably due to the transfer of blood flow from the penis to the pelvic musculature. More invasive and expensive tests such as Doppler ultrasound to assess penile arterial function, dynamic infusion cavernosometry to assess venous leakage syndrome, and penile arteriography are generally reserved for research or penile vascular surgery candidates.

Treatment of Erectile Dysfunction

Multiple effective therapeutic options are now available for the treatment of erectile dysfunction. Treatment should be individualized and based on cause, personal preference, partner issues, cost, and practicality of the therapeutic modality (Table 52.3).

Oral therapy for erectile dysfunction consists of sildenafil, vardenafil, or tadalafil. Sildenafil is a type-5 phosphodiesterase inhibitor that potentiates the penile response to sexual stimulation. It is effective in improv-

ing the rigidity and duration of erection. It is taken 1 hour before sexual activity and has no effect until sexual stimulation occurs. Because absorption is attenuated when sildenafil is ingested with a fatty meal, patients need to be educated about this issue.

Vardenafil is a more potent and specific phosphodiesterase inhibitor. A lower effective dose and better side-effect profile (no effect on color vision) make vardenafil a reasonable option. Tadalafil is a longer acting phosphodiesterase inhibitor with a similar side-effect profile. All three of these agents are contraindicated for concomitant use with nitrate drugs, since the combination can produce profound and fatal hypotension. Choosing between the three currently available phosphodiesterase inhibitors should likely be based on price. There are also labeling differences with the α-blockers that need to be taken into consideration.

Vacuum tumescence devices are an effective and accepted treatment. The apparatus consists of a plastic cylinder with an open end into which the penis is inserted. A vacuum device attached to the cylinder creates negative pressure within the cylinder, and blood

Table 52.3—Treatment Options for Erectile Dysfunction

Treatment	Administration	Applicable Conditions	Onset	Duration of Action	Dosage	Selected Side Effects
Sildenafil*	Oral	N, A?, V?	60 min	4 hours	25–100 mg	Headache, flushing, rhinitis, dyspepsia, transient color blindness; contraindicated with nitrate use; precaution with α-blockers
Vardenafil*	Oral	N, A?, V?	45 min	4 hours	5–20 mg	Headache, flushing, rhinitis, dyspepsia; contraindicated with nitrate use and precaution with α-blockers
Tadalafil*	Oral	N, A?,V?	45–60 min	24–36 hours	5–20 mg	Headache, dyspepsia, flushing, rhinitis; contraindicated with nitrate use and precaution with α-blockers (except tamsulosin)
Vacuum device	External	P, N, V, A?	< 5 min	30 min	—	Petechiae, bruising, painful ejaculation
Papaverine[OL]	Intracavernosal	N, A?, V?	10 min	30–60 min	15–60 mg	Prolonged erection, fibrosis, ecchymosis
Alprostadil	Intracavernosal	N, A?, V?	10 min	40–60 min	5–20 µg	Prolonged erection, pain, fibrosis
Phentolamine[OL]	Intracavernosal	N, A?, V?	10 min	30–60 min	0.5–1 mg	Prolonged erection, fibrosis, headache, facial flushing
MUSE	Intraurethral	N, A?, V?	10–15 min	60–80 min	250–1000 µg	Penile pain or burning, hypotension
Penile prosthesis	Surgical	N, A, V		replacement in 5–10 years		Infection, erosion, mechanical failure
Sex therapy	Counseling	P	weeks	years	weekly	Anxiety

NOTE: A = arteriogenic; min = minutes; MUSE = medicated urethral system for erection; N = neurogenic; P = psychogenic; V = venogenic; ? = possibly.

On July 8, 2005 the U.S. Food and Drug Administration issued a statement approving label changes for all three PDE5 inhibitors that reflect a small number of cases of nonarteritic ischemic optic neuropathy (NAION) that were reported postmarketing. It is not possible at this time to determine causality of PDE5 inhibitors and NAION since other factors are associated with NAION, such as underlying anatomic or vascular risk factors, including but not necessarily limited to: low cup-to-disc ratio ("crowded disc"), age over 50, diabetes mellitus, hypertension, coronary artery disease, hyperlipidemia, and smoking. It is not possible to determine whether these events are related directly to the use of PDE5 inhibitors, to the patient's underlying vascular risk factors or anatomical defects, to a combination of these factors, or to other factors. Men who experience visual changes or loss of vision in one or both eyes are advised to stop the medication and contact their doctor or health care provider immediately.

flows into the penis to produce penile rigidity. A penile constriction ring placed at the base of the penis then traps the blood in the corpora cavernosa to maintain an erection for about 30 minutes. The vacuum device is effective for psychogenic, neurogenic, and venogenic erectile dysfunction, but it requires manual dexterity. Local pain, swelling, bruising, coolness of penile tip, and painful ejaculation are potential side effects. It is important to remove the constriction ring after 30 minutes.

Intracavernous injection of vasoactive drugs such as papaverine, phentolamine, and alprostadil are effective in producing erections adequate for sexual activity. Alprostadil, which is the only agent approved by the FDA for intracavernous injection, produces erections that last 40 to 60 minutes. Phentolamine[OL] is mainly used in combination therapy with papaverine[OL] or alprostadil, or both. Potential side effects are bruising, ecchymoses or hematoma, local pain, fibrosis from repeated injections, and priapism. Alprostadil appears to cause less scarring and priapism than papaverine. If an erection lasts longer than 4 hours, detumescence is necessary by aspiration of blood from the corpora cavernosa or injection of phenylephrine, since there is the potential for intracavernous hypoxia and fibrosis of trabecular smooth muscle, which may prevent future erections. In general, intracavernosal therapy should probably be reserved for patients who fail oral therapy with a phosphodiesterase inhibitor. Alprostadil can also be administered intraurethrally using MUSE (medicated urethral system for erection). This system contains a small pellet of alprostadil that is placed within the urethra and is rapidly absorbed through the urethral mucosa to produce an erection within 10 to 15 minutes. Possible side effects are penile pain, urethral burning, and a throbbing sensation in the perineum.

Testosterone supplementation increases libido and may improve erectile dysfunction in men with true hypogonadism. It is available as an intramuscular injection (testosterone enanthate or cypionate) or topical transdermal patch and gel. Possible side effects associated with testosterone include polycythemia, increase in prostate size, gynecomastia, and fluid retention. It is important to perform a digital rectal

[OL] Not approved by the U.S. Food and Drug Administration for this use.

examination to assess the prostate and obtain a baseline prostate-specific antigen level prior to initiation of therapy. If there is a rise in prostate-specific antigen or hematocrit with testosterone therapy, it usually occurs within 6 months. Therefore, it is advisable to check these levels at 3-month intervals during the first year of therapy, then every 12 months thereafter.

Surgical implantation of a penile prosthesis is another therapeutic option. Mechanical failure, infection, device erosion, and fibrosis are possible complications. However, since the availability of alprostadil and, more recently, phosphodiesterase inhibitors, surgical implantation of a penile prosthesis is rarely used (ie, men with severe arterial occlusive disease). Penile revascularization surgery has limited success.

Psychogenic erectile dysfunction should be referred for further evaluation and treatment.

REFERENCES

■ Bodie J, Lewis J, Schow D, et al. Laboratory evaluations of erectile dysfunction: an evidence based approach. *J Urol.* 2003;169(6):2262–2264.

■ Mulligan T, Reddy S, Gulur PV, et al. Disorders of male sexual function. *Clin Geriatr Med.* 2003;19(3):473–481.

■ Nusbaum MR, Lenahan P, Sadovsky R. Sexual health in aging men and women: adressing the physiologic and psychological sexual changes that occur with age. *Geriatrics.* 2005;60(9):18–23.

■ Padero MC, Bhasin S, Friedman TC. Androgen supplementation in older women: too much hype, not enough data. *J Am Geriatr Soc.* 2002; 50(6):1131–1140.

■ Rajpurkar A, Dhabuwala CB. Comparison of satisfaction rate and erectile function in patients treated with sildenafil, intracavernous prostaglandin E$_1$, and penile implant surgery for erectile dysfunction in urology practice. *J Urol.* 2003;170(1):159–163.

■ Sarrel PM. Sexual dysfunction: treat or refer. *Obstet Gynecol.* 2005;106(4):834–839.

■ Seftel AD. Erectile dysfunction in the elderly: epidemiology, etiology and approaches to treatment. *J Urol.* 2003; 169(6):1999–2007.

KEY POINTS

■ A number of treatment options exist for benign prostatic hyperplasia (BPH), including watchful waiting, drug therapies, minimally invasive procedures, and more extensive operations. The choice is influenced by the extent of symptoms, the presence of complications from outflow obstruction, and the preferences of the patient.

■ The use of 5α-reductase inhibitors for BPH is especially indicated when the prostate gland is large.

■ Recommendations regarding screening for prostate cancer using PSA differ among experts, and patients should be educated about the risks and benefits of this screening strategy so that they can make a well-informed decision.

■ Several treatment options exist for men with localized prostate cancer, including watchful waiting, resection of the gland and seminal vesicles, and radiation therapy. How the patient balances the potential benefits and burdens of the various options will influence the choice of therapy.

■ For patients with chronic prostatitis, efforts should be made to identify the causative organism, and even with a prolonged course of appropriate antibiotics, a cure can be expected in fewer than half the patients.

With advancing age, the prevalence of prostate diseases increases dramatically. The three most common conditions are benign prostatic hyperplasia (BPH), prostate cancer, and prostatitis. Self-reported prostate disease affects about 3 million Americans. BPH develops in over half the men aged 65 years and older and affects the overwhelming majority of men after age 85 years. Prostate cancer is the second leading cause of cancer death in men, and many men have asymptomatic or low-grade tumors that cause few or no health problems. The prevalence of prostatitis is similar to that of ischemic heart disease or diabetes mellitus. The three common prostatic conditions are reviewed herein, with special attention to diagnosis and management.

BENIGN PROSTATIC HYPERPLASIA

Epidemiology

BPH is a noncancerous enlargement of the epithelial and fibromuscular components of the prostate gland. The epithelial component normally makes up 20% to 30% of prostate volume and contributes to the seminal fluid. The fibromuscular component comprises 70% to 80% of the prostate and is responsible for expressing prostatic fluid during ejaculation. Age and long-term androgen stimulation induce BPH development. Microscopic appearance of BPH may occur as early as age 30, is present in 50% of men by age 60, and is present in 90% of men by age 85. In half of these cases, microscopic BPH develops into palpable macroscopic BPH. Of those with macroscopic BPH, only half develop into clinically significant disease brought to medical attention. BPH is one of the most common conditions in aging men; in the United States annually it accounts for more than 1.7 million office visits and 250,000 surgical procedures.

Prostatism, or Lower Urinary Tract Symptoms

The symptoms of BPH are nonspecific; other diseases can result in identical symptoms. The pathophysiology of BPH symptoms is not completely understood, but presumably it involves the periurethral zone of the prostate gland, which results in obstructed urine flow and compensatory responses of the urinary bladder, such as hypertrophy and decreased capacity. The urethral obstruction has both mechanical (obstructing mass) and dynamic (smooth muscle contractions) components. The resulting lower urinary tract symptoms are divided into irritative (frequency, urgency, nocturia) and obstructive (hesitancy, intermittency, weak stream, incomplete emptying) manifestations. The American Urological Association developed a quantitative symptom index for severity assessment and treatment response monitoring, which was adopted by the World Health Organization and is known as the International Prostate Symptom Score (IPSS). Although tracking symptom severity is useful in the longitudinal management of patients, symptom severity has not been found to correlate with prostate size, urine flow rates, or postvoid residual volume. BPH primarily affects quality of life, although complications such as recurrent urinary tract infection, bladder stones, urinary retention, chronic renal insufficiency, and hematuria can develop.

Diagnosis

Differential diagnosis of lower urinary tract symptoms includes endocrine disorders (especially diabetes mellitus), neurologic disorders, urinary tract infections, sexually transmitted diseases, kidney or bladder stones, and medications (especially drugs with anticholinergic and diuretic effects). Digital rectal examination (DRE) may be unremarkable or reveal an enlarged, smooth, rubbery, symmetrical gland. Urinalysis is routinely performed to evaluate for urinary tract infection, hematuria, and glycosuria. A baseline serum creatinine assesses kidney function and the possibility of obstructive uropathy or intrinsic renal disease, or both. Additional optional tests include postvoid residual urine volume, urine flow rates, and pressure flow studies. These tests may be considered when the diagnosis is uncertain or an invasive treatment is being planned.

Treatment Approaches

BPH therapy is patient dependent and driven by the impact of symptoms on the patient's quality of life (see Table 53.1). All patients should be educated regarding life-style modification: fluid adjustments (avoid caffeine) and avoidance of medications (especially anticholinergics) that aggravate symptoms. Patients with mild to moderate symptoms may be satisfied with life-style modification only. Both medical and surgical treatments are also available, with medication the usual first approach. Indications for surgical treatment include patient preference, dissatisfaction with medication, and refractory urinary retention, as well as renal dysfunction, bladder stones, recurrent urinary tract infections, or hematuria if these are clearly due to prostatic obstruction.

Medical Treatment

The two main pharmacologic approaches are α-adrenergic antagonists and 5α-reductase inhibitors.

α-Adrenergic antagonists, or α-blockers, are directed at the dynamic component of urethral obstruction. Smooth muscle of the prostate and bladder neck has a resting tone mediated by α-adrenergic innervation. α-Blockers relax the smooth muscle in the hyperplastic prostate tissue, prostate capsule, and bladder neck, thus decreasing resistance to urinary flow. Of the two major α-adrenergic receptors, α_1 receptors predominate in the prostate, and the α_{1a} subtype comprises 70% of these receptors. α-Blockade development for BPH therapy has progressed from selective α_1 agents (prazosin[OL], alfuzosin) to long-acting selective α_1 agents (terazosin, doxazosin) and now to long-acting α_{1a} subtype selective agents (tamsulosin). The most common adverse effects of α_1 agents are dizziness, mild asthenia (fatigue or weakness), and headaches. Postural hypotension occurs infrequently and can be minimized by careful dose titration.

The enzyme 5α-reductase is required for the conversion of testosterone to the more active dihydrotestosterone. Finasteride is an inhibitor of this enzyme and reduces tissue levels of dihydrotestosterone, thus reducing prostate gland size. Improvements in symptom scores and urine flow rates may not be evident for up to 6 months. Finasteride is most effective in men with larger prostates (>40 g,

Table 53.1—Management Options for Benign Prostatic Hyperplasia

Category	Interventions	Rationale	Comments
Life-style modification	Reduce nighttime fluids to manage nocturia Eliminate bladder irritants (eg, caffeine, alcohol, nicotine)	Factors outside the urinary tract contribute to urinary symptoms	Often sufficient management for mild symptoms Complements management for moderate to severe symptoms
Pharmacologic management	α-Adrenergic antagonists Selective α_1: prazosin[OL], alfuzosin Long-acting selective α_1: terazosin, doxazosin Long-acting selective α_{1A} subtype selective: tamsulosin	Relaxation of the smooth muscle in hyperplastic prostate tissue, prostate capsule, and bladder neck decreases resistance to urinary flow	Adverse effects: dizziness, mild asthenia, headaches, postural hypotension (reduced with careful dose titration, not present with tamsulosin), abnormal ejaculation, rhinitis
	5α-Reductase inhibitors: finasteride, dutasteride	Reduced tissue levels of dihydrotestosterone result in prostate gland size reduction	Most effective for men with larger prostates (> 40 g) Results may not be evident for up to 6 months
Surgery	Transurethral resection of the prostate Transurethral incision of the prostate Open prostatectomy Transurethral vaporization of the prostate Stent placement	Removal or expansion of peri-urethral prostate tissue reduces obstruction to urinary flow	Indicated for BPH-induced recurrent UTI, recurrent or persistent gross hematuria, bladder stones, renal insufficiency

NOTE: BPH = benign prostatic hyperplasia; UTI = urinary tract infection.

[OL] Not approved by the U.S. Food and Drug Administration for this use.

about the size of a plum). Because finasteride reduces serum prostate-specific antigen (PSA) levels an average 50%, baseline serum PSA determination is advocated for men in whom prostate cancer surveillance is planned. Subsequently, after a 6-month trial if continued finasteride therapy is desired, a PSA level on treatment is obtained and then measured annually for cancer surveillance.

When used together over years, the combination of α-adrenergic antagonists with 5α-reductase inhibitors has been shown to be safe and to reduce clinical progression of BPH better than either agent alone. In particular, a lower risk of urinary retention, urinary incontinence, renal insufficiency, and recurrent bladder infections is associated with combination therapy. Also, consistent results from a number of trials demonstrate that the herbal preparation *Serenoa repens,* or saw palmetto, improves urinary symptoms and flow measures in men with BPH. The improvements are similar to those associated with treatment with finasteride, and there are fewer reported adverse effects with *S. repens.* (See also "Complementary and Alternative Medicine," p 74.)

Surgical Treatment

Surgical management includes transurethral resection of the prostate, transurethral incision of the prostate, open prostatectomy, transurethral vaporization of the prostate, and device insertion such as stent placement. Surgical approaches offer the best chance for symptom improvement but also have the highest rates of complications. The benefits of surgical treatments are generally considered equivalent, but complication rates differ. Transurethral resection of the prostate is the standard of care to which other BPH treatments are compared and has an 80% likelihood of successful outcome in properly selected patients. Usually performed under spinal anesthesia, a transurethral resection of the prostate involves the passage of an endoscope through the urethra to remove surgically the inner portion of the prostate. Long-term complications may include retrograde ejaculation, urethral stricture, bladder neck contracture, incontinence, and impotence. Transurethral incision of the prostate is an endoscopic procedure via the urethra to make one to two cuts in the prostate and prostate capsule, relieving urethral constriction. Limited to small prostate glands (<30 g), transurethral incision of the prostate offers lower rates of retrograde ejaculation, bleeding, and contractures. Open prostatectomy involves removal of the inner portion of the prostate through a retropubic or suprapubic incision. It is best used for patients with larger prostates or with complicating conditions such as bladder stones or urethral strictures. Open prostatectomy is associated with incisional morbidity, longer hospitalization, and greater risk of impotence. Transurethral vaporization of the prostate uses a high-energy electrode inserted via the urethra to vaporize the prostate. This approach has little bleeding but creates more prolonged irritative voiding. Prostatic stents are used to maintain expansion of the prostatic urethra and are employed for temporary and permanent uses.

PROSTATE CANCER

Incidence and Epidemiology

Cancer of the prostate is the most common noncutaneous cancer and the second leading cause of cancer deaths among men in the United States. It was estimated that in 2005, 232,090 men would be diagnosed and 30,350 men would die from prostate cancer. The incidence increases with age and is rare in men younger than 40 years. In autopsy studies where the entire prostate is examined, incidental histologic evidence of cancer of the prostate is found in 30% of men over 50 and 80% of men over 80. The incidence of disease varies according to race, with American blacks having the highest risk in the world. Among black men cancer of the prostate occurs at an earlier age, has a higher mortality rate, and tends to be at a more advanced stage of disease at diagnosis. Family history is a contributing factor. Men with one first-degree relative affected have more than a twofold increased risk, and with two first-degree relatives affected, more than an eightfold increased risk. Androgens are necessary for prostate cancer pathogenesis; the disease does not occur in men castrated before puberty. Diets high in total fat consumption are associated with increased risk. The association between cancer of the prostate and early onset of sexual activity, sexually transmitted disease, or vasectomy is inconclusive.

Symptoms

Cancer usually arises in the peripheral zone of the prostate. The majority of patients, especially those with early-stage, potentially curable disease, are asymptomatic. Cancer of the prostate spreads by three routes: direct extension, the lymphatics, and the blood stream. Direct invasion of the urethra and bladder can lead to irritative voiding symptoms, urinary incontinence, and hematuria. Extension of disease to adjacent nerves may cause impotence and pelvic pain. Nodal metastasis may cause extrinsic ureteral obstruction. Leg edema may develop from lymphatic obstruction. Hematogenous metastasis to bone may cause severe local pain, normochromic normocytic anemia, pathologic fractures, and spinal cord compression. Less commonly, hematogenous metastasis involves viscera—namely, the lung, liver, and adrenal glands.

Screening Controversy

The benefit of early detection and the best approach to treatment of prostate cancer are controversial. At the heart of the screening debate is the fact that no direct evidence exists to show that early detection decreases prostate cancer mortality rates. There is a large reservoir of cancer of the prostate that does not need to be diagnosed because the majority of men with prostate cancer die with the disease, not from it. The well-recognized burden of progressive cancer of the prostate is the impetus for early detection and management. The American Urological Association and the American Cancer Society advocate annual screening, recommending the PSA test and DRE beginning at age 50 for men with at least a 10-year life expectancy and earlier (age 40) for men at high risk (black men, first-degree relative affected). Groups that use explicit criteria to develop evidence-based practice guidelines (U.S. Preventive Services Task Force, American College of Physicians, and Canadian Task Force on the Periodic Health Examination) have recommended against routine PSA screening for cancer of the prostate. Guidelines are in agreement that the controversy surrounding screening should be discussed with patients in order to achieve individualized, informed courses of action. The effectiveness of PSA screening is particularly questionable in elderly men.

Screening and Diagnostic Tests

DRE of the prostate allows palpation of the posterior surfaces of the lateral lobes, where cancer most often begins. Cancer characteristically is hard, nodular, and irregular. DRE enhances screening efforts by detecting some cancers with a normal PSA level. DRE is inherently inaccurate because parts of the prostate gland cannot be reached. About half of the cancers thought to be "confined" to the prostate on the basis of DRE are found during surgery to have already spread. DRE produces many false-positive results; about one third of positive DRE tests are shown to be cancer by biopsy. Local extension of cancer of the prostate into the seminal vesicles can often be detected by DRE. Despite its limitations, DRE remains important for screening and staging.

The serum PSA test is not specific for cancer of the prostate. PSA elevations occur in benign conditions of the prostate, namely, hypertrophy and prostatitis, and in transient response to conditions such as ejaculation and prostatic massage. The sensitivity of the PSA test is also imperfect. Declines in PSA values have been associated with acute hospitalization and use of medications such as finasteride and saw palmetto. Normal PSA levels are found in 30% to 40% of men with cancer confined to the prostate (false-negative tests). The reported positive predictive value of PSA in screening studies is 28% to 35%: about one third of men with elevated PSA levels have cancer of the prostate demonstrated by fine-needle biopsy.

Several approaches to improve the accuracy of PSA testing have been developed. PSA density is derived from the PSA concentration divided by the volume of the gland (measured by ultrasound). Cancer of the prostate produces higher PSA levels per unit volume than BPH and should therefore yield a higher PSA density. The PSA rate of change or velocity is more specific for cancer of the prostate than a single PSA measurement. Using a PSA velocity value of ≥ 0.75 ng/mL/year achieves 90% specificity, whereas using a single PSA level >4 ng/mL achieves 60% specificity. This high specificity for PSA velocity is realized even in normal-range serum PSA levels (<4 ng/mL). Another approach involves age-adjusted PSA reference ranges because PSA values increase with age. Finally, one can measure the ratio of free to complexed PSA, recognizing that PSA bound to α_1-antichymotrypsin accounts for a larger proportion of total PSA with cancer of the prostate than with BPH.

Abnormal DRE or PSA tests lead to transrectal ultrasound–guided biopsy of the prostate for pathologic diagnosis. Cancer may appear as a hypoechoic density, but ultrasound is not specific enough to be used as a screening tool. Spring-loaded core needle biopsies are routinely taken from the base, middle, and apex of each lobe (six samples total). Biopsies may also be taken from specific palpable nodules.

Grading

The Gleason grading system is the most commonly used system that is based on the histologic appearance of prostate cancer. The Gleason grade ranges from 1, or well differentiated, to 5, or poorly differentiated. The Gleason score is the sum of the most common Gleason grade observed plus the next most common Gleason grade seen. The Gleason score ranges from 2 to 10. Gleason scores are sometimes grouped as 2–4, well differentiated; 5–7, moderately differentiated; 8–10, poorly differentiated. Well-differentiated tumors have a favorable prognosis; poorly differentiated tumors, an unfavorable prognosis. Most clinically detected tumors are moderately differentiated.

Staging

Staging of cancer of the prostate is necessary for planning disease management. Two classification systems are used: the tumor, regional node, metastasis (TNM) system and the Jewett-Whitmore (ABCD) system (Table 53.2). Usually detected by transurethral resection of the prostate, incidentally discovered cancers are staged according to the amount of tissue involved (T1 or A). Stage T1c reflects the growing number of tumors detected because of an elevated PSA level. Tumors detectable by DRE and confined to the prostate (T2 or B) are subdivided on the basis of the amount of tumor that is palpable. The degree of extension and invasion of surrounding structures stage tumors that extend beyond the prostatic capsule (T3 to T4 or C). Advanced disease (M1 or D) has metastasized.

The initial staging evaluation includes PSA level, DRE findings, and transrectal ultrasonography results. Bone scans may be performed on patients with PSA values greater than 10 ng/mL or complaints of bone pain. For patients electing active treatment, surgical assessment of lymph node involvement (pelvic lymphadenectomy) is performed by itself or in conjunction with prostate surgery or implantation of radioactive seeds. Computed tomography (CT) scans are often employed for active treatment planning.

In the past, CT scans, magnetic resonance imaging scans, pedal lymphangiography, and pelvic lymph node dissection were routinely employed in various combinations to evaluate the extent of cancer of the prostate. These tests should be eliminated in the initial staging evaluation of prostate cancer patients because they have been associated with unacceptably high false-negative and false-positive results. A subset of patients appears to benefit from CT scans combined with fine-needle aspiration. Patients who have a PSA >25 ng/mL, a Gleason score >6, and a palpable abnormality on DRE are currently recommended to undergo a CT scan with fine-needle aspiration if a lymph node larger than 6 mm is present. Many of these patients will be diagnosed with nodal metastasis and thus spared the need for bilateral pelvic lymph-node dissection and its associated morbidity.

The serum PSA level should be used to eliminate the staging radionuclide bone scan. In the asymptomatic, newly diagnosed, previously untreated prostate cancer patient, a PSA concentration ≤10 ng/mL has been associated with rare (0% to 0.8%) findings of skeletal metastases. Adopting recommendations to eliminate the staging radionuclide bone scan in this population will substantially reduce testing, because 50% to 60% of men with newly diagnosed cancer of the prostate have a serum PSA concentration in this range.

Management of Localized Disease

Localized cancer lends itself to cure, but the prevalence of men dying with cancer of the prostate (often asymptomatic) but not from the disease questions the necessity of treatment. No trials have shown that treatment prolongs life when treatment is compared with watchful waiting. Thus, three approaches to

Table 53.2—Staging Systems for Prostate Cancer

TNM Stage	Jewett-Whitmore Stage	Description
T1	A1, A2	Tumor is an incidental finding
T2	B1, B2	Tumor is palpable, confined to prostate
T3	C1, C2	Tumor extends beyond the prostate capsule, may involve seminal vesicles
T4	C2	Tumor invades adjacent structures (eg, bladder neck, rectum, pelvic wall)
N	D1	Lymph node metastasis present
M	D2	Distant metastasis present

NOTE: TNM = tumor, regional node, metastasis.
SOURCE: For further details, see AUA Prostate Cancer Clinical Guidelines Panel. *Report on the Management of Clinically Localized Prostate Cancer.* Baltimore, MD: American Urological Association; 1995.

localized prostate cancer are routinely advocated: watchful waiting, radical prostatectomy, and radiation therapy (see Table 53.3).

Watchful waiting (also called *expectant* or *conservative management; surveillance*) is the approach offered most commonly to men with less than a 10-year life expectancy, who have significant medical comorbidities, or whose tumor is small and well to moderately differentiated. Conservative management studies have shown that 10-year disease-specific survival is 89% to 96% for Gleason score 2–5 tumors, 70% to 82% for Gleason score 6 tumors, 30% to 58% for Gleason score 7 tumors, and 13% to 40% for Gleason score 8–10 tumors. Because most men with cancer of the prostate are asymptomatic, watchful waiting attempts to spare men the burden of unnecessary treatment. However, awaiting symptoms in men with prostate cancer before initiating treatment means sacrificing the opportunity for cure. Patients are offered palliation if and when symptoms develop.

Radical prostatectomy involves the surgical removal of the entire prostate gland and the seminal vesicles. It can be performed through a perineal (incision near the rectum) or retropubic (lower abdominal incision) approach. The perineal approach allows an easier vesicourethral anastomosis and less bleeding, whereas the retropubic approach allows access to the pelvic lymph nodes and spares the neurovascular supply to the corpora cavernosa (with improved potency). The major morbidities of this treatment are urinary incontinence and erectile dysfunction. Surgery is thought to have the highest incidence of post-treatment sexual dysfunction. A population-based study of 1291 men undergoing radical prostatectomy for clinically localized prostate cancer found that 18 months later, 59.9% reported erections not firm enough for sexual intercourse and 8.4% were incontinent. Patients following

Table 53.3—Management Approaches for Localized Prostate Cancer

Management	Description	Comments
Watchful waiting	Prostate cancer is not treated until symptoms develop	Offered to men with less than a 10-year life expectancy; significant medical comorbidities; small, well-differentiated tumors; or unwillingness to bear treatment burdens Awaiting symptoms sacrifices opportunity for cure
Radical prostatectomy	Surgical removal of the entire prostate gland and seminal vesicles	Offered to men with an absence of surgical contraindications Adverse effects realized immediately
External beam radiation therapy	Standard regimen delivers 6000 to 7000 rads of pelvic radiation over a 7-week period	Radiation reaches tissues outside the prostate including pelvic lymph nodes Adverse effects develop over time
Brachytherapy	Radioactive seeds (eg, iridium, palladium) are implanted into the prostate gland using computed tomography scan guidance	Most adverse effects realized immediately

radical prostatectomy are more likely to experience stress incontinence, with symptoms ranging from occasional leakage to no urinary control. Bladder neck contractures also occur, resulting in obstructive voiding symptoms and urinary retention. Both sexual dysfunction and urinary symptoms have a negative impact on quality of life. The relationship between these morbidities and sense of bother is not direct; for example, those with the most leakage may have little bother while those with minimal leakage may report substantial bother. The goal of surgery is cure. Biochemical progression (PSA ≥0.4 ng/mL) has been reported in 40% of men 10 years after radical prostatectomy for localized disease. Actuarial metastasis-free survival at 15 years is 82%. Thus, this treatment can be offered to men with locally confined disease, with greater than a 10-year life expectancy, and without contraindications to operative therapy.

Radiation therapy is provided through external beam radiation or through implantation of radioactive sources (known as *brachytherapy*). The standard regimen of external beam radiation delivers a total of 6000 to 7000 rads over a 7-week period. Pelvic lymph nodes can be radiated as well. Proctitis and urethritis are common acute side effects. Chronic complications include erectile dysfunction, urinary incontinence, and chronic proctitis. The incidence of urinary stress incontinence after radiation therapy is significantly less than with surgery, but the presence of irritative voiding dysfunction is greater. Bowel dysfunction, uncommon after surgery, affects more than half of patients after radiation. Bowel symptoms include diarrhea, rectal urgency, and fecal soiling. The majority of patients classify these bowel symptoms as minor with little to no effect on quality of life. Local control and cancer survival rates are comparable to those of radical prostatectomy. Conformal radiation therapy is a mode of high-precision external-beam radiation that uses high-resolution CT scan data and advanced computer technology to conform the radiation dose to the three-dimensional configuration of the tumor. This new technology shows promise in reducing complications and adverse effects.

Brachytherapy involves retropubic or perineal implantation of radioactive seeds, usually iridium or palladium. Improvements in three-dimensional imaging of the prostate through CT scan or ultrasound guidance have allowed more uniform distribution of seeds throughout the prostate and overcome many of the past limitations of brachytherapy. Potency is better preserved with seed implants. Urinary symptoms include frequency, dysuria, and urge incontinence. Bowel symptoms include rectal urgency and rectal bleeding. The morbidity of seed implants appears to improve over time following the initial seed placement. Currently no evidence suggests that brachytherapy is more effective than external beam radiation or prostatectomy.

Management of Locally Advanced Prostate Cancer

Locally advanced prostate cancer extends beyond the capsule or invades the seminal vesicle, without evidence of distant or nodal metastasis. Radiation therapy is the recommended treatment, and adjuvant androgen deprivation provides additional benefit toward increased survival and freedom from metastases. However, controversy exists as to when androgen deprivation should be initiated. Patients may have a prolonged asymptomatic cancer period, while significant negative quality-of-life changes from long-term androgen deprivation occur, including loss of stamina, increased fatigue, hot flashes, diminished muscle mass, and premature osteoporosis. Patients should therefore be given the choice of early versus delayed androgen deprivation.

Management of Advanced Disease

Advanced disease is treated with androgen ablation and symptom-specific approaches, such as focal radiation therapy to painful bone metastasis. Androgen ablation aims to eliminate prostate cancer growth stimulation and includes orchiectomy or luteinizing hormone-releasing hormone (LHRH) agonists with antiandrogens. Orchiectomy and LHRH agonists are equally effective at reducing androgens to castration levels. Orchiectomy is the oldest, safest, least expensive approach but is rejected by nearly half of U.S. men. LHRH agonists such as leuprolide and goserelin produce castration levels about a month after an initial increase in serum testosterone levels. Antiandrogens (eg, flutamide) are often given before initiation of LHRH agonists to blunt the effects of the initial testosterone increase. Antiandrogens inhibit the binding of androgen to its receptor. After castration a small amount of adrenal androgen exists and may allow continued stimulation of prostate cancer growth. Antiandrogens may be combined with chemical or surgical castration, a practice called *complete androgen ablation*. Survival rates for antiandrogens alone are inferior to those for chemical or surgical castration alone; complete androgen ablation offers slight improvement in survival over that offered by castration only.

Radiation therapy is useful for relieving the pain of isolated bone metastasis and reducing the risk of fracture of bones with significant destruction. Diffuse bone metastases require alternative approaches. Bone-seeking radiopharmaceuticals such as strontium can be beneficial for pain control. Androgen deprivation decreases bone pain in two thirds of symptomatic patients.

PROSTATITIS

Etiology

Prostatitis is an inflammatory condition of the prostate that may represent acute bacterial, chronic bacterial, or nonbacterial causes. The most common sources of acute or chronic infection are ascending urethral infection or reflux of infected urine into the prostatic ducts, or both. Direct extension or lymphatic spread from the rectum or hematogenous spread also occurs. Acute prostatitis is an infectious process that is more common in young men. Pathogens in men 35 years and younger often include *Neisseria gonorrhea* and *Chlamydia trachomatis*. In older men acute prostatitis is associated with indwelling urethral catheter use, and coliforms are the suspected bacterial cause. More than 80% of patients with prostatitis have no identifiable infectious agent.

Diagnosis

Acute bacterial prostatitis is characterized by fever, chills, dysuria, and a tense or boggy, extremely tender prostate. Because bacteremia may result from manipulation of the inflamed gland, minimal rectal examination is indicated. Gram's stain and culture of the urine can identify the causative agent.

Chronic bacterial prostatitis presents classically as recurrent bacteriuria caused by the same organism, although most patients will not have this presentation. Patients have varying degrees of obstructive or irritative voiding symptoms and perineal pain. The prostate often feels normal. First-void or midstream urine is compared with expressed prostatic secretion or urine collected postmassage. The expressed sample should reveal leukocytosis and the causative agent. Sterile expressant with leukocytosis suggests nonbacterial prostatitis.

Treatment

Acute bacterial prostatitis is treated with antibiotics and may require hospitalization. The severe inflammation allows antibiotics to penetrate the prostate, and prompt response to empiric therapy is expected. CT or magnetic resonance imaging should be considered to evaluate for an abscess if recovery is delayed. Antibiotic selection should be based initially on urine Gram's stain results, with subsequent consideration of sensitivity profiles. Fluoroquinolones are highly effective in most cases.

Antibiotics are less effective for chronic bacterial prostatitis because of the poor penetration of the prostate by most of these drugs. Prolonged therapy of 6 to 16 weeks offers a cure rate of 30% to 40%. Continuous low-dose antibiotic suppression therapy can be offered for those with frequent symptomatic relapse. Total prostatectomy offers cure but at a high risk-to-benefit ratio. Transurethral resection of the prostate is safer but cures only one third of patients.

Nonbacterial prostatitis is treated symptomatically. A small percentage of cases may involve occult infections, and empiric antibiotic therapy is often used. Efforts to reduce pain and discomfort include anti-inflammatory agents, sitz baths, fluid adjustments (avoid caffeine), anticholinergic agents, and α-adrenergic antagonists.

REFERENCES

■ AUA Practice Guidelines Committee. AUA guideline on management of benign prostatic hyperplasia (2003). Chapter 1: Diagnosis and treatment recommendations. *J Urol.* 2003;170(2 Pt 1):530–547.

- Holden J, Emery CB. Prostate cancer: Primary care providers play critical role. *Adv Nurse Pract.* 2004;12(4):28–35; quiz 36.

- Penson DF, Litwin MS. The physical burden of prostate cancer. *Urol Clin North Am.* 2003;30(2):305–313.

- Schaeffer AJ, Datta NS, Fowler JE, et al. Advances in the diagnosis and treatment of prostatitis: overview summary statement. *Urology.* 2000; 60(Suppl 6):1–4.

- Wilson SS, Crawford ED. Screening for prostate cancer: current recommendations. *Urol Clin North Am.* 2004;31(2):219–226.

CHAPTER 54—MUSCULOSKELETAL DISEASES AND DISORDERS

KEY POINTS

- Most musculoskeletal complaints in older adults are not caused by true arthritis but rather by disorders resulting from derangement of tendons, bursae, muscles, connective tissue, and nerves. Symptoms typically involve a region of the body rather than discrete joints.

- Among those aged 65 and older, osteoarthritis is the most prevalent articular disease.

- Most blood testing in rheumatologic conditions can, at best, only help confirm the clinical impression or provide prognostic data. Studies show that laboratory testing tends to be overused.

- Well-designed studies have now shown the value of exercise in the management of rheumatoid arthritis, osteoarthritis, polymyositis, and systemic lupus erythematosus. Exercise preserves function, reduces symptoms, and reduces sick days. Prescribed exercise must now be considered an essential part of the treatment of all the rheumatologic disorders.

Musculoskeletal complaints are among the most common reasons that older adults seek medical attention. About 1 in 4 of all patients seen by primary care physicians presents with a musculoskeletal condition. Osteoarthritis (OA), whether based on radiographic findings, clinical symptoms, or self-report, is overwhelmingly prevalent in older persons. Depending upon the source of data and which joint is involved, OA is present in anywhere from 50% to 90% of older adults.

DIAGNOSING MUSCULOSKELETAL DISEASE IN OLDER ADULTS

The rheumatologic disorders can be broadly classified as those that present with predominantly musculoskeletal symptoms and those that present with symptoms suggesting a systemic illness. True joint disease (arthritis) is characterized by symptoms and physical examination findings localized to the joints. A patient's history of joint swelling is strong evidence from the outset that true joint involvement is present. History of pain in a joint with motion or weight bearing is suggestive of arthritis. Further questioning about patterns of joint involvement, the presence of morning stiffness, stiffness after periods of inactivity, the effect of activity, and the effect on sleep can greatly narrow diagnostic possibilities.

Musculoskeletal symptoms that seem to be located in a joint are instead often due to a variety of disorders of periarticular tissues, muscles, nerves, and metabolism. These soft-tissue disorders include chronic postural strain, acute muscular and ligamentous strain, bursitis, and fibromyalgia plus conditions not directly related to joints, such as endocrinopathies and neuropathies. Pain complaints in soft-tissue disorders often involve anatomic regions, such as the shoulder girdle or a whole extremity, and rarely include a history of joint swelling; the patient commonly cannot clearly indicate which joint is involved.

When symptoms of pain and fatigue are generalized and not specifically referable to joints or classic bursal areas, differentiating between inflammatory and noninflammatory conditions is paramount. In the inflammatory disorders that may present with generalized aching and pain, there are usually historical and physical findings that lead to the correct diagnosis. The presence of rash, fever, stomatitis, dysphagia, Raynaud's phenomenon, or true muscle weakness suggests one of the autoimmune rheumatologic disorders. The absence of such symptoms make generalized conditions such as fibromyalgia or regional conditions such as chronic postural strain or myofascial pain more likely.

Laboratory Testing

Laboratory testing plays a small role in the diagnosis of rheumatologic diseases in older adults because of the lack of tests that are specific, the high background incidence of OA, and increased seroreactivity in later life, especially in women. Tests for erythrocyte sedimentation rate (ESR) and rheumatoid factor are neither sensitive nor specific. The antinuclear antibody test has such a high sensitivity in systemic lupus erythematosus (SLE) that a negative test essentially excludes it; however, a positive antinuclear antibody is of very low specificity. A few blood tests are specific. For example, either high titers of anti–double-stranded DNA antibodies or the presence of the anti-Sm antibody is specific for SLE, but unfortunately neither is sensitive. Most blood testing in rheumatologic conditions can, at best, only help confirm the clinical impression or provide prognostic data. Studies show that laboratory testing tends to be overused.

The Role of Exercise in Treatment

The value of exercise in treating older adults has long been understood. Exercise helps preserve muscle and bone mass, reverses the increased fat-to-muscle ratio associated with aging, and preserves physical function. In contrast, traditional thinking in rheumatoid arthritis (RA) as recent as the mid-1980s was that exercise should be avoided and even that total bed rest was a mainstay treatment for severe flares. Conventional wisdom also held that weight bearing in OA would accelerate joint degeneration and that exercise in polymyositis would aggravate muscle inflammation. Increasingly, well-designed studies have disproved these beliefs and have shown the value of exercise in the management of RA, OA, polymyositis, and SLE. Rather than worsening these disorders, exercise preserves function, reduces symptoms, and reduces sick days. Prescribed exercise must be considered an essential part of the treatment of all the rheumatologic disorders.

JOINT DISEASE

Osteoarthritis

Radiologic evidence of OA can be found in nearly 100% of adults aged 65 and over. OA is the major cause of knee, hip, and joint pain, as well as back pain in older adults. Knee pain alone, according to data from NHANES III (the third National Health and Nutrition Examination Survey) affects more than 20% of adults aged 60 or over, with an incidence approaching 30% for those aged 80 and over. Sequential NHANES data suggests that the rising incidence of knee pain can be attributed to the increasing obesity and decreasing physical activity of Americans in recent decades.

OA is a degenerative disease of cartilage that correlates strongly with aging, yet pathologic changes in osteoarthritic cartilage are quite distinct from changes seen in normal aging cartilage. OA is also a heterogenous group of related joint disorders that have a variety of causes; these may be genetic, associated with metabolic disease, or due to joint malformation, joint trauma, or damage from other joint diseases. A wide range of distinct patterns of joint involvement are used to classify OA, including isolated finger interphalangeal joint bony enlargement, severe deterioration of weight-bearing joints, isolated spinal involvement, and generalized axial and peripheral joint degeneration. Primary OA appears to be genetically determined, with dominant expression in woman and recessive expression in men; wrists, elbows, shoulders, and ankles tend not to be affected. Involvement of these joints with OA is suggestive of the presence of another disease or factor contributing to joint degeneration.

Underlying pathology in OA does not feature inflammation, though hypertrophy of synovium and accumulation of joint effusions is typical. Progressive changes in cartilage include poor chondrocyte function and death, altered cartilage composition with poor mechanical properties, cartilage surface fibrillation, and eventual gross cartilage destruction. Associated boney proliferation at the cartilage-bone interface leads to palpable and radiographically distinct osteophytes around affected joints.

Pain and reduced joint motion are the hallmarks of OA, with attendant ligamental instability and muscle atrophy. OA in weight-bearing joints is associated with gait abnormalities, which increase the risk of falling and injury, contributing substantially to OA morbidity, especially in the oldest and most frail patients. Disability can be profound. The ACR diagnostic criteria for OA of the knee and hip are summarized in Table 54.1.

Management of OA usually begins with efforts to control pain. Rarely do analgesics alone accomplish pain control. By the time of clinician evaluation for symptomatic OA, function has likely worsened because of muscle atrophy and limitation of joint motion. These collateral changes put an affected joint at biomechanical disadvantage that both increases pain and predisposes the joint to even more rapid deterioration. Early efforts to strengthen atrophied muscles related to the diseased joint and to improve joint motion are critical. Analgesics play a role in allowing physical therapy to be used effectively in the long-term management of OA. Early referral to a physical therapist for evaluation and to define a set of exercises the patient can do daily at home is usually indicated. With OA of the weight-bearing joints, especially the knees, early remobilization and an ongoing walking exercise program may progressively improve function and reduce pain rather than lead to the often-feared inevitable deterioration of affected joints. Weight loss can

Table 54.1—Diagnostic Criteria for Osteoarthritis

Knee Pain	Hip Pain
plus at least one of the following:	*plus at least two of the following:*
■ Age > 50 years	■ ESR < 20 mm/hour
■ Stiffness < 30 minutes	■ Femoral or acetabular osteophytes
■ Crepitus	■ Joint-space narrowing
■ Osteophytes on radiography:	■ Osteophytes on radiography:
91% sensitive	89% sensitive
86% specific	91% specific

NOTE: ESR = erythrocyte sedimentation rate (Westergren).

SOURCES: Data from Altman R, Asch E, Bloch D, et al. The American College of Rheumatology criteria for the classification and reporting of osteoarthritis of the knee. *Arthritis Rheum.* 1986;29:1039–1049, and Altman R, Alarcon G, Appelrouth D, et al. The American College of Rheumatology criteria for the classification and reporting of osteoarthritis of the hip. *Arthritis Rheum.* 1991;34:505–514.

also help improve function and reduce pain, especially if the lumbar spine or weight-bearing joints are involved. Joint injection with corticosteroids or hyaluronic acid derivatives, and joint lavage can be of temporary benefit with low risk for toxicity. If interest in avoiding knee arthroplasty is high, a cartilage-preserving lateral tibial wedge osteotomy can be considered, provided that the medial knee compartment OA is isolated and the lateral knee compartment is intact. If conservative management proves to be inadequate with knee or hip disease, total arthroplasty is an excellent ultimate solution.

Recommendations about which analgesics to use for OA have changed over the past decade. Research shows that acetaminophen is often as effective as any of the nonsteroidal anti-inflammatory drugs (NSAIDs). Considerable gastrointestinal and renal toxicity can be associated with NSAID use in older adults. The ACR recommends acetaminophen as the first choice analgesic in treating OA. Similar recommendations have been issued by the American Geriatrics Society. Clinical studies over the past 2 years suggest an emerging consensus that NSAIDs may be slightly more effective in treating OA of the knee, especially when analgesia is still required after 3 to 6 months of treatment.

Controversy continues regarding possible kidney and liver damage from acetaminophen. There is no disagreement about the severe hepatic toxicity of acetaminophen overdose; however, hepatotoxicity is not seen when dosing guidelines are followed. Of course, with older adults who are cognitively impaired, inadvertent or accidental overdose of any prescribed medication is always a possibility. Investigators continue to be intrigued about the possibility that chronic acetaminophen use contributes to renal insufficiency.

Possibly because phenacetin was banned by the Food and Drug Administration more than 20 years ago because of the high risk of nephropathy, suspicions about acetaminophen (the active metabolite of phenacetin) persist. Nearly all studies of the renal effects of acetaminophen use have been retrospective and have had numerous methodologic problems. The preponderance of data suggests that the risk of nephropathy from acetaminophen is quite low when it is used in modest doses by those without preexisting kidney disease. Acetaminophen, given under physician supervision, is still the analgesic of choice for patients with existing renal insufficiency, according to the National Kidney Foundation recommendations.

If acetaminophen is initially ineffective, nonacetylated salicylates such as salsalate or magnesium choline salicylate, which have lower gastrointestinal toxicity than most older NSAIDs, can be given. The selective COX-2 inhibitors are more expensive. COX-2 inhibitors have the same risk of unwanted renal effects as the other NSAIDs. They may also be associated with increased risk of myocardial infarction. The COX-2 inhibitors are further discussed in the section on RA (see p 406).

Hyaluronic acid is a major constituent of synovial fluid and contributes to both synovial fluid viscosity and cartilage elasticity. Hyaluronic acid and hyaluronan polymers were approved in 1997 for intra-articular injection for OA of the knee. This therapy is given in a series of weekly injections into the knee, five for hyaluronic acid and three for hyaluronan polymers. The benefits of these preparations typically last for 6 months, which is substantially longer than for corticosteroid injection.

Glucosamine and chondroitin sulfate are components of glycosaminoglycan molecules that are important in maintaining mechanical properties of connective tissue and cartilage. When taken orally, these compounds are absorbed and incorporated into cartilage. Both have been studied separately as treatments for OA, with evidence of benefit. In OA of the knee, the effectiveness of glucosamine is equivalent to that of ibuprofen, with less gastrointestinal toxicity. The therapeutic benefit of chondroitin sulfate does not become apparent for several weeks after it is started, and improvement lasts for several weeks after it is stopped. Long-term studies will be needed before chondroitin sulfate can be considered a disease-modifying drug for OA. Glucosamine and chondroitin sulfate are available in combination as nutriceuticals. Although both compounds are nontoxic, the dosage and bioavailability has not been established; therefore, the benefit seen in therapeutic trials cannot be predicted with these over-the-counter preparations.

Gout

Gout is perhaps the oldest recognized form of arthritis; it was unmistakably described in Hippocrates, and Sydenham's clinical description of his own experience of gout in the late 17th century can hardly be improved upon today. Through the 19th century, the classification of arthritis had rheumatic fever as a distinct form of arthritis, and other forms of joint disease were considered to be subtypes of gout. Hence, terms like *rheumatoid gout* were used for the disease now called *rheumatoid arthritis*. These views prevailed until about 150 years ago when the relationship of classic gout with high levels of uric acid in blood was recognized. Proof of intra-articular monosodium urate crystals as the specific cause of acute gout was not established until the early 1960s.

Gout often presents as acute monarthritis, usually of the first metatarsal phalangeal joint, mid-foot, or ankle. With subsequent attacks, the knee, elbow, or wrist can be involved. Later in the course of untreated disease, attacks tend to be less intense and to last longer, and they may feature simultaneous involvement of more than one joint. Late in untreated disease, chronic low-grade inflammation in multiple joints appears and tophi (gross subcutaneous urate deposits on extensor surfaces) develop. In this late phase of untreated gout, the condition can be mistaken for nodular RA, with the tophi being mistaken for rheumatoid nodules. This can be a sad error, because gout and RA do not occur together, and the two conditions are treated differently. Thus, a strong case is made for microscopic evaluation of samples of joint fluid in the initial evaluation of chronic polyarticular, as well as acute monarticular, arthritis.

With rare exceptions, the clinical emergence of gout is preceded by a period of asymptomatic hyperuricemia. However, hyperuricemia is neither consistently present at the time of an acute gout attack, nor does it confirm a diagnosis of gout. Acute attacks can be precipitated by trauma, acute nonarticular illness requiring hospitalization, dehydration (acute gout is particularly common postoperatively), or medications that can affect serum levels of uric acid.

A diagnosis of gout is most directly and unequivocally established by observing the presence of strongly negatively birefringent needle-shaped crystals in a sample of joint fluid. Needle-shaped urate crystals can often be seen by ordinary or dark field microscopy of joint fluid, but confirmation of negative birefringence requires the use of a polarizing microscope equipped with a compensator plate. Many laboratories and most rheumatologists have access to such a microscope, which is essential in diagnosing pseudogout, described in the next section.

The treatment of gout is biphasic. The acute episode is best managed with a short course of an NSAID. The choice of the NSAID is not critical, because the risk of gastrointestinal toxicity is less likely to emerge during the 10 to 21 days needed for a response during an acute attack. If NSAIDs are contraindicated, colchicine may be an alternative for an acute episode. Drugs such as allopurinol or probenecid, which can acutely lower uric acid levels, should not be used in the management of acute gout, because premature lowering of uric acid level will paradoxically intensify and prolong an acute gout attack.

Once the acute attack has been resolved, attention can be turned to correcting the underlying problem of urate deposition. Urate can accumulate in body tissues because of uric acid overproduction in the body, reduced renal elimination, or both. Ninety percent of chronic hyperuricemia is a consequence of reduced renal excretion that is due to renal disease or drugs, especially diuretics. Uric acid overproduction in older adults is seen in disorders with increased tissue turnover, such as lymphoproliferative disease, chronic hemolytic anemia, and psoriasis, as well as rare genetic enzymatic defects.

Drugs, for example probenecid, that promote renal uric acid excretion can correct hyperuricemia in young adults who have normal kidney function. In older adults, reduced kidney function renders uricosuric drugs less effective. The most effective treatment for uric acid reduction is allopurinol, which acts by blocking the formation of uric acid. The dosage of allopurinol can be adjusted upward from a starting dosage of 100 mg daily, increasing the daily dose by 100 mg at 2- to 4-week intervals until serum uric acid levels are 5 or below. Because of the high likelihood of decreased kidney function with aging, somewhat lower allopurinol doses may be adequate in older patients to reduce uric acid to the desired therapeutic level.

During treatment to lower uric acid levels, the risk of recurrent acute gout attacks is raised. Prophylaxis against acute attacks is advisable for 3 to 6 months while treatment to lower uric acid is introduced and optimized. Although NSAIDs could be used for prophylaxis, the risk of gastrointestinal toxicity with chronic use must be considered. Colchicine can be effective for prophylaxis in older adults at a reduced dosage of 0.6 mg daily. This low dose is well tolerated and does not have an associated risk of gastrointestinal ulceration. Colchicine should be avoided in individuals with hepatic disease or advanced renal insufficiency and is contraindicated if both hepatic and renal diseases are present.

Chondrocalcinosis

Radiographically evident deposition of calcium pyrophosphate dihydrate (CPPD) crystals in articular tissue is markedly related to aging and can be seen in up to 50% of adults aged 90 and over. CPPD crystals can be found in synovial fluid and are associated with several clinical syndromes. CPPD crystals can cause attacks of acute monarthritis, most commonly the knee, wrist, or shoulder, termed *pseudogout* because of the resemblance to acute (urate) gout. CPPD deposition can occur simultaneously in multiple joints and be responsible for chronic polyarticular synovitis reminiscent of RA. Radiographic chondrocalcinosis with or without CPPD crystals in the synovial fluid can also be present in joints with OA without any evidence of inflammation. The coexistence of CPPD crystals and OA is not surprising, because both conditions are common in older adults; however, controversy persists regarding the relationship of the two disorders. Differentiation of CPPD deposition arthropathy from urate gout and RA is important, because the treatment approaches are different.

Acute pseudogout attacks can be treated with a limited course of oral colchicine[OL] or an NSAID in a manner similar to the treatment for acute urate gout. Similarly, intra-articular corticosteroids will halt an attack in patients for whom an NSAID is contraindicated. Parenteral corticosteroids are effective for acute pseudogout when NSAIDs and intra-articular corticosteroid injections are both contraindicated. Given once and possibly again in 1 to 2 days, triamcinolone acetonide 60 mg IM, betamethasone 7 mg IM, or methylprednisolone 125 mg IV have all proved to be safe and effective. Although a single intravenous dose of colchicine of 1 to 2 mg is long acting and can be effective in treating acute pseudogout, the risk of tissue necrosis with accidental extravasation and of bone-marrow suppression in older adults with renal or hepatic impairment suggests this should be considered very carefully in individual cases. Recurrent attacks of pseudogout can be prevented by the use of prophylactic oral colchicine. Any combination of oral and intravenous colchicine is absolutely contraindicated.

SOFT-TISSUE RHEUMATISM

The variety and number of conditions that present with musculoskeletal symptoms is impressive. This section describes the general approach to a patient with a regional musculoskeletal complaint and then discusses a selection of clinically common soft-tissue disorders.

Evaluating Reports of Pain

Most musculoskeletal complaints in older adults are not caused by true arthritis but rather by disorders resulting from derangement of tendons, bursae, muscles, connective tissue, and nerves. Symptoms typically involve a region of the body rather than discrete joints. It makes sense to evaluate a new musculoskeletal complaint as likely soft-tissue rheumatism. The physical examination can begin with observation of the patient performing active range of motion of the affected region. Interpreting abnormal range of motion requires an understanding of the anatomy of the relevant muscles, tendons, bones, and nerves.

The shoulder, for example, is not a simple ball-in-socket joint, but an extremely mobile system of three bones (scapula, clavicle, and humerus) that is attached to the rest of the skeleton only at the sternoclavicular joint. The rest of the shoulder girdle floats and slides over the body and is controlled by a complex set of muscles and associated innervation. To evaluate a painful shoulder, instruct the patient to abduct the shoulder from 0 degrees at the side through 90 degrees to 180 degrees, with hand above the head. Test shoulder internal and external rotation by having the patient put the backs of the hands on the sacrum and then the palms on the occiput. Depending on the result of these active range-of-motion tests, the examiner can further pinpoint the likely site of pathology by selectively moving the shoulder components for the patient. Passive motion is most informative when active motion has been demonstrated to be painful or limited. The glenohumeral joint can be isolated while the patient completely relaxes the shoulder; the examiner holds one hand over the upper scapula to prevent scapular motion and simultaneously slowly abducts, extends, flexes, and rotates the shoulder joint. True shoulder (glenohumeral) joint disease would be indicated if isolated passive joint motion is painful. In the case that active motion proved to be painless, then the examiner can first palpate key periarticular structures and then engage the patient with a series of selective resisted active movements that stress particular anatomic elements of the shoulder apparatus. Figure 54.1 shows an algorithm for evaluating the complaint of shoulder pain. A similar method can be applied to other regions of the musculoskeletal system.

Fibromyalgia

Fibromyalgia is a generalized pain syndrome that occurs at nearly all ages; prevalence rates of 2% to 10%

OL Not approved by the U.S. Food and Drug Administration for this use.

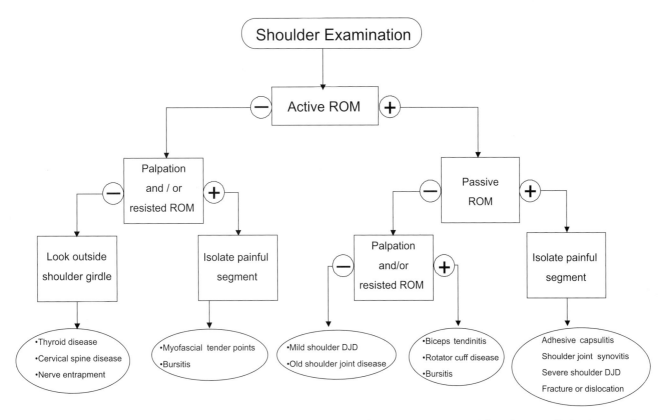

Figure 54.1—Evaluation of shoulder pain. DJD = degenerative joint disease; ROM = range of motion; + = limitation or pain; −
= no limitation or pain.

are similar around the world, independently of nationality or ethnicity and cultural factors. Although there is no pathophysiologic explanation of the condition, the uniform worldwide incidence is persuasive that the condition is real. It was originally termed *fibrositis* in the early 20th century; more recent usage favors the term *fibromyalgia,* because there is no demonstrable inflammation in symptomatic tissues. A conceptual breakthrough was made nearly 30 years ago with seminal publications by Smythe and Moldofsky that demonstrated characteristic changes in sleep polysomnography in individuals who were defined by the classic "fibrositis" tender points (see Figure 54.2). Furthermore, it was found that electroencephalographic (EEG) changes and classic tender points could be induced by experimental disruption of deep sleep in normal volunteers. Researchers also learned that the EEG changes could be normalized and tender points could be resolved by aerobic exercise and by medications that tend to deepen deep sleep. Over the next 15 years, a multitude of symptoms were associated with fibromyalgia that tended to overlap with those of patients with irritable bowel syndrome and chronic fatigue syndrome. Some experts incorporated these symptoms as secondary criteria for diagnosis.

In 1990 the American College of Rheumatology (ACR) issued criteria for fibromyalgia diagnosis that were about 88% sensitive and 81% specific (see the caption for Figure 54.2). The criteria allow for the coexistence of fibromyalgia with other musculoskeletal disorders. With this approach, fibromyalgia is not simply a diagnosis of exclusion. No laboratory studies can help confirm the diagnosis. Despite the skepticism of many observers who believed fibromyalgia to be an artificial construct, research in the past decade has helped to develop an understanding of fibromyalgia as a condition of altered pain processing by the central nervous system. This research has paralleled advances in understanding the neurologic basis of pain itself. These advances have not yet led to new treatment, but there is ground for optimism.

The average age of fibromyalgia patients is around 45 years, and the majority are female. The condition seems to be a primary and persistent disorder that afflicts adults well into their 80s. Research indicates that the distress experienced by fibromyalgia patients diminishes with advancing age, suggesting that management in older adults may be less challenging. Mainstays of treatment have changed little in recent years. Reassurance that the condition is not life threatening and can be improved is indicated. Aerobic exercise is recommended, partly because of the original findings of Smythe and Moldofsky but also because of the deconditioning and muscle weakness seen in

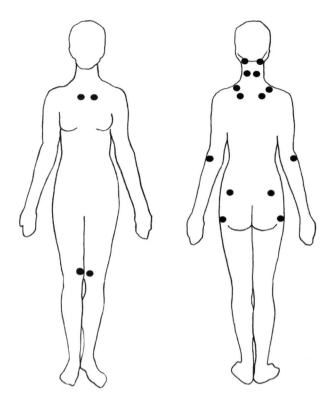

Figure 54.2—Fibromyalgia tender point sites.

For a diagnosis of fibromyalgia, both of the following must be present: (1) a history of widespread pain for at least 3 months; (2) pain in 11 of 18 tender points on digital palpation. For a tender point to be considered positive, the patient must state that the palpation was "painful"; "tender" is not considered synonymous with "painful."

SOURCE: Diagnostic criteria are from Wolfe F, Smythe HA, Yunus MB, et al. The American College of Rheumatology 1990 criteria for the classification of fibromyalgia: report of the multicenter criteria committee. *Arthritis Rheum.* 1990;33:160–172.

fibromyalgia. Analgesics give benefit; the role of narcotics is not yet well defined. Tramadol has been investigated and found to give benefit without serious adverse effects. Tricyclic antidepressants have long been used with benefit, but other antidepressants of different classes are also effective. Also, the muscle relaxant cyclobenzaprine and the benzodiazepine alprazolam[OL] have given benefit. Some patients find benefit from rotating medications every 6 months if tolerance seems to emerge. (See also "Persistent Pain," p 131.)

Myofascial Trigger Points

When examination does not reveal arthritis, tendinitis, bursitis, or nerve impingement as the cause of regional pain, careful palpation may locate indurated, and sometimes crepitant, trigger points. Myofascial trigger

points are distinct from the symmetrical multiple tender points of fibromyalgia in that palpation of trigger points reproduces the pain syndrome. Trigger points are most common over the upper back at upper or medial edges of a scapula. Similar trigger points can sometimes be discovered over the anterior chest, lower back, sacral, and iliac areas. The cause is poorly understood. Anesthetic injection into a trigger point can confirm the diagnosis. Treatment includes repeated ice application to the trigger points or injection with anesthetic or glucocorticoid, or both.

Biceps Tendinitis

Pain in the anterior shoulder with associated exquisite tenderness over the proximal biceps tendon and exacerbation with supination of the forearm (with elbow flexed to 90 degrees) against resistance (Yergason sign) is diagnostic of biceps tendinitis. Also, anterior flexion of the shoulder against resistance is likely to exacerbate the pain in biceps tendinitis. The condition is usually associated with repetitive motions but can be associated with bony impingement problems in the shoulder apparatus. Biceps tendinitis responds well to tendon sheath infiltration with glucocorticoid with or without anesthetic. Steroid iontophoresis can also be effective. Stretching and range-of-motion exercises are indicated during and following healing.

Rotator Cuff Disease

The shoulder rotator cuff is formed superiorly by a common tendinous insertion on the humeral greater tuberosity of the supraspinatus, infraspinatus, and teres minor muscles and inferiorly by the insertion of the subscapularis muscle on the lesser humeral tuberosity. Vascular supply to the upper portions of the rotator cuff is somewhat limited and easily compromised by impingement. Several bursae are associated with the rotator cuff and contribute to symptoms in rotator cuff problems. Rotator cuff disorders tend not to be as acute in older as in younger adults. A history of a recent acute event is not likely to be elicited, but a past episode of a fall with direct blow to the shoulder or falling with the arm outstretched may be recalled. Rotator cuff derangement can involve partial tear or degeneration or complete degenerative destruction. Although trauma is commonly an important factor, tissue ischemia from impingement and changes in bony relationships with advanced shoulder joint degeneration are more likely to be dominant factors in older patients. With complete loss of the rotator cuff, initiation of active abduction of the hanging arm is severely impaired. With partial tear or degeneration, only pain and giving way with the shoulder abducted to 90 degrees may be present. Management of rotator cuff degeneration should include identification of aggravating factors that can be avoided, especially sleeping with the arm outstretched. Initiation of tailored physical therapy to maintain shoulder range of motion is essential. Injection of a mixture of anesthetic and glucocorticoid into related bursal areas can be helpful in relieving pain and allowing progressive physical therapy to be successful. Surgery is an intervention of last resort in the treatment of rotator cuff disorders in older adults.

Lower Cervical Nerve Impingement

Intermittent pain in the shoulder, deltoid, and upper arm area in the absence of shoulder joint or associated musculotendinous structures should raise suspicion of cervical nerve impingement. The C5 level is most commonly involved. A cervical compression test (Spurling maneuver) can help identify cervical nerve impingement. In this maneuver, the seated person tilts and turns the head slightly to the affected side. Steady vertical downward pressure on the top of the head is exerted by the examiner for 10 to 15 seconds. Reproduction of the symptoms on the affected side is a positive test. With more advanced impingement, sensory changes over the upper arm can be demonstrated on examination. Further evaluation would include cervical spine plain radiographs, including oblique views to optimally show the neuroforamina and detect bony impingement. Cervical disk disease can occur and might best be discovered with magnetic resonance imaging. Electrodiagnostic testing may also help sort out more obscure cases. Cervical traction twice daily at home, use of a cervical pillow, and avoidance of aggravating activities are the mainstays of conservative treatment. When muscle spasm is associated with cervical impingement, hot or cold applications plus injection of any identified trigger points can aid in the control of symptoms during recovery. Rarely, surgical intervention is needed for cervical nerve impingement.

Adhesive Capsulitis

Adhesive capsulitis (frozen shoulder syndrome) is an acute process of obscure cause that involves inflammation of the shoulder joint capsule. The condition can follow other shoulder disorders or injury. ESR may acutely increase. Unilateral shoulder involvement can help differentiate this condition from polymyalgia rheumatica. Shoulder pain and tenderness plus severely restricted active and passive range of motion are present. Early intervention with aggressive range-of-motion exercises combined with intra-articular glucocorticoids are important to preserve shoulder motion and reduce inflammation. Although not essential, shoulder arthrography with glucocorticoid and anesthetic injection at the time of arthrogram should be both diagnostic and therapeutic. In addition to intra-articular injection, percutaneous glucocorticoid injections anteriorly, posteriorly, and laterally into the glenohumeral joint capsule and shoulder bursal areas can also be effective. Adhesive capsulitis usually follows a course of several months that includes three phases: freezing, frozen, and thawing. With timely treatment, the outcome should be good, but physical therapy needs to extend well beyond the thawing phase.

Olecranon Bursitis

Enlargement of the olecranon bursa with marked distension due to effusion with or without inflammation and surrounding cellulitis is common regardless of age. In younger adults occupational factors are often present, supporting the notion that olecranon bursitis can have an origin based in repetitive trauma. Olecranon bursitis is also commonly associated with RA and gout, with or without nodules in the former case and tophi in the latter. Infection of the bursa is also common, usually with staphylococci. Evaluation of an inflamed olecranon begins with sterile aspiration of fluid for cultures and cell count. The presence of surrounding cellulitis could be due to infection or acute gout; diagnostic aspiration of the bursa through affected skin mandates initiation of an antibiotic and continuation until culture results are in hand. Antibiotic selection should provide *Staphylococcus aureus* coverage, with modification that is based on culture results. Repeated aspiration during treatment may help recovery from infection. The course of recovery can be prolonged, with frequent relapses. The bursa often spontaneously drains, and complete healing of the cutaneous fistula may require many months. Olecranon bursitis associated with RA or gout is managed in accordance with the underlying disease once infection is excluded. Noninfectious olecranon bursitis suspected to be of traumatic origin should be treated with padding and avoidance of further trauma; aspiration and injection of the bursa could be considered. Close follow-up is indicated because olecranon bursae are so prone to spontaneous infection.

Carpal Tunnel Syndrome

Entrapment of the median nerve where it passes through the carpal tunnel of the wrist is one of the most common nerve-entrapment syndromes in older adults. Symptoms of median nerve compression can occur with wrist synovitis due to RA, gout, or pseudogout. Hypothyroidism and diabetes mellitus are predisposing factors. Amyloidosis is an infrequent but well-known cause of carpal tunnel syndrome. The most common cause, however, is repetitive trauma. Carpal tunnel syndrome presents with nocturnal hand pain, tingling, and numbness involving the median nerve distribution in the hand. Pain during the day, even with radiation proximally to the shoulder, is occasionally seen and can confound diagnosis. In addition to the sensory deficits almost always present, atrophy of the thenar eminence can develop in longstanding median nerve compression. Evaluation should include inquiry into factors in the patient's daily activities that could exacerbate carpal tunnel disease. Untreated or unrecognized hypothyroidism and diabetes should be tested for. A cock-up wrist splint, especially at night, can lessen symptoms. Some clinicians recommend isometric flexion exercises of metacarpal phalangeal joints and the affected wrist joint in which the tense flexor tendons act like a bowstring to stretch the transverse ligament overlying the carpal tunnel. Injection of glucocorticoids into the carpal tunnel, taking care not to inject the median nerve, can be of benefit and is highly recommended by some clinicians. Injection of the wrist joint when carpal tunnel syndrome is related to active wrist synovitis due to RA, gout, or pseudogout is usually quite effective. Surgical release of the transverse ligament can relieve symptoms when conservative measures fail.

Trochanteric Bursitis

Several bursae surround the hip joint and femoral trochanteric areas. Two bursa are of particular interest in soft-tissue rheumatism. The first is the bursa that directly overlies the greater femoral trochanter, and the second is deep to the gluteus maximus and posterior and slightly superior to the trochanter. Presenting symptoms of trochanteric bursitis include hip pain that is localized over the lateral proximal thigh. Pain on the affected side during sleep is usually present. The cause of trochanteric bursitis is not well understood. Significant predisposing factors may include local trauma, strain, and obesity. Treatment in elderly persons should include physical therapy, evaluation of transferring techniques to minimize excessive gluteal muscle stress, stretching exercises, and the use of a pillow positioned posterolaterally behind the involved side to discourage inadvertent resting on the affected bursa during sleep. Infiltration of the trochanteric areas with glucocorticoids is very helpful.

Anserine Bursitis

Several bursae are associated with the knee. In elderly persons the two most important are both associated with knee joint arthritis: the gastrocnemius and semimembranosus bursae in the popliteal fossa (see next section) and the anserine bursa anteromedially distal to the knee. The anserine bursa is located in relation to the insertion of the medial collateral liga-ment on the proximal tibia. Anserine bursitis presents with the complaint of knee pain that may bother the patient especially at night. Palpation over the area of the bursa should reveal marked local tenderness. Swelling, induration, or effusion may exist in association with anserine bursitis. Knee OA may be symptomatic as well. Cold applications may be of benefit. A pillow placed between the knees at night can lessen both nocturnal pain and recurrence in susceptible individuals. Injection of the bursa with a mixture of glucocorticoid and anesthetic is effective and can provide prompt relief.

Popliteal Cyst

A popliteal cyst (Baker cyst) may develop at any age. A symptomatic cyst can present with knee pain with pressure in the posterior knee; occasionally, a popliteal cyst can present with acute rupture. A popliteal cyst develops as an extension of the knee joint synovial space posteriorly into the gastrocnemius and semimembranosus bursae. Knee arthritis is almost always a precursor. Knee effusions in arthritis result in high resting intra-articular pressure that increases many-fold with knee flexion or with weight bearing. High knee synovial pressure tends to force fluid into one of the popliteal bursa. The communication between joint and bursa also tends to behave like a ball valve, with one-way movement of fluid from knee to bursa. This process leads to progressive popliteal cyst formation and enlargement, with eventual emergence of pain behind the knee. In addition to pain, the cyst can become a space-occupying lesion and can impede deep venous return from the lower leg.

Inspection for the presence of a popliteal cyst should be part of the routine knee examination in patients with known OA or who present with knee pain. Often a popliteal cyst is not distinctly palpable. Inspection of both popliteal fossae with the patient standing may reveal asymmetric fullness on one side. Hyperextension of the ankle while the knee is fully extended can accentuate the bulge of a popliteal cyst. Ultrasound examination of the popliteal fossa easily demonstrates the presence of a cyst. Though highly accurate, magnetic resonance imaging of the knee is rarely necessary to evaluate for a popliteal cyst.

A popliteal cyst can rupture spontaneously or with exertion. The result can be dramatic, with acute pain, swelling, warmth, and erythema of the lower leg that mimics all the signs of deep-vein thrombosis. In a few days, bruising can surface in the lower leg and form a bruise below the lateral malleolus on the affected side (crescent sign). Occasionally, true deep-vein thrombosis can develop following acute popliteal cyst rupture. Venography or serial venous Doppler studies, or both, may be required to correctly interpret the course of popliteal cyst rupture. Glucocorticoid injection into the knee may be of benefit with acute cyst rupture, because presumably the same mechanisms that direct fluid from the knee to the popliteal cyst will carry the injected steroid into the area of the ruptured cyst. Similarly, knee arthrocentesis followed by glucocorticoid instillation for a symptomatic, but intact, popliteal cyst may reduce synovial fluid production and intra-articular pressure and give a few months' improvement in popliteal symptoms. In the case of associated knee OA, a series of knee hyalin injections (see the next section) could ameliorate the factors driving popliteal cyst formation. Correction of the underlying knee disease that has led to development of the popliteal cyst is required to control cyst recurrence. Aspiration of the cyst itself, taking care to avoid the popliteal neurovascular bundle, with injection of glucocorticoid directly into the cyst is recommended by some clinicians.

INFLAMMATORY DISORDERS

Polymyalgia Rheumatica

Polymyalgia rheumatica (PMR) is a distinct syndrome that occurs in older adults, as early as age 50 but predominantly after age 60. The onset tends to be insidious, with corresponding delays in diagnosis. The classic symptom of PMR is remarkable proximal limb girdle stiffness and aching pain upon arising in the morning. ESR is so often markedly elevated that a high ESR is one of the essential diagnostic criteria. The syndrome may be accompanied by fatigue, low-grade fever, weight loss, and variable expression of synovitis of proximal joints of the upper, more than lower, extremities. Studies of PMR in recent years have confirmed the presence of synovitis identical to that seen in RA, with synovial thickening, effusions, and lymphocytic synovial infiltration. PMR can progress to chronic polyarthritis that fulfills criteria for RA. Of more immediate clinical importance is the common coexistence of PMR with giant cell arteritis (GCA), a more serious, potentially life-threatening disease. This relationship is discussed in the next section. Even with uncomplicated PMR, treatment with corticosteroids is associated with significant iatrogenic long-term morbidity, including diabetes mellitus, osteoporotic fracture, muscle atrophy, hypertension, glaucoma, and acceleration of cataracts and skin atrophy.

The cause of PMR is unknown. Studies for infectious agents responsible for triggering the syndrome have been inconclusive. Type II HLA gene associations have been found, but associations differ from those for RA.

The standard treatment of PMR is oral prednisone beginning at 15 mg daily. Dramatic improvement is so much to be expected that some have proposed that low-dose corticosteroid responsiveness confirms the diagnosis of PMR. ESR normalization corresponds to initial symptomatic improvement. Prednisone dose can be tapered over succeeding months on the basis of control of symptoms. PMR often runs a course of 2 to 3 years, and many patients are able to discontinue prednisone by then. Unfortunately, mean time to the first adverse event on corticosteroid therapy for PMR is about 1.6 years. Occasional patients with PMR respond to NSAIDs. Though long-term prednisone has significant toxicity, prednisone may be safer in older adults than NSAIDs, provided the prednisone dose can be minimized and parallel efforts are made to protect bone mass. In a randomized trial of methylprednisolone acetate, a dosage of 120 mg IM every 3 to 4 weeks has been found to control PMR with fewer fractures, less weight gain, and lower cumulative dose than a daily oral prednisone regimen.

Giant Cell Arteritis

Giant cell arteritis (GCA) is the most common form of vasculitis to affect older adults. This form of vasculitis predominantly affects proximal branches of the aorta. Therefore, inflammatory and ischemic manifestations are mostly seen in the head and upper extremities. Occasionally, gross inflammation with tender, nodular swelling and erythema of the temporal arteries can be seen. In the absence of gross findings, symptoms of temporal headache, jaw and tongue claudication, and sudden vision loss may be seen. Diagnosis can be confirmed by biopsy of a temporal artery, thus the often-used synonym *temporal arteritis*. ACR criteria for the diagnosis of GCA are available on the ACR Web site (http://www.rheumatology.org/publications/classification). The recognition of GCA is often preceded by several months of a nonspecific systemic illness that includes weight loss, fever, and muscle aching that is indistinguishable from PMR. GCA can also present with sudden blindness with no prior systemic illness or with upper-extremity limb claudication. Other manifestations can include stroke, ischemic necrosis of tongue or scalp, or, rarely, myocardial infarction. Aortic aneurysm, predominantly thoracic, is a late manifestation of GCA even when previously appropriately treated. The incidence of aneurysm in GCA is about 10%, with thoracic and abdominal aneurysm discovery 5.9 and 2.5 years, respectively, after GCA diagnosis.

The cause of GCA is unknown. Infectious agents have long been suspected, but none has yet been confirmed as causative.

The diagnosis of GCA may require a high index of suspicion combined with the finding of an otherwise unexplained elevated ESR above 40 mm/hour. Combined elevation of ESR and C-reactive protein is more specific (97%) than elevated ESR alone for biopsy-positive GCA. Because of the risk of sudden blindness, most clinicians start high-dose oral prednisone as soon as the possibility of GCA is seriously considered, and then proceed to biopsy. Administration of prednisone does not change arterial histology for weeks. Diagnosis can sometimes even be established or reestablished after a few years of prednisone treatment. Arterial involvement is patchy, and diagnostic histologic changes can be missed by biopsy. This oversight can be minimized by biopsy of the symptomatic side and by obtaining a piece of artery several centimeters long. Multiple longitudinal sections as well as cross-sections of artery should be examined by a pathologist. Still, on occasion biopsies are negative in cases in which suspicion remains high.

Because 25% of cases of GCA are associated with PMR, there is a longstanding controversy as to which patients with PMR should undergo temporal artery biopsy. There are no clear data to guide decision making in this situation. One reasonable criterion would be to obtain temporal artery biopsies in cases of PMR in which there are symptoms or physical findings suggestive of arteritis (ie, temporal headache; visual changes; tongue, jaw, or limb claudication; neck or chest pain; or neurologic changes suggestive of central nervous system ischemia). The temporal artery can also be involved with other forms of systemic vasculitis. Vasculitides other than GCA should be considered whenever the temporal artery biopsy shows necrotizing vasculitis but an absence of giant cells.

The treatment of GCA requires high-dose prednisone initially. No other treatment has been so clearly proven to be effective. Clinicians differ on the definition of high dose, with some recommending starting dosages as high as 120 mg daily. There are no data that show dosages above 40 mg daily to be more effective. Older adults are highly susceptible to corticosteroid toxicity, and toxicity increases markedly with total dose. The use of higher doses should be individualized and considered when there is resistance to initial treatment or disease is unusually severe. Response is confirmed when ESR falls rapidly over the first month of therapy. Tapering of the steroid should begin at the rate of 10% to 20% of the total dose per month as soon as the ESR is normalized. Published studies of methotrexate as a steroid-sparing agent have not consistently proved methotrexate to be effective.

Rheumatoid Arthritis

Late-onset RA appears to be clinically different from the same disease with onset earlier in life. The condition in the older adult is more likely to be of rapid onset, involve fewer and more proximal joints, and to be rheumatoid-factor negative. Nodules are less likely and joint destruction may be less severe. Overall prognosis may be better than with earlier onset, seropositive, nodular, erosive disease. Nevertheless, RA is a chronic disease that persists indefinitely, with high risk for progressive joint damage and functional impairment, and more recent reviews confirm that late-onset RA is still a serious disease. Criteria to aid in the diagnosis of RA are listed in Table 54.2.

Treatment is almost always indicated, and therapeutic options have increased since 1998 with the introduction of a variety of entirely new drugs for the management of RA. In more severe cases, consultation with a rheumatologist is indicated.

NSAIDs are often recommended as first-line medications for symptom control in RA. The older nonselective NSAIDs, such as ibuprofen, naproxen, diclofenac, and several others, nonspecifically inhibit both cyclooxygenase isoenzymes.

Selective COX-2 inhibitors introduced in the late 1990's carried the hope that they would be substantially free of antiplatelet effects, gastric toxicity, and renal toxicity. Clinical studies have confirmed that the incidence of serious gastric toxicity was about half that of nonselective COX NSAIDs. However, if COX-2 inhibitors are used concomitantly with mini-dose aspirin, the risk of gastric toxicity becomes similar to that of older NSAIDs. Renal toxicity, unfortunately, has proved to be as serious with the COX-2 inhibitors as with older NSAIDs.

In 2004, evidence suggesting a relationship between the COX-2 inhibitor rofecoxib and increased risk of stroke and myocardial infarction surfaced. In response to this, rofecoxib was withdrawn from the market in late 2004 and valdecoxib, another COX-2 inhibitor, was voluntarily withdrawn from the market in early 2005. Celecoxib is still marketed. The mechanism of increased cardiovascular adverse effects from COX-2 inhibitors is uncertain. The lack of inhibition

---

Table 54.2—Criteria for Diagnosing Rheumatoid Arthritis

The presence of at least four of the following signs and symptoms:

- Morning stiffness for at least 6 weeks
- Arthritis of three or more joint areas for at least 6 weeks
- Arthritis of the hand joints for at least 6 weeks
- Symmetric arthritis for at least 6 weeks
- Subcutaneous rheumatoid nodules
- Elevated serum rheumatoid factor
- Radiographic changes that include erosions or unequivocal bony calcification in periarticular bone

SOURCE: Data from Arnett FC, Edworthy SM, Bloch DA, et al. The American Rheumatism Association 1987 revised criteria for the classification of rheumatoid arthritis. *Arthritis Rheum.* 1988;31:315–324.

of platelet function could be a partial explanation, because older NSAIDs at least reversibly inhibit platelet aggregation.

Certainly, NSAIDs can no longer be considered first-line therapy for arthritis or other chronic, painful conditions. Alternatives to old NSAIDs and selective COX-2 inhibitors might include the relatively selective COX-2 inhibitors: nabumetone, etodolac, and meloxicam. Nabumetone and etodolac were introduced before celecoxib, and meloxicam was introduced in 2004. These three agents have generally less serious gastric adverse effects than older NSAIDs and have less renal toxicity than either older NSAIDs or the selective COX-2 inhibitors. At this time, they are not known to cause an increased risk of stroke and myocardial infarction with long-term use. Therapy with a low-dose corticosteroid such as prednisone may be a preferable option, provided dosages can be limited to 5 mg daily and precautions are taken to preserve bone density. The nonacetylated salicylate salsalate has minimal gastric mucosal toxicity yet has preserved anti-inflammatory activity.

RA is recognized as a lifelong systemic disease associated with progressive joint and extra-articular organ involvement that leads to functional decline and shortened longevity. Mere symptomatic treatment is no longer considered appropriate. Disease-modifying drugs should be considered for treating all cases of RA. Longitudinal studies have confirmed the preservation of function when disease-modifying drugs are instituted early and maintained over the long term.

Parenteral gold, penicillamine, azathioprine, and cyclophosphamide use has markedly declined in the past decade because of the availability of safer effective drugs. Methotrexate has been approved for use in RA for more than a decade and has become established as the disease-modifying agent of choice. When given daily, methotrexate can cause hepatic injury, with cirrhosis and end-stage liver failure. Low-dose, weekly, oral pulse therapy dramatically reduces the risk of hepatic toxicity, provided ethanol intake is completely avoided. Methotrexate can be used in combination with other immunosuppressive agents to yield proven additive or synergistic benefit.

Minocycline[OL] and hydroxychloroquine are well tolerated, have minimal toxicity if used in low dosages, and may be a good choice for mild disease. Sulfasalazine (only the enteric-coated tablets are approved for RA) is more effective than hydroxychloroquine but requires divided daily dosing, has a high incidence of gastrointestinal intolerance, and cannot be given in the presence of sulfa allergy.

Cyclosporine is approved for use in severe RA alone or in combination with methotrexate. Toxicity

remains a concern, and the role of cyclosporine in treating RA is still evolving. Leflunomide is approved both for symptomatic improvement of RA and to prevent radiographic progression in joint damage. Its onset of action (about 4 weeks) is relatively fast compared with that of older disease-modifying drugs.

Several other new drugs have been developed for treatment of RA in the last few years. The group includes etanercept, infliximab, and adalimumab, tumor necrosis factor receptor blockers, which are given parenterally. Infliximab is approved for use only in combination with methotrexate. Clinical trials show marked initial response to these drugs, but they must be continued indefinitely. They are all associated with increased incidence of opportunistic infections and are very expensive. Infliximab has been associated with systemic postinfusion reactions of fever, chills, headache, chest pain, and dyspnea. Anakinra, a recombinant form of the human interleukin-1 receptor antagonist IL-1Ra, is administered as daily subcutaneous injections. Infections during anakinra therapy are mostly bacterial respiratory tract infections with no opportunistic infections. Abatacept, the latest drug approved for the treatment of RA, inhibits T-cell activation. It can be used alone or in combination with other disease-modifying antirheumatic drugs that are not TNF blockers. Adverse events include allergic reactions that are rarely life-threatening and respiratory infections.

Systemic Lupus Erythematosus

Although thought of as a disease in younger women with a higher prevalence among black women, SLE can present in later life. SLE is a multisystem disorder that can have a wide variety of presentations and predominant organ system involvement at any age. SLE is diagnosed with high specificity when any four or more of eleven criteria are documented singly or together at any time during the patient's life (for a detailed description of the ACR criteria, see http://rheumatology.org/publications/classification).

Criteria include malar rash, photosensitivity, stomatitis, nonerosive arthritis, serositis (pleurisy or pericarditis), seizure, nephropathy (urinary casts or heavy proteinuria), cytopenias (leukopenia, hemolytic anemia, or thrombocytopenia), positive antinuclear antibody, and any one of other immunologic abnormalities (anti-double stranded DNA, anti-SM, or false positive test for syphilis). Fever, Raynaud's phenomenon, alopecia, migraine, antiphospholipid syndrome, and Sjögren's syndrome are also often seen in SLE.

It is not surprising that patterns of organ involvement in SLE are different in older adults. Numerous studies suggest that late-onset SLE affects women and men more equally (3:1 in older adults versus 10:1 in young adults); relatively more white than black older

---

[OL] Not approved by the U.S. Food and Drug Administration for this use.

adults are affected. Late-onset SLE is less likely to present with rash, arthritis, Raynaud's phenomenon, nephropathy, and the involvement of the central nervous system and more likely to present with serositis, Sjögren's syndrome, and positive rheumatoid factor. In older adults, SLE onset may be more insidious, involve fewer organ systems, and have fewer relapses. As nephropathy and central nervous system involvement are related to mortality in younger women, late-onset lupus has been sometimes thought of as a milder disease. Despite the impression of milder disease in older adults, immunosuppressive and cytotoxic medications are required as often in managing late-onset SLE.

Hormonal factors may be partly responsible for the differences between early- and late-onset SLE. Estrogens are suspected of being an aggravating factor in young women. Studies of the administration of postmenopausal estrogen for 2 years or more in women is associated with a fivefold increase in SLE risk. The increased risk is somewhat lower if estrogen is combined with a progestational agent. In a population-based study, SLE in women was found to be associated with a doubled overall incidence of cancer.

The treatment of SLE in older adults is similar to the treatment given in early-onset disease. Corticosteroids are less well tolerated by the older adult and should be reserved as much as possible for organ- or life-threatening SLE flares. Hydroxychloroquine has been shown to be of benefit in SLE skin involvement and to reduce the overall number of disease relapses in younger adults. Hydroxychloroquine is well tolerated and has few serious adverse effects in dosages of 5 mg/kg/day or less. Dapsone, azathioprine, and weekly oral methotrexate are used by some clinicians as alternatives to corticosteroids or as corticosteroid-sparing agents. Monthly intravenous pulse cyclophosphamide is reserved for severe or life-threatening disease.

Sjögren's Syndrome and Sjögren's Disease

Sjögren's syndrome with xerostomia and keratoconjunctivitis sicca has been long recognized as occasionally complicating RA. The incidence of Sjögren's syndrome in other connective-tissue diseases is also increased. Dry eye and dry mouth symptoms without confirmation of Sjögren's syndrome occur in up to 40% of older adults who do not have a connective-tissue disease, and these symptoms are undoubtedly contributed to by many of the medications often prescribed to older adults. The treatment of sicca symptoms and uncomplicated Sjögren's syndrome is targeted toward symptoms and includes artificial tears and artificial saliva along with ophthalmologic and

dental preventive care. Pilocarpine 5 mg orally three times a day can help stimulate saliva flow.

Sjögren's disease (SD) is a systemic, multiorgan chronic disease that features lymphocytic infiltration of exocrine glands throughout the body, including lacrimal, salivary, respiratory tree, intestinal tract, pancreatic, hepatic, renal, and vaginal glands. In addition, cutaneous vasculitis and central nervous system involvement are often seen. The involvement of salivary and lacrimal glands is responsible for the sicca symptoms seen in Sjögren's syndrome that is associated with other connective-tissue diseases. The peak onset of SD is in mid-life to early late life.

There is no single diagnostic test for SD. Unexplained interstitial lung disease, renal impairment, hepatic dysfunction, esophageal dysfunction, malabsorption, or central nervous system disease resembling multiple sclerosis should raise the suspicion of SD. Antinuclear, anti-SSA, and anti-SSB antibodies are usually present. Rheumatoid factor and a variety of autoantibodies against gastric parietal cells, mitochondria, smooth muscle, and thyroid are often seen. An ophthalmologic examination can confirm the presence of keratoconjunctivitis, and biopsy of a lip or lacrimal gland can confirm the presence of characteristic lymphocytic infiltration. Biopsy of a rash can verify the presence of cutaneous vasculitis.

Symptomatic and preventive treatment is indicated for sicca symptoms, as described above. Trial therapy with hydroxychloroquine may help stabilize disease activity, as in SLE. Dapsone may be effective for cutaneous vasculitis. Corticosteroids and other cytotoxic drugs should be reserved for organ- or life-threatening disease.

Polymyositis and Dermatomyositis

Polymyositis (PM) is a heterogeneous group of inflammatory diseases of striated muscle that are not unique to older adults; however, late-onset PM is evaluated and treated somewhat differently in older adults. The onset of PM is often insidious. The cardinal symptom is muscle weakness, most marked in proximal muscle groups. Muscle tenderness is usually not prominent. Exercise tolerance is reduced, and an inability to perform simple tasks such as reaching above the head or ascending stairs may be present. Other system involvement is common in PM and reminiscent of other connective-tissue diseases, including rash, arthritis, esophageal dysmotility, and Raynaud's phenomenon. Cardiac involvement is not rare and usually presents with dysrhythmias. Rash may involve the eyelids (heliotrope) or the nose and malar areas, or be more generalized. Rash with dorsal thickening over the interphalangeal joints (Gottron's papules) are distinctly different from the dorsal phalangeal rash of systemic lupus that spares the interphalangeal joints. When rash is present, PM is referred to as dermatomyositis (DM).

In contrast to childhood PM, adult-onset PM affects women more often than men, and blacks more often than whites. Also, esophageal involvement and respiratory failure complicated with bacterial pneumonia are more likely in older PM patients. Up to 50% of cases of late-onset PM, and especially DM, are associated with underlying malignancy. No one cancer type seems most strongly associated: Colon, lung, breast, prostate, uterus, and ovary are all well represented with PM and DM. Ovarian cancer is the most commonly associated gynecologic cancer underlying PM and DM. Mortality in adult PM and DM is usually associated with esophageal disease, respiratory failure with bacterial pneumonia, and malignancy.

Serum levels of muscle enzymes are usually markedly elevated in PM. Electromyography will reveal changes consistent with myositis, provided affected muscle is tested. Paraspinal muscle involvement is typical and should be included in the muscles tested. The diagnosis is confirmed with muscle biopsy that reveals inflammatory cellular infiltrates. The diagnosis of PM or DM in older adults entails a search for underlying malignancy. Minimum evaluation would include chest radiography and colon examination. In women, a pelvic examination and imaging plus mammography is included; in men, a prostate examination and prostate-specific antigen testing.

An important histologic and clinical subtype of PM is inclusion-body myositis. Rimmed vacuoles and an accumulation of amyloid in muscle fibers are seen on muscle biopsy. Inclusion-body myositis predominantly affects men and is more likely to involve distal muscle groups including the volar forearm flexor and ankle dorsi flexor muscles. The onset and progression is slower than in PM. Inclusion-body myositis is also thought to be relatively resistant to anti-inflammatory therapy.

Remission of PM and DM after treatment of an underlying malignancy is seen. Therapy should also generally be directed at the inflammatory process itself. Corticosteroids are almost always the first drug of choice. Prednisone at 1 mg/kg/day is a typical starting dosage. Some clinicians advocate three daily intravenous doses of methylprednisolone, 1000 mg initially for severe disease. In the absence of prospective data, this high-dose regimen should be individualized. Prednisone can be tapered after an initial phase in which muscle strength improves and levels of muscle enzymes return to normal. Rates of tapering of 10% to 20% of the total dose per month are typical. Methotrexate, given parenterally, in a weekly pulse regimen can be combined with corticosteroids. Somewhat higher methotrexate dosages than those used in treating RA are given by some clinicians, up to 50 mg weekly. Methotrexate may also have a steroid-sparing effect in long-term therapy. Weekly oral methotrexate is effective in managing refractory skin manifestations of DM. Azathioprine may also have a steroid-sparing effect, but it is not as well accepted in the treatment of PM. Supervised exercise over 6-week and 6-month study periods has proved to be beneficial in PM, improving function without aggravating the underlying disease.

REFERENCES

■ American Geriatrics Society Panel on Exercise and Osteoarthritis. Exercise prescription for older adults with osteoarthritis pain: consensus practice recommendations. *J Am Geriatr Soc.* 2001;49(6):808–823.

■ Burks K. Osteoarthritis in oder adults: current treatments. *J Gerontol Nurs.* 2005;31(5):11–19; quiz 59–60.

■ Natvig B, Picavet HS. The epidemiology of soft tissue rheumatism. *Best Pract Res Clin Rheumatol.* 2002;16(5):777–793.

■ Salvarani C, Cantini F, Boiardi L, et al. Polymyalgia rheumatica. *Best Pract Res Clin Rheumatol.* 2004;18(5):705–722.

■ Tsai PF, Means KM. Osteoarthritic knee or hip pain: possible indicators in elderly adults with cognitive impairment. *J Gerontol Nurs.* 2005;31(8):39–45.

■ Tutuncu Z, Kavanaugh A. Rheumatic disease in the elderly: rheumatoid arthritis. *Clin Geriatr Med.* 2005;21(3):513–525.

CHAPTER 55—BACK AND NECK PAIN

KEY POINTS

- Back problems are the third most common reason for physician visits by older persons, and degenerative conditions of the spine are the most common cause of these problems.

- Pain that is insidious in onset, progressive in its course, and nonpositional, that is associated with night pain and systemic symptoms or signs, and that persists for more than 1 month should raise concerns about tumor or infection. Nonsystemic causes of pain are characterized by intermittent, often positional pain that is worse at onset and usually improves with time.

- The physical examination of the back, hips, and legs is essential in the assessment of an older patient with back pain. Plain radiographs remain the most useful starting point in a back pain work-up of an older patient.

- Management requires a therapeutic approach that addresses the structural problems most likely to be causing the pain.

- Neck pain is most often due to mechanical disease of the cervical spine and is best diagnosed on physical examination.

Back problems are the third most common reason for physician visits by older persons, and degenerative conditions of the spine are the most common cause of these problems. Less common conditions that can cause back pain, such as tumors, infections, and visceral lesions, occur more often in older than in younger patients and may require emergent treatment. Anatomic abnormalities are commonly found in diagnostic imaging tests of an older person's lumbar spine but may be unrelated to the patient's complaints.

The causes, natural history, and prognosis of back pain in older and younger persons are different. For example, although herniation of the nucleus pulposus of the lumbar disk is a common cause of back pain in younger adults, this herniation is unlikely to occur above the age of 60 because of changes in the water content of the nucleus pulposus. Although the natural history of mechanical lower back pain in younger people has been well outlined in the literature, it has not been well defined in older people. Mechanical instability of the lumbar spine, osteoporotic fractures, lumbar spinal stenosis, and systemic causes of pain are more common in the older age group.

A systematic approach to the diagnosis of lower back pain in older patients requires knowledge of the typical presentation of common back conditions of elderly persons, an understanding of the anatomy of the lumbar spine, the identification of physical findings associated with common abnormalities, and the judicious use of diagnostic imaging studies. (See Table 55.1.)

SYSTEMIC CAUSES OF BACK PAIN

Back pain due to systemic causes merits immediate attention and intervention. The pattern of pain with these conditions can be distinctive. Tumors or infections of the spine usually have an insidious onset of

Table 55.1—Conditions Causing Back Pain in Older Persons

Condition	History	Examination	Laboratory Tests, Imaging
Tumor	Persistent, progressive pain at rest; systemic symptoms	No focal abnormalities	Anemia, elevated ESR, abnormal bone scan or MRI
Infection	Persistent pain, fever; at-risk patient (eg, indwelling catheter)	Tender spine	Elevated ESR, WBC; positive bone scan or MRI
Unstable lumbar spine	Recurring episodes of pain on change of position	Pain going from flexed to extended position	One disc space narrowed and sclerotic spondylolisthesis
Lumbar spinal stenosis	Pain on standing and walking relieved by sitting and lying	Immobile spine; L4, L5, S1 weakness	MRI or CT scan showing stenosis
Sciatica	Pain in the posterior aspect of leg; may be incomplete	Often positive straight leg raise; L4, L5, S1 weakness	Variable diagnostic imaging findings
Vertebral compression fracture	Sudden onset of severe pain; resolves in 4–6 weeks	Pain on any movement of spine; no neurologic deficits	Vertebral end-plate collapse; compression fracture seen on plain film
Osteoporotic sacral fracture	Sudden lower back, buttock, or hip pain	Sacral tenderness	H-shaped uptake on bone scan

NOTE: CT = computed tomography; ESR = erythrocyte sedimentation rare; MRI = magnetic resonance imaging; WBC = white blood cell count.

pain that becomes more and more persistent with time. This pain is usually nonpositional and associated with systemic systems and signs; it often persists through the night. The likelihood of cancer as a cause of back pain increases in patients aged 50 and older, those with a previous history of cancer, and those with pain that persists for longer than 1 month.

Fever, discrete local vertebral tenderness, upper lumbar or thoracic pain, and nonpositional pain may indicate vertebral infection. Approximately 10% of patients with endocarditis have back pain. Infection may produce back pain in patients at risk for endovascular infections, such as those on hemodialysis, with chronic indwelling venous access catheters, with a history of recent or chronic urinary tract infections, or with a history of intravenous drug abuse.

A number of visceral problems, from abdominal aortic aneurysms to intra-abdominal infections or tumor, can present with back pain. Referred pain from these conditions should be suggested by the historical pattern of the pain, the absence of positional changes, and a normal physical examination of the lumbosacral spine.

NONSYSTEMIC CAUSES OF BACK PAIN

Lumbar Spinal Stenosis

Lumbar spinal stenosis results from a narrowing of either the central or lateral aspect of the lumbar spine canal. This narrowing may be due to facet joint osteophytes, encroachment of the annulus fibrosus of the lumbar disc, or hypertrophy of the ligamentum flavum. Diagnostic imaging tests often demonstrate spinal stenosis in patients without back pain or with other causes of pain; the clinician must recognize the characteristic historical and physical features of this condition.

Flexion of the lumbar spine causes an increase in spinal canal volume and decrease in nerve root bulk. Extension of the lumbar spine produces a decreased volume of the spinal canal with an increased nerve root bulk. As a result of these anatomical changes, positions that flex the spine, such as sitting, bending forward, walking uphill, and lying in a flexed position, all relieve symptoms. Extension of the lumbar canal, which occurs with prolonged standing, walking, and walking downhill, exacerbates symptoms.

Lumbar spinal stenosis produces pain either in the back or in the legs, made worse by standing or walking. Pain in the calf when walking can often mimic the claudication of arterial insufficiency and is referred to as *pseudoclaudication*. Continued walking after this point may produce combinations of paresthesia, numb-ness, and weakness in one or both legs. Walking uphill is easier than walking downhill, and walking with an assistive device, such as a shopping cart, which allows some flexion of the lumbar spine, is usually better tolerated. These symptoms are usually progressive and consistent, not intermittent. There is often subtle weakness in the muscles innervated by the L4, L5, and S1 nerve roots. (See Table 55.2 and the assessment section, below.)

Sciatica

Sciatica describes a lancinating pain, usually felt from the buttock down the posterior aspect of the leg to the foot; it may occur only in isolated regions of the distribution of the sciatic nerve. In older persons there are two common patterns of sciatica. Sciatic pain that comes on only with standing and walking and that limits the person's ability to walk at a relatively constant distance is usually a result of lumbar spinal stenosis. Other older patients may develop the relatively sudden onset of sciatic pain, present at rest and exacerbated by sudden maneuvers, such as getting out of a bed or chair. This abrupt and persistent pain, not necessarily related to the erect position, usually resolves spontaneously in several weeks. The diagnosis of sciatica can be confirmed by the demonstration of muscle weakness of the L4, L5, and S1 innervated muscles of the foot, ankle, and hip. (See Table 55.2 and the assessment section, below.)

Unstable Lumbar Spine

Lumbar degenerative disc disease may produce an unstable lumbar spine. Patients with this condition often have episodes of severe pain in the back or in the distribution of the sciatic nerve. This pain usually comes on suddenly, often following abrupt movements. It usually lasts only minutes to hours, but recurs frequently. This pain also comes on with significant flexion or extension of the lumbar spine. On physical examination, the patient often has guarded movements of the lumbar spine and pain when moving from the flexed to the extended position. Diffuse disk space narrowing and vertebral osteophytosis are common in older persons and not related to back pain. When there are significant disk and bone changes at one disk and facet joint level that are out of proportion to the other disk spaces, instability of the lumbar spine may be the cause of the patient's back pain.

Osteoporotic Vertebral Compression Fracture

Vertebral compression fractures are a common cause of back pain in older persons. Many of these fractures,

Table 55.2—Innervation of Lower Extremities

Function	Muscle	Peripheral Nerve	Nerve Root
Great toe dorsiflexion	Extensor hallucis longus	Deep peroneal	L5
Ankle dorsiflexion	Tibialis anterior	Deep peroneal	L4, L5
Ankle eversion	Peroneus longus, brevis	Superficial peroneal	L5, S1
Ankle plantar flexion	Gastrocnemius, soleus	Tibial	S1, S2
Knee extension	Quadriceps	Femoral	L3, L4
Hip flexion	Iliopsoas	Femoral	L2, L3
Hip adduction	Adductor magnus, brevis, longus	Obturator	L3, L4
Hip abduction	Gluteus medius	Superior gluteal	L4, L5
Hip extension	Gluteus maximus	Inferior gluteal	L5, S1

however, are found incidentally and are asymptomatic. The pain from an acute vertebral fracture usually lasts from 2 weeks to 2 months. The onset of pain is abrupt and pain is intense; it is felt deep at the site of the fracture. There is often marked tenderness over the involved vertebra. The pain is usually worse on standing and walking, and relieved with lying down. Although the pain commonly radiates to the flank, abdomen, and legs, neurologic sequelae should not occur in patients with spontaneous osteopenic fractures. Symptomatic fractures most often affect the lower thoracic and lumbar vertebrae.

The acute pain resolves slowly. One study found that analgesic use decreased by 16% by day 5 and 33% by day 14. Patients often have trouble walking for 2 weeks and have approximately 1 month of restricted activity.

The impact of these fractures, and osteoporosis in general, on chronic back pain and the function of older persons is unclear. Some studies have found that multiple fractures are associated with more disability, frailty, and back pain; others have not demonstrated a correlation between osteoporosis and chronic back pain.

Osteoporotic Sacral Fractures

Lower back pain in elderly women may be due to osteoporotic sacral fractures. This pain often occurs spontaneously, usually involving the lower back. Pain can also be felt in the buttock or hip area. Sacral tenderness on physical examination is found in a majority of patients. There is a high incidence of associated additional osteoporotic fractures.

Plain radiographs are usually negative. Technetium bone scans show a characteristic H-shaped uptake over the sacrum. A computed tomography (CT) scan shows displacement of the anterior border of the sacrum. These fractures have an excellent prognosis for recovery, with no neurologic deficits. The pain usually resolves in 4 to 6 weeks.

ASSESSMENT OF BACK PAIN

See Table 55.3.

History

Pain that is insidious in onset, progressive in its course, and nonpositional, that is associated with night pain and systemic symptoms or signs, and that persists for more than 1 month should raise concerns about tumor or infection. Nonsystemic causes of pain are characterized by intermittent, often positional pain that is worse at onset and that usually improves with time.

Diseases of the hip often produce pain in the back and leg in a distribution that resembles that of back disease. Back disease is more apt to cause pain when a patient goes from the supine to the sitting position or when bending or stooping. Hip disease can cause pain after prolonged sitting and when moving from a sitting to a standing position.

Physical Examination

The physical examination of the back, hips, and legs is essential in the assessment of an older patient with back pain. (See Table 55.4.) The finding of subtle but asymmetric weakness of the hip, ankle, and feet muscles innervated by the lumbar and sacral nerves can help elucidate the cause of back and lower extremity pain.

A thorough back examination begins with the patient in the upright position. The back should be moved through all four planes of movement of the lumbar spine, side flexion to the right, side flexion to the left, forward flexion, and extension. Asymmetric limitation of the range of motion of the lumbar spine, or reproduction of the patient's pain with these maneuvers, often indicates mechanical disease of the lumbar spine. The pain of lumbar spinal stenosis is often produced by spinal extension.

The remainder of the examination is performed with the patient in the supine position. A straight leg

Table 55.3—Assessment of Lower Back Pain in Older Persons

Symptoms	Conditions
Acute pain	Vertebral compression fracture
	Disk displacement
	Osteoporotic sacral fracture
	Visceral pain (eg, aortic aneurysm)
Positional pain	Increased with standing and walking and relieved with sitting—lumbar spinal stenosis
	Brought on by bending, lifting, or unguarded movements—unstable lumbar spine
Persistent pain (gradually increasing, nonpositional)	Tumor
	Infection

Table 55.4—Physical Examination of Older Persons With Lower Back Pain

Sign	Condition
Paravertebral muscle spasm	Mechanical disease
Asymmetric range of motion of the lumbar spine	Mechanical disk disease
	Unstable lumbar spine
Spinal tenderness	Vertebral compression fracture
	Infection
Weakness of the L4–L5 and L5–S1 muscles	Mechanical disk disease
	Lumbar spinal stenosis
Normal examination of lumbar spine	Osteoporotic sacral fracture
	Hip disease
	Tumor
	Referred visceral pain

raise test can be informative if positive, but a negative test does not exclude any condition. Each patient with a back complaint should have a complete examination of the hips, as hip disease often mimics back disease. The passive range of motion of the hip should be assessed. The examiner should be able to abduct the hip to 40 degrees before the pelvis starts to tilt. The hip should flex beyond 110 degrees, externally rotate 50 to 60 degrees, and internally rotate 15 to 20 degrees.

The manual examination of the muscles of the lower extremities can be helpful. This examination should distinguish between weakness due to a nerve root problem and weakness due to a peripheral neuropathy. (See Table 55.2). Great toe extension, ankle dorsiflexion, and ankle eversion weakness with no involvement of the hip abductors and hip extensors suggests a peripheral neuropathy rather than lumbar spine disease. A patient with lumbar spine disease is more likely to have weakness of lumbar and sacral innervated hip, as well as of ankle and foot, muscles.

A patient should be closely observed both rising from a chair and walking. Unless the patient has significant sciatica, back disease should not cause a limp. A significant limp suggests hip disease as a cause of the patient's pain.

Laboratory Tests and Imaging

Plain radiographs remain the most useful starting point in a back pain work-up of an older patient. Although these films are not recommended in the initial evaluation of back pain in younger patients, they are appropriate for patients aged 70 and over. This single test can demonstrate degenerative disk and joint disease, vertebral compression fractures, deformities such as spondylolisthesis and scoliosis, systemic disorders such as osteoporosis and Paget's disease, and, in some cases, infectious processes and neoplasms. A complete blood cell count with erythrocyte sedimentation rate is perhaps the most useful screening laboratory test for an underlying systemic disease.

A technetium bone scan is useful in evaluating a suspected infection or neoplasm. CT and magnetic resonance imaging (MRI) have largely replaced myelography in assessing the neural canal. CT imaging is, in many cases, slightly superior in demonstrating the bony architecture of the spine, whereas the MRI is more sensitive to morphology of soft tissue, including disk, ligamentum flavum, neoplasm, and infection. Either CT or MRI studies are necessary to document spinal stenosis should surgical treatment be contemplated.

The utility of diagnostic imaging studies is tempered by the high false-positive rates of these studies in older persons. A diagnostic imaging study simply identifies an anatomic abnormality; it does not demonstrate that this abnormality is the cause of the patient's pain. One study found that 57% of persons aged 60 and older, with no history of lower back pain or sciatica, had abnormal lumbar spine MRIs. Of these persons, 36% had a herniated nucleus pulposus and 21% had lumbar spinal stenosis. Another study found that only 36% of asymptomatic persons had normal disks at all levels; the prevalence of disk abnormalities did increase in older persons. Other studies have shown similarly high rates of abnormal findings in asymptomatic persons. These studies reinforce the need to correlate carefully the patient's history and physical examination with the findings on diagnostic imaging studies.

MANAGEMENT OF BACK PAIN

Management of back pain is hampered by the common difficulty of making a definitive diagnosis. Patients can do well, however, with a therapeutic approach that addresses the structural problems most likely to be causing their pain.

Treatment of an unstable lumbar spine is symptomatic. Nonopioid analgesics are often helpful in the early stages. As soon as the acute symptoms subside, a gentle, progressive exercise program should be initiated that is designed to strengthen and improve the efficiency of the spinal and abdominal musculature. An aquatic program offers the dual benefits of rapid rehabilitation with a low incidence of reinjury. Walking in chest-high water against resistance and performing the flutter kick are two simple aquatic exercises.

Chronic mechanical pain is based on excessive vertebral motion that is more pronounced and repetitive. The pain is usually associated with advanced degenerative disc and facet joint disease. Management is aimed at eliminating or reducing motion. This can be done internally by strengthening the paraspinous and abdominal muscles, thus providing an internal "brace" for the lumbar spine. It must be stressed that this exercise should be a lifetime commitment. Lumbar sacral corsets and braces provide an external method of immobilizing the lumbar spine. The third option, a structural alteration to limit motion, is accomplished by surgical fusion.

Analgesia is the most important goal of treatment of vertebral compression fractures, while trying to avoid the complications of the bed rest required by the patient's pain. Braces and corsets are rarely required, as the natural history of the acute pain is relatively brief.

Corsets may offer symptomatic relief if the pain is persistent. Spinal extension exercises also may be helpful. Calcitonin OL can act as an analgesic and may shorten the period of acute pain.

Vertebroplasty is the percutaneous injection of bone cement into a collapsed vertebra. Although there are encouraging reports of this procedure in patients with substantial vertebral compression lesions, the long-term efficacy of these procedures has not been established in randomized controlled trials. In view of the good short-term natural history of pain following fractures, most clinicians suggest vertebroplasty only for patients with persistent pain despite conservative management with rest, analgesics, and calcitonin.

Because of the mechanical encroachment on lumbar nerve roots which causes lumbar spinal stenosis, conservative therapy is limited. Uncontrolled European studies advocate marked immobilization of the lumbar spine. Epidural corticosteroid injections have been used extensively for the sciatica associated with lumbar spinal stenosis, but a review of controlled trials of this therapy failed to demonstrate efficacy of injection over controls.

Lumbar spinal stenosis is the most common indication for spinal surgery in older adults. Long-term benefit from laminectomy, or laminectomy combined with fusion, is about 50% to 70%, regardless of whether the stenosis is central or lateral. In a prospective study of surgery for spinal stenosis, the ideal candidates for surgery were found to be those patients with severe narrowing of the spinal canal, minimal associated back pain, no coexisting conditions that affect walking, and symptom duration of less than 4 years.

NECK PAIN

Causes

Although neck pain can be due to inflammatory and systemic conditions, it is most often due to mechanical disease of the cervical spine. Inflammatory conditions, such as polymyalgia rheumatica and rheumatoid arthritis, are characterized by morning stiffness, systemic complaints such as fatigue, fever, and weight loss, and muscle and joint complaints elsewhere in the body. Most importantly, these patients do not have the characteristic physical findings of patients with mechanical disease of the cervical spine.

Mechanical disease of the cervical spine can cause neck and occiput pain, scapula and trapezius pain, radicular pain down the arm, as well as spastic paraparesis due to cervical spinal stenosis.

A number of injection studies have demonstrated the referral pain pattern of cervical spine disease. C2–C3 disease is felt in the occiput; C3–C4 and

---

OL Not approved by the U.S. Food and Drug Administration for this use.

C4–C5 problems are referred into the posterior and lateral aspects of the neck. C5–C6 lesions are referred into the trapezius and upper cervical region; C6–C7 disease is felt in the retroscapular region, often felt as far down as the mid- to lower thoracic region. This referral process produces not only pain in these regions but also local muscle spasm and tenderness, often mistaken for "trigger points."

Irritation of a cervical nerve root produces lancinating pain and numbness in the neck and upper scapular region, radiating into the arm in a dermatomal distribution. Characteristic muscle weakness of the upper extremity muscles (see below) confirms the specific nerve root involved.

Narrowing of the cervical canal (cervical spondylosis or cervical spinal stenosis) can produce a syndrome of lower extremity clumsiness and weakness, spasticity of the legs, bladder spasticity, and upper motor neuron signs of the lower extremities (clonus, hyperreflexia, and Babinski's signs). Although progressive signs and symptoms call for an aggressive diagnostic and therapeutic approach, the natural history of this problem can be quite stable, and surgical intervention is not always necessary.

Assessment

Mechanical disease of the cervical spine is best diagnosed on physical examination. There are four planes of movement of the cervical spine: rotation to the right, rotation to the left, flexion, and extension. Mechanical disease of the cervical spine is demonstrated if there is asymmetric limitation of the range of motion of the cervical spine in some but not all of these movements, and if there is weakness of the upper extremity muscles innervated by the cervical nerve root. The shoulder abductor and elbow flexor muscles are innervated by C5 and C6 nerve roots, the wrist extensor and thumb opponens muscles by C6 and C7, and the elbow extensor and finger abductors muscles by C7 and C8. Weakness of the C7- and C8-innervated muscles is most common with cervical disk disease, because the C7–T1 interspace is the most common site of cervical spine lesions. Patients with mechanical disease of the cervical spine often awake in the morning with this discomfort, have difficulty with full rotation of the cervical spine, and have difficulty with such activities as backing an automobile out of a driveway.

Diagnostic Imaging

The role of diagnostic imaging tests in the diagnosis and management of neck pain is unclear. Among persons older than 55 years, 80% have signs of degenerative cervical disk disease on cervical spine radiography. These films, therefore, are often unhelpful in the assessment of neck pain. Although MRIs of the cervical spine more completely define anatomical abnormalities in this region, these abnormalities are quite common in older persons. Anatomical abnormalities call for interventions only if they are consistent with the historical and physical features of the patient's condition.

Management

There is much controversy about the therapy of mechanical disease of the cervical spine. Studies of manipulation, cervical traction, cervical collars, local physical modalities, acupuncture, and injection therapies have not shown consistent efficacy for any of these modalities. Two studies from the Netherlands and Finland have shown promising results for manual therapy and active neck muscle training in the treatment of neck pain. These studies were both done, however, on younger patients. Because many patients notice that their neck pain is worse in the morning, a trial of several weeks of a soft cervical collar to be worn at nighttime is worthwhile before proceeding with more aggressive interventions.

REFERENCES

- Atlas SJ, Deyo RA. Evaluating and managing acute low back pain in the primary care setting. *J Gen Intern Med.* 2001;16(2):120–131.

- Babb A, Carlson WO. Spinal stenosis. *S D Med.* 2006;59(3):103–105.

- Devereaux MW. Neck and low back pain. *Med Clin North Am.* 2003;87(3):643–662.

- Knopp JA, Diner BM, Blitz M, et al. Calcitonin for treating acute pain of osteoporotic vertebral compression fractures: a systematic review of randomized, controlled trials. *Osteoporos Int.* 2005;16(10):1281–1290.

- Papaioannou A, Watts NB, Kendler DL, et al. Diagnosis and managment of vertebral fractures in elderly adults. *Am J Med.* 2002;113(3):220–228.

- Rao R. Neck pain, cervical radiculopathy, and cervical myelopathy: pathophysiology, natural history, and clinical evaluation. *J Bone Joint Surg Am.* 2002;84-A(10):1872–1881.

CHAPTER 56—DISEASES AND DISORDERS OF THE FOOT

KEY POINTS

- Foot problems, both orthopedic problems and skin and nail changes, are common and have important functional consequences for older persons.

- Many orthopedic foot problems can be adequately addressed with orthotics and proper shoes.

- Skin problems may require debridement and topical medications in addition to orthotics and proper footwear.

- Systemic illnesses can be associated with serious foot problems, for which regular podiatric care is advised.

Foot problems lead to some of the most distressing symptoms and disabling conditions affecting older patients. Foot and related problems and their sequelae may be local, or they may be associated with systemic conditions. The ability to remain pain free and ambulatory is a key element in successful aging.

Feet are fairly rigid structures that carry heavy physical workloads, both static and dynamic. The foot, though shaped like a rectangle, bears static forces in a triangular pattern. Flat and hard surfaces force the foot to absorb shock; over the lifespan, the foot is subjected to both prolonged and repetitive micro- and macrotrauma. When the foot is unable to adapt to stress, inflammatory changes in bone and soft tissue are produced that may manifest in one or more of many mechanical disorders, including synovitis, fasciitis, and arthritis. In addition, vascular, neurologic, dermatologic, rheumatologic, and endocrinologic diseases increase the older person's risk of serious foot problems.

ORTHOPEDIC DISORDERS OF THE FOOT

For the older person, disease or decreased activity, or both, may cause osteopenia, progressive loss of muscle mass, and atrophy of tissue, and these may affect the structure and function of the foot. Manifestations of degenerative processes affecting older persons that are specific to the foot include plantar fasciitis, atrophy of the plantar fat pad, and hammertoe (digiti flexus) formation (see Table 56.1 for definitions and descriptions of several foot disorders and deformities). When these and other conditions cause foot pain, the older person's mobility and ambulatory status may be further limited, and as the ambulatory status of the person changes, foot problems may worsen.

Common orthopedic foot disorders in the elderly person are the consequences of severe or repeated trauma, inflammation, metabolic change, strain, obesity, osteoarthritis, rheumatoid arthritis, gout, and osteoporosis. Manifestations of these processes in the foot include stress fractures, tendonitis, residual deformities (including rotational digital deformities), joint swelling, anterior imbalance, bursitis, neuritis, and neuromas. Because even minor trauma can result in a fracture, a stress fracture should be suspected when foot pain is severe, prolonged, and not otherwise explained.

Disorders of the Mid- and Forefoot

Deformities such as flat feet (pes planus), high arched feet (pes cavus), bunions (hallus valgus), and hammertoes create pain and reduce the older person's ability to walk. *Hammertoe* is a general term applied to several types of contracture deformities of the toes. It is usually seen in the lesser toes, but a hallux (great toe) hammertoe may develop in the presence of coexistent neurologic abnormalities. The classic hammertoe is dorsiflexion at the metatarsophalangeal joint and plantar contraction of the proximal interphalangeal joint. Mallet toes and claw toes are different variations. A cock-up toe occurs when the contracture provides no contact between the toe and plane of support.

Rotational deformities and overlapping toes (see Figure 56.1) due to hallux valgus and arthritis are also referred to clinically as hammertoes. These deformities are related to atrophy of interossei muscles of the foot and contractures of the long extensor tendons. The deformities can be classed as flexible, semi-rigid, or rigid, depending on the motion demonstrated and the ability to reduce the deformity. The toes may also become rotated, and with arthritic changes, they may become dislocated and subluxed (as in rheumatoid arthritis). These deformities increase the formation of corns, especially in the presence of ill-fitting footwear or incompatible shoe lasts (the *last* is the model over which shoes are made). In older patients the heads and bases of the phalanges are commonly enlarged, and degenerative changes can often be demonstrated at the tufted end of the distal phalanx.

The management of all deformities should be directed toward relief of pain and improvement of the ability to walk. The choice of management strategies depends on the causes and symptoms. When deformity is noted, shoe modification is important and should include a high toe box (a deep and rounded covering

Table 56.1—A Glossary of Foot Disorders

Disorder	Definition or Description
Calcaneal spur	A calcification of the attachment of the plantar fascia, usually at the medial plantar tuberosity of the calcaneus. The spur projects anteriorly and is the consequence of chronic repetitive trauma or stress resulting from biomechanical and pathomechanical change. When ligamentous calcification occurs, inflammation and associated pain at the attachment are the result. This may be referred to as *heel pain syndrome* and may be related to plantar fasciitis.
Cystic erosion	Areas of radiolucency usually noted with arthritic changes, such as rheumatoid arthritis, and usually occurring in the metatarsal heads with associated joint changes.
Digiti flexus	May be fixed or flexible flexion at the metatarsal phalangeal joints; ie, hammertoe.
Digiti quinti varus	Refers to a valgus displacement or splaying of the fifth metatarsal, with a resulting varus or inward deviation of the fifth toe.
Entrapment syndrome	Occurs when a nerve is compressed by ligamentous or other soft-tissue inflammation, resulting in pain and possibly numbness and neuropathic symptoms. The most common sites are the posterior tibial nerve and the intermetatarsal nerves, plantarly.
Haglund's deformity	A hyperostosis of the posterior and superior portion of the calcaneus, which expands the shape of the calcaneus, which can in turn place pressure on the attachment of the Achilles tendon. The presence of the deformity also can produce a pressure area for the counter of the shoe. It is easily demonstrated on a lateral radiograph of the foot and is clinically significant, with pain associated with tendonitis or bursitis, usually resulting from an incompatibility of foot to shoe last.
Hallux abducto valgus	An alternative clinical diagnosis for hallux valgus, or bunion. There is a varus splaying of the first metatarsal with a valgus and rotational deformity of the phalanges of the great toe.
Hallux limitus and rigidus	A degenerative joint change involving the first metatarsal phalangeal joint, resulting from dorsal spurs, with a marked limitation or absence of any range of motion. The difference between hallux limitus and rigidus is based on the radiographic interpretation and difference in function.
Hallux valgus	Deviation of the tip of the great toe, or main axis of the toe, toward the outer or lateral side of the foot; ie, *bunion.*
Metatarsal prolapse	Marked prominence of the metatarsal head, usually associated with atrophy or posterior displacement, or both, of the anterior plantar fat pad, pes cavus, or digital contractures, which force the metatarsal heads in a plantar projection.
Metatarsalgia	Pain in the forefoot near the heads of the metatarsals.
Morton's syndrome	A congenital shortening of the first metatarsal shaft, which creates an abnormal metatarsal arc. Excessive weight is placed on the second metatarsal head during gait and stance. The dynamics and pathomechanics of the foot are modified and provide one of the causes of hallux valgus, abducto valgus, and rotational deformity of the hallux.
Periostitis	Inflammation of the periosteum.
Pes cavus	Represents a higher than normal arch and is commonly associated with neurologic change. In the older patient, excessive pressure is usually placed on the metatarsal heads. With atrophy of the plantar fat pad and displacement, pressure is increased, which can serve as a predisposing cause for pain and ulceration.
Pes planus	A flattening of the medial longitudinal arch, where the calcaneal pitch on a radiograph is usually below 15 degrees; ie, *flat feet.*
Pes valgo planus	Represents the same clinical picture as pes planus, with an addition of pronation, demonstrated by a lateral deviation of the Achilles tendon and an outward and rotational deformity of the foot, which presents a compensatory deformity due to complex biomechanical imbalance.
Plantar fasciitis	An inflammation and pain involving repetitive microtrauma to the plantar fascia, particularly at its posterior calcaneal attachment; associated with biomechanical and pathomechanical changes in the function of the foot. It is related to calcaneal spurs, ligamentous calcification, and tissue atrophy.
Tailor's bunion	An enlargement of the fifth metatarsal phalangeal joint, usually with a lateral deviation of the fifth metatarsal shaft and head and a medial and rotational deformity of the fifth toe. It is usually associated with a splaying of the fifth metatarsal and can present with bursitis, capsulitis, and degenerative joint change.
Tenosynovitis	Inflammation of a tendon and enveloping sheath.

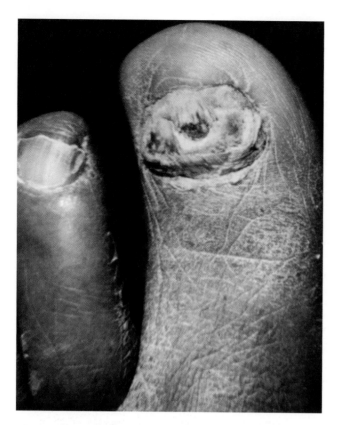

Figure 56.1—Hallux abducto valgus, hammertoe, subluxated second toe, xerosis onychodystrophy, onychodysplasia.

over the toe area). Silicone molds can be used to maintain a more normal position of the toes, acting as a digital brace. Where hyperkeratosis is noted, debridement should be completed to reduce the possibility of ulceration. Padding with materials such as lamb's wool, silicone, or foam can help reduce pressure. For most older patients, nonoperative treatment strategies are effective in controlling the pain associated with the deformity. Surgical revision remains an option when these measures are not successful.

Metatarsalgia refers to pain in the anterior metatarsal area. It can be functional in nature or associated with metatarsophalangeal abnormalities. It can be associated with anterior fat pad atrophy or displacement, retrograde pressure from hammertoe deformities on the metatarsal heads, and other pathomechanical changes. It may also be due to degenerative changes, deformities that increase the angle at which the foot makes contact with the plane of support. It may be associated with obesity, a consequence of the increase in weight bearing and imbalance. Incompatibility of foot to shoe last and ill-fitting footwear are additional possible causes.

Management depends on the cause and includes padding, orthotics such as a metatarsal pad, shoe modifications, physical therapy, local corticosteroid injection, digital molds to help transfer an anteriorly displaced fat pad, and analgesics if the problem is related to degenerative joint changes. A metatarsal bar is a transverse bar used to transfer weight over the metatarsal heads and is usually placed on the plantar surface or sole of the shoe. It may be placed between the insole and outsole.

Heel and Arch Pain

Plantar fasciitis is a common syndrome that causes pain in the sole of the foot. This heel pain is usually due to a strain of the plantar fascial attachment, which inserts on the medial plantar tuberosity of the calcaneus. A calcaneal spur may develop as a result of chronic stress on the attachment. Conservative management is usually effective for the older patient. Oral analgesics, injectable corticosteroids, pressure reduction (heel cups and night splints), and physical medicine are the initial forms of therapy. Orthotics can reduce pressure on the heel by changing biomechanics during the gait cycle and transferring weight elsewhere.

Heel pain may also be caused by the rubbing of the shoe on the back of the heel. This may result in inflammation known as posterior Achilles bursitis. This can occur between the calcaneus and the Achilles tendon or between the tendon and skin. Constant pressure can result in bursal formation. Haglund's deformity or disease, which is an osseous enlargement of the posterior–superior segment of the calcaneus, complicates this condition and its management. Nonoperative management is usually effective.

DISORDERS OF THE SKIN AND NAILS

With aging, the skin, ligaments, muscles, neurovascular structures, and bones undergo changes. The skin is one of the first structures to demonstrate change with aging. Trophic changes, such as a loss of hair below the knee and on the dorsum of the foot and toes, are common. The skin may become atrophic and resemble parchment. It also loses the normal lubricants and becomes xerotic. Brownish pigmentations are often related to the deposition of hemosiderin. A combination of physiologic changes in the skin coupled with continuing repetitive trauma, pressure, and atrophy of soft tissue prompts hyperkeratosis to form as a normal protective function. When the hyperkeratosis becomes excessive, it tends to act as a foreign body, increasing pressure and creating local ischemia, which can lead to tissue breakdown. Localized pressure can create subkeratotic hemorrhage, and the resultant hematoma becomes the predisposing factor for the development of ulcerations.

Hyperkeratosis

Common foot complaints of elderly persons concern the many forms of hyperkeratotic lesions, such as tyloma (calluses) and heloma (corns). The biomechanical and pathomechanical factors that create these problems are associated with compressive, tensile, and shearing stresses. Soft-tissue loss associated with aging and atrophy of the plantar fat pad increases pain and limits ambulation. Contractures, gait changes, deformities, the incompatibility of foot type to the shoe last, and arthritis are additional factors that need consideration. A multiplicity of conditions, including skin tone and elasticity, result in the development of keratotic lesions in elderly persons.

Management should be directed toward the functional and activity needs of the patient. Treatment includes debridement, padding, weight dispersion and diffusion, emollients, shoe modifications and last changes, orthoses, and surgical revision. Keratotic lesions can become primary irritants and can produce local avascularity that can precipitate ulceration. Pressure ulcers in the foot usually begin with subkeratotic hemorrhage. Once debrided and managed properly, they usually heal, but they may recur unless adequate measures are instituted to reduce pressure to the local areas of ulceration. Despite all measures, the problem may persist because of residual deformity and systemic diseases, such as diabetes mellitus. (See also "Pressure Ulcers," p 238.)

Xerosis

Excessive dryness, or xerosis, is associated with a lack of hydration and lubrication and is a related keratin dysfunction. Fissures develop as a result of dryness and associated stress on the heel. Management aims to prevent infection and further complications. A 10%, 20%, or 40% urea cream or solution or 12% ammonium lactate may be helpful as a mild and safe keratolytic. A heel sleeve or pad made with mineral oil or a heel cup can help to minimize trauma to the heel, thus reducing the potential for complications.

Nail Problems

Disorders of the toenails are common in older persons. Toenails undergo changes much more than do fingernails as a consequence of trauma, the environment of the shoe or sock, and the forces associated with ambulation. The toenails undergo degeneration and trophic changes (onychopathy) with thickening or longitudinal ridging (onychorrhexis) that is the consequence of repeated microtrauma, disease, and nutritional impairment. Nail malformation (onychodystrophy and onychodysplasia), subungual hematoma, discoloration, loosening or separation of the nail from the nail bed (onycholysis), nail thickening (onychauxis and onychogryphosis) (see Figure 56.2 and Figure 56.3), and subungual keratosis are all prevalent among older adults. Deformities of the toenails may become more pronounced and may be complicated by xerotic changes in the periungual nail folds as onychophosis

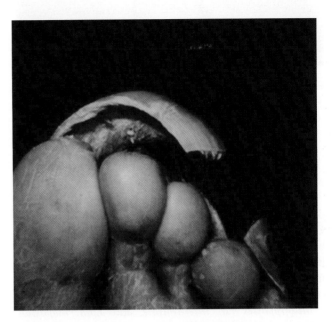

Figure 56.2—Onychauxis, subungual diabetic ulcer, xerosis, with arterial insufficiency and onychomycosis.

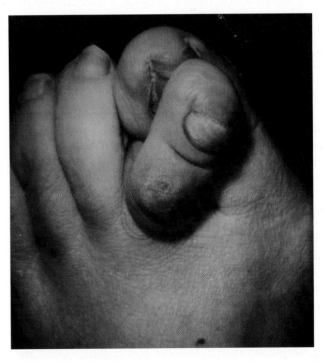

Figure 56.3—Onychogryphosis, onychomycosis, subungual debris, and tinea pedis.

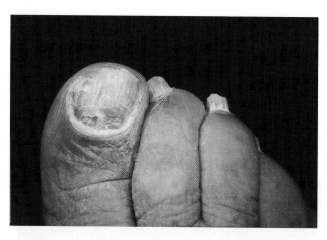

Figure 56.4—Onychomycosis. Nails infected by fungi are often yellow, thickened, and friable, with yellow-brown debris under the nail plate.

(hyperkeratosis) and tinea unguium (onychomycosis) with periungual infection.

Fungal infections account for 20% of all nail disease and are almost exclusively found in adults. Onychomycosis (Figure 56.4) can be caused not only by dermatophytes (fungi that infect keratinized tissues), but also by certain yeasts and nondermatophytic molds. The most common dermatophytes causing onychomycosis are *Trichophyton rubrum*, *Trichophyton mentagrophytes* var. *interdigitale*, and *Epidermophyton floccosum*. *Candida albicans* can infect the nails in chronic mucocutaneous candidiasis; however, other candida species (such as *C. parapsilosis*) can infect the nails of otherwise healthy persons. Nondermatophytic onychomycosis usually occurs in previously diseased nails or aged nails. It can often be difficult to determine whether a positive nondermatophytic nail culture is truly infection or contamination. In most cases of onychomycosis, there is preceding or concomitant tinea pedis.

Onychomycosis can be divided into four clinical subtypes: distal subungual onychomycosis, proximal subungual onychomycosis, white superficial onychomycosis, and candidal onychomycosis. Distal subungual onychomycosis is most common, and proximal subungual onychomycosis is least common. On clinical examination, infected nails have whitish or brownish-yellow discoloration. In response to the infection, hyperproliferation of the nail bed occurs, leading to subungual hyperkeratosis (yellow-brown debris under the nail bed). Diagnosis can be confirmed by potassium hydroxide (KOH) preparation or fungal culture of the nail plate or subungual debris.

A decision to treat is usually made because of the cosmetic concern of a yellow friable nail, other comorbidities (particularly diabetes mellitus, where the break in the epidermal barrier due to the fungal infection can serve as a route for bacterial infections), and occasionally because of pain. Topical agents have not been effective. A topical nail lacquer, ciclopirox (which is applied daily for 1 year) has been made available to treat onychomycosis, but in clinical studies it was found that less than 12% of patients achieved clear or almost clear toenails with its use. Griseofulvin is a systemic medication administered orally, but poor absorption, side effects, and drug interactions have limited adherence and efficacy. Regimens with newer agents, such as oral terbinafine, fluconazole, and itraconazole, have fewer side effects and drug interactions. Fluconazole can be used to treat candidal infections. It is well tolerated and has an excellent safety profile. When prescribing itraconazole, it is imperative to review all other medications the patient is taking; itraconazole interacts with warfarin, digoxin, and many other drugs through the cytochrome P-450 liver enzyme system. Terbinafine is the only orally active fungicidal agent that can be administered orally. It has fewer drug interactions but may interact with tricyclic antidepressants. Regardless, treatment can take 3 to 4 months, and the rate of relapse of onychomycosis is high.

Ingrown toenails are relatively common in elderly persons and are usually the consequence of deformity, disease, or onychopathy (onychodysplasia, or involution) and improper self-care. When the nail penetrates the skin, an abscess may result. If an ingrown nail is not managed early, periungual granulation tissue may form and complicate treatment. Onychia, inflammation of the soft tissue adjacent to the nail plate, is usually precipitated by local trauma or pressure but may be a complication of systemic disease or an early sign of infection. Mild erythema, swelling, and pain are the most prevalent findings. Management includes removing all pressure, applying tepid saline compresses, and using antibiotics if needed. Lamb's wool, tube foam, or shoe modification may reduce pressure. Paronychia, inflammation of the nail matrix plus the deeper and surrounding structures, may develop with infection and abscess of the posterior nail wall. It is a serious problem because of the potential for bone involvement as a result of the close association of the nail with the distal phalanx. Management includes surgical debridement and antibiotic treatment, if needed.

Elderly patients may also develop subungual hemorrhage from direct or constant trauma of the shoes, coagulopathies, or bed covers. Bleeding under the nail may result in an ulcer or loss of the toenail (onycholysis) if it is substantial.

Subungual heloma (also known as a corn or clavus) is usually associated with a subungual exostosis, spur, or hypertrophy of the tufted end of the distal phalanx. Initial management includes debridement and protection of the toe involved, as well as the use of a shoe with a high toe box (deep and rounded). Surgical excision of the osseous deformity may be required if the condition cannot be successfully treated in a conservative manner.

SYSTEMIC DISEASES AND THE FOOT

Diabetes Mellitus

Diabetes is the most important disease affecting foot health in older persons. (See also "Diabetes Mellitus," p 349.) It has been estimated that 50% to 75% of all amputations in diabetic patients could be prevented by periodic assessment, early intervention, and foot health education. The ocular complications of diabetes may affect the ability of the older person to see ingrown toenails, corns, and ulcers. The slower wound healing also contributes to the foot problems common to patients with diabetes.

These problems include neuropathy, vascular insufficiency,, dermopathy, atrophy of the muscles and soft tissues, and deformity. Neuropathy, especially sensory impairment, is a precursor to ulcers. Insensitivity, paresthesias, decreased vibratory sense, and loss of protective sensation are among the most important neuropathic changes.

Arterial insufficiency causes pallor, a loss or decrease in the posterior tibial and dorsalis pedis pulse, dependent rubor, and decreased capillary filling time in the toes. Severe vascular disease may result in rest pain that typically occurs at night. A loss of the plantar metatarsal fat pad is associated with vascular insufficiency and predisposes the patient to ulcerations at the site of bony prominences or deformities of the foot.

Prevention and early recognition are key in managing foot ulcers. Clinicians should examine the feet of diabetic patients at each visit and instruct patients and caregivers in the importance of daily foot inspections. Preventive strategies include optimizing glycemic control, and monitoring and treating peripheral neuropathy, arterial disease, limited joint mobility, bony deformities, hyperkeratosis, and onychodystrophy. Using the Semmes-Weinstein monofilament, assessing vibratory sensation, and monitoring reflex changes all help the clinician to assess the risk for and help prevent foot ulcers in patients with diabetes. Reducing excessive pressure, shock, and shear by accommodating, stabilizing, and supporting deformities by weight diffusion and dispersion is also important in ulcer prevention.

When prevention fails and an ulcer develops, the history should focus on duration, inciting event or trauma, prior ulcerations, wound care, and pressure off-loading procedures. The examination can include an assessment of the location and depth, the presence of infection, ischemic or neuropathic changes, edema, and the presence of a Charcot joint. Imaging is essential to exclude osteomyelitis and may include plain radiography, computed tomography, technetium bone scans, indium scans, and magnetic resonance imaging. Noninvasive vascular studies include Doppler and transcutaneous oxygen tension. Consultation with a vascular specialist may be needed when vascular insufficiency is severe or the wounds are nonhealing.

The general principles of management include debridement, pressure relief, off-loading, avoidance or limitation of weight bearing, proper wound management, management of infection with early antibiotics, management of ischemia, medical management of comorbidities, and hospitalization and surgical management when necessary. Weight bearing can be modified by the use of crutches, wheelchairs, and bed rest, as well as contact casts, walkers, boots, braces, total contact orthosis, modified surgical shoes and boots, and appropriate dressings. A wide variety of dressings and topical agents are available; selection is guided by nature of the ulcer and its complications. Topical agents include saline, antiseptics, topical antibiotics, enzymes, growth factors, and dermal skin substitutes. Empiric antibiotic therapy should be instituted early, especially if infection may become limb threatening. With osteomyelitis or limb-threatening infection, hospitalization is usually indicated. The choice of antibiotic is based on the clinical symptoms, culture and sensitivity, and the presence of deep infection, bone exposure, or sepsis, as well as whether soft tissue or bone is infected.

Peripheral Vascular Disease

Older adults with peripheral vascular disease demonstrate many of the same signs and symptoms as those with diabetes mellitus. (See "Cardiovascular Diseases and Disorders," p 316.) In contrast to neuropathic ulcers, vascular ulcers are extremely painful.

Arthritis

Osteoarthritis is common in older adults. It occurs in weight-bearing joints and causes pain, swelling, stiffness, limitation of movement, and deformity. It may be worsened by chronic trauma, strain, or obesity. Gouty arthritis results early in intense pain and erythema and later in joint damage.

Rheumatoid arthritis affects the hands and feet equally and results in muscle wasting and marked deformity. The metatarsophalangeal joints become dislocated or subluxed; there is increased protrusion of the metatarsal heads, and walking becomes painful. If

SPECIAL SHOES AND ORTHOTICS

Foot pain and stress can be relieved through weight diffusion and weight dispersion. Weight diffusion is accomplished with an increase in the thickness of an orthosis or sole of a shoe that is placed between the foot and the plane of support, such as the floor. Weight dispersion is accomplished by diverting pressure away from painful areas of the foot by making specific adjustments to an orthosis or insole or by some form of internal or external shoe modification. Examples include balance padding, metatarsal padding, and external shoe wedges or bars. The primary treatment goals of both approaches are to relieve pain, restore maximum function, and maintain restored function once it is achieved.

Special footwear and orthotics aim to reduce shock and shear, transfer weight from painful areas, correct or support flexible deformities, accommodate fixed deformities, and control or limit joint motion. Shoes with depth or extra-depth lasts are usually suggested to accomplish these objectives. A *depth shoe* is a shoe that usually has a filler or insole that extends from heel to toe and that provides at least 3/16" of additional depth in the shoe and a high toe box, so that an orthotic or customized insole can be placed in the shoe and prevent the top of the foot from being compressed against the underside of the toe box. An extra-depth shoe provides 1/4" of additional depth, and a super-depth shoe provides an additional 1/2" of depth for total-contact orthoses or inserts. Custom shoes are recommended for patients with severe deformity, amputation, or other foot problems for which special lasts are required.

Shoe modifications that are often useful for older patients include mild calcaneal wedges to limit motion and alter gait, metatarsal bars to transfer weight, Thomas heels to increase calcaneal support, long shoe counters to increase mid-foot support and control foot direction, heel flares to add stability, shank fillers or wedges to produce a total weight-bearing surface, steel plates to restrict motion, and rocker bars to prevent flexion and extension. Additional internal modifications include longitudinal arch pads, wedges, bars, lifts, and tongue or bite pads. Orthoses are available in rigid, semi-rigid, and flexible varieties; they are made from an array of materials, of which plastic, leather, and laminates are the most useful.

Medicare provides for what are termed *therapeutic shoes* (depth, super-depth, or custom) and *multidensity inserts*. To be eligible, patients must have a history of diabetes mellitus or other disease affecting foot health, evidence of a comprehensive management plan for the disease process that specifies that therapeutic shoes are needed, and documentation that he or she has one or more of the following conditions: peripheral neuropathy with evidence of callus formation, a history of pre-ulcerative calluses, a history of a previous ulceration, a foot deformity, previous amputation of all or part of the foot, or poor circulation. Appropriate footwear is effective in the prevention of serious foot complications.

THE ROLE OF THE PRIMARY CLINICIAN IN FOOT CARE

Foot impairment, including diseases and disorders of the foot that are common in elderly patients, may affect the general health and functioning of older patients. Periodic comprehensive podogeriatric assessment is recommended for older patients. Practitioners should be aware of local conditions and the complications of systemic diseases, such as diabetes mellitus, peripheral arterial disease, arthritic changes, neurologic disorders, and mental health symptoms that manifest as foot symptoms and signs. Primary practitioners should recognize common foot problems and should refer patients for podiatric care and management in a timely and appropriate manner. The quality of life for older persons can be significantly improved by early detection and comprehensive management of foot problems.

REFERENCES

■ Edmonds ME, Foster AVM, Sanders L. *Manual of Diabetic Foot Care.* Malden, MA: Blackwell Publishing; 2004.

■ Helfand AE, ed. Clinical podogeriatrics: assessment, education, and prevention. *Clin Podiatr Med Surg.* 2003;20(3).

■ Helfand AE. Foot problems in older patients—a focused podogeriatrics assessment study in ambulatory care. *J Am Podiatr Med Assoc.* 2004;94(3):294–304.

■ Lorimer D, French G, O'Donnell M, et al. *Neale's Common Foot Disorders, Diagnosis and Management.* 6th ed. New York: Churchill Livingstone; 2002.

■ Veves A, Giurini JM, LoGerfo FW. *The Diabetic Foot: Medical and Surgical Management.* Totowa, NJ: Humana Press; 2002.

CHAPTER 57—NEUROLOGIC DISEASES AND DISORDERS

KEY POINTS

- Cerebrovascular disease is the leading cause of disability and death among older persons.

- Control of systolic hypertension is the most important factor in preventing stroke.

- Common causes of late-life seizure include vascular disease, new mass lesions, and alcohol or medication withdrawal.

- Parkinson's disease may be recognized by an insidious onset of asymmetrical tremor or muscular rigidity.

The number of disorders that affect the nervous system increases rapidly with advancing age. Subtle neurologic abnormalities often are detected on examination. In one study of nearly 500 older adults the following signs were found which could not be attributed directly to any specific medical or a neurologic disease: diminished arm swing (present in 29% of those examined), diminished toe vibration sense (21%), hyper-reflexia in arms (10%), unequal nasolabial folds (9%), absent pupillary response (9%), Babinski's sign (7%), diminished toe position sense (7%), and reduction in arm strength (5%). False findings imply that the diagnosis of neurologic disease may be more difficult in the setting of these "normal" signs. Still, a large percentage of elderly persons will have neurologic disease that cause a variety of impairments. The goal of the clinician is to determine the significance of these abnormalities and to make an accurate diagnosis and implement appropriate treatment.

CEREBROVASCULAR DISEASES

Stroke is a leading cause of disability and death among older persons. The incidence of stroke increases with advancing age, approximately doubling with each decade. The incidence of stroke for men is 2.1 per 1000 at ages 55 to 64 years, 4.5 per 1000 at ages 65 to 74 years, and 9.3 per 1000 at ages 75 to 84 years. The incidence of stroke for women is 25% to 30% lower than that for men in comparable age groups, but it surpasses that of men in the age group 85 years and older.

Throughout the latter half of the 20th century the incidence of stroke declined in the United States, Canada, and Western Europe. This drop may be attributable to better control of modifiable risk factors, including hypertension, heart disease, diabetes mellitus, cigarette smoking, elevated blood lipids, and alcohol use. Hypertension is the most prevalent risk factor for stroke, and its treatment results in a substantial reduction in the risk of stroke. Treatment of isolated systolic hypertension in elderly persons reduces the risk of stroke by nearly 40%. (See "Hypertension," p 331.) Heart disease is also an important risk factor for stroke, including atherosclerotic coronary heart disease, left ventricular hypertrophy, valvular heart disease, valve replacement, and valvular and nonvalvular atrial fibrillation. (See "Cardiovascular Diseases and Disorders," p 316.) Several studies have confirmed a two- to fourfold increased risk of stroke in patients with diabetes mellitus. Studies suggest that tight control of blood-sugar levels might reduce the risk of stroke in patients with diabetes mellitus, although the evidence for reduction of other vascular complications (eg, retinopathy, nephropathy) is somewhat more compelling. (See "Diabetes Mellitus," p 349.) Cigarette smoking independently increases the risk of stroke as much as threefold, according to the Framingham Study. The incidence of stroke declines significantly even after 2 years of cessation of smoking, and after 5 years the level of risk returns to that of nonsmokers. Elevated blood lipids and alcohol use are other important risk factors for stroke. (See "Substance Abuse," p 274.)

Besides being the most common acute, serious neurologic disease, stroke also is a leading cause of death. The fatality rate within 1 month of an acute stroke is 20% to 30% across all age groups; mortality is highest among older persons. Survival in part depends on the location and severity of the stroke. The most important predictor is the severity of neurologic signs. The severity of the neurologic deficits following stroke can be quantified by use of an instrument such as the NIH Stroke Scale (see http://www.vh.org/adult/provider/neurology/Stroke/Scaleind.html or http://www.strokecenter.org/trials/scales/nihss.pdf). In general, a score of less than 5 in this scale, which ranges from 0 to 42, is associated with a very good prognosis. Persons with a score greater than 20 have a very poor prognosis and a high likelihood of major complications.

Neurologic causes of death include the brain injury itself or resultant brain edema. Common medical causes of death are myocardial infarction, arrhythmia, heart failure, aspiration pneumonia, and pulmonary embolism. Age in itself does not influence the gross neurologic aspects of stroke, but older age is associated with lesser recovery in activities of daily living. Older stroke patients can benefit from formal rehabilitation.

Internal Carotid Artery Disease

A lesion at the origin of the internal carotid artery, most commonly secondary to atherosclerosis, can lead to transient monocular blindness (amaurosis fugax) or a cerebral hemispheric deficit (eg, focal motor, sensory, or cognitive symptoms or signs) because both the retina and cerebral hemispheres derive their blood supply from the internal carotid artery. Hemispheric deficits include hemiparesis or hemisensory loss, homonomous hemianopia or aphasia, or apraxia. The initial evaluation of patients with these symptoms or signs usually includes a neuroimaging study (computed tomography or magnetic resonance imaging) and noninvasive imaging of the carotid arteries (B-mode ultrasonography and Doppler ultrasonography or magnetic resonance angiography). Data from the North American Symptomatic Carotid Endarterectomy Trial (NASCET) indicate that the optimal treatment for symptomatic carotid stenosis of greater than 70% is carotid endarterectomy, provided the patient has few comorbidities and the institution performs a high number of endarterectomies. The operation can be performed with reasonable safety in elderly persons provided medical comorbidity is relatively low. The optimal treatment for symptomatic carotid stenosis of less than 70% or of asymptomatic carotid stenosis is still not clear; treatment options include carotid endarterectomy or medical management. Medical management should seek to optimize blood pressure, lipid status, and antiplatelet agents.

Aspirin is the mainstay of antiplatelet therapy for atherosclerotic stroke prevention. Studies on the use of aspirin in stroke prevention suggest that higher dosages than 325 mg of aspirin per day do not add therapeutic benefit, but the minimum necessary dosage has not been fully investigated. Many physicians routinely prescribe 81 to 325 mg per day, although even the lower dosage may cause gastrointestinal irritation and blood loss. Patients who fail aspirin monotherapy are usually advanced to other platelet-inhibiting medications. These may include sustained-release dipyridamole combined with aspirin. Clopidogrel 75 mg once daily is an alternative for patients who cannot tolerate aspirin.

The only clear role for warfarin is primary or secondary stroke prevention in the setting of cardioembolic disease. Specific indications include atrial fibrillation, severe valvular disease, and known intracardiac clot secondary to myocardial infarction.

Vertebrobasilar Arterial Diseases

Syndromes associated with vascular lesions in the posterior circulation (vertebral and basilar arteries) result in cranial nerve impairment or dysfunction of the descending motor or ascending sensory tracks within the brain stem. Because of the large number of pathways passing through the brain stem, vertebrobasilar occlusion results in myriad signs, including abnormal eye movements; Horner's syndrome; unilateral or bilateral or crossed motor and sensory abnormalities in the face, arm, or leg; ataxia; dysarthria; dysphagia; and even stupor or coma. Because the thalamus and inferior portions of the cerebral hemispheres also are supplied by the vertebrobasilar system, behavioral and visual symptoms also can occur. Treatment of posterior circulation cerebrovascular disease is medical, as no surgical approach to improving the posterior circulation has been shown to improve outcomes. Although many clinicians prefer warfarin anticoagulation over antiplatelet agents for patients with vertebrobasilar disease, no formal studies have confirmed better clinical outcomes with warfarin. A large trial (Warfarin-Aspirin Recurrent Stroke Study) found aspirin and warfarin to be equally efficacious (unless the cause is cardioembolic, in which case warfarin is superior).

Lacunar Disease

Lacunar disease secondary to occlusion of small penetrating vessels is presumably the consequence of lipohyalinosis (lipid deposition and hyalinization) or local atherosclerosis. Lacunar strokes may result in several well-defined syndromes, including pure motor hemiplegia, pure hemisensory stroke, ataxic hemiparesis, and dysarthria–clumsy hand syndrome. Risk factors include hypertension and diabetes mellitus. The most effective means of managing lacunar disease is aggressive treatment of these risk factors. Although aspirin also is prescribed for stroke prevention in patients who have suffered lacunar strokes, it has not been shown to prevent lacunar strokes specifically. Lacunar strokes may occur independently or concurrently with large-vessel cerebrovascular disease.

Intracerebral Hemorrhage

Intracerebral hemorrhage accounts for 15% to 20% of all strokes. Approximately 80% occur between the ages of 40 and 70. A racial distribution suggests that black Americans and Asian Americans may be at slightly higher risk than white Americans.

The most common risk factor for intracerebral hemorrhage is hypertension, which is present in 75% to 80% of the cases. Excessive use of alcohol is also associated with a higher incidence. Common locations for hypertensive bleeds are the putamen, thalamus, cerebellar hemisphere, pons, and cerebrum. In elderly patients a common cause of cerebral lobar hemorrhage is cerebral amyloid angiopathy, which usually occurs without systemic amyloidosis. In these cases intracranial bleeds tend to be recurrent. Hemorrhage also can complicate the use of antiplatelet agents and anticoagulants. Other secondary causes of intracerebral hemorrhage should not be overlooked. These include trauma, arteriovenous malformations, and aneurysms. Acute treatment is supportive, with interim control of severe hypertension and discontinuation or antiplatelets. Large lobar or intraventricular hemorrhages may be considered for neurosurgical drainage.

Treatment Following Ischemic Stroke

The current protocol for care of the elderly stroke patient includes optimizing hydration status; controlling blood pressure while avoiding acute hypotension; preventing deep-vein thrombosis; detecting and treating coronary ischemia, heart failure, and cardiac arrhythmias; and initiating long-term treatment with antiplatelet agents or oral anticoagulation to prevent recurrent stroke, depending upon the presumed cause. Dehydration on presentation is common, but rehydration must be gradual to reduce the risk of cerebral edema. In patients with clinically evident cerebrovascular disease immediately after the occurrence of an ischemic cerebral infarction, it is appropriate to withhold treatment of hypertension (unless blood pressure is very high, eg, higher than 220/110 mm Hg) until the situation stabilizes. Even when treatment has been withheld temporarily, the eventual goal is to reduce blood pressure gradually while avoiding orthostatic hypotension. The target systolic blood pressure should be 10 to 20 points higher than the patient's baseline pressure; if the baseline is unknown, systolic pressure should not be lowered beyond 160 mm Hg. Patients with acute ischemic stroke who are treated with fibrinolytic agents require careful blood-pressure monitoring, especially over the first 24 hours after treatment is started. Elevated blood pressure should gradually be brought down to the upper end of the normal range. Patients with a history of ischemic heart disease or arrhythmia and patients with large strokes should be monitored by electrocardiography for 48 hours. For large cardioembolic strokes (eg, involving most of the middle cerebral artery territory or involving both middle and anterior cerebral artery territories), one generally waits 48 hours before beginning anticoagulation. Earlier anticoagulation does not improve outcome. Early initiation of aspirin[OL] therapy has a low risk of bleeding side effects and might improve outcome, modestly.

The only therapy approved by the U.S. Food and Drug Administration for ischemic stroke is recombinant tissue–plasminogen (rt-PA) activator (its generic name is alteplase). Infusion of this medication within 3 hours of stroke onset approximately doubles the chances of a favorable outcome at 3 months. The benefits of this treatment, however, must be weighed against the increased the risk of intracranial hemorrhage, which can be fatal or can result in worsened neurologic status. Most hemorrhagic events occur among patients with severe strokes, and outcomes among persons with severe strokes are very poor without treatment. Use of this medication requires careful assessment by a physician experienced in the treatment of stroke. Tissue-plasminogen activator should be considered when patients present within 3 hours of onset of neurologic deficit and computed tomography confirms the absence of intracranial hemorrhage. Major contraindications include infarction of greater than one third of a hemisphere, major surgery within 2 weeks, previous intracranial hemorrhage, sustained systolic blood pressure above 185 or diastolic above 110, symptoms of subarachnoid hemorrhage, recent urinary or gastrointestinal tract bleeding, coagulopathy, thrombocytopenia, or INR above 1.7. The NIH Stroke Scale is helpful for stratifying ischemic stroke patients according to risk and benefit for rt-PA. Scores below 5 generally have a favorable outcome regardless of treatment. Scores higher than 20 have a substantially increased hemorrhagic complication rate. Even though older patients might have a higher rate of bleeding complications than persons younger than 65, the risk is not sufficiently high to preclude treatment. (See also the section on stroke rehabilitation in "Rehabilitation," p 106.)

SUBDURAL HEMATOMA

A collection of blood between the dura and the arachnoid is referred to as a *subdural hematoma*. It is usually due to head trauma, although the trauma may be mild, particularly in older adults. In approximately 15% of cases, the hematomas are bilateral.

Perhaps most relevant in the elderly patient is the chronic subdural hematoma. The incidence of chronic subdural hematoma increases with age, from 0.13 per 100,000 for those in their 20s to 7.4 per 100,000 for those in their 70s. In 50% of chronic subdural hematomas, there is no history of head injury, although other risk factors include clotting disorders, shunting procedures (eg, ventriculo-peritoneal shunting for normal-pressure hydrocephalus may separate the blood vessels from the dura, resulting in tears), and seizures.

The symptoms of chronic subdural hematoma are headache, slight or severe impairment in cognition, and hemiparesis. Some patients may have seizures. Focal neurologic signs (weakness, sensory loss, and change in

---

[OL] Not approved by the U.S. Food and Drug Administration for this use.

sensation) may be present. Neuroimaging studies reveal an extra-axial collection of blood.

The treatment of the hematoma varies depending on whether it is symptomatic or an incidental finding on a neuroimaging study. If symptomatic and the patient's condition is worsening, then removal of the clot may be attempted. If asymptomatic or if the patient's condition is improving, then clinical monitoring is appropriate, as the hematoma may shrink and disappear without surgery.

HEADACHES

There is evidence to suggest that the prevalence of headaches diminishes with age. One study demonstrated that although 74% of men and 92% of women between the ages of 21 and 34 years have headaches, these proportions drop to 22% and 55% after the age of 75 years. Headache is one of the most common medical complaints in young persons, and yet one study suggests that it is the 10th most common symptom in older women and the 14th most common symptom in older men. Headache incidence also declines with age; only 2% of all sufferers of an initial migraine are over the age of 50 years.

Persistent headaches are more likely to represent systemic or intracranial lesions (ie, nonbenign conditions) in older adults than in younger adults. One study demonstrated that among younger patients, 10% of headaches represent systemic or intracranial lesions; in older adults, this proportion was found to be 34%. These nonbenign conditions include intracranial masses (eg, primary or secondary tumors, subdural hematomas), cervical spondylosis, chronic obstructive pulmonary disease, carbon monoxide poisoning, and giant cell arteritis. In addition, many commonly used medications can cause headaches that are dull, diffuse, and nondescript, including vasodilators (eg, nitrates), hypotensives (eg, reserpine, atenolol, and methyldopa), antiparkinsonian agents, and stimulants.

One secondary cause of headache specific to older adults is giant cell (temporal) arteritis. This disease does not appear to occur below the age of 50 and peaks in incidence between the ages of 70 and 80. Women are affected twice as often as men. Pain may be centered at temporal or occipital arteries. Palpation of the scalp arteries may reveal focal tenderness and nodularity. Complaints of visual changes, low-grade fever, polymyalgia, and constitutional symptoms further suggest the diagnosis. Twenty percent of patients suffer visual loss that is generally irreversible. Peripheral markers of inflammation are typically elevated; however, nearly 10% of patients have a normal erythrocyte sedimentation rate. Elevated C-reactive protein may be

more sensitive. Patients with the proper presentation should be promptly evaluated by temporal artery biopsy. Prednisone 40 to 60 mg daily day relieves symptoms within a few days. The dose is gradually tapered with close serologic monitoring.

As in younger persons, the common primary headache disorders may be classified into migraines (with or without aura) and tension-type headaches. Migraines are often unilateral, pulsating headaches of moderate or severe intensity associated with nausea, vomiting, or photophobia. Auras, when they occur, usually precede the headache and are manifested by transient neurologic symptoms that are localizable to the cerebral cortex or brain stem. Visual phenomena are among the most common types of auras. In contrast to migraines, tension-type headaches are often more diffuse, have a pressing or a tight quality, and are not associated with nausea or vomiting.

Headaches in older adults, however, may present in atypical ways. With migraines in particular, auras tend to disappear with age, and in some individuals the reverse occurs (headaches disappear while auras remain). The occurrence of an isolated visual or sensory aura in the absence of a headache can be diagnostically challenging in the sense that these symptoms may be signs of transient ischemic attacks as well.

The treatment of headaches may be categorized as either abortive (ie, treating an attack that has already begun) or preventive. Apart from various over-the-counter preparations, abortive therapies include ergotamines or triptans (eg, sumatriptan), which act by central serotonergic mechanisms. These medications are mild vasoconstrictors and contraindicated in the setting of uncontrolled hypertension, stroke, and coronary artery disease. Generally, safety data in geriatric populations is lacking. Preventive therapies include β-blockers (propranolol, atenolol [OL]), valproic acid, topiramate, tricyclic antidepressants, and calcium channel blockers. The choice of an agent should be guided by an effort to avoid adverse effects and drug interactions.

Older adults may not tolerate headache medications as well as younger patients do; moreover, in some older patients a medication may be contraindicated by comorbidities or existing drug regimens. For example, β-blockers and tricyclic antidepressants, which are often used as preventive therapy, may be associated with lethargy or sedation.

MOVEMENT DISORDERS

A movement disorder may be defined simply as abnormal involuntary movements. These movements are not the result of weakness or sensory deficits; they are the result of dysfunction of the basal ganglia or the extrapyramidal motor system. Movement disorders may

---

[OL] Not approved by the U.S. Food and Drug Administration for this use.

be classified as hyperkinesias (excessive movement) or hypokinesias (paucity of movement). A particular movement disorder (eg, Parkinson's disease) may be characterized by several types of involuntary movements (eg, tremor, bradykinesia). Several movement disorders are especially common among older persons.

Parkinson's Disease

Parkinson's disease is a progressive neurodegenerative disease in which cell death in the substantia nigra and consequent reduction in brain dopamine levels results in a constellation of signs, including tremor at rest, bradykinesia, rigidity, and postural instability. The pathologic hallmark of the disease is the Lewy body, an intracellular inclusion body found in the substantia nigra.

The incidence increases dramatically with age, and the incidence among people in their 70s and 80s in the United States is approximately 200 cases per 100,000 (0.2%). The incidence among those in their 70s and 80s in other countries (Iceland, India, Scotland, Australia) has been estimated to be even higher, approaching 1000 to 2000 per 100,000 (1% to 2%). The disease most commonly appears between the ages of 50 and 79 years. In a small proportion of cases, the disease clusters within families and has a genetic basis. In a small number of these families, the disease has been linked to a region on the long arm of chromosome 4 that encodes the neuronal protein α-synuclein. In addition, environmental toxins (eg, manganese and pesticides) have been associated with some forms of the disease.

The disease begins insidiously and asymmetrically. The clinical manifestations include tremor, usually in one hand or sometimes in both, classically involving the fingers in a pill-rolling motion. The tremor (usually 3 to 5 Hz) is present at rest and usually decreases with active, purposeful movement. Muscular rigidity is usually readily evident on passive movement of a limb. Passive movement may demonstrate a smooth resistance or superimposed ratchet-like jerks (cogwheel phenomenon). The term *bradykinesia* is often used to describe either a slowness in initiating movement (ie, a paucity of spontaneous movements) or movements themselves that are slow, and the term *freezing* is used to describe sudden interruption of movement. Other clinical features of Parkinson's disease may include the following:

- tachykinesia: the tendency for movements to become smaller and faster;
- tachyphemia: the tendency to speak more and more rapidly until all of the words run together into a mumble;
- micrographia: the tendency to make loops that become smaller and tighter when drawing loops across a page, to exhibit handwriting that is very small;
- festinating gait: to take steps that inadvertently quicken and become smaller, and
- impaired finger tapping: in which the amplitude lessens and the movements become more rapid until the fingers seem stuck together.

Postural abnormalities are evident in the standing and sitting positions, and an erect posture is not readily assumed or maintained. The head tends to fall forward on the trunk. The tendency to fall forward (propulsion) or backward (retropulsion) results from the loss of postural reflexes. Bradykinesia prevents the patient from stopping the fall, either by taking a step or moving the arms. The face can become mask-like, with lack of expression and diminished eye blinking.

Mood abnormalities, usually depression or anxiety, are common, as are cognitive impairment and dementia. These may place severe restrictions on the medications that might be used to relieve the tremor, bradykinesia, and rigidity.

One of the diagnostic challenges may be distinguishing mild early parkinsonism from the changes that often accompany normal aging (slowing down, loss of balance, stiffness, difficulty walking, stooped posture). However, the bradykinesia and rigidity of Parkinson's disease are usually asymmetric at onset, with one side slightly affected and the other remaining normal. In addition, tremor at rest is not a feature of normal aging, and although elderly persons may complain of stiffness, true extrapyramidal rigidity is otherwise uncommon.

The diagnosis is made clinically. Neuroimaging should be considered in atypical presentations such as the abrupt onset of tremor, focal weakness, sensory disturbances, or reflex abnormalities not attributed to muscle tone asymmetry.

Treatment programs must be individualized. This caution applies especially to elderly patients, who have reduced tolerance for dopaminergic and anticholinergic agents, the mainstays of parkinsonism therapy. Nonpharmacologic therapy includes a regular exercise program. Many elderly patients benefit from a course of physical therapy aimed at restoring their confidence in walking and maintaining balance, as well as teaching them simple tricks to help them manage unpredictable and disabling freezing episodes, and, when needed, selecting a cane or walker of the appropriate size and weight. A home visit by an occupational therapist may help to plan the appropriate placement of wall rails, grab bars, and other such assistive devices that reduce the possibility of falling.

Treatment of the motor manifestations of parkinsonism is important, but many elderly patients also complain of difficulty with constipation and insomnia. Constipation is particularly bothersome to elderly patients taking levodopa, which tends to exacerbate the constipation associated with reduced levels of physical activity. Treatment includes a diet rich in fruit and fiber, prune and other juices, frequent consumption of liquids, and use of osmotic laxatives. Elderly Parkinson's disease patients with insomnia should also be given individualized treatment. Some patients wake up at night because of a low dopamine state, which results in feelings of stiffness and malaise that are severe enough to awaken the patient. Higher bedtime doses of levodopa or even sustained-release forms of levodopa are appropriate. Patients may also experience insomnia because they are sleeping too much during the day, which may be a side effect of levodopa therapy. In these cases, it may be important to reduce the dosage of levodopa and correct the reversed sleep-wake cycle. Because urinary urgency may be a feature of Parkinson's disease, this may be the cause of the frequent night-time awakenings.

The major factor influencing the treatment of elderly patients with Parkinson's disease is their propensity to develop confusion and psychosis on antiparkinsonian medications. In general, the therapeutic regimen should be kept simple. Rather than prescribing small doses of multiple medications, prescribe higher doses of one or two medications; toxic side effects are less likely to occur. Levodopa provides the most improvement in the motor manifestations of Parkinson's disease relative to its toxic side effects on the central nervous system, whereas those with anticholinergic properties (agents such as trihexyphenidyl and amantadine) provide the least benefit. The dopamine agonists (bromocriptine, ropinirole, pramipexole) fall in between. Although psychosis may be treated effectively with clozapine, olanzapine, or quetiapine, which have fewer extrapyramidal side effects than other antipsychotic agents, confusion and disorientation may be treated more simply by lowering the doses of antiparkinsonian medications. In this setting, anticholinergic medications should be the first to be discontinued, followed by selegiline, dopamine agonists, and, finally, levodopa.

The most effective step in treating patients with Parkinson's disease is to accomplish dopamine replacement by using levodopa combined with carbidopa. Levodopa is converted to dopamine in both the central nervous system and the periphery. To reduce peripheral conversion, levodopa is combined with carbidopa (a peripheral decarboxylate inhibitor), which does not cross the blood-brain barrier. Treatment usually begins with a half tablet of the 25:100 combination (ie, 25 mg carbidopa to 100 mg levodopa) once or twice a

day. Every 1 to 2 weeks, the dose can be increased by one half to one tablet, to reach a dose of one full tablet three times a day, if needed and if side effects are tolerable. If disabling bradykinesia, rigidity, postural instability, or tremor are still present, the dose can be gradually increased further, with cautious observation of side effects. Older adults, particularly if cognitively impaired, rarely tolerate more than 1000 mg per day of levodopa. Common adverse effects include nausea, abdominal cramping, orthostatic hypotension, and confusion. A controlled-release form (25:100 and 50:200) generally requires a slightly higher total daily dose. By approximately 5 years of levodopa therapy, half of patients will develop dyskinesias from the drug. Because of this, less effective dopamine agonists should be considered for initial therapy when the patient's life span is projected to be significantly more than 5 years such that dyskinesias will likely develop.

For patients with milder disease and no signs of dementia, dopamine agonists may be used initially as monotherapy. A cautious induction period with each is required, as nausea, orthostatic hypotension, and confusion are common side effects. Bromocriptine is begun with 1.25 mg per day and gradually increased by 1.25-mg increments every 2 to 5 days, to a total daily dose of 10 to 30 mg. Other newer dopamine agonists include ropinirole (given in starting dosages of 0.25 mg three times per day and increased as needed to dosages of 3 mg per day) and pramipexole (given in starting dosages of 0.125 mg three times per day and increased as needed to dosages of 4.5 mg per day). All dopamine agonists, and to a lesser extent levodopa, have been associated with sudden sleep attacks in which patients may fall asleep abruptly while driving. Patients should be warned of this rare but potentially serious adverse effect of therapy. As Parkinson's disease progresses, patients eventually require a switch from dopamine agonists to levodopa. Later in the disease when the response to levodopa becomes variable, dopamine agonists may be reintroduced to manage periods of off-time.

Selegiline in dosages of 5 mg twice a day (8 AM and noon) may be used in an early stage to slow disease progression. Likewise, rasagiline, a novel, second-generation, selective, irreversible monoamine oxidase type B inhibitor, can be used as monotherapy or as adjunctive therapy for Parkinson's disease. Rasagiline has been shown to be well tolerated at 1 mg once daily and to improve symptoms and motor fluctuations in patients with early and moderate to advanced Parkinson's disease. Importantly, use of rasagiline has not been associated with significant cognitive or behavioral adverse changes in mentation, behavior, or mood.

Amantadine, a drug particularly useful for treating tremor, is generally prescribed at 100 mg two to three times daily; the dosage should be adjusted in renal impairment. Amantadine's mild anticholinergic effects appear to play a role in its antiparkinsonian effects. It also promotes dopamine release in the corpus striatum. Elderly patients often develop cognitive side effects, including hallucinations. Tolcapone and entacapone are new drugs for Parkinson's disease and are used as adjunctive treatment usually in combination with levodopa and carbidopa for patients with severe Parkinson's disease who are not responding satisfactorily to, or are not appropriate candidates for, other adjunct therapies.

Surgical options are increasingly being utilized for Parkinson's disease patients who have symptoms uncontrollable by medical therapies. Depending on a patient's most troubling symptoms, brain stimulators or stereotactic lesioning may be considered. Subthalamic nucleus stimulation is achieved by attaching an embedded pacemaker-like generator to a wire with the tip located deep to the thalamus. High-frequency stimulation results in improvement in tremor, akinesia, rigidity, and gait. Several sites have been identified which, when lesioned, can help certain symptoms of Parkinson's disease. Lesioning of the pallidum is often successful in the treatment of contralateral dyskinesias. Lesioning of the ventral intermediate nucleus of the thalamus has been successful in the treatment of contralateral tremor. Generally, the morbidity of these procedures is low among patients in otherwise fair to good health who do not have dementia.

Multiple System Atrophy

A histopathologic understanding of three parkinsonisms—olivopontocerebellar atrophy, Shy-Drager syndrome, and striatonigral degeneration—has permitted these overlapping syndromes to be carried under the rubric multiple system atrophy (MSA). Sometimes called a *Parkinson's plus disease*, MSA is characterized by parkinsonism (rigidity, tremor, bradykinesia, and postural instability) plus autonomic symptoms, cerebellar signs, and sometimes myoclonus. Other features that may accompany MSA are upper motor signs, severe dysarthria, stridor, dystonia, and an amyotrophic lateral sclerosis (ALS)–like picture. The diagnosis is clinical and can initially be indistinguishable from idiopathic Parkinson's disease. The mean age of onset for MSA is 55. It has a slight male preponderance and is progressive to death in approximately 7 years.

Autonomic symptoms are often the first to allow MSA to be differentiated from Parkinson's disease. Patients complain of dizziness, lightheadedness, or syncope on standing, and of postexertional weakness, gait unsteadiness, and dimming of vision. Impaired temperature control, reduced sweating, sphincter disturbance with urinary or fecal incontinence, diarrhea, constipation, impotence, iridic atrophy, impaired eye movements, Horner's syndrome, and anisocoria may also occur.

Orthostatic hypotension is often the most disabling symptom. Nonpharmacologic treatment of the autonomic dysfunction includes eating small meals, getting up slowly, and avoiding excessive straining at stool. Compressive clothing and elastic stockings, increased salt and fluid intake, and sleeping in a reverse Trendelenburg position may ameliorate some of the orthostatic symptoms. Drugs that are sometimes useful in treating the orthostatic hypotension include midodrine and fludrocortisone [OL]. Use of these medications occasionally results in supine hypertension, which requires close blood-pressure monitoring. Levodopa may initially help the rigidity, bradykinesia, and postural instability. Unfortunately, dopamine replacement often worsens the orthostatic hypotension.

Progressive Supranuclear Palsy

Progressive supranuclear palsy accounts for approximately 4% of cases of parkinsonism. It is marked by supranuclear gaze palsy, square wave jerks (defined below), and cognitive impairment. Onset usually occurs during the late 50s or early 60s. The pathogenesis is unknown. The disease usually progresses rapidly, with marked incapacity occurring within 3 to 5 years and death within 10 years, generally as a result of intercurrent infection or other complications of immobility.

This disease derives its name from progressive impairments of voluntary gaze. The majority of patients develop eye movement restrictions at approximately year 4 of the disease course. Patients are unable to voluntarily look downward or upward (upward gaze is less severely involved). Limitation of voluntary gaze is termed *supranuclear*. Because the vestibular nuclei are still able to direct eye movements, when the examiner abruptly tips the head, the eyes can be driven to look downward or upward. In addition to gaze palsy, patients with progressive supranuclear palsy often exhibit macro-square wave jerks. During fixation, small brief saccadic-appearing eye movements occur every few seconds. These eye movements are involuntary and give the appearance of scanning eye movements around a small target.

As the disease progresses out of the early stages, it differentiates from the appearance of idiopathic Parkinson's disease. Resting tremor is usually mild, and the rigidity is more pronounced at the neck and trunk. Axial rigidity is often striking, giving patients a hyperextended neck with contracted facial muscles bearing an expression of sustained surprise. Gait is disturbed early in the course, with frequent falls in the majority of patients. Cognition is often affected, with personality changes, impaired judgment, and some-

---

[OL] Not approved by the U.S. Food and Drug Administration for this use.

times inappropriate laughing and crying. Unlike MSA, other than urinary incontinence, autonomic dysfunction is atypical.

No fully effective treatment is available. Treatment with levodopa may be partially effective at reducing the rigidity, although the dramatic response to levodopa that is experienced by patients with Parkinson's disease is usually lacking. Generally, any improvement is transient.

Drug-Induced Movement Disorders

A variety of different types of involuntary movements may arise as a result of the use of medications. It is important to distinguish acute drug effects, chronic but reversible drug effects, and chronic and irreversible drug effects. One acute drug effect that may happen with antipsychotic medications is an acute dystonic reaction resulting in oral, lingual, or nuchal dystonia. If it is severe enough, treatment with intravenous diphenhydramine or lorazepam may be required, although this approach in older adults should be exercised with caution, given the propensity for this agent to produce somnolence or confusion. Fortunately, acute dystonia occurs less frequently in older than in younger adults. Chronic reversible drug effects (effects that resolve upon discontinuation of the causative medication) include action tremor (eg, lithium, theophylline, valproic acid), parkinsonism (antipsychotic, antiemetic medications, metoclopramide), chorea (estrogen, antiepileptic medications), or dystonia (dopamine replacement therapy in Parkinson's disease). Chronic irreversible drug effects or tardive phenomena often begin after the medication (usually an antipsychotic medication) has been in use for weeks to months. Movements may include orobuccal dyskinesias, dystonia, akathisia (sensation of needing to move), myoclonus, and tics. Advanced age and duration of treatment with antipsychotic medications are the only well-established risk factors for developing tardive movement disorders. Once the diagnosis of a tardive phenomenon is established, the clinician should attempt to reduce the dosage of medication or discontinue it. Treatment for tardive dyskinesia or tardive dystonia includes anticholinergic agents (trihexyphenidyl), baclofen[OL], reserpine[OL], or clozapine[OL], each of which must be used with caution in older adults. In cases of severe tardive dystonia in which there is neck jerking or sustained eye closure, intramuscular injections of botulinum toxin[OL] may reduce the frequency and severity of movements.

[OL] Not approved by the U.S. Food and Drug Administration for this use.

Essential Tremor

Essential tremor is the most common form of abnormal tremor. The tremor is an action tremor, which is present when the limbs are in active use (eg, while writing or while holding a cup). The tremor most commonly involves the arms, although the head and voice are also commonly involved. Other areas of the body may include the chin, tongue, and legs. The tremor is often slightly worse in one arm than in the other. One of the striking features of the tremor is that it has a varying amplitude so that during some moments the tremor is mild or even absent and during others it is severe. The tremor disappears when the arms are relaxed, that is, when the person is sitting with hands in the lap or when standing or walking with arms held at the sides. Functionally, the tremor may interfere with many daily activities, such as eating, writing, or fastening buttons. Stress or anxiety can exacerbate the tremor. The frequency of the tremor is in the 4- to 12-Hz range; because age is inversely related to the frequency of the tremor, older persons have slower tremor, which is often in the 4- to 8-Hz range.

The prevalence of the disorder increases with advancing age, with as many as 1% to 5% of persons aged 60 years and older affected. The age of onset seems to have a bimodal distribution, with peaks in the teens and 20s and in the 50s through the 70s. The prevalence rates among men and women are similar, although head tremor may be more common among women.

Between 17% and 100% of affected persons report having an affected relative, which suggests that there is a familial form of the tremor. In some families, many individuals are affected over several generations. Familial forms of the tremor have been linked to regions on chromosomes 2p and 3q. There are no apparent clinical differences between the familial and sporadic forms of essential tremor. The cause of the sporadic form of the illness is not known; age is the only known risk factor for essential tremor.

It may be difficult to distinguish essential tremor from several other conditions. Physiologic tremor, which is present in all people, varies in amplitude, and it may be more noticeable in some individuals. It may also be enhanced by anxiety, stimulants, hypoglycemia, medications, or certain illnesses (eg, hyperthyroidism). The tremor is often faster than that of essential tremor (8 to 12 Hz) and the amplitude lower. Although patients with Parkinson's disease most typically have a tremor at rest, they may also have an action tremor. In addition, if essential tremor is severe enough, it may even be present at rest. However, other features of Parkinson's disease (bradykinesia and rigidity) should not be present in persons with essential tremor.

The main indications for treatment of essential tremor are embarrassment and disability. The latter may manifest itself either as difficulty performing certain tasks (eg, eating and writing), modification in the way the task is performed (eg, only drinking with a straw out of closed cups), and even avoidance of certain tasks. Initial therapy includes β-blocking agents (eg, propranolol, atenolol[OL]), primidone[OL], phenobarbital[OL], diazepam[OL], and newer agents, including gabapentin[OL] and clozapine[OL]. The response to these agents is variable (ie, some patients experience moderate improvement, whereas others experience none), and the tremor is rarely reduced to asymptomatic levels. Some patients with severe, medically refractory tremor may undergo deep brain (thalamic) stimulator surgery in which the ventral intermediate (VIM) nucleus of the thalamus is stimulated at high frequency with an implanted electrode. The treatment has been shown to be effective in controlling tremor.

EPILEPSY

A seizure is a paroxysmal excessive or hypersynchronous cerebral neuronal discharge, or both, that results in a transient change in motor function, sensation, or mental state. Recurrent seizures are the defining feature of epilepsy. Depending on whether the seizure discharges involve only a portion of the cortex or the entire cortex, seizures are broadly classified as partial or generalized. Partial seizures are subdivided on the basis of whether or not the seizure is associated with impairment of consciousness. Simple partial seizures do not impair consciousness and most often are associated with focal rhythmic motor twitching. Complex partial seizures are associated with alteration of consciousness and commonly amnesia for the event. Automatisms and other motor manifestations may occur with complex partial seizures. Generalized seizures in older adults are almost invariably convulsive ("grand mal").

New-onset seizures occur in a bimodal pattern with respect to age, with an initial peak in incidence within the first year of life and a second peak after the age of 60 years. Disease-specific causes of epilepsy are more common in older adults, and one-half or more of older adult patients with new-onset epilepsy have an underlying cause. Common causes include vascular disease, space-occupying lesions, brain trauma, alcohol withdrawal, and neurodegenerative diseases. Related to this is the observation that the incidence of partial seizures increases in older adults, whereas the incidence of generalized tonic-clonic seizures remains constant with respect to age. Beyond the age of 65, approximately one half of new-onset cases of epilepsy have a complex partial pattern. This pattern may be explained by the greater incidence of underlying focal lesions in older age groups.

Because of this propensity for new-onset cases of epilepsy to be harbingers of focal lesions, the work-up of older adults to exclude an underlying treatable cause is particularly important. The neurologic history and examination should aim to clinically characterize the seizure and localize its source, as well as elicit other signs of a focal lesion or a metabolic disturbance (eg, uremia, hepatic failure). Blood studies (blood urea nitrogen; serum levels of sodium, glucose, magnesium, calcium; and liver function tests), magnetic resonance imaging, and electroencephalography play important roles.

The treatment of epilepsy in older adults is particularly challenging. The prevalence of adverse drug-disease and drug-drug interactions increases with age. One example of a drug-disease interaction is that between anticonvulsants such as divalproex sodium and hepatic disease, given the tendency of divalproex and other anticonvulsants such as carbamazepine to exacerbate preexisting liver dysfunction, particularly in the older patient. In terms of drug-drug interactions, cimetidine and propranolol increase the serum concentrations of phenytoin and carbamazepine, respectively. Age-related changes in renal and hepatic function may alter drug metabolism significantly, so that older adults must often be placed on lower doses of antiepileptic drugs (AEDs). A sizable fraction of many AEDs is bound to plasma proteins. Since aging causes a reduced synthesis of albumin, it may be important to monitor free (unbound) levels of AEDs (eg, phenytoin). Older persons may be particularly sensitive to medication side effects. For example, AEDs may intensify an underlying dementia or exacerbate mild cognitive decline. Management questions invariably arise when treating older adults with AEDs. Even an experienced neurologist may seek the assistance of a clinical pharmacist to resolve issues of drug interactions, dosages, and side effects. Finally, there are a variety of reasons why older adults may have difficulty with adherence. It is particularly important in treating older adults to involve caregivers so that the goals of the treatment, side effects, and monitoring of progress may be understood.

There are a variety of AEDs, and most must be started slowly and the dose increased gradually (see Table 57.1). Reduction in seizure frequency and severity and the onset of side effects are the parameters that should be followed, not the blood level. If monotherapy has not adequately controlled the seizures and the dose has been maximized, then monotherapy with another agent should be tried before resorting to add-on therapy. Epilepsy surgery

---

[OL] Not approved by the U.S. Food and Drug Administration for this use.

Table 57.1—Antiepileptic Therapy in Older Adults

Drug	Dosage (*mg*)	Target Blood Level (*μg/mL*)	Comments (Metabolism, Excretion)
Carbamazepine	200–600 bid	4–12	Many drug interactions; mood stabilizer; occasional hyponatremia; thrombocytopenia, SIADH, leukopenia; sustained-release form available (L, K)
Gabapentin	300–600 tid	n.a.	Used as adjunct to other agents; adjust dose on basis of creatinine clearance (K)
Lamotrigine	100–300 bid	2–4	When used with valproic acid, begin at 25 mg qod, titrate to 25–100 mg bid (L, K)
Levetiracetam	500–1500 bid	n.a.	Adjust dose on basis of creatinine clearance (K)
Oxcarbazepine	300–1200 bid	n.a.	Many drug interactions; can cause hyponatremia, leukopenia (L)
Phenobarbital	30–60 bid–tid	20–40	Many drug interactions; not recommended for de novo use in older adults (L)
Phenytoin	200–300 qd	5–20*	Many drug interactions; exhibits nonlinear pharmacokinetics (L)
Tiagabine	2–12 bid–tid	n.a.	Adverse-event profile in older adults less well described (L)
Topiramate	25–100 qd–bid	n.a.	May affect cognitive functioning at high doses (L, K)
Valproic acid	250–750 tid	50–100	Can cause weight gain; several drug interactions; mood stabilizer; follow LFTs and platelets (L)
Zonisamide	100–400 qd	n.a.	Anorexia; contraindicated in patients with sulfonamide allergy

NOTE: bid = twice a day; K = metabolized via kidneys; L = metabolized via liver; LFTs = liver functions tests; n.a. = not available; qod = every other day; SIADH = syndrome of inappropriate secretion of antidiuretic hormones; tid = three times a day.

* Phenytoin is extensively bound to plasma albumin. In cases of hypoalbuminemia or marked renal insufficiency, calculate adjusted phenytoin concentration (C):

$$C_{adjusted} = \frac{C_{observed} \ (\mu g/mL)}{0.2 \times albumin \ (g/dL) + 0.1}$$

If creatinine clearance < 10 mL/min, use:

$$C_{adjusted} = \frac{C_{observed} \ (\mu g/mL)}{0.1 \times albumin \ (g/dL) + 0.1}$$

Obtaining a free phenytoin level is an alternate method for monitoring phenytoin in cases of hypoalbuminemia or marked renal insufficiency.

SOURCE: Adapted from Reuben DB, Herr K, Pacala JT, et al. *Geriatrics At Your Fingertips: 2006.* 8th ed. New York: American Geriatrics Society; 2006:141–142. Adapted with permission.

has become an increasingly common choice of patients whose seizures have proven refractory to pharmacologic management. The utility of surgery in elderly patients is not known. Discontinuing AEDs should be considered if the patient has not had a seizure for several years, particularly if the original seizure activity was a single or poorly characterized event.

MOTOR NEURON DISEASE

Amyotrophic lateral sclerosis (ALS) is a neurodegenerative condition involving both upper and lower motor neuron cell bodies; it is characterized clinically by a progressive weakness and wasting of skeletal muscles, often in combination with bulbar palsy and respiratory failure. The incidence increases with age but reaches a plateau in the 60s. To date, age remains the single most clearly identifiable risk factor for this progressive and fatal disorder.

Patients commonly present with gait disturbance, falls, foot drop, weakness in grip, dysphagia, or dysarthria. On neurologic examination, patients may have a combination of upper motor neuron signs (hyperreflexia, clonus, extensor plantar responses) and lower motor neuron signs (weakness, atrophy fascicula-

tions). Although cranial nerves may be involved, with weakness of the face tongue and pallet, the extraocular movements are usually spared. The electromyogram demonstrates findings consistent with diffuse denervation (diffuse fibrillation potentials, positive sharp waves) and poor recruitment of motor units. The differential diagnosis includes lesions at the level of the foramen magnum or the high cervical cord and vitamin-B_{12} deficiency. The prognosis is poor, with the average survival on the order of 2 to 3 years. The presence of bulbar signs carries a poorer prognosis.

Although most new cases of ALS occur in older adults, the incidence and prevalence of this disorder relative to other more common neurologic disorders is low. Therefore, gait disturbance and focal motor weakness may be attributed to the more common cerebrovascular diseases or to cervical radiculomyelopathy rather than to ALS. Older adults are also more likely to have coexisting neuropathology, adding to the challenge of and delay in diagnosing ALS. One study showed that those over the age of 65 years were diagnosed after 19 months, in comparison with those who were less than 65 years of age, who were diagnosed after 3 months.

The treatment is mostly supportive. Riluzole, which has demonstrated modest effects upon survival or time to tracheostomy, is now in widespread use. The action of riluzole is thought to protect against glutamate toxicity, which may be involved in the pathogenesis of ALS.

MYELOPATHY

In older persons, myelopathy or spinal cord dysfunction is most often the result of compression of the spinal cord. Most commonly affected is the cervical region. Intrinsic spinal cord lesions are often the result of spinal cord tumors or vascular events (infarcts or hemorrhages). Extrinsic compressive lesions are more prevalent; common causes among older patients are cervical spondylosis (with resultant osteophyte formation and degenerative disc disease), disc prolapse or herniation, rheumatoid arthritis resulting in vertebral body subluxation, or spinal metastases. Nearly 80% of patients aged 70 years or older have radiographic evidence of osteophyte formation with significant narrowing of the spinal canal; the majority of these cases are asymptomatic. Spinal stenosis is a congenitally, abnormally narrow spinal canal. When disc protrusion occurs in a patient with spinal stenosis, it further compromises the capacity of a spinal canal that is already limited. Narrowing of the cervical canal may lead to neck stiffness and pain; radicular pain, sensory loss, or weakness in the arm; and weakness and upper motor neuron signs (hyperreflexia, spasticity, Babinski's sign) in the lower extremities. Narrowing of the lumbar canal may lead to lower back pain, to radicular pain, sensory loss, or weakness in the legs, and to upper motor neuron signs in the legs. Other symptoms of spinal cord compression include gait disturbance, falls, or complaints of "numb, clumsy hands." On examination, the patient may exhibit spastic paraparesis (symmetric or asymmetric), sensory loss at a particular cord level, or problems with micturition.

Magnetic resonance imaging is the key diagnostic step. If the patient cannot tolerate this procedure because of the presence of metallic objects, a pacemaker, or severe claustrophobia, then spinal computed tomography with intrathecal contrast should be performed.

Conservative management, particularly if neck pain is an associated feature, includes activity modification, neck immobilization with a cervical collar, massage, heat treatment, physical therapy, and medications (muscle relaxants and pain medications, including nonsteroidal anti-inflammatory agents). Decompressive surgery is recommended for persistent pain or a progressive neurologic deficit. Older patients are more prone to have multiple levels of involvement, and some studies have suggested that their prognosis after surgery is poorer than that of younger patients.

RADICULOPATHY

Radiculopathy results from compression of a spinal root as it exits the spinal cord. Among older adults, this may be the result of herniated discs or osteophyte formation. Symptomatic nerve root compression may result in complaints of pain radiating down the neck, back, arm, or leg, and on neurologic examination, this may be accompanied by motor and sensory deficits as well as diminution of reflexes in the distribution of a particular spinal root or roots. (See also "Back and Neck Pain," p 410.)

PERIPHERAL NEUROPATHY

The prevalence of peripheral neuropathy in older adults has been estimated to be as high as 20%, and some degree of subclinical decrement in peripheral nerve function on electromyography is probably universal in healthy older adults. Peripheral neuropathy may be particularly devastating in older adults because of gait impairment due to sensory and motor deficits and thus a propensity to fall. In developed countries, diabetic neuropathy is the most common form of neuropathy; up to 60% of patients who have diabetes mellitus and who are over the age of 60 years have a peripheral neuropathy. Several types of neuropathy are associated with diabetes mellitus, including a distal symmetric neuropathy, asymmetric neuropathies that may involve cranial nerves, roots, or plexus, and mononeuropathy multiplex. Other common causes of peripheral neuropathy in older adults are medications (eg, amiodarone, colchicine, phenytoin, lithium, vincristine, isoniazid), alcohol abuse, and nutritional deficiencies (eg, of vitamins B_6 and B_{12} as well as of thiamine, folate, and niacin), renal disease (ie, uremia), monoclonal gammopathy (eg, multiple myeloma), and neoplasm (eg, infiltration of peripheral nerves by malignant cells, paraneoplastic syndromes associated with oat cell carcinoma of the lung, breast cancer, ovarian cancer, renal cell carcinoma, and prostate cancer).

The treatment of the neuropathy depends on the cause, ranging from withdrawal of the causative agent (alcohol, medications) to nutritional supplementation (nutritional deficiency), or treatment of the primary cancer (neoplastic neuropathy). There is some evidence that optimizing glucose control may lessen the severity of diabetic neuropathy. Treatment of neuropathic pain includes the use of tricyclic antidepressants, anticonvulsant medications (eg, carbamazepine [OL],

---

OL Not approved by the U.S. Food and Drug Administration for this use.

gabapentin^{OL}—both are off-label uses except for specific neuropathies), and selective serotonin-reuptake inhibitors. Topical agents include capsaicin cream and local anesthetic medications. Another alternative may include the antidepressant duloxetine. Duloxetine is a serotonin-norepinephrine reuptake inhibitor (SNRI) in the same class as the antidepressant venlafaxine. It has recently been approved by the U.S. Food and Drug Administration for the management of neuropathic pain.

MYOPATHY

Myopathies are characterized by proximal muscle weakness, wasting, and diminished or absent reflexes, and they may be accompanied by elevations in serum enzymes (creatinine kinase) and a myopathic pattern on electromyogram and on muscle biopsy (ie, fiber degeneration follows a random pattern). Older adults may attribute mild or moderate muscle weakness to aging and therefore may not immediately consult a physician. Proximal muscle weakness, which results in difficulty rising from a chair, difficulty in climbing stairs, or difficulty washing the hair, is particularly likely to be attributed to aging or arthritis.

The most common myopathies in older adults are polymyositis, endocrine myopathies, toxic myopathies, and myopathies associated with carcinoma. Polymyositis is a disorder of skeletal muscle of diverse causes characterized by an infiltration of the muscles with lymphocytes. Muscle biopsy usually shows signs of degeneration, regeneration, and infiltration by lymphocytes. Treatment with prednisone should be used with caution in older adults because of its propensity to produce psychosis. In thyrotoxic myopathy, weakness and wasting are greatest in the pelvic girdle muscles and to some extent in the muscles of the shoulder region. Reflexes may be normal, and the diagnosis is made by the distribution of muscle weakness in a patient with thyrotoxicosis. Improvement of the myopathy follows treatment of the underlying endocrine disorder. Hypothyroidism may also cause a myopathy that improves with thyroid replacement therapy. Myopathy may occasionally be the result of a remote effect of a cancer (ie, a paraneoplastic disorder), with complaints of weakness often preceding the establishment of a diagnosis of cancer. Several drugs cause myopathy, including corticosteroids, lipid-lowering agents, procainamide, and diuretics that produce hypokalemia.

RESTLESS LEGS SYNDROME

See "Sleep Problems" (p 232).

REFERENCES

- Alexander NB, Goldberg A. Gait disorders: search for multiple causes. *Cleve Clin J Med.* 2005;72(7):586, 589–590, 592–594.

- Ferris A. Robertson RM, Fabunmi R, et al; American Heart Association. American Stroke Association. American Heart Association and American Stroke Association national survey of stroke risk awareness among women. *Circulation.* 2005;111(10):1321–1326.

- Thomas E, Boardman HF, Croft PR. Why do older people report fewer headaches? *Gerontology.* 2005;51(5):322–328.

- Toure JT, Brandt NJ, Limcangco MR, et al. Impact of second-gneration antipsychotics on the use of antiparkinson agents in nursing homes and assisted-living facilities. *Am J Geriatr Pharmacother.* 2006;4(1):25–35.

CHAPTER 58—HEMATOLOGIC DISEASES AND DISORDERS

KEY POINTS

- The reserve capacity of hematopoiesis diminishes with advancing age.

- The possibility of a multifactorial cause should be considered when a patient with anemia of chronic disease has a hemoglobin below 10 g/dL.

- Concentrations of coagulation enzymes increase with age and lead to increased hypercoagulability.

- Polycythemia vera, essential thrombocythemia, and idiopathic myelofibrosis occur primarily in older persons and have a slow rate of spontaneous transformation to leukemia.

Hematopoiesis is regulated by a complex series of interactions between hematopoietic cells, their stromal microenvironment, and diffusible regulatory molecules that affect cellular proliferation. The orderly development of the hematopoietic system in vivo and the maintenance of homeostasis require that a strict balance be maintained between self-renewal, differentiation, maturation, and cell loss. Within the hematopoietic system, populations of terminally differentiated cells are continually entering the peripheral blood, to be replaced by cells from a transit or amplification compartment. Evaluation of the effect of age on hematopoiesis at the organ or cellular level demonstrates evidence of a diminished reserve capacity. Abnormalities in function, not evidenced in the basal state, become apparent in the stimulus-driven state. In addition to being lower, the aged response tends to be more variable. Given a comparable stress, hematologic abnormalities are likely to occur earlier and to be of greater severity in elderly than in younger persons. Thus, the rate of return of the hemoglobin to normal following phlebotomy is blunted, and the ability to mount a granulocyte response to infection is reduced. Numerous animal studies have shown a reduced ability of the aged hematopoietic system to respond to stimulation. Studies in humans have not been as conclusive. (See also "Biology," p 7.)

Although, there is no significant change in basal blood cell counts with aging, there does tend to be a modest increase in the prevalence of anemia. This is particularly noted in men 75 years and older, who in cross-sectional studies have significantly lower values than their younger counterparts (65 or younger). This large effect has not been noted in longitudinal studies. The mechanism for the difference is unclear but is thought to reflect the presence of comorbid illness or reduced erythropoietin (EPO) drive, or both, as a result of declines in androgen concentrations. There does not appear to be an impaired ability of older persons to increase their hematocrit in response to exogenous EPO or increase their granulocyte count following the administration of granulocyte colony-stimulating factor. There is also little evidence to suggest that leukocyte counts are consistently lower in older persons with bacterial infections or in response to a surgical insult. Thus, the severity of neutropenia following chemotherapy in older cancer patients is greater in those who are underweight and malnourished than in those who are not. Age appears to reduce the hematopoietic reserve capacity. This, however, is of clinical relevance only in the presence of other comorbidities (occult or latent) that also adversely effect functioning. In several observational studies, protein energy malnutrition has been reported as being in part responsible for age-related anemia. Thus, the evidence is that aging and illness combined lead to significant abnormalities.

Aging does not appear to affect the circulating concentrations of EPO and colony-stimulating factors; the increase in response to anemia or infection in older people is equal to that noted in their younger counterparts. However, in response to stress, the blunted hematopoietic response seen with age has been attributed to an impaired ability to release growth factors.

This might explain the age-related reduced neutrophil response to infection seen in animal studies and may contribute to increased infection-induced morbidity with aging. The production of certain growth factors, particularly interleukin-6, appears to increase with aging. (See Table 44.1, p 305.) This has led to the notion that aging is accompanied by dysregulation of growth factor production, with overproduction of some and underproduction of other cytokines. An important question is whether aging affects the ability of the hematopoietic system to respond to injected growth factors such as EPO and granulocyte colony-stimulating factor. Current information suggests that in the absence of comorbidity, the response is unaffected by age.

ANEMIA

Clearly, the most common age-related hematologic abnormality, anemia, occurs in both older men and women. Studies have shown a high prevalence of anemia in hospitalized older persons, patients attending geriatric clinics, and institutionalized older persons. However, if stringent criteria are employed for the selection of apparently normal subjects, the prevalence drops. An analysis of the second National Health and Nutrition Education Survey demonstrated a significant reduction in hemoglobin levels with advancing age in apparently healthy men and a minimal although significant decrease in older women. There are few reports on the incidence of new cases of anemia in the elderly population. In the general population, the annual incidence of anemia is estimated to be 1% to 2%. Compared with this, the incidence of anemia in a well-defined population of elderly (>65 years of age) whites attending the Mayo Clinic was reported to be four- to sixfold higher. Anemia was diagnosed in accordance with World Health Organization criteria, if the hemoglobin concentration was <13 g/dL in men and <12 g/dL in women. In this study, in every age group over 65 years, the incidence of anemia in men was higher than that in women. It has been suggested that reduced sensitivity to EPO occurs because of declines in testosterone concentrations. In several studies, the prevalence rate before age 80 is reported as being 8% to 10% in women and 12% to 14% in men. In the over-80-year cohort, the prevalence of anemia is 12% to 16% in women and 18% to 22% in men. At the time of diagnosis, >50% of the patients had mild anemia (hemoglobin >11.0 g/dL for women, and >12.0 g/dL for men), and only 2% had a hemoglobin concentration lower than 10 g/dL. In over 80% of patients, the anemia was normocytic, with the cause either being multifactorial or anemia of chronic disease. Significantly, despite an exhaustive work-up, in 16% of the elderly persons the cause of the anemia remained uncertain. Whether this subset of patients represents the true anemia of aging remains unclear.

Presentation of Anemia

The presence of multiple pathologies in older persons often makes the evaluation of anemia difficult. In hospitalized patients, multiple disorders can contributed to the anemia. A classic example is a patient with active rheumatoid disease who has lost blood from aspirin ingestion. Similarly, protein-energy malnutrition or blood loss will markedly aggravate the anemia associated with neoplasia. Iron deficiency and vitamin-B_{12} deficiency may coexist, presenting confusing red blood cell indices. The possibility of a multifactorial causation—including blood loss, malnutrition, folate deficiency, or hemolysis—should always be considered when the anemia of chronic disease or inflammation is associated with a hemoglobin below 10 g/dL. In this circumstance, laboratory investigations commonly give equivocal results; hence, a bone marrow examination may be required. Clinical judgment is critically important in deciding how aggressive the work-up for anemia ought to be.

Work-up of Anemia

For practical purposes, we recommend 12 g/dL as a lower limit of normal for hemoglobin for both elderly men and elderly women. Attempting to define the cause of anemia when the hemoglobin concentration is between 12 and 14 g/dL rarely yields a cause. Even at a level of 12 g/dL, a decision as to how aggressively evaluate a patient with borderline low hematocrit must rest on clinical judgment. The complex nature of the problems that present in older persons, together with the high risk of simultaneous multiple pathologies, makes this decision much more critical. On the other hand, once a decision has been made to investigate low hemoglobin in an older person, the principles involved in assessment and evaluation are very similar to those that would be used in patients of any age.

The causes of the various anemias seen in elderly persons are summarized in Table 58.1. The initial approach to the patient with anemia must include a complete history and physical examination, as well as a complete blood cell count to allow evaluation of the production rate of red blood cells. Microcytosis (mean corpuscular volume [MCV] <84) indicates an impairment of hemoglobin synthesis, and macrocytosis (MCV >100) may be caused by reticulocytosis or more commonly by an abnormality in nuclear maturation. Red cell production is estimated from the reticulocyte production index. Hemolytic anemia usually has a reticulocyte index greater than 3, whereas a failure of production is indicated by a reticulocyte index of less than 2. Decreased production is caused by the hypoproliferative anemias or by ineffective erythropoiesis. An elevated lactate dehydrogenase (LDH) level and indirect hyperbilirubinemia result from the increased destruction of red cell precursors in the marrow and may be used to distinguish ineffective erythropoiesis from hypoproliferative anemia. A rational approach to the laboratory work-up of anemia is illustrated in Figure 58.1. A significantly elevated reticulocyte count, indirect hyperbilirubinemia, and an elevated LDH level are diagnostic of hemolytic anemia. A low reticulocyte count, elevated indirect bilirubin, and an elevated LDH level suggest ineffective erythropoiesis. In older persons with ineffective erythropoiesis, macrocytosis strongly suggests vitamin-B_{12} or folate deficiency, and microcytosis should suggest sideroblastic anemia.

The Hypoproliferative Anemias

Iron is the only nutrient that limits the rate of erythropoiesis. Thus, inadequate iron supply for erythropoiesis, the commonest cause of anemia in older persons, results in a hypoproliferative anemia. This is diagnosed by the presence of a decreased serum

Table 58.1—Physiologic Classification of Anemia

Hypoproliferative	Ineffective	Hemolytic
■ Iron-deficient erythropoiesis	■ Macrocytic	■ Immunologic
Iron deficiency	Vitamin B_{12}	Idiopathic
Chronic disease	Folate	Secondary
■ Erythropoietin lack	Myelodysplastic syndrome (refractory anemia)	■ Intrinsic
Renal	■ Microcytic	Metabolic
Endocrine	Thalassemia	Abnormal hemoglobin
■ Stem-cell dysfunction	Sideroblastic	■ Extrinsic
■ Aplastic anemia	■ Normocytic	Mechanical
	Myelodysplastic syndrome	

SOURCE: Data from Chatta GS, Lipschitz DA. Aging and hematopoiesis. In: Hazzard WR, Blass JP, Ettinger WH Jr., et al., eds. *Principles of Geriatric Medicine and Gerontology.* 5th ed. New York: McGraw-Hill Health Professions Division; 2003:763–770.

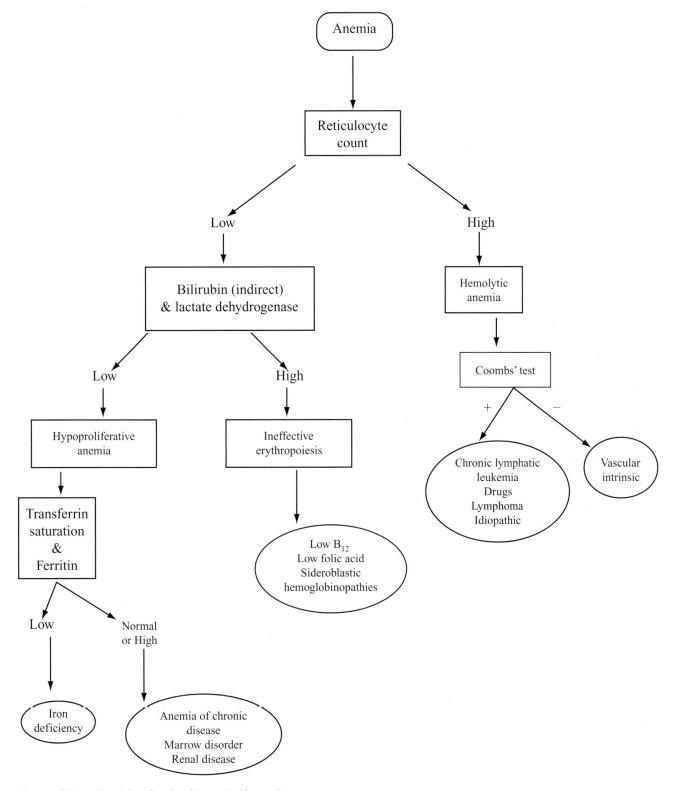

Figure 58.1—Algorithm for the diagnosis of anemia.

iron and a reduced transferrin saturation (serum iron divided by the total iron binding capacity, or TIBC, expressed as a percentage). Absolute iron deficiency (blood loss) is the commonest cause of iron-deficient erythropoiesis in younger persons. In the elderly person, the cause is more likely to be the "anemia of chronic disease" or anemia associated with inflammation. Iron-deficient erythropoiesis in these disorders results from a defective ability of the reticuloendothelial system to reutilize iron derived from senescent red cells. Thus, tissue iron stores are normal or increased, resulting in a serum ferritin concentration above 50 ng/mL and a reduction in the TIBC. This contrasts with a low serum ferritin and high TIBC, which reflect absent iron stores in blood-loss anemia. Blood-loss anemia, the anemia of inflammation and chronic disease, and the anemia associated with protein-energy malnutrition are the most prevalent anemias in elderly populations. Nutritional iron deficiency is very rare in the elderly age group, despite the prominence of other nutritional problems. When unexplained iron deficiency does occur, it is almost exclusively due to blood loss from the gastrointestinal tract. Angiodysplasia of the large bowel and diverticular disease are common causes but should be considered only once a neoplasm has been excluded. Rarely, iron deficiency can result from malabsorption or urinary losses of iron, which occur in the face of intravascular hemolysis.

The pathophysiology of the anemia of chronic disease is complex and is due to an inability of macrophages to release iron from the breakdown of senescent red cells. As a consequence, the serum iron falls and, as with blood-loss anemia, there is inadequate iron supply for erythropoiesis. In contrast to blood-loss anemia, in which iron stores are absent, in the anemia of chronic disease iron stores are normal or increased. Laboratory features include a mild anemia, a low serum iron, low transferrin saturation, and normal to increased iron stores (ferritin >100 ng/mL). The term *anemia of chronic disease* is often used to explain an anemia associated with some other major disease process. Examples include cancer, collagen vascular disorders, rheumatoid arthritis, and inflammatory bowel disease. Occasionally, the anemia may be the initial manifestation of an occult disease. It is critical that this condition be distinguished from iron-deficiency (blood-loss) anemia, to avoid unnecessary gastrointestinal tests to identify a cause for blood loss and to prevent the inappropriate prescription of oral iron therapy.

Decreased EPO production accounts for the anemia of end-stage renal disease. EPO has been in clinical use since 1985 for patients with end-stage renal disease. In some instances, the anemia of cancer and chronic diseases is associated with inappropriately low EPO levels. Many cancer patients have anemia independently of any myelosuppressive therapy. The anemia is characterized by an inability to use iron stores and an inadequate EPO response. In addition, a component of the erythroid suppression is mediated by cytokines like interleukin-1, tumor necrosis factor alpha, and transforming growth factor beta. The precise incidence of cancer-related anemia is not known. However, a number of studies have documented a decrease in transfusion frequency, following treatment with EPO. Depending on symptoms, erythroid support is recommended for hemoglobin levels below 11 g/dL. EPO treatment should be instituted after excluding hemolysis and iron deficiency. Typically, the starting dose of EPO ranges from 20,000 to 40,000 units subcutaneously every week. If required, the dosage can be escalated to 60,000 units per week. Conversely, some patients require treatment only every 2 to 3 weeks. Hemoglobin levels should be monitored weekly, to avoid the vascular sequelae of an iatrogenic polycythemia. A target hemoglobin of 12 to 13 gm/dL is usually safe. Most patients respond within 4 to 6 weeks. Iron should be added to the regimen if ferritin levels fall below 50 ng/mL. If there is no reticulocyte response after 4 to 6 weeks of EPO treatment, therapy should be discontinued. Although it is difficult to prospectively identify responders, it has been reported that patients with endogenous EPO levels of <200 mU/mL are most likely to respond to treatment with EPO.

Marrow failure due to interference with the proliferation of hematopoietic cells occurs in elderly persons. The disorder is generally associated with suppression of all marrow elements and is suggested by the presence of peripheral pancytopenia. Common causes include drugs, immune damage to the stem-cell population, intrinsic marrow lesions, and marrow replacement by malignant cells or fibrous tissue. The latter is usually associated with a myelophthisic blood picture (nucleated red cells, giant platelets, and metamyelocytes on smear) as a reflection of the disruption of marrow stromal architecture. The presence of pancytopenia and the absence of iron-deficient erythropoiesis is an indication for bone marrow aspiration and biopsy. Occasionally isolated suppression of erythropoiesis occurs, which is referred to as *pure red cell aplasia*. This disorder may be drug-related or may be caused by benign or malignant abnormalities of lymphocytes, including thymoma. These patients present with isolated anemia, an elevated serum iron, and absent erythroid precursors on bone marrow examination.

Ineffective Erythropoiesis

Macrocytic anemias in the elderly person result from vitamin-B_{12} and folate deficiency. The prevalence of pernicious anemia increases with advancing age. The disorder results from malabsorption of vitamin B_{12} as a consequence of the action of antibodies against gastric parietal cells and intrinsic factor. Atrophic gastritis and decreased secretion of intrinsic factor occur, resulting in failure of vitamin-B_{12} absorption. Pernicious anemia occurs most commonly in persons over the age of 60 and is more common in women. Although cobalamin deficiency is common with aging, anemia secondary to this is rare (see the section below on vitamin B_{12}, folate and homosysteine). The presence of pancytopenia, macrocytosis, hypersegmented neutrophils in the peripheral smear, a decreased reticulocyte index, an increased LDH level, and indirect hypobilirubinemia suggests a diagnosis of megaloblastic anemia. The bone marrow classically shows giant metamyelocytes, hypersegmented neutrophils, and enlarged erythroid precursors with more hemoglobin than would be expected from the immaturity of their nuclei (nuclear cytoplasmic dissociation). Chronic pancreatitis and diseases of the distal ileum (blind loop syndrome) may also cause vitamin-B_{12} deficiency. The Schilling test is able to distinguish a deficiency of intrinsic factor (malabsorption corrected by ingested vitamin B_{12} and intrinsic factor) from an abnormality in the ability of the ileum to absorb the vitamin B_{12}–intrinsic factor complex (absorption still impaired with intrinsic factor plus vitamin B_{12}). Folate deficiency of sufficient severity to cause anemia in the elderly person is rare. Alcohol and various other drugs are also known to interfere with folate absorption and metabolism. Vulnerability to deficiency is significantly greater when folate requirements are increased as a result of inflammation, neoplastic disease, or hemolytic anemia.

The myelodysplastic syndromes (MDS) are a group of stem-cell disorders characterized by disordered hematopoiesis that occur primarily in the elderly age group. Refractory anemia and refractory anemia with ringed sideroblasts account for 25% to 30% of the MDS syndromes. Refractory anemia commonly presents as a macrocytic anemia with marrow erythroid hyperplasia and relatively normal myeloid and megakaryocytic lineages. Cytogenetic abnormalities are relatively common in MDS, and one of particular interest in elderly patients is deletion of the long arm of chromosome 5 (5q−). The median age at presentation is 66 years, and the 5q− syndrome is characterized by macrocytic anemia, modest leukopenia, normal or increased platelet counts, marrow erythroid hypoplasia or hyperplasia, and female preponderance. Treatment of MDS in the elderly person tends to be supportive. The 5q− syndrome has a relatively good prognosis with a low propensity for transformation to an acute leukemia. Di Guglielmo's syndrome is another stem-cell disorder that is more common in older people; patients present with anemia that is characterized by megaloblastic erythroid precursors, dysplastic myeloid cells, and hyperplasia in the marrow. The disease usually evolves into an erythroleukemia, with an associated pancytopenia and the presence of nucleated red cells, and immature myeloid and megakaryocytic precursors in the circulation. Treatment is usually supportive.

Hemolytic Anemias

The causes of hemolytic anemia in elderly persons are somewhat different than in younger persons. Although most patients with congenital disorders will have been previously identified, an occasional older patient with congenital hemolytic anemia may present for the first time with symptoms related to cholelithiasis. Autoimmune hemolytic anemia is the commonest cause in the elderly age group: the diagnosis is made by the presence of a positive Coombs' test. In younger persons, a cause of the autoimmune hemolysis is only rarely identified. In the elderly person, on the other hand, the anemia is more likely to be associated with a lymphoproliferative disorder (non-Hodgkin's lymphoma or chronic lymphocytic leukemia), collagen vascular disease, or drug ingestion. Corticosteroids and splenectomy are usually effective in patients with red cell antibodies of the immunoglobulin G (IgG) type. Patients with red cell antibodies of the IgM variety are more likely to be refractory to such treatment. A disorder of some importance in older adults is microangiopathic hemolytic anemia, secondary to either disseminated intravascular coagulation (DIC) or occurring as a manifestation of the syndrome of thrombotic thrombocytopenic purpura (TTP). DIC is usually associated with severe infections or disseminated neoplasm and presents not only with hemolysis but also a consumptive coagulopathy. The presence of red cell fragmentation, thrombocytopenia, a prolonged prothrombin time and prolonged partial thromboplastin time, and hemosiderinuria suggests this diagnosis. Treatment of DIC entails treating the underlying disorder, as well as blood product support (including fresh frozen plasma and cryoprecipitate as needed). TTP is characterized by the pentad of fever, intravascular hemolysis, thrombocytopenia, neurologic symptoms, and renal dysfunction. In contrast to DIC, in TTP both the prothrombin time and partial thromboplastin time are normal. Early diagnosis is imperative, as TTP responds very well to treatment with plasmapheresis.

VITAMIN B_{12}, FOLATE, AND HOMOCYSTEINE

Older persons are more likely than younger persons to have lower levels of vitamin B_{12} and folate. In epidemiologic studies, approximately 10% of apparently healthy persons aged 70 and over were found to have vitamin-B_{12} levels that are deficient, and 5% to 10% were found to have low folate values. These low values may be clinically important. Methylmalonic acid levels are increased in the urine and serum, marrow deoxyuridine suppression is abnormal, and excretion of formiminoglutamic acid is increased. These tests tend to indicate functional abnormalities as a direct consequence of low vitamin B_{12} or folate. Pernicious anemia is rarely caused by vitamin-B_{12} deficiency. Atrophic gastritis leading to vitamin-B_{12} malabsorption is the likely cause in the majority of cases. This can also contribute to low folate levels in older persons. However, alcohol abuse, drug interactions with folate absorption, and inadequate dietary intake are the most common causes of low folate levels. Low vitamin-B_{12} and folate levels are not necessarily accompanied by macrocytosis or evidence of megaloblastic anemia. There is some evidence to suggest that low vitamin-B_{12} levels may contribute to cognitive decline in older persons. There is no question that severe vitamin B_{12}-deficiency can result in cognitive loss and significant neurologic deficits. In the older population with low vitamin-B_{12} levels, there is little evidence at the current time to indicate an important relationship between the vitamin and dementia. Nevertheless, aggressive replacement must always be undertaken when a demented patient presents with low levels of vitamin B_{12} or folate.

Low levels of vitamin B_{12} or folate are accompanied by increased levels of homocysteine. In recent years a great deal of attention has focused on the role of raised homocysteine levels in coronary artery disease risk. It is clear that deficiencies of vitamin B_{12} and folate are common in older persons and that the reductions have clinical relevance. Empiric prescription of vitamin B_{12} or folate for older persons with ischemic heart disease may be reasonable. Even in patients with atrophic gastritis, oral vitamin B_{12} is generally adequate; 10% will be absorbed by mass action alone and not require the presence of intrinsic factor. Thus, a daily dose of 1 mg vitamin B_{12} will replete a person with levels in the low-to-normal range. Parenteral replacement should be used in severe deficiencies with vitamin B_{12}, that is, levels below 100 pg/mL. It has been suggested that in elderly patients with low normal (<350 pg/mL) B_{12} level, methylmalonic acid (MMA) levels be checked to exclude metabolically active B_{12} deficiency. Kidney failure can artificially raise the serum MMA level. Those patients with low-normal B_{12} levels and macrocytosis (with or without anemia) or neurologic changes should be considered for vitamin replacement, particularly if the MMA level is elevated.

PLATELETS AND COAGULATION

Platelet counts do not change with aging, but the concentrations of a large number of coagulation enzymes have been shown to increase with age. These include factors VII, VIII, and fibrinogen. In centenarians, highly significant increases in the concentrations of these factors are noted, as are levels of factors IX, X, and thrombin-antithrombin complexes. Fibrin formation is also increased, as evidenced by higher concentrations of fibrinopeptide A. In addition, elevated levels of D-dimers suggest increased hyperfibrinolysis. These facts suggest that aging may be accompanied by increased hypercoagulability. Hyperhomocysteinemia, secondary to low B_{12} levels, is also more common in the elderly age group and may be an additional factor associated with hypercoagulability. However, the very high level of clotting factors and evidence of hypercoagulability in remarkably healthy centenarians have also led to the suggestion that elevated coagulation factors may not be markers of increased risks of thrombosis.

Bleeding diatheses are not uncommon in older persons. Unexplained bruises, repeated nosebleeds, gastrointestinal losses, or excessive blood loss during surgery or following dental extraction are common presentations. In these patients, screening platelet counts and coagulation studies should be obtained. Tests of platelet aggregation are useful in detecting disorders of platelet function. Thrombocytopenia is a common cause of bleeding problems in older persons. A level less than 150,000 mL is considered significant, but bleeding usually occurs at much lower levels. Common causes include decreased production of platelets in the bone marrow, sequestration in enlarged spleens, and increased peripheral destruction. Decreased production of platelets occurs in the leukemias, marrow aplasia, or most commonly in older persons in association with drugs that suppress platelet production. The major cause of increased peripheral destruction is immune thrombocytopenia. A lymphoma, collagen vascular disease, or a drug-induced cause is common in older persons with autoimmune thrombocytopenia. Treatment of thrombocytopenia depends upon the cause. For decreased production, platelet transfusion should be considered if there is significant blood loss, irrespective of the platelet count. Generally, bleeding occurs when the count drops to 20,000 per μL or less. Since the immune thrombocytopenia is usually secondary in older persons, the initial approach is to identify and treat the primary cause. If no cause is found, a trial of corticosteroids is warranted. Isolated thrombocytopenia in the elderly person should prompt a work-up to exclude MDS, particularly when the low platelet count is thought to be secondary to inadequate production.

DIC and TTP are also important causes of thrombocytopenia in the elderly age group, which ought to be recognized and treated appropriately.

Platelet function disorders (thrombopathy), although uncommon, can cause significant bleeding in older persons on aspirin therapy. Aspirin irreversibly acetylates cyclooxygenase, affecting arachidonic acid metabolism. The net effect is significant loss of platelet function. In the rare circumstance, spontaneous bleeding may occur or may be precipitated by injury or surgery. Platelet transfusions may be needed.

Bleeding can also occur because of clotting factor deficiencies, which in the elderly person are usually acquired and caused by the presence of circulating clotting factor inhibitors. The most common is an acquired inhibitor to factor VIII. The onset is often sudden, titers to anti-factor VIII antibodies can be very high, and presentation is with bleeding into joints and muscle, similar to that in hemophilia A. Treatment involves factor replacement; depending on the severity, prednisone or cyclophosphamide may also be needed. Deficiency of the vitamin K–dependent clotting factors tends to occur in older persons with major illnesses. Disorders of the hepatobiliary tree, antibiotics that neutralize bowel bacteria (a major source of the vitamin), malabsorption, and severe malnutrition are the causes. Even if the patient was not prescribed warfarin, inappropriate use must be considered. The deficits are readily treated with vitamin K. (See the anticoagulation information in the Appendix, p 453). Liver disease must always be considered in patients who present with excessive bleeding. The prothrombin time is prolonged even in mild to moderate liver disease. The partial thromboplastin time remains normal until liver disease becomes severe. With the exception of factor VIII (which is produced by endothelial cells), liver disease causes reductions in all clotting factors. Liver disease is also associated with DIC. Fibrin degradation products are not cleared as well, and platelet function may be affected. The treatment of a bleeding diathesis in liver disease is fresh frozen plasma. A bleeding disorder will be thought of only if it is appropriately included in a differential diagnosis. This particularly applies to chronic blood loss from the gastrointestinal system. In those in whom endoscopic evaluation does not identify a cause, careful evaluation of platelets, including platelet functions and coagulation, should always be considered.

CHRONIC MYELOPROLIFERATIVE DISORDERS

The Philadelphia chromosome–negative chronic myeloproliferative disorders—polycythemia vera (PV), essential thrombocythemia (ET), idiopathic myelofibrosis (IMF)—have overlapping clinical features but exhibit different natural histories and different therapeutic requirements. All three disorders occur primarily in the elderly age group and are characterized by the involvement of a multipotent hematopoietic progenitor cell, marrow hypercellularity, overproduction of one or more marrow lineages, thrombotic and hemorrhagic diatheses, exuberant extramedullary hematopoiesis, and a slow rate of spontaneous transformation to acute leukemia. Thus PV, ET, and IMF have a long natural history, distinguishing them from chronic myeloid leukemia, the Philadelphia chromosome–positive myeloproliferative disorder, which progresses and transforms much more rapidly. The main cause of morbidity and mortality in PV and ET is thrombosis, which occurs more commonly in older patients or in those with previous vascular complications. Severe bleeding is rare and limited to patients with a very high platelet count or to those taking antiplatelet drugs. Cytotoxic therapy is effective in preventing thrombosis but increases the risk of leukemic transformation. Since there is no curative therapy for PV and ET, the goals of therapy are to minimize thrombotic risk and prevent progression to marrow fibrosis or acute leukemia, or both.

Several different treatment strategies for PV have been tested in randomized clinical trials. In the PV Study Group (PVSG-01) trial, 431 patients were randomized to one of the following: phlebotomy alone, 32P plus phlebotomy, or chlorambucil plus phlebotomy. The median survival in the three arms was 13.9 years, 11.8 years, and 8.9 years, respectively. In the phlebotomy-only arm, thrombotic deaths were higher, particularly in the first 2 to 3 years. In the other two arms, there was a higher incidence of leukemic transformation. The risk of thrombotic events is highest in patients aged 60 years or older and those with a prior history of thrombosis. The PVSG currently recommends:

- phlebotomy in all patients to keep the hematocrit below 0.45;
- myelosuppressive agents like 32P or busulfan in patients at high risk of thrombosis (>60 years of age) and in those with excessive phlebotomy requirements;
- anagrelide, an antiplatelet agent for symptomatic thrombocytosis.

Finally, given the results of the European Collaboration on Low-dose Aspirin in Polycythemia Vera trial, in all patients with PV an antithrombotic strategy with low-dose aspirin is recommended. In this trial, 531 patients with PV with a hematocrit in the 0.46 range were randomized to no aspirin or low-dose aspirin. In the aspirin arm there was a 59% reduction in cardiovascular mortality, with a nonsignificant risk of increased bleeding.

The incidence of thrombotic and hemorrhagic complications in ET was recently analyzed in 1850 patients from 21 retrospective cohort studies. Rates of thrombosis and hemorrhage ranged from 7% to 17% and 8% to 14%. Age over 60 years, a prior thrombotic event, and a long duration of thrombocytosis are the major risk factors for thrombotic events. A very high platelet count (1500 × 109/L) is a risk factor for bleeding. Consensus-based practice guidelines for ET include, first, observation in asymptomatic low-risk patients with platelet counts below 1500 × 109/L, and second, hydroxyurea plus aspirin in high-risk patients, which has been shown to be superior in a recent randomized clinical trial. Anagrelide, a new antiplatelet agent, is very effective at reducing high platelet counts. However, its efficacy as compared with hydroxyurea in reducing thrombotic events remains to be proven in a randomized controlled trial.

ET, like PV, has a long natural history with a low incidence of leukemic transformation. On the other hand, IMF progresses much more rapidly, with median survival in the 3.5- to 5.5-year range. Neoangiogenesis is a hallmark of IMF and is characterized by increased microvessel density in the marrow. It is also the basis of thalidomide-based trials in IMF, preliminary results from which look promising.

REFERENCES

- Balducci L. Epidemiology of anemia in the elderly: information on diagnostic evaluation. *J Am Geriatr Soc.* 2003;51(3 Suppl):S2–S9.

- Chatta GS, Lipschitz DA. Aging and hematopoiesis. In: Hazzard WR, Blass JP, Ettinger WH Jr., et al., eds. *Principles of Geriatric Medicine and Gerontology.* 5th ed. New York: McGraw-Hill Health Professions Division; 2003:763–770.

- Clark R, Grimley Evans J, Schneede J, et al. Vitamin B_{12} and folate deficiency in later life. *Age Ageing.* 2004;33(1):34–41.

- Penninx BW, Pahor M, Woodman RC, et al. Anemia in old age is associated with increased mortality and hospitalization. *J Gerontol A Biol Sci Med Sci.* 2006;61(5):474–479.

CHAPTER 59—ONCOLOGY

KEY POINTS

- Older patients and black Americans of all ages are more likely to develop cancer and present with more advanced disease.

- Epidemiologic data have not supported the long-held clinical dogma that cancers in older people are less aggressive or slower growing.

- Age-associated resistance to chemotherapy has not been demonstrated; further, acute toxicities (nausea, vomiting, and hair loss) are less prominent in older patients.

- Surgery, radiation, chemotherapy, and biologic therapy are safe and effective treatment modalities for older cancer patients when appropriate precautions are taken on the basis of the patient's comorbidities, vital organ functions, and medications.

Prevalence studies indicate that cancer is primarily a burden for geriatric populations. In fact, the median age for cancer in the United States is 70 years. Though cancer has long been recognized as a disease of older people, emphasis on geriatric issues and cancer is a recent development.

Three questions have arisen that form the underpinnings of this new emphasis:

- Why are tumors more common in elderly people?

- Is there a difference in tumor aggressiveness with advancing age?

- Should treatment be different for the older patient?

Experimental data and clinical experience have indicated that tumors are not resistant to treatment by virtue of age alone. However, age is associated with slight reductions in certain organ functions, and these deficiencies in physiologic reserve might be magnified by comorbid conditions. Cancer treatments, especially chemotherapy, may therefore be associated with an increase in adverse events, and treatment should be tailored to the individual, taking into consideration potential increased toxicities and balancing this with expectations of survival in the context of comorbidities.

A review of the National Cancer Institute's Surveillance, Epidemiology and End Results (SEER) data revealed that more than 50% of all cancers are diagnosed in patients aged 65 years and older, and this older patient population incurs more than 60% of all cancer deaths. The data also reveal important trends. Whereas between 1968 and 1985, cancer mortality decreased 23% in patients younger than 55 years (primarily reflecting advances in the therapy of acute leukemias, Hodgkin's disease, non-Hodgkin's lymphomas, and testicular cancers), cancer mortality for those aged 55 years and older increased by 17%. Thus, in the older age groups, we are faced with an increasingly prevalent disease for which modern therapies have not improved overall survival. We have much to learn about providing optimal management of cancer in elderly adults, but an emphasis on disease prevention and screening remains a logical priority.

CANCER BIOLOGY AND AGING

Explaining the Increased Prevalence of Cancer With Age

There are at least three reasons for the increased prevalence of cancer with age. First, cancers, particularly those that occur after menopause, are thought to develop over a long period, perhaps decades. This is best exemplified by the current understanding of colon cancer, which has been shown to develop because of an accumulation of several damaging genetic events occurring in a stochastic manner over time. Thus, if mutations are acquired at a constant rate, older people are more likely to have lived long enough to develop the 8 to 10 genetic lesions it takes to develop a malignancy. In contrast, lymphomas are just as likely to occur in young as in old people. Lymphocytes normally undergo gene rearrangements and mutations to generate antigen receptors, and these processes appear to be particularly vulnerable to errors that may lead to lymphoma at any age.

A second reason for the greater prevalence of cancer with advancing age is that DNA repair mechanisms are thought to decline with age. As a consequence, cells may accumulate damage. Normally, a dividing cell pauses in G1 (the gap after mitosis [M] and before DNA replication [S]) and in G2 (the gap after S and before M) to take inventory and repair any damage before proceeding to the next phase. These are the G1 and G2 checkpoints. Older cells may fail to detect or repair damage and fail to control DNA replication accurately. This leads to aneuploidy and to uncontrolled proliferation. In younger people, these aberrations may trigger the death of the cell; in older people, the errors may be tolerated and fail to signal cell death. Cells without functioning checkpoints are vulnerable to loss of growth control.

A third contribution to increased cancer incidence in older people may be a decline in the function of the immune system, particularly in cellular immunity. A number of findings suggest that the immune system can recognize and control certain cancers. A decline in immune function may lead to the emergence of a cancer in an older person that was controlled when that person was younger.

The Different Characteristics of Cancer With Age

There has been a long-held but incompletely documented clinical dogma that cancers in older people are less aggressive or slower growing. However, epidemiologic data from tumor registries or large clinical trials have not supported this notion. Such data may be confounded by geriatric problems that shorten survival independently of the cancer (eg, comorbidity, multiple medications, physician or family bias regarding diagnosis and treatment in elderly adults, and age-associated life stresses). These factors may counter any primary influence that aging might have on tumor aggressiveness. However, there is experimental support for the contention that there is reduced tumor aggressiveness with age. Data obtained from laboratory animals with a wide range of tumors under highly controlled circumstances demonstrate slower tumor growth, fewer experimental metastases, and longer survival in old mice. Tumor growth involves several levels of interaction between the tumor and the host. It may be that tumor angiogenesis is impaired in older people, thereby controlling the rate of tumor growth. The clinical importance of this is limited, inasmuch as it is difficult to know in any given patient whether the course of the disease will be characterized by an indolent or aggressive pattern of growth.

Breast cancer is the most notable clinical example of age-associated decline in tumor aggressiveness. Older patients are more likely to have more favorable histologic types, higher levels of estrogen and progesterone receptor expression, lower growth fraction, and less frequent metastases. In a published series on breast cancer patients with primary tumors of 1 cm (diameter) or less, the single most important predictor of metastasis to axillary nodes has consistently been found to be patient age: patients under the age of 50 years have the highest likelihood of spread, whereas those over the age of 70 years have the lowest likelihood of spread. Stage for stage, older patients seem to have longer survival than younger patients.

By contrast, Hodgkin's disease seems to be a more aggressive disease in older patients. The most likely reason for the age-associated differences in prognosis is that Hodgkin's disease is a different disease in patients aged 45 years and older than in younger patients. Incidence data demonstrate two distinct peak incidence rates, one at age 32 years and one at age 84 years. The frequency of particular histologic subtypes of Hodgkin's disease is different in younger and older patients; nodular sclerosis is the most common subtype in younger patients, mixed cellularity is the most common in older patients. In all reported treatment series, older age is an independent prognostic factor. Additional study is necessary to document age-associated differences in tumor cell biology.

Acute leukemia, like Hodgkin's disease, appears to be a different disease in older people; the MDR1 drug resistance pump is more commonly expressed, patients respond less well to treatment, and survival is shorter than in younger patients. However, for most cancer types, the molecular biology and clinical behavior of the tumor is similar across the age span.

Ethnic Differences in Cancer Incidence and Mortality

As the demographics of the U.S. population changes, additional information is needed on incidence and natural history differences in cancers occurring in different ethnic and racial groups. The U.S. Census Bureau estimates that by 2050, Hispanic Americans will account for nearly 25% of the population and black Americans, Asian Americans, and Native Americans combined will total another 25%. Overall, black Americans have the highest cancer incidence and mortality rates. Cancer incidence among black Americans is 10% higher than among white Americans, 50% to 60% higher than among Hispanic Americans and Asian

Americans, and more than twice as high as among Native Americans. The cancer death rate for black Americans is about 30% higher than for white Americans and more than twice as high as for Hispanic Americans, Asian Americans, and Native Americans. For the period from 1992 to 1998, 5-year survival for all cancers was 64% for white Americans and 53% for black Americans.

The factors contributing to the ethnic differences are not defined. However, certain data suggest that when the quality of the health care delivered to white and black Americans is similar, disease outcomes in the two groups are comparable. Specific incidence, diagnosis, and survival data for common cancers in different ethnic groups are provided in Table 59.1 and Table 59.2.

PRINCIPLES OF CANCER MANAGEMENT

Current forms of cancer treatment include surgery, radiation, cytotoxic chemotherapy, hormone manipulation, and biologic therapy. Age alone does not preclude any of these approaches, but because of normal changes with age in certain organs and also age-associated conditions (comorbidities), special considerations are warranted.

Randomized clinical trials are the most reliable instrument to study medical intervention, and treatment decisions are best founded on the results of such work. However, despite efforts from the cooperative

Table 59.1—Ethnic and Racial Differences in Cancer Incidence, United States, 1996–2000 *(per 100,000 population)*

Site	White Americans		Black Americans		Hispanic Americans		Asian Americans	
	Male	Female	Male	Female	Male	Female	Male	Female
All	555.9	431.8	696.8	406.3	419.3	312.2	392.0	306.9
Breast	—	140.8	—	121.7	—	89.8	—	97.2
Colon	64.1	46.2	72.4	56.2	49.8	32.9	57.2	38.8
Lung	79.4	51.9	120.4	54.8	46.1	24.4	62.1	28.4
Prostate	164.3	—	272.1	—	137.2	—	100.0	—

SOURCE: Data from: Ward E, Jemal A, Cokkinides V, et al. Cancer disparities by race/ethnicity and socioeconomic status. *CA Cancer J Clin.* 2004;54(2):78–93.

Table 59.2—Racial Differences in Cancer Diagnosis and Survival

Site	Advanced Disease at Diagnosis (%)		5-Year Survival (%)	
	White Americans	Black Americans	White Americans	Black Americans
Breast	33	43	88	74
Colon	19	24	63	53
Lung	38	40	15	12
Head and neck	55	73	60	36
Bladder	21	35	83	64
Endometrial	22	39	86	60

SOURCE: Data from: Jemal A, Tiwari RC, Murray T, et al. Cancer statistics, 2004. *CA Cancer J Clin.* 2004;54(1):8–29.

oncology groups, patients entered onto trials are by and large younger and presumably healthier than the typical geriatric patient with the same disorder. Furthermore, common end points of these trials are length of survival (for therapeutic interventions) or disease-specific deaths (for prevention studies), and these end points are not always the most appropriate outcomes for older patients (because of their inherently limited life expectancies on the basis of age alone).

Clinical researchers are starting to address issues of geriatric oncology. New, more geriatrics-oriented trials focus more on reducing symptoms and improving quality-of-life than on life expectancy. Surveys have indicated that older patients, when fully informed, most often choose life-extending treatments, even at the risk of toxicity. It is the physician and the patient's family that are most focused on quality-of-life issues. Furthermore, for the most part, tumors are not more resistant to treatment in older patients. In addition, acute toxicities (nausea, vomiting, hair loss) are less prominent in older patients than in younger ones. Thus, although quality of life remains a primary treatment consideration, efforts at extending life should not be denied older patients on the basis of their age alone.

Cancer Screening

Screening is designed to detect disease in asymptomatic individuals with the hope that early-stage disease is more readily curable. Thus, to be useful, screening needs to identify mainly people who actually have disease, and the disease needs to have been shown to be more readily cured when found in asymptomatic people than in symptomatic people. Screening for colon cancer, cervical cancer, and probably breast cancer has been shown to save lives. Controlled prospective randomized trials are the only method of documenting the value of screening, and the study populations must be followed for many years to document the survival advantage of to the screened group.

A screening test is evaluated on the basis of its ability to distinguish people with authentic disease from those without disease. (For the terms used to assess screening tests, see the Appendix, p 464.) Screening is of greatest value when the disease being sought is common in the population being screened and the test being used is highly specific. The use of weakly specific tests in populations with low disease prevalence does not save lives. In some instances, more harm is done through morbidities and mortality associated with the diagnostic evaluation of positive screening tests than the good associated with early detection of cancer.

Screening is subject to three main types of bias: lead time, length, and selection biases. These biases can make a test appear to be effective when it actually is not. Lead time bias occurs when the underlying disease is not able to be affected by treatment. It results in earlier diagnosis but does not alter the time of death. Thus, the person spends more time as a patient, but the course of the disease is basically unaltered.

Length bias occurs when a test identifies clinically slowly progressive or nonprogressive disease that would never have become a symptomatic problem for the patient. Screening for prostate cancer is affected by length bias. Elevated prostate-specific antigen levels can detect cancers that will never cause the patient's death. This leads to overdiagnosis, the detection of "disease" that is of no consequence, also called *pseudodisease*.

Selection bias is based on the observation that people willing to be screened for cancer may not reflect the population as a whole. Volunteers may be more health conscious or have other personal habits that favorably influence prognosis. Thus, their outcome from screening may be better than what would be seen in a random population.

In addition to these biases, two additional issues are barriers to screening older people for cancers. First, most of the large cancer clinical studies that have documented the efficacy of screening have systematically omitted the study of older people. Thus, it is not clear whether the benefits of a particular screening test initiated at age 50 extends to people at age 70 or 75. For prostate cancer, it is believed that screening is not indicated for someone with less than 10 years' life expectancy. For men without other comorbidities, this rule would suggest that men older than age 80 should not be screened. Data are not available in other cancers.

Multiple guidelines for screening are available for health care providers, as well as patient-specific information to help individuals decide what type of health promotion activities they want to engage in. The decisions about whether to adhere to these guidelines are often difficult for the older individual or the power of attorney (POA) to make. Guidelines for overall health screening decisions can help direct health care providers and the patient or POA in this decision process. An individualized approach is critical when working with older individuals in the area of health promotion and should drive the decision process.

Chemotherapy

Aging may be associated with changes in key pharmacologic parameters of antineoplastic agents and in the susceptibility to end-organ toxicity (see Table 59.3).

The most consistent pharmacokinetic change of aging is a progressive delay in renal excretion because of a reduction in glomerular filtration rate. The more prolonged half-life of renally excretable agents may account in part for more severe toxicity. In a study of women aged 65 and older with metastatic breast cancer, doses of methotrexate and cyclophosphamide were modified according to the creatinine clearance. As a consequence, the myelotoxicity was markedly reduced without compromise of the therapeutic effect.

Owing to differences in their pharmacokinetics and pharmacodynamics, certain drugs may be particularly suitable for treating older patients. Oral etoposide provides valuable palliation for small cell cancer of the lung and large cell lymphoma, with minimal risk of complications. Fludarabine, which is very active in lymphoproliferative neoplasms, induces apoptosis of cancer cells, a process that may be altered in malignancies developing in older people. Vinorelbine and gemcitabine are two newer agents that are active against lung and breast cancer and are well tolerated and effective in older patients.

Hormonal Therapy

Hormonal treatment is effective in cancers of the breast, the prostate, and the endometrium. Tamoxifen, a selective estrogen receptor modulator, has antagonistic and partial agonistic effects. It is a useful therapy in adjuvant treatment of breast cancer and also has estrogen-like positive effects on cardiovascular risk factors and bone disease. Other more selective drugs in this category, such as raloxifene, are in clinical testing. Although inactive as a single agent, tamoxifen is synergistic with chemotherapy in the management of malignant melanoma. Currently used hormonal agents are listed in Table 59.4. Most of these are well tolerated by older adults and commonly are the treatment of choice in this age group. Diethylstilbestrol is an estrogenic compound with serious cardiovascular risks (stroke, heart attack, thromboembolism) when used to treat prostate cancer in older men.

Biologic Therapy

Modulation of immune response is a particularly attractive option in treating the older adult, whose natural defenses against cancer may be impaired by immune senescence. Only a limited number of options are clinically available, and these are clearly inadequate to restore a normal immune response in the older adult.

Recombinant α-interferon at moderate dosages (eg, 3 million units, three times weekly) is reasonably well tolerated by patients of all ages. At higher doses α-interferon causes myelodepression, severe fatigue,

Table 59.3—Chemotherapy Issues in Geriatric Oncology

Issue	Comments
General	Comorbidities and multiple medications add complexity
Pharmacokinetic changes	A progressive delay with age in the elimination of renally excreted drugs, due to a reduction in glomerular filtration rate, may account in part for more severe toxicity
Pharmacodynamic changes	Possible enhanced resistance with age to antitumor agents Increased expression of the multidrug resistance gene has been reported in some older patients Other proteins that result in drug efflux have been shown to have prognostic importance, but age-associated changes have not been described Increased tumor hypoxia with age has been observed in a murine model
Toxicity	Mucositis, cardiotoxicity, and peripheral and central neurotoxicity become more common and more severe with aging Cardiotoxicity is a complication of anthracyclines and anthraquinone, mitomycin C, and high-dose cyclophosphamide; the incidence of cardiotoxicity also increases with age Peripheral neurotoxicity with vincristine is more common and more severe in older patients The incidence of cerebellar toxicity from high-dose cytosine arabinoside increases with age
Myelotoxicity	Chemotherapy-related myelotoxicity may become more severe and more prolonged with aging, but moderately toxic treatment regimens, such as CMF (cyclophosphamide, methotrexate, fluorouracil), cisplatin and fluorouracil, and cisplatin and etoposide are tolerated by many patients aged 70 and older without life-threatening neutropenia or thrombocytopenia However, infections are markedly increased among older acute leukemia patients undergoing intensive induction treatment; in these cases it is possible that the disease itself, rather than an age-associated change in "marrow reserve," is responsible for the depletion of hemopoietic stem cells
Recent advances	Granulocyte colony-stimulating factor and granulocyte-macrophage colony-stimulating factor have reduced the incidence of neutropenic infections in patients receiving intensive treatment, and their effectiveness does not appear to be diminished with advancing patient age Certain new drugs or new formulations may be particularly suitable to the aged patient, eg, oral etoposide and fludarabine, gemcitabine, vinorelbine, capecitabine, paclitaxel protein-bound particles, and liposomal doxorubicin

Table 59.4—Hormonal Agents Commonly Used in Treating Cancer

Site	Hormonal Agents
Breast	Antiestrogens: tamoxifen, toremifene
	Progestational agents: medroxyprogesterone acetate
	Aromatase inhibitors: aminoglutethimide, letrozole, anastrozole, exemestane
Prostate	LH-RH analogs: goserelin, leuprolide
	Estrogens: diethylstilbestrol
	Antiandrogens: flutamide, bicalutamide
Endometrium	Progestational agents
	Antiestrogens

flu-like illness, malaise, fever, neuropathy, and abnormalities of liver enzymes. Delirium, depression, and dementia after α-interferon use have been reported in people aged 65 and older. More information on the safety of this compound in the elderly patient would be desirable. This is particularly important because interferon has been shown to be effective therapy for chronic myeloid leukemia, hairy cell leukemia, and multiple myeloma, hematologic malignancies that occur more commonly among elderly people. Interferon may also prolong survival after chemotherapy for follicular lymphoma. It is being tested at higher, more toxic doses in patients with stage II melanoma after surgical resection of the primary lesion. About 15% of patients with metastatic melanoma may experience a partial response from α-interferon.

Interleukin-2 is used to treat metastatic melanoma and renal cancer. When administered daily at 3 million units per square meter, it may produce partial responses in about 15% of patients and complete remissions in about 5% of patients, many of these responses are long lasting. Interleukin-2 can produce severe dose-related toxicity, including capillary leak syndrome, hypotension, acute respiratory distress syndrome, cardiac arrhythmias, peripheral edema, renal failure (prerenal), cholestatic liver dysfunction, skin rashes, and thrombocytopenia. These complications tend to appear gradually in less severe form; generally, patients do not suddenly deteriorate. The toxicities reverse completely within a few days of stopping the drug. It is a strong clinical impression that interleukin-2 toxicities are less severe and develop later in older patients.

Monoclonal antibodies directed against CD20 (rituximab) expressed on B-cell lymphomas and against HER-2/*neu* (trastuzumab) expressed on breast cancer and other epithelial malignancies are effective treatments. In most patients, the antibodies are given just before combination chemotherapy; the antibodies appear to augment the response to the drugs. These humanized antibodies generally have mild toxicities. Patients may develop hypotension or shortness of breath with the first infusion because of complement fixation. Symptoms clear when the infusion rate is slowed, and such symptoms rarely recur. Other antibodies against cancers are in development.

Radiation Therapy

Radiation therapy provides palliation for virtually all cancers, and it may be part of a treatment plan for lymphomas and cancers of the prostate, bladder, cervix, esophagus, breast, and head and neck area. In combination with cytotoxic chemotherapy, radiation therapy has allowed organ preservation in cancers of the anus, bladder, and larynx, and in extremity sarcomas. A central issue for radiation therapy in the older patient is safety. There has been a trend for almost five decades to use radiation therapy as an alternative to surgery in poor surgical candidates, mainly patients aged 65 and older, with the implied expectation that such an approach is less toxic. In fact, published reports have indicated that radiation therapy is both safe and effective in older patients. However, concern remains when treatment involves irradiation of the whole brain (fear of neurologic sequelae, including dementia) or pelvis (fear of marrow aplasia or myelodysplasia or radiation enteritis), but no systematic investigation has categorically substantiated these concerns.

Advances in radiation therapy include techniques that allow a more restricted radiation field, especially partial brain irradiation, new applications of brachytherapy (insertion of radiation sources into the tumor bed), the development of radiosurgery (gamma ray knife, a precisely focused external beam of radiation) that allows destruction of small lesions (diameter ≤4 cm) of the central nervous system without craniotomy, and the development of new radiosensitizers.

Surgery

Concerns related to cancer surgery in the older adult are safety and rehabilitative potential. Several reports indicate that age itself is not a risk factor for elective cancer surgery, but the length of hospital stay and the time to full recovery become more prolonged with advancing age of the patient. Similar results have been reported both from referral centers and community hospitals.

Advances in anesthesia and surgery have benefited the older patient. Included among these are new endoscopic procedures that provide valuable palliation for the many tumors of the gastrointestinal tract, and the more widespread use of spinal anesthesia for major abdominal interventions, with a substantial decline in perioperative complications and mortality. More widespread use of laparoscopic surgical techniques and application of laser and photodynamic therapy is also broadening the surgical armamentarium and providing more older patients with potential palliation and cure.

The trend to manage cancer without deforming surgery may preclude the need for complex rehabilitation and may be of special value for older people. Organ preservation without compromise of treatment outcome is obtainable for cancer of the anus and of the larynx, and is being studied for cancers of the oropharynx, the esophagus, the bladder, and the vulva. Also, the use of initial (neoadjuvant) chemotherapy before primary surgery has been shown to be effective in patients with large primary breast and lung cancers. Such an approach results in less extensive and potentially more curative surgical procedures.

See also "Perioperative Care" (p 92).

Quality-of-Life Issues

Several studies have determined that the perception of quality of life is highly subjective and is poorly reproduced by external observers, even if there is a close relationship to the patient. Furthermore, there is considerable discrepancy between the clinician's determination of the patient's quality of life and the patient's own assessment, even when the clinician is very familiar with the patient's physical condition; clinicians tend to underestimate the patient's quality of life.

Early assessments of quality of life focused on functional status and freedom from pain, but these factors, although important, are inadequate to evaluate far-reaching consequences of serious diseases on all domains of life. In the past decade several instruments for the measurement of quality of life have been validated and successfully used to study specific problems, such as the effects on quality of life of intensive care, the consequences of limb amputation, of partial and total mastectomy, and of iatrogenic impotence. These instruments are questionnaires requesting a person to rate his or her own well-being in several dimensions with a categorical or a visual analogue scale. Unfortunately, these instruments have not been adjusted for the special needs of the older adult. It is reasonable to assume that the importance of some factors, such as professional or job satisfaction, may decline with age, while the importance of others, including social support and the perception of family burden, may become more prominent.

Other problems related to assessing quality of life include the complexity of some questionnaires, which may overburden some older people. In addition, little progress has been made in the assessment of quality of life in cognitively impaired people. Studies of pain in demented people have demonstrated the reliability of repetitive behavioral testing in the assessment of dis-

comfort, even in patients with cognitive impairment. Perhaps the same principles may be applied to the assessment of quality of life in demented patients.

At present, the main application of quality-of-life assessment in clinical decision making concerns the choice between interventions yielding comparable survival. An area of potential use is in medical decisions involving limited survival benefits at the price of a decline in quality of life. At present, the value of this trade-off is evaluated with measures known as "quality of life adjusted survival" or "quality-adjusted time without symptoms or toxicity," both of which include complex interviews of limited application to people aged 70 and older.

SPECIFIC CANCERS

Breast Cancer

Controversy surrounds several critical issues in the management of this most common malignancy in older women. These issues include the following.

Postoperative Irradiation After Lumpectomy

Although irradiation after lumpectomy is safe in women aged 65 and older, it may be a source of significant inconvenience and cost to the patient. The value of postoperative irradiation has been questioned because the local recurrence rate of breast cancer may decrease with age, and the inconvenience of daily radiation treatment protocols may outweigh the limited benefits for some.

Need for Axillary Lymphadenectomy

Given the benefits regardless of nodal status of adjuvant tamoxifen in all postmenopausal women with estrogen-receptor positive breast cancer, axillary dissection when the axilla is clinically negative may add unnecessary morbidity. This is particularly true if the procedure requires general anesthesia. However, proponents of lymphadenectomy claim that the procedure not only has a staging function but also may improve the curability of breast cancer or reduce the duration of adjuvant tamoxifen treatment. In some centers, axillary dissection is being replaced by biopsy of the *sentinel node*, the first lymph node draining the area of the breast that harbors the cancer. This is determined at surgery by injecting a dye into the site of the resected lump and removing the first node that turns blue. Early data suggest that sentinel node sampling is just as accurate as axillary dissection but considerably less toxic.

Adjuvant Hormonal Treatment

A meta-analysis of randomized trials established that adjuvant treatment with tamoxifen for at least 2 years prolongs both the disease-free survival and the overall survival of postmenopausal women. The benefits and risks of more prolonged treatment, especially for women over 70, are still controversial. Letrozole and anastrozole, aromatase inhibitors, are believed to be more effective than tamoxifen in the treatment of early state breast cancer for women with estrogen-receptor positive tumors. In addition, these drugs provide a definite, if small, overall survival advantage compared with tamoxifen for women with advanced breast cancer.

Initial Management of Metastatic Breast Cancer

Women aged 65 and older with metastatic, hormone receptor-positive breast cancer are likely to have effective palliation with hormonal therapy, such as tamoxifen. Hormonal treatment has also been shown to benefit older patients with hormone receptor–poor tumors, but chemotherapy has been shown to be safe and effective in this group of patients, as well.

Lung Cancer

Lung cancer is becoming increasingly common in older women for reasons that are not completely understood. The increase may be due to the more widespread smoking among women. In addition, some data suggest that women are at greater risk of developing lung cancer per unit of tobacco exposure. Lung cancer currently is the leading cause of cancer death in men and women. Early recognition and surgical resection remain the best chance for cure. For patients with lesions in a location that precludes surgery, occasionally localized radiation results in long-term survival. Over the past decade chemotherapy has been shown to produce clinical responses and provide effective palliation for a portion of the patients with metastatic disease. Patients live longer but the added increment is measured in weeks to months. New chemotherapeutic agents, such as vinorelbine and gemcitabine, and more established agents such as paclitaxel or docetaxel used in lower-dose weekly schedules, have proved to be effective treatments for older patients with lung cancer.

Colon Cancer

Two thirds of colon cancer cases are in persons aged 65 years and over. With advancing age, right-sided lesions and presentations with anemia rather than pain are more likely. Colonoscopy has become the mainstay of diagnosis, primarily because it enables the gastroenterologist to directly visualize and biopsy the entire colon. Surgical excision may be adequate for lesions confined to the colon, but if extension to regional nodes is observed, postoperative adjuvant chemotherapy (usually 5-fluorouracil plus leucovorin) has been found to reduce recurrence by 40% to 50%. Survival of patients with metastases to the liver or other organs remains disappointing, despite the appearance of new drugs, such as irinotecan, capable of inducing partial remissions in a subset of patients. New drugs that target a tyrosine kinase (an integral enzyme for cellular proliferation) within tumor cells and neutralize vascular endothelial growth factor (thought to promote angiogenesis) are currently in development, and these offer great promise. Surgical excision of solitary hepatic lesions has been shown to offer survival advantage for selected patients, primarily those with smaller lesions, five or fewer lesions confined to a single hepatic lobe, and a longer interval from original tumor resection until the diagnosis of hepatic metastasis.

Prostate Cancer

See "Prostate Disease" (p 423).

Hematologic Malignancies

Leukemias

Acute myeloid leukemia (AML) after myelodysplastic syndromes, as occurs more commonly among elderly patients, is more likely to be refractory to treatment and to have a smoldering course, requiring only supportive care. What is not clear is whether the prevalence of unfavorable cytogenetic abnormalities and of multilineage neoplastic involvement increases with age in de novo AML. The subset of myelodysplasia patients who do not have excess blasts or overt leukemia but are neutropenic and have recurrent infections may benefit from intermittent granulocyte colony-stimulating factor.

In a trial with older patients with AML, the effectiveness of delayed treatment was found to be much inferior to that of immediate treatment. Although this study established the value of timely chemotherapy, the choice of treatment (whether full-dose induction or low-dose cytarabine) remains controversial. In one study, the survival of older patients with leukemia treated with low-dose cytarabine was found to be superior to the survival of those receiving standard induction, because of lower treatment-related mortality. Others have obtained different results and claimed the superiority of standard treatment.

Chronic Lymphocytic Leukemia

Chronic lymphocytic leukemia (CLL) is the most common form of leukemia in the Western world; about 12,500 cases are diagnosed each year in the United States. The incidence is declining for unknown reasons. The median age at diagnosis is 61 years. The diagnosis is most often made incidentally when a peripheral white blood cell count reveals leukocytosis with a small lymphocyte count above 4,000/μL. Treatment is generally withheld until it is required to control a life-threatening or symptomatic complication. The major complications of CLL are infection and marrow failure. Because about 25% of patients develop autoimmune anemia or thrombocytopenia some time in the course of CLL, the mechanism of any decline in peripheral blood cell counts must be investigated. Autoimmune mechanisms can be treated with glucocorticoids or splenectomy, whereas marrow infiltration by tumor cells requires antitumor therapy. Chlorambucil and fludarabine are the two most active agents. Median survival varies with the stage of disease. Once anemia or thrombocytopenia develops as a consequence of marrow failure, median survival is about 18 months.

Non-Hodgkin's Lymphoma

The prognosis of low- and intermediate-grade non-Hodgkin's lymphoma worsens with age, but the explanation remains unclear. It is possible that older patients have more aggressive variants or, equally likely, that older patients are increasingly susceptible to the complications of intensive treatment.

The treatment of older patients with intermediate-grade large-cell lymphoma is controversial. As many as 30% of such patients obtain a durable complete remission with standard treatment (CHOP, ie, cyclophosphamide, doxorubicin, vincristine, prednisone). Administration of lower-than-normal dosages results in a poorer outcome. Whether hematopoietic growth factors can lessen the hematopoietic toxicity of treatment has not been specifically addressed in the aged population. The outcome of CHOP treatment in the most common form of lymphoma (diffuse large B-cell lymphoma) appears to be significantly improved by the addition of rituximab, a monoclonal antibody directed at CD20 expressed on B cells.

Hodgkin's Disease

Hodgkin's disease exhibits a curious bimodal age-incidence curve, with a second peak late in life. There have been earlier reports that older patients with advanced disease respond less well to therapy and that their survival is shorter. Several factors may contribute: more extensive disease at presentation, biologic differences from authentic Hodgkin's disease, greater toxicity with standard treatment regimens, or the provision of less aggressive treatment. Each of these factors may be involved. Most older patients tolerate full doses of ABVD (ie, doxorubicin, bleomycin, vinblastine, dacarbazine) without life-threatening bone-marrow toxicity.

Multiple Myeloma

Multiple myeloma is diagnosed in about 14,400 people each year in the United States. The median age at diagnosis is 68 years; it is rare in people younger than 40 years. Black Americans have twice the incidence of white Americans. The classic triad of myeloma is marrow plasmacytosis (>10%), lytic bone lesions, and a serum or urine, or both, monoclonal gammopathy. Monoclonal gammopathy is common in older people, estimated at 6% of those aged 70 or older. Distinguishing myeloma from monoclonal gammopathy of uncertain significance is important. When an abnormal paraprotein is discovered on serum immunoelectrophoresis, the best diagnostic test to identify myeloma is a skeletal survey. However, if the skeletal survey is normal, a bone marrow biopsy is still indicated to determine the presence of marrow plasmacytosis. Patients with monoclonal gammopathy of uncertain significance do not have lytic bone lesions and usually do not have the other features of myeloma, including hypercalcemia, renal failure, anemia, or susceptibility to infection, and marrow plasma cells are less than 10% of the total cell number. Patients with myeloma require treatment when the lytic bone lesions become symptomatic or progressive, recurrent infections occur, or the serum paraprotein increases. Standard treatment consists of intermittent pulses of an oral alkylating agent and prednisone given for 4 to 7 days every 4 to 6 weeks. Supportive care includes bisphosphonates to decrease bone turnover, erythropoietin and other hematinics for the anemia, intravenous immunoglobulin for recurrent infections, radiation to specific symptomatic bone lesions, maintenance of hydration to preserve renal function, and adequate analgesia.

PRINCIPLES OF MANAGEMENT

Both the incidence and prevalence of cancer increase with age, and older people more often present with advanced-stage disease. Efforts to screen the older population for common cancers (such as colon, breast, and prostate) before they experience symptoms are likely to discover earlier and more curable lesions.

Older patients may have less physiologic reserve than younger patients, but unless a specific comorbid illness is influencing baseline organ function, cancer treatments with curative or palliative potential should be offered to most patients in most settings, regardless of age. Curative surgical procedures may require more prolonged convalescence, but recovery from most procedures is expected. Radiation therapy is safe and effective in the same settings it is used in younger patients. Chemotherapy may need to be adjusted to the individual patient's level of tolerance of the adverse effects, but usually the changes should be made based on toxicities actually encountered rather than on toxicities anticipated. Biologic therapies are usually safe; some produce less toxicity in older than in younger patients.

See also "Dermatologic Diseases and Disorders" (p 284) for the diagnosis and treatment of skin cancers, and "Persistent Pain" (p 131) and "Palliative Care" (p 125) for the management of pain and end-of-life care.

REFERENCES

- American Geriatrics Society Ethics Committee. Health Screening Decisions for Older Adults: AGS Position Paper. *J Am Geriatr Soc.* 2003;51(2):270–271.

- Bach PB, Schrag D, Brawley OW, et al. Survival of blacks and whites after a cancer diagnosis. *JAMA.* 2002; 287(16):2106–2113.

- Balducci L, Lyman GH, Ershler WB et al., eds. *Comprehensive Geriatric Oncology.* 2nd ed. Philadelphia: Lippincott Williams and Wilkins; 2004.

- Muss HB, Longo DL, eds. Cancer in the elderly. *Semin Oncol.* 2004;31:125–296.

APPENDIX CONTENTS

ANTICOAGULATION

Warfarin Therapy

Prescribing Warfarin

- For anticoagulation in nonacute conditions, initiate therapy by giving warfarin (Coumadin, Carfin, Sofarin) 2–5 mg/day as fixed dose [T: 1, 2, 2.5, 3, 4, 5, 6, 7.5, 10]; reduce dose if INR > 2.5 on day 3.
- Half-life is 31–51 hours; steady state is achieved on day 5–7 of fixed dose.
- Warfarin therapy is implicated in **many** adverse drug-drug interactions.
- Some drugs that **increase** INR in conjunction with warfarin:

alcohol (with concurrent liver disease)	clofibrate	NSAIDs
amiodarone	clotrimazole	piroxicam
androgens	fluconazole	propafenone
antibiotics (many)	flu vaccine	propranolol
acetaminophen (> 1.3 g/day > 1 week)	isoniazid	sulindac
acetylsalicylic acid or aspirin (> 3 g/day)	ketoprofen	tolmetin
chloral hydrate	metolazone	trimethoprim
cimetidine	miconazole	

- Some drugs that **decrease** INR in conjunction with warfarin

barbiturates	dicloxacillin	rifampin
carbamazepine	etretinate	sucralfate
cholestyramine	griseofulvin	trazodone
cyclosporine	nafcillin	vitamin K

Indications for Anticoagulation in the Absence of Active Bleeding or Severe Bleeding Risk

Condition	Target INR	Duration of Therapy
Hip or major knee surgery	2.0–3.0	At least 7–10 days
Idiopathic venous thromboembolism (includes pulmonary embolism)	2.0–3.0	At least 6–12 months*
Atrial fibrillation	2.0–3.0	Indefinitely
Mitral valvular heart disease with history of systemic embolization or left atrial diameter > 5.5 cm	2.0–3.0	Indefinitely
Cardiomyopathy with ejection fraction < 25%	2.0–3.0	Indefinitely
Mechanical aortic valve with normal left atrial size and sinus rhythm	2.0–3.0**	Indefinitely
Mechanical aortic valve with enlarged left atrium or atrial fibrillation or both	2.5–3.5**†	Indefinitely
Mechanical mitral valve	2.5–3.5**†	Indefinitely
Caged ball or caged disk valve	2.5–3.5‡	Indefinitely
Bioprosthetic heart valve	2.0–3.0	3 months
Acute myocardial infarction complicated by severe left ventricular dysfunction, heart failure, previous emboli, mural thrombus on echocardiography	2.0–3.0	1–3 months

* For first event of idiopathic deep-vein thrombosis or pulmonary embolism, consider indefinite anticoagulation, particularly after cases of life-threatening embolism or in patients with thrombophilia such as Factor V Leiden mutations.

** If additional risk factors are present or if there is systemic embolism despite anticoagulation treatment, target INR is 2.5–3.5 and aspirin 80–100 mg/day should be added.

† Alternative target INR 2.0–3.0 with addition of aspirin 80–100 mg/day.

‡ With addition of aspirin 80–100 mg/day.

Treatment of Warfarin Overdose

INR	Clinical Situation	Action
≥ 3.5 and < 5.0	No significant bleeding	Omit next warfarin dose or lower dose or both
≥ 5.0 and < 9.0	No significant bleeding	Omit next 1–2 doses of warfarin and restart therapy at lower dose; alternatively, omit 1 dose and give VK 1–2.5 mg po
≥ 9.0	No significant bleeding	Discontinue warfarin and give VK 3–10 mg po; give additional VK po if INR is not substantially reduced in 24–48 hours. Restart warfarin at lower dose when INR is therapeutic.
Any elevation	Serious bleeding	Discontinue warfarin; give VK 10 mg by slow IV infusion, supplemented with fresh frozen plasma or prothrombin complex concentrate depending on urgency of situation; check INR every 6 hours; repeat VK every 12 hours as needed
Any elevation	Life-threatening bleeding	Discontinue warfarin; give VK 10 mg by slow IV infusion, supplemented with prothrombin complex concentrate; repeat this treatment as needed

NOTE: IV = intravenous; po = by mouth; VK = vitamin K.

SOURCE: Data from American College of Chest Physicians Consensus Panel on Antithrombotic Therapy: Ansell J, Hirsch J, Pollar L, et al. The pharmacology and management of the vitamin K antagonists.. In: Seventh ACCP Conference on Antithrombotic and Thrombolytic Therapy. *Chest.* 2004; 126:2045–2335.

Acute Anticoagulation

Anticoagulants for Deep-Vein Thrombosis or Pulmonary Embolism Prophylaxis and Treatment

Class, Agent	Prophylaxis Dosage By Condition Type	Treatment Dosage	Comments
Heparin			
Unfractionated heparin (Hep-Lock)	General surgery: 5000 U SC 2 h before and q 12 h after surgery	5000 U/kg IV bolus followed by 15 mg/kg/h IV*	Bleeding, anemia, thrombocytopenia, hypertransaminasemia, urticaria (L, K)
Low-Molecular-Weight Heparin			
Enoxaparin (Lovenox)	THA, HFX: 30 mg SC q 12 h or 40 mg SC qd KR: 30 mg SC q 12 h AS: 40 mg SC qd	Outpatient treatment of DVT: 1 mg/kg SC q 12 h; inpatient treatment of DVT ± PE: 1 mg/kg SC q 12 h or 1.5 mg/kg SC qd*	Bleeding, anemia, hyperkalemia, hypertransaminasemia, thrombocytopenia, thrombocytosis, urticaria, angioedema (K)
Dalteparin (Fragmin)	Low-risk THA: 2500–5000 U SC before surgery, 5000 U SC qd after surgery Abdominal surgery: 2500–5000 U SC before and after surgery	DVT: 100 U/kg SC q 12 h; also indicated for anticoagulation in acute coronary syndrome	Same (K)
Tinzaparin (Innohep)	NA	175 anti-Xa IU/kg SC qd*	Same (K)
Heparinoid			
Danaparoid (Orgaran)	THA, HFX, HIT: 750 anti-Xa U SC bid	NA	Same as LMWH (K)
Factor Xa Inhibitor			
Fondaparinux (Arixtra)	THA, HFX, KR: 2.5 mg SC qd beginning 6–8 h after surgery	Weight < 50 kg: 5 mg SC qd; weight 50–100 kg: 7.5 mg SC qd; weight > 100 kg: 10 mg SC qd	Contraindicated if CrCl <30 mL/min (K)

(table continued on next page)

Anticoagulants for Deep-Vein Thrombosis or Pulmonary Embolism Prophylaxis and Treatment (continued)

Class, Agent	Prophylaxis Dosage By Condition Type	Treatment Dosage	Comments
Direct Thrombin Inhibitors			
Argatroban	HIT: 2 μg/kg/min IV infusion	HIT: 2 μg/kg/min IV infusion	Decrease dosage if hepatic impairment (L)
Lepirudin (Refludan)	HIT: 4 mg/kg bolus, then 0.15 mg/kg/h	HIT: 4 mg/kg bolus, then 0.15 mg/kg/h	Decrease bolus to 0.2 mg/kg if CrCl < 60
Thrombolytics			
Streptokinase (Kabikinase, Streptase)	NA	250,000 U IV over 30 min, then 100,000 U/h for 24 h†	Risk of hemorrhage increased with age and higher BMI; HTN, hallucination, agitation, confusion, serum sickness (L)

NOTE: AS = aortic stenosis; bid = twice a day; BMI = body mass index; CrCl = creatinine clearance; d = day(s); DVT = deep-vein thrombosis; H = hepatic elimination; h = hour(s); HFX = hip fracture surgery; HIT = heparin-induced thrombocytopenia; HTN = hypertension; IV = intravenous(ly); K = renal elimination; KR = knee replacement; LMWH = low-molecular-weight heparin; NA = not applicable; q = each, every; SC = subcutaneous(ly); THA = total hip arthroplasty (hip replacement).

* Also indicated for anticoagulation in acute coronary syndrome.

† Dose in acute myocardial infarction is 1.5 million U IV over 60 minutes.

Source: Reuben DB, Herr KA, Pacala JT, et al. *Geriatrics At Your Fingertips 2006*. 8th ed. New York: The American Geriatrics Society; 2006:18–20. Reprinted with permission.

ASSISTED LIVING FACILITIES POSITION STATEMENT

Health Care Systems Committee, American Geriatrics Society

Background

The American Geriatrics Society (AGS) believes that Assisted Living Facilities (ALF) can offer seniors an environment that could enhance their health status over other possible living arrangements. This Position Statement is to provide policymakers, administrators, health care professionals, and consumers with guidance for achieving optimum outcomes with regards to ALFs.

Positions

The following principles are essential to realizing the potential benefits of ALFs.

1. ALFs have a responsibility to provide complete information to prospective residents to assure that an appropriate match is made between resident and facility.

> **Rationale:** Consumers of ALFs need to have detailed information regarding the services provided and any associated costs. In contrast to nursing facilities whose primary payor are the states through Medicaid, ALF payors tend to be the residents themselves. As a result, ALFs are subject to less state and federal regulation and are more affected by market pressures. In order for consumers to make optimal decisions, ALFs need to disclose fully the services provided, the limitations of their facility, how much functional decline they can handle effectively, and especially the criteria residents must continue to meet to remain in the ALF. In addition, the staffing levels and expertise should be discussed with all potential ALF residents.

> **Reference:** Hawes C, Phillips C, Rose M. (2000) High Service or High Privacy Assisted Living Facilities, their Residents and Staff: Results from a National Survey. Miriam Rose, Myers Research Institute. U.S Department of Health and Human Services, Office of the Assistant Secretary for Planning and Evaluation, Office of Disability, Aging, and Long-Term Care Policy (ASPE) and Research Triangle Institute, November.

2. Residents entering an ALF should have a baseline evaluation, completed within 30 days of their admission, of their physical, medical and psychosocial needs, and a detailed review of all medications, prescription, nonprescription, herbal and other remedies, completed by a qualified, licensed practitioner experienced in the care of older adults. This culturally sensitive evaluation should be the basis for the development of a care plan that indicates resident physical and psychosocial needs along with resident preferences for treatment and strategies for meeting identified needs. This care plan should be available to the resident and to the ALF staff. The ALF should clearly indicate, preferably prior to admission, the specific elements of the care plan that the ALF will meet and is willing to accommodate as well as the responsibility of the resident/family.

> **Rationale:** A resident's move to assisted living is a critical life-change event. This event offers a special opportunity for a comprehensive review of the resident's health and social needs. This move to an ALF often signals some medical, cognitive or functional need for the senior, which makes a comprehensive assessment all the more crucial at this transition of care. It also offers the opportunity to provide optimum interventions designed to maintain independence and prevent pre-existing conditions from deteriorating.

3. ALF staff should be knowledgeable and skilled in carrying out important components of geriatric care, including, but not limited to, safe medication administration, falls prevention, incontinence care, communication techniques, dementia care, skin care, and able to recognize the changes that can signal acute illness, delirium, and depression.

> **Rationale:** Staffing levels and expertise do vary between ALFs. In a national study of ALFs, 40% reported having full-time registered nurse staff, 55% had a registered nurse either full or part time, and 71% had a registered nurse or licensed practical nurse on staff full or part time. About half (52%) used outside agencies to supply registered or licensed practical nurses. Staff working on-site should be sufficient in numbers and experience to meet the ongoing needs of the residents at all times. Staff should be knowledgeable regarding safe medication administration, falls prevention, incontinence care, communication techniques, dementia care, skin care, and recognition of the changes that can signal acute illness/delirium.

Reference: Phillips, Munoz, Sherman et al. (2003) Effects of Facility Characteristics on Departures from Assisted Living: Results from a National Study. *Gerontologist* 42 (5): 690–696.

Reference: Ambulatory Geriatric Clinical Care and Services Position Statement. Developed by the AGS Health Care Systems Committee and approved May 2000 by the AGS Board of Directors. *Journal of the American Geriatrics Society*, 48:845-846.

4. A primary care provider (includes geriatric nurse practitioners as well as physicians) experienced in geriatrics care should be available within each ALF to help direct staff in optimizing outcomes for each resident.

Rationale: The benefit of clinical leadership within long-term-care facilities was noted in 1978 in the *Journal of the American Geriatrics Society* and later supported by a 1993 AGS position statement on the Physician's Role in the Long-Term Care Facility, which illustrated the importance of this involvement. This benefit is true in all long-term-care facilities, including ALFs, extended-care units, skilled nursing facilities, intermediate care facilities, and residential units caring for frail residents. More recently the work of the Assisted Living Workgroup highlighted the link between these clinical services and outcome for ALF residents.

Reference: Ingman SR, Lawson IR, Carbon D. (1978) Medical Direction in Long-term Care. *Journal of the American Geriatrics Society* 26(4);157–166.

Reference: Assisted Living Workgroup Report to US Senate Special Committee on Aging 2003. Available at: www.aahsa.org/alw.htm (accessed November 2005).

5. ALFs need to become aligned with other facilities, providers, and systems of care to produce optimum outcomes for seniors.

Rationale: A comprehensive system of care is able to accommodate seniors with varied needs as they traverse through different levels of health and function in their aging lifetime. Key to coordination of care is communication at each transition of care.

Reference: Improving the Quality of Transitional Care for Persons with Complex Care Needs Position Statement. Developed by the AGS Health Care Systems Committee and approved May 2002 by the AGS Board of Directors. The American Geriatrics Society, New York, NY.

6. ALF resources need to be within the reach of those living in rural and low-income communities.

Rationale: The lack of noninstitutional, long-term-care services in many rural areas may explain why residents of nursing homes in rural areas tend to be younger and less disabled than their urban counterparts. Part of this can be accomplished with continued funding of the 1915[c] Home and Community Based Services waiver program to provide needed services. The 1915[c] Home and Community Based Services waiver is the primary Medicaid funding vehicle for low-income persons requiring assisted-living services.

Reference: Spector W, et al. (1996) Appropriate placement of nursing home residents in lower levels of care. *Millbank Quarterly.* 74:139–160.

Credits

American Geriatrics Society and approved by the AGS Board of Directors in May 2004. Written by the AGS Health Care Systems Committee, with special thanks to Drs. Richard Stefanacci, Leslie Wooldridge, and Kenneth Brummel-Smith. AGS, The Empire State Building, 350 Fifth Avenue, Suite 801, New York, NY 10118.

SOURCE: American Geriatrics Society. Assisted Living Facilities: American Geriatrics Society Position Paper, AGS Health Care Systems Committee. *J Am Geriatr Soc.* 2005;53(3):536–537. Reprinted by permission of Blackwell Science, Inc.

DEPRESSION: THE GERIATRIC DEPRESSION SCALE (SHORT FORM)

Choose the best answer for how you felt over the past week.

1. Are you basically satisfied with your life?	yes/**no**
2. Have you dropped many of your activities and interests?	**yes**/no
3. Do you feel that your life is empty?	**yes**/no
4. Do you often get bored?	**yes**/no
5. Are you in good spirits most of the time?	yes/**no**
6. Are you afraid that something bad is going to happen to you?	**yes**/no
7. Do you feel happy most of the time?	yes/**no**
8. Do you often feel helpless?	**yes**/no
9. Do you prefer to stay at home, rather than going out and doing new things?	**yes**/no
10. Do you feel you have more problems with memory than most?	**yes**/no
11. Do you think it is wonderful to be alive now?	yes/**no**
12. Do you feel pretty worthless the way you are now?	**yes**/no
13. Do you feel full of energy?	yes/**no**
14. Do you feel that your situation is hopeless?	**yes**/no
15. Do you think that most people are better off than you are?	**yes**/no

NOTE: Score bolded answers. One point for each of these answers. Cut-off: normal = 0–5; above 5 suggests depression. For additional information on administration and scoring, refer to the following references:

1. Sheikh JI, Yesavage JA. Geriatric Depression Scale: recent evidence and development of a shorter version. *Clin Gerontol.* 1986;5:165–172.
2. Yesavage JA, Brink TL, Rose TL, et al. Development and validation of a geriatric depression rating scale: a preliminary report. *J Psych Res.* 1983;17:27.

SOURCE: Courtesy of Jerome A. Yesavage, MD.

FALLS: GUIDELINES FOR PREVENTION

Recommendations from the American Geriatrics Society

The aim of this guideline is to assist health care professionals in their assessment of fall risk and in their management of older patients who are at risk of falling and those who have fallen. The Panel on Falls Prevention assumes that health care professionals will use their general clinical knowledge and judgment in applying the general principles and specific recommendations of this document to the assessment and management of individual patients. Decisions to adopt any particular recommendation must be made by the practitioner in light of available evidence and resources. (The key to strength of recommendations, indicated by letters A–D, is located in the note on next page.)

Assessment

Approach to older persons as part of routine care (not presenting after a fall):

■ All older persons who are under the care of a health professional or their caregivers should be asked at least once a year about falls.

■ All older persons who report a single fall should be observed as they stand up from a chair without using their arms, walk several paces, and return (ie, the "Get Up and Go Test"). Those demonstrating no difficulty or unsteadiness need no further assessment.

■ Persons who have difficulty or demonstrate unsteadiness performing this test require further assessment.

Approach to older persons presenting with one or more falls or who have abnormalities of gait or balance or both, or who report recurrent falls:

■ Older persons who present for medical attention because of a fall, report recurrent falls in the past year, or demonstrate abnormalities of gait or balance, or both, should have a fall evaluation performed. This evaluation should be performed by a clinician with appropriate skills and experience, which may necessitate referral to a specialist (eg, geriatrician).

■ A fall evaluation is defined as an assessment that includes the following: a history of fall circumstances, medications, acute or chronic medical problems, and mobility levels; an examination of vision, gait and balance, and lower extremity joint function; an examination of basic neurologic function, including mental status, muscle strength, lower extremity peripheral nerves, proprioception, reflexes, tests of cortical, extrapyramidal, and cerebellar function; and assessment of basic cardiovascular status, including heart rate and rhythm, postural pulse and blood pressure, and, if appropriate, heart rate and blood-pressure responses to carotid sinus stimulation.

Multifactorial Interventions

■ Among *community-dwelling* older persons (ie, those living in their own homes), multifactorial interventions should include: gait training and advice on the appropriate use of assistive devices (B); review and modification of medication, especially psychotropic medication (B); exercise programs, with balance training as one of the components (B); treatment of postural hypotension (B); modification of environmental hazards (C); and treatment of cardiovascular disorders, including cardiac arrhythmias (D).

■ In *long-term care and assisted-living settings*, multifactorial interventions should include: staff education programs (B); gait training and advice on the appropriate use of assistive devices (B); and review and modification of medications, especially psychotropic medications (B).

■ The evidence is insufficient to make recommendations for or against multifactorial interventions in *acute hospital* settings.

Single Intervention: Exercise

- Although exercise has many proven benefits, the optimal type, duration, and intensity of exercise for falls prevention remain unclear (B).

- Older people who have had recurrent falls should be offered long-term exercise and balance training (B).

- Tai Chi C'uan is a promising type of balance exercise, although it requires further evaluation before it can be recommended as the preferred balance training (C).

Single Intervention: Environmental Modification

- When older patients at increased risk of falls are discharged from the hospital, a facilitated environmental home assessment should be considered (B).

Single Intervention: Medications

- Patients who have fallen should have their medications reviewed and altered or stopped, as appropriate, in light of their risk of future falls. Particular attention to medication reduction should be given to older persons taking four or more medications and to those taking psychotropic medications (C).

Single Intervention: Assistive Devices

- Studies of multifactorial interventions that have included assistive devices have demonstrated benefit. However, there is no direct evidence that the use of assistive devices alone will prevent falls. Therefore, while assistive devices may be effective elements of a multifactorial intervention program, their isolated use without attention to other risk factors cannot be recommended (C).

Single Intervention: Behavioral and Educational Programs

- Although studies of multifactorial interventions that have included behavioral and educational programs have demonstrated benefit, when used as an isolated intervention, health or behavioral education does not reduce falls and should not be done in isolation (B).

NOTE:

Key to Strength of Recommendation: A: Directly based on Class I evidence; B: Directly based on Class II evidence or extrapolated recommendation from Class I evidence; C: Directly based on Class III evidence or extrapolated recommendation from Class I or II evidence; D: Directly based on Class IV evidence or extrapolated recommendation from Class I, II, or III evidence.

Key to Categories of Evidence: Class I: Evidence from at least one randomized controlled trial or a meta-analysis of randomized controlled trials; Class II: Evidence from at least one controlled study without randomization or evidence from at least one other type of quasi-experimental study; Class III: Evidence from nonexperimental studies, such as comparative studies, correlation studies, and case-control studies; Class IV: Evidence from expert committee reports or opinions and/or clinical experience of respected authorities.

SOURCE: Adapted from American Geriatrics Society, British Geriatrics Society, and American Academy of Orthopaedic Surgeons Panel on Falls Prevention. Guidelines for the prevention of falls in older persons. *J Am Geriatr Soc* 2001;49(5):664–672. Reprinted by permission of Blackwell Science, Inc.

INCONTINENCE: BEHAVIORAL PREVENTION AND MANAGEMENT

Behavioral treatment for urinary incontinence depends on careful instruction of the patient. The following tools are examples of patient education materials for bladder training, bladder urge control, and pelvic muscle (Kegel's) exercises that have been found to be clinically useful. See "Urinary Incontinence" (p 171) for discussion of the use of behavioral approaches.

Bladder Training

Bladder training involves following a strict schedule for bathroom visits during the day. The schedule starts with bathroom visits every 2 hours or so, but the time between visits is gradually increased. The longer stretch of time between bathroom visits gives you increased bladder control and independence.

If you have a habit of using the bathroom more than once every 2 hours due to urgency—with or without urge incontinence—you may benefit from bladder training. Bladder training has been shown to be effective for both stress and urge incontinence.

Goals

Bladder training has several goals. It helps you

- Lengthen the amount of time between bathroom visits.

- Increase the amount of urine that the bladder can comfortably hold.

- Improve self-control over bladder urges by voiding on a schedule, not when the urge strikes.

- Reduce or eliminate incontinence.

- Increase independence in bladder management.

How To Do Bladder Training

Bladder training requires motivation for starting and maintaining a schedule for voids. Each week, as incontinence decreases, the schedule is changed slightly so that your bathroom visits occur less often. Bladder training will take between 6 and 8 weeks for success, but noticeable improvements will occur early in the program.

- Start with a Bladder Diary. Record your bathroom visits and urine leaks on the Bladder Diary for 48 hours. Measure the urine you produce during bathroom visits with a calibrated cup. This will help determine the amount of urine your bladder is able to hold.

- Review the Bladder Diary with your clinician, who will set a bladder training schedule according to the amount of time between your usual bathroom visits. For many people, the bathroom visits are scheduled for every 1 to 2 hours.

- For the first week, use the bathroom strictly according to the schedule. If a strong bladder urge strikes, use the Bladder Urge Control Procedure (below) to regain control and wait until the next scheduled time to void. If the urge is too strong and it cannot be entirely suppressed, use the bathroom, but then resume the bladder schedule.

- Each week, increase the time between bathroom visits by 30 minutes, as tolerated. As incontinence decreases week by week, the schedule can be further increased. For many individuals, bathroom visits every 3 to 6 hours is desirable. For most older persons, every 3 to 4 hours is optimal.

- Monitor the number of urine leaks each day and for the entire week. Also monitor the amount of each leak. For example, a person may have two leaks a day, but instead of large leaks that saturate a pad, they are small dribbles that slightly dampen the pad. This is considered good improvement.

- If the number of urine leaks does not lessen in 1 week, then maintain the same bladder training schedule for another week. Adjust the schedule in the next week when urine leaks decrease.

Bladder Urge Control Procedures

When a bladder urge strikes, you may be tempted to rush to the bathroom to prevent incontinence. This response can cause more harm than good, since the already overactive bladder becomes more stimulated and irritated with the rushed movement to the toilet. To get control over the bladder, practice the Bladder Control Procedure when the urge strikes. In this procedure, you

- Stand quietly or sit still. This prevents overstimulation of the bladder.

- Take slow, relaxed breaths.

- Contract the pelvic floor muscles repeatedly (see pelvic muscle exercises below). This helps keep the urethra closed to prevent urine from leaking. This also calms the bladder through special signals that are carried to the brain.

- Concentrate on making the urge go away. Use mental imagery and self-talk to help suppress the urge. Think to yourself, "I am in control of my bladder and this bladder has one job only and that is to hold urine until I am ready to go to the toilet." Imagine the urge as a wave that has peaked and now is fading away.

- Use mental distraction to reduce the awareness of the discomfort of the urge. Hum a tune or do mathematical calculations (subtract 7 from 100, then continue subtracting 7).

- When the urge subsides, do not use the toilet until the next scheduled void.

- If the urge does not completely subside, you may use the toilet.

When used with every urge, this procedure becomes more effective and gives you greater control over your bladder. Be encouraged by even small improvements in your symptoms. Although progress may seem slow, you are developing entirely new habits for bladder control. These healthy bladder habits will remain an important part of your life style. This takes both time and patience, but the rewards are worth the effort.

Pelvic Muscle (Kegel's) Exercises

Pelvic muscles, like other muscles, can become weak or damaged. Pelvic muscle exercises strengthen weak muscles around the bladder.

- Start by doing your pelvic muscle exercises 3 to 4 times each week. Usually it takes about 10 minutes to do the exercises. Your clinician will give you exact instructions about how many times you should perform the exercises and the number of times a day.

- Practice anywhere and any time. It is usually best to begin practicing them when lying on your bed. Once you have mastered the exercises lying down, practice them sitting in a chair. Then advance to practicing them standing. Soon you will be able to do them anywhere.

- Never use your stomach, thigh, or buttock muscles. To find out whether you are also contracting your stomach muscles, place your hand on your abdomen while you squeeze your pelvic muscle. If you feel your abdomen move, then you are also using these muscles.

- Avoid holding your breath. Inhale and exhale slowly while counting. In time, you will learn to practice effortlessly.

- If you forget to do your exercises for several days, do not be discouraged. When you have realized you have forgotten, begin your program again as instructed. Do not try to make up for lost days by doing more exercises or you will have sore muscles.

After 4 to 6 weeks of following your prescribed exercise routine, you will begin to notice that you are having fewer urinary accidents. After 3 months, you will see an even bigger difference. It may help to keep a diary of the times you practice your exercises and the times that you leak urine. This will give you a picture of the progress you are making. If you are having problems, your clinician may suggest biofeedback, weighted vaginal cones, or electrostimulation to help you with pelvic muscle exercises.

SOURCE: Adapted from Busby-Whitehead J, Kinkade J, Granville L. *Urinary Incontinence: Management in Primary Practice*. Tool Kit 2, Practicing Physician Education Project, Robinson BE, ed. New York: The John A. Hartford Foundation and The American Geriatrics Society; 2000. Reprinted with permission.

NUTRITION SCREENING: DETERMINE YOUR NUTRITIONAL HEALTH CHECKLIST

The nutrition screen is based on these warning signs of poor nutrition:

Disease

Eating poorly

Tooth loss, mouth pain

Economic hardship

Reduced social contact

Multiple medicines

Involuntary weight loss or gain

Need for assistance in self-care

Elderly (age > 80)

The mnemonic DETERMINE represents the warning signs and the questions in the screen.

Read the statements below. Circle the number in the "YES" column for those that apply to you or someone under your care. For each "YES" answer, score the number listed. Total your nutrition score.

	YES
1. I have an illness or condition that made me change the kind and/or amount of food I eat.	2
2. I eat fewer than 2 meals per day.	3
3. I eat few fruits or vegetables, or milk products.	2
4. I have 3 or more drinks of beer, liquor, or wine almost every day.	2
5. I have tooth or mouth problems that make it hard for me to eat.	2
6. I don't always have enough money to buy the food I need.	4
7. I eat alone most of the time.	1
8. I take 3 or more different prescribed or over-the-counter drugs a day.	1
9. Without wanting to, I have lost or gained 10 pounds in the last 6 months.	2
10. I am not always physically able to shop, cook, and/or feed myself.	2
TOTAL _____	

NOTE: Scoring: 0–2 = good; 3–5 = moderate nutritional risk; 6 or more = high nutritional risk.

SOURCE: DETERMINE Your Nutritional Health Checklist. Reprinted with permission of the Nutrition Screening Initiative, a project of the American Academy of Family Physicians, the American Dietetic Association, and the National Council on Aging, Inc., and funded in part by a grant from Ross Products Division, Abbott Laboratories Inc.

TERMS USED TO INTERPRET SCREENING AND DIAGNOSTIC TESTS

Term	Definition, Description
Positive test	Condition present = true positive (a)
	Condition absent = false positive (b)
Negative test	Condition present = false negative (c)
	Condition absent = true negative (d)
Sensitivity	Proportion of persons with the condition who test positive: $a\ /\ (a + c)$
Specificity	Proportion of persons without the condition who test negative: $d\ /\ (b + d)$
Positive predictive value	Proportion of persons with a positive test who have the condition: $a\ /\ (a + b)$
Negative predictive value	Proportion of persons with a negative test who do not have the condition: $d\ /\ (c + d)$
Positive predictive value (PPV)	Depends on sensitivity and specificity of the test and the prevalence of the disease: PPV = $prevalence \times sensitivity\ /\ (prevalence \times sensitivity) + (1 - prevalence)(1 - specificity)$

NOTE: For conditions, like cancer, that are relatively uncommon in asymptomatic people, a test for a low prevalence condition that is only modestly specific will result in many more positive tests than there are individuals who actually have cancer. This is the main difficulty with screening, as a positive test must be followed by more specific tests that are usually more invasive and associated with morbidity.

RESOURCES

What Can You Find on the AGS Website?
http://www.americangeriatrics.org
e-mail: info.amger@americangeriatrics.org

- **What is the American Geriatrics Society?** AGS mission and goals, current activities, history, AGS staff/contact information, list of Board of Directors and Committee Chairs and their affiliations.

- **All New MyAGS: An AGS Members Only Resource**
  Created by the American Geriatrics Society, My AGS offers members access to exclusive members only tools and resources while enabling them to navigate the regular AGS website at the same time. Resources include one click access to the Journal of the American Geriatrics Society, Access to the Online Members Directory, free support materials for the American Board of Internal Medicine (ABIM) geriatrics modules under the ABIM Self-Evaluation Process, AGS Legislative Toolkit, AGS Practice Management Toolkit and more.

- Information on all AGS publications, including the *Geriatrics Review Syllabus: A Core Curriculum in Geriatric Medicine (GRS), Geriatric Nursing Review Syllabus, GRS Teaching Slides, Case-Based Geriatrics Review, Doorway Thoughts,* and *Geriatrics At Your Fingertips.*

- **Geriatrics-For-Specialists Website**—To respond to the need for better geriatric training, the American Geriatrics Society (AGS), with funding from the John A. Hartford Foundation, established the Geriatrics for Specialists Project. Launched in 1994, the project is expanding geriatrics expertise in 10 surgical and related medical specialties.

- **Professional Education** opportunities, including free online CME opportunities, information on the **Geriatrics Recognition Award (GRA)**, and listings of continuing education courses and AGS co-sponsored events.

- **Patient Education**—Link to the AGS Foundation for Health in Aging (FHA) which strives to make trustworthy and practical health care information available to the public. Its many pamphlets, fact sheets, consumer tools, books and website are designed to inform your patients about multiple chronic illnesses and promote disease prevention and healthy living.

- **Public Policy**—an overview of AGS public policy and legislative activities.

- **Council of State Affiliates Representatives (COSAR)**—information on AGS state affiliates promoting geriatrics at the local level.

- **Links** to dozens of aging/health/education-related Web sites.

- **AGS Annual Meeting Information**

- **Junior Faculty Development Opportunities**—An updated listing of junior faculty award opportunities, including the **Hartford Geriatrics Health Outcomes Research Scholars Award Program** and the **T. Franklin Williams Research Scholars Award**.

- Access to other AGS publications including the *Journal of the American Geriatrics Society,* the *Annals of Long-Term Care: Clinical Care and Aging,* the **AGS Newsletter**, and full-text versions of AGS Position Papers, Statements, and Guidelines.

Directory of Agencies and Organizations for Geriatric Clinicians

While this list represents a comprehensive guide to organizations that address the clinical care needs of older people, it is not a resource of all social service agencies and organizations assisting older citizens. If you have questions that do not specifically relate to one of the following organizations, please contact your state and/or area agency on aging as listed by the Administration on Aging (AOA). These agencies provide information on, and refer callers to, local services for senior citizens. To locate state and area agencies on aging, visit the AOA Web site at http://www.aoa.dhhs.gov/agingsites/state.html or call the Eldercare Locator service (1-800-677-1116) operated by the National Association of Area Agencies on Aging.

Note: The organizations on this list are arranged in categories in the following order:
- *GENERAL AGING*
- *END-OF-LIFE ISSUES*
- *EDUCATION*
- *LEGAL ISSUES AND ELDER ABUSE*
- *RESOURCES ON SPECIFIC HEALTH PROBLEMS:*

Cancer	Neurologic Problems
Complementary and Alternative Medicine	Nutritional Concerns
Diabetes Mellitus	Pain
Digestive Problems	Psychological Problems
Head and Neck Problems	Sexuality and Sexual Concers
Hearing Problems	Sight Problems
Heart and Circulation Problems	Skin Problems
Joint, Muscle, and Bone Problems	Urinary Problems
Lung and Breathing Problems	
Memory and Thinking Problems	

GENERAL AGING

Administration on Aging
330 Independence Avenue, SW
Washington, DC 20201
Tel: (202) 619-0724
Fax: (202) 401-7620 or (202) 537-3555
Web site: http://www.aoa.gov
E-Mail: aoainfo@aoa.gov or aoainfo@aoa.hhs.gov

National Aging Information Center (NAIC)
(A Service of the Administration on Aging)
330 Independence Avenue, SW, Room 4656
Washington, DC 20201
Telephone: (202) 619-7501
TTY: (202) 401-7575
Fax: (202) 401-7620
Web site: http://www.aoa.gov/naic
E-Mail: naic@aoa.gov

Agency for Health Care Research and Quality (AHRQ), formerly the Agency for Health Care Policy and Research
540 Gaither Road
Rockville, MD 20850
Tel: (301) 427-1364
On-line retrieval:
http://www.ahrq.gov

Aging Network Services
Topaz House
4400 East-West Hwy., Suite 907
Bethesda, MD 20814
Tel: (301) 657-4329
Fax: (301) 657-3250
Web site:
http://www.agingnets.com
E-Mail: ans@agingnets.com

Alliance for Aging Research
2021 K Street, NW, Suite 305
Washington, DC 20006
Tel: (202) 293-2856
Fax: (202) 785-8574
Web site: www.agingresearch.org
Email: info@agingresearch.org

American Academy of Home Care Physicians
PO Box 1037
Edgewood, MD 21040
Tel: (410) 676-7966
Fax: (410) 676-7980
Web site: www.aahcp.org
E-Mail: aahcp@comcast.net

American Association of Homes & Services for the Aging
2519 Connecticut Avenue, NW
Washington, DC 20008-1520
Tel: (202) 783-2242
Fax: (202) 783-2255
Web site: www.aahsa.org
E-Mail: info@aahsa.org

American Association of Retired Persons
601 E Street, NW
Washington, DC 20049
Tel: (800)424-3410 or (888) OUR-AARP (687-2277)
Web site: www.aarp.org
E-Mail: member@aarp.org

American College of Health Care
Administrators
300 N. Lee Street, Suite 301
Alexandria, VA 22314
Tel: (703) 739-7900 or (888)
88-ACHCA (882-2422)
Fax: (703) 739-7901
Toll Free: (888) 888-ACHCA
(22422)
Web site: www.achca.org
E-Mail: info@achca.org

American Federation for Aging
Research
70 West 40th St., 11th Floor
New York, NY 10018
Tel: (212) 703-9977
Fax: (212) 832-2298
(212)-997-0030
Web site: www.afar.org
E-Mail: info@afar.org

American Geriatrics Society
The Empire State Building
350 Fifth Avenue, Suite 801
New York, NY 10118
Tel: (212) 308-1414
Fax: (212) 832-8646
Web site:
www.americangeriatrics.org
E-Mail:
info.amger@americangeriatrics.org

American Health Care Association
1201 L Street, NW
Washington, DC 20005
Tel: (202) 842-4444
Fax: (202) 842-3860
Toll Free for Publications Only
(800) 321-0343
Web site: www.ahca.org

American Hospital Association
1 North Franklin
Chicago, IL 60606
Tel: (312) 422-3000
Fax: (312) 422-4796
Web site: www.aha.org

American Medical Directors
Association
10480 Patuxent Parkway, Suite 760
Columbia, MD 21044
Tel: (410) 740-9743
Toll Free: (800) 876-2632
Fax: (410) 740-4572
Web site: www.amda.com
Email: info@amda.com

American Occupational Therapy
Association
4720 Montgomery Lane, PO Box
31220
Bethesda, MD 20824-1220
Tel: (301) 652-2682 or (800)
372-8555
Fax: (301) 652-7711
Web site: www.aota.org

American Red Cross
American Red Cross National
Headquarters
2025 E. Street, NW
Washington, DC 20006
Tel: (202) 303-4498
Web site: www.redcross.org

American Senior Fitness Association
PO Box 2575
New Smyrna Beach, FL 32170
Tel: (800) 243-1478
Web site: www.seniorfitness.net
E-Mail: sfa@ucnsb.net

American Seniors Housing
Association
1850 M Street, NW, Suite 540
Washington, DC 20036
Tel: (202) 974-2300
Fax: (202) 775-0112
Web site: www.nmhc.org
E-Mail: info@nmhc.org

American Social Health Association
Hotlines under the auspices of the
ASHA American Social Health
Association
CDC National AIDS Hotline
(English)—Toll Free (800)
342-AIDS PO Box13827
CDC National AIDS Hotline
(Spanish)—Toll Free: (800)
344-7432
CDC National AIDS Hotline—TTY
Toll Free: (800) 243-7889 Tel:
(919) 361-8400
CDC National STD Hotline—Toll
Free: (800) 227-8922 Fax: (919)
361-8425
CDC National Immunization
Information Hotline—Toll Free:
(800) 232-2522
Web site: www.ashastd.org

American Society on Aging
833 Market Street, Suite 511
San Francisco, CA 94103-1824
Tel: (415) 974-9600 or (800)
537-9728
Fax: (415) 974-0300
Web site: www.asaging.org
E-Mail: info@asaging.org

American Society of Consultant
Pharmacists
1321 Duke Street
Alexandria, VA 22314-3516
Tel: (703) 739-1300
Fax: (703) 739-1321
Toll Free Tel: (800) 355-2727
Toll Free Fax: (800) 707-ASCP
Fast Fax: (800) 220-1321 or (703)
739-1321
Web site: www.ascp.com
E-Mail: info@ascp.com

Assisted Living Federation of
America
11200 Waples Mill Road, Suite 150
Fairfax, VA 22030
Tel: (703) 691-8100
Fax: (703) 691-8106
Web site: www.alfa.org
E-Mail: info@alfa.org

B'nai B'rith
International Headquarters
2020 K Street, NW, 7th Floor
Washington, DC 20006
Tel: (202) 857-6600
Fax: (202) 857-1099
Toll Free: (888) 388-4224
Senior Housing
Tel: (202) 857-6581
Fax: (202) 857-0980
E-Mail: senior@bnaibrith.org

Catholic Charities
1731 King Street, Suite 200
Alexandria, VA 22314
Tel: (703) 549-1390
Fax: (703) 549-1656
Web site:
www.catholiccharitiesusa.org

Children of Aging Parents
PO Box 167
Richboro, PA 18954
Tel: (800) 227-7294
Toll Free Information/Referral:
(800) 227-7294
Web site: www.caps4caregivers.org
Email: info@caps4caregivers.org

CDC National Prevention
Information Network
For information on HIV, AIDS,
STD, TB
PO Box 6003
Rockville, MD 20849-6003
Tel: (301) 562-1098
Toll Free Tel: (800) 458-5231
Toll Free Fax: (888) 282-7681
Toll Free TTY: (800) 243-7012
Web site: www.cdcnpin.org
E-Mail: info@cdcnpin.org

Commission on Accreditation for
Rehabilitation Facilities (CARF)
4891 East Grant Road
Tucson, AZ 85712
Tel: (520) 325-1044 or
(888) 281-6531
Fax: (520) 318-1129
Web site: www.carf.org

Department of Veteran Affairs
Office of Public Affairs
810 Vermont Avenue, NW
Washington, DC 20420
Tel: (202) 273-5700
Fax: (202) 273-6705
Web site: www.va.gov

Disabled American Veterans
807 Maine Avenue, SW
Washington, DC 20024
Tel: (202) 554-3501
Fax: (202) 554-3581
Web site: www.dav.org

Family Caregivers Alliance
180 Montgomery St., Suite 1100
San Francisco, CA 94104
Tel: (415) 434-3388 or
(800) 455-8106
Fax: (415) 434-3508
Toll Free: (800) 445-8106
Web site: www.caregiver.org.
E-Mail: info@caregiver.org

Gerontological Society of America
1030 15th Street NW, Suite 250
Washington, DC 20005
Tel: (202) 842-1275
Fax: (202) 842-1150
Web site: www.geron.org
Email: geron@geron.org

Healthcare Information and
Management Systems Society
230 East Ohio Street, Suite 500
Chicago, IL 60611-3269
Tel: (312) 664-4467
Fax: (312) 664-6143
Web site: www.himss.org
Email: himss@himss.org

Interfaith Caregivers Alliance
One West Armour Blvd.
Suite 202
Kansas City, MO 64111
Tel: (816) 931-5442
Fax: (816) 931-5202
Web site:
www.interfaithcaregivers.org
E-Mail: info@interfaithcaregivers.org

Joint Commission on Accreditation
of Healthcare Organizations
(JCAHO)
One Renaissance Boulevard
Oakbrook Terrace, IL 60181
Tel: (630) 792-5000
Fax: (630) 792-5005
Web site: www.jcaho.org

Medicare Hotline
Toll Free English & Spanish:
(800) MEDICARE (633-4227)
7500 Security Boulevard Baltimore,
MD 21244-1850
Web site: www.medicare.gov

National Adult Day Services
Association
2519 Connecticut Ave., NW
Washington, DC 20008
Tel: (202) 508-1205 or
(800) 558-5301
Fax: (202) 783-3255
Web site: www.nadsa.org
info@nadsa.org

National Asian Pacific Center on
Aging
Melbourne Tower, Suite 914
1511 Third Avenue
Seattle, WA 98101
Tel: (206) 624-1221
Fax: (206) 624-1023
Web site: www.napca.org

National Association of Area
Agencies on Aging
1730 Rhode Island Ave., NW
Suite 1200
Washington, DC 20036
Tel: (202) 872-0888
Fax: (202) 872-0057
Web site: www.n4a.org
E-Mail: rseay@n4a.org
Toll Free Eldercare Locator:
(800) 677-1116, operated as a
cooperative partnership of the
Administration on Aging, the
National Association of Area
Agencies on Aging, and the
National Association of State Units
on Aging.

National Association of Directors of
Nursing Administration
10101 Alliance Road, #140
Cincinnati, OH 45242
Tel: (513) 791-3679
Fax: (513) 791-3699
Toll Free: (800) 222-0539
Web site: www.nadona.org
Email: info@nadona.org

National Association for Home Care
228 7th Street, SE
Washington, DC 20003
Tel: (202) 547-7424
Fax: (202) 547-3540
Web site: www.nahc.org

National Association of Professional
Geriatric Care Managers
1604 North Country Club Road
Tucson, AZ 85716
Tel: (520) 881-8008
Fax: (520) 325-7925
Web site: www.caremanager.org

National Association for the Support
of Long Term Care
1321 Duke Street, Suite 304
Alexandria, VA 22314
Tel: (703) 549-8500
Fax: (703) 549-8342
Web site: www.NASL.org

National Caucus and Center on
Black Aged, Inc.
1220 L Street, NW, Suite 800
Washington, DC 20005
Tel: (202) 637-8400
Fax: (202) 347-0895
Web site: www.ncba-aged.org
E-Mail: info@ncba-aged.org

National Citizens' Coalition for
Nursing Home Reform
801 L Street, NW Suite 801
Washington, DC 20036-2211
Tel: (202) 332-2275
Fax: (202) 332-2949
Web site: www.nccnhr.org
E-Mail: nccnhr1@nccnhr.org

National Council on the Aging
300 D Street, SW, Suite 801
Washington, DC 20024
Tel: (202) 479-1200
Fax: (202) 479-0735
Web site: www.ncoa.org
E-Mail: info@ncoa.org

National Council on Patient
Information and Education
4915 Saint Elmo Avenue
Suite 505
Bethesda, MD 20814-6053
Tel: (301) 656-8565
Fax: (301) 656-4464
Web site: www.talkaboutrx.org
Email: ncpie@ncpie.info

National Family Caregivers
Association
10400 Connecticut Avenue # 500
Kensington, MD 20895-3944
Tel: (301) 942-6430
Fax: (301) 942-2302
Toll Free: (800) 896-3650
Web site: www.nfcacares.org
E-mail: info@nfcacares.org

National Health Information Center
PO Box 1133
Washington, DC 20013-1133
Tel: (301) 565-4167
Toll Free: (800) 336-4797
Fax: (301) 884-4256
Web site:
http://www.health.gov/nhic
E-Mail: info@nhic.org

National Indian Council on Aging
10501 Montgomery Boulevard NE
Suite 210
Albuquerque, NM 87111-3846
Tel: (505) 292-2001
Fax: (505) 292-1922
Web site: www.nicoa.org
E-Mail: dave@nicoa.org

National Institute on Aging
Building 31, Room 5C27
31 Center Drive MSC 2292
Bethesda, MD 20892-2292
Tel: toll free (800) 222-4225 or
(301) 496-1752
Fax: (301) 496-1072
Web site: www.nih.gov/nia

National Institute on Disability and
Rehabilitation Research
ABLEDATA
8630 Fenton Street
Suite 930
Silver Spring, MD 20910
Tel: (301) 608-8998
Fax: (301) 608-8958
Toll Free: (800) 227-0216
Web site: www.abledata.com
Email: adaigle@macroint.com

National Rehabilitation Information
Center
4200 Forbes Boulevard, Suite 202
Lanham, MD 20706
Toll Free: (800) 346-2742
Fax: (301) 459-5900 or
(301) 459-5984
Web site: www.naric.com
Email: naricinfo@heitechservices.com

National Subacute Care Association
7315 Wisconsin Avenue, Suite 424E
Bethesda, MD 20814
Tel: (301) 961-8680
Fax: (301) 961-8681
Web site: www.nsca.net
E-Mail: nsca@tiac.net

Projecto Ayuda
1452 West Temple Street, Suite 100
Los Angeles, CA 90026
Tel: (213) 487-1922
Fax: (213) 202-5905

United Seniors Health Cooperative
409 Third Street SW
Washington, DC 20024
Tel: (202) 479-6973
Fax: (202) 479-6660
Web site: unitedseniorshealth.org

Visiting Nurse Associations of
America
99 Summer St., Suite 1700
Boston, MA 02110
Tel: (617) 737-3200
Fax: (617) 227-4843
(617) 737-1144
Web site: www.vnaa.org
Email: vnaa@vnaa.org

Well Spouse Foundation
63 West Main St., Suite H
Freehold, NJ 07728
Tel: (732) 577-8899 or
(800) 838-0879
Fax: (732) 577-8644
Toll Free: (800) 838-0879
Web site: www.wellspouse.org
E-Mail: info@wellspouse.org

END-OF-LIFE ISSUES

Americans for Better Care of the
Dying
3720 Upton St. NW, Rm. B147
Washington, DC 20016
Tel: (202) 895-2660
Fax: (202) 966-5410
Web site: www.abcd-caring.com
E-Mail: info@abcd-caring.org

Center to Improve Care of the
Dying
Rand Corporation
1200 South Hayes Street
Arlington, VA 22202
Tel: (703) 413-1100
Web site: www.medicaring.org

Choice in Dying, Inc.
1035 30th Street, NW
Washington, DC 20007
Tel: (202) 338-9790
Fax: (202) 338-0242
Toll Free: (800) 989-WILL (9455)
Web site: partnershipforcaring.org

Compassion in Dying
6312 SW Capital Hwy, Suite 415
Portland, OR 97239
Tel: (503) 221-9556
Fax: (503) 228-9160
Web site:
www.compassionindying.org
E-Mail:
info@compassionandchoices.org

GriefNet
Internet Address: www.rivendell.org

Hospice Association of America
228 Seventh Street, SE
Washington, DC 20003
Tel: (202) 546-4759
Fax: (202) 547-9559
Web site: www.hospice-america.org

Hospice Education Institute
3 Unity Square, PO Box 98
Machiasport, ME 04655
Tel: (207) 255-8800
Fax: (207) 255-8000
Toll Free for Publications:
(800) 331-1620
Hospice Link Referral Service—Toll
Free: (800) 331-1620
Web site: www.hospiceworld.org
E-Mail: info@hospiceworld.org

Hospice Foundation of America
2001 S Street NW, Suite 300
Washington, DC 20009
Tel: (202) 638-5419
Toll Free: (800) 854-3402
Fax: (202) 638-5312
Web site:
www.hospicefoundation.org
E-Mail: hfa@hospicefoundation.org

The Last Acts Campaign
Barksdale Ballard & Co.
1951 Kidwell Drive, Suite 205
Vienna, VA 22182
Tel: (703) 827-8771
Fax: (703) 827-0783
Web site: www.lastacts.org

Life With Dignity
1744 Riggs Place NW Suite 300
Washington, DC 20009
Tel: (202) 986-0118
Web site: www.lifewithdignity.org
E-Mail: lwdfdn@aol.com

National Hospice and Palliative Care
Organization
1700 Diagonal Road, Suite 625
Alexandria, VA 22314
Tel: (703) 837-1500
Fax: (703) 837-1233
Web site: www.nhpco.org
E-Mail: nhpco_info@nhpco.org

EDUCATION

Association for Gerontology in
Higher Education
1030 15th Street, NW, Suite 240
Washington, DC 20005-1503
Tel: (202) 289-9806
Fax: (202) 289-9824
Web site: www.aghe.org

Association of American Medical
Colleges
2450 N Street, NW
Washington, DC 20037-1126
Tel: (202) 828-0400
Fax: (202) 828-1125
Web site: www.aamc.org
Email: rsherrod@aamc.org

LEGAL ISSUES AND ELDER ABUSE

Legal Services for the Elderly
130 West 42nd Street, 17th Floor
New York, NY 10036
Tel: (212) 391-0120
Fax: (212) 719-1939
E-Mail: hn4923@handsnet.org

National Academy of Elder Law
Attorneys
1604 North Country Club Road
Tucson, AZ 85716
Tel: (520) 881-4005
Fax: (520) 325-7925
Web site: www.naela.org
E-Mail: info@naela.com

National Center on Elder Abuse
A consortium of the following six
partners with NASUA the lead
agency:
National Association of State Units
on Aging (NASUA)
Commission on Legal Problems of
the Elderly of the American Bar
Association (ABA)
The Clearinghouse on Abuse and
Neglect of the Elderly of the
University of Delaware CANE)
The San Francisco Consortium for
Elder Abuse Prevention of the
Goldman Institute on Aging
(GIOA)
The National Association of Adult
Protective Services Administrators
(NAAPSA)
The National Committee to Prevent
Elder Abuse (NCPEA)
1201 15th Street, NW, Suite 350
Washington, DC 20005
Tel: (202) 898-2586
Fax: (202) 898-2583
Web site: www.elderabusecenter.org
E-Mail: ncea@nasua.org

National Association of State Units
on Aging
1201 15th Street, Suite 350
Washington, DC 20005
Tel: (202) 898-2578
Fax: (202) 898-2583
Web site: www.nasua.org
E-Mail: info@nasua.org

National Clearinghouse on Elder
Abuse (Literature)
University of Delaware
College of Human Resources,
Education and Public Policy
Department of Consumer Studies
211 Allison Annex
Newark, DE 19716
Tel: (302) 831-3525
Fax: (302) 831-6081

National Committee for Prevention
of Elder Abuse (Research)
Institute on Aging
UMASS Memorial Health Care
119 Belmont Street
Worcester, MA 01605
Tel: (508) 334-6166
Fax: (508) 334-6906
Web site:
www.preventelderabuse.org

National Senior Citizens Law
Center
1101 14th Street, NW, Suite 400
Washington, DC 20005
Tel: (202) 289-6976
Fax: (202) 289-7224
Web site: www.nsclc.org
E-Mail: nsclc@nsclc.org

RESOURCES ON SPECIFIC HEALTH PROBLEMS

Cancer

American Cancer Society, Inc.
National Headquarters
1599 Clifton Road, NE
Atlanta, GA 30329
Tel: (404) 320-3333
Fax: (404) 329-5787
Toll Free National Cancer
Information Center:
(800) 227-2345
Web site: www.cancer.org

National Cancer Institute
Public Inquiries Office
Building 31, Room 10A31
31 Center Drive, MSC 2580
Bethesda, MD 20892-2580
Tel: (301) 435-3848
Toll Free: (800) 4-CANCER
(422-6237)
Web site: www.nci.nih.gov
E-Mail: cancergovstaff@mail.nih.gov

Complementary and Alternative Medicine

Department of Health and Human
Services, Public Health Service
Healthfinder
PO Box 1133
Washington, DC 20013-1133
Web site: www.healthfinder.gov
E-Mail: healthfinder@nhic.org

The Evidence-Based
Complementary and Alternative
Web site for Health Care
Professionals
19 Russell Street
Toronto, ON M5S 2S2
Fax: (416) 978-1833
Web site: www.camline.org
E-Mail: cam.line@utoronto.ca

HerbMed by the Alternative
Medicine Foundation, Inc.
PO Box 60016
Potomac, MD 20859
Tel: (301) 340-1960
Fax: (301) 340-1936
Web site: www.herbmed.org
Email: info@amfoundation.org

National Center for Complementary
and Alternative Medicine
NCCAM Clearinghouse
PO Box 7923
Gaithersburg, MD 20898
Toll Free: (888) 644-6226
Tel: (301) 519-3153
TTY: (866) 464-3615
Fax: (866) 464-3616
Web site: www.nccam.nih.gov
E-Mail: info@nccam.nih.gov

Natural Medicines Comprehensive
Database
3120 W. March Lane
PO Box 8190
Stockton, CA 95208
Tel: (209) 472-2244
Fax: (209) 472-2249

WebMD Inc.
Corporate Headquarters
669 River Drive
Elmwood Park, NJ 07407
Tel: (201) 703-3400
Fax: (201) 703-3401
Web site: www.WebMD.com

Diabetes Mellitus

American Diabetes Association
Attn: Customer Service
1701 North Beauregard Street
Alexandria, VA 22311
Tel: (703) 549-1500
Fax: (703) 549-6995
Toll Free: (800) DIABETES
(232-3472)
Web site: www.diabetes.org
E-Mail:
customerservice@diabetes.org

National Diabetes Information
Clearinghouse
1 Information Way
Bethesda, MD 20892-3560
Tel: (301) 654-3327 or
(800) 860-8747
Fax: (301) 907-8906
Web site: www.niddk.nih.gov
E-Mail: ndic@info.niddk.nih.gov

Digestive Problems

American Liver Foundation
75 Maiden Lane, Suite 603
New York, NY 10038
Toll Free: (800) GO LIVER
(465-4837)
Web site: www.liverfoundation.org
E-Mail: info@liverfoundation.org

National Digestive Disease
Information Clearinghouse
2 Information Way
Bethesda, MD 20892-3570
Tel: (301) 654-3810 or
(800) 891-5389
Fax: 703-738-4929
Web site: www.niddk.nih.gov
E-Mail: nddic@info.niddk.nih.gov

United Ostomy Association
19772 MacArthur Boulevard
Suite 200
Irvine, CA 92612-2405
Tel: (949) 660-8624
Fax: (949) 660-9262
Toll Free: (800) 826-0826
Web site: www.uoa.org
E-Mail: info@uoa.org

Head and Neck Problems

American Academy of
Otolaryngology—Head and Neck
Surgery, Inc.
1 Prince Street
Alexandria, VA 22314-3357
Tel: (703) 836-4444
Fax: (703) 683-5100
TTY: (703) 519-1585
Web site: www.entnet.org

American Council for Headache
Education
19 Mantua Road
Mt. Royal, NJ 08061
Tel: (856) 423-0258
Toll Free: (800) 255-ACHE (2243)
Fax: (856) 423-0082
Web site: www.achenet.org
E-Mail: achehg@talley.com

American Dental Association
211 East Chicago Avenue
Chicago, IL 60611
Tel: (312) 440-2500
Fax: (312) 440-2800
Web site: www.ada.org

American Society for Geriatric
Dentistry
401 North Michigan Avenue
Chicago, IL 60611
Tel: (312) 527-6764
Fax: (312) 673-6663
Web site: www.foscod.org
E-Mail: SCD@SCDonline.org

National Headache Foundation
428 West St. James Place, 2nd
Floor
Chicago, IL 60614-2750
Tel: (773) 388-6399
Toll Free: (888) NHF-5552
Fax: (773) 525-7357
Web site: www.headaches.org
E-Mail: info@headaches.org

National Institute of Dental &
Craniofacial Research
National Institute of Health
Bethesda, MD 20892-2190
Tel: (301) 496-4261
Fax: (301) 496-9988
Web site: www.nidcr.nih.gov
E-Mail: nidcrinfo@mail.nih.gov

Hearing Problems

American Tinnitus Association
65 SW Yamhill Street
Portland, OR 97204
Tel: (503) 248-9985
Fax: (503) 248-0024
Toll Free: (800) 634-8978
Web site: www.ata.org
E-Mail: tinnitus@ata.org

Better Hearing Institute
515 King Street, Suite 420
Alexandria, VA 22314
Toll Free: (800) EARWELL
(327-9355) or (703) 684-3391
Fax: (703) 750-9302
Web site: www.betterhearing.org
E-Mail: mail@betterhearing.org

International Hearing Society
16880 Middlebelt Road, Suite 4
Livonia, MI 48154
Tel: (734) 522-7200
Fax: (734) 522-0200
Toll Free Hearing Aid
Helpline: (800) 521-5247
Web site: www.ihsinfo.org

National Institute on Deafness and
Other Communication Disorders
National Institute of Health
31 Center Drive, MSC 2320
Bethesda, MD 20892-2320
Tel: (301) 496-7243
Fax: (301) 402-0018
Toll Free NIDCD Information
Clearinghouse: (800) 241-1044
Web site: www.nidcd.nih.gov
E-Mail: nidcdinfo@nidcd.nih.gov

Self Help for Hard of Hearing
People
7910 Woodmont Avenue, Suite
1200
Bethesda, MD 20814
Tel: (301) 657-2248
Fax: (301) 913-9413
TTY: (301) 657-2249
Web site: www.shhh.org
E-Mail: national@shhh.org

Heart and Circulation Problems

American Association of
Cardiovascular and Pulmonary
Rehabilitation
National Office
401 North Michigan Avenue, Suite
2200
Chicago, IL 60611
Tel: (312) 321-5146
Web site: www.aacvpr.org
E-Mail: aacvpr@smithbucklin.com

American Heart Association
7272 Greenville Avenue
Dallas, TX 75231
Tel: (214) 373-6300
Toll Free Tel: (800) 242-8721
Web site: www.americanheart.org
AHA's Stroke Connection:
(800) 553-6321

Courage Stroke Network
3915 Golden Valley Road
Golden Valley, MN 55422
Tel: (763) 520-0520 or
(800) 553-6321
Fax: (763) 520-0577

National Heart, Lung and Blood
Institute
Office of Prevention, Education and
Control
31 Center Drive, MSC 2480
Bethesda, MD 20892-2480
Tel: (301) 496-5437
Fax: (301) 402-2405
Web site: www.nhlbi.nih.gov
E-Mail: nhlbiinfo@nhlbi.nih.gov

National Institute of Neurological
Disorders and Stroke
NIH Neurological Institute
PO Box 5801
Bethesda, MD 20824
Toll Free: (800) 352-9424 or
(301) 496-5751
Web site: www.ninds.nih.gov

National Stroke Association
9707 E. Easter Lane
Englewood, CO 80112
Tel: (303) 649-9299
Fax: (303) 649-1328
Toll Free: (800) STROKES
(787-6537)
Web site: www.stroke.org

Joint, Muscle, and Bone Problems

American Academy of Orthopedic
Surgeons
6300 North River Road
Rosemont, IL 60018-4262
Tel: (847) 823-7186
Toll Free: (800) 346-AAOS (2267)
Fax: (847) 823-8125
Web site: www.aaos.org
E-Mail: custserv@aaos.org

American Podiatric Medical
Association
9312 Old Georgetown Road
Bethesda, MD 20814
Tel: (301) 571-9200
Fax: (301) 530-2752
Toll Free for Patient Education
Literature only: (800) FOOT-CARE
Web site: www.apma.org
E-Mail: askapma@apma.org

Arthritis Foundation
PO Box 7669
Atlanta, GA 30357
Tel: (404) 872-7100
Toll Free Information:
(800) 283-7800
Fax: (404) 872-0457
Web site: www.arthritis.org
E-Mail: help@arthritis.org

Lupus Foundation of America
2000 L Street, NW, Suite 710
Washington, DC 20036
Tel: (202) 349-1155
Toll Free Line for Information
Packet: English (800) 558-0121,
Spanish (800) 558-0231
Fax: (202) 349-1156
Web site: www.lupus.org

National Arthritis and
Musculoskeletal and Skin Diseases
Information Clearinghouse
National Institutes of Health
1 AMS Circle
Bethesda, MD 20892-3675
Tel: (301) 495-4484
Toll Free: (877) 22-NIAMS
(226-4267)
Fax: (301) 718-6366
Web site: www.nih.gov/niams
E-Mail: niamsinfo@mail.nih.gov

National Osteoporosis Foundation
1232 22nd Street NW
Washington, DC 20037-1292
Tel: (202) 223-2226
Fax: (202) 223-2237
Toll Free Info: (800) 223-9994
Web site: www.nof.org
E-Mail: customerservice@nof.org

Lung and Breathing Problems

American Association of
Cardiovascular and Pulmonary
Rehabilitation
401 North Michigan Avenue, Suite
2200
Chicago, IL 60611
Tel: (312) 321-5196
Web site: www.aacvpr.org
E-Mail: aacvpr@smithbucklin.com

American Lung Association
61 Broadway, 6th Floor
New York, NY 10019
Tel: (212) 315-8700
Fax: (212) 265-5642
Toll Free: (800) LUNG-USA
(800-586-4872)
Web site: www.lungusa.org
E-Mail: info@lungusa.org

National Heart, Lung and Blood
Institute
Office of Prevention, Education and
Control
31 Center Drive, MSC 2480
Bethesda, MD 20892-2480
Tel: (301) 496-5437
Fax: (301) 402-2405
Web site: www.nhlbi.nih.gov
E-Mail: nhlbiinfo@nhlbi.nih.gov

Memory and Thinking Problems

Alzheimer's Association
225 North Michigan Avenue
Floor 17
Chicago, IL 60601
Toll Free Information:
(800) 272-3900
Tel: (312) 335-8700
TTY: (312) 335-8882
Fax: (312) 335-1110
Web site: www.alz.org
E-Mail: info@alz.org
Safe Return Program
(identification tags, medical alert
bracelets): (888) 572-8566

Alzheimer's Disease Education and
Referral Center
PO Box 8250
Silver Spring, MD 20907-8250
Tel: (301) 495-3311
Fax: (301) 495-3334
Toll Free Information Service:
(800) 438-4380
Web site: www.alzheimers.org
E-Mail: adear@alzheimers.org

Neurologic Problems

American Academy of Neurology
1080 Montreal Avenue
St. Paul, MN 55116
Tel: (651) 695-2717 or
(800) 879-1960
Fax: (651) 695-2791
Web site: www.aan.com
E-Mail: memberservices@aan.com

American Parkinson's Disease
Association
1250 Hylan Boulevard
Suite 4B
Staten Island, NY 10305-1946
Tel: (718) 981-8001
Toll Free Information Hotline:
(800) 223-2732
Fax: (718) 981-4399
Web site: www.apdaparkinson.org
E-Mail: apda@apdaparkinson.org

Epilepsy Foundation of America
4351 Garden City Drive
Landover, MD 20785
Tel: (301) 459-3700
Toll Free Information & Referral:
(800) 332-1000
Fax: (301) 577-2684
Web site: www.efa.org

Huntington's Disease Society of
America
505 Eighth Avenue, Suite 902
New York, NY 10018
Tel: (212) 242-1968
Fax: (212) 239-3430
Toll Free Hotline: (800) 345-4372
Web site: www.hdsa.org
E-Mail: hdsainfo@hdsa.org

National Institute of Neurological
Disorders and Stroke
NIH Neurological Institute
PO Box 5801
Bethesda, MD 20824
Toll Free: (800) 352-9424 or
(301) 496-5751
Web site: www.ninds.nih.gov
(for other stroke information, see
Heart & Circulation)

Parkinson's Disease Foundation
1359 Broadway, Suite 1509
New York, NY 10018
Tel: (212) 923-4700
Toll Free: (800) 457-6676
Fax: (212) 923-4778
Web site: www.pdf.org
E-Mail: info@pdf.org

Nutritional Concerns

Food and Nutrition Information
Center
US Department of Agriculture
National Agriculture Library
Building
10301 Baltimore Avenue
Room 304
Beltsville, MD 20705-2351
Tel: (301) 504-5719
Fax: (301) 504-6409
Web site:
http://www.nal.usda.gov/fnic
E-Mail: fnic@nal.usda.gov

Meals On Wheels Association of
America
203 S. Union Street
Alexandria, VA 2231
Tel: (703) 548-5558
Fax: (703) 548-8024
Web site: www.mowaa.org
E-Mail: mowaa@tbq.dqsys.com

Pain

American Chronic Pain Association
PO Box 850
Rocklin, CA 95677
Tel: (916) 632-0922
Fax: (916) 632-3208
Web site: www.theacpa.org
E-Mail: acpa@pacbell.net

American Geriatrics Society
The Empire State Building
350 Fifth Avenue, Suite 801
New York, NY 10118
Tel: (212) 308-1414
Fax: (212) 832-8646
Web site:
www.americangeriatrics.org
E-Mail:
info.amger@americangeriatrics.org

American Pain Society
4700 West Lake Avenue
Glenview, IL 60025
Tel: (847) 375-4715
Fax: (847) 375-7777
Web site: www.ampainsoc.org
E-Mail: info@ampainsoc.org

City of Hope Pain Resource Center
City of Hope National Medical
Center
Dept. of Nursing Research &
Education
1500 East Duarte Road
Duarte, CA 91010
Tel: (626) 359-8111 ext. 3829
Web site: www.cityofhope.org
E-Mail: media@coh.org

National Chronic Pain Outreach
Association
PO Box 274
Millboro, VA 24460-9606
Tel: (540) 862-9437
Fax: (540) 862-9485
Email: ncpoa@cfw.com
Web site: www.chronicpain.org

Psychological Problems

American Association for Geriatric
Psychiatry
7910 Woodmont Avenue, Suite
1050
Bethesda, MD 20814-3004
Tel: (301) 654-7850
Fax: (301) 654-4137
Web site: www.aagpgpa.org
E-Mail: main@aagpgpa.org

National Alliance for the
Mentally Ill
Colonial Place Three
2107 Wilson Blvd.
Suite 300
Arlington, VA 22201-3042
Tel: (703) 524-7600
Fax: (703) 524-9094
Toll Free: (800) 950-6264
Web site: www.nami.org

National Institute of Mental Health
Information Resources & Inquiries
6001 Executive Blvd., Room 8184,
MSC 9663
Bethesda, MD 20892-9663
Tel: (301) 443-4513
Fax: (301) 443-5158
Web site: www.nimh.nih.gov
E-Mail: nimhinfo@nih.gov

National Mental Health Association
2001 N. Beauregard Street, 12th
Floor
Alexandria, VA 22311
Tel: (703) 684-7722
Fax: (703) 684-5968
Toll Free Information:
(800) 969-NMHA (6642)
Web site: www.nmha.org

Sexuality and Sexual Concerns

American College of Obstetricians
and Gynecologists
409 12th Street, SW PO Box
96920
Washington, DC 20090-6920
Tel: (202) 638-5577
Fax: (202) 484-1595
Web site: www.acog.com
E-Mail: resources@acog.org

American Urological Association
1000 Corporate Boulevard
Linthicum, MD 21090
Tel: (410) 689-3700 or (866)
RING AUA (746-4282)
Fax: (410) 689-3800
Web site: www.auanet.org
E-Mail: aua@auanet.org or
executiveadministration@auanet.org

Hysterectomy Educational
Resources and Services Foundation
422 Bryn Mawr Avenue
Bala Cynwyd, PA 19004
Tel: (610) 667-7757
Fax: (610) 667-8096
Web site: www.hersfoundation.com
E-Mail: HERSFdn@earthlink.net

Sexuality Information and
Education Council of the
United States
130 West 42nd Street, Suite 350
New York, NY 10036
Tel: (212) 819-9770
Fax: (212) 819-9776
Web site: www.siecus.org
E-Mail: siecus@siecus.org

Sight Problems

American Academy of
Ophthalmology
PO Box 7424
San Francisco, CA 94120
Tel: (415) 561-8500
Fax: (415) 561-8533
Toll Free: (800) 222-3937
Web site: www.eyenet.org
E-Mail: comm@aao.org

American Foundation for the Blind
11 Penn Plaza, Suite 300
New York, NY 10001
Tel: (212) 502-7600
Toll Free: (800) AFB LINE
(232-5463)
Fax: (212) 502-7777
Web site: www.afb.org
E-Mail: afbinfo@afb.net

American Optometric Association
243 North Lindbergh Blvd.
St. Louis, MO 63141
Tel: (314) 991-4100
Fax: (314) 991-4101
Toll Free: (800) 365-2219
Web site: www.aoanet.org

Better Vision Institute
1700 Diagonal Road, Suite 500
Arlington, VA 22314
Tel: (703) 548-4560
Toll Free: (800) 642-3253
Fax: (703) 548-4580
Web site: www.visionsite.org
E-Mail: vca@visionsite.org

Foundation for Glaucoma Research
490 Post Street, Suite 1472
San Francisco, CA 94104
Tel: (415) 986-3162 or
(800) 826-6693
Fax: (415) 986-3763
Web site: www.glaucoma.org or
info@glaucoma.org

National Eye Institute
Information Office
2020 Vision Place
Bethesda, MD 20892-3655
Tel: (301) 496-5248
Fax: (301) 402-1065
Web site: www.nei.nih.gov
E-Mail: 2020@nei.nih.gov

Prevent Blindness America
211 West Wacker Drive, Suite 1700
Chicago, IL 60606
Toll Free: (800) 331-2020
Web site: www.preventblindness.org
E-Mail: info@preventblindness.org

Skin Problems

American Academy of Dermatology
1350 First St., NW, Suite 870
Washington, DC 20005-2355
Tel: (202) 842-3555
Toll Free: (888) 462-DERM (3376)
Fax: (202) 842-4355
Web site: www.aad.org
E-Mail: yurbikas@aad.org

American Academy of Facial Plastic
and Reconstructive Surgery
310 South Henry Street
Alexandria, VA 22314
Tel: (703) 299-9291
Fax: (703) 299-8898
Toll Free: (800) 332-FACE
Web site: www.aafprs.org
E-Mail: info@aafprs.org

American Social Health Association
Herpes Resource Center
PO Box 13827
Research Triangle Park, NC 27709
Tel: (919) 361-8400
Fax: (919) 361-8425
Web site: http://www.ashastd.org
E-Mail: phidra@ashastd.org

National Arthritis and
Musculoskeletal and Skin Diseases
Information Clearinghouse
National Institutes of Health
1 AMS Circle
Bethesda, MD 20892-3675
Tel: (301) 495-4484
Toll Free: (877) 22-NIAMS
(226-4267)
Fax: (301) 718-6366
Web site: www.nih.gov/niams
E-Mail: niamsinfo@mail.nih.gov

The Skin Cancer Foundation
245 5th Avenue, Suite 1403
New York, NY 10016
Tel: (212) 725-5176
Toll Free: (800) SKIN-490
(754-6490)
Fax: (212) 725-5751
Web site: www.skincancer.org
E-Mail: info@skincancer.org

Urinary Problems

National Association for Continence
(NAFC)
PO Box 1019
Charleston, SC 29402
Tel: (843) 377-0900
Toll Free: (800) BLADDER
(252-3337)
Fax: (843) 377-0905
Web site: www.nafc.org
E-Mail: memberservices@nafc.org

National Kidney and Urologic
Diseases Information Clearinghouse
3 Information Way
Bethesda, MD 20892-3560
Tel: (800) 891-5390
Fax: (703) 738-4929
Web site: www.niddk.nih.gov
E-Mail: nkudic@info.niddk.nih.gov

National Kidney Foundation
30 East 33rd Street
Suite 1100
New York, NY 10016
Tel: (212) 889-2210
Toll Free: (800) 622-9010
Fax: (212) 689-9261
Web site: www.kidney.org
E-Mail: info@kidney.org

The Simon Foundation for
Continence
PO Box 815
Wilmette, IL 60091
Tel: (847) 864-3913
Toll Free: (800) 23-SIMON
(237-4666)
Fax: (847) 864-9758
Web site: www.simonfoundation.org
E-Mail:
simoninfo@simonfoundation.org

NORMAL LABORATORY VALUES*
FOR BLOOD, PLASMA, AND SERUM CHEMISTRIES, HEMATOLOGY, AND URINE
Referenced in the Questions and Critiques

BLOOD, PLASMA, SERUM CHEMISTRIES

Aminotransferase, alanine (ALT, SGPT)   0–35 U/L

Aminotransferase, aspartate (AST, SGOT)   0–35 U/L

Bicarbonate (CO_2)   21–30 mEq/L

Blood gas studies:

  PO_2 83–108 mm Hg

  PCO_2 Female: 32–45 mm Hg; Male: 35–48 mm Hg

  pH   7.35–7.45

  Oxygen saturation   95%–98%

Calcium   8.8–10.3 mg/dL

Calcium, ionized   4.5–5.6 mEq/L

Carcinoembryonic antigen   < 2.5 ng/mL

Chloride   98–106 mEq/L

Cholesterol:

  Total   Recommended: < 200 mg/dL; Moderate risk: 200–239 mg/dL; High risk: ≥ 240 mg/dL

  High-density lipoprotein (HDL)   Female: < 35 mg/dL; Male: < 29 mg/dL

  Low-density lipoprotein (LDL)   Recommended: < 130 mg/dL; Moderate risk: 130–159 mg/dL; High risk: ≥ 160 mg/dL

Creatinine   0.7–1.5 mg/dL

Creatine kinase   Female: 26–140 U/L; Male: 38–174 U/L

Digoxin (therapeutic level)   0.8–2.0 ng/mL

Folate   2.2–17.3 ng/mL

Glucose   Fasting: 70–105 mg/dL; 2-h postprandial: < 140 mg/dL

Iron   50–150 µg/dL

Iron-binding capacity, total   250–450 µg/dL

Lactate dehydrogenase   60–100 U/L

Magnesium   1.8–3.0 mg/dL

Parathyroid hormone   10–65 pg/mL

Phosphatase, acid   0.5–5.5 U/L

Phosphatase, alkaline   20–135 U/L

Phosphorus (age 60 and over)   Female: 2.8–4.1 mg/dL; Male: 2.3–3.7 mg/dL

Potassium   3.5–5 mEq/L

Prostate-specific antigen   < 4 ng/mL, normal; > 10 ng/mL, abnormal; 4–10 ng/mL, equivocal

Protein, total   6.4–8.3 g/dL

  Albumin   3.5–5.5 g/dL

  Globulin   2.0–3.5 g/dL

Rheumatoid factor, latest test   > 1:80 is abnormal

Sodium   136–145 mEq/L

Testosterone:

  Women   < 3.5 nmol/L

  Men   10–35 nmol/L

Thyrotropin (TSH)   0.5–5.0 µU/mL

Thyroxine (T_4)   Total, 5–12 µg/dL; free, 0.9–2.4 ng/dL

Triglycerides   Recommended: < 250 mg/dL

Urea nitrogen (BUN)   8–20 mg/dL

Uric acid   2.5–8.0 mg/dL

Vitamin B_{12} 190–900 pg/mL

HEMATOLOGY

Erythrocyte count   Female: 4.2–5.4 × 10^6/µL; Male: 4.7–6.1× 10^6/µL

Erythrocyte sedimentation rate (Westergren)   0–35 mm/h

Ferritin   Female: 10–120 ng/mL; Male: 20–150 ng/mL

Hematocrit   Female: 33%–43%; Male: 39%–49%

Hemoglobin   Female: 11.5–15.5 g/dL; Male: 14.0–18.0 g/dL

Hemoglobin A_{1c} 5.3%–7.5%

Leukocyte count and differential   4800–10,800/µL; 54%–62% segmented neutrophils, 3%–5% band forms, 23%–33% lymphocytes, 3%–7% monocytes, 1%–3% eosinophils, < 1% basophils

Mean corpuscular hemoglobin   28–32 pg

Mean corpuscular volume   86–98 fL (86–98 mm^3)

Platelet count   150,000–450,000/µL

URINE

Creatinine clearance   90–140 mL/min

Creatinine, urine   Female: 11–20 mg/kg per 24 h; Male: 14–26 mg/kg per 24 h

Urine, postvoid residual volume   < 50 mL, normal; > 200 mL, abnormal; 50–200 mL, equivocal

---

* Note: As normal ranges vary among laboratories, data in this table may not conform with all laboratories' data.

QUESTIONS

Directions: Each of the questions or incomplete statements below is followed by four or five suggested answers or completions. Select the ONE answer or completion that is BEST in each case and circle or place an "X" through the letter you have selected for each answer on the answer sheet. Answer sheets for self-assessment are available to download at: http://www.americangeriatrics.org/products/gnrs_2.shtml. The repeated questions with answers and supporting critiques are located on p 505. The table of Normal Laboratory Values on the facing page may be consulted for any of the questions in this book.

1. A 76-year-old woman comes to the office for follow-up evaluation of hypertension. Her blood pressure was 148/82 mm Hg at a recent examination. She returned for repeat measurements on two occasions; the average of all these readings is 146/83 mm Hg. She is in good general health and has no history or evidence of coronary artery disease or diabetes mellitus. Her current medications are a daily multivitamin and a calcium supplement. She lives alone, eats out frequently, and does not participate in a regular exercise program. She does not smoke or consume alcohol.

   Evaluation to date has not identified a secondary cause for hypertension. She is obese (BMI [kg/m^2] = 31), and her waist circumference is 92 cm.
   Laboratory studies:
   Fasting glucose   115 mg/dL
   Total cholesterol   220 mg/dL
   High-density lipoprotein 42 mg/dL
   Triglycerides   200 mg/dL

   Which of the following is most appropriate regarding management of her hypertension?

   (A) Recommend lifestyle interventions for 6 months.
   (B) Begin a β-blocker.
   (C) Begin a thiazide-type diuretic.
   (D) Begin an angiotensin-converting enzyme inhibitor.
   (E) Begin a calcium channel blocker.

2. A 78-year-old thin woman comes to the office because she has acute lower back pain that began when she tried to open a stuck window. The pain is so severe that she has difficulty standing or sitting. The pain lessens when she lies down, and increases when she rolls to the side. The pain does not radiate to her legs.

   On physical examination, there is marked tenderness in the mid-lumbar spine area and moderate paravertebral muscle spasm in the lumbar region. Bilateral straight leg raise tests are normal. She has full motor strength of the proximal and distal muscles of both lower legs.

   Radiography of the lumbar spine shows diffuse disk space narrowing and vertebral osteophytosis throughout the lumbar region.

   What is the most likely diagnosis?

   (A) Herniated lumbar disk at L-4, L-5
   (B) Instability of the lumbar spine
   (C) Lumbar spinal stenosis
   (D) Vertebral compression fracture
   (E) Ruptured abdominal aortic aneurysm

3. A 72-year-old woman is brought to the office by her daughter, with whom she lives. The patient has asthma. The daughter has just been diagnosed with influenza, by a nasal swab antigen test. The mother has consistently refused to get the influenza vaccine because she says she "always got the flu from the shot," but she agrees to be immunized now.

   In addition to immunization, prophylaxis using which of the following would best prevent influenza in this patient?

   (A) Amantadine
   (B) Rimantadine
   (C) Oseltamivir
   (D) Zanamivir

4. An 80-year-old man has hypertension, heart failure, osteoarthritis, and visual and hearing impairments. He is enrolled in the traditional Medicare Parts A and B programs and is considering taking out a supplemental insurance policy.

Which of the following services are not covered under traditional Medicare Parts A and B and should be considered by a patient when selecting supplemental insurance?

(A) Cataract surgery
(B) Cochlear implant
(C) Hearing aid
(D) Diagnostic audiogram
(E) Evaluation by an ophthalmologist

5. A 79-year-old patient comes to the office at the insistence of family members who believe that she has been behaving differently over the past 2 years. She is a college-educated former teacher who has been retired for 10 years and lives with her husband. She has a history of well-controlled hypertension, mild macular degeneration, and mild osteoarthritis. She used to play golf and bridge, but now she seems less interested in these activities and is less social with family and friends. Her family reports that she takes initiative less often than before and is more easily distracted once she starts an activity. She now occasionally says things, such as criticizing family members, which surprise and concern her family. The patient says that she is fine and has no complaints. When asked about the symptoms her family describes, she answers that sometimes she does not want to do things as often as before, but that she still enjoys playing golf and bridge. She denies any depressive symptoms. Physical examination, including a complete neurologic examination, is within normal limits. Her score on the Mini–Mental State Examination is 29 of 30.

Which of the following is the most appropriate next step?

(A) Reassure the patient and family that her function is appropriate for her age.
(B) Obtain neuroimaging.
(C) Order formal neuropsychologic testing.
(D) Have the patient return in 2 weeks for repeat testing.

6. An 87-year-old woman is admitted to your service at a skilled nursing facility. She has an ischemic cardiomyopathy with a left ventricular ejection fraction of 15% and a progressive dementia. She does not understand her condition or the possible outcomes with treatments and therefore lacks decisional capacity.

She has no advance directives. She has outlived most of her friends, was never married, and has no children, although she does have a niece. The niece, although caring, has never discussed illness or end-of-life decisions with her aunt. You do know that the patient was combative with hospital care, needing both chemical and physical restraints during the hospitalization prior to this admission. You are discussing care options with the niece. You have told her, considering her aunt's cardiac and functional level, that attempting resuscitation would be a relatively futile procedure, and on this basis she has agreed with a do-not-attempt-resuscitation–do-not-intubate order. You then turn the conversation to the available treatment options for an exacerbation of her aunt's heart failure. You give her the option of sending her aunt to the hospital or having her remain in the nursing home and receive the maximum monitoring, treatment, and palliation available in that setting.

In guiding the niece as to how she should make this decision, it is appropriate that you tell her which of the following?

(A) Look at the benefits and burdens of these treatments for all demented patients.
(B) Consult a lawyer before making this type of decision.
(C) Look at benefits and burdens of this intervention for her aunt.
(D) Use the substituted-judgment standard.

7. A 71-year-old woman just moved to an assisted living facility. Her husband died 8 months ago, and she recently moved to the city to be near her daughter. She has a 45-year history of generalized anxiety disorder, for which she has taken diazepam 10 mg daily for the past 30 years. She asks for a prescription to continue the diazepam.

Which of the following is most appropriate at this time?

(A) Continue diazepam.
(B) Immediately discontinue diazepam.
(C) Substitute buspirone for diazepam.
(D) Substitute venlafaxine for diazepam.

8. A 72-year-old man moves into an assisted living facility. Results of his initial examination are normal except for hypertension and he has no symptoms.

Laboratory studies:

Hemoglobin	12.0 g/dL
Mean corpuscular volume	90.0 fL
Mean corpuscular hemoglobin	90.0 pg/cell
Serum protein	9.5 g/dL (elevated)
Serum immunoglobulins	
IgG	2500 mg/L (elevated)
IgA	230 mg/dL (normal)
IgM	150 mg/dL (normal)
Serum protein electrophoresis	monoclonal M spike

Bone marrow biopsy reveals 8% plasma cells. Skeletal survey is normal.

What is the most appropriate management now?

(A) Reassessment in 1 year
(B) Chemotherapy
(C) Radiation therapy
(D) Bone marrow transplantation

9. A 94-year-old woman who lives in a nursing home is referred for evaluation of increasing lower extremity edema. The patient has a history of coronary artery disease, including two myocardial infarctions and coronary artery bypass at age 79, and she has type 2 diabetes mellitus, hypertension, moderate Alzheimer's disease, depression, and severe osteoarthritis of both hips. She has an indwelling Foley catheter for urinary incontinence. Over the past few weeks, the nursing-home staff has noted progressive swelling of both legs up to the level of the mid-thigh. The patient is wheelchair bound and requires assistance with most activities. Current medications include aspirin, lisinopril, furosemide, metformin, nortriptyline, donepezil, and haloperidol. Additional history is fragmentary, but the nursing-home staff reports no recent complaints of chest pain or shortness of breath. The patient's living will specifies no cardiopulmonary resuscitation and no artificial life support.

On physical examination, the patient is frail, alert, pleasant, and oriented only to name. She responds to questions but with inconsistent answers. Heart rate is 84 per minute and regular, blood pressure is 130/70 mm Hg, and respiratory rate is 18 per minute. There is no jugular venous distention. A few bibasilar crackles are heard. She has a regular, grade I-II/IV systolic murmur and an S_4, with no S_3. The abdomen is not tender and has no masses. There is moderate to marked edema to the level of the mid thigh bilaterally. She has no focal neurologic deficits.

Laboratory studies:

Hemoglobin	11.3 g/dL
Leukocyte count	5400/µL
Platelet count	217,000/µL
Creatinine	1.0 mg/dL
Blood urea nitrogen	24 mg/dL
Glucose	124 mg/dL
Serum electrolytes	normal
Albumin	3.4 g/dL
Liver enzymes	mildly elevated

Which of the following is the most appropriate approach to managing this patient's edema?

(A) Obtain a B-type natriuretic peptide level and an echocardiogram.
(B) Obtain a plasma D-dimer level and lower extremity venous Doppler ultrasonography.
(C) Apply bilateral lower extremity pneumatic compression device.
(D) Apply support stockings and elevate her legs.
(E) Restrict dietary sodium moderately and increase diuretic dosage.

10. A 73-year-old black man comes to the office with a painless lesion on his left heel. He states that the lesion has slowly been getting bigger, but he is not sure how long he has had it. He does not recall trauma and reports no drainage or bleeding. History includes chronic venous insufficiency with venous stasis ulcers and osteoarthritis of the knees. He ambulates with a four-point cane. When he watches television, he sits in a recliner to keep his legs elevated. On examination, his left plantar heel has a firm, black raised plaque with irregular margins. It measures 4.5 × 3.7 cm. The patient has 1+ pulses bilaterally and normal sensation.

Which of the following is the most appropriate next step?

(A) Radiography of the foot
(B) Shave biopsy of the lesion
(C) Incisional biopsy of the lesion
(D) Arterial Doppler ultrasonography
(E) Bone scan

11. A 75-year-old man comes to the office because he has excessive daytime sleepiness and insomnia characterized by awakenings throughout the night. He also has disagreeable leg sensations during the day that are relieved only when he moves his legs. His partner confirms that the patient kicks frequently when he is asleep.

Which of the following treatments is most likely to help this patient?

(A) Ropinirole 0.25 mg at bedtime
(B) Celecoxib 200 mg at bedtime
(C) Mirtazapine 15 mg at bedtime
(D) Modafinil 100 mg twice daily
(E) Zolpidem 10 mg at bedtime

12. A 74-year-old man with a history of coronary artery disease had three-vessel coronary artery bypass 3 days ago. He was extubated on postoperative day 1. He now requires evaluation because he remains agitated despite chemical and physical restraints. He pulls at the oxygen tubing despite wrist restraints. Because of his confusion, ambulation has been limited and the Foley catheter is continued. Vital signs are normal. Recommendations include removal of the Foley catheter and obtaining a urinalysis and urine culture.

Which of the following may significantly reduce his agitation and promote resolution of the delirium?

(A) Limit mobility to chair transfers until delirium clears.
(B) Remove the wrist restraints.
(C) Place him in a geri-chair near the nurse's station.
(D) Assist with feeding.

13. A 75-year-old patient comes to the office for his annual check-up. He had complained of hearing loss for several years but until recently had declined to visit an audiologist because he did not think his hearing was bad enough. The audiology report indicates that he has a mild to moderate bilaterally symmetric sensorineural hearing loss with good word recognition scores. During today's interview, he does not seem to follow the discussion, even though he is wearing his new hearing aids. He states that he rarely uses the hearing aids because they do not seem to work in the situations that are most difficult for him. His wife agrees, but also mentions that he has not returned to the audiologist for his follow-up visit.

Which of the following is the most appropriate recommendation?

(A) Return to the audiologist for a hearing aid check, and counseling.
(B) Return these hearing aids to the audiologist to exchange for more effective aids.
(C) Substitute an assistive listening device for hearing aids in the situations that are most difficult for him.
(D) Schedule a cochlear implant evaluation.
(E) Screen for hearing handicap with the Hearing Handicap Inventory for the Elderly—Screening Version (HHIE–S)

14. In which of the following settings is the prevalence of depressive symptoms and diagnosable major depression highest?

(A) Community
(B) Outpatient medical clinic
(C) General hospital
(D) Long-term-care facility

15. Which of the following describes expected age-related changes in pulmonary function?

(A) Stable total lung capacity; decreased vital capacity, decreased forced vital capacity, decreased FEV_1, and increased residual volume
(B) Decreased total lung capacity, decreased forced vital capacity, decreased FEV_1, and decreased residual volume
(C) Increased total lung capacity, increased forced vital capacity, increased FEV_1, and increased residual volume
(D) Decreases in all volumes
(E) Decreased lung capacity, decreased residual volume, increased forced vital capacity, and increased FEV_1

16. A 68-year-old man comes to the office because of lower urinary symptoms associated with benign prostatic hyperplasia. He awakens once or twice each night to urinate; the frequency of his nocturia has increased gradually over the past 4 years. He has no other urinary tract symptoms. He has coronary heart disease that is well managed with metoprolol 100 mg and aspirin 81 mg daily.

On physical examination, blood pressure is 140/70 mm Hg, and pulse is 55 per minute. On digital rectal examination, the prostate is not enlarged, has no nodules, induration, or asymmetry. Prostate-specific antigen (PSA) level is 6 ng/mL (increased from 2.5 ng/mL at age 65 and 3 ng/mL at age 67).

What is the most appropriate next step in the evaluation of this patient?

(A) Remeasure the PSA level.
(B) Refer to a urologist for a prostate biopsy.
(C) Order a transrectal ultrasound.
(D) Order a bone scan.

17. On your monthly visit of an 85-year-old man in the nursing home, he feels well. He has a history of hypertension, stable kidney insufficiency, and coronary artery disease, with myocardial infarction 2 years ago (ejection fraction, 35%). He takes aspirin 81 mg daily, furosemide 20 mg twice daily, metoprolol 25 mg twice daily, and pravastatin 40 mg daily.

On examination, blood pressure is 165/79 mm Hg, consistent with readings over the past few visits.

Laboratory studies:
Sodium	137 mEq/L
Potassium	4.3 mEq/L
Urea nitrogen	25 mg/dL
Creatinine	2.3 mg/dL (stable)

Which of the following is the most appropriate intervention?

(A) Add lisinopril.
(B) Increase metoprolol.
(C) Substitute hydrochlorothiazide for furosemide.
(D) Add amlodipine.

18. A 69-year-old woman with mild mental retardation comes to the office with one of her residential caregivers, who describes gradually worsening anger, agitation, and isolation over the past 12 months. Approximately 6 months ago she began treatment with a selective serotonin-reuptake inhibitor, but her response has been negligible despite titration of the medication to the maximum recommended dose. She has no previous history of emotional or behavioral problems. She takes acetaminophen for mild pain due to degenerative arthritis, and she has bilateral cataracts but is reluctant to proceed with surgery.

She has enjoyed working in a noncompetitive setting for over 20 years, but this activity is now in jeopardy because her visual impairment interferes with the work. She has no supportive family and only a small network of peer friendships. She is her own guardian and has always been involved in decisions about her life and health.

Which of the following is the most appropriate next step in caring for this patient?

(A) Begin psychotherapy, focusing on helping her with health care decisions.
(B) Begin a medication to augment the antidepressant.
(C) Add an atypical antipsychotic agent to decrease her agitation.
(D) Arrange for neuropsychological testing.
(E) Discontinue the antidepressant and begin a medication for anxiety.

19. An 82-year-old woman who lives in a long-term-care facility is evaluated for agitation that occurs during the day and when she awakens from sleep. She has mild Alzheimer's dementia. She spends most of the day sitting in front of the television in a lounge with low lights, occasionally dozing off. The patient is mobile and fully participates in all basic activities of daily living. Review of her medications and physical examination reveal no apparent cause for the agitation. Mental status examination reveals only mild cognitive impairment.

Which of the following nonpharmacologic interventions is most likely to benefit this patient?

(A) Ask staff to exercise the patient twice daily.

(B) Ask staff to discourage the patient from watching television and to introduce nighttime diapers.

(C) Ask staff to keep the patient in a bright environment during the day and a quiet, dark environment at night without interruptions.

(D) Ask staff to prevent daytime napping and implement enforced sleeping hours, with restriction of evening fluid intake.

(E) Provide the patient with a soft nightlight, familiar items and photographs at the bedside, and orienting objects, such as a clock.

20. The primary care provider for a 79-year-old woman with advanced dementia is called by the police when the patient is found dead at home. She lived with her son, who had called paramedics when he discovered that she was not responsive. The paramedics found an elderly woman lying almost naked on her bed, and they were concerned about her appearance. They described a thin woman with feces on her buttocks and abdomen, elongated fingernails and toenails caked with dirt, two large pressure sores (stage IV on her buttock and stage III on her right shoulder), and matted, dirty hair.

It has been difficult to care for her. Her son always reported that she did not want him to bring her to the doctor, and she had refused a home-health aide when she was in an earlier stage of dementia. On her last visit to the office, 18 months ago, she was found to have lost a substantial amount of weight and was disheveled and somewhat dirty. Home-health care was initiated, but her son refused their services when they came to his house, saying that he was able to care for her and that she did not want anyone else to help.

For religious reasons, the son wants the death certificate signed as soon as possible so that she can be buried within 24 hours. The police request direction about what to do next. Which of the following is the most appropriate response?

(A) Request transport of the body to an emergency department for further evaluation.

(B) Sign the death certificate.

(C) Release the body to the mortuary and make a referral to Adult Protective Services.

(D) Request an evaluation by a coroner or medical examiner.

21. A 72-year-old black American woman cares for her 75-year-old black American husband with Alzheimer's disease in their own home.

Which of the following factors is the strongest predictor of whether the husband will be placed in a nursing home within the next year?

(A) The wife's age
(B) The husband's racial background
(C) The wife's racial background
(D) The husband's hallucinations and delusions
(E) The husband's dependence in one or more activities of daily living

22. A 75-year-old woman comes to the office because of pain and swelling of the right forefoot that have progressed over the past 3 weeks. She relates going on a 2-mile walk prior to the onset of symptoms. The symptoms began as a mild ache but have become increasingly intense with her usual walking. Two weeks ago she visited the local emergency department for the pain; radiographs demonstrated normal metatarsophalangeal joints and no fractures. She has tried nonsteroidal anti-inflammatory agents, ice, and warm compresses without relief.

On physical examination, vital signs are normal. She has good pedal pulses and normal sensation. The right foot is tender to palpation at the midshaft of the second metatarsal. There is no pain with range of motion to the second metatarsophalangeal joint. There is callus on the plantar aspect of the second metatarsophalangeal joint. Ankle joint range of motion is less than 5 degrees with maximal dorsiflexion. A moderate hallux valgus and bunion are present.

What is the most likely diagnosis?

(A) Stress fracture
(B) Gout
(C) Morton's neuroma
(D) Ganglion cyst
(E) Degenerative joint disease

23. A 75-year-old man returns to the office for a follow-up visit after a 6-week trial of St. John's wort 300 mg two to three times daily. At the initial visit, he met criteria for major depressive disorder but denied having recurrent thoughts of death or suicidal ideation. He has a history of hypertension, which is well controlled on a low-salt diet and hydrochlorothiazide 12.5 mg daily, and osteoarthritis, for which he occasionally takes acetaminophen. He has no history of mental health problems. He was reluctant to take a prescription antidepressant but suggested trying St. John's wort. At follow-up, there is no apparent improvement in his depression, and he now agrees to begin treatment with sertraline.

    Which of the following is the best recommendation with respect to the St. John's wort?

    (A) Continue St. John's wort and begin sertraline.
    (B) Discontinue St. John's wort and begin sertraline after 4 weeks.
    (C) Discontinue St. John's wort and begin sertraline the next day.
    (D) Discontinue St. John's wort and begin sertraline in 1 week.

24. An 82-year-old man is admitted with acute right upper quadrant pain and an impacted gall stone. An open cholecystectomy is planned once the patient has been stabilized and fully assessed.

    The patient resides at home with his wife. His past medical history includes: a 50-pack-per-year cigarette history and current smoking; chronic obstructive pulmonary disease for 5 years, stable on an ipratropium-albuterol metered-dose inhaler and occasional short courses of oral corticosteroids. He has no prior cardiac history and is taking no medications other than his pulmonary drugs.

    On physical examination he has a body mass index (kg/m^2) of 34, blood pressure 132/78 mm Hg, heart rate 88, respiratory rate 18; he is

afebrile. Lung examination shows distant breath sounds with end expiratory wheezes throughout both lung fields. The remainder of his examination is unremarkable.

Other assessments show:

FEV$_1$	30% of predicted
Electrocardiogram	normal
Chest x-ray	hyperlucent lung fields, no infiltrates, and no changes of the cardiac silhouette
Arterial blood gas (room air)	pH 7.42, PCO_2 48 mm Hg, PO_2 68 mm Hg, HCO_3 31 mEq/L
Blood urea nitrogen	34 mg/dL
Serum albumin	2.9 gm/dL

What conveys the greatest risk for postoperative respiratory failure in this patient?

(A) Age greater than 69 years
(B) History of chronic obstructive pulmonary disease
(C) Obesity
(D) Upper abdominal surgery
(E) Albumin less than 3.0 mg/dL

25. A 76-year-old man comes to the emergency department following the abrupt onset of rectal bleeding. He has a history of coronary heart disease, heart failure, renal insufficiency, gastroesophageal reflux disease, and degenerative joint disease. Daily medications include metoprolol, furosemide, potassium chloride, simvastatin, celecoxib, and lansoprazole. The bleeding stops spontaneously. Diagnostic colonoscopy, performed after oral cleansing with polyethylene glycol and electrolyte solution, demonstrates residual blood in the ascending colon, scattered diverticula in the sigmoid colon, and multiple, 5-mm, flat cherry-red lesions in the cecum.

    What is the most likely cause for bleeding in this patient?

    (A) Angiodysplasia
    (B) Nonspecific colitis
    (C) Aortoenteric fistula
    (D) Upper gastrointestinal lesion

26. An 81-year-old female resident of an assisted-living facility comes to the emergency department with complaints of fatigue, nausea, and frequent urination. She has a history of hypertension, osteoporosis with spine compression fractures, osteoarthritis, and macular degeneration. The patient has previously been independent in instrumental activities of daily living, except for medications, and she uses a walker for ambulation. She is admitted to an Acute Care for the Elderly (ACE) unit with urosepsis.

Which of the following is a component of this type of intervention?

(A) An environment that promotes mobility and orientation
(B) A care map to outline her current medications
(C) A protocol outlining the length of stay for urosepsis
(D) A discussion with her family about the need for restorative care
(E) A teaching session on health promotion interventions

27. The most commonly overlooked aspect of the care of patients with hip fracture on discharge from a subacute unit and arrival in the rehabilitation setting is:

(A) Deep-vein thrombosis prophylaxis
(B) Delirium prevention
(C) Osteoporosis treatment
(D) Nutritional support

28. A 70-year-old woman comes to the office for management of osteoporosis. She has a history of nephrolithiasis. She went through menopause approximately 18 years ago and takes the following medications: alendronate 70 mg weekly, calcium carbonate 1500 mg daily, and vitamin D 800 IU daily. She drinks three glasses of milk and several servings of yogurt and cheese daily. Her bone mineral density, as measured by dual energy x-ray absorptiometry (DEXA), reveals a T score of –3.0 at the hip and –2.5 at the lumbar spine.

Laboratory studies:
Ionized calcium	6.1 mEq/L
Phosphorus	2.7 mg/dL

Parathyroid hormone	62 pg/mL
Serum creatinine	0.9 mg/dL
Thyrotropin	2.1 µU/mL

What is the most likely cause of this patient's hypercalcemia?

(A) Primary hyperparathyroidism
(B) Milk-alkali syndrome
(C) Humoral hypercalcemia of malignancy
(D) Granulomatous disease

29. An 87-year old woman comes to the office because of short-term memory loss persisting for several months, which is getting worse according to her husband. She has some college education. She has a history of hypertension, which is well controlled with hydrochlorothiazide, 25 mg daily. She is otherwise in good health. She sleeps and eats normally and has no day-to-day problems except for occasional difficulty locating her car in the parking lot. Physical and neurologic examination reveal nothing remarkable. There is no evidence of sadness or anhedonia. She scores 25 of 30 points on the Mini–Mental State Examination, losing 3 points on recall and 2 on orientation.

What is the most likely cause of the memory complaint?

(A) Benign senescent forgetfulness
(B) Mild cognitive impairment
(C) Dementia
(D) Minor depression
(E) Major depression

30. A 68-year-old man comes to the office for follow-up management after external-beam radiation treatment to his prostate for a moderately differentiated adenocarcinoma (Gleason grades 3 and 4). Bone scan is negative for metastatic lesion. Before treatment, his prostate-specific antigen (PSA) level had increased from 3.0 to 21 over 3 years. After radiation treatment, his PSA level fell to 4.0, but over the next 6 months it increased to 7.0. He has begun combined androgen blockade with flutamide and leuprolide, as prescribed by his urologist.

Which of the following additional treatments might you discuss with the urologist to prevent metastatic disease?

(A) Orchiectomy
(B) Ketoconazole
(C) Zoledronic acid
(D) Cyclophosphamide

31. A 75-year-old woman comes to the office for a routine visit. She has a history of hypertension, osteoporosis, chronic obstructive pulmonary disease, osteoarthritis, and insomnia. Two months ago she began celecoxib 100 mg daily for arthritis and diphenhydramine at bedtime for sleep. Other medications include lisinopril 40 mg daily, hydrochlorothiazide 25 mg daily, salmeterol two inhalations twice daily, ipratropium three inhalations four times daily, atenolol 75 mg daily, calcium carbonate 500 mg three times daily, vitamin D 200 IU daily, alendronate 70 mg weekly, and a multivitamin daily.

    On examination, blood pressure is 178/92 mm Hg; this is consistent with home readings the patient has taken over the past month. At office visits 3 and 6 months ago, systolic blood pressure was between 148 and 152 mm Hg, and diastolic pressure was between 80 and 85 mm Hg.

    Which of the following is the most appropriate intervention?

    (A) Substitute furosemide for hydrochlorothiazide.
    (B) Substitute acetaminophen for celecoxib.
    (C) Increase atenolol.
    (D) Substitute ramipril for lisinopril.
    (E) Substitute zolpidem for diphenhydramine.

32. An 82-year-old nursing-home resident is hospitalized with pneumonia. She has a history of hypertension and is functionally impaired from a debilitating stoke. On admission, the nurses note her to be pleasant, alert, and oriented to person, place, and time. On examination on her second hospital day, vital signs are stable and physical examination is consistent with pneumonia and old stroke. She awakens when called by name but closes her eyes for prolonged periods during conversation. She complains of feeling tired and does not want to talk much. She is distracted by the voices in the hallway, so that questions must be repeated several times. She slurs her words more than

before and has significant difficulty with word finding. An antibiotic for the pneumonia is the only new medication.

Which of the following best explains her symptoms?

(A) Alzheimer's disease
(B) Dementia with Lewy bodies
(C) Delirium
(D) Depression
(E) Stroke

33. A 67-year-old man comes to the office with his family to obtain an additional medical opinion. He has lost 18.2 kg (40 lb) in the past 6 months, is weak, spends most of his time in bed, has given up participating in family activities, and is no longer interested in watching sporting events on television. His family is concerned that he has a serious, undiagnosed medical problem. He tends to sit quietly and let his family answer questions, but when pressed, he indicates that he cannot swallow solids or liquids because his throat is blocked. His family reports that he eats and drinks small amounts. He believes he has cancer that the doctors have yet to find. According to the medical records he provides, radiography and computed tomography of the chest are normal, and upper endoscopy is unremarkable. Several sets of blood work have been obtained, none of which indicate dehydration, anemia, or hepatic or renal dysfunction.

    Which of the following is the most likely explanation for these findings?

    (A) Occult lung cancer
    (B) Vascular dementia
    (C) Alzheimer's disease
    (D) Major depression with psychotic features
    (E) Panic disorder

34. The daughter of a 91-year-old patient who saw an article on the Internet requests a physical therapy referral for progressive resistance training to help her mother stay independent.

    Which of the following statements is true regarding progressive resistance training?

(A) Physical disability, as measured by standardized scales, will improve.
(B) Gains in strength are common.
(C) Health-related quality of life improves.
(D) Injury due to the exercises is rare.
(E) The patient's advanced age is a contraindication.

35. A 74-year-old man comes to the office because he has a 3-month history of generalized itching. The itching has worsened as the weather has gotten colder. The patient states that this happens every winter. History includes hypertension, for which he has taken lisinopril for the past 4 years. He does not take any other agents or over-the-counter medications. He has been using a moisturizing cream with little relief. On examination, there is diffuse skin involvement with dry scaling on the trunk and extremities. The shins resemble "cracked porcelain" with red fissures that form an irregular reticular pattern.

Which of the following is the most likely cause of the itching?

(A) Drug eruption
(B) Xerosis
(C) Scabies
(D) Psoriasis
(E) Contact dermatitis

36. Which of the following statements regarding calorie restriction is correct?

(A) Calorie restriction has been shown consistently to increase life span in mice.
(B) Animal studies have demonstrated positive effects of calorie restriction on fertility.
(C) Calorically restricted rodents, nonhuman primates, and healthy men demonstrate lower fasting insulin levels and lower body temperature.
(D) Calorie restriction is most beneficial when initiated late in life.
(E) Calorically restricted mice live longer, are more fit, and are more likely to reproduce than control mice with unlimited access to food.

37. A 69-year-old man comes to the office because of difficulty swallowing solids and liquids. The dysphagia has progressed slowly over 8 months,

and he has lost 20 pounds. He reports no pain. Barium radiograph demonstrates a narrowed distal esophageal segment 4.1 cm long and no dilated esophageal segment proximal to this narrowed portion. Esophageal manometry demonstrates failure of the lower esophageal sphincter to relax with swallowing, and aperistalsis of the esophageal body.

Which diagnostic procedure should be performed first?

(A) Esophagoscopy
(B) Endoscopic ultrasonography
(C) Computed tomography
(D) Chest magnetic resonance imaging
(E) Laparotomy

38. A preoperative medical consultation is requested for an obese 72-year-old man admitted for coronary artery bypass grafting scheduled for the next day. He has known three-vessel coronary artery disease. He has been complaining of a headache but is otherwise considered a good candidate for the procedure.

On examination, he has tenderness over the right temporal artery and a right carotid bruit. Laboratory studies reveal a Westergren sedimentation rate of 82 mm/hr. Giant cell (temporal) arteritis is suspected.

Which of the following is the most appropriate initial step?

(A) High-dose corticosteroids
(B) Etanercept
(C) Temporal artery biopsy
(D) Coronary artery bypass graft
(E) Methotrexate

39. An 88-year-old woman living in an assisted living facility comes to the office for a follow-up visit. She has poorly controlled stage 2 hypertension, gastroesophageal reflux disease, depression, and hypothyroidism. She has lived alone since her husband's death 2 years ago. Medications include hydrochlorothiazide 50 mg daily, lisinopril 10 mg twice daily, diltiazem 30 mg four times daily, esomeprazole 20 mg daily, citalopram 40 mg daily, levothyroxine 0.1 mg daily, and aspirin 81 mg daily. Metoprolol 50 mg twice daily was added to her regimen 2 months ago, when her blood-pressure reading

was 168/81 mm Hg. She has no new symptoms and has had no blood-pressure readings since her visit 2 months ago.

On physical examination, blood pressure is found to be 165/78 mm Hg and heart rate is 68 per minute. There are no orthostatic blood-pressure changes. She has grade 1 hypertensive retinopathy and a laterally displaced point of maximal impulse with an apical fourth heart sound. On a Mini-Mental State Examination, she recalls only 1 of 3 objects at 3 minutes and performs a normal clock-drawing test. She reports three positive responses on the Geriatric Depression Scale. Echocardiogram shows left ventricular hypertrophy. Recent laboratory studies demonstrate normal electrolytes and renal function (calculated creatinine clearance is 43 mL/min) and thyrotropin level of 3.8 μU/mL. Medications are set up in pill boxes for her and she has a visit from the nursing assistant at least three times a day for medication reminders. She takes these most of the time with these reminders. The nursing assistant also reports that she is drinking at least two glasses of wine daily.

Which of the following best explains the persistence of her poorly controlled blood pressure?

(A) Pseudohypertension
(B) Nonadherence to medication
(C) Alcohol intake
(D) Hyperaldosteronism
(E) Renovascular hypertension

40. An 89-year-old woman, recently admitted to a nursing facility, is found to be frequently incontinent of urine and occasionally incontinent of stool, on initial assessment for the Minimum Data Set. She has Alzheimer's disease and lumbosacral spinal stenosis and has been taking a cholinesterase inhibitor and acetaminophen. The patient's family states that her incontinence has gradually worsened over the past 5 years, and its current severity was an important factor in placing her in the facility. The patient is unable to give a detailed history and denies bladder problems. Observations by the nursing staff suggest a diagnosis of overactive bladder with urge incontinence.

Examination reveals no evidence of severe atrophic vaginitis, pelvic prolapse, or fecal impaction. Catheterization a few minutes after an episode of incontinence reveals a residual volume of 40 mL. Urinalysis of a specimen obtained by catheterization shows 3+ bacteria and 5 to 10 leukocytes per high-power field, and the culture grows over 100,000 colony-forming units of *Escherichia coli*.

Which of the following is the most appropriate next step for managing her incontinence?

(A) A trial of oxybutynin, 2.5 mg three times daily
(B) A trial of long-acting tolterodine, 4 mg daily
(C) A 7- to 10-day course of ciprofloxacin
(D) Initiation of a prompted voiding program
(E) Simple cystometric testing

41. A 75-year-old smoker who recently had a myocardial infarction comes to the office for advice on life-style changes. History includes chronic obstructive pulmonary disease with a moderately impaired FEV_1.

In such patients, smoking cessation is associated with which of the following?

(A) Improved cognition
(B) Cessation of a decline in FEV_1
(C) Reduction in all-cause mortality
(D) Lung cancer risk that is the same as a nonsmoker

42. A 75-year-old man cares for his wife, who has Alzheimer's disease, in their own home. Because his wife needs increasing help with activities of daily living, the husband reluctantly decides to place her in a nursing home.

Which of the following factors predicts a more successful transition for the husband after his wife enters the nursing home?

(A) An ambivalent marital relationship
(B) The husband's anticipating loneliness after placement
(C) The husband's having a sense of identity outside of his caregiving role
(D) The husband's volunteering at the nursing home at which his wife resides

43. A generally healthy 74-year-old woman returns to the office for follow-up of incontinence. She is physically active and extremely bothered by

the incontinence. Her symptoms include continuous dribbling and urgency with incontinence during most activities. In the past 15 years, she has had two bladder suspension surgeries that only transiently improved her symptoms of stress incontinence.

On examination she has a positive cough test for stress incontinence, both standing before voiding and supine after voiding. Mild vaginal atrophy and a moderate cystocele are noted on pelvic examination. Postvoid residual urine is 30 mL, and urinalysis is negative. During the last 6 months she underwent a course of biofeedback and has been regularly using pelvic muscle exercises and bladder-training techniques. She uses estrogen vaginal cream twice weekly. She tolerated oxybutynin 2.5 mg three times daily with no amelioration of symptoms; when the dosage was raised to 5 mg three times daily, she had dry mouth, dry eyes, and constipation with no improvement in symptoms.

Which of the following is the most appropriate next step for this patient?

(A) Refer her to a urogynecologist for consideration of surgical intervention.
(B) Increase the estrogen cream to 5 times per week.
(C) Add vaginal cones to enhance her pelvic muscle exercises.
(D) Begin long-acting tolterodine, 4 mg daily.
(E) Begin pseudoephedrine, 30 mg three times daily.

44. A daughter comes with her mother to her mother's clinic appointment and requests that you fill out conservatorship papers. The mother is an 84-year-old woman who has been living on her own since the death of her husband 7 years ago. You have followed her for the past 3 years in your office for type 2 diabetes, atrial fibrillation (for which she receives an anticoagulant), and moderate aortic stenosis. During this time you have noted an increase in nonadherence with her medication regimen. She had a hospital admission 1 month ago for dehydration, partially due to hyperglycemia, and her INR was noted to be 1.2. She was unclear as to whether she had been taking her pills correctly when in hospital. Now she assures you that she has that "all taken care of" but does

not give you specifics on how she obtains her medications nor how she remembers to take them. She does know that she needs to get tested for her warfarin regularly. The daughter states that her mother does not eat correctly, rarely showers, and refuses to allow others to help her.

Her Folstein Mini–Mental State Examination (MMSE) score is 25 (errors were in recall, orientation, and the three-step command). Her Executive Interview (EXIT 25) score of 9, demonstrating difficulty with sequencing, intrusions, perseveration, and self-monitoring, suggests mild to moderate impairment in executive functioning.

The most important aspect of this patient and her examination that would persuade you that she may or may not need a conservator is which of the following?

(A) The EXIT 25 score of 9
(B) The MMSE score of 25
(C) The daughter's concern
(D) The functional ability of the patient
(E) The hospitalization

45. A 79-year-old man comes to the office for a follow-up visit. He lives at home with his son, who moved in last year to care for his father in exchange for room and board. In response to questions about his home situation, he reports that his son "treats me pretty rough sometimes." The patient does not want to be separated from his son and does not want to move out of his own house. The son works full time and drinks heavily at home. Sometimes he does not provide dinner for his father and has left him for prolonged periods without helping him change his clothes or ensuring that he has food. The patient has a history of severe osteoarthritis of the knees and left hip, heart failure, and diabetes mellitus. He ambulates using a walker with moderate assistance from another person, is unable to transfer independently, and is afraid of falling.

Physical examination reveals significant peripheral neuropathy and multiple bruises on his forearms. Heart rate is 80 per minute and regular. He has crackles at the bases of both lungs. Cognitive examination is normal, but he is depressed. His diaper is wet, and the skin in his perianal area is covered with dried feces.

Which of the following is the most appropriate next step in assisting this patient?

(A) Admit him to a nursing home.
(B) Notify Adult Protective Services of possible mistreatment.
(C) Request visiting nurse services for home safety evaluation.
(D) Initiate therapy with a selective serotonin-reuptake inhibitor.
(E) Request meals-on-wheels.

46. Which of the following is the strongest predictor for failure to achieve independent ambulation after surgical repair of a hip fracture?

(A) Cognitive status
(B) Age
(C) Incontinence
(D) Premorbid functional status
(E) Depression

47. Which of the following statements is true with regard to assisted-living facilities?

(A) Meals, laundry service, housekeeping, and skilled nursing services are usually provided.
(B) Rates at assisted-living facilities average $200 a day.
(C) Medicare pays for individuals to reside at assisted-living facilities.
(D) Long-term-care insurance may cover the cost of assisted living.

48. A 72-year-old man comes to the emergency department because of constant right lower quadrant abdominal pain that has been present for almost 48 hours. He has nausea and anorexia but no fever, chills, vomiting, diarrhea, hematochezia, hematuria, or dysuria.

On physical examination his abdomen is soft to palpation and tender in the right lower quadrant, with voluntary guarding. Bowel sounds are hypoactive. Rectal examination is negative for occult blood.

Laboratory values include hemoglobin of 12.6 g/dL and leukocyte count of 14,800/μL

(neutrophils 88%, bands 7%, monocytes 4%, lymphocytes 8%). Amylase and liver chemistries are normal. Abdominal radiograph reveals a nonspecific gas pattern.

What is the most appropriate next step to establish the diagnosis?

(A) Ultrasound of the abdomen
(B) Gastrografin (meglumine diatrizoate) enema
(C) Computed tomography of abdomen
(D) Small bowel series
(E) Colonoscopy

49. During a routine office visit, a 75-year-old man complains of erectile dysfunction. He had a myocardial infarction 8 years ago. He has a history of well-controlled hypertension for 15 years, rare episodes of angina with severe exertion, hyperlipidemia, and benign prostatic hyperplasia. Medications are enalapril, hydrochlorothiazide, doxazosin, aspirin, lovastatin, and a nitroglycerin patch. Physical examination is notable for blood pressure of 130/80 mm Hg and somewhat decreased peripheral pulses. There is no evidence of Peyronie's disease.

Which of the following is the best treatment for erectile dysfunction for this patient?

(A) Intracavernosal injections of alprostadil
(B) Oral yohimbine
(C) Oral sildenafil
(D) Intramuscular testosterone every 2 weeks
(E) Vacuum tumescent device

50. Which of the following is true regarding osteoporosis in older men?

(A) Androgen levels have been correlated to bone mass and fractures in older men.
(B) Estrogen levels are an important determinant of osteoporosis in men.
(C) Osteoporosis is more likely to be primary or idiopathic in older men than in older women.
(D) No treatment benefit has been documented for alendronate in older men with idiopathic osteoporosis.
(E) Outcome after hip fracture is better for older men than for older women.

51. A 65-year-old woman comes to the office for a physical examination, during which a 2 × 2 cm smooth, ovoid nodule is palpated in the left lobe of the thyroid gland. The nodule moves easily with swallowing and is not associated with cervical lymphadenopathy. She has no history of radiation exposure to the head or neck. Serum thyrotropin and serum free thyroxine levels are normal.

Which of the following is the most appropriate next step?

(A) Referral for fine-needle aspiration biopsy
(B) Referral for possible left thyroid lobectomy
(C) Thyroid uptake and scan
(D) Reexamination in 6 months

52. A 79-year-old man comes to the office because he has had a generalized, throbbing, almost constant headache for the past 3 weeks. He has no previous history of headache. No obvious factor precipitated the headache, although the patient notes that chewing food seems to accentuate jaw pain. Two days ago he lost vision in his left eye for 5 minutes; this resolved spontaneously. Earlier today he suddenly lost hearing in his left ear. His current medications include aspirin and folic acid. Neurologic examination is normal except for the hearing loss.

Which of the following is the most appropriate treatment?

(A) Azathioprine
(B) Clopidogrel
(C) Heparin
(D) Phenytoin
(E) Prednisone

53. A 60-year-old man is brought to the office by his family because he has difficulty walking and is becoming increasingly confused. He has a history of alcoholism. On examination, he is unable to move his eyes horizontally, and he has upbeat nystagmus, dysmetria of the extremities, and severe ataxia.

Which of the following vitamins is most likely to be deficient in this patient?

(A) Vitamin B_1
(B) Vitamin B_6
(C) Vitamin B_{12}
(D) Vitamin E
(E) Vitamin K

54. A 76-year-old woman who lives with her husband in a retirement community comes to the office because she has nearly fallen on three occasions during the previous 6 months. In each instance she averted the fall by grabbing hold of something. She has moderate visual impairment due to macular degeneration and osteoarthritis involving several joints, especially the left hip and knee. She takes pride in not having to take any medications. She has 1 mixed drink before dinner almost every day, while socializing with other residents, and has a glass of wine with dinner 2 to 3 times each week. Alcohol, combined with impaired vision and the effects of arthritis on balance and gait, is suspected as a possible cause of the near-falls. She has not been treated previously for an alcohol-use disorder.

Which of the following is the most appropriate first step in the care of this patient?

(A) Treat with naltrexone, 50 mg once daily for 12 weeks.
(B) Treat with disulfiram, 200 mg once daily until drinking is reduced.
(C) Provide information about risks and advise her to reduce her drinking.
(D) Refer to an age-specific residential treatment center.
(E) Refer to a self-help group such as Alcoholics Anonymous.

55. A 76-year-old woman is undergoing treatment for major depression that began 6 months after her husband died. She has had three episodes of depression since age 58. Her previous most recent episode was 4 years ago, when her husband was diagnosed with colon cancer. At that time she tolerated and responded to sertraline 50 mg daily; this regimen is resumed for the current episode of depression. After 3 weeks of treatment she feels significantly better, and after 4 months she reports that she is back to normal. She has no significant side effects.

Which of the following is most appropriate in management of this patient?

(A) Discontinue sertraline and monitor her closely.
(B) Taper sertraline slowly over the next few months.
(C) Continue sertraline at half the current dose.
(D) Continue sertraline at the current dose.

56. An 84-year-old woman is referred for evaluation of anemia. The patient has a history of anemia, hypertension, osteoarthritis, and renal insufficiency. Her hemoglobin was 10 g/dL until 9 months ago, when it dropped to 6.8 g/dL. At that time there was no evidence of bleeding, and ferritin, serum iron, iron-binding capacity, and B_{12} and folic acid levels were normal. With transfusion, her hemoglobin stabilized between 9 and 10 g/dL. The patient has no history of weight loss, hematochezia, melena, or hematuria. She complains of pain in her neck, knees, and wrists. Medications include enalapril and acetaminophen. Physical examination is within normal limits.

Laboratory tests:
Hemoglobin	8.9 g/dL
Mean corpuscular volume	87 fL
Leukocyte count	3700/μL
Platelet count	150,000/μL
Westergren erythrocyte sedimentation rate	77 mm/h
Reticulocyte count	0.9%
Folic acid	1.3 ng/mL (normal)
Thyrotropin	2.1 μU/mL
Iron	89 μg/dL
Iron-binding capacity	234 μg/dL
Serum calcium	9.2 mg/dL
Serum albumin	4.0 g/dL
Blood urea nitrogen	32 mg/dL
Serum creatinine	1.8 mg/dL

Which of the following is the most appropriate next step?

(A) Serum erythropoietin level
(B) Chest radiograph and liver function tests
(C) Serum and urine protein electrophoresis and immunofixation
(D) Bone marrow biopsy

57. An 86-year-old widowed white man is brought to the emergency department after a neighbor found him sleeping in his car with the engine on while it was parked in the garage. The patient's physical and cognitive examinations are unremarkable. Laboratory tests are remarkable only for slightly elevated liver function. His affect is restricted. The patient denies any suicide attempt and explains that he fell asleep after he drove back home. He refuses to allow his son, who lives out of state, to be contacted because "he does not want him to be bothered." Similarly, he refuses to talk to the psychiatric triage nurse, insisting that he should go home now.

Which of the following is the most appropriate next step in the management of this patient?

(A) Discharge with follow-up the next day with his primary care provider.
(B) Initiate involuntary psychiatric evaluation.
(C) Admit the patient to a general medical unit for further observation.
(D) Keep the patient in the emergency department for further observation.
(E) Call the patient's son to discuss your concerns.

58. A 70-year-old woman describes early morning awakening and daytime fatigue for the past 8 months. She is generally healthy and has no symptoms of anxiety or depression. Over the past year she has been retiring as early as 7 PM. Despite recent efforts to retire later in the evening, she continues to awaken regularly at 3 AM.

Which of the following most likely accounts for this patient's sleep disturbance?

(A) Breathing-related sleep disorder
(B) Circadian rhythm advance
(C) Periodic limb movements
(D) Restless legs syndrome
(E) Sleep apnea

59. An 87-year-old man who is an established patient comes to the office because over the past year he has noted increasing shortness of breath with activity. He reports that 2 years ago he could easily walk 1 mile, but now he has to stop and rest after walking one block. He also becomes "winded" after climbing one flight of stairs. He has no chest discomfort or palpitations but often becomes lightheaded when he

stands up, and he felt as though he was going to "pass out" on at least two occasions. History includes type 2 diabetes mellitus and depression. He does not smoke or drink alcohol. He is the primary caregiver for his wife, who is disabled with advanced Parkinson's disease. Current medications include glyburide, aspirin, atorvastatin, and paroxetine.

On physical examination, heart rate is 70 per minute and regular, blood pressure is 140/60 mm Hg, respiratory rate is 18 per minute, and body mass index (kg/m^2) is 25. He has a flat affect. Examination of the neck shows no jugular venous distention, normal thyroid, and delayed carotid upstrokes bilaterally. He has a III/VI late-peaking systolic ejection murmur and S$_4$ gallop, with no S$_3$. His Mini–Mental State Examination score is 28 of 30, with no focal deficits.

Laboratory studies:

Hemoglobin	13.8 g/dL
Hematocrit	41%
Leukocyte count	6500/μL
Platelet count	180,000/μL
Creatinine	1.0 mg/dL
Blood urea nitrogen	22 mg/dL
Albumin	3.8 g/dL

Electrocardiography shows sinus rhythm and left ventricular hypertrophy with repolarization abnormality. Echocardiography shows moderate left ventricular systolic dysfunction (ejection fraction 35%) and a heavily calcified aortic valve (estimated area 0.6 cm^2).

Which of the following is the most appropriate management for this patient?

(A) Aortic valve replacement
(B) Balloon aortic valvuloplasty
(C) Percutaneous coronary angioplasty, if indicated
(D) Angiotensin-converting enzyme inhibitor and titration to tolerance
(E) Digoxin

60. A 75-year-old woman comes to the office because she has had repeated episodes of profound dizziness and near loss of consciousness, along with at least two episodes in which she found herself on the floor but was unaware of how she fell. She denies any confusion after the episode or any significant trauma. She has hypertension, and her daily medication is amlodipine 5 mg.

On physical examination, blood pressure is 152/84 mm Hg and heart rate is 76 per minute when she is supine. In upright posture, blood pressure is 146/86 mm Hg and heart rate is 86 per minute. There is no jugular venous distension or carotid bruit. Lungs are clear. There is a slightly delayed carotid upstroke and a II/VI systolic murmur at the base with an intact S$_2$ but no gallop.

Which of the following is the most appropriate next step in the evaluation of this patient to stratify her risk for adverse outcomes?

(A) Blood tests
(B) Electrocardiography
(C) Holter monitoring
(D) Event monitor
(E) Tilt-table test

61. A 69-year-old man comes to the office because for the past several weeks he has had recurrent spells of room-spinning vertigo that last for about 4 minutes. The spells occur spontaneously, are unassociated with positional changes, and are accompanied occasionally by double vision and sometimes by weakness on the right side. Several times, he has had sudden drop attacks, after which he has mild weakness of both legs lasting several minutes. He has a history of diabetes mellitus and coronary artery disease.

Which of the following is the most likely cause of the vertigo?

(A) Vestibular neuronitis
(B) Vertebrobasilar insufficiency
(C) Labyrinthitis
(D) Migraine-associated vertigo
(E) Ménière's disease

62. An 80-year-old woman comes to the office because she recently has had difficulty eating and swallowing solid foods. She notes that when she prepares to swallow, the food scrapes her cheeks and roof of her mouth. The patient has hypertension, diabetes mellitus, a recent history of kidney stones, and depression. Current medications include hydrochlorothiazide and metformin. For the

first time in many years, her last dental examination revealed several cavities, located at the roots of the teeth.

Which of the following is the most likely cause of her symptoms?

(A) Aging
(B) Salivary duct stones
(C) Metformin
(D) Hydrochlorothiazide

63. A 78-year-old woman comes to the office because she has heavy vaginal bleeding after no bleeding for many years. She has been on continuous estrogen replacement therapy for the past 30 years. Physical examination, including pelvic, reveals severe arthritis. She requests evaluation with the least invasive test, because she has severe arthritis.

What is the best evaluation for this patient?

(A) Coagulopathy work-up
(B) Vaginal ultrasound to assess endometrial thickness
(C) Endometrial biopsy
(D) Hysteroscopy
(E) Dilation and curettage

64. An 81-year-old woman with a history of "bad nerves" comes to the office for a second opinion because she is "tired of being sick all my life." She has a history of headaches, back pain, and joint pain, for which she had taken nonsteroidal anti-inflammatory drugs (NSAIDs) intermittently for decades. She also has nausea, bloating, and stomach ache that persisted after she discontinued NSAIDs. She cannot tolerate certain foods, has difficulty swallowing, and at times is unable to speak. She has had gastroenterology, neurology, and rheumatology consultations, and different tests were recommended, but no medications were prescribed. She sleeps and eats well, and enjoys crafts and spending time with family and friends. At this visit she appears upset and tearful.

Which of the following is most likely?

(A) Major depressive disorder
(B) Generalized anxiety disorder
(C) Somatization disorder
(D) Hypochondriasis
(E) Pain disorder

65. An 87-year-old resident of an Alzheimer's assisted-living unit is evaluated because she has fallen twice in the past month. She has a history of dementia, urge urinary incontinence, and hypertension. She has had no recent acute illness or changes in medication. She takes vitamin E 400 units twice daily, galantamine 8 mg twice daily, enteric-coated aspirin 81 mg daily, sustained-release tolterodine 4 mg daily, and hydrochlorothiazide 25 mg daily. Unless redirected, she spends most of the day walking. It is difficult to get her to finish her meals.

On examination, she is alert, oriented to place but not date, and thin, and she appears tired. She has normal gait speed, with normal foot clearance and arm swing, but she turns quickly and reaches for the wall to steady herself.

Which of the following would be part of a treatment plan to reduce this patient's risk of falling?

(A) Medication with quetiapine 25 mg daily
(B) Scheduled brief rest periods during the day
(C) Use of hip protectors during the day
(D) Use of a lap tray to prevent her from getting up

66. A 72-year-old woman has a 15-year history of type 2 diabetes mellitus. She also has a history of coronary artery disease and heart failure. She began taking glipizide 8 years ago for her diabetes. Over the past 2 years she has required additional therapy. Initially, she did well on a combination of glipizide and NPH insulin at bedtime. Over the past 6 months, glipizide was stopped, and she has required twice-daily doses of NPH and regular insulin, given before breakfast and dinner. Despite increasing doses of insulin, her hemoglobin A_{1C} has increased to 9% and she now has hypoglycemia before lunch and during the night. Serum creatinine is 1.6 mg/dL.

Which of the following is the best management step?

(A) Add metformin.
(B) Add rosiglitazone.
(C) Replace the regular insulin with insulin lispro.
(D) Restart the glipizide.

67. A 65-year-old postmenopausal woman comes to the office for advice on physical activity to decrease her likelihood of having vertebral fractures and disability. Her mother has severe osteoporosis and back deformity with kyphosis.

Which of the following has been shown to reduce the likelihood of osteoporotic vertebral fractures?

(A) Daily high-intensity running program
(B) Progressive back extensor resistive exercise program 5 times each week
(C) High-intensity strength training exercises twice weekly
(D) Walking at an average pace 1 hour three times each week
(E) Household chores

68. A 79-year-old woman comes to the emergency department with palpitations and shortness of breath of 2 hours' duration. She has a history of hypertension, type 2 diabetes mellitus, mild restrictive lung disease, gastroesophageal reflux disease, and positional tremor. The patient relates that she was sitting in a chair when she noted the sudden onset of "heart racing," followed a few minutes later by difficulty breathing. She reports no chest discomfort, diaphoresis, dizziness, or syncope. When the symptoms did not resolve after an hour, her son brought her to the emergency department.

On physical examination, the patient is in mild respiratory distress. Heart rate ranges from 130 to 150 per minute and is irregular, blood pressure is 140/70 mm Hg, and respiratory rate is 22 per minute. Her neck is supple, with normal jugular venous pressure and no thyromegaly. Bibasilar crackles are heard. The heart is irregularly irregular, with a II/VI systolic ejection murmur and no S_3 or S_4 gallop. She has a moderate positional tremor.

Laboratory studies:
Cardiac biomarker
  proteins   normal
Creatinine   0.8 mg/dL
Blood urea nitrogen   17 mg/dL
Hemoglobin   13.1 g/dL
Hemoglobin A_{1C} 7.3%
Thyrotropin   2.0 μU/mL

Total cholesterol   198 mg/dL
  High-density
  lipoprotein   55 mg/dL
  Low-density lipoprotein 113 mg/dL
  Triglycerides   150 mg/dL

Electrocardiography reveals atrial fibrillation with rapid ventricular response, left ventricular hypertrophy with repolarization abnormality, and no ischemic changes. Chest radiograph shows mild cardiomegaly with mild pulmonary vascular redistribution. Adenosine-thallium stress test reveals a left ventricular ejection fraction of 67% with no evidence of ischemia. Echocardiogram demonstrates moderate left ventricular hypertrophy, mild left atrial enlargement, normal left ventricular systolic function, and mild left ventricular diastolic dysfunction.

The patient is treated with intravenous diltiazem with subsequent reversion to sinus rhythm (85 per minute). Intravenous furosemide results in a net diuresis of 1160 cc, and her shortness of breath resolves. Myocardial infarction is excluded by normal serial troponin levels.

Which of the following are appropriate discharge medications for this patient?

(A) Aspirin, warfarin, amiodarone, and angiotensin-converting enzyme inhibitor
(B) Warfarin, diltiazem, β-blocker, and angiotensin-receptor blocker
(C) Aspirin, β-blocker, angiotensin-converting enzyme inhibitor, and statin
(D) Warfarin, β-blocker, angiotensin-converting enzyme inhibitor, and angiotensin-receptor blocker
(E) Diltiazem, β-blocker, angiotensin-converting enzyme inhibitor, and statin

69. A 72-year-old man comes to the office because he has had itching and burning of his feet for 2 months. He also notes a strong odor when he removes his socks. He wears shoes with rubber soles. History includes hypertension, osteoarthritis, and childhood asthma. On examination, the lateral borders of both feet show erythema and scaling in a moccasin distribution. The toe web spaces are normal.

Which of the following is the most appropriate next step?

(A) Examine skin scrapings on a saline wet mount slide.
(B) Culture skin scrapings.
(C) Examine potassium hydroxide stain of scrapings of the rash.
(D) Do a punch skin biopsy.

70. A 76-year-old man with Alzheimer's disease is brought to the office for a follow-up visit. For the past few weeks he has had difficulty staying asleep at night. He goes to bed at 9 PM, sleeps until about 2 AM, and awakens to go to the bathroom. He remains awake for several hours, during which he is often disoriented, paces the house, and wakes his wife. He and his wife are fatigued, and he is more withdrawn during the day. He requires help with instrumental activities of daily living (IADLs), needs reminders with some basic ADLs, and is independent with feeding, toileting, and ambulation. His general health is good. There is no evidence of sadness or anhedonia, and he is eating well. He has well-controlled hypertension on a diuretic and takes an oral hypoglycemic agent for mild type 2 diabetes mellitus. He had a transurethral resection of the prostate 1 year ago for prostatic hyperplasia and has had no recurrence. At his last office visit, he was counseled about sleep hygiene, but this intervention has failed.

Which of the following, given at bedtime, is the most appropriate first-line pharmacologic treatment?

(A) Zolpidem, 5 to 10 mg
(B) Melatonin, 0.3 to 5 mg
(C) Zaleplon, 5 to 10 mg
(D) Trazodone, 25 to 50 mg
(E) Lorazepam, 1 mg

71. Which of the following is correct regarding the use of occlusive dressings in the treatment of pressure ulcers?

(A) They promote a mildly alkaline pH.
(B) They maintain a relatively high oxygen tension on the wound surface.
(C) They are more likely than nonocclusive dressings to preserve cytokines.
(D) They are associated with more pain from partial-thickness wounds than nonocclusive dressings.

72. An 85-year-old woman is evaluated because she has lost 2.7 kg (6 lb) since admission to a nursing home 1 month ago after a stroke. Her admission weight was 120 pounds and her height 64 inches. She has mild cognitive impairment. The staff reports that she takes a long time to chew her food and that she pockets food in her cheek. She denies pain with chewing or swallowing, and she is not depressed. Examination indicates that her denture fits well and that she has no oral lesions. Her gag reflex is intact.

Which of the following is the most appropriate first step?

(A) Request swallowing evaluation.
(B) Order a nutritional supplement.
(C) Discuss feeding tube placement with her family.
(D) Order mirtazapine.
(E) Initiate therapy with megestrol acetate.

73. A 70-year-old woman is concerned about vaginal discomfort and pain and occasional bleeding with intercourse. She had a hysterectomy and oophorectomy for fibroids at age 56, and estrogen receptor−positive breast cancer at age 65. The breast cancer was treated with lumpectomy and radiation, with no evidence of recurrence. She has never taken hormone replacement therapy. She is on no medications other than ibuprofen as needed for joint pains. In former years, sexual activity was mutually pleasurable to her and her husband. Her husband has recently started taking sildenafil.

Physical examination is remarkable for vaginal atrophic changes and mild difficulty introducing a regular-size speculum. No masses are present.

Which of the following is the best therapeutic choice for this patient?

(A) Oral conjugated estrogen
(B) Oral esterified estrogen and methyltestosterone
(C) Oral fluoxetine
(D) Water-soluble lubricant
(E) Intramuscular testosterone

74. A 72-year-old man comes to the office for a first visit. He runs 5 miles daily and occasionally has soreness in his knees that responds to aspirin. He takes several over-the-counter health preparations, including a multiple vitamin, calcium 500 mg, and a fish oil extract. On questioning, the patient describes an increasing sense of urinary urgency and nocturia, one or two times a night, over the past 2 years. He is bothered enough by the symptoms to consider treatment.

On physical examination, blood pressure is 110/70 mm Hg and heart rate is 60 per minute. Digital rectal examination reveals a normal prostate. Urinalysis and blood urea nitrogen and creatinine levels are normal; prostate-specific antigen level is 1.5 ng/mL.

Which of the following is most appropriate at this time?

(A) Obtain a transrectal ultrasound study.
(B) Initiate treatment with tamsulosin, 0.4 mg daily.
(C) Initiate treatment with oxybutynin, 2.5 mg three times daily.
(D) Initiate treatment with finasteride, 5 mg daily.

75. The daughter of a 93-year-old woman with Alzheimer's disease calls to discuss the patient's weight loss. The patient lives with her daughter and has had dementia for more than 6 years. Her average adult weight was 72.7 kg (160 lb). In recent years, she has weighed approximately 63.6 kg (140 lb); the community health nurse reports that she weighed 55.5 kg (122 lb) last week. The patient has not walked in at least 3 months and has required assistance for all of her activities of daily living, including feeding, for the past year. According to recent laboratory studies, her albumin level is 2.1 g/dL and total cholesterol is 93 mg/dL. Additional laboratory tests are unremarkable.

When last examined, the patient was frail but well cared for and did not engage with you or her daughter.

What is the most appropriate response to this patient's weight loss?

(A) Prescribe nutritional supplements.
(B) Arrange for placement of a gastrostomy tube.
(C) Prescribe megestrol 400 mg oral suspension daily.
(D) Arrange swallowing evaluation.
(E) Recommend hospice care.

76. A 73-year-old man fractures his hip while roller blading. He undergoes total hip arthroplasty and is discharged to a skilled nursing facility on the third postoperative day. At initial nursing evaluation, his right heel is erythematous and has a "mushy" feel to it. The history and physical examination notes indicate that the extremities are "within normal limits." Three days later nursing notes document a blister on the heel. There is no notation that the physician is called. A physician progress note the following day does not document examination of the patient's extremities. Two days later the blister opens and reveals a large ulcer with necrotic tissue. The physician is called and gives treatment orders for wet-to-dry dressings. The patient's family calls the state health department and a survey is done, the results of which document a pattern of poor skin care in the facility. The patient has an extended stay in the nursing facility and is ultimately discharged to an assisted-living facility. He files a lawsuit against the hospital, doctors, and nursing facility.

Which of the following may affect the outcome of this case?

(A) Wet-to-dry dressings have not been found efficacious in recent studies.
(B) Nursing homes are rarely defendants in lawsuits related to pressure ulcers.
(C) Lack of detail about skin condition in nursing-home charts deters lawsuits.
(D) Plaintiffs have introduced survey results to show a pattern of poor care in a facility.

77. Which antihypertensive class is less effective as a single agent in black than in white Americans?

(A) Angiotensin-converting enzyme inhibitors
(B) Calcium channel blockers
(C) Centrally acting agents
(D) Diuretics

78. An 89-year-old woman comes to the office complaining of feeling short of breath when climbing the stairs for the previous 2 weeks. Her lung examination is notable for bibasilar crackles. Electrocardiography showed changes of an inferior wall myocardial infarction of indeterminate age, chest radiography revealed some fluid at the bases, and echocardiography showed an ejection fraction of 35%. Her creatinine level was 2.2. She is placed on a loop diuretic, and at follow-up 2 weeks later, she is asymptomatic.

In addition to a β-blocker, which of the following classes of medication should be added at this time?

(A) Calcium channel blocker
(B) Long-acting nitrate
(C) Digoxin
(D) Angiotensin-converting enzyme inhibitor
(E) Aldactone

79. A 68-year-old woman residing in a long-term-care facility is evaluated because of recent onset of dizziness, difficulty with ambulation, and mental status changes. History includes epilepsy, seasonal allergies, overactive bladder, recently diagnosed depression, and osteoporosis. Medications include phenytoin 300 mg daily, alendronate 70 mg weekly, tolterodine 2 mg twice daily, fexofenadine 60 mg daily, and calcium carbonate 500 mg three times daily; 2 weeks ago she began fluoxetine 20 mg daily.

Laboratory studies from 1 month ago:
Phenytoin concentration   13.7 μg/mL
Sodium   138 mEq/L
Potassium   4.0 mEq/L
Urea nitrogen   15 mg/dL
Creatinine   1.0 mg/dL
Albumin   2.6 g/dL

Which of the following is the most appropriate next intervention?

(A) Obtain an unbound (free) phenytoin concentration.
(B) Discontinue tolterodine.
(C) Discontinue fexofenadine.
(D) Discontinue fluoxetine.

80. A 71-year-old woman comes to the office for a routine physical examination. History includes pedal edema due to venous insufficiency, episodic insomnia due to situational anxiety, and mild acid reflux disease. She has no fatigue, poor appetite, or gastrointestinal symptoms. Medications include garlic capsules 270 mg each morning, *Ginkgo biloba* 40 mg one or two times daily, kava 150 mg one to two capsules at bedtime as needed, and valerian 1.5 g at bedtime as needed for sleep.

Physical examination is normal. Laboratory results are normal except for an alanine aminotransferase level of 210 IU/L and an aspartate aminotransferase level of 250 IU/L. Previous liver function tests were normal. The patient is advised to discontinue all supplements pending further evaluation of the transaminase abnormalities.

Of the supplements used by this patient, which one is the most likely cause of the laboratory abnormalities?

(A) Garlic
(B) *Ginkgo biloba*
(C) Kava
(D) Valerian

ANSWER: C

The Food and Drug Administration has issued a consumer advisory notice about the potential risk of hepatic toxicity associated with use of kava (also known as kava kava). Kava comes from the dried root of *Piper methysticum*. It is used for anxiety, insomnia, restlessness, and stress. Kavapyrones, the active constituents in kava, have centrally acting relaxant properties for skeletal muscle. The sale of products containing kava is restricted in several countries because of associated adverse hepatic effects. In 11 patients who developed liver failure that was associated with kava use and who underwent liver transplantation, doses (when known) ranged from 60 to 240 mg daily. Kava products may differ in the amounts and distribution of kavapyrones present. Patients with evidence of liver disease or hepatic abnormalities and patients at risk for liver disease should avoid these herbal therapies.

Garlic, *Ginkgo biloba*, and valerian have not been associated with liver function abnor

81. A 75-year-old woman comes to the office because she has a painless blurring in her right eye that has progressed over the past few months. She is more sensitive to light and complains of glare and haloes. Ten years ago she had cataract surgery with intraocular lens implantations to both eyes with good results. She was recently diagnosed with type 2 diabetes, and her eye examination did not reveal any diabetic retinopathy.

Which of the following is the most likely cause of her symptoms?

(A) Vitreous hemorrhage
(B) Macular degeneration
(C) Opacified posterior lens capsule
(D) Diabetic macular edema

82. A 75-year-old woman comes to the office because she has fatigue, difficulty falling asleep, and frequent headaches. She has no history of hypertension. She is the primary caregiver for her 79-year-old husband; he has Alzheimer's disease (Mini–Mental State Examination score of 14 of 30) and has recently developed behavioral problems related to repetitive questions and demands. On examination, the patient's blood pressure is 168/95 mm Hg.

Which of the following is the most helpful intervention for her at this time?

(A) Prescribe a calcium channel blocker.
(B) Prescribe lorazepam.
(C) Prescribe sertraline.
(D) Refer to a psychiatrist for psychotherapy.
(E) Provide counseling about community services related to dementia caregiving.

83. An 87-year-old woman with Alzheimer's disease comes to the office with her daughter for advice on managing care. She lives with her daughter, who works during the day. Over the past year she has become increasingly dependent in her instrumental activities of daily living. Four months ago, the daughter noticed that her

mother was forgetting to eat the prepared lunch and neglecting to take her afternoon medications. She began to sleep more during the day and was awake and confused at night. The mother and daughter are committed to keeping the mother at home as long as possible. They are not willing to hire caregivers at home because they find them too unreliable.

Which of the following would be most appropriate to suggest as the next step in managing the mother's care?

(A) Nursing-home placement
(B) Enrollment in adult day care
(C) Referral to home-health care
(D) Referral to respite care
(E) Assisted-living placement

84. A 77-year-old man comes to the office because of insomnia and nocturia. He lives alone in a continuing-care community that he joined 8 months ago. On a medical history form, he describes himself as a social drinker. Other than a recent hospitalization for pancreatitis, he has been healthy. Alcohol use is considered as a potential cause of or contributor to the pancreatitis and the sleep and urinary symptoms.

Which of the following is the most appropriate next step?

(A) Measurement of carbohydrate-deficient transferrin serum level
(B) Measurement of alanine and aspartate aminotransferase
(C) Close-ended questions about symptoms and consequences of drinking
(D) Close-ended questions about quantity and frequency of drinking
(E) Screening questionnaire with items on quantity, frequency, and effects of drinking

85. An 82-year-old man comes to the office for a routine physical examination. He has a history of hypertension and atrial fibrillation. He reports episodes of dizziness and has occasional diarrhea but no melena or hematochezia. Medications include atenolol, digoxin, and warfarin. He was the primary caregiver for his wife; she died 1 year ago after a long struggle with cancer. He admits to being fatigued and to having a poor appetite, but he does not think that he is depressed. On examination, blood

pressure and heart rate are well controlled; his blood pressure is 138/70 mm Hg, pulse is 60 per minute, respiratory rate is 14 per minute, and temperature is 36.7°C (98°F). He has lost 6.4 kg (14 lb; 6% of his body weight) over the past 6 months. The rest of the physical examination shows no substantial changes from the previous visit.

Which of the following is most likely to reveal the cause of this man's weight loss?

(A) Fecal occult blood testing
(B) Serum digoxin level
(C) Geriatric depression screen
(D) Home visit
(E) Chest radiography

86. A 90-year-old resident of a skilled nursing facility has fallen three times in the past month. She has a history of dementia, hypertension, atrial fibrillation, osteoarthritis, and transient ischemic attacks. She walks with a walker. Medications include hydrochlorothiazide 25 mg daily, atenolol 50 mg daily, warfarin 2 mg daily, celecoxib 100 mg daily, calcium carbonate 600 mg twice daily, a multivitamin daily, donepezil 10 mg daily, and lorazepam 0.25 mg twice daily as needed.

Which of the following should be done first to assess her risk for future falls?

(A) Order 24-hour cardiac monitoring.
(B) Measure her blood pressure when she is lying down, sitting, and standing.
(C) Review the circumstances of her falls.
(D) Ask the physical therapist to evaluate her gait, transfers, and walker.

87. A man inquires about whether his 80-year-old aunt can receive house calls for her medical care. She lives by herself in a second-floor apartment in a building with no elevator. She has morbid obesity, coronary artery disease, heart failure, adult-onset diabetes mellitus, hyperlipidemia, asthma, and chronic back pain. She is independent in activities of daily living, but can walk only 10 feet with a walker. She cannot negotiate steps, which constitute the only access to her apartment; she never leaves her apartment, other than when she is hospitalized. Her nephew brings her meals and assists in other instrumental activities of daily living.

For health coverage, she has traditional Medicare Parts A and B and no supplemental insurance.

How would Medicare compensate for a house call to this patient?

(A) Medicare Part A would pay on a capitation basis.
(B) Medicare Part A would pay on a fee-for-service basis.
(C) Medicare Part B would pay on a capitation basis.
(D) Medicare Part B would pay on a fee-for-service basis.
(E) Medicare would not pay for physician home visits.

88. Which of the following structures is most susceptible to age-related histopathologic changes that result in sensorineural hearing loss and dizziness?

(A) Inner ear
(B) Central auditory system
(C) Ossicles
(D) Tympanitic membrane
(E) External auditory canal

89. A 92-year-old woman is being treated with paroxetine for major depression following successful surgery for uncomplicated hip fracture. Her overall physical and cognitive status is otherwise good. She has mild hypertension and osteoarthritis, and she takes a thiazide diuretic and acetaminophen. Ten days after paroxetine is started, the patient's daughter calls to report that her mother is lethargic and confused.

Which of the following metabolic disturbances is the most likely cause of this patient's delirium?

(A) Hyponatremia
(B) Hypernatremia
(C) Hypoglycemia
(D) Hyperglycemia

90. An 86-year-old woman comes to the office because she has pelvic pressure, especially when moving her bowels. She has class III heart failure. On pelvic examination, she is found to have grade III uterine prolapse.

Which of the following is the most appropriate next step in her management?

(A) Refer for hysterectomy.
(B) Prescribe Kegel's exercises.
(C) Prescribe the use of a pessary.
(D) Prescribe topical estrogen.

91. A 78-year-old man comes to the office for a 6-month follow-up visit. He has a history of well-controlled stage 1 hypertension, benign prostatic hyperplasia, and osteoarthritis. His prostate and musculoskeletal symptoms are stable. Medications are lisinopril 10 mg daily, hydrochlorothiazide 25 mg daily, ibuprofen 200 mg three times daily (begun at his last visit), and saw palmetto.

On physical examination, his blood pressure is 152/78 mm Hg, and heart rate is 82 per minute with a regular rhythm. He has joint deformities in both hands consistent with osteoarthritis; there is no acute inflammation. He has 1+ bilateral lower extremity edema to the mid-shin; the edema was not evident at his last visit.

Which of the following is the best approach to management of this patient?

(A) Recommend compression stockings.
(B) Discontinue ibuprofen.
(C) Increase the hydrochlorothiazide.
(D) Begin a loop diuretic.
(E) Increase the lisinopril dosage.

92. A 73-year-old woman comes to the office because of pain in her right shoulder for the past 6 weeks. The pain is often worse when she wakes up in the morning and with prolonged sitting and standing; lying down relieves the pain. She feels spasm and notes tenderness in her right shoulder. It bothers her particularly when she backs her car out of the driveway in the morning. She has had no weight loss, fatigue, general malaise, or other systemic symptoms.

On physical examination, there is good mobility of the right shoulder with no pain. She has moderate spasm and tenderness in the right trapezius region, asymmetric loss of movement of the cervical spine, and mild weakness of the right elbow extensor and right finger abductors.

What is the most likely cause of this patient's pain?

(A) Fibromyalgia
(B) Metastatic cancer affecting the right scapula
(C) Rotator cuff tendonitis of the right shoulder
(D) Acromioclavicular disease of the right shoulder
(E) Cervical disk disease

93. The effect of physical activity on bone density is most highly correlated with which of the following?

(A) Frequency of activity
(B) Duration of activity
(C) Intensity of activity
(D) Type of activity
(E) Volume of aerobic activity

94. An 84-year-old woman comes to the office accompanied by her daughter for evaluation of progressive weight loss. The patient thinks she has good nutrient intake. She denies problems sleeping, depressive symptoms, change in bowel habits, or other active medical problems. She has had no serious illness or surgery in the past 5 years. She takes a daily multivitamin but is on no other regular medicines. She has lived alone since her husband's death 7 years ago. The daughter states that her mother is less active socially than before and spends most of her time reading, knitting, or watching television. The daughter is convinced that her mother has cancer; her father also started losing weight before metastatic cancer was diagnosed. A mammogram done 6 months ago and a screening colonoscopy done 2 years ago were normal.

The patient weighs 54.5 kg (120 lbs; body mass index 22 [kg/m^2]), 12% less than the prior year. The remainder of the physical examination is normal. Mini–Mental State Examination score is 28 of 30, and Yesavage Geriatric Depression Scale (short form) score is 2 (not depressed). Stool guaiac, urinalysis, complete blood cell count, electrolytes, and liver, renal, and thyroid function tests are normal, as is chest radiography. Electrocardiography reveals normal sinus rhythm.

Which of the following is now indicated?

(A) Computed tomographic scan of the abdomen
(B) Upper and lower endoscopy
(C) Upper gastrointestinal study with small bowel follow-through
(D) No further diagnostic testing

95. An 86-year-old woman comes to the office because she has mid-back pain at rest and with activity that has worsened over the past few months. She has longstanding osteoporosis with previous compression fractures at T10 and L1. She reports no other symptoms. Medications include calcium, vitamin D, and risedronate. After her last compression fracture 2 years ago, she was started on calcitonin, but it was discontinued after 1 month because of continued back pain and the development of rhinitis. Acetaminophen and over-the-counter nonsteroidal anti-inflammatory agents around the clock provided no relief. After her last visit 3 months ago, she began acetaminophen with hydrocodone (750 mg/7.5 mg), 1 tablet every 6 hours. This regimen provided better pain control initially, but she now rates her pain as 7 out of 10 on most days and states that it limits many of her activities, including bathing and dressing.

Physical examination reveals moderate kyphosis and mild tenderness to palpation over her mid-spine and the surrounding paraspinous muscles. Neurologic examination demonstrates intact lower extremity reflexes, strength, and sensation. Radiography of her thoracic and lumbar spine shows severe degenerative disc disease along with the old compression fractures at T10 and L1; no new vertebral fractures or other processes are visualized.

What is the most appropriate management strategy for this patient?

(A) Increase the acetaminophen with hydrocodone to 1 tablet every 4 hours around the clock.
(B) Switch to immediate-release oxycodone.
(C) Evaluate for kyphoplasty.
(D) Refer for physical therapy.
(E) Add cyclobenzaprine.

96. In a nursing facility, which of the following is the best approach to identify residents at risk

for development of pressure ulcers and to monitor existing pressure ulcers?

(A) Develop risk and monitoring scales specific to that facility.
(B) Implement the Braden scale and the Pressure Ulcer Scale for Healing (PUSH).
(C) Implement the Braden and Norton scales.
(D) Implement the PUSH tool and the Pressure Sore Status Tool (PSST).

97. In a patient with psychosis associated with Alzheimer's disease, pharmacotherapy is begun with an atypical antipsychotic.

Which of the following is more likely with an atypical than with a conventional antipsychotic agent?

(A) Greater likelihood of remission of psychotic symptoms
(B) Reduced rate of falls and injury
(C) Reduced incidence of tardive dyskinesia
(D) Lower incidence of somnolence
(E) Absence of QTc prolongation

98. A 67-year-old woman with recently diagnosed metastatic ovarian cancer comes to the office for a follow-up visit. She has new symptoms of nausea and vomiting. Several months ago, the patient underwent debulking surgery and chemotherapy, but there was extensive carcinomatosis on follow-up imaging 3 months later, and her CA-125 level has remained high. At her last appointment, she acknowledged that her cancer will not be cured and stated that she is reluctant to undergo further invasive procedures or to be rehospitalized. Her current nausea and vomiting started 2 days ago. She has been unable to tolerate any oral intake and has not had a bowel movement in 4 days. Her only medications are acetaminophen with codeine as needed and docusate sodium stool softener every morning.

On examination, the patient appears thin and uncomfortable. She is afebrile. Blood pressure is 98/60 mm Hg, and pulse is 105 per minute. Cardiopulmonary examination is unremarkable aside from tachycardia. The abdomen is markedly distended with decreased bowel sounds, tympany on percussion, and diffuse tenderness on palpation. Rectal examination is normal, with no stool in the vault.

In addition to providing the patient with morphine, which of the following is the most appropriate management strategy for this patient?

(A) Diverting colostomy
(B) Nasogastric suctioning
(C) Octreotide
(D) Atropine
(E) Ondansetron

99. An 84-year-old woman living in a retirement home has over the past week become increasingly agitated, especially at night. She climbs out of bed, and on at least one occasion she fell, sustaining a bruise on her hip. She has a 2-year history of cognitive decline consistent with Alzheimer's disease. She has type 2 diabetes mellitus treated with glyburide and chronic obstructive pulmonary disease treated with a salmeterol inhaler. Staff at her retirement home report that she has been a poor sleeper since she was admitted 18 months earlier, but she is otherwise cooperative and cheerful. On examination, she appears fearful and complains of criminals coming into her room at night to attack her.

Which of the following is the best initial management strategy?

(A) Use of side rails on her bed at night
(B) Music therapy in the evening
(C) Physical examination and routine laboratory testing
(D) Treatment of hip pain with acetaminophen
(E) Use of bright-light therapy to improve sleep

100. A 79-year-old woman comes to the office because of pain, swelling, stiffness, and mild erythema of her right forefoot. She is healthy and takes no medications other than vitamins and calcium. The patient recalls an injury 4 months earlier, in which a package of frozen chicken fell on the foot from a top-loading freezer compartment of her refrigerator. She recalls that the foot swelled immediately and became discolored and painful. At the local hospital emergency department, radiographs of her right foot showed no evidence of fracture. She was advised to take anti-inflammatory medications, apply ice to the area, and rest and elevate the foot. Although the discoloration from the original injury subsided, the swelling has persisted and the pain is now excruciating.

On physical examination, there is exquisite pain on palpation of the right forefoot. The skin over the metatarsal area is warm, erythematous, and dry. The toes are cool to touch, with mild cyanosis over the dorsum. Neurologic findings are normal. Pedal pulses are palpable. Repeat radiographs reveal periarticular soft-tissue swelling and patchy osteoporosis involving the metatarsals and metatarsal phalangeal articulations. Serologic tests for antinuclear antibody and rheumatoid factor are negative, and electromyography and nerve conduction velocity studies are normal.

Which of the following is the most likely diagnosis?

(A) Tarsal tunnel syndrome
(B) Raynaud's phenomenon
(C) Rheumatoid arthritis
(D) Reflex sympathetic dystrophy
(E) Stress fracture

QUESTIONS, ANSWERS, AND CRITIQUES

Directions: Each of the questions or incomplete statements below is followed by four or five suggested answers or completions. Select the ONE answer or completion that is BEST in each case and circle or place an "X" through the letter you have selected for each answer on the answer sheet. Answer sheets for self-assessment are available to download at: http://www.americangeriatrics.org/products/gnrs_2.shtml. The table of Normal Laboratory Values on p 478 may be consulted for any of the questions in this book.

1. A 76-year-old woman comes to the office for follow-up evaluation of hypertension. Her blood pressure was 148/82 mm Hg at a recent examination. She returned for repeat measurements on two occasions; the average of all these readings is 146/83 mm Hg. She is in good general health and has no history or evidence of coronary artery disease or diabetes mellitus. Her current medications are a daily multivitamin and a calcium supplement. She lives alone, eats out frequently, and does not participate in a regular exercise program. She does not smoke or consume alcohol.

   Evaluation to date has not identified a secondary cause for hypertension. She is obese (BMI [kg/m²] = 31), and her waist circumference is 92 cm.
   Laboratory studies:

Fasting glucose	115 mg/dL
Total cholesterol	220 mg/dL
High-density lipoprotein	42 mg/dL
Triglycerides	200 mg/dL

   Which of the following is most appropriate regarding management of her hypertension?

   (A) Recommend lifestyle interventions for 6 months.
   (B) Begin a β-blocker.
   (C) Begin a thiazide-type diuretic.
   (D) Begin an angiotensin-converting enzyme inhibitor.
   (E) Begin a calcium channel blocker.

   ANSWER: A

   The initial assessment and evaluation of this patient confirmed that she met criteria for stage 1 essential hypertension. In addition, the constellation of this patient's findings (central obesity, hypertension, hypertriglyceridemia, low level of high-density lipoprotein, and impaired fasting glucose level) satisfies criteria for the metabolic syndrome. The most appropriate management of this patient's hypertension is a 6-month trial of lifestyle interventions. Most older adults with hypertension are sedentary, overweight, insulin resistant, and salt sensitive, so the blood-pressure reduction that follows effective lifestyle changes may be even greater among older patients. The Trial of Nonpharmacologic Interventions in the Elderly (TONE) demonstrated that relatively modest reductions in dietary sodium (average decrease of 40 mmol/day) and body weight (average reduction of 4.7 kg) lowered blood pressure to a degree comparable to that achieved with a single antihypertensive drug (average reduction of 5 mm Hg systolic and 3 mm Hg diastolic). The Dietary Approaches to Stop Hypertension (DASH) study demonstrated similar findings. Exercise training is an effective intervention to lower blood pressure in hypertensive patients; it confers additional benefits with respect to improving insulin sensitivity and the lipid profile.

   None of the medications listed in the other options is indicated for initial treatment of stage 1 hypertension. If lifestyle interventions do not lower systolic blood pressure to 140 mm Hg after 6 months, then adding a medication should be considered. A thiazide-type diuretic would be the best option to select at that time.

   Patients with stage 1 hypertension and features of the metabolic syndrome are at greater risk of cardiovascular events. The role of more aggressive treatment of the lipid abnormalities (with statins or other drugs) or insulin resistance (with insulin-sensitizing drugs) is not yet clear. The lifestyle interventions for blood pressure will confer similar benefits on manifestations of the metabolic syndrome.

2. A 78-year-old thin woman comes to the office because she has acute lower back pain that began when she tried to open a stuck window. The pain is so severe that she has difficulty standing or sitting. The pain lessens when she lies down, and increases when she rolls to the side. The pain does not radiate to her legs.

On physical examination, there is marked tenderness in the mid-lumbar spine area and moderate paravertebral muscle spasm in the lumbar region. Bilateral straight leg raise tests are normal. She has full motor strength of the proximal and distal muscles of both lower legs.

Radiography of the lumbar spine shows diffuse disk space narrowing and vertebral osteophytosis throughout the lumbar region.

What is the most likely diagnosis?

(A) Herniated lumbar disk at L-4, L-5
(B) Instability of the lumbar spine
(C) Lumbar spinal stenosis
(D) Vertebral compression fracture
(E) Ruptured abdominal aortic aneurysm

ANSWER: D

This patient's clinical presentation is typical for vertebral compression fracture. The acute onset of lower back pain in an elderly woman after trying to open a window is a classic scenario. Spasm of the paravertebral muscles and tenderness of the lumbar spine are also typical. Vertebral compression fractures rarely cause neurologic signs, and the absence of leg weakness also favors this diagnosis. Compression fractures of the vertebrae may not be apparent on plain radiographs of the spine for up to 4 weeks after the injury. Technetium bone scans and magnetic resonance imaging identify compression fractures earlier than plain radiographs.

Herniation of the lumbar disk is rare in persons older than 55 years, as the nucleus pulposus of the disk loses water content with age, becomes less gel-like, and does not herniate outside the lumbar disk space. In addition, disk herniation is likely to cause mild weakness of the L-4, L-5 innervated muscles of the legs with a positive straight leg raise test.

Instability of the lumbar spine can cause acute lower back pain but does not usually cause pain when the patient rolls to the side.

Severe pain from sitting or standing is rare. Radiography of the lumbar spine will often demonstrate one disk space that is narrowed and sclerotic out of proportion to other disk spaces.

The pain of lumbar spinal stenosis develops after prolonged standing and walking and is relieved when the patient sits. Lumbar spinal stenosis does not cause acute lower back pain or pain from rolling side to side.

Although a visceral source should always be considered in patients with acute onset of back pain, this patient's presentation is not consistent with a ruptured aneurysm. Ruptured aneurysm is associated with persistent and severe pain that is not relieved by lying down. Tenderness and muscle spasm in the lumbar spine are uncommon in a patient with a ruptured aneurysm.

3. A 72-year-old woman is brought to the office by her daughter, with whom she lives. The patient has asthma. The daughter has just been diagnosed with influenza, by a nasal swab antigen test. The mother has consistently refused to get the influenza vaccine because she says she "always got the flu from the shot," but she agrees to be immunized now.

In addition to immunization, prophylaxis using which of the following would best prevent influenza in this patient?

(A) Amantadine
(B) Rimantadine
(C) Oseltamivir
(D) Zanamivir

ANSWER: C

Both neuraminidase inhibitors, oseltamivir and zanamivir, are available for treatment of influenza. Only oseltamivir is approved for prophylaxis of influenza. Unlike amantadine and rimantadine, which cover only influenza A, neuraminidase inhibitors protect against both influenza A and B. Oseltamivir is preferred because it is administered orally, whereas zanamivir requires an inhalation device, which is often difficult for older adults to use, and zanamivir can trigger bronchospasm in patients with reactive airway disease.

Oseltamivir and zanamivir should be considered in older adults even if the documented strain is influenza A, because amantadine causes marked adverse effects and requires dose adjustment to prevent kidney failure. Rimantadine has fewer adverse effects and does not need adjustment for reduced kidney function, but it is more expensive than amantadine. In recent years, the CDC has recommended against use of amantadine and rimantadine because of resistance.

The effect of neuraminidase inhibitors on such secondary end points as hospitalization and death has been examined only in a few small studies. Thus, in patients without a strict contraindication, drug prophylaxis does not replace the vaccine, which has proven efficacy for preventing hospitalization and death. Furthermore, the vaccine's protective efficacy lasts several months, whereas chemoprophylaxis is useful only for as long as it is taken (usually 2 weeks).

4. An 80-year-old man has hypertension, heart failure, osteoarthritis, and visual and hearing impairments. He is enrolled in the traditional Medicare Parts A and B programs and is considering taking out a supplemental insurance policy.

Which of the following services are not covered under traditional Medicare Parts A and B and should be considered by a patient when selecting supplemental insurance?

(A) Cataract surgery
(B) Cochlear implant
(C) Hearing aid
(D) Diagnostic audiogram
(E) Evaluation by an ophthalmologist

ANSWER: C

Medicare Part A primarily covers acute care related to hospitalization; Part B provides coverage for outpatient and clinician services comprising diagnosis and treatment (including surgery) of medical illness. Medicare provides coverage for cataract surgery and diagnostic evaluations of hearing and visual deficits. Medicare covers cochlear implants for patients with bilateral severe or profound sensorineural hearing impairment who have limited benefit from hearing or vibrotactile aids. Parts A and B do not cover many types of medical equipment, including hearing aids and eyeglasses, or many

preventive services. Diagnostic services, including diagnostic tests and consultation with specialists, are partially or completely covered by Part B.

5. A 79-year-old patient comes to the office at the insistence of family members who believe that she has been behaving differently over the past 2 years. She is a college-educated former teacher who has been retired for 10 years and lives with her husband. She has a history of well-controlled hypertension, mild macular degeneration, and mild osteoarthritis. She used to play golf and bridge, but now she seems less interested in these activities and is less social with family and friends. Her family reports that she takes initiative less often than before and is more easily distracted once she starts an activity. She now occasionally says things, such as criticizing family members, which surprise and concern her family. The patient says that she is fine and has no complaints. When asked about the symptoms her family describes, she answers that sometimes she does not want to do things as often as before, but that she still enjoys playing golf and bridge. She denies any depressive symptoms. Physical examination, including a complete neurologic examination, is within normal limits. Her score on the Mini–Mental State Examination is 29 of 30.

Which of the following is the most appropriate next step?

(A) Reassure the patient and family that her function is appropriate for her age.
(B) Obtain neuroimaging.
(C) Order formal neuropsychologic testing.
(D) Have the patient return in 2 weeks for repeat testing.

ANSWER: C

Executive function refers to the area of cognition responsible for regulation of complex goal-directed behavior. Problems with executive functioning may manifest as lack of initiative, difficulty maintaining attention and focus, perseveration, lack of insight, poor judgment, disinhibition, and changes in personality. Loss of executive control is associated with functional decline. The Mini–Mental State Examination (MMSE) assesses a number of different cognitive functions, such as orientation, registration, recall, attention and calculation, language, and visual-spatial skills. Although a score of 29 is reassuring, the MMSE incompletely assesses executive functioning. Because the patient's symptoms may indicate a problem in this area, neuropsychologic testing of executive function would be more likely to determine if dysfunction exists. Simple office-based assessment of executive functioning is possible, although normal results may not obviate further testing by a neuropsychologist. The clock-drawing test assesses executive control and visual-spatial skills, both of which are incompletely assessed by the MMSE. The test involves asking the patient to draw a clock face, to put in all the numbers, and to set the hands at a particular time (commonly 1:45, 2:50, and 11:10). Word-list generation or the use of standardized questionnaires, such as the Executive Interview (EXIT) test of executive function, would also be appropriate.

Given the family's description, and level of concern, the possibility of cognitive problems is sufficiently strong that reassurance without further assessment would be inappropriate in spite of the near-normal MMSE. Neuroimaging with computed tomography or magnetic resonance imaging is not the most appropriate next step for this patient, since the nature of her cognitive problems has not yet been elucidated adequately. Testing results are unlikely to change over the next 2 weeks.

6. An 87-year-old woman is admitted to your service at a skilled nursing facility. She has an ischemic cardiomyopathy with a left ventricular ejection fraction of 15% and a progressive dementia. She does not understand her condition or the possible outcomes with treatments and therefore lacks decisional capacity. She has no advance directives. She has outlived most of her friends, was never married, and has no children, although she does have a niece. The niece, although caring, has never discussed illness or end-of-life decisions with her aunt. You do know that the patient was combative with hospital care, needing both chemical and physical restraints during the hospitalization prior to this admission. You are discussing care options with the niece. You have told her, considering her aunt's cardiac and functional level, that attempting resuscitation would be a

relatively futile procedure, and on this basis she has agreed with a do-not-attempt-resuscitation–do-not-intubate order. You then turn the conversation to the available treatment options for an exacerbation of her aunt's heart failure. You give her the option of sending her aunt to the hospital or having her remain in the nursing home and receive the maximum monitoring, treatment, and palliation available in that setting.

In guiding the niece as to how she should make this decision, it is appropriate that you tell her which of the following?

(A) Look at the benefits and burdens of these treatments for all demented patients.
(B) Consult a lawyer before making this type of decision.
(C) Look at benefits and burdens of this intervention for her aunt.
(D) Use the substituted-judgment standard.

ANSWER: C

The cascade of decision making for incapacitated patients is (1) the patient's expressed wishes, (2) substituted judgment, and (3) beneficence. In this case, the patient has not given any specific directions before becoming incapacitated. In order to make the decision by substituted judgment, the decision maker must have a sense of the patient's values, preferences, and thoughts about issues of health care and end of life. The niece does not have this information, and there is no one else who could be of assistance in this.

Therefore, the appropriate standard for decision making is beneficence; that is, looking at the potential benefits and burdens of treatment is the standard for decision making. This decision must be made on the basis of the possible benefits and burdens for this particular patient in this particular circumstance. Hospitalization may be more or less traumatic for different demented patients; therefore, a general statement should not be made of the relative burden of hospitalization that would hold up for all patients with dementia. For this patient, the possible advantages of hospitalization include increased cardiac monitoring and intravenous positive inotropic agents. These could potentially be life prolonging. This must be weighed against her difficulties with coping with the strange and confusing environment of the hospital and the functional loss that would occur if chemical and physical restraints were used, all of which would affect her quality of life. Consulting a lawyer in this case would not be helpful, as the timeline for decision making would likely preclude a lawyer's involvement, and a lawyer would have no additional information about the patient's wishes.

7. A 71-year-old woman just moved to an assisted living facility. Her husband died 8 months ago, and she recently moved to the city to be near her daughter. She has a 45-year history of generalized anxiety disorder, for which she has taken diazepam 10 mg daily for the past 30 years. She asks for a prescription to continue the diazepam.

Which of the following is most appropriate at this time?

(A) Continue diazepam.
(B) Immediately discontinue diazepam.
(C) Substitute buspirone for diazepam.
(D) Substitute venlafaxine for diazepam.

ANSWER: A

Given that this is the woman's first contact with the physician, that she is adjusting to a move to a new city after her husband's death, and that there is no imminent risk from continuing the diazepam, it is prudent to maintain the diazepam for now. It is also appropriate to arrange a follow-up appointment with her to discuss the possibility of withdrawing diazepam in the future, at which point it would be important to establish whether she still has generalized anxiety disorder, whether she currently has symptoms of depression, and whether she has a recent history of falls or cognitive impairment. It would also be important to determine whether she previously tried withdrawing the diazepam and, if so, whether this was associated with exacerbation or recurrence of anxiety.

If she is relatively asymptomatic and has not recently tried discontinuing the diazepam, then a slow withdrawal of the drug, by 1 mg per week, would be appropriate. If the history or attempt at withdrawal suggests that she needs ongoing treatment, appropriate options are to continue diazepam at the lowest effective dose,

cognizant of the potential risks as she grows older; to substitute buspirone for diazepam if she does not have significant depressive symptoms; or to substitute with an antidepressant that is effective in generalized anxiety disorder, especially if she has comorbid depressive symptoms. Citalopram, escitalopram, sertraline, or venlafaxine are suitable antidepressants. Buspirone and antidepressant medications have a delayed onset of action and do not suppress withdrawal symptoms of benzodiazepines. Thus, if one of these medications is substituted for the benzodiazepine, it needs to be given at a therapeutic dose for 4 weeks before the benzodiazepine is gradually withdrawn. Despite this approach, some patients are less satisfied with the anxiolytic effects of buspirone than with a benzodiazepine.

8. A 72-year-old man moves into an assisted living facility. Results of his initial examination are normal except for hypertension and he has no symptoms.

Laboratory studies:
Hemoglobin	12.0 g/dL
Mean corpuscular volume	90.0 fL
Mean corpuscular hemoglobin	90.0 pg/cell
Serum protein	9.5 g/dL (elevated)
Serum immunoglobulins	
IgG	2500 mg/L (elevated)
IgA	230 mg/dL (normal)
IgM	150 mg/dL (normal)
Serum protein electrophoresis	monoclonal M spike

Bone marrow biopsy reveals 8% plasma cells. Skeletal survey is normal.

What is the most appropriate management now?

(A) Reassessment in 1 year
(B) Chemotherapy
(C) Radiation therapy
(D) Bone marrow transplantation

ANSWER: A

This patient has a monoclonal gammopathy of undetermined significance (MGUS). MGUS occurs in up to 2% of patients 50 years old, and in up to 4% of patients older than age 70. In a

35-year follow-up series, MGUS was found to progress to multiple myeloma, IgM lymphoma, primary amyloidosis, macroglobulinemia, chronic lymphocytic leukemia, or plasmacytoma in 115 of 1384 patients. In 32 additional patients, the monoclonal protein concentration increased to more than 3 g/dL, or the percentage of plasma cells in the bone marrow increased to more than 10% (smoldering multiple myeloma) without progression to overt myeloma or related disorders. The cumulative probability of progression was 12% at 10 years, 25% at 20 years, and 30% at 25 years. The risk of progression of MGUS to multiple myeloma or related disorders is about 1% per year. Thus, treatment is not warranted at this time.

The 5-year survival rate for multiple myeloma is between 25% and 30%, and is usually lower in older patients. Clinical progression to multiple myeloma is associated with anemia in 66% of patients, chronic renal insufficiency in 25%, hypercalcemia in 20%, bone pain in 60%, and lytic lesions in 70%. Prognostic markers include elevated β_2-microglobulin, lactate dehydrogenase level, and chromosome 13 abnormalities. Most elderly patients cannot undergo bone marrow transplantation. Treatment usually includes melphalan and prednisone, high-dose dexamethasone, or dexamethasone plus thalidomide. Radiation therapy would be appropriate for painful bone lesions.

9. A 94-year-old woman who lives in a nursing home is referred for evaluation of increasing lower extremity edema. The patient has a history of coronary artery disease, including two myocardial infarctions and coronary artery bypass at age 79, and she has type 2 diabetes mellitus, hypertension, moderate Alzheimer's disease, depression, and severe osteoarthritis of both hips. She has an indwelling Foley catheter for urinary incontinence. Over the past few weeks, the nursing-home staff has noted progressive swelling of both legs up to the level of the mid-thigh. The patient is wheelchair bound and requires assistance with most activities. Current medications include aspirin, lisinopril, furosemide, metformin, nortriptyline, donepezil, and haloperidol. Additional history is fragmentary, but the nursing-home staff reports no recent complaints of chest pain or shortness of breath. The patient's living will specifies no cardiopulmonary resuscitation and no artificial life support.

On physical examination, the patient is frail, alert, pleasant, and oriented only to name. She responds to questions but with inconsistent answers. Heart rate is 84 per minute and regular, blood pressure is 130/70 mm Hg, and respiratory rate is 18 per minute. There is no jugular venous distention. A few bibasilar crackles are heard. She has a regular, grade I-II/IV systolic murmur and an S_4, with no S_3. The abdomen is not tender and has no masses. There is moderate to marked edema to the level of the mid thigh bilaterally. She has no focal neurologic deficits.

Laboratory studies:

Hemoglobin	11.3 g/dL
Leukocyte count	5400/μL
Platelet count	217,000/μL
Creatinine	1.0 mg/dL
Blood urea nitrogen	24 mg/dL
Glucose	124 mg/dL
Serum electrolytes	normal
Albumin	3.4 g/dL
Liver enzymes	mildly elevated

Which of the following is the most appropriate approach to managing this patient's edema?

(A) Obtain a B-type natriuretic peptide level and an echocardiogram.
(B) Obtain a plasma D-dimer level and lower extremity venous Doppler ultrasonography
(C) Apply bilateral lower extremity pneumatic compression device.
(D) Apply support stockings and elevate her legs.
(E) Restrict dietary sodium moderately and increase diuretic dosage.

ANSWER: E

The cause of this patient's lower extremity edema is likely multifactorial. Potential contributing factors include worsening heart failure, venous thromboembolic disease, chronic venous insufficiency, excess dietary sodium, and medication side effects. Because of the patient's dementia and physical disabilities, conservative management, emphasizing comfort measures, is appropriate. To this end, a trial of moderate sodium restriction and increased diuretic dosage is the most appropriate course. The results of B-type natriuretic peptide level testing and echocardiography are unlikely to affect management significantly. D-dimer has low specificity in this setting, and the patient is a poor candidate for anticoagulation, even if venous Doppler ultrasonography indicates the presence of deep-vein thrombosis. Support stockings and elevation of the legs are noninvasive and nonpharmacologic, but may be difficult to implement in an elderly patient with dementia and severe osteoarthritis of the hips; in addition, they are unlikely to be effective as the sole treatment for edema. Pneumatic compression devices would also be difficult to implement and probably ineffective in this patient.

10. A 73-year-old black man comes to the office with a painless lesion on his left heel. He states that the lesion has slowly been getting bigger, but he is not sure how long he has had it. He does not recall trauma and reports no drainage or bleeding. History includes chronic venous insufficiency with venous stasis ulcers and osteoarthritis of the knees. He ambulates with a four-point cane. When he watches television, he sits in a recliner to keep his legs elevated. On examination, his left plantar heel has a firm, black raised plaque with irregular margins. It measures 4.5 × 3.7 cm. The patient has 1+ pulses bilaterally and normal sensation.

Which of the following is the most appropriate next step?

(A) Radiography of the foot
(B) Shave biopsy of the lesion
(C) Incisional biopsy of the lesion
(D) Arterial Doppler ultrasonography
(E) Bone scan

ANSWER: C

As this patient's raised lesion has grown and has irregular margins, acral lentiginous melanoma (ALM) should be suspected, and the lesion should be biopsied. ALM can occur on the palm, sole, nail bed, and mucous membrane. It is a variant of melanoma (other variants are lentigo maligna melanoma, superficial spreading melanoma, and nodular melanoma). Black persons have a lower incidence of melanoma than white persons. In black persons, ALM

most commonly appears on the acral surface of the foot. Blacks with cutaneous melanoma are more likely to present with advanced disease, with a median survival of 45 months. White persons with melanoma are 3.6 times more likely to present with early disease and have a median survival of 135 months. Diagnosis in black persons may be delayed for many reasons, such as infrequent inspection of the feet compared with other parts of the body, low suspicion for melanoma in black persons, and atypical presentation. In a retrospective case review, ALM was misdiagnosed as wart, callous, fungal disorder, foreign body, crusty lesion, sweat gland condition, blister, nonhealing wound, mole, and keratoacanthoma. Subungual ALM was misdiagnosed as subungual hematoma, onychomycosis, ingrown toenail, and defective or infected toenail.

When melanoma is suspected, the best approach is excisional biopsy, which permits measurement of thickness. Shave biopsy is contraindicated when melanoma is suspected. Incisional biopsy through most of the dark, raised area is appropriate when the lesion is large or in an area where excisional biopsy cannot be performed, such as the face, hands, or feet. Melanoma should be in the differential diagnosis of heel ulcers; it would be a mistake to manage this raised lesion as a pressure ulcer with dry dressing and avoidance of weight bearing. Radiography or a bone scan of the foot to look for fracture or chronic osteomyelitis is not appropriate, as the physical examination does not suggest fracture or an infected wound. Arterial Doppler ultrasonography would be done for an ischemic heel ulcer, but this patient has pulses (although diminished), and the lesion's irregular margins indicate possible melanoma.

11. A 75-year-old man comes to the office because he has excessive daytime sleepiness and insomnia characterized by awakenings throughout the night. He also has disagreeable leg sensations during the day that are relieved only when he moves his legs. His partner confirms that the patient kicks frequently when he is asleep.

Which of the following treatments is most likely to help this patient?

(A) Ropinirole 0.25 mg at bedtime
(B) Celecoxib 200 mg at bedtime
(C) Mirtazapine 15 mg at bedtime
(D) Modafinil 100 mg twice daily
(E) Zolpidem 10 mg at bedtime

ANSWER: A

Periodic limb movements are a major cause of insomnia in older persons. The distinctive periodic motor output, in which the legs kick at 20- to 40-second intervals throughout the night, may be related to changes in arterial blood pressure or supraspinal factors that lead to brief arousals and fragmented sleep. The prevailing hypothesis is that a deficit in dopaminergic transmission contributes to this disorder, since affected patients have lower binding of the D2 receptor in the basal ganglia, and treatment with dopamine agonists is effective. Periodic limb movements can be treated with dopaminergic agents, such as ropinirole, pramipexole, or levodopa-carbidopa[OL], which decrease both the number of kicks and arousals during the night.

The cyclooxygenase inhibitor celecoxib[OL] is not indicated for periodic limb movements. Antidepressants, such as mirtazapine[OL], and hypnotics, such as zolpidem[OL], have not been shown to benefit patients with periodic limb movements. Modafinil[OL] may improve daytime drowsiness but does not help the nighttime awakenings and limb movements.

12. A 74-year-old man with a history of coronary artery disease had three-vessel coronary artery bypass 3 days ago. He was extubated on postoperative day 1. He now requires evaluation because he remains agitated despite chemical and physical restraints. He pulls at the oxygen tubing despite wrist restraints. Because of his confusion, ambulation has been limited and the Foley catheter is continued. Vital signs are normal. Recommendations include removal of the Foley catheter and obtaining a urinalysis and urine culture.

Which of the following may significantly reduce his agitation and promote resolution of the delirium?

(A) Limit mobility to chair transfers until delirium clears.
(B) Remove the wrist restraints.
(C) Place him in a geri-chair near the nurse's station.
(D) Assist with feeding.

ANSWER: B

A multifaceted targeted intervention is most effective in preventing and treating delirium in hospitalized patients. All potential contributors to delirium should be identified and addressed if possible. Nonpharmacologic strategies are extremely important and often overlooked. Physical restraints may precipitate or contribute significantly to the agitation. If there are no major concerns for traumatic withdrawal of life-saving devices such as endotracheal tubes, removing the restraints and allowing the patient to move at will can greatly reduce anxiety. The patient may require close monitoring and perhaps supervision from the family. Family members may provide a calming effect if they are educated about delirium and its reversibility.

Limiting mobility in any respect is detrimental at this point. The patient needs ambulation at least three times daily. Programs that focus on early mobilization of postoperative hip fracture patients show better outcomes. Although nutritional intake is extremely important in the overall care of this patient, it is feasible that the patient would not require assistance if the restraints were removed and the patient were allowed to feed himself. Spoon-feeding an agitated patient may increase agitation. Placing the restrained patient near the nurse's station will not improve his delirium.

13. A 75-year-old patient comes to the office for his annual check-up. He had complained of hearing loss for several years but until recently had declined to visit an audiologist because he did not think his hearing was bad enough. The audiology report indicates that he has a mild to moderate bilaterally symmetric sensorineural hearing loss with good word recognition scores. During today's interview, he does not seem to follow the discussion, even though he is wearing his new hearing aids. He states that he rarely uses the hearing aids because they do not seem to work in the situations that are most difficult

---

OL-Not approved by the U.S. Food and Drug Administration for this use.

for him. His wife agrees, but also mentions that he has not returned to the audiologist for his follow-up visit.

Which of the following is the most appropriate recommendation?

(A) Return to the audiologist for a hearing aid check, and counseling.
(B) Return these hearing aids to the audiologist to exchange for more effective aids.
(C) Substitute an assistive listening device for hearing aids in the situations that are most difficult for him.
(D) Schedule a cochlear implant evaluation.
(E) Screen for hearing handicap with the Hearing Handicap Inventory for the Elderly—Screening Version (HHIE–S)

ANSWER: A

Success with hearing aids depends in large part on whether audiologic rehabilitation is undertaken to help hearing-impaired persons recover lost physical, psychologic, or social skills. Patients should return to the audiologist within 3 weeks to ensure that the characteristics and fit of a new hearing aid are adequate and that the patient can operate the hearing aid appropriately. An individualized orientation is critical for identifying hearing aid components, teaching care and maintenance, setting realistic expectations, and counseling to facilitate adjustment. The orientation may include training for auditory visual integration, which focuses on combining visual and auditory input to promote receptive communication.

It is premature to return the hearing aid before adjustments are attempted to optimize audibility and speech understanding. All hearing aid companies offer a free trial period (excluding some minimal expenditures) to ensure customer satisfaction.

Assistive listening devices are used to complement, not replace, hearing aids. They use remote microphone technology to overcome communication problems created by noise or distance. The microphone is placed 3 to 6 inches from the sound source, which overcomes the negative effects of distance on speech understanding. Different assistive devices offer sound enhancement, television or media enhancement, telecommunications, and signal-alerting

technology, and they can be purchased without a prescription. Audiologists can help patients identify the most appropriate assistive listening device.

Individuals with mild to moderate sensorineural hearing impairment are not candidates for cochlear implants, because they have a relatively large amount of residual hearing and can benefit from hearing aids.

The Hearing Handicap Inventory for the Elderly—Screening Version is used to identify individuals at risk for hearing impairment who may require follow-up. This patient has already had a complete audiologic evaluation, so functional screening is not appropriate. He should be referred back to the audiologist, and his wife should accompany him if possible.

14. In which of the following settings is the prevalence of depressive symptoms and diagnosable major depression highest?

(A) Community
(B) Outpatient medical clinic
(C) General hospital
(D) Long-term-care facility

ANSWER: D

The cross-sectional prevalence of major depression among older persons is between 1% and 3% in the community, 10% and 12% in primary (ambulatory) care, 10% and 15% in acute (medical-surgical hospital) care, and 15% and 25% in chronic or long-term (nursing-home) care. In all these settings, the prevalence of significant depressive symptoms is two to three times higher than the prevalence of diagnosable major depression, ranging from 10% in the community to 40% in nursing homes. The higher prevalence of depression in treatment settings has been attributed to the association of depression with physical illness and disability. The prevalence of major depression is 13% in patients with diabetes mellitus, 16% in those with coronary artery disease, 17% in those with arthritis, and 22% in those with acute stroke. Depression is also associated with Alzheimer's and Parkinson's diseases, other neurodegenerative disorders, cancer, thyroid disease, end-organ failure, hip fracture, vitamin B_{12} deficiency, fibromyalgia, chronic fatigue syndrome, irritable bowel syndrome, and chronic pain. In controlled studies, depressed patients with medical illness have been found to respond to antidepressant treatment or psychotherapy similarly to depressed patients without comorbid medical illness.

15. Which of the following describes expected age-related changes in pulmonary function?

(A) Stable total lung capacity; decreased vital capacity, decreased forced vital capacity, decreased FEV_1, and increased residual volume
(B) Decreased total lung capacity, decreased forced vital capacity, decreased FEV_1, and decreased residual volume
(C) Increased total lung capacity, increased forced vital capacity, increased FEV_1, and increased residual volume
(D) Decreases in all volumes
(E) Decreased lung capacity, decreased residual volume, increased forced vital capacity, and increased FEV_1

ANSWER: A

With normal aging there is a loss of static elastic recoil of the lung that is balanced by an increased stiffness of the thoracic cage; this generally results in a maintenance of total lung capacity at volumes equal to those of younger adults. The loss of elastic recoil and an increase in closing volume result in a predictable increase in residual volume (the volume of air remaining in the lungs after the forced vital capacity maneuver). Consequently, there is a reduction in vital capacity, which is the difference between total lung capacity and residual volume. The FEV_1 reaches a maximal volume in young adulthood and then declines steadily over a person's life.

16. A 68-year-old man comes to the office because of lower urinary symptoms associated with benign prostatic hyperplasia. He awakens once or twice each night to urinate; the frequency of his nocturia has increased gradually over the past 4 years. He has no other urinary tract symptoms. He has coronary heart disease that is well managed with metoprolol 100 mg and aspirin 81 mg daily.

On physical examination, blood pressure is 140/70 mm Hg, and pulse is 55 per minute. On digital rectal examination, the prostate is not enlarged, has no nodules, induration, or asymmetry. Prostate-specific antigen (PSA) level is 6 ng/mL (increased from 2.5 ng/mL at age 65 and 3 ng/mL at age 67).

What is the most appropriate next step in the evaluation of this patient?

(A) Remeasure the PSA level.
(B) Refer to a urologist for a prostate biopsy.
(C) Order a transrectal ultrasound.
(D) Order a bone scan.

ANSWER: A

This patient has had a relatively orderly progression of his prostate-specific antigen (PSA) level, with a sudden rise. Serial PSA levels can vary for several reasons, including subclinical prostatitis and vigorous prostatic massage. Often the cause is unknown. Any single abnormal PSA level should be confirmed 4 to 6 weeks later before proceeding with work-up for prostate cancer.

Referral to a urologist is appropriate if the increase in PSA level is confirmed. Transrectal ultrasound is not a diagnostic test for prostate cancer and should be used as part of a transrectal prostate biopsy. A bone scan is used to stage known prostate cancer.

17. On your monthly visit of an 85-year-old man in the nursing home, he feels well. He has a history of hypertension, stable kidney insufficiency, and coronary artery disease, with myocardial infarction 2 years ago (ejection fraction, 35%). He takes aspirin 81 mg daily, furosemide 20 mg twice daily, metoprolol 25 mg twice daily, and pravastatin 40 mg daily.

On examination, blood pressure is 165/79 mm Hg, consistent with readings over the past few visits.

Laboratory studies:
Sodium	137 mEq/L
Potassium	4.3 mEq/L
Urea nitrogen	25 mg/dL
Creatinine	2.3 mg/dL (stable)

Which of the following is the most appropriate intervention?

(A) Add lisinopril.
(B) Increase metoprolol.
(C) Substitute hydrochlorothiazide for furosemide.
(D) Add amlodipine.

ANSWER: A

This patient has structural heart disease from myocardial infarction and longstanding hypertension but no symptoms of heart failure. Despite his kidney insufficiency (estimated creatinine clearance of 25 mL/min), the use of an angiotensin-converting enzyme (ACE) inhibitor is indicated. ACE inhibitors improve survival and reduce morbidity after myocardial infarction. Kidney function may deteriorate acutely when an ACE inhibitor is initiated, and patients with chronic kidney insufficiency are especially susceptible. A transient 10% to 20% increase in serum creatinine can be anticipated when ACE inhibitor therapy is started and is not a reason to discontinue therapy. Serum creatinine and electrolytes should be evaluated before and 1 to 2 weeks after starting therapy.

Given this patient's kidney function, hydrochlorothiazide will probably not be effective for reducing blood pressure. Increasing metoprolol or adding amlodipine may reduce his blood pressure, but, given his history of myocardial infarction, lisinopril is the best choice.

18. A 69-year-old woman with mild mental retardation comes to the office with one of her residential caregivers, who describes gradually worsening anger, agitation, and isolation over the past 12 months. Approximately 6 months ago she began treatment with a selective serotonin-reuptake inhibitor, but her response has been negligible despite titration of the medication to the maximum recommended dose. She has no previous history of emotional or behavioral problems. She takes acetaminophen for mild pain due to degenerative arthritis, and she has bilateral cataracts but is reluctant to proceed with surgery.

She has enjoyed working in a noncompetitive setting for over 20 years, but this activity is now in jeopardy because her visual impairment interferes with the work. She has no supportive family and only a small network of peer friend-

ships. She is her own guardian and has always been involved in decisions about her life and health.

Which of the following is the most appropriate next step in caring for this patient?

(A) Begin psychotherapy, focusing on helping her with health care decisions.
(B) Begin a medication to augment the antidepressant.
(C) Add an atypical antipsychotic agent to decrease her agitation.
(D) Arrange for neuropsychological testing.
(E) Discontinue the antidepressant and begin a medication for anxiety.

ANSWER: A

Older persons with mental retardation have limitations in insight, judgment, coping ability, and family support systems. It is likely that, as this patient's sensory impairment worsened, she was less able to cope with work and with the associated stress of needing to make health care decisions. A course of psychotherapy focusing on health care decisions and her fears and expectations is the best choice of the options listed. The ideal outcome would be for her to choose treatment for the visual impairment that has radically changed her environment.

Augmenting her current antidepressant treatment is less than ideal, given the limited clinical evidence that she is depressed or that it would best be treated with medication.

Adding a low-dose atypical antipsychotic to decrease agitation may be appropriate in some situations, but at this point it is more prudent to avoid a medication with potentially serious adverse effects. Typical and atypical antipsychotic medications may succeed in decreasing some target behaviors, but at the cost of dampening all behavior.

Although some psychologic testing might be beneficial, it is inappropriate to defer active treatment while trying to arrange for a battery of neuropsychological tests. The most pertinent testing would offer insight into her cognitive and adaptive skills and information regarding her mood and behavior. Much of this could be assessed by gathering information on the patient and spending time in therapy with her.

Given the clinical picture, the patient seems anxious. However, beginning a benzodiazepine anxiolytic medication at this point could worsen her mood and behavior and cause serious adverse effects.

19. An 82-year-old woman who lives in a long-term-care facility is evaluated for agitation that occurs during the day and when she awakens from sleep. She has mild Alzheimer's dementia. She spends most of the day sitting in front of the television in a lounge with low lights, occasionally dozing off. The patient is mobile and fully participates in all basic activities of daily living. Review of her medications and physical examination reveal no apparent cause for the agitation. Mental status examination reveals only mild cognitive impairment.

Which of the following nonpharmacologic interventions is most likely to benefit this patient?

(A) Ask staff to exercise the patient twice daily.
(B) Ask staff to discourage the patient from watching television and to introduce nighttime diapers.
(C) Ask staff to keep the patient in a bright environment during the day and a quiet, dark environment at night without interruptions.
(D) Ask staff to prevent daytime napping and implement enforced sleeping hours, with restriction of evening fluid intake.
(E) Provide the patient with a soft nightlight, familiar items and photographs at the bedside, and orienting objects, such as a clock.

ANSWER: C

Disrupted, brief sleep at night is common in the long-term-care setting, and patients are commonly asleep during the day. According to actigraphic data (from a device usually worn on the wrist that measures activity), nursing-home patients are rarely asleep or awake for a full hour throughout the night and day. Low lighting, noise, and interruptions by staff to wake and turn patients are partially responsible for poor sleep consolidation. Patients in nursing homes need to be in bright environments during the day and in a quiet, dark environment at night. Awakenings at night are often accom-

panied by agitation and may result in greater daytime agitation. Even severely demented nursing-home patients spontaneously change shoulder and hip position throughout the night, obviating the need to awaken them to prevent bedsores related to incontinence.

Exercise may be generally helpful, but it does not address the environmental concerns and nighttime awakening that are likely responsible for this patient's agitation. Similarly, removing the television does not address the daytime low light and napping. Fluid restriction, enforced sleep hours, and prevention of napping are not reasonable expectations of the staff and generally are difficult to enforce in a long-term-care facility. The provision of a nightlight, orienting objects, and a familiar nonthreatening environment is useful in dementia syndromes and delirium, especially for patients with "sundowning" or loss of orientation, which is not the case with this patient.

20. The primary care provider for a 79-year-old woman with advanced dementia is called by the police when the patient is found dead at home. She lived with her son, who had called paramedics when he discovered that she was not responsive. The paramedics found an elderly woman lying almost naked on her bed, and they were concerned about her appearance. They described a thin woman with feces on her buttocks and abdomen, elongated fingernails and toenails caked with dirt, two large pressure sores (stage IV on her buttock and stage III on her right shoulder), and matted, dirty hair.

It has been difficult to care for her. Her son always reported that she did not want him to bring her to the doctor, and she had refused a home-health aide when she was in an earlier stage of dementia. On her last visit to the office, 18 months ago, she was found to have lost a substantial amount of weight and was disheveled and somewhat dirty. Home-health care was initiated, but her son refused their services when they came to his house, saying that he was able to care for her and that she did not want anyone else to help.

For religious reasons, the son wants the death certificate signed as soon as possible so that she can be buried within 24 hours. The police request direction about what to do next. Which of the following is the most appropriate response?

(A) Request transport of the body to an emergency department for further evaluation.
(B) Sign the death certificate.
(C) Release the body to the mortuary and make a referral to Adult Protective Services.
(D) Request an evaluation by a coroner or medical examiner.

ANSWER: D

This may be a case of fatal neglect and should be reported to the coroner or medical examiner for expert postmortem evaluation and autopsy. Some signs of neglect may be difficult to distinguish from chronic illness. For example, dehydration, malnutrition, and pressure sores may be unavoidable as persons with multiple medical problems become more debilitated. In cases of medical neglect, however, the caregiver fails to seek appropriate medical care for the patient. It is important in these circumstances for the clinician to confer with the coroner or medical examiner's office about appropriateness of care. The medical examiner may perform an autopsy or toxicology screening and may look for evidence to support or refute the possibility of fatal neglect.

A death certificate should not be signed under these circumstances. First, it has been 18 months since the patient's last examination, suggesting that she has not been under active care. Also, there is reason to suspect neglect: the person is found in filthy conditions with severe pressure sores and possible malnutrition. Although extenuating circumstances may explain the situation (in this case, a person who refused care), it is not within the clinician's purview to make this determination.

Once a patient is pronounced dead, it is not necessary or appropriate to bring the body to an emergency department if abuse or neglect is suspected. Similarly, it is not appropriate to make a referral to Adult Protective Services once a person has died.

21. A 72-year-old black American woman cares for her 75-year-old black American husband with Alzheimer's disease in their own home.

Which of the following factors is the strongest predictor of whether the husband will be placed in a nursing home within the next year?

(A) The wife's age
(B) The husband's racial background
(C) The wife's racial background
(D) The husband's hallucinations and delusions
(E) The husband's dependence in one or more activities of daily living

ANSWER: D

Considerable research has focused on identifying risk factors for nursing-home placement. Caring for a spouse or other relative with dementia is stressful. Behavioral problems, such as asking the same question repetitively, wandering, and psychotic symptoms, appear to be particularly potent predictors of nursing-home placement. In one study, the presence of a behavior problem shortened a demented person's stay in the community by about 2 years.

Other risk factors include the caregiver's being over 75 years old, the demented person's living alone, one or more dependencies in activities of daily living, and more advanced cognitive impairment. Race and ethnicity may play a protective role in placement decisions. Black or Hispanic Americans with dementia are less likely than white Americans with dementia to be placed in a nursing home.

22. A 75-year-old woman comes to the office because of pain and swelling of the right forefoot that have progressed over the past 3 weeks. She relates going on a 2-mile walk prior to the onset of symptoms. The symptoms began as a mild ache but have become increasingly intense with her usual walking. Two weeks ago she visited the local emergency department for the pain; radiographs demonstrated normal metatarsophalangeal joints and no fractures. She has tried nonsteroidal anti-inflammatory agents, ice, and warm compresses without relief.

On physical examination, vital signs are normal. She has good pedal pulses and normal sensation. The right foot is tender to palpation at the midshaft of the second metatarsal. There is no pain with range of motion to the second metatarsophalangeal joint. There is callus on the plantar aspect of the second metatarsophalangeal joint. Ankle joint range of motion is less than 5 degrees with maximal dorsiflexion. A moderate hallux valgus and bunion are present.

What is the most likely diagnosis?

(A) Stress fracture
(B) Gout
(C) Morton's neuroma
(D) Ganglion cyst
(E) Degenerative joint disease

ANSWER: A

In 95% of cases, stress fracture appears in the lower extremities, is generally the sequelae of overuse, and occurs when repetitive, subthreshold stress exceeds the bones' reparative capacity. In the foot, stress fractures affect the second to fourth metatarsals approximately 90% of the time. Postmenopausal women often have osteoporosis or osteopenia. As a result, women are more likely than men to have stress fractures.

The hallmark finding is pinpoint tenderness on the affected metatarsal with surrounding edema. Initial radiographs are often normal; abnormal findings may not be evident until 3 to 6 weeks after injury. When present, the typical radiographic changes are a linear cortical lucent region with periosteal and endosteal thickening. Fractures that occurred several weeks earlier will also have bone callus formation about the fracture site. A three-phase bone scan is the gold standard for diagnosis when radiographs are normal. Hallux valgus deformities suggest lack of normal weight-bearing force under the first metatarsal and often result in increased pressure to the adjacent lesser metatarsals, as manifested in this patient by the plantar callus under the second metatarsophalangeal joint. Additionally, an Achilles tendon contracture induces "toe-walking" and subsequent increased forefoot pressure. The increased weight-bearing pressure, along with prolonged repetitive stress, increases risk for stress fracture.

Gout affects joints and would induce pain with toe range of motion. Morton's neuroma elicits pain with palpation in the intermetatarsal space and not the bone. It can also cause shooting, burning pain to the distal toes to which it provides innervation. A ganglion cyst rarely is painful and would be visible as a soft palpable mass. Degenerative joint disease, like gout, is painful with range of motion.

23. A 75-year-old man returns to the office for a follow-up visit after a 6-week trial of St. John's wort 300 mg two to three times daily. At the initial visit, he met criteria for major depressive disorder but denied having recurrent thoughts of death or suicidal ideation. He has a history of hypertension, which is well controlled on a low-salt diet and hydrochlorothiazide 12.5 mg daily, and osteoarthritis, for which he occasionally takes acetaminophen. He has no history of mental health problems. He was reluctant to take a prescription antidepressant but suggested trying St. John's wort. At follow-up, there is no apparent improvement in his depression, and he now agrees to begin treatment with sertraline.

Which of the following is the best recommendation with respect to the St. John's wort?

(A) Continue St. John's wort and begin sertraline.
(B) Discontinue St. John's wort and begin sertraline after 4 weeks.
(C) Discontinue St. John's wort and begin sertraline the next day.
(D) Discontinue St. John's wort and begin sertraline in 1 week.

ANSWER: D

St. John's wort inhibits neuronal reuptake of serotonin, norepinephrine, and dopamine. Case reports of St. John's wort used concurrently with a selective serotonin-reuptake inhibitor (SSRI) describe symptoms characteristic of central serotonin excess. In one case, a patient developed nausea, anxiety, restlessness, and irritability after taking St. John's wort for 2 days with ongoing sertraline treatment. Another patient became incoherent, groggy, and lethargic following a single dose of paroxetine 20 mg added to ongoing use of St. John's wort 600 mg per day. The patient had previously been treated with paroxetine for 8 months without adverse effect.

The active constituents of St. John's wort are thought to be hypericin and hyperforin. The elimination half-lives of hypericin and hyperforin are 43 hours and 9 hours, respectively. Since it takes five half-lives to eliminate about 95% of a medication, the risk of developing central serotonin excess may be minimized by waiting 7 to 10 days before starting an SSRI following use of St. John's wort.

24. An 82-year-old man is admitted with acute right upper quadrant pain and an impacted gall stone. An open cholecystectomy is planned once the patient has been stabilized and fully assessed.

The patient resides at home with his wife. His past medical history includes: a 50-pack-per-year cigarette history and current smoking; chronic obstructive pulmonary disease for 5 years, stable on an ipratropium-albuterol metered-dose inhaler and occasional short courses of oral corticosteroids. He has no prior cardiac history and is taking no medications other than his pulmonary drugs.

On physical examination he has a body mass index (kg/m^2) of 34, blood pressure 132/78 mm Hg, heart rate 88, respiratory rate 18; he is afebrile. Lung examination shows distant breath sounds with end expiratory wheezes throughout both lung fields. The remainder of his examination is unremarkable.
Other assessments show:

FEV$_1$	30% of predicted
Electrocardiogram	normal
Chest x-ray	hyperlucent lung fields, no infiltrates, and no changes of the cardiac silhouette
Arterial blood gas (room air)	pH 7.42, PCO_2 48 mm Hg, PO_2 68 mm Hg, HCO_3 31 mEq/L
Blood urea nitrogen	34 mg/dL
Serum albumin	2.9 gm/dL

What conveys the greatest risk for postoperative respiratory failure in this patient?

(A) Age greater than 69 years
(B) History of chronic obstructive pulmonary disease
(C) Obesity
(D) Upper abdominal surgery
(E) Albumin less than 3.0 mg/dL

ANSWER: D

Respiratory failure is a recognized postoperative complication for older patients undergoing surgery, but age alone is not a major risk factor for postoperative pulmonary complications. The relative risk for pulmonary complication related to advanced age is approximately doubled. Comorbidities and the type of surgery to be performed play a much larger role in predicting postoperative pulmonary complications. Smoking multiplies the relative risk by approximately 3 and chronic obstructive pulmonary disease by 3 to 4. Obesity has not been found to be a risk factor for postoperative pulmonary complications in older patients; however, the presence of obesity-associated obstructive sleep apnea may confer added risk. Albumin levels less than 3.0 gm/dL increase the risk by 2.5 and blood urea nitrogen greater than 30 mg/dL by 2.3.

The strongest predictor of postoperative respiratory failure remains the type of surgery being performed. Upper abdominal surgery confers a 4.2-fold increased risk of respiratory failure during the postoperative period. Repair of an abdominal aneurysm increases the risk of postoperative respiratory failure by 14, thoracic surgery by 8. Emergency surgery also adds significantly to the risk of postoperative respiratory failure.

The risk of postoperative respiratory failure can be predicted in men undergoing noncardiac surgery by using the Arozullah Multifactorial Risk Index. This index assigns points on the basis of the type of surgery, emergent versus nonemergent surgery, albumin, blood urea nitrogen, functional status, history of chronic obstructive pulmonary disease, and age. Patients are assigned to one of five postoperative respiratory risk categories on the basis of total points. By the use of criteria set forth in the Arozullah Index, the patient in this case would score a total of 34 points, which would assign a 10.1% risk of postoperative respiratory failure.

25. A 76-year-old man comes to the emergency department following the abrupt onset of rectal bleeding. He has a history of coronary heart disease, heart failure, renal insufficiency, gastroesophageal reflux disease, and degenerative joint disease. Daily medications include metoprolol, furosemide, potassium chloride, simvastatin, celecoxib, and lansoprazole. The bleeding stops spontaneously. Diagnostic colonoscopy, performed after oral cleansing with

polyethylene glycol and electrolyte solution, demonstrates residual blood in the ascending colon, scattered diverticula in the sigmoid colon, and multiple, 5-mm, flat cherry-red lesions in the cecum.

What is the most likely cause for bleeding in this patient?

(A) Angiodysplasia
(B) Nonspecific colitis
(C) Aortoenteric fistula
(D) Upper gastrointestinal lesion

ANSWER: A

The incidence of lower gastrointestinal bleeding increases more than 200-fold between ages 20 and 80. Angiodysplasia, also called *arteriovenous malformation* or *vascular ectasia,* is the source of lower gastrointestinal bleeding in up to 20% of older patients and occurs with equal frequency in men and women. Two thirds of cases are found in persons older than age 70. More than half are located in the cecum and proximal ascending colon, but they may occur throughout the gastrointestinal tract, usually are multiple, and are 5 to 10 mm wide. They are dilated, thin-walled vessels in the mucosa and submucosa that are lined by endothelium or by smooth muscle. In more than 90% of cases, bleeding stops spontaneously. Typically, diagnosis is by direct visualization by colonoscopy, but mesenteric angiography is more sensitive than colonoscopy and can detect angiodysplasia deep in the submucosa that may not be visible grossly.

Diverticular disease is the cause in up to 37% of older patients with brisk rectal bleeding. The prevalence of diverticular disease is age dependent, increasing to 30% by age 60 and to 65% by age 85. Diverticula occur at weak points in the bowel wall, usually in the sigmoid colon, where blood vessels penetrate the circular muscle of the bowel. Diverticular bleeding is usually painless and self-limited, and it rarely coexists with acute diverticulitis.

Diverticular bleeding and angiodysplasia are responsible for almost 60% of cases of lower gastrointestinal bleeding in older adults. Other sources of bleeding include colorectal neoplasms, an upper gastrointestinal source, colitis (from ischemia, inflammation, infection, or radiation), solitary rectal ulcers, and hemorrhoids. Aortoenteric fistula is a less common cause.

Approximately 10% of cases of major lower intestinal bleeding and 20% of cases of minor bleeding in elderly persons are caused by benign or malignant neoplasm. In 15% of older adults, the source of lower gastrointestinal bleeding is in the upper gastrointestinal tract. Upper intestinal endoscopy may be necessary to reveal the source of bleeding.

An infectious cause should be excluded in an older patient with acute bloody diarrhea. *Salmonella* organisms and *Escherichia coli* O157:H7 serotypes are common in elderly patients. *Clostridium difficile*–induced diarrhea rarely causes bleeding.

Nonsteroidal anti-inflammatory agents have been implicated as a cause of nonspecific colitis, exacerbation of idiopathic inflammatory bowel disease, and diverticular bleeding.

26. An 81-year-old female resident of an assisted-living facility comes to the emergency department with complaints of fatigue, nausea, and frequent urination. She has a history of hypertension, osteoporosis with spine compression fractures, osteoarthritis, and macular degeneration. The patient has previously been independent in instrumental activities of daily living, except for medications, and she uses a walker for ambulation. She is admitted to an Acute Care for the Elderly (ACE) unit with urosepsis.

Which of the following is a component of this type of intervention?

(A) An environment that promotes mobility and orientation
(B) A care map to outline her current medications
(C) A protocol outlining the length of stay for urosepsis
(D) A discussion with her family about the need for restorative care
(E) A teaching session on health promotion interventions

ANSWER: A

This patient was fortunate to have an Acute Care for the Elderly (ACE) unit in her area. In several major hospital studies, ACE units show promise in preserving activities of daily living. These units focus on multidisciplinary approaches to care of the hospitalized older adult. Components of an ACE unit include an environment that promotes mobility and orientation, nursing initiated protocols for independent self-care, strong interdisciplinary planning with early social work screening, and medical care review to promote optimal regimens. Some studies suggest that ACE units are associated with less functional decline in activities of daily living at discharge and a trend toward decreased length of hospitalization. However, it has also been shown that admission to an ACE unit early on in the hospital course is important, as there is little benefit once a patient has been stabilized on another unit. The multidisciplinary nature of the care and the emphasis on function as well as disease have made ACE units a unique model for the care of hospitalized older adults.

27. The most commonly overlooked aspect of the care of patients with hip fracture on discharge from a subacute unit and arrival in the rehabilitation setting is:

    (A) Deep-vein thrombosis prophylaxis
    (B) Delirium prevention
    (C) Osteoporosis treatment
    (D) Nutritional support

    ANSWER: C

    The medical consultation for patients with hip fractures is multifaceted, and its emphasis depends on the patient's phase of illness. One neglected area has been the evaluation and treatment of osteoporosis. Several studies suggest that few patients with hip fracture receive evaluation and adequate treatment for osteoporosis, even though they are at risk of another osteoporotic fracture. Only 12% to 24% of patients with hip fracture report having had dual radiographic absorptiometry. Vitamin D and calcium were reported to be prescribed in only 3% to 27% of fracture patients. Antiresorptive agents were used more frequently (12% to 79% of patients) than vitamin D and calcium, although fewer than 10% of patients received bisphosphonates. Up to 40% of patients with hip fracture received no osteoporosis therapy, and only 13% received therapy that

followed guidelines of the National Osteoporosis Foundation. A system to ensure evaluation and management of osteoporosis appears to be needed.

Prevention of venous thromboembolism and delirium as well as nutritional support should be addressed during the acute phase of the hospital stay. These issues should have been resolved before the patient is discharged from a subacute setting.

28. A 70-year-old woman comes to the office for management of osteoporosis. She has a history of nephrolithiasis. She went through menopause approximately 18 years ago and takes the following medications: alendronate 70 mg weekly, calcium carbonate 1500 mg daily, and vitamin D 800 IU daily. She drinks three glasses of milk and several servings of yogurt and cheese daily. Her bone mineral density, as measured by dual energy x-ray absorptiometry (DEXA), reveals a T score of −3.0 at the hip and −2.5 at the lumbar spine.

    Laboratory studies:
Ionized calcium	6.1 mEq/L
Phosphorus	2.7 mg/dL
Parathyroid hormone	62 pg/mL
Serum creatinine	0.9 mg/dL
Thyrotropin	2.1 µU/mL

    What is the most likely cause of this patient's hypercalcemia?

    (A) Primary hyperparathyroidism
    (B) Milk-alkali syndrome
    (C) Humoral hypercalcemia of malignancy
    (D) Granulomatous disease

    ANSWER: A

    The patient's history of nephrolithiasis coupled with her fairly severe bone loss (despite intake of alendronate, calcium, and vitamin D) raises concern for secondary causes of osteoporosis, such as hyperthyroidism, hyperparathyroidism, Cushing's syndrome, or glucocorticoid therapy. This patient has evidence of hypercalcemia. In the ambulatory care setting, the most common cause of hypercalcemia is primary hyperparathyroidism. Primary hyperparathyroidism is more common in women, and the prevalence increases with age (the incidence in postmenopausal women is fivefold higher than in the general population).

The serum parathyroid hormone level is the key to diagnosis of primary hyperparathyroidism. In this case, the parathyroid hormone level is inappropriately normal in the context of hypercalcemia. The low serum phosphorus level also suggests hyperparathyroidism.

Although this patient's high intake of calcium supplements and dairy products suggests milk-alkali syndrome, the preserved renal function and the high-normal parathyroid hormone level do not support this diagnosis (parathyroid hormone would be suppressed in milk-alkali syndrome). Similarly, humoral hypercalcemia of malignancy and granulomatous disease are unlikely, since the parathyroid hormone level would be low or undetectable in these conditions.

29. An 87-year old woman comes to the office because of short-term memory loss persisting for several months, which is getting worse according to her husband. She has some college education. She has a history of hypertension, which is well controlled with hydrochlorothiazide, 25 mg daily. She is otherwise in good health. She sleeps and eats normally and has no day-to-day problems except for occasional difficulty locating her car in the parking lot. Physical and neurologic examination reveal nothing remarkable. There is no evidence of sadness or anhedonia. She scores 25 of 30 points on the Mini–Mental State Examination, losing 3 points on recall and 2 on orientation.

What is the most likely cause of the memory complaint?

(A) Benign senescent forgetfulness
(B) Mild cognitive impairment
(C) Dementia
(D) Minor depression
(E) Major depression

ANSWER: B

This patient complains of memory loss that, according to her husband, appears to be worsening. There are no other cognitive complaints, and there are no other obvious medical problems. She continues to show a reasonable level of day-to-day functioning.

Examination reveals abnormalities on the Mini–Mental State Examination (MMSE), especially the inability to recall three objects. There is no evidence of depressive symptoms. Given the absence of depressive or other psychiatric symptoms and the absence of a medical problem to explain the memory loss, the differential diagnosis focuses on age-related benign memory loss, mild cognitive impairment, and a dementia syndrome.

Mild cognitive impairment is most likely since the patient has a subjective memory complaint that is confirmed by an informant, and she has measurable memory impairment on the MMSE. The memory decline cannot be ascribed to aging alone, even in an 87-year-old woman, given her good health and level of education. She does not meet criteria for dementia because the cognitive decline affects only memory and she is functionally intact. Although the type of cognitive impairment can be determined on clinical grounds, identifying the cause may require a limited laboratory and imaging work-up, even though in most similar cases laboratory (thyroid tests, vitamin B_{12}, and metabolic panel) and brain imaging studies are normal.

Diagnosing mild cognitive impairment and differentiating it from usual aging are important for two reasons. First, since mild cognitive impairment progresses to Alzheimer-type dementia at the rate of about 10% to 15% per year, patients should be followed closely for further decline (especially if they drive), and appropriate treatment should be instituted as needed. Second, ongoing clinical trials are examining the efficacy of several medications in preventing progression of mild cognitive impairment to dementia. Already, in some memory clinics, patients with mild cognitive impairment are treated with cholinesterase inhibitors and vitamin E, although current data do not yet support this practice.

30. A 68-year-old man comes to the office for follow-up management after external-beam radiation treatment to his prostate for a moderately differentiated adenocarcinoma (Gleason grades 3 and 4). Bone scan is negative for metastatic lesion. Before treatment, his prostate-specific antigen (PSA) level had increased from 3.0 to 21 over 3 years. After

radiation treatment, his PSA level fell to 4.0, but over the next 6 months it increased to 7.0. He has begun combined androgen blockade with flutamide and leuprolide, as prescribed by his urologist.

Which of the following additional treatments might you discuss with the urologist to prevent metastatic disease?

(A) Orchiectomy
(B) Ketoconazole
(C) Zoledronic acid
(D) Cyclophosphamide

ANSWER: C

In many cases, prostate cancer progresses slowly and can be considered more as a chronic illness than a life-threatening disease. This patient is at high risk of metastases because he had a pretreatment PSA level above 20 and a combined Gleason grade of 7. Despite treatment with external-beam radiation, the PSA level increased, suggesting residual disease. Residual or recurrent disease can be treated by salvage surgery or androgen ablation. Because the patient was started on combined androgen ablation with flutamide and leuprolide, orchiectomy is not currently needed. Ketoconazole and chemotherapy should be considered only if androgen ablation fails.

The role of bisphosphonates such as zoledronic acid and pamidronate in prostate cancer is expanding. Bisphosphonates may help prevent osteoporosis and bone metastases and may lessen bone pain. Osteoporosis is a complication of androgen-deprivation therapy in men with prostate carcinoma. Androgen deprivation, from bilateral orchiectomy or treatment with a gonadotropin-releasing hormone agonist, decreases bone mineral density and increases fracture risk. Other factors, including diet and life style, may contribute to bone loss. Intravenous pamidronate, a second-generation bisphosphonate, prevents bone loss during androgen-deprivation therapy. Zoledronic acid, a more potent third-generation bisphosphonate, prevents bone loss and increases bone mineral density during androgen deprivation-therapy. Its use for prevention of bone metastases from prostate cancer is off label.

In addition, bisphosphonates may have a direct antitumor effect, possibly related to inhibition of tumor cell adhesion and spread to bone, induction of apoptosis, anti-angiogenic properties, or increased T-cell counts. Although data are limited, both pamidronate and zoledronic acid have been shown to decrease skeletal-related events in prostate cancer patients. More research is needed before bisphosphonates are used for their anticancer properties. The role of bisphosphonates in treating bone pain in metastasis is more controversial, because some data suggest that they are not as effective as chemotherapy or targeted radiation therapy.

Treatment with cyclophosphamide[OL] is well tolerated in prostate cancer but response rates are low.

31. A 75-year-old woman comes to the office for a routine visit. She has a history of hypertension, osteoporosis, chronic obstructive pulmonary disease, osteoarthritis, and insomnia. Two months ago she began celecoxib 100 mg daily for arthritis and diphenhydramine at bedtime for sleep. Other medications include lisinopril 40 mg daily, hydrochlorothiazide 25 mg daily, salmeterol two inhalations twice daily, ipratropium three inhalations four times daily, atenolol 75 mg daily, calcium carbonate 500 mg three times daily, vitamin D 200 IU daily, alendronate 70 mg weekly, and a multivitamin daily.

On examination, blood pressure is 178/92 mm Hg; this is consistent with home readings the patient has taken over the past month. At office visits 3 and 6 months ago, systolic blood pressure was between 148 and 152 mm Hg, and diastolic pressure was between 80 and 85 mm Hg.

Which of the following is the most appropriate intervention?

(A) Substitute furosemide for hydrochlorothiazide.
(B) Substitute acetaminophen for celecoxib.
(C) Increase atenolol.
(D) Substitute ramipril for lisinopril.
(E) Substitute zolpidem for diphenhydramine.

[OL]Not approved by the U.S. Food and Drug Administration for this use.

ANSWER: B

The recent addition of celecoxib is the most likely cause of her increased blood pressure. Traditional (nonselective) nonsteroidal anti-inflammatory drugs (NSAIDs) can increase blood pressure, especially in patients with hypertension. Emerging data indicate that cyclooxygenase-2 selective agents such as celecoxib may increase blood pressure to a similar extent as nonselective NSAIDs. Because this patient's hypertension is uncontrolled despite three medications, it would be prudent to initiate a different pain medication.

Hydrochlorothiazide is less effective in patients with kidney disease (creatinine clearance under 30 mL/min), but because this patient has no signs of kidney disease, changing hydrochlorothiazide to furosemide will likely not improve blood-pressure control. In addition, furosemide is a less potent antihypertensive than the thiazide diuretics. Because angiotensin-converting enzyme inhibitors have similar efficacy at equipotent dosages, substituting ramipril for lisinopril would not be effective. Increasing the atenolol dosage may improve blood-pressure control. But, because this patient has chronic obstructive pulmonary disease, it would be prudent to keep the β-blocker dosage low to avoid loss of β_1 selectivity that may occur with higher dosages.

Although diphenhydramine may have adverse effects in elderly adults (dry mouth, constipation, urinary retention particularly in men with benign prostatic hyperplasia), it is not likely that stopping the diphenhydramine will improve her blood-pressure control.

32. An 82-year-old nursing-home resident is hospitalized with pneumonia. She has a history of hypertension and is functionally impaired from a debilitating stoke. On admission, the nurses note her to be pleasant, alert, and oriented to person, place, and time. On examination on her second hospital day, vital signs are stable and physical examination is consistent with pneumonia and old stroke. She awakens when called by name but closes her eyes for prolonged periods during conversation. She complains of feeling tired and does not want to talk much. She is distracted by the voices in the hallway, so that questions must be repeated several times. She slurs her words more than

before and has significant difficulty with word finding. An antibiotic for the pneumonia is the only new medication.

Which of the following best explains her symptoms?

(A) Alzheimer's disease
(B) Dementia with Lewy bodies
(C) Delirium
(D) Depression
(E) Stroke

ANSWER: C

This patient has an acute change in cognition with fluctuating signs. Her inattention, lethargy, and change in cognition or speech are the cardinal features of delirium, which can often be identified by careful observation. A cognitive assessment, such as the Mini–Mental State Examination, should be completed to formally assess her cognitive status, and a delirium tool can be used to confirm the diagnosis. The Confusion Assessment Method is simple and widely used for detection of delirium in hospitalized older persons. It assesses for presence of an acute change in mental status with a fluctuating course, inattention, and presence of either disorganized thinking or altered level of consciousness.

The patient has no history of dementia, and inattention and lethargy are generally not features of dementia.

In hospitalized persons with lethargy and psychomotor retardation, delirium is often misdiagnosed as depression. Many studies show that among the majority of hospital psychiatric consultations for depression, the true diagnosis is delirium. The recognition of delirium is poor among nurses and physicians, especially if baseline cognitive and functional status is not available.

Although a second stroke may explain the word-finding difficulties and lethargy, there are no other overt neurologic signs to indicate stroke.

33. A 67-year-old man comes to the office with his family to obtain an additional medical opinion. He has lost 18.2 kg (40 lb) in the past 6 months, is weak, spends most of his time in bed, has given up participating in family activities, and is no longer interested in

watching sporting events on television. His family is concerned that he has a serious, undiagnosed medical problem. He tends to sit quietly and let his family answer questions, but when pressed, he indicates that he cannot swallow solids or liquids because his throat is blocked. His family reports that he eats and drinks small amounts. He believes he has cancer that the doctors have yet to find. According to the medical records he provides, radiography and computed tomography of the chest are normal, and upper endoscopy is unremarkable. Several sets of blood work have been obtained, none of which indicate dehydration, anemia, or hepatic or renal dysfunction.

Which of the following is the most likely explanation for these findings?

(A) Occult lung cancer
(B) Vascular dementia
(C) Alzheimer's disease
(D) Major depression with psychotic features
(E) Panic disorder

ANSWER: D

In older adults, the presentation of major depression with psychotic features is often masked by concomitant physical symptoms. Although major depression can coexist with panic disorder, the latter involves multiple acute episodes of physical symptoms with intense fear of impending doom. In contrast, this patient has a sustained conviction of a physical abnormality not supported by medical evidence. The patient's conviction alone, however, is not sufficient to make the diagnosis of major depression with psychotic features. Patients with occult malignancy can present with weight loss and poorly articulated physical complaints. An important diagnostic clue is the presence of other signs and symptoms suggesting major depression: psychomotor retardation, loss of interest, loss of energy, social withdrawal, and increased time in bed. These symptoms are more likely to reflect depression than physical impairment, because he has lost interest in activities (for example, watching sports on television) that are unaffected by physical limitation from weight loss and weakness. A primary psychiatric concern is also suggested by his delusional belief that he cannot swallow.

This is contradicted by the family, as well as by his examination.

Recognizing the presence of psychosis (somatic delusion) in this patient has important implications for further management. Major depression with psychotic features responds poorly to pharmacotherapy with an antidepressant alone, requiring the addition of an antipsychotic agent. However, the addition of an antipsychotic does not always enhance efficacy and has the potential to increase side effects. Although it has limited availability and less acceptability to patients, electroconvulsive therapy is the treatment of choice for older patients who have major depression with psychotic features.

The history does not suggest cognitive impairment, and thus vascular dementia and Alzheimer's disease are unlikely.

34. The daughter of a 91-year-old patient who saw an article on the Internet requests a physical therapy referral for progressive resistance training to help her mother stay independent.

Which of the following statements is true regarding progressive resistance training?

(A) Physical disability, as measured by standardized scales, will improve.
(B) Gains in strength are common.
(C) Health-related quality of life improves.
(D) Injury due to the exercises is rare.
(E) The patient's advanced age is a contraindication.

ANSWER: B

Muscle weakness is common in old age and is associated with physical disability and an increased risk of falls. Progressive resistance training exercises (that is, movements performed against a specific external force that is regularly increased during training) are designed to increase strength in older people.

In almost 70 trials with nearly 4000 subjects, progressive resistance training was found to have a large positive effect on strength. Some measures of functional limitation, such as gait, showed modest improvements. However, there is no evidence that progressive resistance training has an effect on health-related quality-of-life measures or on physical disability as measured by standardized scales. In most of the studies, musculoskeletal injuries were detected.

Patients at advanced age may benefit from exercise interventions. The patient's underlying health status is a better determinant of outcome than age. Extremely disabled patients may not gain much in terms of functional improvement, and healthy persons may not need such exercises. However, other patients, especially those with deconditioning, are likely to see some benefits.

35. A 74-year-old man comes to the office because he has a 3-month history of generalized itching. The itching has worsened as the weather has gotten colder. The patient states that this happens every winter. History includes hypertension, for which he has taken lisinopril for the past 4 years. He does not take any other agents or over-the-counter medications. He has been using a moisturizing cream with little relief. On examination, there is diffuse skin involvement with dry scaling on the trunk and extremities. The shins resemble "cracked porcelain" with red fissures that form an irregular reticular pattern.

Which of the following is the most likely cause of the itching?

(A) Drug eruption
(B) Xerosis
(C) Scabies
(D) Psoriasis
(E) Contact dermatitis

ANSWER: B

Xerosis (dry skin) is the most common cause of generalized itching in older patients. Clinically the skin is dry and scaly; in more severe cases the skin becomes inflamed, with fissuring and cracking of the stratum corneum that resembles cracked porcelain (erythema craquelé; in French *craquelé* means "marred with cracks"). Xerosis gets worse in winter, with low environmental humidity. It can be reduced by using a humidifier in the bedroom, decreasing the frequency of baths, using warm instead of hot water, and using only mild and moisturizing soaps (eg, Dove, Basis, Aveeno) or avoiding soaps altogether. The patient should be instructed in the use of emollients on wet skin,

especially with lactic acid (5% or 12%) and urea (10% to 20%), which loosen retained layers of stratum corneum and decrease the scaliness. Ammonium lactate cream 5% contains urea and is available over the counter; the 12% formulation requires a prescription. Oils in the bath prolong hydration of the stratum corneum, but they are not advisable for older patients as they make the tub surface slippery and may increase the risk of falling. A mild topical corticosteroid may be helpful in some cases.

In an older patient with generalized pruritus, it is important to exclude other causes, including drug eruptions, scabies, systemic disease (diabetes mellitus or liver and kidney disorders), or lymphoproliferative disease (lymphoma or leukemia). Drug eruptions can present with all kinds of rashes and should be in the differential diagnosis of any symmetric eruption. They usually occur within the first week of initiating a new drug, although reactions to penicillins can be delayed. It is important to get a good drug history, including over-the-counter drugs and food additives. This patient's history of rash with cold weather makes xerosis more likely than drug eruption.

Scabies is a skin infestation by mites. It is characterized by burrows: gray or skin-colored ridges, 0.5 to 1.0 cm long, that end with a minute papule or vesicle. There may be secondary urticarial papules, eczematous plaques, excoriations, and superimposed bacterial infection. In psoriasis, the lesions are well-demarcated erythematous plaques with adherent silvery scales, and they usually involve elbows, knees, scalp, and trunk (extensor surfaces). Contact dermatitis is a type IV hypersensitivity reaction after contact with an antigen and is characterized by pruritus and burning of the skin. It causes inflammation of the skin and can be acute, subacute, or chronic. The acute form presents with erythematous patches with vesicles, erosions, and crusts. Subacute contact dermatitis presents with patches of mild erythema, dry scales, and sometimes small papules. Chronic contact dermatitis may have patches of lichenification (thickening) with satellite small papules, excoriation, or mild erythema. In contact dermatitis there is a history of exposure to an external agent, rather than a seasonal predilection.

36. Which of the following statements regarding calorie restriction is correct?

(A) Calorie restriction has been shown consistently to increase life span in mice.

(B) Animal studies have demonstrated positive effects of calorie restriction on fertility.

(C) Calorically restricted rodents, nonhuman primates, and healthy men demonstrate lower fasting insulin levels and lower body temperature.

(D) Calorie restriction is most beneficial when initiated late in life.

(E) Calorically restricted mice live longer, are more fit, and are more likely to reproduce than control mice with unlimited access to food.

ANSWER: C

Calorie restriction has been shown to slow aging and extend life span in yeast, flies, worms, rats, and mice. Animals on a calorically restricted diet receive a well-balanced diet, yet eat less than control animals allowed unlimited access to the same food. Although most calorically restricted animals live longer, the impact of calorie restriction varies considerably in mice. For example, calorie restriction increases the life span of C57BL/6 mice, but not DBA/2 mice. The physiologic effects of calorie restriction are complex. Although restricted animals seem more fit, are more active, develop fewer tumors, and have fewer of the neurologic and endocrine abnormalities typically observed in control animals with unlimited access, they are more susceptible to bacterial infections and have reduced fertility. Human calorie restriction is probably unrealistic, yet two of the most robust markers of calorie restriction in rodents (reduced body temperature and reduced plasma insulin) have also been observed in caloric-restricted rhesus monkeys and in older men studied as part of the Baltimore Longitudinal Study of Aging. Studies of *Drosophila* spp. indicate that the life span can be extended even if calorie restriction is instituted late in life.

37. A 69-year-old man comes to the office because of difficulty swallowing solids and liquids. The dysphagia has progressed slowly over 8 months, and he has lost 20 pounds. He reports no pain. Barium radiograph demonstrates a narrowed distal esophageal segment 4.1 cm long and no dilated esophageal segment proximal to this narrowed portion. Esophageal manometry demonstrates failure of the lower esophageal sphincter to relax with swallowing, and aperistalsis of the esophageal body.

Which diagnostic procedure should be performed first?

(A) Esophagoscopy
(B) Endoscopic ultrasonography
(C) Computed tomography
(D) Chest magnetic resonance imaging
(E) Laparotomy

ANSWER: A

Achalasia is an esophageal motor disorder characterized clinically by dysphagia to liquids and solids, radiographically by esophageal dilatation with smooth "bird beak" distal narrowing, and manometrically by incomplete or absent relaxation of the lower esophageal sphincter and aperistalsis of the esophageal body. Most affected patients have primary or idiopathic achalasia, a disorder of unknown cause characterized pathologically by myenteric lymphocyte inflammation with injury to and progressive depletion of myenteric ganglion cells. However, some patients have pseudoachalasia associated with malignancy, which has clinical, radiographic, and manometric findings often indistinguishable from primary achalasia.

The peak incidence of pseudoachalasia is between ages 60 and 80 (initial onset of primary achalasia has a nearly uniform age distribution between ages 10 and 70). In older adults, recent-onset dysphagia, findings of achalasia on barium studies, and a narrowed distal esophageal segment longer than 3.5 cm with little or no proximal dilatation are highly suggestive of pseudoachalasia caused by an occult malignancy, even in the absence of other suspicious radiographic findings. The most common mechanism for pseudoachalasia is direct involvement of the esophageal myenteric plexus by neoplastic cells. Rarely, a distant neoplasm may cause this syndrome as a paraneoplastic process. Pseudoachalasia is most often associated with adenocarcinoma of the gastroesophageal junction. It has also been associated with malignancy of the esophagus, lung, liver, prostate, breast, and pancreas, as well as with lymphoma and mesothelioma.

Esophagoscopy detects mucosal or structural abnormalities of the esophagus and proximal stomach. It is useful for detection of pseudoachalasia, placement of manometry catheters, and dilatation of peptic strictures. All patients with achalasia should have esophagoscopy with biopsy of any suspicious area. Large endoscopic biopsies may not demonstrate the presence of malignancy. If endoscopic biopsy is nondiagnostic, endoscopic ultrasound, computed tomography, and laparotomy may be appropriate.

Pneumatic dilatation, thought to cause a controlled tear of the lower esophageal sphincter by vigorous stretching, is successful in 70% to 90% of patients. Generally, if there is no durable response after three treatments, an alternative therapy should be attempted. Surgical management consists of myotomy of the abnormal lower esophageal sphincter. Success rates approach 90% for relief of dysphagia.

38. A preoperative medical consultation is requested for an obese 72-year-old man admitted for coronary artery bypass grafting scheduled for the next day. He has known three-vessel coronary artery disease. He has been complaining of a headache but is otherwise considered a good candidate for the procedure.

On examination, he has tenderness over the right temporal artery and a right carotid bruit. Laboratory studies reveal a Westergren sedimentation rate of 82 mm/hr. Giant cell (temporal) arteritis is suspected.

Which of the following is the most appropriate initial step?

(A) High-dose corticosteroids
(B) Etanercept
(C) Temporal artery biopsy
(D) Coronary artery bypass graft
(E) Methotrexate

ANSWER: A

Temporal arteritis is characterized by intense inflammation that can compromise blood flow to critical structures in the head and neck, and can result in headache and visual impairment.

Although the head and neck can be investigated with vascular imaging (such as magnetic resonance imaging or ultrasound), biopsy is the diagnostic procedure of choice to detect arteritis in cranial vessels. Further, the type of arteritis (giant cell, polyarteritis) can be distinguished only by biopsy and has important therapeutic implications. Clinical subtypes of giant cell arteritis can be distinguished by the predominant anatomic involvement: cranial giant cell arteritis with ischemic complications in the eye, the face, and the central nervous system; large-vessel giant cell arteritis with occlusions in the subclavian or axillary vessels; and aortic giant cell arteritis. Arteritis can also involve coronary arteries, and giant cell arteritis can result in ostial lesions.

The appropriate initial step is treatment with high-dose corticosteroids, even before definitive diagnosis with temporal artery biopsy. Methotrexate and etanercept are anti-inflammatory agents more appropriately used as disease-modifying agents in rheumatoid arthritis. Surgery should be delayed until the disease is well controlled.

39. An 88-year-old woman living in an assisted living facility comes to the office for a follow-up visit. She has poorly controlled stage 2 hypertension, gastroesophageal reflux disease, depression, and hypothyroidism. She has lived alone since her husband's death 2 years ago. Medications include hydrochlorothiazide 50 mg daily, lisinopril 10 mg twice daily, diltiazem 30 mg four times daily, esomeprazole 20 mg daily, citalopram 40 mg daily, levothyroxine 0.1 mg daily, and aspirin 81 mg daily. Metoprolol 50 mg twice daily was added to her regimen 2 months ago, when her blood-pressure reading was 168/81 mm Hg. She has no new symptoms and has had no blood-pressure readings since her visit 2 months ago.

On physical examination, blood pressure is found to be 165/78 mm Hg and heart rate is 68 per minute. There are no orthostatic blood-pressure changes. She has grade 1 hypertensive retinopathy and a laterally displaced point of maximal impulse with an apical fourth heart sound. On a Mini-Mental State Examination, she recalls only 1 of 3 objects at 3 minutes and performs a normal clock-drawing test. She reports three positive responses on the Geriatric Depression Scale. Echocardiogram shows left ventricular hypertrophy. Recent laboratory studies demonstrate normal electrolytes and renal function (calculated creatinine clearance is 43 mL/min) and thyrotropin level of 3.8 μU/mL. Medications are set up in pill boxes for her and she has a visit from the nursing assistant at least three times a day for medication reminders. She takes these most of the time with these reminders. The nursing assistant also reports that she is drinking at least two glasses of wine daily.

Which of the following best explains the persistence of her poorly controlled blood pressure?

(A) Pseudohypertension
(B) Nonadherence to medication
(C) Alcohol intake
(D) Hyperaldosteronism
(E) Renovascular hypertension

ANSWER: C

Resistant hypertension is defined in the Seventh Report of the Joint National Committee on Prevention, Detection, Evaluation, and Treatment of High Blood Pressure as "failure to reach goal blood pressure in patients who are adhering to full doses of an appropriate three-drug regimen that includes a diuretic." Causes of resistant hypertension include inaccurate blood-pressure measurement (pseudohypertension), volume overload, drug-induced effect, inadequate dosing of antihypertensive drugs, diet and alcohol intake and incorrect combinations of therapies, as well as secondary causes of hypertension (eg, renovascular disease, sleep apnea, hyperaldosteronism, chronic kidney disease, and pheochromocytoma). Although there are several clues to suggest that this patient's poorly controlled blood pressure persists because she does not adhere to the medication regimen, her living in an assisted living facility and the involvement of a nursing assistant make this far less likely. The risk factors for nonadherence in this patient include: multiple medications are administered at different times throughout the day, she may have short-term memory

impairment (forgetfulness is a major contributor to nonadherence), and a history of depression. However, her physical examination reflects the reduced heart rate that would be expected after the addition of the β-blocker at her last visit. Laboratory evidence of adequate thyroid hormone replacement suggests she is taking her thyroid medication.

Ethanol intake is more likely to be the cause of her persistent hypertension. The prevalence of hypertension, stroke, cardiomyopathy, and arrhythmias is higher with excessive alcohol consumption. A principal mechanism by which ethanol exerts these cardiovascular effects is through modulation of blood pressure. Reducing excessive alcohol intake can likewise reduce blood pressure up to 4 mm Hg, on average, which could substantially affect the rates of stroke and ischemic heart disease.

Although pseudohypertension needs to be considered in older patients with resistant hypertension, the constellation of physical (hypertensive retinopathy) and echocardiographic findings indicates target-organ damage from established hypertension. Renovascular hypertension is the most common of the secondary causes of hypertension among older patients. This patient's pattern of hypertension is not consistent with this possibility: She has normal renal function and no evidence of or risk factors for coronary or peripheral vascular disease. The normal electrolyte pattern makes hyperaldosteronism unlikely. Pheochromocytoma is a rare cause of secondary hypertension, and the patient has none of the symptoms that would typically accompany this condition.

40. An 89-year-old woman, recently admitted to a nursing facility, is found to be frequently incontinent of urine and occasionally incontinent of stool, on initial assessment for the Minimum Data Set. She has Alzheimer's disease and lumbosacral spinal stenosis and has been taking a cholinesterase inhibitor and acetaminophen. The patient's family states that her incontinence has gradually worsened over the past 5 years, and its current severity was an important factor in placing her in the facility. The patient is unable to give a detailed history and denies

bladder problems. Observations by the nursing staff suggest a diagnosis of overactive bladder with urge incontinence.

Examination reveals no evidence of severe atrophic vaginitis, pelvic prolapse, or fecal impaction. Catheterization a few minutes after an episode of incontinence reveals a residual volume of 40 mL. Urinalysis of a specimen obtained by catheterization shows 3+ bacteria and 5 to 10 leukocytes per high-power field, and the culture grows over 100,000 colony-forming units of *Escherichia coli*.

Which of the following is the most appropriate next step for managing her incontinence?

(A) A trial of oxybutynin, 2.5 mg three times daily
(B) A trial of long-acting tolterodine, 4 mg daily
(C) A 7- to 10-day course of ciprofloxacin
(D) Initiation of a prompted voiding program
(E) Simple cystometric testing

ANSWER: D

The most appropriate intervention for this patient is a trial of prompted voiding. From 25% to 40% of similar patients respond well to this behavioral protocol, and responsiveness can generally be determined within 3 to 5 days. Some patients benefit from the addition of a bladder-relaxant drug such as oxybutynin or tolterodine, but, because of potential adverse effects, these drugs should be used as an adjunct to a toileting program. Cholinesterase inhibitors can worsen urge incontinence. Bladder-relaxant drugs may worsen cognitive impairment or precipitate delirium in patients with dementia. They should therefore be used only in patients who have bothersome overactive bladder symptoms that do not respond to a toileting program alone. Eradicating bacteriuria, even in the presence of pyuria, does not improve the severity of incontinence in chronically incontinent nursing-home patients who have no other symptoms of infection. Moreover, treating asymptomatic bacteriuria is not recommended in the nursing home. Simple cystometry would not benefit the patient, as it would not change the initial approach to management.

41. A 75-year-old smoker who recently had a myocardial infarction comes to the office for advice on life-style changes. History includes chronic obstructive pulmonary disease with a moderately impaired FEV_1.

In such patients, smoking cessation is associated with which of the following?

(A) Improved cognition
(B) Cessation of a decline in FEV_1
(C) Reduction in all-cause mortality
(D) Lung cancer risk that is the same as a nonsmoker

ANSWER: C

Although most smokers who have a myocardial infarction want to quit, after 4 years half will still be smoking. Several studies have demonstrated a 25% to 50% reduction in all-cause mortality in older adults who quit smoking. Other retrospective studies show that the risk of recurrent coronary artery disease in a smoker who quits equals that of a nonsmoker 3 years after cessation of smoking.

No evidence indicates that current smokers who quit will have less cognitive decline. FEV_1 will continue to decline, but rates of decline will be similar to those of persons who have never smoked. In persons who quit smoking, deaths due to chronic obstructive pulmonary disease have been shown to statistically increase, but deaths due to all causes (including cardiovascular and cancer) decrease. Men without coronary disease who quit at age 65 years gain an average of 1.4 to 2 years of life; women gain 2.7 to 3.7 years of life. In the smoker who quits, the risk of lung cancer declines more slowly than the risk of coronary artery disease but approaches that of the nonsmoker by 10 years.

42. A 75-year-old man cares for his wife, who has Alzheimer's disease, in their own home. Because his wife needs increasing help with activities of daily living, the husband reluctantly decides to place her in a nursing home.

Which of the following factors predicts a more successful transition for the husband after his wife enters the nursing home?

(A) An ambivalent marital relationship
(B) The husband's anticipating loneliness after placement
(C) The husband's having a sense of identity outside of his caregiving role
(D) The husband's volunteering at the nursing home at which his wife resides

ANSWER: C

The decision to place a family member in a nursing home is almost always wrenching. Even when the patient has significant functional deficits, difficult-to-manage behavioral problems, or other features that increase the likelihood of placement, caregivers usually have some doubt or guilt about the decision they have made.

Caregivers display a continuum of reactions to the transition. Some seem to make the transition less traumatically than others. Once the person with dementia is out of the home, the caregiver may not know what to do with the sudden increase in free time and may have a sense of guilt or obligation to visit the person in the nursing home. In some situations, the well spouse spends virtually all of his or her waking time at the nursing home, with little or no social life beyond the facility. Other spouses seem to avoid the facility, sometimes out of guilt or worry that their presence will kindle uncomfortable questions from the demented person about why he or she cannot "go home."

Of the options given, a sense of identity outside of the caregiving role has the most support in the literature for predicting a successful transition for the caregiver. This sense of identity can take a number of forms, such as involvement in civic groups, volunteering, or assisting others who are caring for loved ones with dementia.

43. A generally healthy 74-year-old woman returns to the office for follow-up of incontinence. She is physically active and extremely bothered by the incontinence. Her symptoms include continuous dribbling and urgency with incontinence during most activities. In the past 15 years, she has had two bladder suspension surgeries that only transiently improved her symptoms of stress incontinence.

On examination she has a positive cough test for stress incontinence, both standing before voiding and supine after voiding. Mild vaginal atrophy and a moderate cystocele are noted on pelvic examination. Postvoid residual urine is 30 mL, and urinalysis is negative. During the last 6 months she underwent a course of biofeedback and has been regularly using pelvic muscle exercises and bladder-training techniques. She uses estrogen vaginal cream twice weekly. She tolerated oxybutynin 2.5 mg three times daily with no amelioration of symptoms; when the dosage was raised to 5 mg three times daily, she had dry mouth, dry eyes, and constipation with no improvement in symptoms.

Which of the following is the most appropriate next step for this patient?

(A) Refer her to a urogynecologist for consideration of surgical intervention.
(B) Increase the estrogen cream to 5 times per week.
(C) Add vaginal cones to enhance her pelvic muscle exercises.
(D) Begin long-acting tolterodine, 4 mg daily.
(E) Begin pseudoephedrine, 30 mg three times daily.

ANSWER: A

This patient's history and physical examination findings are most compatible with a diagnosis of intrinsic sphincter deficiency (type 3 stress incontinence), with an additional component of overactive bladder. Patients with intrinsic sphincter deficiency typically have a history of one or more lower urinary tract surgeries, report nearly continuous leakage of urine while active, and have a positive cough test for stress incontinence—sometimes even in the supine position with only a small amount of urine in the bladder. Although symptoms may improve with conservative therapy consisting of topical estrogen, pelvic muscle exercises, and bladder training, along with a bladder relaxant for overactive bladder, patients with intrinsic sphincter deficiency generally require surgical intervention. Some patients benefit from periurethral injections of collagen, but many require a pubovaginal sling procedure.

This patient will not benefit from a higher dose of topical estrogen, as the dose she has been on for 6 months has probably had its effect on the vaginal and urethral epithelium. Furthermore, it may be that estrogen is not effective for stress, urge, or mixed urge-stress urinary incontinence. Vaginal cones can be effective, but there is no evidence that they add benefit to a well-performed and practiced pelvic muscle exercise program. Some patients respond better to one bladder relaxant than another, and long-acting tolterodine has fewer adverse effects than short-acting oxybutynin. However, this patient's predominant problem is probably intrinsic sphincter deficiency, not overactive bladder. Thus, a trial of a different bladder relaxant would unlikely benefit her most bothersome symptoms. Symptoms of overactive bladder are relieved in some patients after surgery for stress incontinence. Adding the α-agonist pseudoephedrine may benefit patients with stress incontinence, but it is unlikely to have a major impact in a patient with intrinsic sphincter deficiency.

44. A daughter comes with her mother to her mother's clinic appointment and requests that you fill out conservatorship papers. The mother is an 84-year-old woman who has been living on her own since the death of her husband 7 years ago. You have followed her for the past 3 years in your office for type 2 diabetes, atrial fibrillation (for which she receives an anticoagulant), and moderate aortic stenosis. During this time you have noted an increase in nonadherence with her medication regimen. She had a hospital admission 1 month ago for dehydration, partially due to hyperglycemia, and her INR was noted to be 1.2. She was unclear as to whether she had been taking her pills correctly when in hospital. Now she assures you that she has that "all taken care of" but does not give you specifics on how she obtains her medications nor how she remembers to take them. She does know that she needs to get tested for her warfarin regularly. The daughter states that her mother does not eat correctly, rarely showers, and refuses to allow others to help her.

Her Folstein Mini–Mental State Examination (MMSE) score is 25 (errors were in recall, orientation, and the three-step command). Her Executive Interview (EXIT 25) score of 9, demonstrating difficulty with sequencing, intrusions, perseveration, and self-monitoring,

suggests mild to moderate impairment in executive functioning.

The most important aspect of this patient and her examination that would persuade you that she may or may not need a conservator is which of the following?

(A) The EXIT 25 score of 9
(B) The MMSE score of 25
(C) The daughter's concern
(D) The functional ability of the patient
(E) The hospitalization

ANSWER: D

The most important factor in assessing this (or any other) patient for the need for a conservator is whether her decisions place her at significant risk. If she has the decisional capacity to understand the risks and benefits of her decisions, then she is competent to make these decisions. If she does not have this decisional capacity and makes decisions that place her at risk, then conservatorship is warranted. Although specific neuropsychologic testing can clarify the areas of deficit and support the need for a conservator, a person's demonstrated inability to care for him or herself is the gold standard for legal action.

The MMSE is a good indicator of decreased cognitive function in key areas that may affect decisional capacity, such as memory and language, but only when it demonstrates severe impairment (MMSE score of 10 or less) can it be said to demonstrate cognitive function below which the person is highly unlikely to still have the ability to safely make decisions and care for him or herself.

For tests of executive function, the correlation with impaired decision making may be higher, but even then, a score of 15 or higher on the EXIT 25 is needed in order to have a high predictive value for incompetence.

The mere fact of hospitalization is not sufficient evidence. There may have been problems causing both temporary mental status problems and dehydration, such as an infection, which could explain her medication nonadherence. The daughter's opinion, although important, should not be the sole determinant for this decision. Both of these factors may be used to correlate with other evidence to support the decision.

45. A 79-year-old man comes to the office for a follow-up visit. He lives at home with his son, who moved in last year to care for his father in exchange for room and board. In response to questions about his home situation, he reports that his son "treats me pretty rough sometimes." The patient does not want to be separated from his son and does not want to move out of his own house. The son works full time and drinks heavily at home. Sometimes he does not provide dinner for his father and has left him for prolonged periods without helping him change his clothes or ensuring that he has food. The patient has a history of severe osteoarthritis of the knees and left hip, heart failure, and diabetes mellitus. He ambulates using a walker with moderate assistance from another person, is unable to transfer independently, and is afraid of falling.

Physical examination reveals significant peripheral neuropathy and multiple bruises on his forearms. Heart rate is 80 per minute and regular. He has crackles at the bases of both lungs. Cognitive examination is normal, but he is depressed. His diaper is wet, and the skin in his perianal area is covered with dried feces.

Which of the following is the most appropriate next step in assisting this patient?

(A) Admit him to a nursing home.
(B) Notify Adult Protective Services of possible mistreatment.
(C) Request visiting nurse services for home safety evaluation.
(D) Initiate therapy with a selective serotonin-reuptake inhibitor.
(E) Request meals-on-wheels.

ANSWER: B

This patient is being neglected by his son. The son assumed responsibility for providing care when he moved into his father's house with the promise that he would help him in exchange for housing and food. He therefore has an obligation to ensure that his father's basic needs are met. Although not all states have mandatory reporting requirements, all states have a mechanism by which a health care provider may report possible mistreatment. The agency that takes this report (Adult Protective Services) is required to investigate and assess for abuse. It is not the clinician's role to determine whether abuse or neglect has occurred; rather, the clinician makes a report when he or she has reasonable suspicion of mistreatment. The Adult Protective Service worker will then go to the victim's home and attempt to interview both the alleged victim and perpetrator. The worker may find that the patient is eligible for home-health services such as meals-on-wheels, a home-health aide or homemaker, and other community-based programs that will allow him to remain clean and safe. Since the patient is cognitively intact and understands his situation, he will decide upon his living situation for himself and cannot be admitted to a nursing home against his will.

In this scenario, risk factors for neglect include the patient's physical dependence and depression. As a person becomes more dependent on another for care, the risk of neglect rises. Some have theorized that depression is linked to neglect because depression may impair executive function and therefore interfere with the victim's ability to make good decisions. Neglect may also be a causative factor in depression. Depression should be treated, but not before the safety of the patient's circumstances are more thoroughly probed. There is conflicting information as to whether gender and race are associated with neglect. Many victims of neglect are also cognitively impaired.

Few studies have examined risk factors that make a caregiver more likely to be abusive. One small study examined characteristics of caregivers who were known to actively abuse or passively neglect an older person who was dependent on them. The older persons were physically dependent but did not have dementia. Of the nine caregivers who were proven to be physical abusers, seven used alcohol heavily, which indicates that it is important to identify alcoholism in the caregiver. In the present case, it may be appropriate to refer the son to a program such as Alcoholics Anonymous, but the more immediate need is to protect the patient.

46. Which of the following is the strongest predictor for failure to achieve independent ambulation after surgical repair of a hip fracture?

(A) Cognitive status
(B) Age
(C) Incontinence
(D) Premorbid functional status
(E) Depression

ANSWER: D

Functional status before the fracture is the best predictor of rehabilitation outcomes: if the patient did not walk independently before the fall, it is unlikely he or she will walk independently after the fracture repair, even with rehabilitation.

Advanced age is a known risk factor for poor outcome. However, studies in patients over age 90 have shown that outcomes in this group can be good. Age probably serves as a marker for more serious functional deficits, rather than as an independent risk factor.

The presence of dementia or cognitive impairment is generally considered a negative predictor of rehabilitation outcomes, but some studies have shown that rehabilitation can improve functional performance in patients who can follow at least one-step commands.

Incontinence is a common secondary effect of immobility and may cause falls. However, it does not appear to be as significant as premorbid mobility in determining dependence in other activities of daily living.

Depression is a common sequela of disabling conditions and is known to affect rehabilitation outcomes. However, it is treatable when recognized, and treatment leads to improved rehabilitation outcomes. Depression is not as strong a risk factor as premorbid ·functional status.

47. Which of the following statements is true with regard to assisted-living facilities?

(A) Meals, laundry service, housekeeping, and skilled nursing services are usually provided.
(B) Rates at assisted-living facilities average $200 a day.
(C) Medicare pays for individuals to reside at assisted-living facilities.
(D) Long-term-care insurance may cover the cost of assisted living.

ANSWER: D

A wide range of services are available for residents of assisted-living facilities. Some of the services that may be included are three meals a day served in a community dining area, housekeeping services, transportation, assistance with activities of daily living, access to medical services, 24-hour staffing, emergency alert systems in each domicile, health promotion and exercise classes, medication management, laundry service, and social and recreational activities. These services may be included in the daily rate or cost extra, or they may not be available, as determined by each facility. Skilled nursing services are not provided. In contrast, at nursing homes, skilled nursing services, meals, laundry services, housekeeping, and medical services are usually provided.

Medicare does not pay for assisted-living facilities; financing is the responsibility of the individual or his or her family. Daily rates range from $15 to $200. Private long-term-care insurance policies may cover the cost of assisted-living facilities or personal services, such as home-health aides. Although the number of policies sold is increasing rapidly, few persons, in absolute numbers, currently carry long-term-care insurance.

48. A 72-year-old man comes to the emergency department because of constant right lower quadrant abdominal pain that has been present for almost 48 hours. He has nausea and anorexia but no fever, chills, vomiting, diarrhea, hematochezia, hematuria, or dysuria.

On physical examination his abdomen is soft to palpation and tender in the right lower quadrant, with voluntary guarding. Bowel sounds are hypoactive. Rectal examination is negative for occult blood.

Laboratory values include hemoglobin of 12.6 g/dL and leukocyte count of 14,800/μL (neutrophils 88%, bands 7%, monocytes 4%, lymphocytes 8%). Amylase and liver chemistries are normal. Abdominal radiograph reveals a nonspecific gas pattern.

What is the most appropriate next step to establish the diagnosis?

(A) Ultrasound of the abdomen
(B) Gastrografin (meglumine diatrizoate) enema
(C) Computed tomography of abdomen
(D) Small bowel series
(E) Colonoscopy

ANSWER: C

Appendicitis accounts for 5% of all acute abdominal conditions in patients aged 60 years and older. Older patients often have delayed and atypical presentations, leading to increased incidence of perforation and intra-abdominal infection. Perforation occurs in up to 72% of older patients, possibly because of delayed diagnosis or more rapid progression of disease. Comorbidity in older patients increases the operative risks and postoperative complications. Often there is no fever and no or minimal pain.

The incidence of appendicitis in the growing older population seems to be increasing. Approximately 10% of patients with appendicitis are elderly, but this age group accounts for more than 50% of deaths associated with appendicitis and for a disproportionately high rate of postoperative morbidity.

The most common reasons for delay in diagnosis include delayed patient presentation to the clinician (often more than 2 days after symptoms begin), systemic disease masking symptoms of acute appendicitis, mild and less specific symptoms, lack of leukocytosis, and failure to include appendicitis in the differential diagnosis. Misdiagnosis occurs in up to 50% of cases. Conditions that are confused with appendicitis include bowel obstruction, diverticulitis, cecal carcinoma, Meckel's diverticulitis, typhlitis, Crohn's disease (which has a second peak incidence in older patients), acute cholecystitis, pancreatitis, obstructing urolithiasis, and perforated duodenal ulcer (which rarely presents with right lower quadrant pain).

Abdominal radiographs are not sensitive in the emergency department evaluation of adult patients with nontraumatic abdominal pain. Computed tomography has 90% to 98% sensitivity for detecting acute appendicitis and may help in distinguishing between appendicitis and inflammatory and neoplastic conditions with which it might be confused. Ultrasonography has a sensitivity of only 53%. Gastrografin enema, small bowel series, and colonoscopy would not be the most appropriate next step in this clinical scenario. Each of these would not help diagnose the condition and may be associated with complications, including perforation.

49. During a routine office visit, a 75-year-old man complains of erectile dysfunction. He had a myocardial infarction 8 years ago. He has a history of well-controlled hypertension for 15 years, rare episodes of angina with severe exertion, hyperlipidemia, and benign prostatic hyperplasia. Medications are enalapril, hydrochlorothiazide, doxazosin, aspirin, lovastatin, and a nitroglycerin patch. Physical examination is notable for blood pressure of 130/80 mm Hg and somewhat decreased peripheral pulses. There is no evidence of Peyronie's disease.

Which of the following is the best treatment for erectile dysfunction for this patient?

(A) Intracavernosal injections of alprostadil
(B) Oral yohimbine
(C) Oral sildenafil
(D) Intramuscular testosterone every 2 weeks
(E) Vacuum tumescent device

ANSWER: E

Given the clinical and medication history of this patient, the best option is a vacuum device because of its safety profile. The disadvantages of a vacuum device are relative lack of spontaneity, penile reddening, and cooler penile temperature in some patients.

Sildenafil, vardenafil, and tadalafil are phosphodiesterase inhibitors for the treatment of erectile dysfunction. Although these agents have not been directly compared, they seem to have different durations of effect, with tadalafil lasting 24 to 36 hours. Phosphodiesterase inhibitors are contraindicated in patients on regular or intermittent nitrate therapy because they can potentiate fatal episodes of hypotension. The concurrent use of phosphodiesterase inhibitors with α-blockers is complicated. Use of sildenafil with α-blockers is listed as a precaution, vardenafil is absolutely contraindicated, and tadalafil is contraindicated except with tamsulosin 0.4 mg. Headache, flushing, and changes in color vision may also occur with these agents.

Intracavernosal injection of alprostadil (10 to 20 μg) is effective in producing erections, but it can be associated with penile pain, burning, and hematomas. It would not be the first choice of therapy for this patient because his aspirin use puts him at risk for hematomas or bleeding.

Yohimbine (5 to 25 mg), an α_2-blocker, can be associated with elevated blood pressure, which this patient already has, as well as nausea and dizziness. In randomized, double-blind controlled trials, it has not been found to work better than placebo.

Testosterone replacement (200 mg) may benefit patients with low libido but may not restore erectile function. Adverse effects can include polycythemia, gynecomastia, and fluid retention. It should not be administered to men with prostate cancer but does not seem to exacerbate symptoms of benign prostatic hyperplasia.

50. Which of the following is true regarding osteoporosis in older men?

   (A) Androgen levels have been correlated to bone mass and fractures in older men.
   (B) Estrogen levels are an important deter-minant of osteoporosis in men.
   (C) Osteoporosis is more likely to be primary or idiopathic in older men than in older women.
   (D) No treatment benefit has been documented for alendronate in older men with idiopathic osteoporosis.
   (E) Outcome after hip fracture is better for older men than for older women.

ANSWER: B

Osteoporosis is an important problem for older men. Hypogonadism can be associated with increased fracture risk, and androgen replacement in hypogonadal men can delay loss of bone mass. However, androgen levels do not predict risk of fracture in older men. The Framingham cohort demonstrated that

hypogonadism related to aging has little influence on bone mineral density, but serum estradiol levels have a strong and positive association with bone mineral density. Clinical studies have further shown that levels of estradiol and estrone in older men are related to osteoporosis. Men with lower levels appear more susceptible to lower bone mineral density, and estrogen appears to have an independent effect in this regard when multivariate analyses are performed.

Men with osteoporosis should undergo evaluation for secondary causes. In 40% to 60% of cases, a contributing factor can be identified (such as hypogonadism, glucocorticoid therapy, gastrointestinal disease); this identification seems to be greater than in studies of women. Older men with osteoporosis can benefit from treatment with a number of modalities, including bisphosphonates. For reasons that are not entirely clear, the mortality associated with hip fracture is higher among older men than among older women. In one report of 363 patients with hip fractures, the 12-month mortality was 32% in men and 17% in women.

51. A 65-year-old woman comes to the office for a physical examination, during which a 2 × 2 cm smooth, ovoid nodule is palpated in the left lobe of the thyroid gland. The nodule moves easily with swallowing and is not associated with cervical lymphadenopathy. She has no history of radiation exposure to the head or neck. Serum thyrotropin and serum free thyroxine levels are normal.

Which of the following is the most appropriate next step?

   (A) Referral for fine-needle aspiration biopsy
   (B) Referral for possible left thyroid lobectomy
   (C) Thyroid uptake and scan
   (D) Reexamination in 6 months

ANSWER: A

Palpable thyroid nodules are found in up to 7% of the general adult population. The prevalence is higher in women and older adults. The clinical challenge is to distinguish the few nodules that are malignant (and require surgical resection) from the vast majority that are benign.

In addition to measurement of serum thyrotropin level, fine-needle aspiration biopsy is well established as the initial procedure of choice for evaluating a thyroid nodule. It is an outpatient procedure with 85% sensitivity and 90% specificity for malignant thyroid lesion when an adequate specimen is interpreted by an experienced cytopathologist. Repeat biopsy is indicated if the initial aspirate is not diagnostic.

Radioisotope imaging studies (such as iodine 123 thyroid uptake scan) lack sensitivity and accuracy. The iodine scan separates cold nodules, which are more likely to be malignant, from hot nodules, which are rarely malignant. Imaging would not add much in this case, because the normal serum thyrotropin level suggests that the nodule is cold, thus requiring further evaluation by fine-needle aspiration.

52. A 79-year-old man comes to the office because he has had a generalized, throbbing, almost constant headache for the past 3 weeks. He has no previous history of headache. No obvious factor precipitated the headache, although the patient notes that chewing food seems to accentuate jaw pain. Two days ago he lost vision in his left eye for 5 minutes; this resolved spontaneously. Earlier today he suddenly lost hearing in his left ear. His current medications include aspirin and folic acid. Neurologic examination is normal except for the hearing loss.

Which of the following is the most appropriate treatment?

(A) Azathioprine
(B) Clopidogrel
(C) Heparin
(D) Phenytoin
(E) Prednisone

ANSWER: E

This man has characteristic symptoms of giant cell (temporal) arteritis, a disorder primarily seen in persons above age 50. Headache is the most common presenting symptom; it is typically throbbing and may be most prominent in the temporal region. Various neurologic complications can develop in the setting of giant cell arteritis, including sudden vision loss due to anterior ischemic optic neuropathy and sudden hearing loss due to acute auditory nerve infarction. Jaw claudication is common.

Prominent elevation of the erythrocyte sedimentation rate and C-reactive protein level is characteristic, and diagnosis is confirmed with temporal artery biopsy.

Treatment is initiated with high doses of oral corticosteroids, typically 40 to 60 mg of prednisone daily. Treatment with higher doses or with intravenous methylprednisolone is suggested for patients with an acute neurologic syndrome. Azathioprine is not effective in the acute management of giant cell arteritis. Medications used to treat thrombotic or embolic cerebrovascular disease, such as clopidogrel and heparin, are not appropriate for giant cell arteritis. The anticonvulsant drug phenytoin has no effect on the inflammation that characterizes giant cell arteritis.

53. A 60-year-old man is brought to the office by his family because he has difficulty walking and is becoming increasingly confused. He has a history of alcoholism. On examination, he is unable to move his eyes horizontally, and he has upbeat nystagmus, dysmetria of the extremities, and severe ataxia.

Which of the following vitamins is most likely to be deficient in this patient?

(A) Vitamin B_1
(B) Vitamin B_6
(C) Vitamin B_{12}
(D) Vitamin E
(E) Vitamin K

ANSWER: A

Wernicke's encephalopathy is associated with ocular motor abnormalities (often inability to move the eyes), nystagmus, ataxia, global confused state, vestibular paresis, hypotension, and hypothermia. It occurs secondary to deficiency in vitamin B_1 (thiamine). Older patients are at risk for Wernicke's encephalopathy especially if there is a history of alcohol abuse or malnutrition. Other conditions that place patients at risk are prolonged intravenous feeding, intravenous hyperalimentation, hyperemesis gravidarum, anorexia (which can be associated with dementia or depression), prolonged fasting, refeeding after starvation, and gastric plication. Treatment consists of intravenous thiamine. Often the nystagmus and eye abnormalities resolve with treatment, and there may be some resolution of the gait imbalance, but the confusion and memory deficit may remain. The other vitamins are not usually deficient in patients with alcoholism.

54. A 76-year-old woman who lives with her husband in a retirement community comes to the office because she has nearly fallen on three occasions during the previous 6 months. In each instance she averted the fall by grabbing hold of something. She has moderate visual impairment due to macular degeneration and osteoarthritis involving several joints, especially the left hip and knee. She takes pride in not having to take any medications. She has 1 mixed drink before dinner almost every day, while socializing with other residents, and has a glass of wine with dinner 2 to 3 times each week. Alcohol, combined with impaired vision and the effects of arthritis on balance and gait, is suspected as a possible cause of the near-falls. She has not been treated previously for an alcohol-use disorder.

Which of the following is the most appropriate first step in the care of this patient?

(A) Treat with naltrexone, 50 mg once daily for 12 weeks.
(B) Treat with disulfiram, 200 mg once daily until drinking is reduced.
(C) Provide information about risks and advise her to reduce her drinking.
(D) Refer to an age-specific residential treatment center.
(E) Refer to a self-help group such as Alcoholics Anonymous.

ANSWER: C

Brief intervention is effective and can be conducted in primary care settings. It typically involves informing patients about potential problems associated with their drinking and specifically advising them to reduce consumption of alcohol.

Naltrexone, an opioid antagonist, reduces craving and the emotional response to the pleasurable effects of alcohol. Naltrexone has been shown to decrease alcohol use by social drinkers, including those at risk of harm from their drinking. Its greatest benefit may be for social drinkers who have not responded to nonpharmacologic therapy or who regularly drink heavier amounts. Outcomes are best when naltrexone is given as an adjunct to a comprehensive treatment plan, rather than as monotherapy. This patient has not received previous treatment for drinking, and her drinking is limited to about 7 to 10 alcoholic beverages per week. Moreover, she takes pride in the fact that she does not take any medications.

This patient can be described as a drinker at risk for harm from her drinking; it is unlikely that she is alcohol dependent. The American Society of Addiction Medicine regards residential treatment centers as an appropriate option for treating alcohol dependence. Such centers are not usually necessary for the management of nondependent drinking, even when it places a person at risk for harm, in part because the centers focus on overcoming dependence and preventing relapses. Self-help groups such as Alcoholics Anonymous focus on helping participants overcome dependence and maintain sobriety.

Disulfiram is recommended only for treatment of alcohol dependence. Moreover, it is not used routinely in older patients because the disulfiram-ethanol reaction may pose cardiovascular risks.

55. A 76-year-old woman is undergoing treatment for major depression that began 6 months after her husband died. She has had three episodes of depression since age 58. Her previous most recent episode was 4 years ago, when her husband was diagnosed with colon cancer. At that time she tolerated and responded to sertraline 50 mg daily; this regimen is resumed for the current episode of depression. After 3 weeks of treatment she feels significantly better, and after 4 months she reports that she is back to normal. She has no significant side effects.

Which of the following is most appropriate in management of this patient?

(A) Discontinue sertraline and monitor her closely.
(B) Taper sertraline slowly over the next few months.
(C) Continue sertraline at half the current dose.
(D) Continue sertraline at the current dose.

ANSWER: D

In most older patients, depression should be managed as a chronic relapsing and remitting illness that requires treatment for acute episodes and prophylaxis to prevent relapse or recurrence. In younger and older patients with recurrent depression, maintenance of antidepressant treatment at full therapeutic dose is necessary to prevent recurrence. Older patients with a first episode of depression (late-onset depression) are also likely to have recurrence, and most need long-term treatment. Even in younger patients with a first episode of depression, AHCPR-AHRQ guidelines recommend a minimum of 3 months of acute treatment followed by 6 to 9 months of continuation treatment before discontinuation is attempted under close monitoring.

This patient has been treated for 4 months and tolerates the antidepressant well. It would be inappropriate to discontinue her medication, even if it were done slowly to prevent discontinuation symptoms or rebound relapse. In studies comparing long-term use of antidepressants given at half the dose or at the full dose required for initial remission, older patients treated with half the dose had more brittle remission with more residual symptoms. Similarly, trials to prevent recurrence show weaker benefits with long-term individual psychotherapy than with long-term antidepressant medications. No data support the belief that it is safer to discontinue antidepressant medications in patients in whom reactive depression is associated with a psychosocial stressor (for example, grief associated with a spouse's death) than in a patient who appears to have an endogenous depression. The contrast between reactive and endogenous depression is flawed: recent research has shown that patients genetically predisposed to depression tend to react more negatively to psychosocial stressors. Conversely, antidepressant medication appears to buffer these patients against the impact of stressors.

56. An 84-year-old woman is referred for evaluation of anemia. The patient has a history of anemia, hypertension, osteoarthritis, and renal insufficiency. Her hemoglobin was 10 g/dL until 9 months ago, when it dropped to 6.8 g/dL. At that time there was no evidence of bleeding, and

ferritin, serum iron, iron-binding capacity, and B_{12} and folic acid levels were normal. With transfusion, her hemoglobin stabilized between 9 and 10 g/dL. The patient has no history of weight loss, hematochezia, melena, or hematuria. She complains of pain in her neck, knees, and wrists. Medications include enalapril and acetaminophen. Physical examination is within normal limits.
Laboratory tests:

Hemoglobin	8.9 g/dL
Mean corpuscular volume	87 fL
Leukocyte count	3700/µL
Platelet count	150,000/µL
Westergren erythrocyte sedimentation rate	77 mm/h
Reticulocyte count	0.9%
Folic acid	1.3 ng/mL (normal)
Thyrotropin	2.1 µU/mL
Iron	89 µg/dL
Iron-binding capacity	234 µg/dL
Serum calcium	9.2 mg/dL
Serum albumin	4.0 g/dL
Blood urea nitrogen	32 mg/dL
Serum creatinine	1.8 mg/dL

Which of the following is the most appropriate next step?

(A) Serum erythropoietin level
(B) Chest radiograph and liver function tests
(C) Serum and urine protein electrophoresis and immunofixation
(D) Bone marrow biopsy

ANSWER: C

Anemia is best considered in terms of the bone marrow, the organ of erythropoiesis. Anemia may be due to hypoproliferative erythropoiesis, ineffective erythropoiesis, or a consumptive (hemolytic) process. The laboratory tests most useful in identifying the cause are mean corpuscular volume and corrected reticulocyte count. A reticulocyte count in the normal range cannot be considered normal in the setting of anemia, where the normal bone marrow can increase erythrocyte production by a factor of 10. Therefore, the reticulocyte count must be corrected for the degree of anemia. In this case, the corrected reticulocyte count is the product of the uncorrected reticulocyte percentage and the patient's hemoglobin divided by normal hemoglobin (11.5 in a woman). This would equal 0.69, which is an inadequate erythroid response. In this case, the patient has a reticulocytopenic anemia that is normocytic; that is, the mean corpuscular volume is in the normal range. These two findings indicate that the anemia is hypoproliferative. This is the most common type of anemia in elderly persons, and it is most commonly caused by iron deficiency or anemia of chronic inflammation. Other causes include chronic kidney failure, pure erythrocyte aplasia, marrow-infiltrative disorders, and multiple myeloma.

Several features in this case suggest multiple myeloma, most obviously the longstanding history of mild renal insufficiency. The patient's arthritic symptoms may represent bone disease or, less likely, amyloidosis. The initial laboratory findings also support a diagnosis of multiple myeloma, given the high erythrocyte sedimentation rate and the normal serum calcium level despite renal insufficiency. Thus, it would be appropriate to pursue a diagnosis of multiple myeloma. Erythropoietin level, liver function tests, and chest radiography are not appropriate tests for multiple myeloma. Bone marrow biopsy may not lead to the diagnosis, since the disease is often patchy; a negative bone marrow biopsy does not exclude multiple myeloma. Serum and urine protein electrophoresis and immunofixation are positive in 85% to 90% of persons with multiple myeloma. False-negative studies in the serum and urine do not exclude the diagnosis, but occur in only 10% to 15% of patients. Urine and serum studies are necessary since, in some patients, only light chains are produced, and these would be detected in the urine as Bence-Jones protein rather than in the serum as monoclonal immunoglobulin.

57. An 86-year-old widowed white man is brought to the emergency department after a neighbor found him sleeping in his car with the engine on while it was parked in the garage. The patient's physical and cognitive examinations are unremarkable. Laboratory tests are remarkable only for slightly elevated liver function. His affect is restricted. The patient denies any suicide attempt and explains that he fell asleep after he drove back home. He refuses to allow his son, who lives out of state, to be contacted because "he does not want him to be bothered." Similarly, he refuses to talk to the psychiatric triage nurse, insisting that he should go home now.

Which of the following is the most appropriate next step in the management of this patient?

(A) Discharge with follow-up the next day with his primary care provider.
(B) Initiate involuntary psychiatric evaluation.
(C) Admit the patient to a general medical unit for further observation.
(D) Keep the patient in the emergency department for further observation.
(E) Call the patient's son to discuss your concerns.

ANSWER: B

This patient presents with a psychiatric emergency, since the circumstances and presence of several major risk factors make suicide a strong possibility. His refusal of further evaluation for depression and suicidality does not leave the clinician any choice. White men 85 years and older have the highest suicide rate among all demographic groups in the United States. Widowhood and lack of social support increase the risk of suicide. In addition, this patient's blunted affect suggests depression, and his elevated liver function suggests that he may be drinking. Depression and alcoholism are strongly linked to suicide completion in late life.

It would be helpful to obtain additional clinical information from a family member, but it is inappropriate (and possibly illegal) to call the patient's son without his permission. Keeping the patient in the emergency department or admitting him to a general medical unit for further observation creates a significant risk. He may elope, try to hurt himself in the hospital, or be discharged at a later time without ever having been evaluated properly. Even if he agrees to follow-up the next day with his primary care provider, this strategy is dangerous: he may not go, or if he goes, he may deny being depressed and suicidal, and kill himself. In several psychological autopsy studies, more than two thirds of elderly persons who completed suicide had been seen by a primary care provider within 1 month of killing themselves; up to one half had been seen within 1 week, and one fourth had been seen within 24 hours.

58. A 70-year-old woman describes early morning awakening and daytime fatigue for the past 8 months. She is generally healthy and has no symptoms of anxiety or depression. Over the past year she has been retiring as early as 7 PM. Despite recent efforts to retire later in the evening, she continues to awaken regularly at 3 AM.

Which of the following most likely accounts for this patient's sleep disturbance?

(A) Breathing-related sleep disorder
(B) Circadian rhythm advance
(C) Periodic limb movements
(D) Restless legs syndrome
(E) Sleep apnea

ANSWER: B

Integration of circadian rhythms depends on the suprachiasmatic nucleus of the anterior hypothalamus, which deteriorates with age, particularly in women. As people age, the circadian rhythm advances so that sleepiness occurs earlier in the evening (perhaps at 7 PM or 8 PM), and awakening occurs spontaneously about 8 hours later. Most older adults try to correct the problem by retiring later in the evening, but they nevertheless wake up as core body temperature rises in the early morning hours. Another common pattern is for older adults to nap during the late afternoon or early evening and then have initial insomnia and wake up too early in the morning. Changes in circadian rhythm may also be responsible for daytime agitation in dementia patients who reside in long-term-care facilities.

Treatment of this advanced sleep phase involves delaying the sleep cycle with bright light late in the day, ideally from 7 PM to 9 PM. Also, older adults should try to be outdoors as late in the day as possible before the sun goes down. This strategy will delay the circadian rhythm, so patients will become sleepy later in the evening and sleep later in the morning. In the absence of sunlight, a bright-light box is effective for light exposure later in the day. Normal room light is not bright enough to be effective.

Sleep apnea and breathing-related disorders are more likely to produce excessive daytime sleepiness, rather than the pattern of insomnia seen in this case. Periodic limb movements and restless legs syndrome are both characterized by brief arousals throughout the night and reduced total sleep time. Early-morning awakening is not characteristic of either of these disorders.

59. An 87-year-old man who is an established patient comes to the office because over the past year he has noted increasing shortness of breath with activity. He reports that 2 years ago he could easily walk 1 mile, but now he has to stop and rest after walking one block. He also becomes "winded" after climbing one flight of stairs. He has no chest discomfort or palpitations but often becomes lightheaded when he stands up, and he felt as though he was going to "pass out" on at least two occasions. History includes type 2 diabetes mellitus and depression. He does not smoke or drink alcohol. He is the primary caregiver for his wife, who is disabled with advanced Parkinson's disease. Current medications include glyburide, aspirin, atorvastatin, and paroxetine.

On physical examination, heart rate is 70 per minute and regular, blood pressure is 140/60 mm Hg, respiratory rate is 18 per minute, and body mass index (kg/m^2) is 25. He has a flat affect. Examination of the neck shows no jugular venous distention, normal thyroid, and delayed carotid upstrokes bilaterally. He has a III/VI late-peaking systolic ejection murmur and S_4 gallop, with no S_3. His Mini–Mental State Examination score is 28 of 30, with no focal deficits.

Laboratory studies:

Hemoglobin	13.8 g/dL
Hematocrit	41%
Leukocyte count	6500/μL
Platelet count	180,000/μL
Creatinine	1.0 mg/dL
Blood urea nitrogen	22 mg/dL
Albumin	3.8 g/dL

Electrocardiography shows sinus rhythm and left ventricular hypertrophy with repolarization abnormality. Echocardiography shows moderate left ventricular systolic dysfunction (ejection fraction 35%) and a heavily calcified aortic valve (estimated area 0.6 cm^2).

Which of the following is the most appropriate management for this patient?

(A) Aortic valve replacement
(B) Balloon aortic valvuloplasty
(C) Percutaneous coronary angioplasty, if indicated
(D) Angiotensin-converting enzyme inhibitor and titration to tolerance
(E) Digoxin

ANSWER: A

This patient has severe symptomatic aortic stenosis with moderate left ventricular dysfunction. The only effective treatment for this condition is aortic valve replacement (AVR). Early and long-term results of AVR in older persons are excellent, with significant improvement and restoration of normal age-adjusted life expectancy for most patients. Angiography is indicated before AVR to exclude significant coronary artery disease, which is common even in asymptomatic patients. If present, coronary bypass grafting should be performed at the time of AVR. Contraindications to AVR include moderate or severe dementia, advanced chronic lung disease, or other terminal illness.

Balloon aortic valvuloplasty provides short-term palliation for some patients with severe aortic stenosis, but restenosis occurs within 6 to 12 months in most cases and long-term outcomes are poor. Coronary angioplasty is an effective therapy for obstructive coronary artery disease but has no impact on the prognosis of patients with severe aortic stenosis. Angiotensin-converting enzyme inhibitors and digoxin may provide palliation for patients with severe aortic stenosis, but these and other medications do not alter the natural history of the disease, which is characterized by progressive clinical deterioration following the onset of symptoms.

60. A 75-year-old woman comes to the office because she has had repeated episodes of profound dizziness and near loss of consciousness, along with at least two episodes in which she found herself on the floor but was unaware of how she fell. She denies any confusion after the episode or any significant trauma. She has hypertension, and her daily medication is amlodipine 5 mg.

On physical examination, blood pressure is 152/84 mm Hg and heart rate is 76 per minute when she is supine. In upright posture, blood pressure is 146/86 mm Hg and heart rate is 86 per minute. There is no jugular venous distension or carotid bruit. Lungs are clear. There is a slightly delayed carotid upstroke and a II/VI systolic murmur at the base with an intact S_2 but no gallop.

Which of the following is the most appropriate next step in the evaluation of this patient to stratify her risk for adverse outcomes?

(A) Blood tests
(B) Electrocardiography
(C) Holter monitoring
(D) Event monitor
(E) Tilt-table test

ANSWER: B

Risk stratification is an essential initial step in management of the patient with unexplained syncope. The most important risk factor is the presence of structural heart disease as identified through history, physical examination, electrocardiography, or echocardiography. Electrocardiography is the most likely of the options given to aid in risk stratification, and thus prognosis and diagnosis. Although the electrocardiogram is most commonly normal after a syncopal episode, it may reveal a definitive diagnosis, such as Mobitz type II second- or third-degree atrioventricular block, alternating left and right bundle branch block, ventricular tachycardia, pacemaker malfunction, paroxysmal supraventricular tachycardia, sinus bradycardia, sinoatrial block, or pauses, if associated with symptoms. Such findings occur in fewer than 5% of patients, as arrhythmias resulting in syncope are often self-limited, but other electrocardiographic rhythm and conduction abnormalities or the presence of pathologic Q waves can indicate a myocardial infarction and thus structural heart disease that will guide further evaluation.

Blood tests have an extremely low yield for patients with unexplained syncope. For example, hypoglycemia does not result in a transient loss of consciousness, but rather requires intervention in order to reverse the metabolic derangement that could be contributing to symptoms. Unless it uncovers frequent ventricular ectopy or nonsustained ventricular tachycardia, short-term continuous electrocardiographic monitoring, such as telemetry or Holter monitor or an event monitor, is not useful for identifying the cause of syncope, since weeks, months, or even years may pass before the next arrhythmia-related event. Also, most arrhythmias detected in patients with syncope are brief and result in no symptoms.

Triage decisions and management should be based on preexisting cardiac disease or electrocardiographic abnormalities, which are important predictors of arrhythmic syncope and mortality, rather than on symptoms. A tilt-table test would be an appropriate evaluation only after structural heart disease has been excluded.

61. A 69-year-old man comes to the office because for the past several weeks he has had recurrent spells of room-spinning vertigo that last for about 4 minutes. The spells occur spontaneously, are unassociated with positional changes, and are accompanied occasionally by double vision and sometimes by weakness on the right side. Several times, he has had sudden drop attacks, after which he has mild weakness of both legs lasting several minutes. He has a history of diabetes mellitus and coronary artery disease.

Which of the following is the most likely cause of the vertigo?

(A) Vestibular neuronitis
(B) Vertebrobasilar insufficiency
(C) Labyrinthitis
(D) Migraine-associated vertigo
(E) Ménière's disease

ANSWER: B

Transient ischemia within the vertebrobasilar system is a common cause of spontaneous attacks of vertigo in older patients. Typically, the vertigo begins abruptly, lasts several minutes, and is often associated with other neurologic symptoms. In any older patient with brief episodes of vertigo, and especially in patients with risk factors for cerebrovascular disease (such as diabetes mellitus, hypertension, hypercholesterolemia, peripheral vascular disease, coronary artery disease), transient ischemic attacks must be excluded. Diplopia, unilateral or bilateral weakness, and drop attacks (sudden falls without loss of consciousness) are also signs

of posterior circulation insufficiency; other signs and symptoms include visual hallucinations, vision loss, visceral sensations, headache, dysarthria, and ataxia. Magnetic resonance imaging, magnetic resonance angiography of the brain and neck (to look for evidence of cerebrovascular atherosclerotic disease) if possible, and diffusion-weighted imaging (to look for evidence for an ischemic infarct) are appropriate. Management could include antiplatelet drugs such as clopidogrel[OL], combination aspirin and slow-release dipyridamole[OL], or warfarin[OL] if there is evidence for emboli.

Vestibular neuronitis produces a spontaneous episode of vertigo that lasts for several days and crescendos over several hours, often with nausea and vomiting. It is thought to occur secondary to viral infection of the eighth cranial nerve. The term *labyrinthitis* is sometimes used by clinicians interchangeably with *vestibular neuronitis*, but it can also refer to a bacterial infection that extends from the middle ear (for example, otitis media or cholesteatoma). It is unusual for migraine-associated vertigo to present first in older age, and with several focal neurologic complaints. Ménière's disease is associated with hearing loss, aural fullness, tinnitus, and episodic rotational vertigo usually of about 20 minutes' to several hours' duration.

62. An 80-year-old woman comes to the office because she recently has had difficulty eating and swallowing solid foods. She notes that when she prepares to swallow, the food scrapes her cheeks and roof of her mouth. The patient has hypertension, diabetes mellitus, a recent history of kidney stones, and depression. Current medications include hydrochlorothiazide and metformin. For the first time in many years, her last dental examination revealed several cavities, located at the roots of the teeth.

Which of the following is the most likely cause of her symptoms?

(A) Aging
(B) Salivary duct stones
(C) Metformin
(D) Hydrochlorothiazide

OL Not approved by the U.S. Food and Drug Administration for this use.

ANSWER: D

Saliva has multiple functions in the oral cavity: It is a protective cleanser with antibacterial activity, a buffer that inhibits demineralization, a lubricant, and a transport medium to taste sensors. These functions are seriously altered in xerostomia. Although older adults are likely to have a decreased amount of active glandular tissue, numerous clinical studies have demonstrated that salivary flow does not decrease significantly with age. Signs and symptoms of xerostomia include intra-oral dryness or burning, alterations in tongue surface, dysphagia, cheilosis, alterations in taste, difficulty with speech, and development of root caries.

The causes of salivary stones (sialoliths) are largely unknown; theories range from autoimmune to inflammatory causes. Salivary stones are unrelated to kidney stones. Salivary stones do not cause severe xerostomia, as the stones are usually local, affecting one gland (commonly the submandibular gland). Sialoliths usually occur unilaterally, so saliva is still present in other major and minor salivary glands.

Many conditions and treatments may contribute to xerostomia, including radiation, chemotherapy, psychologic stressors, endocrine disorders, and nutritional disorders. Xerostomia is a side effect of more than 200 commonly used drugs. Antihypertensive medications (especially diuretics) and antidepressants (especially tricyclic antidepressants) reduce saliva flow. Metformin is not known to decrease salivary flow.

Treatment for patients with xerostomia includes scrupulous oral hygiene, with use of a soft toothbrush and fluoride rinses, reduced consumption of alcohol, frequent intake of water, saliva substitutes, and avoidance of highly acidic foods.

63. A 78-year-old woman comes to the office because she has heavy vaginal bleeding after no bleeding for many years. She has been on continuous estrogen replacement therapy for the past 30 years. Physical examination, including pelvic, reveals severe arthritis. She requests evaluation with the least invasive test, because she has severe arthritis.

What is the best evaluation for this patient?

(A) Coagulopathy work-up
(B) Vaginal ultrasound to assess endometrial thickness
(C) Endometrial biopsy
(D) Hysteroscopy
(E) Dilation and curettage

ANSWER: B

Causes of postmenopausal bleeding (bleeding after 1 year of amenorrhea) include vaginal atrophy, trauma, infection, cervical cancer, endometrial cancer, endometrial or cervical polyps, and endometrial hyperplasia. Bleeding can occur with the start of continuous combined hormone replacement therapy. From 75% to 86% of women report amenorrhea after 1 year of continuous combined therapy. Endometrial assessment is recommended during the first year only if the bleeding is unusually heavy or prolonged. The endometrium should be evaluated if there is bleeding after 1 year.

Endometrial biopsy, hysteroscopy, dilation and curettage, and transvaginal ultrasonography are all effective for evaluating vaginal bleeding. Transvaginal ultrasound is the least invasive diagnostic test for endometrial hyperplasia or cancer detection. Its specificity is about 63% for women on combination hormone replacement therapy. An endometrial thickness (endometrial stripe) measuring 4 mm or less is normal. If results are abnormal, endometrial biopsy should be obtained. Endometrial biopsy is done in the office and is 85% to 95% sensitive for endometrial hyperplasia or cancer. If office-based endometrial biopsy is unobtainable as a consequence of the inability to enter the endometrial cavity (because of stenotic os) or functional impairment (such as debilitating arthritis), transvaginal ultrasound may be useful.

Dilation and curettage is the gold standard for evaluating postmenopausal bleeding. The procedure is usually done in the operating room in women with a negative or nondiagnostic endometrial biopsy or in women with abnormal ultrasound findings in whom an office endometrial biopsy is not possible.

Hysteroscopy is often performed along with dilation and curettage. It does not add to the diagnostic accuracy for endometrial hyperplasia or cancer but may increase the sensitivity for sessile or pedunculated intraluminal masses.

Coagulopathy work-up is done in addition to evaluation of vaginal bleeding only if the patient has other symptoms or signs suggesting coagulopathy.

64. An 81-year-old woman with a history of "bad nerves" comes to the office for a second opinion because she is "tired of being sick all my life." She has a history of headaches, back pain, and joint pain, for which she had taken nonsteroidal anti-inflammatory drugs (NSAIDs) intermittently for decades. She also has nausea, bloating, and stomach ache that persisted after she discontinued NSAIDs. She cannot tolerate certain foods, has difficulty swallowing, and at times is unable to speak. She has had gastroenterology, neurology, and rheumatology consultations, and different tests were recommended, but no medications were prescribed. She sleeps and eats well, and enjoys crafts and spending time with family and friends. At this visit she appears upset and tearful.

Which of the following is most likely?

(A) Major depressive disorder
(B) Generalized anxiety disorder
(C) Somatization disorder
(D) Hypochondriasis
(E) Pain disorder

ANSWER: C

This is a typical case of somatization disorder. Patients often present with an "organ recital," involving, at a minimum, pain in at least four areas of the body, two gastrointestinal complaints, one genitourinary or sexual and one pseudoneurologic symptom other than pain, with a duration longer than 6 months and debut prior to age 30. In somatization disorder, multiple symptoms are not fully explained by the physical findings.

Hypochondriasis refers to preoccupation with having a disease based on misinterpretation of symptoms. Diagnosis of major depressive disorder requires depressed mood or anhedonia, and a constellation of symptoms, such as changes in sleep and appetite, that this patient does not display. Generalized anxiety disorder refers to excessive worry about multiple issues, including safety of self or others, and is associated with fatigue, restlessness, insomnia, problems concentrating, appetite change, and

muscular tension. This patient is concerned about multiple somatic complaints for which no medical cause has been found. In pain disorder, pain is the only focus of clinical attention, and psychologic factors have an important role in onset, exacerbation, and maintenance of pain.

65. An 87-year-old resident of an Alzheimer's assisted-living unit is evaluated because she has fallen twice in the past month. She has a history of dementia, urge urinary incontinence, and hypertension. She has had no recent acute illness or changes in medication. She takes vitamin E 400 units twice daily, galantamine 8 mg twice daily, enteric-coated aspirin 81 mg daily, sustained-release tolterodine 4 mg daily, and hydrochlorothiazide 25 mg daily. Unless redirected, she spends most of the day walking. It is difficult to get her to finish her meals.

On examination, she is alert, oriented to place but not date, and thin, and she appears tired. She has normal gait speed, with normal foot clearance and arm swing, but she turns quickly and reaches for the wall to steady herself.

Which of the following would be part of a treatment plan to reduce this patient's risk of falling?

(A) Medication with quetiapine 25 mg daily
(B) Scheduled brief rest periods during the day
(C) Use of hip protectors during the day
(D) Use of a lap tray to prevent her from getting up

ANSWER: B

This assisted-living resident has dementia and walks excessively throughout the day. She becomes fatigued by this activity, and she may not be eating or drinking sufficiently. It is likely that fatigue is contributing to her risk of falls. Her difficulty getting up from a chair and turning suggests impairment of lower extremity strength and balance. Having regular rest periods throughout the day would be an important component of a treatment plan to reduce her risk of falling again. During these times, she could be offered snacks and drinks to increase her caloric intake and improve hydration. Her deficits in lower extremity strength and balance would best be addressed initially by a physical therapy evaluation and individualized treatment.

Quetiapine and other atypical antipsychotic medications are not indicated. They would not decrease her walking behavior and would be likely to increase her risk for falls as a consequence of adverse effects (postural hypotension, dizziness, and somnolence). Consistent use of hip protectors during the day may help prevent a hip fracture but would not be part of a plan to prevent falls. A regular group exercise program might be a component of a fall prevention plan for her, once she has been evaluated by physical therapy and has responded to scheduled rest periods. Although an individualized exercise program would be more likely to improve her strength and balance, a supervised group exercise program might help maintain gains and could serve as a distractor to keep her from walking during that time. The use of a lap tray is a physical restraint and should be avoided. A trial of providing food and drink during rest periods and while she is "on the go" should be attempted prior to any use of restraints.

66. A 72-year-old woman has a 15-year history of type 2 diabetes mellitus. She also has a history of coronary artery disease and heart failure. She began taking glipizide 8 years ago for her diabetes. Over the past 2 years she has required additional therapy. Initially, she did well on a combination of glipizide and NPH insulin at bedtime. Over the past 6 months, glipizide was stopped, and she has required twice-daily doses of NPH and regular insulin, given before breakfast and dinner. Despite increasing doses of insulin, her hemoglobin A_{1C} has increased to 9% and she now has hypoglycemia before lunch and during the night. Serum creatinine is 1.6 mg/dL.

Which of the following is the best management step?

(A) Add metformin.
(B) Add rosiglitazone.
(C) Replace the regular insulin with insulin lispro.
(D) Restart the glipizide.

ANSWER: C

This case illustrates a common problem in type 2 diabetes mellitus: over time, oral agents no longer control hyperglycemia and insulin therapy becomes necessary. As insulin deficiency progresses, more sophisticated insulin regimens are needed to control hyperglycemia while minimizing hypoglycemia.

In this patient, as the dose of insulin was increased, hypoglycemia developed and hemoglobin A_{1C} increased further. Insulin lispro is a rapidly absorbed insulin analogue. Peak serum levels after subcutaneous injection occur earlier and are shorter than with regular insulin. In both types 1 and 2 diabetes mellitus, insulin lispro is less likely than regular insulin to produce postprandial hypoglycemia. Therefore, substituting lispro for regular insulin will minimize hypoglycemia and is the best option.

The use of metformin in patients with heart failure or renal impairment (serum creatinine higher than 1.5 mg/dL in men or 1.4 mg/dL in women) significantly predisposes to lactic acidosis, a potentially fatal complication. Thiazolidinediones (rosiglitazone, pioglitazone) cause plasma volume expansion and may exacerbate this patient's heart failure. These drugs should not be used in patients with New York Heart Association class III or IV heart failure. Adding rosiglitazone (without modification of the insulin regimen) would not solve this patient's problem with hypoglycemia before lunch and during the night, even if her volume status were carefully monitored. She was previously resistant to the glipizide so restarting it would be unlikely to be effective.

67. A 65-year-old postmenopausal woman comes to the office for advice on physical activity to decrease her likelihood of having vertebral fractures and disability. Her mother has severe osteoporosis and back deformity with kyphosis.

Which of the following has been shown to reduce the likelihood of osteoporotic vertebral fractures?

(A) Daily high-intensity running program
(B) Progressive back extensor resistive exercise program 5 times each week
(C) High-intensity strength training exercises twice weekly
(D) Walking at an average pace 1 hour three times each week
(E) Household chores

ANSWER: B

Aerobic, weight-bearing, and resistance exercises all increase the bone mineral density of the vertebrae in postmenopausal women. The best evidence comes from a well-done prospective trial on strengthening back musculature, which showed sustained reduction in fracture over 10 years. Women between the ages of 48 and 65 (mean age 55) were randomly assigned to a progressive resistive back-strengthening exercise program for 2 years or to a control group. At 10-year follow-up, the exercise group had significantly better back muscle strength and greater vertebral bone mineral density than the control group, and the control group had a 2.7-fold greater risk of vertebral fracture.

A prospective observational cohort study of older women showed that hip fractures were associated with higher levels of leisure time, sports activity, and household chores, and fewer hours of sitting daily. Furthermore, vertebral fractures were more likely in the moderately or vigorously active women. Total physical activity, hours of household chores per day, and hours of sitting per day were not significantly associated with wrist or vertebral fractures.

In women followed for 12 years in the Nurses Health Study, walking for at least 4 hours each week was associated with a 41% lower risk of hip fracture than walking less than 1 hour each week. However, vertebral fractures were not included in the analysis.

High-intensity strength training can increase muscle mass, muscle strength, dynamic balance, and bone density in postmenopausal women. However, fracture rates over time have not been reported, and there is no convincing evidence that high-intensity exercise (such as running) is superior to lower intensity activity (such as walking).

68. A 79-year-old woman comes to the emergency department with palpitations and shortness of breath of 2 hours' duration. She has a history of hypertension, type 2 diabetes mellitus, mild restrictive lung disease, gastroesophageal reflux disease, and positional tremor. The patient relates that she was sitting in a chair when she noted the sudden onset of "heart racing," followed a few minutes later by difficulty breathing. She reports no chest discomfort,

diaphoresis, dizziness, or syncope. When the symptoms did not resolve after an hour, her son brought her to the emergency department.

On physical examination, the patient is in mild respiratory distress. Heart rate ranges from 130 to 150 per minute and is irregular, blood pressure is 140/70 mm Hg, and respiratory rate is 22 per minute. Her neck is supple, with normal jugular venous pressure and no thyromegaly. Bibasilar crackles are heard. The heart is irregularly irregular, with a II/VI systolic ejection murmur and no S_3 or S_4 gallop. She has a moderate positional tremor.

Laboratory studies:

Cardiac biomarker proteins	normal
Creatinine	0.8 mg/dL
Blood urea nitrogen	17 mg/dL
Hemoglobin	13.1 g/dL
Hemoglobin A_{1C}	7.3%
Thyrotropin	2.0 µU/mL
Total cholesterol	198 mg/dL
High-density lipoprotein	55 mg/dL
Low-density lipoprotein	113 mg/dL
Triglycerides	150 mg/dL

Electrocardiography reveals atrial fibrillation with rapid ventricular response, left ventricular hypertrophy with repolarization abnormality, and no ischemic changes. Chest radiograph shows mild cardiomegaly with mild pulmonary vascular redistribution. Adenosine-thallium stress test reveals a left ventricular ejection fraction of 67% with no evidence of ischemia. Echocardiogram demonstrates moderate left ventricular hypertrophy, mild left atrial enlargement, normal left ventricular systolic function, and mild left ventricular diastolic dysfunction.

The patient is treated with intravenous diltiazem with subsequent reversion to sinus rhythm (85 per minute). Intravenous furosemide results in a net diuresis of 1160 cc, and her shortness of breath resolves. Myocardial infarction is excluded by normal serial troponin levels.

Which of the following are appropriate discharge medications for this patient?

(A) Aspirin, warfarin, amiodarone, and angiotensin-converting enzyme inhibitor
(B) Warfarin, diltiazem, β-blocker, and angiotensin-receptor blocker
(C) Aspirin, β-blocker, angiotensin-converting enzyme inhibitor, and statin
(D) Warfarin, β-blocker, angiotensin-converting enzyme inhibitor, and angiotensin-receptor blocker
(E) Diltiazem, β-blocker, angiotensin-converting enzyme inhibitor, and statin

ANSWER: C

This patient has new-onset atrial fibrillation and heart failure with preserved left ventricular systolic function ("diastolic" heart failure), as well as a history of hypertension and diabetes. Data from the Heart Outcomes Prevention Evaluation (HOPE) study and the Heart Protection Study indicate that older adults with diabetes or vascular disease benefit from routine treatment with an angiotensin-converting enzyme (ACE) inhibitor (ramipril) and a statin (simvastatin), even when left ventricular function and fasting lipid profile are normal or near normal. In addition, despite this patient's "negative" stress test, her age and risk factors place her at moderate risk for coronary heart disease and stroke, thus justifying the addition of aspirin to her regimen. Although the value of β-blocker therapy in patients with diastolic heart failure is unproven, β-blockers are effective anti-ischemic, antihypertensive, and rate-controlling agents, and they may reduce the risk of recurrent atrial fibrillation. Warfarin is indicated in the management of chronic or paroxysmal atrial fibrillation, but long-term use of this drug following a single episode of atrial fibrillation that resolves within 24 hours is unproven. Intravenous diltiazem is an effective agent for controlling heart rate in patients with acute atrial fibrillation and rapid ventricular response, but β-blockers are preferable for long-term treatment. Angiotensin-receptor blockers have been shown to reduce admissions but not mortality in patients with diastolic heart failure; by contrast, the ACE inhibitor ramipril reduced both mortality and morbidity in diabetic patients in the HOPE study, so ACE inhibitors are preferable to angiotensin-receptor blockers in this population. Amiodarone is not indicated in patients with transient atrial fibrillation.

69. A 72-year-old man comes to the office because he has had itching and burning of his feet for 2 months. He also notes a strong odor when he removes his socks. He wears shoes with rubber soles. History includes hypertension, osteoarthritis, and childhood asthma. On examination, the lateral borders of both feet show erythema and scaling in a moccasin distribution. The toe web spaces are normal.

Which of the following is the most appropriate next step?

(A) Examine skin scrapings on a saline wet mount slide.
(B) Culture skin scrapings.
(C) Examine potassium hydroxide stain of scrapings of the rash.
(D) Do a punch skin biopsy.

ANSWER: C

Scaliness in a moccasin distribution is characteristic of tinea pedis; therefore, the best approach is to demonstrate hyphae with a potassium hydroxide stain. Cultures or skin biopsy are not necessary. Tinea pedis can also present with peeling, fissures, and maceration of the web spaces. Because the web spaces can be the port of entry for skin bacteria, especially staphylococci and streptococci, it is important to look between the toes, especially in patients with diabetes mellitus or recurrent lower-extremity cellulitis. Tinea pedis of the moccasin type or chronic hyperkeratotic type is more common in atopic individuals and is most often caused by *Trichophyton rubrum*. This patient has a history of childhood asthma, which is associated with atopy.

Tinea pedis should be treated with a topical broad-spectrum antifungal preparation containing imidazoles. A cream or solution should be applied twice daily and continued for 2 weeks after the rash has resolved. Keratolytic agents (salicylic acid, lactic acid, hydroxy acid) with plastic occlusion help reduce the hyperkeratosis. Moccasin-type tinea pedis is often associated with tinea unguium of the nails, which is a source of reinfection. If there is a nail reservoir, it should be eradicated with a systemic antifungal agent, such as itraconazole or terbinafine, if contraindications or cost are not an issue for the patient.

To minimize recurrence of tinea pedis, the patient should wash his feet daily with benzoyl peroxide bar, dry between the spaces well, and avoid thick socks and shoes that increase sweating. If the patient has frequent recurrences, indefinite use of a topical antifungal agent may be needed.

Use of topical steroids alone may initially improve the rash by reducing the inflammation, but the fungal infection will continue to spread. A combination antifungal-steroid agent may be used when there is prominent inflammation, but topical steroids should be used with caution as they can cause atrophy of the skin and other complications. Allergic contact dermatitis to rubber chemicals can cause a rash of the soles, mostly on the pressure points, while the proximal parts of the toes and the toe webs are spared. This rash can be misdiagnosed as fungal infection. A potassium hydroxide stain will be negative in allergic contact dermatitis.

70. A 76-year-old man with Alzheimer's disease is brought to the office for a follow-up visit. For the past few weeks he has had difficulty staying asleep at night. He goes to bed at 9 PM, sleeps until about 2 AM, and awakens to go to the bathroom. He remains awake for several hours, during which he is often disoriented, paces the house, and wakes his wife. He and his wife are fatigued, and he is more withdrawn during the day. He requires help with instrumental activities of daily living (IADLs), needs reminders with some basic ADLs, and is independent with feeding, toileting, and ambulation. His general health is good. There is no evidence of sadness or anhedonia, and he is eating well. He has well-controlled hypertension on a diuretic and takes an oral hypoglycemic agent for mild type 2 diabetes mellitus. He had a transurethral resection of the prostate 1 year ago for prostatic hyperplasia and has had no recurrence. At his last office visit, he was counseled about sleep hygiene, but this intervention has failed.

Which of the following, given at bedtime, is the most appropriate first-line pharmacologic treatment?

(A) Zolpidem, 5 to 10 mg
(B) Melatonin, 0.3 to 5 mg
(C) Zaleplon, 5 to 10 mg
(D) Trazodone, 25 to 50 mg
(E) Lorazepam, 1 mg

ANSWER: D

Mild sleep disturbances affect up to 20% of outpatients with dementia. Usually the disturbance is not associated with depression or other psychiatric symptoms and is thus a primary sleep disorder. Most common are early insomnia and middle insomnia, as with this patient. The sleep problems often adversely affect the patient and exhaust caregivers. If left untreated, sleep problems can slowly lead to full reversal of the sleep cycle, which is difficult to treat. Sleep hygiene interventions are only modestly successful and are often difficult for the caregiver to implement. Bright-light therapy may improve sleep disturbance in patients with dementia, but the equipment is expensive and there is no third-payer support; it is also difficult to implement outside institutional settings. Therefore, pharmacologic management is often necessary. Although there are no controlled trials to guide decision making, trazodone is preferred by most experts given its low adverse-effect profile (including dizziness, excessive sedation, confusion, and hypotension), potential antidepressant activity, and low cost. Starting doses of 25 to 50 mg are recommended, and doses as high as 150 to 200 mg may be needed. Melatonin is unproven in this setting and anecdotally appears to have limited efficacy. Newer agents such as zolpidem and zaleplon, which are schedule IV agents, are best reserved as second-line agents. Benzodiazepines, such as lorazepam, and related compounds lead to disinhibition and agitation and cause falls; they are reserved for short-term treatment of more severe forms of sleep disturbance in patients with dementia. Over-the-counter medications containing the antihistamine diphenhydramine should be avoided because its anticholinergic activity can worsen dementia. Any evidence of sleep apnea, depression, psychosis, or mania should be investigated as the cause of the sleep disorder and treated. Sleep apnea in particular appears to be more common than previously thought, even in non-overweight patients with dementia. It should be assessed with a sleep laboratory study and treated appropriately with weight loss and a continuous positive airway pressure device.

71. Which of the following is correct regarding the use of occlusive dressings in the treatment of pressure ulcers?

   (A) They promote a mildly alkaline pH.
   (B) They maintain a relatively high oxygen tension on the wound surface.
   (C) They are more likely than nonocclusive dressings to preserve cytokines.
   (D) They are associated with more pain from partial-thickness wounds than nonocclusive dressings.

ANSWER: C

Understanding the effect of occlusive dressings has been an important development in successful wound care. By offering an occluded, moist environment, occlusive dressings maintain a mildly acidic pH and a relatively low oxygen tension on the wound surface. The steep oxygen gradient stimulates angiogenesis, an important factor in wound healing. Low oxygen tension also provides optimal conditions for proliferation of fibroblasts and formation of granulation tissue. Cytokines encourage granulation-tissue formation and epithelialization and are more likely to be preserved in an occluded wound environment. Moisture also facilitates epidermal migration, angiogenesis, and connective-tissue synthesis. Moisture supports autolysis of necrotic material by providing the solute for enzymatic debridement. Wound desiccation should be avoided, as it leads to cell death. Occlusive dressings better limit the pain associated with partial-thickness wounds than do nonocclusive dressings.

72. An 85-year-old woman is evaluated because she has lost 2.7 kg (6 lb) since admission to a nursing home 1 month ago after a stroke. Her admission weight was 120 pounds and her height 64 inches. She has mild cognitive impairment. The staff reports that she takes a long time to chew her food and that she pockets food in her cheek. She denies pain with chewing or swallowing, and she is not depressed. Examination indicates that her denture fits well and that she has no oral lesions. Her gag reflex is intact.

Which of the following is the most appropriate first step?

   (A) Request swallowing evaluation.
   (B) Order a nutritional supplement.
   (C) Discuss feeding tube placement with her family.
   (D) Order mirtazapine.
   (E) Initiate therapy with megestrol acetate.

ANSWER: A

Weight loss is a clinically important sign of nutritional risk in the nursing-home population, and regular assessment of weight change is an important element of quality nursing-home care. Weight change is reported in the Minimum Data Set, and national nursing-home quality measures consider prevalence of weight loss. This resident's history of stroke places her at high risk for a swallowing disorder; the prolonged eating and pocketing of food further point toward this possibility. An intact gag reflex does not preclude the presence of a swallowing disorder. The evaluation may vary from bedside assessment to endoscopy. The tests have a wide range of sensitivity, specificity, and inter-rater reliability. Bedside assessment is generally considered the simplest and most efficient initial screen. Videofluoroscopy allows visualization of the trajectory of different types of food and liquids. Some swallowing difficulties may be resolved by change in diet consistency or patient position during feeding.

Initiating a nutritional supplement or placing a feeding tube is inappropriate in the absence of a swallowing evaluation. Recent literature has focused on the lack of evidence supporting tube feeding for persons with advanced dementia. However, this resident has mild cognitive impairment, and the cause of weight loss is most likely a swallowing disorder related to stroke. If alternative options are not effective, placement of a feeding tube may be appropriate after discussion with the resident and family. Mirtazapine may increase appetite among depressed persons but would not be the best initial choice in this nondepressed person. The evidence for efficacy of megestrol acetate in nursing homes is mixed, but it would not be considered a first-line therapy in this resident.

Megestrol acetate has been associated with fluid retention, exacerbation of heart failure, adrenal suppression, vaginal bleeding or discharge, thromboembolism, and delirium.

73. A 70-year-old woman is concerned about vaginal discomfort and pain and occasional bleeding with intercourse. She had a hysterectomy and oophorectomy for fibroids at age 56, and estrogen receptor–positive breast cancer at age 65. The breast cancer was treated with lumpectomy and radiation, with no evidence of recurrence. She has never taken hormone replacement therapy. She is on no medications other than ibuprofen as needed for joint pains. In former years, sexual activity was mutually pleasurable to her and her husband. Her husband has recently started taking sildenafil.

Physical examination is remarkable for vaginal atrophic changes and mild difficulty introducing a regular-size speculum. No masses are present.

Which of the following is the best therapeutic choice for this patient?

(A) Oral conjugated estrogen
(B) Oral esterified estrogen and methyltestosterone
(C) Oral fluoxetine
(D) Water-soluble lubricant
(E) Intramuscular testosterone

ANSWER: D

About one third of sexually active women age 65 and older report dyspareunia. Causes include inadequate vaginal lubrication (most commonly due to estrogen deficiency), irritation and dryness of the external genitalia, vulvovaginitis, local trauma (such as from episiotomy scars), urethritis, improper intromission (often related to angle of penile entry), anorectal disease, altered anatomy of the female genital tract (such as retroverted or prolapsed uterus), and arthritis.

In women who are appropriate candidates, estrogen, either systemically or locally (in the form of a cream or estradiol-releasing vaginal ring or pellet), is the best choice, as the major cause of dyspareunia is loss of lubrication due to estrogen deficiency. Some women may require both systemic and local application of estrogen for best effect. The use of estrogen for the

shortest possible duration is advisable. With this patient's history of breast cancer, however, most clinicians would hesitate to use estrogen, including locally, as topical estrogen cream can have systemic effects. The use of combined estrogen and testosterone or testosterone alone enhances libido and may improve vaginal lubrication. This patient, however, does not have low libido, and these agents may cause virilization, hepatic dysfunction, and worsened lipid parameters. In this patient, the best option with the least risk to the patient is the use of a water-soluble lubricant.

This patient has no history of depression. In addition, fluoxetine and other selective serotonin-reuptake inhibitors can cause anorgasmia and loss of libido.

74. A 72-year-old man comes to the office for a first visit. He runs 5 miles daily and occasionally has soreness in his knees that responds to aspirin. He takes several over-the-counter health preparations, including a multiple vitamin, calcium 500 mg, and a fish oil extract. On questioning, the patient describes an increasing sense of urinary urgency and nocturia, one or two times a night, over the past 2 years. He is bothered enough by the symptoms to consider treatment.

On physical examination, blood pressure is 110/70 mm Hg and heart rate is 60 per minute. Digital rectal examination reveals a normal prostate. Urinalysis and blood urea nitrogen and creatinine levels are normal; prostate-specific antigen level is 1.5 ng/mL.

Which of the following is most appropriate at this time?

(A) Obtain a transrectal ultrasound study.
(B) Initiate treatment with tamsulosin, 0.4 mg daily.
(C) Initiate treatment with oxybutynin, 2.5 mg three times daily.
(D) Initiate treatment with finasteride, 5 mg daily.

ANSWER: B

This patient's evaluation is consistent with mild to moderate benign prostatic hyperplasia. Further evaluation is not needed before proceeding with medical treatment or watchful waiting.

An α-blocker such as tamsulosin is the recommended initial treatment for men with small prostates and primarily irritative symptoms; symptoms may improve within several weeks. Finasteride is most effective in men with large prostates and primarily obstructive symptoms; clinical improvement takes several months. Further, a recent report suggests that treatment with finasteride may lower the overall risk of prostate cancer but increase the risk of aggressive prostate cancer. Although this risk can be managed with careful monitoring and should not preclude its use in appropriate patients, it reinforces the practice of initiating treatment with an α-blocker in men with small prostates.

This patient's symptoms are relatively mild for surgery to be considered. Oxybutynin is used for the management of urge urinary incontinence, not obstructive uropathy, and might precipitate urinary retention in this patient.

75. The daughter of a 93-year-old woman with Alzheimer's disease calls to discuss the patient's weight loss. The patient lives with her daughter and has had dementia for more than 6 years. Her average adult weight was 72.7 kg (160 lb). In recent years, she has weighed approximately 63.6 kg (140 lb); the community health nurse reports that she weighed 55.5 kg (122 lb) last week. The patient has not walked in at least 3 months and has required assistance for all of her activities of daily living, including feeding, for the past year. According to recent laboratory studies, her albumin level is 2.1 g/dL and total cholesterol is 93 mg/dL. Additional laboratory tests are unremarkable. When last examined, the patient was frail but well cared for and did not engage with you or her daughter.

What is the most appropriate response to this patient's weight loss?

(A) Prescribe nutritional supplements.
(B) Arrange for placement of a gastrostomy tube.
(C) Prescribe megestrol 400 mg oral suspension daily.
(D) Arrange swallowing evaluation.
(E) Recommend hospice care.

ANSWER: E

In this patient with end-stage dementia, the time course is consistent with adult failure-to-thrive syndrome, and no readily reversible cause of weight loss has been identified. No interventions have been shown consistently to make a significant difference in such cases. There is little harm in a trial of oral supplements, but supplements are costly. Artificial feeding and hydration via gastrostomy have adverse effects and have not been shown to improve most outcomes of interest. Careful hand feeding is usually preferable and may be more efficacious. Megestrol suspension is approved for use in AIDS wasting syndrome; one study of megestrol for long-term-care patients showed an association with deep-vein thrombosis with its use. Other medications have not made a substantial difference for patients in this situation. It is unlikely that this patient can participate in a swallowing evaluation. As this patient likely has a prognosis of less than 6 months, it is appropriate to refer her to hospice after a plan of care is agreed upon. The most appropriate response to her weight loss is to meet with her family to clarify her goals and preferences in the context of her terminal condition.

76. A 73-year-old man fractures his hip while roller blading. He undergoes total hip arthroplasty and is discharged to a skilled nursing facility on the third postoperative day. At initial nursing evaluation, his right heel is erythematous and has a "mushy" feel to it. The history and physical examination notes indicate that the extremities are "within normal limits." Three days later nursing notes document a blister on the heel. There is no notation that the physician is called. A physician progress note the following day does not document examination of the patient's extremities. Two days later the blister opens and reveals a large ulcer with necrotic tissue. The physician is called and gives treatment orders for wet-to-dry dressings. The patient's family calls the state health department and a survey is done, the results of which document a pattern of poor skin care in the facility. The patient has an extended stay in the nursing facility and is ultimately discharged to an assisted-living facility. He files a lawsuit against the hospital, doctors, and nursing facility.

Which of the following may affect the outcome of this case?

(A) Wet-to-dry dressings have not been found efficacious in recent studies.
(B) Nursing homes are rarely defendants in lawsuits related to pressure ulcers.
(C) Lack of detail about skin condition in nursing-home charts deters lawsuits.
(D) Plaintiffs have introduced survey results to show a pattern of poor care in a facility.

ANSWER: D

Since the passage of nursing-home reform legislation in 1987 and the publication of Omnibus Budget Reconciliation Act of 1987 (OBRA-87) regulations in 1992, the risk of litigation for negligent care involving pressure ulcers has increased. Although OBRA-87 has increased the awareness of good skin care and the importance of prevention of pressure ulcers, it has also helped spotlight the problem. Legislating good skin care has thus opened up opportunities for lawsuits.

Critically ill patients are among the most vulnerable for developing pressure ulcers. In pressure ulcer−related lawsuits, hospitals have been the defendants in almost one fourth of cases. In this scenario, pressure-related deep-tissue damage occurred while the patient was in the hospital but was not readily apparent without an examination. Once pressure-related deep-tissue injury was identified by nursing-home staff, the plan of care should have been modified to address this issue.

One of the most important aspects of medical malpractice involving pressure ulcers is documentation. Coordination of documentation is also important. In this case, the nurses documented evidence of a pressure ulcer, but the physician's notes did not corroborate these findings, and there was no evidence that the physician had been notified by the nursing staff.

Standard of care is essentially a legal concept that reflects common and expected practices in the community. It does not necessarily reflect the latest information offered in the literature. Despite the literature supporting moisture-retentive dressings in wound care, many clinicians still consider wet-to-dry dressings to be the standard of care.

By law, all nursing homes that accept Medicaid and Medicare payments must be surveyed by state inspectors at least every 15 months, and more frequently for cause. Survey results are public documents, and plaintiffs can easily obtain them. Plaintiffs have been successful in introducing survey results to show a pattern of poor care in a facility.

77. Which antihypertensive class is less effective as a single agent in black than in white Americans?

(A) Angiotensin-converting enzyme inhibitors
(B) Calcium channel blockers
(C) Centrally acting agents
(D) Diuretics

ANSWER: A

Hypertension is more prevalent and often more severe in African-descended populations living outside Africa than in any other population. Black patients generally respond well to diuretic therapy, with the fall in blood pressure exceeding that seen with monotherapy with an angiotensin-converting enzyme (ACE) inhibitor or a β-blocker. This increased efficacy of diuretics suggests an important role for volume in the genesis of hypertension in black patients and is consistent with the observation that blacks have a higher frequency of salt sensitivity (as defined by a rise in blood pressure with salt loading) than whites. Hypertension also appears to be less angiotensin II−dependent in blacks than in whites. Although black patients do not respond well to ACE inhibitors or β-blockers when these agents are given as monotherapy, either drug is effective when given in combination with a diuretic.

Black patients are also more responsive to calcium channel blockers than to monotherapy with ACE inhibitors or β-blockers. This relative advantage may apply only to the use of calcium channel blockers as monotherapy. There is no difference in the efficacy of centrally acting agents in blacks and whites.

78. An 89-year-old woman comes to the office complaining of feeling short of breath when climbing the stairs for the previous 2 weeks. Her lung examination is notable for bibasilar crackles. Electrocardiography showed changes of an inferior wall myocardial infarction of indeter-

minate age, chest radiography revealed some fluid at the bases, and echocardiography showed an ejection fraction of 35%. Her creatinine level was 2.2. She is placed on a loop diuretic, and at follow-up 2 weeks later, she is asymptomatic.

In addition to a β-blocker, which of the following classes of medication should be added at this time?

(A) Calcium channel blocker
(B) Long-acting nitrate
(C) Digoxin
(D) Angiotensin-converting enzyme inhibitor
(E) Aldactone

ANSWER: D

According to a review of randomized clinical trials on use of angiotensin-converting enzyme (ACE) inhibitors in renal insufficiency, no patient should be denied a long-term trial of ACE inhibitor therapy because of preexisting renal insufficiency. Additional diuretics are not indicated for long-term use because there is no evidence of hypervolemia, and their use may worsen the renal insufficiency. Since this patient has no signs of left ventricular diastolic dysfunction, atrial fibrillation, or ischemia, there is no indication for a calcium channel blocker, digitalis, or nitrate therapy in treatment of her heart failure. Aldactone might be beneficial after maximizing the ACE therapy.

79. A 68-year-old woman residing in a long-term-care facility is evaluated because of recent onset of dizziness, difficulty with ambulation, and mental status changes. History includes epilepsy, seasonal allergies, overactive bladder, recently diagnosed depression, and osteoporosis. Medications include phenytoin 300 mg daily, alendronate 70 mg weekly, tolterodine 2 mg twice daily, fexofenadine 60 mg daily, and calcium carbonate 500 mg three times daily; 2 weeks ago she began fluoxetine 20 mg daily.

Laboratory studies from 1 month ago:
Phenytoin concentration	13.7 μg/mL
Sodium	138 mEq/L
Potassium	4.0 mEq/L
Urea nitrogen	15 mg/dL
Creatinine	1.0 mg/dL
Albumin	2.6 g/dL

Which of the following is the most appropriate next intervention?

(A) Obtain an unbound (free) phenytoin concentration.
(B) Discontinue tolterodine.
(C) Discontinue fexofenadine.
(D) Discontinue fluoxetine.

ANSWER: A

This patient's symptoms are consistent with phenytoin toxicity. Because phenytoin is highly bound to albumin, patients with reduced albumin may have a total plasma concentration within the therapeutic range and an elevated unbound concentration; the unbound concentration of phenytoin is what determines efficacy and toxicity. After adjustment for her low albumin, her phenytoin concentration 1 month ago was 18.3 μg/mL (corrected phenytoin level = observed phenytoin level/0.25 × albumin level + 0.1) or 13.7/(0.25)(2.6) + 0.1 = 18.3, which is on the high side of the therapeutic range of 10 to 20 μg/mL.

Fluoxetine, which was added 2 weeks ago, can inhibit metabolism of phenytoin by its action on the cytochrome P-450 2C9 enzyme. This can lead to increased phenytoin concentrations. Thus, her total and unbound phenytoin concentration is now likely to be higher than 18.3 μg/mL. The appropriate action would be to obtain an unbound (free) phenytoin concentration, or if it is not available, a total concentration and then to perform the adjustment for low albumin. Although fluoxetine is probably not the best antidepressant for her given its potential for interaction with phenytoin, it is premature to reduce the fluoxetine dosage until her symptoms are confirmed to be due to phenytoin toxicity. In any case, a better option for this patient would be to change to any of the other selective serotonin-reuptake inhibitors that all have less of an effect on 2C9 phenytoin metabolism.

Many medications can affect the central nervous system in frail older adults and should be suspected in a person with unexplained cognitive changes. Both tolterodine and fexofenadine have minimal effect on the central nervous system, but could cause problems for individual frail older patients. Given this patient's presentation, these agents would be low in the differential diagnosis as a cause of her symptoms.

80. A 71-year-old woman comes to the office for a routine physical examination. History includes pedal edema due to venous insufficiency, episodic insomnia due to situational anxiety, and mild acid reflux disease. She has no fatigue, poor appetite, or gastrointestinal symptoms. Medications include garlic capsules 270 mg each morning, *Ginkgo biloba* 40 mg one or two times daily, kava 150 mg one to two capsules at bedtime as needed, and valerian 1.5 g at bedtime as needed for sleep.

Physical examination is normal. Laboratory results are normal except for an alanine aminotransferase level of 210 IU/L and an aspartate aminotransferase level of 250 IU/L. Previous liver function tests were normal. The patient is advised to discontinue all supplements pending further evaluation of the transaminase abnormalities.

Of the supplements used by this patient, which one is the most likely cause of the laboratory abnormalities?

(A) Garlic
(B) *Ginkgo biloba*
(C) Kava
(D) Valerian

ANSWER: C

The Food and Drug Administration has issued a consumer advisory notice about the potential risk of hepatic toxicity associated with use of kava (also known as kava kava). Kava comes from the dried root of *Piper methysticum*. It is used for anxiety, insomnia, restlessness, and stress. Kavapyrones, the active constituents in kava, have centrally acting relaxant properties for skeletal muscle. The sale of products containing kava is restricted in several countries because of associated adverse hepatic effects. In 11 patients who developed liver failure that was associated with kava use and who underwent liver transplantation, doses (when known) ranged from 60 to 240 mg daily. Kava products may differ in the amounts and distribution of kavapyrones present. Patients with evidence of

liver disease or hepatic abnormalities and patients at risk for liver disease should avoid these herbal therapies.

Garlic, *Ginkgo biloba*, and valerian have not been associated with liver function abnormalities.

81. A 75-year-old woman comes to the office because she has a painless blurring in her right eye that has progressed over the past few months. She is more sensitive to light and complains of glare and haloes. Ten years ago she had cataract surgery with intraocular lens implantations to both eyes with good results. She was recently diagnosed with type 2 diabetes, and her eye examination did not reveal any diabetic retinopathy.

Which of the following is the most likely cause of her symptoms?

(A) Vitreous hemorrhage
(B) Macular degeneration
(C) Opacified posterior lens capsule
(D) Diabetic macular edema

ANSWER: C

At the time of cataract surgery with an intraocular lens implant, the posterior capsule of the natural lens is left in place. Over time the capsule can opacify. With the styles of intraocular lens implanted 10 years ago, up to 33% opacification can occur, causing a gradual loss of vision, glare, and, in some cases, haloes around lights. Lysing the capsule with an Nd:YAG laser resolves symptoms permanently, and often instantly.

A vitreous hemorrhage occurs acutely and causes immediate symptoms of visual loss. Macular degeneration and diabetic macular edema often cause a distortion of central vision rather than a generalized blurring. Haloes and glare are not common symptoms of either.

82. A 75-year-old woman comes to the office because she has fatigue, difficulty falling asleep, and frequent headaches. She has no history of hypertension. She is the primary caregiver for her 79-year-old husband; he has Alzheimer's disease (Mini–Mental State Examination score of 14 of 30) and has recently developed behavioral problems related to repetitive questions

and demands. On examination, the patient's blood pressure is 168/95 mm Hg.

Which of the following is the most helpful intervention for her at this time?

(A) Prescribe a calcium channel blocker.
(B) Prescribe lorazepam.
(C) Prescribe sertraline.
(D) Refer to a psychiatrist for psychotherapy.
(E) Provide counseling about community services related to dementia caregiving.

ANSWER: E

Providing direct, daily care for a spouse with dementia is stressful and affects the mental and physical health of the caregiver. The stress is compounded when the demented spouse develops behavioral problems, such as repetitive questions, demands, threats, or physical aggression. The behavioral problems are often the turning point that leads to placement in an assisted-living facility or nursing home.

This patient's symptoms are suggestive of caregiver stress. Although treatment of specific symptoms of anxiety or depression with medication or psychotherapy is reasonable, the coincidence of her symptoms with her husband's increased behavioral problems suggests that the most helpful intervention would be to reduce her burden as a caregiver. The use of community respite programs and educational groups for caregivers have both been demonstrated to reduce the sense of burden reported by caregivers and in turn may reduce the behavioral problems exhibited by the demented spouse. If her blood pressure remains elevated, consideration of treatment is indicated.

83. An 87-year-old woman with Alzheimer's disease comes to the office with her daughter for advice on managing care. She lives with her daughter, who works during the day. Over the past year she has become increasingly dependent in her instrumental activities of daily living. Four months ago, the daughter noticed that her mother was forgetting to eat the prepared lunch and neglecting to take her afternoon medications. She began to sleep more during the day and was awake and confused at night. The mother and daughter are committed to keeping

the mother at home as long as possible. They are not willing to hire caregivers at home because they find them too unreliable.

Which of the following would be most appropriate to suggest as the next step in managing the mother's care?

(A) Nursing-home placement
(B) Enrollment in adult day care
(C) Referral to home-health care
(D) Referral to respite care
(E) Assisted-living placement

ANSWER: B

This patient does not require nursing-home care at this time. She may qualify for personal home care, but other, community-based alternatives can be offered initially. Adult day health care, where available, is an excellent alternative for older adults who need monitoring and some care during the day when primary caregivers are working or need respite. The services may range from nonskilled care, including bathing and grooming, to highly skilled care, including wound care management. Often activities are geared toward clients with dementia to keep them stimulated and awake during the day, so that they are less likely to be awake during the night. The charges for adult day health care are often based on a sliding scale. Transportation may be provided by the centers.

Home-care agencies do not provide long-term intervention or nonskilled services in the home. Respite care would only provide very short-term relief and would not be in the daughter's home. Assisted living does not make sense because it removes the patient from her daughter's home.

84. A 77-year-old man comes to the office because of insomnia and nocturia. He lives alone in a continuing-care community that he joined 8 months ago. On a medical history form, he describes himself as a social drinker. Other than a recent hospitalization for pancreatitis, he has been healthy. Alcohol use is considered as a potential cause of or contributor to the pancreatitis and the sleep and urinary symptoms.

Which of the following is the most appropriate next step?

(A) Measurement of carbohydrate-deficient transferrin serum level
(B) Measurement of alanine and aspartate aminotransferase
(C) Close-ended questions about symptoms and consequences of drinking
(D) Close-ended questions about quantity and frequency of drinking
(E) Screening questionnaire with items on quantity, frequency, and effects of drinking

ANSWER: E

A screening questionnaire offers the best approach to assessing alcohol use disorders because it combines accuracy and convenience. The standardized wording is useful for this potentially sensitive topic and reduces the potential for biasing responses. The Michigan Alcoholism Screening Test—Geriatric Version (MAST–G) and the Alcohol-Related Problems Survey (ARPS) were both designed to identify problems in older persons. ARPS distinguishes between nonhazardous and hazardous or harmful drinking by correlating range of drinking with age-related physiologic changes, decreasing health and functional status, and medication use. Both the MAST–G and the ARPS are available in short and self-report forms. Other screening questionnaires, such as CAGE (Cut down, Annoyed by criticism, Guilty feelings about drinking, Eye-opener) or the Alcohol Use Disorders Identification Test (AUDIT), detect cases that meet *Diagnostic and Statistical Manual of Mental Disorders* (*DSM*) criteria for current or past alcohol dependence or abuse, but may not yield information about current drinking or problems not specifically defined by *DSM* criteria.

Close-ended questions about symptoms and consequences of drinking may yield some information relevant to current or past dependence or abuse. However, such questions fail to yield information about the quantity and frequency of drinking. Likewise, close-ended questions about quantity and frequency of alcohol use may yield information about current drinking, but not about symptoms or consequences of drinking. Depending on their wording, close-ended questions may also prompt denial of drinking.

Carbohydrate deficient transferrin is a marker for heavy, regular alcohol use. It is 60% to 75% sensitive and 70% to 80% specific for detecting daily use that exceeds 50 g of ethanol, and its sensitivity improves with increased alcohol consumption. However, the utility of the test may be limited in older people, in whom alcohol-related problems may develop at much lower levels of daily use. A disproportionate increase in aspartate compared with alanine aminotransferase, such that the ratio of aspartate to alanine exceeds 2.0, is suggestive of alcoholic hepatitis. However, the sensitivity and specificity of alanine and aspartate aminotransferases are lower for detecting other alcohol-related problems in older people.

85. An 82-year-old man comes to the office for a routine physical examination. He has a history of hypertension and atrial fibrillation. He reports episodes of dizziness and has occasional diarrhea but no melena or hematochezia. Medications include atenolol, digoxin, and warfarin. He was the primary caregiver for his wife; she died 1 year ago after a long struggle with cancer. He admits to being fatigued and to having a poor appetite, but he does not think that he is depressed. On examination, blood pressure and heart rate are well controlled; his blood pressure is 138/70 mm Hg, pulse is 60 per minute, respiratory rate is 14 per minute, and temperature is 36.7°C (98°F). He has lost 6.4 kg (14 lb; 6% of his body weight) over the past 6 months. The rest of the physical examination shows no substantial changes from the previous visit.

Which of the following is most likely to reveal the cause of this man's weight loss?

(A) Fecal occult blood testing
(B) Serum digoxin level
(C) Geriatric depression screen
(D) Home visit
(E) Chest radiography

ANSWER: B

Anorexia, fatigue, diarrhea, and dizziness are common effects of digoxin toxicity and may result in significant weight loss. Other adverse effects include bradycardia, ventricular arrhythmias, apathy, nausea, confusion, visual disturbances, and depression. There is some controversy surrounding digoxin levels, as some patients may have toxicity at laboratory-established normal levels. Higher levels correlate with more adverse reactions. Clinically, if subacute digoxin toxicity is suspected, a trial of tapering off the drug without testing may also be reasonable.

Medication review should be part of the assessment of weight loss. Fecal occult blood testing to screen for malignancy or hemorrhage is reasonable, but these diagnoses are not as likely as digoxin toxicity. The Geriatric Depression Scale may be positive, but depression should not be considered endogenous until digoxin toxicity is excluded. Depression will likely be refractory until the toxicity resolves. A home visit may determine if the patient is caring for himself and has quality nutritional resources available. However, any poor home conditions may be due to digoxin-related fatigue and apathy. There is little in this case to suggest that chest radiography will be helpful.

86. A 90-year-old resident of a skilled nursing facility has fallen three times in the past month. She has a history of dementia, hypertension, atrial fibrillation, osteoarthritis, and transient ischemic attacks. She walks with a walker. Medications include hydrochlorothiazide 25 mg daily, atenolol 50 mg daily, warfarin 2 mg daily, celecoxib 100 mg daily, calcium carbonate 600 mg twice daily, a multivitamin daily, donepezil 10 mg daily, and lorazepam 0.25 mg twice daily as needed.

Which of the following should be done first to assess her risk for future falls?

(A) Order 24-hour cardiac monitoring.
(B) Measure her blood pressure when she is lying down, sitting, and standing.
(C) Review the circumstances of her falls.
(D) Ask the physical therapist to evaluate her gait, transfers, and walker.

ANSWER: C

The first step in investigating falls by nursing-home residents is to review the circumstances of the fall. Given this patient's dementia, it is likely that she does not remember the falls. Nursing staff should be asked about times and locations of the falls, her activity at the time of the falls, whether any environmental hazards were involved, and whether the patient lost consciousness. The circumstances of the falls will direct further investigation and treatment of risk factors. For example, if the patient falls after going to bed because side rails are raised, the management would be to leave the side rails down or place the bed on the floor.

If there was loss of consciousness, the physician and staff would be directed toward a work-up of syncope, including 24-hour heart monitoring. If there was no apparent loss of consciousness, then other risk factors should be investigated.

A major risk factor for falls is taking four or more medications on a regular basis. Classes of high-risk medications include anticholinergics, antipsychotic medications, antidepressants, sedatives, narcotic pain medications, medications for anxiety, antihypertensives, and diuretics. Medications are more likely to cause problems when a new one has been added, the patient has an acute illness or change in condition, or the patient has been recently discharged from the hospital. Reviewing and, if possible, reducing the number or dosage of medications should be done regularly.

Symptomatic or asymptomatic orthostatic hypotension may occur in more than 50% of frail elderly nursing-home residents and may have contributed to this patient's falls. In evaluating her fall risk, the clinician should measure her blood pressure when she is measured lying down, sitting, and standing and should do this several times during the day to check for postural changes. A drop in systolic pressure of 20 mm Hg or more 3 minutes after standing is positive. Measurement of the patient's blood pressure would be a useful step after exploring the circumstances of her falls, which may reveal solely an environmental cause.

Decreased mobility with abnormal gait and transfers is another important risk factor for falls. Physical therapy, followed by regular supervised exercise, can help nursing-home residents improve mobility. After a fall, assistive devices (canes, walkers, wheelchairs) should be checked to make sure they are in good repair. Nonetheless, evaluation by physical therapy would not be the first action to evaluate this patient's fall risk.

87. A man inquires about whether his 80-year-old aunt can receive house calls for her medical care. She lives by herself in a second-floor apartment in a building with no elevator. She has morbid obesity, coronary artery disease, heart failure, adult-onset diabetes mellitus, hyperlipidemia, asthma, and chronic back pain. She is independent in activities of daily living, but can walk only 10 feet with a walker. She cannot negotiate steps, which constitute the only access to her apartment; she never leaves her apartment, other than when she is hospitalized. Her nephew brings her meals and assists in other instrumental activities of daily living. For health coverage, she has traditional Medicare Parts A and B and no supplemental insurance.

How would Medicare compensate for a house call to this patient?

(A) Medicare Part A would pay on a capitation basis.
(B) Medicare Part A would pay on a fee-for-service basis.
(C) Medicare Part B would pay on a capitation basis.
(D) Medicare Part B would pay on a fee-for-service basis.
(E) Medicare would not pay for physician home visits.

ANSWER: D

Medicare considers patients to be homebound if they have medical conditions that make leaving their home a "considerable and taxing effort." Homebound patients are normally unable to leave home for nonmedical reasons. Thus, this patient would be eligible for home-care coverage. Part A compensates home-care agencies for nonphysician home services on a fixed-fee basis. Part B reimburses physicians on a fee-for-service basis for home visits. A physician may also bill an additional monthly for oversight of the care plan if he or she documents spending at least 30 minutes each month on overseeing all the home care provided to the patient. Traditional Medicare is not a capitation program.

88. Which of the following structures is most susceptible to age-related histopathologic

changes that result in sensorineural hearing loss and dizziness?

(A) Inner ear
(B) Central auditory system
(C) Ossicles
(D) Tympanitic membrane
(E) External auditory canal

ANSWER: A

The inner ear contains the vestibular (balance) and auditory systems and lies in the petrous portion of the temporal bone. The neuronal and sensory cells in the balance and hearing mechanisms of the inner ear are nonmitotic; they are highly differentiated cells that cannot reproduce during adulthood. Their life span is determined by the ability to maintain structural organization within their environment. Degenerative changes occur throughout the auditory and vestibular systems of the inner ear. Age-related changes are especially prominent in the sensory receptors of the vestibular system, namely, the cristae of the semicircular canals and the maculae of the saccule and utricle. Further, there is a reduction in the hair cell population of the semicircular canals and the utricular and saccular maculae. The vasculature of the vestibular system also appears to change with age. The organ of Corti is the inner-ear structure most susceptible to age-related histopathologic changes. The basilar membrane, upon which the sensory hair cells of the inner ear lie, runs through the cochlea from its base to the apex. Degenerative changes are greatest along the basilar membrane, most notably the basal section that is responsive to high frequencies, thus contributing to the high-frequency hearing loss related to age. There is also an age-associated loss of nerve fibers and ganglion cells, which is most pronounced in the basal turn of the cochlea.

The central auditory system relays information from the cochlea and eighth nerve to the auditory cortex. The central auditory system undergoes degenerative changes, but it is responsible for auditory processing, not balance.

The middle ear consists of the tympanic membrane, the tympanic cavity (an air-filled space containing a chain of three ossicles—the malleus, incus, and stapes), and the eustachian tube. Hearing loss due to damage to middle-ear structures is conductive, not sensorineural.

The eustachian tube connects the tympanic cavity to the nasopharynx. The outer ear comprises the external auditory meatus or canal and the pinna. Excessive build-up of cerumen in the external auditory canal is common in older adults and can result in conductive, not sensorineural, hearing loss.

89. A 92-year-old woman is being treated with paroxetine for major depression following successful surgery for uncomplicated hip fracture. Her overall physical and cognitive status is otherwise good. She has mild hypertension and osteoarthritis, and she takes a thiazide diuretic and acetaminophen. Ten days after paroxetine is started, the patient's daughter calls to report that her mother is lethargic and confused.

Which of the following metabolic disturbances is the most likely cause of this patient's delirium?

(A) Hyponatremia
(B) Hypernatremia
(C) Hypoglycemia
(D) Hyperglycemia

ANSWER: A

Hyponatremia is a frequent, under-recognized, and potentially serious complication of treatment with selective serotonin-reuptake inhibitors (SSRIs) or venlafaxine in older patients. It is typically due to a transient syndrome of inappropriate antidiuretic hormone secretion (SIADH). During the first 2 weeks of treatment with an SSRI, plasma sodium concentrations decrease in almost half of older depressed patients, and 10% to 20% may become hyponatremic. Increased risk of SSRI-induced SIADH and hyponatremia is associated with older age, being female, lower baseline sodium level, lower body mass index, and concurrent use of a diuretic medication. Many affected patients are asymptomatic; symptomatic patients have nausea, anorexia, fatigue, or confusion, which can be mistaken for depressive symptoms or medication side effects. In patients at risk, it is prudent to monitor sodium before and 1 or 2 weeks after initiating treatment with an SSRI. At minimum, sodium

level should be obtained in all elderly patients who exhibit abrupt changes in mental status (such as lethargy or confusion) upon initiation of an SSRI.

Hypernatremia or an acute change in glucose level is highly unlikely to be associated with SSRI treatment.

90. An 86-year-old woman comes to the office because she has pelvic pressure, especially when moving her bowels. She has class III heart failure. On pelvic examination, she is found to have grade III uterine prolapse.

Which of the following is the most appropriate next step in her management?

(A) Refer for hysterectomy.
(B) Prescribe Kegel's exercises.
(C) Prescribe the use of a pessary.
(D) Prescribe topical estrogen.

ANSWER: C

Genital prolapse is a downward displacement of one or all pelvic organs. The most common symptoms and signs include pelvic pressure, difficulty with rectal emptying, and a palpable mass. There may also be voiding dysfunction. Grade I prolapse involves extension of the cervix to the mid-vagina; in grade II prolapse the cervix approaches the hymenal ring; in grade III prolapse the cervix is at the hymenal ring; and in grade IV prolapse the cervix is beyond the ring.

Grades I and II prolapse can be treated with topical estrogen cream and Kegel's exercises to strengthen the pelvic floor musculature. Surgery, typically with general anesthesia, can be considered for more severe prolapse. Pessaries can be used to delay or avoid surgery in patients who have comorbid medical conditions or who do not want surgery. Patients must be fitted with a pessary. There are several types, including a ring pessary for mild to moderate prolapse, a Gellhorn pessary for moderate to severe prolapse, and a cube pessary for women in whom perivaginal muscle tone cannot support other types of pessaries. The cube pessary must be removed daily to prevent infection and erosions; the other types may be left in place for weeks, because they allow for drainage of vaginal secretions. The patient should be seen within 1 week of insertion and then regularly, depending on individual circumstances and the pessary type.

Topical estrogen cream alone does not help in the management of genital prolapse. Kegel's or pelvic muscle exercises are likely to have little effect in patients with grade III prolapse. Stool softeners and laxatives have no role in management of genital prolapse.

91. A 78-year-old man comes to the office for a 6-month follow-up visit. He has a history of well-controlled stage 1 hypertension, benign prostatic hyperplasia, and osteoarthritis. His prostate and musculoskeletal symptoms are stable. Medications are lisinopril 10 mg daily, hydrochlorothiazide 25 mg daily, ibuprofen 200 mg three times daily (begun at his last visit), and saw palmetto.

On physical examination, his blood pressure is 152/78 mm Hg, and heart rate is 82 per minute with a regular rhythm. He has joint deformities in both hands consistent with osteoarthritis; there is no acute inflammation. He has 1+ bilateral lower extremity edema to the mid-shin; the edema was not evident at his last visit.

Which of the following is the best approach to management of this patient?

(A) Recommend compression stockings.
(B) Discontinue ibuprofen.
(C) Increase the hydrochlorothiazide.
(D) Begin a loop diuretic.
(E) Increase the lisinopril dosage.

ANSWER: B

Many agents can directly or indirectly increase blood pressure, including sympathomimetic agents, corticosteroids, nonsteroidal anti-inflammatory drugs (NSAIDs), selective cyclooxygenase (COX) 2 inhibitors, excessive alcohol use, and some alternative and over-the-counter drugs (decongestants and ephedra). Although secondary causes of hypertension are uncommon in older adults (more than 90% develop essential hypertension), the effect of medications on blood pressure should always be considered, even in patients who are receiving antihypertensive medications for established hypertension. There are no reported effects of saw palmetto on blood pressure, nor any interactions with antihypertensive medications.

Renal prostaglandins regulate renal hemodynamics, sodium excretion, and renin release. The blood-pressure−elevating effects of NSAIDs are well established and believed to be due to the renal effects of decreasing prostaglandin production, resulting in sodium retention and a decrease in glomerular filtration rate. Although reports are conflicting, most clinical studies have demonstrated blood-pressure increases during chronic COX-2 inhibitor therapy that are comparable to the increases observed with NSAID use. Because most antihypertensive drugs (except calcium channel antagonists) require the production of vasodilating renal prostaglandins, the blood-pressure−elevating effects of COX-2 inhibitors have been reported more commonly in patients also receiving ACE inhibitors or β-blockers.

Increasing the thiazide-type diuretic or increasing the lisinopril dosage should not be considered until the effect of discontinuing the NSAID is clear. Lower extremity edema could be managed by compression stockings or a loop diuretic, but given the likelihood that it developed as a consequence of the NSAID, discontinuing the medication is the best initial approach.

92. A 73-year-old woman comes to the office because of pain in her right shoulder for the past 6 weeks. The pain is often worse when she wakes up in the morning and with prolonged sitting and standing; lying down relieves the pain. She feels spasm and notes tenderness in her right shoulder. It bothers her particularly when she backs her car out of the driveway in the morning. She has had no weight loss, fatigue, general malaise, or other systemic symptoms.

On physical examination, there is good mobility of the right shoulder with no pain. She has moderate spasm and tenderness in the right trapezius region, asymmetric loss of movement of the cervical spine, and mild weakness of the right elbow extensor and right finger abductors.

What is the most likely cause of this patient's pain?

(A) Fibromyalgia
(B) Metastatic cancer affecting the right scapula
(C) Rotator cuff tendonitis of the right shoulder
(D) Acromioclavicular disease of the right shoulder
(E) Cervical disk disease

ANSWER: E

The trapezius area is the site of referred pain from the C-6, C-7 and C-7, C-8 cervical spine regions. Spasm of the trapezius muscle often occurs when the cervical spine is irritated. Asymmetry of motion (rotation to the right, rotation to the left, flexion, and extension) indicates mechanical displacement in the cervical spine. The elbow extensor and finger abductors are both innervated by C-7, C-8. The site of this person's pain, along with the asymmetric loss of range of motion of the cervical spine and weakness in the C-7, C-8–innervated muscle of the arm, suggests cervical disk disease.

This patient's physical findings indicate that there is a mechanical cause of her trapezius muscle spasm. Fibromyalgia refers to diffuse musculoskeletal pain without a clear mechanical or inflammatory cause. Significant fatigue occurs in 90% of patients with fibromyalgia, and sleep disturbances, lightheadedness, dizziness, and other systemic symptoms are common.

Although the scapula can be a site for metastatic cancer, a patient with cancer is likely to have gradually worsening persistent pain that is unrelated to position and movement.

A patient with rotator cuff tendonitis should have a "painful arc" on abduction of the shoulder and pain on resisted movement of the affected tendon. The completely normal physical examination of the shoulder excludes rotator cuff tendonitis. Although irritation of the acromioclavicular disease can produce pain between the shoulder and the neck, this pain should be brought on with abduction of the shoulder between 90 degrees and 160 degrees. The normal shoulder examination makes acromioclavicular disease less likely. Acromioclavicular disease does not usually cause weakness of the elbow extensor and finger abductors.

93. The effect of physical activity on bone density is most highly correlated with which of the following?

(A) Frequency of activity
(B) Duration of activity
(C) Intensity of activity
(D) Type of activity
(E) Volume of aerobic activity

ANSWER: D

The health benefits of physical activity are generally proportional to the amount of physical activity. When activity is performed above minimum thresholds for frequency, duration, and intensity, health benefit depends mainly upon the volume (energy expenditure) of aerobic activity. The dose-response relationship between physical activity and disease risk varies by disease in a manner that is incompletely understood. Cardiovascular disease risk decreases with volume of aerobic activity over a wide range of volume. Furthermore, it has been demonstrated that the beneficial effects of physical activity on health are independent of other risk factors. In particular, beneficial effects have been found to be independent of body mass index. Blood pressure shows little dose-response effect, as most of the effect of physical activity on blood pressure occurs at low levels of activity. The effect of activity on bone density is less related to volume of aerobic activity and more related to the type of activity, with resistance training and high-impact activities correlating with benefit.

94. An 84-year-old woman comes to the office accompanied by her daughter for evaluation of progressive weight loss. The patient thinks she has good nutrient intake. She denies problems sleeping, depressive symptoms, change in bowel habits, or other active medical problems. She has had no serious illness or surgery in the past 5 years. She takes a daily multivitamin but is on no other regular medicines. She has lived alone since her husband's death 7 years ago. The daughter states that her mother is less active socially than before and spends most of her time reading, knitting, or watching television. The daughter is convinced that her mother has cancer; her father also started losing weight before metastatic cancer

was diagnosed. A mammogram done 6 months ago and a screening colonoscopy done 2 years ago were normal.

The patient weighs 54.5 kg (120 lbs; body mass index 22 [kg/m^2]), 12% less than the prior year. The remainder of the physical examination is normal. Mini–Mental State Examination score is 28 of 30, and Yesavage Geriatric Depression Scale (short form) score is 2 (not depressed). Stool guaiac, urinalysis, complete blood cell count, electrolytes, and liver, renal, and thyroid function tests are normal, as is chest radiography. Electrocardiography reveals normal sinus rhythm.

Which of the following is now indicated?

(A) Computed tomographic scan of the abdomen
(B) Upper and lower endoscopy
(C) Upper gastrointestinal study with small bowel follow-through
(D) No further diagnostic testing

ANSWER: D

When older patients have involuntary weight loss, the potential causes are often readily identifiable by history and physical examination alone. When this is not the case, a more thorough diagnostic evaluation is warranted. Data suggest that the probable cause is usually identified by a focused evaluation that begins with the same basic panel of tests as this patient obtained. Additional tests are warranted only if abnormalities are identified with initial testing. If focused evaluation is unrevealing, watchful waiting is more appropriate than extensive undirected testing. In the case presented, the initial evaluation did not identify any abnormalities, so efforts to address her known risk factors for weight loss, such as social isolation and low level of physical activity, would probably provide more benefit to her than additional diagnostic testing.

95. An 86-year-old woman comes to the office because she has mid-back pain at rest and with activity that has worsened over the past few months. She has longstanding osteoporosis with previous compression fractures at T10 and L1. She reports no other symptoms. Medications include calcium, vitamin D, and risedronate. After

her last compression fracture 2 years ago, she was started on calcitonin, but it was discontinued after 1 month because of continued back pain and the development of rhinitis. Acetaminophen and over-the-counter nonsteroidal anti-inflammatory agents around the clock provided no relief. After her last visit 3 months ago, she began acetaminophen with hydrocodone (750 mg/7.5 mg), 1 tablet every 6 hours. This regimen provided better pain control initially, but she now rates her pain as 7 out of 10 on most days and states that it limits many of her activities, including bathing and dressing.

Physical examination reveals moderate kyphosis and mild tenderness to palpation over her mid-spine and the surrounding paraspinous muscles. Neurologic examination demonstrates intact lower extremity reflexes, strength, and sensation. Radiography of her thoracic and lumbar spine shows severe degenerative disc disease along with the old compression fractures at T10 and L1; no new vertebral fractures or other processes are visualized.

What is the most appropriate management strategy for this patient?

(A) Increase the acetaminophen with hydrocodone to 1 tablet every 4 hours around the clock.
(B) Switch to immediate-release oxycodone.
(C) Evaluate for kyphoplasty.
(D) Refer for physical therapy.
(E) Add cyclobenzaprine.

ANSWER: B

The World Health Organization pain management ladder recommends beginning with nonopioid analgesia for mild pain and advancing to combination (nonopioid-opioid) analgesia and then opioid therapy for control of moderate to severe pain. Acetaminophen and combination medication failed to relieve this patient's pain. The dose ceiling of the nonopioid component of the combined nonopioid-opioid agents limits their use. In this case, the acetaminophen with hydrocodone dose (750 mg/7.5 mg) cannot be increased to 1 tablet every 4 hours, as this would exceed the maximum dose of acetaminophen (4000 mg per day). Given her persistent pain and functional status limitations, opioid analgesia should be started and titrated until she is comfortable.

Kyphoplasty is a minimally invasive procedure typically performed by a spine surgeon. A needle is introduced into the vertebral body, a balloon tamp is placed to reduce the fracture, and polymethylmethacrylate, a cement-like material, is injected to fill the void. The procedure reduces pain from vertebral fractures in patients with subacute osteoporotic fractures that are less than 3 months old. This patient's vertebral fractures are too old, and because of this, she is not a candidate for this procedure.

Physical therapy is often a useful adjunct in the management of pain. Therapy might include modalities such as strengthening and stretching, heat, ultrasound, and evaluation for transcutaneous electrical nerve stimulation. This patient would likely benefit from physical therapy, but given the severity of her current symptoms, it is essential to get her pain under control first.

Patients with back pain from vertebral fractures may also have surrounding muscle spasm. This patient's symptoms suggest a degree of paraspinous muscle spasm. Although a muscle relaxant (eg, cyclobenzaprine) might provide some benefit, her primary symptoms appear to be related to her vertebral fractures, and she needs to have this pain controlled first. In addition, because muscle relaxants have significant adverse effects (drowsiness, dizziness, confusion), if they are used at all, they need to be started at a low dose and titrated as needed.

96. In a nursing facility, which of the following is the best approach to identify residents at risk for development of pressure ulcers and to monitor existing pressure ulcers?

(A) Develop risk and monitoring scales specific to that facility.
(B) Implement the Braden scale and the Pressure Ulcer Scale for Healing (PUSH).
(C) Implement the Braden and Norton scales.
(D) Implement the PUSH tool and the Pressure Sore Status Tool (PSST).

ANSWER: B

Developing and validating institution-specific scales is not practical when validated scales already exist. Risk assessment using a standardized scale should be performed on all nursing-home residents upon admission, readmission, return from hospitalization, when there is a significant change in condition, and during quarterly assessments. The two most widely used tools to assess risk are the Norton scale and the Braden scale.

The Norton scale comprises five clinical categories (physical condition, mental state, activity, mobility, and incontinence). The Braden scale comprises six clinical categories (sensory perception, moisture, activity, mobility, nutrition, and friction and shear). A score of 16 or lower on the Norton scale or 18 or lower on the Braden scale indicates increased risk for development of pressure ulcers.

The most widely used validated instruments for assessing the healing of pressure ulcers are the time-consuming Pressure Sore Status Tool (PSST) and the briefer Pressure Ulcer Scale for Healing (PUSH). The PSST is made up of 13 wound characteristics, including depth, size, undermining, type of exudates, and edema. The PUSH tool assesses size of ulcer, exudate amount, and tissue type.

97. In a patient with psychosis associated with Alzheimer's disease, pharmacotherapy is begun with an atypical antipsychotic.

Which of the following is more likely with an atypical than with a conventional antipsychotic agent?

(A) Greater likelihood of remission of psychotic symptoms
(B) Reduced rate of falls and injury
(C) Reduced incidence of tardive dyskinesia
(D) Lower incidence of somnolence
(E) Absence of QTc prolongation

ANSWER: C

Although conventional and atypical antipsychotic agents are similarly effective for the treatment of psychotic symptoms in elderly adults with dementia, their adverse effects differ. Atypical antipsychotics are the treatment of choice for psychosis in Alzheimer's disease because they have lower rates of extrapyramidal symptoms, especially tardive dyskinesia. Tardive dyskinesia is a syndrome of choreiform movements that may emerge after sustained antipsychotic therapy. It is often disfiguring and, in elderly adults, can affect dentition, swallowing, and respiration. Tardive dyskinesia is much more common in elderly than in younger patients treated with antipsychotics. With conventional antipsychotics (eg, haloperidol), the 1-year incidence of tardive dyskinesia is over 30% in older patients and around 5% in younger patients. With atypical antipsychotics, the 1-year incidence of tardive dyskinesia in older patients decreases to less than 5%.

Both conventional and atypical antipsychotic agents are associated with sedation and, less commonly, falls and injury in older patients with dementia. All antipsychotic agents may prolong the QTc interval, although the clinical impact of this is unclear.

98. A 67-year-old woman with recently diagnosed metastatic ovarian cancer comes to the office for a follow-up visit. She has new symptoms of nausea and vomiting. Several months ago, the patient underwent debulking surgery and chemotherapy, but there was extensive carcinomatosis on follow-up imaging 3 months later, and her CA-125 level has remained high. At her last appointment, she acknowledged that her cancer will not be cured and stated that she is reluctant to undergo further invasive procedures or to be rehospitalized. Her current nausea and vomiting started 2 days ago. She has been unable to tolerate any oral intake and has not had a bowel movement in 4 days. Her only medications are acetaminophen with codeine as needed and docusate sodium stool softener every morning.

On examination, the patient appears thin and uncomfortable. She is afebrile. Blood pressure is 98/60 mm Hg, and pulse is 105 per minute. Cardiopulmonary examination is unremarkable aside from tachycardia. The abdomen is markedly distended with decreased bowel sounds, tympany on percussion, and diffuse tenderness on palpation. Rectal examination is normal, with no stool in the vault.

In addition to providing the patient with morphine, which of the following is the most appropriate management strategy for this patient?

(A) Diverting colostomy
(B) Nasogastric suctioning
(C) Octreotide
(D) Atropine
(E) Ondansetron

ANSWER: C

This patient has classic signs and symptoms of intestinal obstruction. Cancer patients may develop a bowel obstruction for various reasons, including intraluminal obstruction (eg, by tumor mass), direct infiltration of the bowel wall (eg, colon carcinoma), external compression of the lumen, carcinomatosis causing dysmotility (eg, ovarian cancer), and intra-abdominal adhesions (eg, from postoperative changes). Symptoms of obstruction are generally due to the normal physiologic processes of the intestine (peristalsis and secretion of fluid, electrolytes, and enzymes) plus the inflammatory process caused by the obstruction.

Bowel obstruction in patients with advanced cancer can be managed with conservative therapy. This patient does not wish to undergo further procedures or hospitalization, and her request should be honored. Thus, surgery is not an option, and placement of a nasogastric tube, which may be uncomfortable, should be avoided. Opioids such as morphine and antiemetics such as prochlorperazine relieve pain and nausea, respectively. Ondansetron, a selective serotonins 5-HT(3)-type receptor antagonist, will also relieve nausea and vomiting, but other, less expensive antiemetics should be tried first. Antisecretory agents such as antimuscarinic anticholinergic drugs (eg, scopolamine or atropine) and somatostatin analogs (eg, octreotide) are effective in the management of intestinal obstruction. Octreotide has fewer adverse effects than antimuscarinic agents and has been shown to have superior improvement in symptoms. It can be administered subcutaneously or intravenously with minimal adverse effects.

The care plan for this patient with metastatic ovarian cancer has shifted from a focus on cure to comfort. She is an ideal candidate for home hospice and its multidisciplinary approach to terminal illness. Home hospice nurses can manage an octreotide pump, and the Medicare hospice benefit would cover this treatment.

99. An 84-year-old woman living in a retirement home has over the past week become increasingly agitated, especially at night. She climbs out of bed, and on at least one occasion she fell, sustaining a bruise on her hip. She has a 2-year history of cognitive decline consistent with Alzheimer's disease. She has type 2 diabetes mellitus treated with glyburide and chronic obstructive pulmonary disease treated with a salmeterol inhaler. Staff at her retirement home report that she has been a poor sleeper since she was admitted 18 months earlier, but she is otherwise cooperative and cheerful. On examination, she appears fearful and complains of criminals coming into her room at night to attack her.

Which of the following is the best initial management strategy?

(A) Use of side rails on her bed at night
(B) Music therapy in the evening
(C) Physical examination and routine laboratory testing
(D) Treatment of hip pain with acetaminophen
(E) Use of bright-light therapy to improve sleep

ANSWER: C

This patient's 1-week history of agitation and psychosis is suggestive of delirium. In older adults with dementia, recent behavioral changes should precipitate review of their medical status and medications to exclude potential causes of an intercurrent delirium. Many common causes can be ruled out with physical examination, routine blood work, urinalysis, chest radiograph if indicated, and review of recent medication changes.

   Use of side rails or any type of physical restraint may increase her risk of harm, leading to entrapment or death. Music therapy is a nonpharmacologic intervention that has been studied in randomized controlled trials. If physical examination and other investigations exclude delirium, this type of intervention could be considered for reducing agitation. Treatment of pain with non-narcotic analgesic medication is an important aspect of management and may contribute to a decrease in agitation. For this

patient, however, the behavioral change clearly preceded the fall. The use of bright lights has been shown to improve sleep-wake cycle disturbances in some studies but not consistently. It is unlikely to be helpful for this patient who also demonstrates psychotic behaviors.

100. A 79-year-old woman comes to the office because of pain, swelling, stiffness, and mild erythema of her right forefoot. She is healthy and takes no medications other than vitamins and calcium. The patient recalls an injury 4 months earlier, in which a package of frozen chicken fell on the foot from a top-loading freezer compartment of her refrigerator. She recalls that the foot swelled immediately and became discolored and painful. At the local hospital emergency department, radiographs of her right foot showed no evidence of fracture. She was advised to take anti-inflammatory medications, apply ice to the area, and rest and elevate the foot. Although the discoloration from the original injury subsided, the swelling has persisted and the pain is now excruciating.

On physical examination, there is exquisite pain on palpation of the right forefoot. The skin over the metatarsal area is warm, erythematous, and dry. The toes are cool to touch, with mild cyanosis over the dorsum. Neurologic findings are normal. Pedal pulses are palpable. Repeat radiographs reveal periarticular soft-tissue swelling and patchy osteoporosis involving the metatarsals and metatarsal phalangeal articulations. Serologic tests for antinuclear antibody and rheumatoid factor are negative, and electromyography and nerve conduction velocity studies are normal.

Which of the following is the most likely diagnosis?

(A) Tarsal tunnel syndrome
(B) Raynaud's phenomenon
(C) Rheumatoid arthritis
(D) Reflex sympathetic dystrophy
(E) Stress fracture

ANSWER: D

The most common cause of reflex sympathetic dystrophy is trauma resulting from fractures, dislocations, sprains, amputations, crush injuries, or even minor cuts of the toes or feet.

Other causes include surgery, diabetes mellitus, hemiparesis, venipuncture, infections, and neoplasms. The signs and symptoms of reflex sympathetic dystrophy—pain, swelling, stiffness, and skin discoloration—are usually sufficient for diagnosis. Three-phase bone scan demonstrates diffuse uptake in the blood flow, pool, and delayed phases, and can confirm the diagnosis. Radiographs show patchy osteoporosis, which may progress to a ground-glass appearance. Diagnostic criteria are pain and tenderness in the extremity, soft-tissue swelling, decreased motor function, trophic skin changes, vasomotor instability, and patchy osteoporosis.

Tarsal tunnel syndrome is a compression syndrome of the posterior tibial nerve. Percussion of the posterior tibial nerve may produce a positive Tinel's sign that radiates to the top of the forefoot. There usually is decreased sensation. Raynaud's phenomenon is characterized by episodic pallor of the digits with paresthesia, followed by cyanosis, and finally rubor, warmth, and a throbbing sensation (white-blue-red skin changes). With osteoporosis, radiographs show trabecular bone resorption and intracortical tunneling. With stress fractures, radiographs may initially be normal, but the fracture site should be visible 4 to 6 weeks after injury. Rheumatoid arthritis can affect the joints of the foot, with erythema, joint swelling, and pain or passive and active range of motion. However, there would be no cyanosis on examination, and the radiographs would show changes characteristic of rheumatoid arthritis, not osteoporosis.

INDEX

Page references followed by *t* and *f* indicate tables and figures, respectively. Those numbers preceded by "q" indicate the question number (not the page number) and critiques.

swallowing and, 168–169
theories of, 8t, 9–10
traits of, 8
Agitated delirium, 226, 228t, q99
Agitation
in dementia, 213–214, 219–220, 260
in depression, 261t
in hospitalized patients, q12
in mental retardation, q18
treatment strategies for, 261t, q19
Agoraphobia, 261t
AHRQ. *See* Agency for Healthcare Research and Quality
AICDS. *See* Automatic implantable cardioverter-defibrillators
AIDS (acquired immunodeficiency syndrome), 313
AIDS wasting syndrome, q75
Albumin, 163–164, 306
Albuterol (Proventil, Ventolin), 302t
Albuterol-ipratropium (Combivent), 302t
Alcohol, q54
benefits of, 277
and blood-pressure control, q39
nutrient interactions, 164t
warfarin interactions, 453
Alcohol abuse, 231
Alcohol dependency, 231, 275
Alcohol-related dementia, 277
Alcohol-Related Problems Survey (ARPS), q84
Alcohol Use Disorders Identification Test (AUDIT), 278, q84
Alcoholics Anonymous, 279, q54
Alcoholics Victorious, 279
Alcoholism, 275, 276
in Alzheimer's disease, 277
at-risk drinking, 277
and continence, 171–172, 172t, 173t
and delirium, 227t
heavy drinking, 276
low-risk or moderate use, 275
and mental health problems, 277
and physical disability, 277
screening for, 61, 61t
and sleep apnea, 232
social drinking, q84
Aldosterone antagonists, 324–325
Aldosteronism, primary, 345–346, 345t
Alendronate, 199–200, 200t
ALFs. *See* Assisted-living facilities
Alfuzosin, 390, 390t
Alginate, 244t
Alkaline phosphatase, 344, 361
Alkalosis, 368
Allergic conjunctivitis, 144
Allopurinol, 299t, 399
Allostasis, 8
Allostatic load, 8
α-Adrenergic agonists
adverse effects of, 143t
and continence, 172t
for glaucoma, 143, 143t

α-Blockers
for benign prostatic hyperplasia, 390, 390t, q74
and continence, 172t
for hypertension, 335
α-Interferon, 446–447
Alprazolam, 71, 227t, 402
Alprostadil, 386, 387t, 388, q49
ALS. *See* Amyotrophic lateral sclerosis
Alteplase, 425
Altered mental status, 220. *See also* Delirium
Alternative medicine, 74–79
Alzheimer's Association, 210
Alzheimer's disease, 204, q83. *See also* Dementia
deaths due to, 5–6, 6t
gait findings in, 183, 184t
genetic testing and, 27
progression of, 207, 208t
protective factors for, 205, 205t
psychosis associated with, q97
risk factors for, 205, 205t
Alzheimer's type dementia, q70
behavioral disturbances in, 215
complementary and alternative medicine for, 77
depression in, 216
diagnostic features of, 206t
differential diagnosis of, 207
mild, q19
pharmacologic treatment of, 211
Amantadine, 227t, 428–429
Amaryl (glimepiride), 355t
Ambulatory electrocardiography monitoring, 159
Ambulatory loop recorders, 159
American Academy of Family Physicians, 88
American Academy of Family Practitioners, 164–165
American Academy of Neurology, 53t
American Academy of Ophthalmology, 140
American Academy of Orthopaedic Surgeons, 53t
American Cancer Society, 392
American College of Cardiology
ACC/AHA Class I indications for early invasive treatment of unstable angina or non-Q-wave myocardial infarction, 319, 319t
ACC/AHA class I indications for permanent pacemaker implantation, 328, 329t
ACC/AHA guideline for perioperative cardiovascular evaluation for noncardiac surgery, 93
ACC/AHA guidelines for coronary revascularization, 319, 319t
ACC/AHA indications for AICDs, 327t
American College of Obstetrics and Gynecology, 376
American College of Physicians, 88, 392
American College of Rheumatology, 401, 402f

American College of Sports Medicine, 53t, 54, 57
American Diabetes Association, 53t
American Dietetic Association, 164–165
American Geriatrics Society (AGS)
activity recommendations, 53t
assisted-living facilities position statement, 456–457
guidelines for improving diabetes care, 351
guidelines for research using cognitively impaired persons as subjects, 24, 24t
recommendations for prevention of falls, 459–460
Website, 465
American Heart Association
ACC/AHA Class I indications for early invasive treatment of unstable angina or non-Q-wave myocardial infarction, 319, 319t
ACC/AHA class I indications for permanent pacemaker implantation, 328, 329t
ACC/AHA guideline for perioperative cardiovascular evaluation for noncardiac surgery, 93
ACC/AHA guidelines for coronary revascularization, 319, 319t
ACC/AHA indications for AICDs, 327t
activity recommendations, 53t
guidelines for prophylactic antibiotics to prevent bacterial endocarditis, 326
recommendations for endocarditis prophylaxis, 312
Web site, 94
American Indians, 17
American Medical Association (AMA), 45, 83, 84
American Medical Directors Association, 116
American Society of Anesthesiologists (ASA), 93, 93t
American Urogynecologic Association, 380, 380t
American Urological Association, 389, 392
Amiloride, 299t
Aminoglutethimide, 446, 447t
Amiodarone, 328, 453
Amitriptyline, 138, 227t, 299t
AML. *See* Acute myeloid leukemia
Amoxicillin, 67. *See also* Antibiotics
Amphetamine, 299t
Amphotericin B, 299t
Ampicillin, 67, 299t
Amputation, 109–110
assessment for, 110
epidemiology, 109–110
rehabilitation for, 110
Amyloidosis, 371
Amyotrophic lateral sclerosis (ALS), 432
Anagrelide, 441
Anakinra, 407
Analgesia. *See also* Pain management; Palliative care
for back pain, 414
narcotic, 172t

prevalence of, 4, 4f
pseudogout, 400
rheumatoid, 399, 406, 406t, 421–422
Arthroplasty, total hip and knee, 109
Artificial sphincters, 179t, 180
Ascites, 72
Asian Americans
    cancer incidence and mortality in, 444, 444t
    complementary and alternative medicine use by, 75
Asmanex (mometasone), 302t
Aspiration, 169
Aspiration pneumonia, 104, 167, 169
Aspirin therapy
    for angina pectoris and non-Q-wave MI, 318
    for atrial fibrillation, q68
    for MI, stroke, and vascular death, 318
    perioperative, 94
    for peripheral vascular disease, 330
    preventive, 61t, 62, 64t, 65, 424
    underprescribing, 70
    warfarin interactions, 453
Assessing Care of Vulnerable Elders (ACOVE) project, 70
Assessment, 41–46. See also Screening
    at admission to hospital, 85, 86t
    "brown-bag" evaluation, 72
    cognitive, 44
    comprehensive geriatric assessment (CGA), 45–46, 106
    in elder mistreatment, 81–82
    of falls risk, 189, 190t
    financial, 82
    functional, 185
    genetic testing, 27
    home care, 119–121
    of hospitalized patients, 84–89
    medications review, 86t
    nutrition, 43, 163–165
    of older drivers, 45
    Outcome and Assessment Information Set (OASIS), 103, 119
    physical, 42–44, 81–82, 86t
    preoperative, 93–97
    psychologic, 44, 82
    rapid screening followed by, 41, 42t
    routine office visits, 41
    sleep evaluation, 230
    social, 44
Assisted-living facilities (ALFs), 3, 124, 456–457, q8, q47
    agencies and organizations, 467
    prevention of falls in, 459
Assistive devices, 110–111
    hearing aids, 148–150, 149–150, 149t
    listening devices, 148, 149t, 150, q13
    low-vision aids, 145
    for preventing falls, 193t, 460
Asthma, 301
Asthmatic COPD, 303
Astigmatism, 140
Astroglide, 383
At-risk drinking, 277

At-risk use, 275
Atenolol, 319
Atherosclerosis
    diabetes mellitus complications, 351–352
    prevention of, 64t
Atherosclerotic vascular disease, 329
Atorvastatin, 322t
Atrial fibrillation, 327–328
    discharge medications for, q68
    in hospitalized patients, 85t, 88
    indications for anticoagulation in, 453t
    paroxysmal, 328
    postoperative, 97
Atrovent (ipratropium), 302t
Attention screening examination, 222t
Attitudes regarding disclosure and consent, 50
Attitudes toward North American health services, 49
Audiometry, 154
AudioScope, 43
AUDIT. See Alcohol Use Disorders Identification Test
Auditory system changes, 146
Autoimmune thrombocytopenia, 440
Autolytic debridement, 243, 243t
Automatic implantable cardioverter-defibrillators (AICDs), 327, 327t
Autonomy, 20, 26
Avandamet (rosiglitazone and metformin), 356t
Avandaryl (rosiglitazone and glimepiride), 356t
Avandia (rosiglitazone), 355t
Aventyl, 135t, 253t. See also Nortriptyline
Avoidant personality disorder features of, 267, 268t therapeutic strategies for, 270, 271t
Axillary lymphadenectomy, 448
Azathioprine, 408, 409
Azmacort, 302t. See also Triamcinolone

B

Back examination, 412–413, 413t
Back pain, 410
    assessment of, 412–414, 413t
    causes of, 410–411, 410t, 411–412
    management of, 414, q95
Baclofen (Lioresal), 135t, 299t, 430
Bacteremia, 307–308
Bacterial endocarditis, 326
Bacteriuria, 180, 310
Baker cyst, 404–405
Balance testing, 43
Balance training, 192
    osteoporosis, falls, fractures and, 56–57
    for preventing falls, 193t
    recommended amounts, 54–55
Balanced Budget Act of 1997 (BBA 97), 38–39, 102–103, 113
Balanced Budget Revision Act of 1999, 39

Barbiturates, 227t, 453
BARD1, 12
Basal cell carcinoma, 292–293, 293f
bcl-2, 13
Beclomethasone (Beclovent, Vanceril, QVAR), 299t, 302t
Bedsores, 239. See also Pressure ulcers
Befuddlement, 220
Behavior(s)
    adaptive behavioral difficulties, 281
    anxious or fearful, 267, 268t
    in dementia, 213–220
    dramatic, emotional, or erratic, 267, 268t
    healthy, 19–20
    maladaptive, 282–283
    odd or eccentric, 267, 268t
    pain, in cognitively impaired persons, 133, 134t
Behavioral disorders. See also Personality disorders
    in dementia, 212, 216, 217t
    in dementia with manic features, 216–217, 217t
    manic-like syndromes in dementia, 216–217
    in mental retardation, 282
    REM sleep behavior disorder, 233
Behavioral treatments
    for aggression or agitation in dementia, 220
    for anxiety disorders, 262
    for dementia care, 215–216, 215t
    for depression, 250t
    for incontinence, 175t, 176–177, 177t, 178t, 461–462
    for insomnia, 219, 219t
    for preventing falls, 460
Bell's palsy, 314
Beneficence, 20, 21, 22–23, 23t, q6
Benign growths, 291–292
Benign positional vertigo, 152
    Epley's maneuver for, 155, 155f
    management of, 155
Benign prostatic hyperplasia, 389–391, q16
    complementary and alternative medicine for, 78
    International Prostate Symptom Score (IPSS), 389
    management options, 390, 390t, q74
Bentyl, 172t
Benzodiazepines
    for anxiety disorders, 261, 261t
    chronic use of, 236–238
    and delirium, 227t
    drug interactions, 71t
    for dyspnea, 130
    for insomnia, 236, 237t
    for mania and manic-like symptoms, 256t
    pharmacodynamics, 69
    for substance abuse, 280
Benztropine, 227t
Bereavement, 231, 249
Bereavement therapy, 250t
Best-interest standard, 22–23
β-Agonists, 301, 302t

Calcium pyrophosphate dihydrate (CPPD) crystals, 400
California Healthcare Foundation, 351
Caloric restriction, 13–14, q36
  theory of aging, 8t, 10
CAM. See Complementary and alternative medicine; Confusion Assessment Method
Canadian Task Force, 64
Canadian Task Force on the Periodic Health Examination, 392
Cancer
  basal cell carcinoma, 292–293, 293f
  biology of, 443–444
  bladder, 65t, 444, 444t
  breast, 61t, 62, 443, 444, 444t, 446, 447t, 448–449
  cervical, 61t, 62
  characteristics of, 443–444
  colon, 64t, 79, 366–367, 444, 444t, 449
  colorectal, 61t, 62, 366
  complementary and alternative medicine for, 78–79
  endometrial, 444, 444t, 446, 447t
  esophageal, 360
  head and neck, 444, 444t
  incidence of, 444
  lung, 65t, 79, 444, 444t, 449
  metastatic breast, 449
  metastatic ovarian, q98
  mortality with, 444
  oral, 61t, 297–298
  ovarian, 65t, q98
  pancreatic, 65t
  prevalence of, 4, 4f, 442, 443
  prevention of, 64t
  principles of management of, 444–448, 450–451
  prostate, 64t, 78–79, 391–395, 393t, 394t, 444, 444t, 446, 447t, q30
  quality-of-life issues, 448
  recommendations for prevention of, 61t
  renal, 447
  resources, 471
  screening for, 445
  skin, 64, 64t, 476
  squamous cell carcinoma, 292, 297–298
  thyroid, 340–341
  vulvar, 379
Candida, 309–310
Candida albicans, 420
Candida parapsilosis, 420
Candidiasis, 290
  chronic mucocutaneous, 420
  oral, 298
Canes, 110
Capacity to Consent to Treatment Instrument, 22
Capitation structures, 28
Capsaicin cream, 76
Captopril, 299t
Carbamazepine (Tegretol, Epitol)
  for behavioral disturbances in dementia with manic features, 216–217, 217t
  for bipolar disorder, 255–256
  drug interactions, 72

for epilepsy, 431–432, 432t
for mania and manic-like symptoms, 256t
for persistent pain, 135t, 138
warfarin interactions, 453
Carbidopa, 427. See also Levodopa-carbidopa
Carbonic anhydrase inhibitors, 143t
Cardiac arrhythmias, 159t, 161, 328
Cardiac asthma, 301
Cardiac care, preoperative, 93–94, 95f
Cardiac disorders. See specific disorders
Cardiac pacing, 192
Cardiobacterium, 312
Cardiomyopathy, 453t
Cardiovascular diseases and disorders, 316–331. See also specific disorders
  activity recommendations for, 53t
  complementary and alternative medicine for, 76–77
  and continence, 171–172, 173t
  postoperative problems, 97
  preventing and managing risk factors, 351–352, 352t
Cardiovascular system
  ACC/AHA guideline for perioperative cardiovascular evaluation for noncardiac surgery, 93
  age-related changes in, 316t
  preoperative assessment and management, 93–94
Caregiver stress, q82
Caregivers, 209–210, q42
  dementia caregiver counseling, 250t
  home care support, 121
Caregiving, 16, 80, 80t
Caries, 294–295
Carotid endarterectomy, 424
Carotid sinus hypersensitivity, 161
Carotid stenosis, 424
Carpal tunnel syndrome, 403–404
Cataract, 140–141
Cataract surgery, q4, q81
Catheters, 180–181
CCAs. See Calcium channel blockers
CCRCs. See Continuing-care retirement communities
Ceftriaxone, 67
Celecoxib, 406–407, q31
Celexa, 252t. See also Citalopram
Cell death, 13
Cellular changes, 10
Cellular defense mechanisms, 12–13
Cellulitis, 242t
Centers for Medicare & Medicaid Services (CMS), 30, 38, 104, 113, 238
  average adjusted per capita cost for FFS medicare beneficiaries, 38
  capitation payments, 38–39
  demonstration projects, 39
  medication quality indicators, 70
Central auditory system, q88
Cephulac (lactulose), 99t
Cerebellar ataxia, 183, 184t
Cerebral insufficiency, 211

Cerebrovascular diseases, 423–425
  and continence, 171–172, 173t
  deaths due to, 5–6, 6t
  gait findings in, 183, 184t
Cervical cancer screening, 61t, 62
Cervical disk disease, q92
Cervical spine disease, 414–415
CGA. See Comprehensive geriatric assessment
Chamomile, 77
Charles Bonnet syndrome, 266
Checklist of Nonverbal Pain Indicators, 133
Chemical pneumonitis, 169
Chemoprophylaxis
  potential beneficial services lacking evidence, 64, 64t
  recommended services, 61t, 65
  services that have been demonstrated not to be beneficial, 65, 65t
Chemoreceptor trigger zone, 137–138
Chemosensory perception, 299
Chemotherapy, 445–446, 446t
Cherry angiomas, 291–292
Chiropractic manipulation, 75
Chlamydia pneumoniae, 309f
Chlamydia trachomatis, 395
Chloral hydrate, 227t, 453
Chlordiazepoxide, 227t
Chlorpheniramine, 299t
Cholesterol, 164
  activity recommendations for, 53t
  high-density lipoprotein (HDL), 353
  low-density lipoprotein (LDL), 317, 321, 353
Cholestyramine, 453
Choline, 163t
Choline magnesium trisalicylate (Tricosal, Trilisate), 135t
Cholinesterase inhibitors, 210–211, 212
Chondrocalcinosis, 400
Chondroitin, 76, 398
Chorea, 430
Choroidal neovascularization, 141, 141f
Chromium, 78
Chromosomal alterations theory of aging, 8t, 9
Chromosome 5, 439
Chronic conditions
  Medicare beneficiaries with chronic conditions and self-reporting fair or poor health, 4, 4f
  prevalence of, 4, 4f
Chronic cough, 301
Chronic hypnotic use, 236–238
Chronic kidney disease, 368, 370
  early referral to nephrologist and pre-ESRD care for, 375
  symptoms of, 369
Chronic kidney failure, 374–376
Chronic lower respiratory disease, 5–6, 6t
Chronic lymphocytic leukemia, 450
Chronic mucocutaneous candidiasis, 420
Chronic myeloproliferative disorders, 441–442

Counseling, 62–63, q82
  dementia caregiver counseling, 250t
  recommended services, 61t
COX-2 inhibitors, q91
  contraindications to, 138–139
  for osteoarthritis, 398
  for pain, 134
  for rheumatoid arthritis, 406–407
CPP32, 13
CPPD (calcium pyrophosphate dihydrate)
    crystals, 400
Creatinine, serum, 369
Creatinine clearance (CrCl), 68, 369, 370
Crescentic glomerulonephritis, 371, 373
Cromolyn (Intal), 302t
Cross-cultural health care, 47
Crutches, 110
Cruzan v. Director, Department of Health of
    Missouri, 24, 25
Cultural aspects, 46–51
Cultural competence, 51
Cultural identity, 47
Culture-specific health risks, 49
Current Procedural Terminology, 28
Cushing's disease, 197t, 345
Cutaneous horns, 292
Cyanocobalamin, 67
Cyclobenzaprine, 402
Cyclophosphamide, 446t
Cyclosporine
  and osteoporosis, 197t
  for psoriasis, 289
  for rheumatoid arthritis, 407
  warfarin interactions, 453
Cymbalta, 254t. See also Duloxetine
Cyproheptadine, 166
Cystatin C, 369
Cysteine proteases, 13
Cystic erosion, 417t
Cystometry, 176
Cytochrome P-450 2D6, 72
Cytochrome P-450 3A4, 71–72

D

daf-2, 13
Daily metabolic requirements, 89
Dalteparin (Fragmin), 318–319, 454t
Danaparoid (Organan), 454t
Dapsone, 408
Darifenacin, 177–178, 177t
Darvon (propoxyphene), 138
Day care, adult, 122
Day hospitals, 122
Daytime napping, q19
Daytime sleepiness, excessive, 230–231, q11
DDIs. See Drug-drug interactions
Death
  ability to predict time of, 25
  causes of, 5–6, 6t
  interventions that may hasten, 25
  Oregon Death with Dignity Act, 25
Debridement, 243, 243t

Decision making
  about institutionalization, 122
  approaches to, 49–50
  end-of-life, 24–26, 50
  medical decisions, 21, 22t
  for patients who lack decisional capacity,
    22–23, 23t, q6
  role of incapacitated patient in, 23
Decisional capacity, 21–24, 22t
  assessment of, 21
  decision making for patients who lack,
    22–23, 23t, q6
  standardized tests of, 22
  temporary loss of, 23–24
Decubitus ulcers, 239. See also Pressure ulcers
Deep-vein thrombosis, 330
  anticoagulants for, 454t–455t
  methods to reduce impact on
    rehabilitation, 105t
Defecography, 362
Dehydroepiandrosterone (DHEA), 75, 346
Delirium, 220–229, q89
  agitated, 226, 228t, q99
  and continence, 171–172, 173t
  diagnosis of, 221–222, 221t, q32
  differential diagnosis of, 209, 221–222
  Hospital Elder Life Program (HELP), 91
  in hospitalized patients, 87, 91, q12, q32
  management of, 225t, 226–227, 227t
  palliation of, 129
  postoperative, 96, 98–99, 224
  prevention of, 91, 227–229
  psychotic symptoms in, 265
  and rehabilitation, 104–105
  reversible causes of, 223–224, 224t
Delirium Index, 223
Delirium Rating Scale, 223
Deltasone, 135t. See also Prednisone
Delusions, 263
  in dementia, 213, 218–219, 218t, 265
  in depression, 265
  evaluation of, 263, 263f
  mood congruent, 265
Dementia, 204–212. See also Alzheimer's
    disease
  activity recommendations for, 53t
  aggression in, 219–220
  agitation in, 213–214, 219–220, 260
  alcohol-related, 277
  Alzheimer's type, 77, 206t, 207, 211, 215,
    216, q19, q70
  antipsychotic agents for, 218, 218t
  anxiety in, 260
  assessment of, 205–206
  behavioral disturbances in, 215, 216, 217t
  behavioral disturbances with manic features
    in, 216–217, 217t
  behavioral interventions for, 215–216,
    215t
  community services related to caregiving
    for, q82
  complementary and alternative medicine
    for, 77
  and continence, 171–172, 173t
  delusions in, 213, 218–219, 218t
  depression in, 216

depressive features of behavioral
    disturbances in, 216, 217t
  diagnostic features of, 206t
  differential diagnosis of, 206–209
  drug interactions, 72
  end-stage, q75
  ethical issues in, 26–27
  and falls, q65
  frontotemporal, 206t, 207
  hallucinations in, 213, 218–219, 218t,
    266–267
  hypersexuality in, 219
  with Lewy bodies, 206t, 207, 215,
    266–267
  manic-like behavioral syndromes in,
    216–217
  with mental retardation, 281, 282–283
  mood disturbances in, 216
  mood stabilizers for, 216–217, 217t
  progression of, 207, 208t
  psychosis in, 213, 218–219, 218t
  and rehabilitation, 105
  reversible, 220
  screening for, 44, 64, 64t
  sleep disturbances in, 219, 233
  vascular, 206, 206t, 207
Dementia caregiver counseling, 250t
Demerol, 138. See also Meperidine
Demographics, 1–7
  nursing-home population, 113
Dental anatomy, 295f
Dental care counseling, 61t, 63
Dental caries, 294–295
Dental pulp changes, 294, 295t
Dentures, 296–297
Depakote, 256t. See also Divalproex sodium
Dependency
  drug and alcohol, 231 (See also Substance
    abuse)
  opioid, 137
Dependent personality disorder
  features of, 267, 268t
  therapeutic strategies for, 270, 271t
Depression, 247–258
  activity recommendations for, 53t
  agitation in, 261t
  in Alzheimer's dementia, 216
  complementary and alternative medicine
    for, 77
  in dementia, 216
  diagnostic criteria for, 248, 248t
  differential diagnosis of, 209, 248–249
  Duke Somatic Algorithm for Geriatric
    Depression, 251
  Geriatric Depression Scale (short form),
    458
  geriatric syndrome of late-life depression,
    247–248, 250, 250t
  guidelines for treatment of, q55
  in hospitalized patients, 85t, 87
  interventions for, 85t
  major, q33, q55
  mixed with anxiety, 260, 261t
  palliation of, 129–130
  prevalence of, q14
  psychotherapy for, 250, 250t

Doxepin, 227t, 299t
DPP-4 inhibitors, 356t
Dressings, 243, 244–246, 244t
    occlusive, q71
DRGs. *See* Diagnostic related groups
Drinking. *See also* Alcoholism
    at-risk, 277, q54
    heavy, 276
    social, q84
Drinking Problems Index, 278
Driving, 28, 45
Dronabinol, 129, 166
Droperidol, 128–129, 128t
Drug dependency, 231. *See also* Substance
    abuse opioid, 137
Drug-disease interactions, 72
Drug-drug interactions (DDIs), 71–72, 71t
Drug eruptions, q35
Drug-induced esophageal injury, 359–360
Drug-induced movement disorders, 430
Drug-nutrient interactions, 164, 164t
Drug use, 275, 276
Drugs. *See also* Pharmacotherapy; *specific*
        drugs
    absorption of, 67
    adverse drug events (ADEs), 69, 70–71,
        70t, 72, 360, 361t
    adverse drug reactions (ADRs), 70
    bioavailability of, 67
    clearance of, 68
    distribution of, 67–68
    elimination of, 68–69
    half-life of, 68
    herbal preparations, 76
    hydrophilic, 67–68
    inhaled medications, 301, 302t
    lipophilic, 67–68
    medications associated with incontinence,
        171–172, 172t
    medications to avoid, 138–139
    metabolism of, 68
    to reduce or eliminate in management of
        delirium, 227t
    that interfere with gustation (taste) and
        olfaction (smell), 299t
    toxicity, 152
Dry-eye syndrome, 144
Dry mouth, 129, 297
Dry skin, q35
DSM-IV. See Diagnostic and Statistical
    Manual of Mental Disorders
Dual-energy radiographic absorptiometry
    (DXA), 197–198
Duke Somatic Algorithm for Geriatric
    Depression, 251
Dulcolax (bisacodyl), 99t
Duloxetine (Cymbalta), 254t
    for depression, 253
    for depressive features of behavioral
        disturbances in dementia, 216, 217t
    for persistent pain, 138
    for stress and mixed urge and stress
        incontinence, 178t, 179
Duragesic (fentanyl), 136t

Dutasteride, 390–391, 390t
Dysergastic reaction, 220
Dyslipidemia, 321
    complementary and alternative medicine
        for, 76–77
    drug regimens for, 322t
    screening for, 61, 61t
    treatment indications for, 321t
Dyspareunia, 382, 383, q73
Dyspepsia, 360
Dysphagia, 168–169, 357–358, q37, q62
    oropharyngeal, 168, 169, 357–358
    secondary to stroke, 169
Dyspnea, 130–131, 300–301
Dystonia, drug-induced, 430
Dystrophy
    onychodystrophy, 418f
    reflex sympathetic, q100
    vulvar, 379

E

Eating and feeding problems, 167–171, q62
Eccentric behaviors, 267, 268t
Echocardiography, 318
    stress echocardiography, 318
    in syncope, 160
    transthoracic, 312
Eczema craquelé, 285–286, 286t
Edentulism, 61t, 296–297
Education, 2
    agencies and organizations, 470
    for preventing falls, 460
Effexor, 254t. *See also* Venlafaxine
Eikenella, 312
Elder mistreatment, 80–84, q20, q45
    agencies and organizations, 470–471
    financial, 82
    of hospitalized patients, 85t, 89
    institutional, 83
    interventions for, 83, 85t
    key indicators of, 81, 81t
    medical-legal interface, 83–84
    physical assessment for, 81–82
    prevention of, 80
    psychologic assessment for, 82
    questions to guide intervention, 83
    risk factors for, 80, 80t
    screening for, 81, 81t, 89
Electrical stimulation, 178, 178t
Electrocardiography, q60
    ambulatory monitoring, 159
    in nystagmus, 154
    in syncope, 158–159
Electroconvulsive therapy
    for bipolar disorder, 257
    for depression, 130
    for psychotic depression, 255
Electroencephalography, 401
Electrolyte balance
    hormonal regulation of, 344–345
    in hospitalized patients, 89
Electrolyte disturbances, 367–368
    postoperative disorders, 97–98
Electronystagmography (ENG), 154

Electrophysiologic studies, 160
EM. *See* Elder mistreatment
Emergencies and urgencies, hypertensive, 336
Emotion-oriented psychotherapy, 209
Emotional disorders, 77
Emphysema, 303
Enalapril, 299t
Encephalopathy
    toxic or metabolic, 220
    Wernicke's, q53
End-of-life care, 50. *See also* Hospice care;
        Palliative care
    agencies and organizations, 470
    decisions, 24–26, 25–26
    intensity of, 50
    overall care near death, 126
End-stage dementia, q75
End-stage renal disease, 375–376
Endocarditis
    bacterial, 326
    infective, 311–312
Endocrine abnormalities, postoperative, 98
Endocrine disorders, 337–349
Endometrial biopsy, q63
Endometrial cancer
    hormonal agents for, 446, 447t
    racial differences in diagnosis and survival,
        444, 444t
Endoscopic gastrostomy, percutaneous, 169–170
Endoscopic palliation, 360
Endoscopic retrograde
    cholangiopancreatography, 361
Endoscopic ultrasonography, 361
Enemas, 99t
Energy modalities, 76
Energy requirements
    age-related changes in, 162
    estimation of, 162, 162t
    in hospitalized patients, 89
Enoxaparin, 318–319, 454t
Ensure HP, 170t
Ensure Plus HN, 170t
Entacapone, 429
Enterobacter, 309
Entrapment syndrome, 417t
Environmental modifications, 111
    for dementia, 210
    for falls, 460
    for home care, 120–121
    for preventing falls, 192, 193t
Enzymatic debridement, 243, 243t
Epidermophyton floccosum, 420
Epilepsy, 431–432
Epinephrine, 143t
Epitol, 256t. *See also* Carbamazepine
Eplerenone, 324–325
Epley's maneuver, 155, 155f
Eptifibatide, 319
Equinovarus, 182t
Erectile dysfunction, 384–386
    causes of, 384–385, 385t
    psychogenic, 385, 388
    treatment of, 387–388, 387t, q49

Erythema craquelé, q35

Erythrocyte sedimentation rate, 397

Erythromycin, 71
    drug interactions, 178

Erythroplakia, 298, 298*f*

Erythropoiesis, ineffective, 436*t*, 438–439

Erythropoietin, 375, 435
    for anemia, 438
    decreased production of, 438

Escherichia coli, 309, 310, 314, q25

Escitalopram, 216, 217*t*, 252*t*

Eskalith, 256*t*. *See also* Lithium carbonate

Esophageal cancer, 360

Esophageal dysphagia, 168

Esophageal injury, drug-induced, 359–360

Esophagoscopy, q37

Esophagus, 357–360

Essential fatty acids, 76

Essential thrombocythemia (ET), 441, 442

Essential tremor, 430–431

Estrogen deficiency, 196

Estrogen replacement therapy, 347–348, 377
    adverse effects of, 430
    for cancer, 446, 447*t*
    for female sexual dysfunction, 382–383, 383, 384*t*
    for menopausal symptoms, 378
    for osteoporosis, 200*t*, 201–202, q50
    for urinary incontinence, 178*t*, 179
    for urogenital atrophy, 378

Eszopiclone, 219, 236, 237*t*

Ethacrynic acid, 299*t*

Ethambutol, 299*t*

Ethanol, 67, q39

Ethical issues, 20–28
    in dementia, 26–27
    in institutionalization, 122
    in malnutrition, 167
    in nursing-home care, 27–28

Ethnic differences
    in cancer incidence and mortality, 444, 444*t*
    difficulty in ADLs and IADLs of Medicare beneficiaries, 5, 5*f*
    in functional limitations, 5
    health stresses and longevity, 17
    in hypertension, q77
    in perceived health of Medicare beneficiaries, 4, 5*t*

Etodolac, 407

Etoposide, 446, 446*t*

Etretinate, 453

European Society of Cardiology, 53*t*

Eustachian tube, q88

Euthanasia, 25

Executive function testing, 44, q5, q44

Executive Interview 25-item examination (EXIT 25), 22, q5, q44

Exemestane, 446, 447*t*

Exenatide (Byetta), 356*t*

Exercise(s). *See also* Physical activity
    for falls, 460
    for gait disorders, 186
    group, 186
    for musculoskeletal disease, 397
    for osteoporosis prevention and treatment, 198–199
    pelvic muscle (Kegel's), 177*t*, 178–179, 178*t*, 380, 462
    for polymyositis and dermatomyositis, 409
    for preventing falls, 193*t*
    progressive resistance training, q34
    for prostate cancer, 78–79
    to reduce risk of osteoporosis, 197*t*
    to reduce risk of osteoporotic vertebral fractures, q67
    resistance training, 54, 55, 193*t*, q34, q67
    for sleep disorders, 77
    for type 2 diabetes mellitus, 78

Exercise: A Guide from the National Institute on Aging, 57

Exercise: Getting Fit for Life (National Institute on Aging), 57

Exercise stress testing, 317–318

Expectant or conservative management, 393

External beam radiation therapy, 394, 394*t*, q30

Extremity deformities, 183, 184*t*

Exubera (inhaled insulin), 356*t*

Eyedrops for glaucoma, 143, 143*t*

Ezetimibe, 322*t*

F

Faces Pain Scale, 132

Facial nerve palsy, 314

Factor VII, 440

Factor VIII, 440

Factor IX, 440

Factor X, 440

Factor Xa inhibitor, 454*t*

Failure-to-thrive syndrome, q75

Fainting. *See* Dizziness; Syncope

Falls, 187–194
    activity recommendations for, 53*t*
    assessment of, 189, 190*t*, 191*f*, 459, q86
    and balance training, 56–57
    clinical guidelines for, 194
    diagnostic approach to, 189–190
    guidelines for prevention of, 459–460
    in hospitalized patients, 85*t*, 86–87
    interventions for, 85*t*, 192, 193*t*, 459, 460
    management of, 189, 190*t*, 191*f*
    prevention of, 61*t*, 188, 190–193, 459–460, q54
    risk of, q65, q86

Family, communication with, 209–210

Farsightedness, 140

Fatty acids, essential, 76

FDA. *See* Food and Drug Administration

Fecal impaction, 362

Fecal incontinence, 362–363, q40

Fecal occult blood testing, 61*t*, 62

Federal financing of health care, 38–40

Fee for service (FFS)
    discounted FFS, 33
    home-health care, 37
    hospice care, 38
    inpatient care, 35
    Medicare, 30–32, 31*t*, 33–34, 34*t*, 35, 38
    nursing-home care, 37
    outcomes, 103
    outpatient care, 33–34
    postacute rehabilitation, 35
    private plans, 38
    structures, 28

Feeding, 169–170

Feeding problems, 167–171

Feeding tubes
    complications with, 170
    jejunostomy, 170
    percutaneous endoscopic gastrostomy (PEG), 169–170
    solutions used in, 169, 170*t*

Feelings, 127

Female androgen deficiency syndrome, 383

Female sexual dysfunction, 382–383
    evaluation and treatment of, 383–384, 384*t*

Female sexuality, 382–384

Femoral neck fracture, 108

Fenofibrate, 322*t*

Fenoprofen, 299*t*

Fentanyl (Duragesic), 136*t*

Festinating gait, 427

Festination, 182*t*

Fever
    in frail, older residents of long-term-care facilities, 306, 306*t*
    redefinition of, 306

Fever of unknown origin (FUO), 314, 314*t*
    antibiotic therapy for, 307, 307*t*
    evaluation of, 315*t*

FFS. *See* Fee for service

FiberCon (polycarbophil), 99*t*

Fibrinogen, 440

Fibromyalgia, 400–402, 401, 402*f*

Fibrositis, 401

Financial assessment, 82

Financial mistreatment, 82

Financing
    federal, 38–40
    health care, 28, 29–40, 30*f*
    home-care certification, 119, 120*t*
    home-health care, 36–37, 121
    for home visits, 119, 120*t*
    hospice care, 37–38
    inpatient care, 34–35
    for nurse practitioners, 117–118
    nursing-home care, 37, 112–113
    postacute rehabilitation, 35–36

Finasteride, 390–391, 390*t*

Fine-needle aspiration biopsy, q51

Finger tapping, 427

Fitness, low, 56

5q- syndrome, 439

Flat feet, 417*t*

Flavoxate, 178

Fleet (bisphosphate emollient enema), 99*t*

Flexibility training, 54

Flexible sigmoidoscopy, 61*t*, 62

Flovent (fluticasone), 302*t*

Flu vaccine, 453

Fluconazole, 453
Fludarabine, 446
Fludrocortisone, 193*t*
Fluid disturbances, 367–368
Fluid management, 89
Fluid needs, 162
Flunisolide (AeroBid), 299*t*, 302*t*
Fluoride
 for osteoporosis, 202
 recommended dietary allowances, 163*t*
Fluoroquinolones, 67
Fluorouracil, 446*t*
Fluoxetine (Prozac), 251, 252*t*, q79
 for depressive features of behavioral
  disturbances in dementia, 216, 217*t*
 drug interactions, 72, 178
Flurazepam, 67, 227*t*
Flurbiprofen, 299*t*
Flutamide, 446, 447*t*
Fluticasone (Flovent), 302*t*
Fluticasone priopionate and salmeterol
 (Advair), 302*t*
Fluvastatin, 322*t*
Fluvoxamine, 251–252
Foam island, 244*t*
FOBT. *See* Fecal occult blood testing
Folate, 439–440
 drug interactions, 164*t*
 recommended dietary allowances, 163*t*
Folate deficiency, 438–439, 440
Folstein Mini-Mental State Examination
 (MMSE), 22, 44, 88, 205, 222, 222*t*,
 q5, q32, q44
Fondaparinux (Arixtra), 454*t*
Food(s). *See also* Nutrition
 calcium-containing, 199*t*
 for sleep disorders, 77
Food and Drug Administration (FDA), 67,
 79
Food guide pyramid, 162
Foot care, 422
Foot diseases and disorders, 416–422, 417*t*
Foot drop, 182*t*
Foot slap, 182*t*
Foradil (formoterol), 302*t*
Forefoot disorders, 416–418, q100
Foreign-born persons, 3
Forgoing and discontinuing interventions,
 24–25
Formality, 47
Formoterol (Foradil), 302*t*
Foster care, adult, 124
Fractures
 and balance training, 56–57
 femoral neck, 108
 of hip, 108–109, q27, q46
 osteoporotic, 410*t*, q67
 prediction of, 196–198
 risk factors for, 196–197
 stress, q22
 vertebral, 203
Fragile X syndrome, 282*t*
Fragmin, 454*t*. *See also* Dalteparin

Freezing, 427
Frontal lobe damage, 282*t*
Frontotemporal dementia
 behavioral disturbances in, 215
 diagnostic features of, 206*t*
 differential diagnosis of, 207
Frozen shoulder syndrome, 403
Functional abilities
 assessment of, 42–43, 185, q44
 Functional Activities Questionnaire, 205
 Functional Ambulation Classification scale,
  185
 Functional Independence Measure (FIM),
  102
 "functional reach" test, 189
 impairments in hospitalized patients, 85*t*,
  86
 performance-based assessment of, 185
 rapid screening followed by assessment and
  management, 41, 42*t*
 and rehabilitation outcome, q46
 self-reported functional limitations of
  Medicare beneficiaries, 5, 5*f*
 trends in, 4
FUO (fever of unknown origin), 314, 314*t*
 antibiotic therapy for, 307, 307*t*
 evaluation of, 315*t*
Furosemide, 324

G

G-regulatory proteins, 13
Gabapentin (Neurontin)
 for epilepsy, 431–432, 432*t*
 for persistent pain, 135*t*, 138
Gait, festinating, 427
Gait apraxia, 183
Gait impairment, 181–187
 associated findings, 183, 184*t*
 glossary, 182*t*
 interventions for, 193*t*
Gait speed, 43
Galantamine, 210, 211
Gallstones, 361, q24
Gardnerella vaginosis, 378
Garlic, q80
Gastric complications, NSAID-induced, 360
Gastroesophageal reflux disease (GERD),
 358–359
Gastrointestinal diseases and disorders,
 357–367
 and continence, 171–172, 173*t*
 infections, 314
 postoperative concerns, 98
Gastroprotective agents, 70
Gastrostomy
 contraindications to, 170
 percutaneous endoscopic, 169–170
Gauze packing, 244*t*
Gaze-evoked nystagmus, 153
Gaze limitation, 429
GDS. *See* Geriatric Depression Scale
Gemcitabine, 446
Gemfibrozil, 299*t*, 322*t*

Gender differences
 in drug metabolism, 68
 in life expectancy, 1, 2*t*
Gender issues, 50
Gene expression, 11–12
Gene mutations, 14
Generalized anxiety disorder, 260, 261*t*, q7
Genetic testing, 27
Genital prolapse, 380, 381, q90
Genitourinary imaging, 370–371
Genu recurvatum, 182*t*
GERD. *See* Gastroesophageal reflux disease
Geriatric Depression Scale (short form,
 GDS), 44, 60, 458
Geriatric Evaluation and Management
 (GEM) units, 90–91
Geriatric Institutional Assessment Profile
 (GIAP), 90
Geriatric Interdisciplinary Team Training,
 104
Geriatric nurse practitioners (GNPs), 116
Geriatric Resource Nurse (GRN) model, 90
Geriatric screening. *See* Screening
Geriatric syndrome of late-life depression,
 247–248
Get Up and Go test, 190
Giant cell arteritis, 405–406, q38, q52
GIAP. *See* Geriatric Institutional Assessment
 Profile
Ginkgo biloba, 77, 211, q80
Glaucoma, 140, 143
 eyedrops for, 143, 143*t*
 primary open-angle (POAG), 143
 screening for, 140, 143
Gleason grading system, 392
Glimepiride (Amaryl), 355*t*
Glipizide (Glucotrol), 355*t*
Glipizide and metformin (METAGLIP), 355*t*
Glomerular filtration rate, 68, 96
Glomerulonephritis
 acute or subacute, 373
 crescentic, 371, 373
 mesangioproliferative, 373
Glucocorticoids
 and osteoporosis, 197*t*
 to reduce risk of osteoporosis, 197*t*
 subclinical hypersecretion, 345–346
Glucophage, 355*t*. *See also* Metformin
Glucosamine supplementation, 75, 76, 398
Glucose blood levels, 61*t*, 64*t*
Glucose intolerance, 350
Glucose management, postoperative, 98
α-Glucosidase inhibitors, 355*t*
Glucotrol (glipizide), 355*t*
Glucovance (glyburide and metformin), 355*t*
Glutathione, 77
Glyburide (Diaβeta, Micronase, Glynase),
 355*t*
Glyburide and metformin (Glucovance), 355*t*
Glynase (glyburide), 355*t*
Glyset (miglitol), 355*t*
GNPs. *See* Geriatric nurse practitioners

Goserelin, 446, 447*t*
Gottron's papules, 408–409
Gout, 399
Gram-negative rods, 309, 309*f*
Grand mal seizures, 431
Granisetron, 128*t*, 129
Granulation, 242*t*
Granulocyte colony-stimulating factor, 446*t*
Granulocyte-macrophage colony-stimulating factor, 446*t*
Grapefruit juice, 72
Grief, 16
Griseofulvin, 453
GRN model. *See* Geriatric Resource Nurse model
Group exercise, 186
Group homes, 124
Group therapy, 209
Growth hormone, 348–349
Growth hormone deficiency, 348
Growth hormone supplementation, 348–349
Guardians, 23
Guide to Community Preventive Services, 59
Gustation (taste), 299*t*
Gynecologic diseases and disorders, 376–381

H

HAART. *See* Highly active antiretroviral therapy
Habit training, 177, 177*t*, 178*t*
Haemophilus influenzae, 308, 309*f*, 312
Haglund's deformity, 417*t*, 418
Hair, 284
Hallucinations, 263
in dementia, 213, 218–219, 218*t*, 265
evaluation of, 263, 263*f*
isolated, syndromes of, 266–267
in Lewy body dementia, 266–267
Hallucinosis, organic, 266–267
Hallux abducto valgus, 417*t*, 418*f*
Hallux limitus and rigidus, 417*t*
Hallux valgus, 417*t*
Haloperidol
for agitated delirium, 228*t*
for delirium, 129
dosing and side effects, 265*t*
for nausea and vomiting, 128–129, 128*t*
Hammertoes, 416, 418*f*
Harris Hip Questionnaire, 106
Hartford Institute for Geriatric Nursing Nurses Improving Care for Health System Elders (NICHE) program, 89–90
Try This, 41
HCFA (Health Care Financing Administration). *See now* Centers for Medicare & Medicaid Services (CMS)
HDL (high-density lipoprotein) cholesterol, 353. *See also* Cholesterol
Head and neck cancer, 444, 444*t*
Head and neck resources, 472
Head-shaking test, 154
Headaches, 426, q38, q52

Healing
monitoring, 245
Pressure Ulcer Scale for Healing (PUSH), 245, q96
Health beliefs, 49
Health care
financing of, 28, 38–40
trends in, 4, 6–7
Health care agent or proxy, 21, 22
Health Care Financing Administration (HCFA). *See now* Centers for Medicare & Medicaid Services (CMS)
Health insurance. *See also* Medicaid; Medicare
coverage for older Americans, 29–30, 31*t*
coverage for rehabilitation care, 102–103
supplemental, q4
Health maintenance organizations (HMOs), 29–30
home-health care, 37
inpatient care, 34
Medicare, 30, 31*t*, 32, 33, 33*t*, 34, 34*t*, 37, 38
nursing-home care, 37
outpatient care, 32
social health maintenance organizations (SHMOs), 123
Health risks, culture-specific, 49
Healthcare Employers' Data Information System (HEDIS), 39
Healthy behaviors, 19–20
Healthy People 2010, 57, 238
Hearing, 146
Hearing aids, 148–150, q4, q13
costs of, 149*t*, 150
styles of, 149–150, 149*t*
Hearing assessment, q13
rapid screening followed by assessment and management, 41, 42*t*
testing, 43–44, 60, 61*t*
Hearing Handicap Inventory for the Elderly—Screening Version, 147, q13
Hearing impairment, 145–151, q13, q52
interventions for, 193*t*
rehabilitation of, 148, 148*t*
resources, 472–473
screening for, 60, 61*t*, 147
sensorineural, q88
strategies to enhance communication with hearing-impaired persons, 147–148, 148*t*
Heart changes, 316*t*
Heart disease
deaths due to, 5–6, 6*t*
ischemic, 316–321
management of, q17
prevalence of, 4, 4*f*
and rehabilitation, 105
resources, 473
valvular, 325–327
Heart failure, 321–325
activity recommendations for, 53*t*
and continence, 171–172, 173*t*
diastolic, q68
postoperative, 97
treatment of, q78

Heart-healthy diet, 76
Heart valves
bioprosthetic, 453*t*
indications for anticoagulation, 453*t*
mechanical, 453*t*
prosthetic, 313
Heat-shock factor (HSF1), 12, 14
Heat-shock protein, 12
Heat-shock protein 70F, 14
Heavy drinking, 276
HEDIS. *See* Healthcare Employers' Data Information System
Heel pain, 417*t*, 418
Heel pressure ulcers, 240, 240*t*
Height, 61*t*
Helicobacter pylori infection, 360, 361
Heloma, subungual, 420–421
HELP. *See* Hospitalized Elderly Longitudinal Project
Hematologic diseases and disorders, 434–442
Hematologic malignancies, 449–450
screening for, 65*t*
Hematoma, subdural, 425–426
Hematopoiesis, 434–435
Hematuria, 369
Hemiparesis, 183, 184*t*
Hemiplegia, 183, 184*t*
Hemolytic anemia, 436, 436*t*, 439
Hemorrhage, intracerebral, 424–425
Heparin
for acute MI, 319–320
for deep-vein thrombosis, 454*t*
low-molecular weight, 454*t*
and osteoporosis, 197*t*
perioperative, 96
for pulmonary embolism, 454*t*
Heparinoid, 454*t*
Herbal preparations, 76
Herpes zoster, 289–290, 289*f*
post-herpetic neuralgia, 290
reactivated, 313–314
Herpes zoster ophthalmicus, 144–145
HHRGs. *See* Home Health Related Groups
HIAP (human inhibitor of apoptosis protein), 13
High-density lipoprotein (HDL) cholesterol, 353. *See also* Cholesterol
High T$_4$ syndrome, 340
Highly active antiretroviral therapy (HAART), 313
Hip fracture, 108–109, q27, q46
Hip pain, q99
Hip protectors, 194
Hip surgery
indications for anticoagulation, 453*t*
for osteoarthritis, 186
total hip and knee arthroplasty, 109
Hispanic Americans
alcohol abuse and dependence among, 276
alcohol use among, 276
CAM use, 75
cancer incidence and mortality in, 444, 444*t*

perceived health of Medicare beneficiaries, 4, 5t

poverty rates, 2

Histamine H$_2$-blocking agents, 227t, 359

History of immigration or migration, 48

History of traumatic experiences, 48

Histrionic personality disorder
features of, 267, 268t
therapeutic strategies for, 270, 271t

HIV infection, 313

HMG-CoA reductase inhibitors
drug regimens for dyslipidemia, 322t
for osteoporosis, 202
perioperative, 94
underprescribing, 70

HMOs. *See* Health maintenance
organizations

Hodgkin's disease, 443–444, 450

Home hazards, 192

Home-health care, 36–37, 119–122
agencies and organizations, 469
billing codes and reimbursement for, 119, 120t
codes, reimbursement, and requirements in certification, 119, 120t
Medicare benefits, 102
office-based house-call programs, 121
rehabilitation outcomes, 104
trends in use, 6–7

Home Health Compare, 37

Home Health Related Groups (HHRGs), 119

Home hospital, 123

Homeostenosis, 8, 93

Homocysteine, 439–440

Hormesis, 8

Hormonal regulation of water and electrolyte balance, 344–345

Hormonal therapy
for breast cancer, 449
for cancer, 446, 447t

Hormone replacement therapy, 65t. *See also*
Estrogen replacement therapy
for osteoporosis, 201–202
and postmenopausal bleeding, 381

Horner's syndrome, 424

Hospice care, 37–38, 126, q75. *See also*
End-of-life care; Palliative care
access to, 126
agencies and organizations, 470
services, 126, 127t

Hospital-acquired pneumonia, 308, 309f

Hospital care, 84–92. *See also* Acute care;
Discharge planning
Acute Care for Elders (ACE) units, 91
assessment at admission, 85, 86t
day hospitals, 122
delirium in hospitalized patients, q12, q32
"early" discharges from, 35, 36t
financing, coverage, and costs of, 34–35
Geriatric Evaluation and Management (GEM) units, 90–91
hazards and opportunities to address, 84, 84t

home hospital, 123

Nurses Improving Care for Health System Elders (NICHE) program, 89–90
nursing care, 89–90
outcomes, 103
rehabilitation outcomes, 103
sleep disturbances in, 233–234
transitions from, 91–92
trends in discharges from, 6

Hospital Elder Life Program (HELP), 91, 228

Hospitalized Elderly Longitudinal Project (HELP), 126

Hot flushes, 377–378

House-call programs, q87
office-based, 121

Housing, sheltered, 125

HSF1. *See* Heat-shock factor

Humalog (insulin lispro), 356t

Humulin (insulin), 356t

Hurley Discomfort Scale, 133

Hutchinson's sign, 144, 289

Hyaluronic acid, 398

Hydralazine, isosorbide dinitrate plus, 325

Hydrocephalus, normal-pressure
and continence, 171–172, 173t
gait findings in, 183, 184t

Hydrochlorothiazide, 299t, 334, q62

Hydrocodone (Lorcet, Lortab, Vicodin, Vicoprofen), 136t, q95

Hydrocolloids, 244t

Hydrocortisone, 98

Hydrogel dressings, 244t

Hydromorphone (Dilaudid, Hydrostat), 136t, 299t

Hydrostat, 136t. *See also* Hydromorphone

Hydroxychloroquine, 407, 408

Hydroxyzine, 129

Hyoscyamine, 178

Hyperadrenocorticoidism, 345

Hypercalcemia, 343–344, q28
and continence, 171–172, 173t
differential diagnosis of, 343, 343t

Hypercholesteremia. *See* Lipids, serum

Hyperglycemia
management of, 354
permissive moderate, 98

Hypericum perforatum (St. John's wort), 254t

Hyperkalemia, 368

Hyperkeratosis, 419–420

Hypernatremia, 367–368

Hyperopia, 140

Hyperparathyroidism
primary, 197t, q28
screening for, 197t
secondary, 196

Hypersexuality, 219

Hypertension, 331–337
activity recommendations for, 53t
classification of, 331, 331t
complementary and alternative medicine for, 76–77

emergencies and urgencies, 336
follow-up visits, 335–336, 335t
nonpharmacologic therapy for, 333, 333t
pharmacologic treatment of, 333–335
postoperative, 97
prevalence of, 4, 4f
resistant, q39
screening for, 60, 61t
treatment of, 332–336, 333t, q1

Hyperthyroidism, 340
diagnostic algorithm for, 341f
screening for, 64t, 197t

Hypertriglyceridemia, 317

Hypnotics
chronic use of, 236–238
and delirium, 227t
effects on continence, 172t
sedative, 172t

Hypoadrenocorticoidism, 345

Hypoalbuminemia, 163–164

Hypochondriasis, 272, 272t

Hypogonadism, 197t, 346–347, 388

Hypokalemia, 368

Hyponatremia, 367–368, q89

Hypophosphatemia, 203

Hypoproliferative anemia, 436–438, 436t, q56

Hypotension
asymptomatic, 324
orthostatic, 155, 161, 429, q86
postprandial, 161
postural, 193t

Hypothyroidism, 338–340
screening for, 64t
subclinical, 338, 339f

Hysteroscopy, q63

I

IADLs. *See* Instrumental activities of daily living

Ibandronate, 200t, 201

Ibuprofen, 406, q91

ICE. *See* Interleukin-1 converting enzyme

ICF. *See International Classification of Functioning, Disability, and Health* (WHO)

ICH-1, 13

Identity, cultural, 47

Idiopathic myelofibrosis, 441, 442

IGF-1. *See* Insulin-like growth factor 1

Imaging. *See also specific modalities*
of brain, 206
in dementia, 206
in gait impairment, 185
genitourinary techniques, 370–371

Imidazole, 67, q69

Imipramine, 178, 179, 227t, 299t

Immigration issues, 48

Immobility
in hospitalized patients, 85t, 86–87
interventions for, 85t
prevention of, 61t

Immune function changes, 305, 305t

Immune senescence, 305

Immune thrombocytopenia, 440

Immunizations, 61*t*, 63–64

Implantable cardioverter-defibrillators, 327, 327*t*

Implantable loop recorders, 159–160

Impulse-control disorders, 282

Incidentalomas, adrenal, 345–347, 345*t*

Incompetence, 21

Incontinence
  fecal, 362–363
  urinary (*See* Urinary incontinence)

Indinavir, 67

Infections
  antibiotic management of, 306–307, 307*t*
  and back pain, 410*t*
  bone and joint, 313
  control of, 245–246
  diagnosis of, 306–307
  gastrointestinal, 314
  management of, 306–307
  predisposition to, 305–306
  presentation of, 306
  prosthetic device, 312–313
  vulvovaginal, 378

Infectious diarrhea, 314

Infectious diseases, 304–315

Infectious Diseases Society of America, 308

Infective endocarditis, 311–312

Inflammation, vulvovaginal, 378

Inflammatory disorders, 405–409

Influenza, 309
  deaths due to, 5–6, 6*t*
  interventions for, 85*t*
  vaccination against, 61*t*, 63, 89, q3

Informed consent for research, 24

Ingrown toenails, 420

Inhaled insulin (Exubera), 356*t*

Inhaled medications, 301, 302*t*

Injury
  counseling to encourage prevention of, 61*t*, 63
  deaths due to, 5–6, 6*t*
  drug-induced esophageal injury, 359–360
  recommendations for prevention of, 61*t*

Inner ear, q88

Innohep (tinzaparin), 454*t*

Inpatient care. *See also* Hospital care
  fee for service, 35
  financing, coverage, and costs of, 34–35
  managed care, 34–35
  rehabilitation outcomes, 103

Insomnia, 229, 230–231, q11, q70, q84. *See also* Sleep problems
  behavioral management of, 219, 219*t*
  in dementia, 219
  prescription medications for, 236, 237*t*
  rebound, 231

Institute for Clinical Systems Improvement, 53*t*

Institute of Medicine Food and Nutrition Board, 162

Institutional mistreatment, 83

Institutionalization, 122

Instrumental activities of daily living (ADLs), 43, 43*t*
  difficulty of Medicare beneficiaries in, 5, 5*f*
  self-reported functional limitations of Medicare beneficiaries, 5, 5*f*

Insulin (Humulin, Novolin, NPH), 356*t*, q66
  inhaled (Exubera), 356*t*
  long-acting (Ultralente), 356*t*
  zinc (Lente), 356*t*

Insulin aspart (NovoLog), 356*t*

Insulin detemir (Levemir), 356*t*

Insulin glargine (Lantus), 356*t*

Insulin glulisine (Apidra), 356*t*

Insulin-like growth factor 1 (IGF-1), 14

Insulin lispro (Humalog), 356*t*, q66

Insulin receptor, 14

Insulin receptor substrate (IRS), 14

Insulin therapy, q66
  postoperative, 98
  preparations, 356*t*

Insurance. *See also* Health insurance; Medicaid; Medicare supplemental, q4

Intal (cromolyn), 302*t*

α-Interferon, 446–447

Interleukin-1 converting enzyme, 13

Interleukin-2, 447

Internal carotid artery disease, 424

International Classification of Functioning, Disability, and Health (ICF) (WHO), 101, 102*f*

International Continence Society, 380, 380*t*

International Prostate Symptom Score (IPSS), 389

Interpersonal therapy, 250*t*

Intertrigo, 287, 287*f*

Intestinal obstruction, q98

Intracellular volume, 89

Intracerebral hemorrhage, 424–425

Intraocular lens implantation, q81

Intrinsic sphincter deficiency, q43

Ipratropium (Atrovent), 302*t*

IPSS. *See* International Prostate Symptom Score

Iron therapy
  for anemia, 98
  drug interactions, 164*t*

Irritable bowel syndrome, 362, 364

IRS. *See* Insulin receptor substrate

Ischemic heart disease, 316–321

Ischemic stroke, 425

Isoniazid, 164*t*, 311, 453

Isosorbide dinitrate plus hydralazine, 325

Itching, generalized, q35

Itraconazole, 72

J

J-curve hypothesis, 335

Januvia (sitagliptan), 356*t*

Jejunostomy feeding tubes, 170

Jevity 1.2, 170*t*

Jewett-Whitmore (ABCD) staging system, 392–393, 393*t*

Jobst stockings, 193*t*

Joint diseases, 397–400

Joint problems
  infections, 313
  resources, 473
  total hip and knee arthroplasty, 109

Judgment, substituted, 22, 23*t*

Justice, 20, 21

K

K-Y jelly, 383

Kabikinase (streptokinase), 455*t*

Kadian, 136*t*. *See also* Morphine

Kava, q80

Kegel's exercises
  for incontinence, 177*t*, 178–179, 178*t*, 462
  for vaginal prolapse, 380

Ketoconazole, 72, 178

Ketoprofen, 453

Kidney biopsy, 370–371

Kidney diseases and disorders, 371–374
  infection during rehabilitation, 105*t*
  Modification of Diet in Renal Disease (MDRD), 96
  postoperative disorders, 97–98
  prevalence of, 4, 4*f*
  resources, 476
  vascular, 373–374

Kidney failure, chronic, 374–376

Kidney transplantation, 375–376

Kidneys, 96

Kingella, 312

Klebsiella, 308, 309

Klonopin, 135*t*, 256*t*. *See also* Clonazepam

Knee arthroplasty, 109

Knee osteoarthritis, 76, 398. *See also* Osteoarthritis

Knee pain, 397

Knee surgery
  indications for anticoagulation, 453*t*
  for osteoarthritis, 186

Koebner's phenomenon, 288

L

Labetalol, 299*t*

Laboratory testing
  in back pain, 413–414
  in falls, 190
  in gait impairment, 185
  in malnutrition, 163–164
  in musculoskeletal disease, 396–397
  services that have been demonstrated not to be beneficial, 65, 65*t*

Labyrinthitis, 152, q61

Lactulose (Cephulac), 99*t*

Lacunar disease, 424

Lamotrigine
  for bipolar disorder, 257
  for epilepsy, 431–432, 432*t*

Micronase (glyburide), 355t
Micronutrient requirements
  age-related changes in, 162
  recommended dietary allowances, 163t
Microvascular complications of diabetes
    mellitus, 353–354
Micturition, 171
Middle ear, q88
Midfoot disorders, 416–418
Midodrine, 193t
Miglitol (Glyset), 355t
Migration, 48
Mild cognitive impairment, 208t, q18, q19,
    q29
  diagnostic features of, 206t
  differential diagnosis of, 207
Milk of Magnesia (magnesium hydroxide),
    99t
Mind-body interventions
  for lower back pain, 76
  for lung cancer, 79
  for menopausal symptoms, 78
Mineral oil-nutrient interactions, 164t
Mini-Cog Assessment Instrument for
    Dementia, 44, 88, 205
Mini-Mental State Examination (MMSE), 22,
    44, 88, 205, 222, q5, q32, q44
  attention test items, 222t
Mini-Nutritional Assessment (MNA-SF), 165
Minimal-change disease, 371
Minimum Data Set (MDS), 114, 163, 167
Minocycline, 407
Miotics, 143t
MiraLax (polyethylene glycol), 99t
Mirtazapine (Remeron, Sol-tabs), 254t
  for depression, 216, 217t, 253
  for insomnia, 212, 236, 237t
  for sleep problems, 219, 236
  for undernutrition syndromes, 166
Mistreatment, elder, 80–84, q20, q45
  agencies and organizations, 470–471
  financial, 82
  of hospitalized patients, 85t, 89
  institutional, 83
  interventions for, 83, 85t
  key indicators of, 81, 81t
  medical-legal interface, 83–84
  physical assessment for, 81–82
  prevention of, 80
  psychologic assessment for, 82
  questions to guide intervention, 83
  risk factors for, 80, 80t
  screening for, 81, 81t, 89
Mitochondrial DNA (mtDNA), 11
Mitomycin C, 446t
Mitral regurgitation, 326
Mitral stenosis, 326–327
Mitral valvular heart disease, 453t
MMSE. See Mini-Mental State Examination
MNA-SF. See Mini-Nutritional Assessment
MND. See Motor neuron disease
Mobility aids, 110–111, 187

Mobility and movement, 426–431
  activities of daily living (ADLs), 42–43,
    43t
  instrumental activities of daily living
    (IADLs), 5, 5f, 43, 43t
  periodic leg movements during sleep,
    232–233, q11
  and pressure ulcers, 241
  rapid screening followed by assessment and
    management, 41, 42t
  restless legs syndrome, 232–233, q11
  Tinetti Performance-Oriented Mobility
    Assessment, 43
Modafinil (Provigil), 254t
Moderators, stress, 18–20
Modification of Diet in Renal Disease
    (MDRD), 96
Mometasone (Asmanex), 302t
Mono-Gesic (salsalate), 135t
Monoamine oxidase inhibitors, 253
Monoclonal gammopathy of undetermined
    significance, q8
Mood disorders, 247–258. See also
    Depression
  psychotic symptoms in, 265
  screening for, 248
Mood disturbances
  in dementia, 216
  in Parkinson's disease, 427
Mood stabilizers
  for behavioral disturbances in dementia
    with manic features, 216–217, 217t
  for personality disorders, 271
Moraxella catarrhalis, 308
Morbidity, 6
Morphine (MSIR, Roxanol, MSContin,
    Kadian), 299t
  for dyspnea, 130–131
  for persistent pain, 136t
  pharmacokinetics, 69
Morton's syndrome, 417t
Motor neuron disease, 432–433
Motor vehicle crashes, 61t
Movement disorders, 426–431, 430
MSAs. See Medical savings accounts
MSContin, 136t. See also Morphine
MSIR, 136t. See also Morphine
Mucocutaneous candidiasis, chronic, 420
Multiple myeloma, 197t, 450, q8, q56
Multiple sclerosis, 171–172, 173t
Multiple system atrophy, 429
Muscle strengthening, 192, 193t
Muscle weakness, q34
Musculoskeletal diseases and disorders,
    396–409
  complementary and alternative medicine
    for, 75–76
  and continence, 171–172, 173t
  and rehabilitation, 105
  resources, 473
MUSE (medicated urethral system for
    erection), 387t, 388
Music therapy, 77
Mycobacterium tuberculosis, 310–311

Mycoplasma pneumoniae, 309f
Myelodysplastic syndromes (MDS), 439, 449
Myelofibrosis, idiopathic, 441, 442
Myelography, 413
Myelopathy, 433
Myocardial infarction
  acute, 317, 319–320, 453t
  chemoprophylaxis of, 61t, 64t
  coronary revascularization after, 320–321
  indications for anticoagulation in, 453t
  management of, q17
  non-Q-wave, 318–319, 319t
  recurrent, 61t
  risk stratification after, 320, 320t
  screening for, 64t
  treatment after, 320, q78
Myofascial trigger points, 402
Myopathy, 183, 184t, 434
Myopia, 140

N

Nabumetone, 299t, 407
Nafcillin, 453
Nail disorders, 418–421
Nalbuphine, 138
Naloxone, 280
Naltrexone, q54
Naproxen, 406
Narcissistic personality disorder
  features of, 267, 268t
  therapeutic strategies for, 270, 271t
Narcotic analgesics, 70, 172t
Narcotics Anonymous, 279
Nasal pillows, 303
Nateglinide (Starlix), 355t
National Center on Elder Abuse, 83, 84
National Cholesterol Education Program
    Expert Panel (3rd Report), 53t
National Council on Aging, Inc., 164–165
National Health and Nutrition Examination
    Surveys (NHANES), 165, 166t
National Institute on Aging, 57
National Osteoporosis Foundation, 197
Native Americans, 75, 444
Nausea and vomiting
  palliation of, 128–129
  postoperative nausea, 98
  treatment of, 128, 128t
Nearsightedness, 140
Neck pain, 410, 414–415
Necrosis, 242t
Nedocromil (Tilade), 302t
Needle suspension, 179t
Nefazodone
  drug interactions, 72
  metabolism of, 68
Neglect, q20, q45. See also Elder
    mistreatment
  self-neglect, 82–83, 89
Neisseria gonorrhea, 395
Nelfinavir, 299t

Neovascularization
    choroidal, 141, 141*f*
    in diabetic retinopathy, 142, 142*f*
Nephritis
    acute interstitial, 373
    acute or subacute glomerulonephritis, 373
    crescentic glomerulonephritis, 371, 373
    deaths due to, 5–6, 6*t*
    mesangioproliferative glomerulonephritis, 373
    pyelonephritis, 310
Nephrologists, 375
Nephropathy
    diabetic, 371
    membranous, 371
    minimal-change, 371
    obstructive, 373
Nephrosis, 5–6, 6*t*
Nephrotic syndrome, 371
    deaths due to, 5–6, 6*t*
Nepro, 170*t*
Neuralgia, post-herpetic, 290
Neurodermatitis, 286
Neuroendocrinologic theory of aging, 8*t*
Neuroimaging, 154
Neurologic diseases and disorders, 423–434
    complementary and alternative medicine for, 77
    and continence, 171–172, 173*t*
    resources, 474
Neurologic testing, 160
Neurontin, 135*t*. *See also* Gabapentin
Neuropsychiatric concerns, preoperative, 96
Neuropsychologic testing, q5
Niacin, 163*t*, 164*t*, 322*t*
NICHE Ready Sheet, 90
Nifedipine, 67, 71, 299*t*
Nighttime awakening, q19
NIH Stroke Scale, 107, 423, 425
Nitrates, 71*t*, 318, 320
Nitrazepam, 69
Nitroglycerin, 97, 318, 319
Nocturia, q84
Nocturnal penile tumescence testing, 386
Nodular thyroid disease, 340–341
Non-Hodgkin's lymphoma, 450
Nonadherence, 72–73
Nonmaleficence, 20–21
Nonsteroidal anti-inflammatory drugs (NSAIDs)
    blood pressure effects of, q91
    and continence, 172*t*
    contraindications to, 138–139
    gastric complications of, 360
    for gout, 399
    for incontinence, 178
    kidney diseases associated with, 374
    for osteoarthritis, 398
    for pain, 134
    for pseudogout, 400
    for rheumatoid arthritis, 406, 407
    risk factors for upper GI adverse events with, 360, 361*t*
    warfarin interactions, 453

Nonverbal communication, respectful, 48
Norpace, 172*t*
Norpramin, 135*t*, 253*t*. *See also* Desipramine
Norton Scale, 239, q96
Nortriptyline (Aventyl, Pamelor), 253*t*
    for depression, 252
    for depression in dementia, 216
    for depressive features of behavioral disturbances in dementia, 216, 217*t*
    for persistent pain, 135*t*, 138
Novolin (insulin), 356*t*
NovoLog (insulin aspart), 356*t*
NPH (insulin), 356*t*
NSAIDs. *See* Nonsteroidal anti-inflammatory drugs
Numeric Rating Scale, 132
Nurse practitioners (NPs), 116–118
Nurses Improving Care for Health System Elders (NICHE) program, 89–90
Nursing care
    Geriatric Resource Nurse (GRN) model, 90
    for hospital patients, 89–90
    trends in use, 6–7
Nursing-home acquired pneumonia, 308
Nursing-home care, 37, 112–118
    ethics in, 27–28
    institutional mistreatment, 83
    outcomes, 103
    physician responsibilities in, 116, 116*t*
    risk factors for, q21
    sleep in, 234, q19
    standard of care in, q76
    transition to, q42
    treatment decisions in, 27
    trends in use, 3
    weight loss in, q72
Nursing Home Compare, 37
Nutriceuticals, 67
Nutrition, 165–166
    age-related changes in, 162–163
    assessment of, 43
    intake, 163
    requirements, 162*t*
    resources, 474
    risk factors for, 164, 165*t*
    undernutrition, 165
Nutrition screening, 163–165
    DETERMINE Your Nutritional Health Checklist, 463
    rapid screening, 41, 42*t*
Nutrition Screening Initiative, 164–165
Nutritional interventions, 166–167
    for hospitalized patients, 85*t*, 88–89
    for preventing pressure ulcers, 240
    to reduce risk of osteoporosis, 197*t*
Nutritional supplementation, 64*t*
    for hospitalized patients, 89
    for pressure ulcers, 245
Nystagmus, 153–154

O

OASIS. *See* Outcome and Assessment Information Set

Obesity, 56, 165–166
    activity recommendations for, 53*t*
    drug interactions, 72
    prevalence of, 165, 166*t*
    recommendations for prevention of, 61*t*
    screening for, 60, 61*t*
OBRA. *See* Omnibus Budget Reconciliation Act
Obsessive-compulsive disorder, 259
    features of, 267, 268*t*
    therapeutic strategies for, 261*t*, 270, 271, 271*t*
Obstructive nephropathy, 373
Obstructive sleep apnea, 303
Occlusive dressings, q71
Occlusive peripheral vascular disease, 329–330
Occult gastrointestinal bleeding, 364–365
Octreotide, q98
Odynophagia, 358
Office-based house-call programs, 121
Office visits, routine, 41
Ofloxacin, 299*t*
Olanzapine (Zyprexa), 212, 266
    for agitated delirium, 228*t*
    dosing and side effects, 265*t*
    for mania, 257
    for mania and manic-like symptoms, 256*t*
    for Parkinson's disease and hallucinations, 266
    for psychosis in dementia, 218, 218*t*
    side effects of, 265
Olecranon bursitis, 403
Olfactory dysfunction, 299, 299*t*
Omega-3-acid ethyl esters, 322*t*
Omeprazole, 359
Omnibus Budget Reconciliation Act of 1987 (OBRA-87), 83, 114, 116, 167, 180, q76
Oncology, 442–451
Ondansetron, 128*t*, 129
Onychauxis, 419, 419*f*
Onychia, 420
Onychodysplasia, 418*f*
Onychogryphosis, 419, 419*f*
Onycholysis, 419, 420
Onychomycosis, 419*f*, 420, 420*f*
Onychopathy, 419
Onychophosis, 419–420
Onychorrhexis, 419
Opacified posterior lens capsule, q81
Operative therapy, 92–93. *See also* Surgery
Ophthalmic corticosteroids, 144
Opioids
    addiction to, 137
    adverse effects of, 137–138
    barriers to use, 137
    and delirium, 227*t*
    dependence on, 137
    for dyspnea, 130–131
    for pain, 134–136
    for persistent pain, 136*t*

pseudo-addiction to, 137
tolerance to, 137
Optic neuropathy, anterior ischemic, 143–144, 144*f*
Oral cancer, 61*t*, 297–298
Oral corticosteroids, 303
Oral diseases and disorders, 294–300
Oral mucosal problems, 297–299
Oral nutrition, 166
Orasone, 135*t*. *See also* Prednisone
Oregon Death with Dignity Act, 25
Organic brain syndrome, 220
Organic hallucinosis, 266–267
Organic personality disorders, 269–270
Orgaran (danaparoid), 454*t*
Oropharyngeal dysphagia, 168, 169, 357–358
Orthopedic foot disorders, 416–418
Orthostatic hypotension, 429, q86
management and treatment of, 155, 161
Orthotics, 111, 186–187, 422
Oseltamivir, 63, 309, q3
Osmolite, 170*t*
Osteoarthritis, 396, 397–398, q31
activity recommendations for, 53*t*
complementary and alternative medicine for, 75–76
diagnostic criteria for, 397, 398*t*
hip and knee replacement surgery for, 186
of knee, 76
Osteomalacia, 197*t*, 203
Osteomyelitis, 313
Osteoporosis, 194–203
activity recommendations for, 53*t*
and balance training, 56–57
hormone replacement therapy for, 201–202
management of, q28
medications to prevent and treat, 199, 200*t*
in men, q50
modifications to reduce risk of, 196–197, 197*t*
prevention of, 61*t*
sacral fractures of, 410*t*, 412
screening for, 61*t*, 62, 197, 197*t*
secondary causes of, 197, 197*t*
treatment of, 198–202, q27
vertebral compression fractures of, 410*t*, 411–412, q67
Outcome and Assessment Information Set (OASIS), 103, 119
Outpatient care, 29–34
rehabilitation outcomes, 103
of substance abuse, 279
Ovarian cancer, 65*t*, q98
Overactive bladder, q40
Overdose, warfarin, 454*t*
Overflow incontinence, 173*t*, 174, 180
Overprescribing, 72
Overweight, 165, 166*t*
Oxazepam, 68
Oxcarbazepine, 431–432, 432*t*
Oxidative stress theory of aging, 8*t*, 9

Oxybutynin, 177–178, 177*t*, 227*t* for urge incontinence, 177*t*
Oxycodone (OxyIR, OxyContin), 136*t*, q95
Oxygen therapy, 130

P

PACE. *See* Program for All-inclusive Care of the Elderly
Pacemakers, 328, 329*t*
Paget's disease, 197*t*, 344
Pain
arch pain, 418
back pain, 410–411, 410*t*, 411–412, 412–414, 413*t*, q95
Checklist of Nonverbal Pain Indicators, 133
in cognitively impaired persons, 133, 134*t*
evaluation of, 400, 400*f*
Faces Pain Scale, 132
gait findings in, 183, 184*t*
heel pain, 417*t*, 418
hip pain, q99
knee pain, 397
lower back pain, 76, 410, 412, 413*t*, q2
McGill Pain Questionnaire, 132
neck pain, 410, 414–415
persistent, 131–139
phantom pain, 110
resources, 474–475
shoulder pain, 400, 401*f*, q92
Pain Disability Scale, 132
Pain disorder, 272, 272*t*
Pain management, 133–139, q95. *See also* Analgesia; Palliative care
activity recommendations for, 53*t*
aggressive, 25
for back pain, 414, q95
complementary and alternative medicine, 76
fundamental approaches to treatment, 133
for phantom pain, 110
pharmacotherapy, 133–137, 135*t*–136*t*
postoperative, 99–100
Painful swallowing, 358
Palliative care, 25, 125–131. *See also* Analgesia; Hospice care; Pain management
agencies and organizations, 470
endoscopic, 360
of nonpain symptoms, 128–131
Palsy
facial nerve (Bell's), 314
progressive supranuclear, 429–430
Pamelor, 135*t*, 253*t*. *See also* Nortriptyline
Pamidronate, 202, q30
Pancreatic cancer screening, 65*t*
Panic attacks, 258
Panic disorder, 258–259, 261*t*
Pantothenic acid, 163*t*
Pap smear, 61*t*, 62, 377
Papaverine, 386, 387*t*
for erectile dysfunction, 388

Paranoid personality disorder
features of, 267, 268*t*
therapeutic strategies for, 270, 271, 271*t*
Paraparesis, 183, 184*t*
Paraplegia, 183, 184*t*
Parathyroid gland disorders, 341–344
Parathyroid hormone
for osteoporosis, 200*t*, 202
secondary hyperparathyroidism, 196
Parkinsonism, 183, 184*t*
Parkinson's disease, 427–429
complementary and alternative medicine for, 77
and continence, 171–172, 173*t*
Parkinson's plus disease, 429
Paroxetine (Paxil), 251, 252, 252*t*
for depression, q89
for depressive features of behavioral disturbances in dementia, 216, 217*t*
drug interactions, 72
Paroxysmal atrial fibrillation, 328
Passive-aggressive personality disorder
features of, 267, 268*t*
therapeutic strategies for, 270, 271*t*
Patient-clinician communication, 41–42
addressing the health provider, 47
addressing the patient, 47
Patient-controlled analgesia (PCA), 100
Pauci-immune crescentic glomerulonephritis, 373
Paxil, 252*t*. *See also* Paroxetine
PC-SPES, 78–79
PCA. *See* Patient-controlled analgesia
Pediculosis capitis, 291
Pediculosis corporis, 291
Pedometers, 57
PEG. *See* Percutaneous endoscopic gastrostomy
Pelvic examination, 377
Pelvic floor support disorders, 379–381
Pelvic muscle exercises (PME) (Kegel's)
for incontinence, 177*t*, 178–179, 178*t*, 462
for vaginal prolapse, 380
Pelvic organ prolapse, 379–380, 380*t*, q90
Penile brachial pressure index, 386–387
Penile prosthesis, 387*t*, 388
Pentamidine, 299*t*
Pentoxifylline, 299*t*
Peptic ulcer disease, 360–361
Percutaneous endoscopic gastrostomy, 169–170
Percutaneous transluminal coronary angioplasty (PTCA), 319, 321, 330
Performance-based functional assessment, 185
Performance-Oriented Mobility Assessment, 43
Periodic limb movement disorder, 232–233, q11
Periodic limb movements during sleep, 232–233
Periodontal anatomy, 295*f*

Postprandial hypotension, 161
Posttraumatic stress disorder, 260, 261t
Postural abnormalities, 427
Postural awareness, 193t
Postural hypotension, 193t
Postvoiding residual volume (PVR), 176
Potassium, 71t, 164t
Potassium hydroxide, q69
Poverty rates, 2
Power of attorney, 445
PPD skin tests, 311
PPOs. *See* Preferred provider organizations
PPS. *See* Prospective payment system
Prader-Willi syndrome, 282t
Pramipexole, 232–233, 428
Pramlintide (Symlin), 356t
Prandin (repaglinide), 355t
Pravastatin, 322t
Prayer, 75
Prazosin, 390, 390t
Pre-ESRD care, 375
Prealbumin, 163–164
Precose (acarbose), 355t
Prednisolone, 71
Prednisone (Deltasone, Liquid Pred, Orasone)
    for giant cell arteritis, 406, q52
    perioperative, 98
    for persistent pain, 135t
    for polymyalgia rheumatica, 405
    for polymyositis and dermatomyositis, 409
Preferred provider organizations (PPOs), 38
Pregabalin (Lyrica), 135t
Prehypertension, 331, 331t
Preoperative assessment and management, 93–97
Preoperative cardiac care, 93–94, 95f
Presbycusis, 146–147
Presbyesophagus, 168–169
Prescription drugs. *See* Drugs; Pharmacotherapy
Pressure Sore Status Tool (PSST), 245, q96
Pressure stockings, 193t
Pressure Ulcer Scale for Healing (PUSH), 245, q96
Pressure ulcers, 238–246, q96
    Braden Scale, 239, 240, q96
    dressings for, 243, 244t
    guidelines for preventing, 239–240
    of heel, 240, 240t
    management of, 241–246, 242t
    Norton Scale, q96
    occlusive dressings for, q71
    prevention of, 239–240, 240–241, 240t, q76
    during rehabilitation, 104
    risk-assessment scales, 239–240
    staging system for, 241–243, 242t, 245
    support surfaces for persons at risk of, 241, 241t
    surgical repair of, 243
Presyncope, 151, 152

Prevention, 59–66. *See also* Screening
    delivery of services, 65–66
    of elder mistreatment, 80
    of falls, 188, 190–193
    of hip fracture recurrence, 108–109
    physical activity effects, 52
    potentially beneficial services lacking evidence, 64, 64t
    of pressure ulcers, 239–240, 240–241, 240t
    recommended services, 60–64, 61t
    services not indicated in older adults, 65–66
    services that have been demonstrated not to be beneficial, 65, 65t
    services to consider, 64–65
Preventive rehabilitation ("Prehab"), 104
Primary care providers, 119
Primary open-angle glaucoma (POAG), 143
Primidone, 227t
Private FFS plans, 38
Private practice model, 117
Probenecid, 399
Problem solving, 250t
Problem substance use, 275
Procainamide, 299t
Prochlorperazine, 128–129, 128t, 299t
Productivity, 18
Progestational agents, 446, 447t
Progesterone, 219
Program for All-inclusive Care of the Elderly (PACE), 37, 122–123
Progressive resistance training, q34
Progressive supranuclear palsy, 429–430
Prokinetic agents, 128–129, 128t
Promethazine, 130, 299t
Prompted voiding, 177, q40
    for stress and mixed urge and stress incontinence, 178t
    for urge incontinence, 177t
Propafenone, 299t, 453
Propantheline, 178
Propoxyphene (Darvon), 138
Propranolol, 299t, 453
Proprioceptive deficits, 183, 184t
Propulsion, 182t
Prospective payment system (PPS), 103, 119
Prostaglandin E$_1$, 386
Prostaglandins, 143t
Prostate cancer, 391–395, q30
    complementary and alternative medicine for, 78–79
    ethnic and racial differences in, 444, 444t
    hormonal agents for, 446, 447t
    localized disease, 393–394, 394t
    screening for, 64t, 392
    staging, 392–393, 393t
Prostate disease, 389–396
Prostate-specific antigen
    screening, 64t
    serum levels, 392, 393, q16, q30
Prostatectomy
    open, 390t

postprostatectomy stress UI, 180
    radical, 393–394, 394t
Prostatism, 389
Prostatitis, 395
Prostheses
    heart valves, 453t
    infections, 312–313
    penile, 387t, 388
Protein-energy undernutrition, 165
Protein requirements
    estimation of, 162t
    in hospitalized patients, 89
Proteinuria, 369–370
Proteus, 309
Proton-pump inhibitors, 359
Proventil (albuterol), 302t
Provider-sponsored organizations (PSOs), 38
Provigil (modafinil), 254t
Prozac, 252t. *See also* Fluoxetine
Pruritus, 288, q35
Pseudo-addiction, 137
Pseudoachalasia, q37
Pseudoclaudication, 411
Pseudodisease, 445
Pseudogout, 400
Pseudomembranous colitis, 365–366
Pseudomonas, 308
Pseudomonas aeruginosa, 309
Psoriasis, 288–289, 289f, q35
PSOs. *See* Provider-sponsored organizations
PSST. *See* Pressure Sore Status Tool
Psychiatric diseases and disorders, 231. *See also specific disorders*
    and continence, 171–172, 173t
    and mental retardation, 281–282
    resources, 475
Psychiatric emergency, q57
Psychoactive medications, 211–212
Psychodynamic therapy, short-term, 250t
Psychogenic dizziness, 156
Psychogenic erectile dysfunction, 385, 388
Psychologic assessment, 44
Psychosis
    associated with Alzheimer's disease, q97
    and continence, 171–172, 173t
    in dementia, 213, 218–219, 218t
    schizophrenia-like, 263f, 264
Psychosocial problems, 14–20, 231
Psychostimulants, 130
Psychotherapy, q18
    emotion-oriented, 209
    for late-life depression, 250, 250t
    for personality disorders, 270
Psychotic depression
    diagnosis of, 248
    electroconvulsive therapy for, 255
Psychotic disorders, 262–267
Psychotic symptoms, 213
    in delirium, 265
    major depression with, q33
    in mood disorder, 265

Rosacea, 285, 285*f*
Rosiglitazone (Avandia), 355*t*
Rosiglitazone and glimepiride (Avandaryl), 356*t*
Rosiglitazone and metformin (Avandamet), 356*t*
Rosuvastatin, 322*t*
Rotator cuff disease, 402–403
Rotator cuff tendonitis, q92
Roxanol, 136*t*. *See also* Morphine
Rule of double effect, 25

S

S-adenosylmethionine (SAM-e), 77
Saccharomyces boulardii, 366
Sacral fractures, osteoporotic, 410*t*, 412
Safe Return, 210
Safety, 210
Salflex (salsalate), 135*t*
Salicylates, 164*t*, 398
Salivary function, 297
Salivary glands, 294, 295*t*, 297
Salivary stones, q62
Salmeterol (Serevent), 302*t*
Salsalate (Disalcid, Mono-Gesic, Salflex), 135*t*
Saquinavir, 299*t*
Sarcopenia, 55
Saw palmetto, 78, 391
Scabies, 290–291, q35
Scheduled toileting, 177*t*, 178*t*
Schilling test, 439
Schizoid personality disorder
    features of, 267, 268*t*
    therapeutic strategies for, 270, 271*t*
Schizophrenia, 263–265
Schizophrenia-like psychosis, 263*f*, 264
Schizophrenia-like syndromes, 263–265
Schizotypal personality disorder
    features of, 267, 268*t*
    therapeutic strategies for, 270, 271*t*
Sciatica, 410*t*, 411
Scissoring, 182*t*
Screening
    attention screening examination, 222*t*
    cancer, 445
    colonoscopic, 366–367
    for dementia, 44
    for elder mistreatment, 81, 81*t*
    for glaucoma, 140, 143
    Hearing Handicap Inventory for the
        Elderly—Screening Version, 147, q13
    for hearing loss, 147
    for hormone hypersecretion in adrenal
        incidentalomas, 345–346, 345*t*
    nutrition, 163–165
    potential beneficial services lacking
        evidence, 64, 64*t*
    for prostate cancer, 392
    questionnaires, q84
    rapid, 41, 42*t*
    recommended services, 60–62, 61*t*
    for secondary osteoporosis, 197, 197*t*

services that have been demonstrated not
    to be beneficial, 65, 65*t*
services to consider, 64–65
terms to interpret tests, 464*t*
for urinary incontinence, 174, 175*t*
vestibular examination, 153–154
Seborrheic dermatitis, 284–285
Seborrheic keratoses, 291, 291*f*
Sedating antidepressants, 236, 237*t*
Sedative hypnotics, 172*t*
Seizures, 159*t*
    epilepsy, 431–432
    during rehabilitation, 105*t*
Selection bias, 445
Selective estrogen receptor modulators
    (SERMs), 200*t*, 201, 202
Selective serotonin-reuptake inhibitors
    (SSRIs), q89
    for anxiety, 258, 261*t*
    for depression, 251–252, 252*t*, 254
    for depressive features of behavioral
        disturbances in dementia, 216, 217*t*
    for mood disturbances in dementia, 216
    nutrient interactions, 164*t*
Selegiline, 428
Selenium, 163*t*
Self-care
    activities of daily living (ADLs), 43*t*
    decisions of, 21, 22*t*
    for lower back pain, 76
Self-efficacy beliefs, 17–18, 17*t*
Self-neglect, 82–83, 89
Semi-starvation, 165
Senescence. *See also* Aging
    clonal, 10
    DNA mutations or deletions during,
        10–11
    gene expression during, 11–12
    immune, 305
Senna (Senokot), 99*t*
Sensorineural hearing loss, q88
Sensory impairment. *See also* Hearing
        impairment; Visual impairment
    in hospitalized patients, 85*t*, 87
    interventions for, 85*t*
    and rehabilitation, 105
Sentinel node, 448
Sepsis, 307–308
Septicemia, 5–6, 6*t*
Serenoa repens (saw palmetto), 391
Serevent (salmeterol), 302*t*
SERMs. *See* Selective estrogen receptor
    modulators
Seroquel, 256*t*. *See also* Quetiapine
Serotonergic antagonists, 128–129, 128*t*
Serotonin norepinephrine-reuptake inhibitors,
    216, 217*t*, 261*t*
Sertraline (Zoloft), 251, 252, 252*t*
    for anxiety, 258
    for depression, 216, q55
    for depressive features of behavioral
        disturbances in dementia, 216, 217*t*
    Duke Somatic Algorithm for Geriatric
        Depression, 251

Serum albumin, 306
Serum cholesterol, 164
Serum creatinine, 369
Serum digoxin levels, q85
Serum lipids, 61, 61*t*, 64*t*
Serum PSA test, 392, 393
Sex therapy, 387*t*
Sexual function disorders, 382–388, 475
Sexuality
    female, 382–384
    male, 384–388
    resources, 475
SF-36 Health Survey, 45, 106
Sharp debridement, 243, 243*t*
Sheltered housing, 125
Shigella, 314
Shingles, 144–145
    reactivated, 313–314
SHMOs. *See* Social health maintenance
    organizations
Shoes, 330, 422
    multidensity inserts, 422
    therapeutic, 422
Short Form-36 Health Survey (SF-36), 45,
    106
Shortness of breath, q59, q68, q78
Shoulder pain, 400, 401*f*, q92
Sialoliths, q62
Side rails, q99
Sight problems. *See* Visual impairment
Sigmoidoscopy, flexible, 61*t*, 62
Sildenafil, 386, 387, 387*t*
Silver dressings, 244*t*, 245–246
Simvastatin, 322*t*, 330
Sinusitis, 4, 4*f*
Sirtuin-activating compounds, 13–14
Sitagliptan (Januvia), 356*t*
Sjögren's disease, 408
Sjögren's syndrome, 408
Skilled nursing facilities, 102, 103, q6
Skin cancer
    resources, 476
    screening for, 64, 64*t*
Skin care, 240, q76
Skin inspection, 64*t*
Skin problems. *See* Dermatologic diseases and
    disorders
SLE. *See* Systemic lupus erythematosus
Sleep
    age-related changes in, 230, q58
    changes with dementia, 233, q70
    evaluation of, 230
    in hospitals, 233–234
    in long-term-care settings, q19
    measures to improve, 234, 234*t*, 235–236,
        235*t*, q19, q58
    in nursing homes, 234, q19
    periodic limb movements during, 232–233
    REM sleep behavior disorder, 233
Sleep apnea, 231–232
    obstructive, 303
Sleep-disordered breathing, 231, 232

T

T₃. *See* Triiodothyronine

T₄. *See* Thyroxine

Tachyarrhythmias, ventricular, 161

Tachykinesia, 427

Tachyphemia, 427

Tacrine, 210

Tadalafil, 387, 387t

Tai Chi Chuan, 57, 192
    for osteoarthritis, 75
    for preventing falls, 193t

Tailor's bunion, 417t

Tamoxifen, 446, 447t

Tamsulosin, 390, 390t, q74

Tardive dyskinesia, 430, q97

Tardive dystonia, 430

Tarsal tunnel syndrome, q100

Taste dysfunction, 299t

Taste perception, 299

Teaching nursing homes, 117

Teams, rehabilitation, 104

Technetium bone scan, 413

Teeth, 294, 295f

Tegretol, 135t, 256t. *See also* Carbamazepine

Telemedicine, 123

Telomerase, 11

Telomeres, 11

Temazepam, 236, 237t

Temporal arteritis, 405, q38, q52

Temporal lobe lesions, 282t

Tenosynovitis, 417t

Terazosin, 390, 390t

Terfenadine, 299t

Teriparatide, 200t

Terminal illness. *See* End-of-life care;
    Palliative care

Terminology
    to interpret screening and diagnostic tests,
      464t
    preferred terms for cultural identity, 47

Testamentary competence, 21

Testosterone, 346–347

Testosterone replacement therapy, 346, q49

Testosterone supplementation, 347
    benefits and risks of, 347, 347t
    for erectile dysfunction, 388
    for female sexual dysfunction, 383, 384t

Tetanus booster, 61t

Tetanus vaccination, 64

Tetracyclines, 299t

Thallium perfusion scintigraphy, 317–318

Theophylline, 68, 164t, 430

Thiamin, 163t

Thiazolidinediones, 172t, 355t

Thinking problems. *See* Cognitive impairment

Thiopental, 67

Thrombin-antithrombin complex, 440

Thrombocythemia, essential, 441, 442

Thrombocytopenia, 440

Thromboembolism
    pulmonary, 303–304
    venous, 109, 453t

Thrombolytics, 455t

Thrombopathy, 441

Thyroid cancer, 340–341

Thyroid disorders, 338–341
    screening for, 64t

Thyroid hormone replacement, 197t

Thyroid nodules, 340, 342f, q51

Thyroid-stimulating hormone (TSH), 340,
    341f

Thyrotoxicosis
    apathetic, 340
    T₃, 340

Thyroxine (T₄)
    high T₄ syndrome, 340
    low T₄ syndrome, 338

Thyroxine (T₄) replacement, 339

Tiagabine, 431–432, 432t

Tilade (nedocromil), 302t

Tilt-table testing, 160

Tiludronate, 202

Timed Get Up and Go (TUG) test, 43, 185,
    190

Timed voiding, 177

Timolol, 143t

Tinea pedis, 419f, q69

Tinea unguium, 420

Tinetti Performance-Oriented Mobility
    Assessment, 43

Tinzaparin (Innohep), 454t

Tiotropium (Spiriva), 302t

Tirofiban, 319

Tissue-plasminogen activator (rt-PA), 425

Tocainide, 299t

α-Tocopherol, 163t. *See also* Vitamin E

Toenail deformities, 419–420

Toileting, scheduled, 177t, 178t

Tolcapone, 429

Tolerance, 137. *See also* Dependency

Tolmetin, 453

Tolterodine, 177–178, 177t

Tooth dentin changes, 294, 295t

Toothlessness, 296–297

Topiramate, 431–432, 432t

Toremifene, 446, 447t

Total hip and knee arthroplasty, 109

Total iron binding capacity, 438

Toxic or metabolic encephalopathy, 220

Tradition, 49

Tramadol (Ultram), 402
    contraindications to, 138
    drug interactions, 72
    for persistent pain, 136t

Transdermal fentanyl (Duragesic), 136t

Transient ischemic attack, 61t

Transitions
    from hospital care, 91–92
    planning for, 100

Transparent film, 244t

Transplantation, renal, 375–376

Transrectal ultrasound-guided biopsy, 392

Transthoracic echocardiography, 312

Transurethral incision of the prostate, 390t,
    391

Transurethral resection of the prostate, 390t,
    391

Transurethral vaporization of the prostate,
    390t, 391

Transvaginal ultrasound, q63

Trastuzumab, 447

Traumatic experiences
    history of, 48
    posttraumatic stress disorder, 260, 261t

Trazodone (Desyrel), 254t
    for anxiety disorders, 261t
    for depressive features of behavioral
      disturbances in dementia, 216, 217t
    distribution of, 67
    for insomnia, 236, 237t
    for sleep problems, 219, 236, q70
    warfarin interactions, 453

Tremor, essential, 430–431

Trendelenburg gait, 182t

Triamcinolone (Azmacort), 302t, 400

Triazolam, 227t, 236

Trichophyton mentagrophytes var. *interdigitale*,
    420

Trichophyton rubrum, 420, q69

Tricosal (choline magnesium trisalicylate),
    135t

Tricyclic antidepressants, 251, 252, 253t
    for depressive features of behavioral
      disturbances in dementia, 216, 217t
    for persistent pain, 135t, 138

Trifluoperazine, 299t

Trigger points, myofascial, 402

Trihexyphenidyl, 430

Triiodothyronine (T₃), 338

Triiodothyronine (T₃) thyrotoxicosis, 340

Trilisate (choline magnesium trisalicylate),
    135t

Trimethoprim, 164t, 453

Trimethoprim-sulfamethoxazole (TMP-SMX),
    310

Trochanteric bursitis, 404

Trospium, 177t, 178

Truth telling, 26

Try This (Hartford Institute for Geriatric
    Nursing), 41

Tube-feeding solutions, 169, 170t

Tuberculosis, 310–311

Tumor, regional node, metastasis (TNM)
    staging system, 392–393, 393t

Tumors, 410t

Turn en bloc, 182t

Two Cal HN, 170t

Tylenol, 135t. *See also* Acetaminophen

Tzanck smear, 290

U

UI. *See* Urinary incontinence

Ulcers
    arterial, 286–287, 287t
    peptic ulcer disease, 360–361

INDEX OF *GRS6* EDITORS AND AUTHORS

GRS6 EDITORIAL BOARD

CHIEF EDITORS

Peter Pompei, MD
Editor in Chief, Syllabus
Associate Professor of Medicine
Stanford University School of Medicine
Stanford, CA

John B. Murphy, MD
Editor in Chief, Questions
Director of Graduate Medical Education, Lifespan
Associate Director, Division of Geriatrics, Department
   of Medicine
Professor of Medicine and Family Medicine
Brown Medical School
Office of Graduate Medical Education
Providence, RI

SYLLABUS EDITORS

Colleen Christmas, MD
Assistant Professor of Medicine
Johns Hopkins University School of Medicine
Division of Geriatric Medicine and Gerontology
Baltimore, MD

Steven R. Counsell, MD
Mary Elizabeth Mitchell Professor of Geriatrics
Director, Indiana University Geriatrics Program
Indiana University School of Medicine
Indianapolis, IN

G. Paul Eleazer, MD
Director, Division of Geriatrics
University of South Carolina, School of Medicine
Columbia, SC

Anne R. Fabiny, MD
Assistant Professor of Medicine
Harvard Medical School
Boston, MA

Susan K. Schultz, MD
Associate Professor, Department of Psychiatry
University of Iowa College of Medicine
Iowa City, IA

QUESTION EDITORS

William J. Burke, MD
Professor and Vice Chair, Psychiatry
University of Nebraska Medical Center
Omaha, NE

Alison A. Moore, MD, MPH
Associate Professor of Medicine
David Geffen School of Medicine at UCLA
Division of Geriatrics
Los Angeles, CA

Gail M. Sullivan, MD, MPH
Associate Professor of Medicine
Associate Director for Education
UConn Center on Aging
University of Connecticut School of Medicine
Farmington, CT

CONSULTING EDITOR FOR PHARMACOTHERAPY

Todd P. Semla, MS, PharmD
Clinical Pharmacy Specialist
Department of Veterans Affairs
Pharmacy Benefits Management & Strategic Health
   Group
Hines, IL
Associate Professor
Department of Psychiatry and Behavioral Sciences
The Feinberg School of Medicine
Northwestern University
Chicago, IL

CONSULTING EDITOR FOR ETHNOGERIATRICS

Carmel Bitondo Dyer, MD
Associate Professor of Medicine
Baylor College of Medicine
Director, Geriatrics Program
Harris County Hospital District
Houston, TX

SPECIAL ADVISORS

James T. Pacala, MD, MS
Associate Professor
Distinguished University Teaching Professor
Department of Family Medicine and Community
   Health
University of Minnesota Medical School
Minneapolis, MN

Stephanie Studenski, MD, MPH
Professor, Department of Medicine (geriatrics)
Staff Physician, VA Pittsburgh GRECC
Pittsburgh, PA

CONSULTING QUESTION REVIEWERS

Itamar B. Abrass, MD
Professor and Division Head,
Gerontology and Geriatric Medicine
University of Washington
Harborview Medical Center
Seattle, Washington

Jane F. Potter, MD
Harris Professor of Geriatric Medicine
Chief, Section on Geriatrics and Gerontology
Department of Internal Medicine
University of Nebraska Medical Center
Omaha, Nebraska

GRS6 CHAPTER AUTHORS

Sumaira Z. Aasi, MD
Assistant Professor
Department of Dermatology
Yale University School of Medicine
New Haven, CT

Harold P. Adams, Jr., MD
Professor and Director
Division of Cerebrovascular Diseases, Department of
  Neurology
University of Iowa Hospitals and Clinics
Iowa City, IA

Reva N. Adler, MD, MPH
Medical Director, STAT Centre and At-home
  Supports
Vancouver Hospital & Vancouver Community Health
  Services
Clinical Associate Professor, Division of Geriatric
  Medicine
University of British Columbia
Vancouver, BC

Marc E. Agronin, MD
Director of Mental Health Services
Miami Jewish Home and Hospital for the Aged
Assistant Professor of Psychiatry
Miller School of Medicine at the University of Miami
Miami, FL

Cathy A. Alessi, MD
Associate Director
Clinical Programs: Geriatric Research, Education and
  Clinical Center, Sepulveda Division
Veterans Administration Greater Los Angeles
  Healthcare System
Professor, University of California, Los Angeles
Multicampus Program in Geriatric Medicine and
  Gerontology
Sepulveda, CA

Neil B. Alexander, MD
Professor, Division of Geriatric Medicine
Department of Internal Medicine
Research Professor, Institute of Gerontology
University of Michigan
Director, VA Ann Arbor Health Care System Geriatric
  Research, Education and Clinical Center
Ann Arbor, MI

Wilbert S. Aronow, MD
Clinical Professor of Medicine
Divisions of Cardiology, Geriatrics, and
  Pulmonary/Critical Care
Westchester Medical Center and New York Medical
  College
Valhalla, NY
Adjunct Professor of Geriatrics and Adult
  Development
Mount Sinai School of Medicine
New York, NY

Priscilla Faith Bade, MD, MS
Associate Professor of Internal Medicine
University of South Dakota School of Medicine
Rapid City, SD

Cynthia Barton, RN, MSN
Gerontological Nurse Practitioner
Memory and Aging Center
Assistant Clinical Professor, School of Nursing
University of California, San Francisco
San Francisco, CA

Marc R. Blackman, MD
Chief, Endocrine Section
Laboratory of Clinical Investigation
National Center for Complementary and Alternative
  Medicine
National Institutes of Health
Bethesda, MD

Caroline S. Blaum, MD, MS
Associate Professor of Internal Medicine
Division of Geriatric Medicine
University of Michigan
Research Scientist, Ann Arbor DVAMC Geriatric
    Research, Education and Clinical Center
Ann Arbor, MI

Harrison G. Bloom, MD
Senior Associate
International Longevity Center, USA
Associate Clinical Professor
Brookdale Department of Geriatrics and Adult
    Development
Mount Sinai School of Medicine
New York, NY

Chad Boult, MD, MPH, MBA
Professor of Public Health
Director, Lipitz Center for Integrated Health Care
Johns Hopkins Bloomberg School of Public Health
The Johns Hopkins University
Baltimore, MD

Cynthia J. Brown, MD
GRECC Investigator
Medical Director
Falls Prevention and Mobility Clinic
Birmingham/Atlanta VA Geriatric Research, Education
    and Clinical Center
Assistant Professor
University of Alabama at Birmingham
Birmingham, AL

David M. Buchner, MD, MPH
Chief, Physical Activity and Health Branch, Division of
    Nutrition and Physical Activity
Centers for Disease Control and Prevention
Atlanta, GA

Lynda C. Burton, ScD
Associate Professor
Department of Health Policy and Management
The Johns Hopkins Bloomberg School of Public
    Health
Baltimore, MD

David Bush, MD
Director, Cardiac Catheterization Laboratory
Johns Hopkins Bayview Medical Center
Associate Professor of Medicine
Division of Cardiology
The Johns Hopkins University School of Medicine
Baltimore, MD

Erin L. Cassidy, PhD
Research Associate
Department of Psychiatry and Behavioral Sciences
Stanford University School of Medicine
Palo Alto, CA

Gurkamal S. Chatta, MD
Associate Professor of Medicine
Division of Hematology-Oncology
University of Pittsburgh
Pittsburgh, PA

Colleen Christmas, MD
Assistant Professor of Medicine
Division of Geriatric Medicine and Gerontology
The Johns Hopkins University School of Medicine
Baltimore, MD

Anne L. Coleman, MD, PhD
Professor of Ophthalmology and Epidemiology
Frances and Ray Stark Chair of Ophthalmology
Jules Stein Eye Institute
University of California, Los Angeles
Los Angeles, CA

Leo M. Cooney, Jr., MD
Humana Foundation Professor of Geriatric Medicine
Chief, Section of Geriatric Medicine
Yale University School of Medicine
New Haven, CT

G. Willy Davila, MD
Chairman, Department of Gynecology
Head, Section of Urogynecology and Reconstructive
    Pelvic Surgery
Cleveland Clinic Florida
Ft. Lauderdale, FL

Margaret A. Drickamer, MD
Associate Professor of Medicine (Geriatrics)
Yale University School of Medicine
New Haven, CT

Catherine E. DuBeau, MD
Associate Professor of Medicine
Section of Geriatrics
University of Chicago
Chicago, IL

Pamela W. Duncan, PhD
Professor, College of Medicine
Career Health Scientist—Department of Veteran
 Affairs
Director of Department of Veterans Affairs Center of
 Excellence in Rehabilitation Outcomes
Department of Aging and Geriatrics Research
Co-Director, Institute of Aging
Department of Aging and Geriatric Research
University of Florida
Gainseville, FL

G. Paul Eleazer, MD
Director, Division of Geriatrics
University of South Carolina School of Medicine
Columbia, SC

E. Wesley Ely, MD, MPH
Associate Professor of Medicine
Associate Director of Aging Research
Tennessee Valley Geriatric Research, Education and
 Clinical Center
Allergy, Pulmonary and Critical Care
Vanderbilt University School of Medicine
Nashville, TN

William B. Ershler, MD
Director Institute for Advanced Studies in Aging and
 Geriatric Medicine
Washington, DC

Terry T. Fulmer, PhD, RN
The Erline Perkins McGriff Professor and Dean
College of Nursing
New York University
New York, NY

Angela Gentili, MD
Associate Professor of Internal Medicine
Director, Geriatrics Fellowship Training Program
VA Medical Center/Virginia Commonwealth
 University
Richmond, VA

Thomas M. Gill, MD
Associate Professor of Medicine
Yale University School of Medicine
New Haven, CT

Lisa J. Granville, MD
Professor and Associate Chair
Department of Geriatrics
Florida State University College of Medicine
Tallahassee, FL

David A. Gruenewald, MD
Associate Professor of Medicine
Division of Gerontology and Geriatric Medicine
Department of Medicine
University of Washington School of Medicine
Staff Physician, Geriatrics Research, Education and
 Clinical Center
VA Puget Sound Health Care System
Seattle, WA

Arthur E. Helfand, DPM
Professor Emeritus
Temple University School of Podiatric Medicine
Retired Chair, Department of Community Health,
 Aging & Health Policy
Adjunct Professor, Department of Medicine
Temple University School of Medicine
Philadelphia, PA

Kenneth W. Hepburn, PhD
Professor and Associate Dean for Research
School of Nursing
University of Minnesota
Minneapolis, MN

Kevin Paul High, MD, MSc
Associate Professor of Medicine
Sections of Infectious Diseases and
 Hematology/Oncology
Wake Forest University School of Medicine
Winston Salem, NC

Gordon L. Jensen, MD, PhD
Director, Vanderbilt Center for Human Nutrition
Professor of Medicine
Vanderbilt University Medical Center
Nashville, TN

Donald A. Jurivich, DO
Chief, Section of Geriatric Medicine
Vitoux Associate Professor of Medicine
University of Illinois at Chicago Medical School
Chicago, IL

Jennifer M. Kapo, MD
Assistant Professor of Clinical Medicine
Division of Geriatrics
University of Pennsylvania
Philadelphia, PA

Judith D. Kasper, PhD
Professor, Department of Health Policy and
 Management
The Johns Hopkins University Bloomberg School of
 Public Health
Baltimore, MD

Jurgis Karuza, PhD
Visiting Professor of Rochester Medical Center
Rochester, NY
Professor and Chair, Psychology Department
State University College at Buffalo
Buffalo, NY

Paul R. Katz, MD
Professor of Medicine
Chief, Division of Geriatrics
University of Rochester School of Medicine and
    Dentistry
Rochester, NY

Catherine Lee Kelleher, MD
Nephrology Division
Denver Health Medical Center
University of Colorado Medical Center
Denver, CO

Gary J. Kennedy, MD
Professor of Psychiatry and Behavioral Science
Albert Einstein College of Medicine
Director, Division of Geriatric Psychiatry
Montefiore Medical Center
Bronx, NY

Anne M. Kenny, MD
Associate Professor of Medicine
UConn Center on Aging
University of Connecticut Health Center
Farmington, CT

Douglas P. Kiel, MD, MPH
Associate Professor of Medicine
Harvard Medical School Division on Aging
Director, Medical Research
HRCA Research and Training Institute
Boston, MA

Kurt Kroenke, MD
Professor of Medicine
Indiana University School of Medicine
Senior Scientist
Regenstrief Institute for Health Care
Indianapolis, IN

C. Seth Landefeld, MD
Professor of Medicine
Chief, Division of Geriatrics
Director, UCSF/Mount Zion Center on Aging
University of California, San Francisco
Associate Chief of Staff, Geriatrics and Extended Care
San Francisco VA Medical Center
San Francisco, CA

Melinda S. Lantz, MD
Director of Psychiatry
Jewish Home and Hospital
Assistant Professor, Department of Geriatrics and
    Adult Development
Mount Sinai School of Medicine
New York, NY

Robert Dean Lindeman, MD
Professor Emeritus of Medicine
University of New Mexico School of Medicine
Albuquerque, NM

David A. Lipschitz, MD, PhD
Professor of Geriatrics
Chair, Donald W. Reynolds Department of Geriatrics
University of Arkansas for Medical Sciences
Little Rock, AR

Dan L. Longo, MD
Scientific Director
National Institute on Aging
Baltimore, MD

Courtney H. Lyder, ND, GNP
University of Virginia Medical Center Professor
Chairman, Department of Acute and Specialty Care
University of Virginia School of Nursing
Charlottesville, VA

Constantine G. Lyketsos, MD, MHS
Professor of Psychiatry and Behavioral Sciences
Co-Director, Division of Geriatric Psychiatry and
    Neuropsychiatry
The Johns Hopkins University and Hospital
Baltimore, MD

William L. Lyons, MD
Assistant Professor
Section of Geriatrics and Gerontology
Department of Internal Medicine
University of Nebraska Medical Center
Omaha, NE

Edward R. Marcantonio, MD, SM
Associate Professor of Medicine
Harvard Medical School
Director of Research
Division of General Medicine and Primary Care
Beth Israel Deaconess Medical Center
Boston, MA

Coleman O. Martin, MD
Clinical Associate
Department of Neurology
University of Iowa Hospitals and Clinics
Iowa City, IA

Alvin M. Matsumoto, MD
Professor, Department of Medicine
University of Washington School of Medicine
Division of Gerontology and Geriatric Medicine
Director, Clinical Research Unit
Associate Director, Geriatric Research, Education, and
    Clinical Center
VA Puget Sound Health Care System
Seattle, Washington

Robert McCann, MD
Professor of Medicine
University of Rochester School of Medicine and
    Dentistry
Highland Hospital Department of Medicine
Rochester, NY

Barbara E. Moquin, PhD(c), MSN, APRN
Senior Nurse Specialist (Research)
National Center for Complementary and Alternative
    Medicine
National Institutes of Health
Division of Intramural Research
Bethesda, MD

R. Sean Morrison, MD
Hermann Merkin Professor of Palliative Care
Professor of Geriatrics and Medicine
Vice-Chair for Research
Brookdale Department of Geriatrics and Adult
    Development
Mount Sinai School of Medicine
New York, NY

Thomas Mulligan, MD
Ruth S. Jewett Professor of Medicine
Chief, University of Florida Division of Geriatrics
Director, Geriatrics Research, Education and Clinical
    Center
North Florida/South Georgia Veterans Health System
Gainesville, FL

David W. Oslin, MD
Associate Professor
Geriatric and Addiction Psychiatry
University of Pennsylvania
Philadelphia, PA

Stacie T. Pinderhughes, MD
Assistant Professor
Albert Einstein College of Medicine
Medical Director
Harlem Community Hospice of Continuum
    Healthcare
New York, NY

Peter Pompei, MD
Associate Professor of Medicine
Stanford University School of Medicine
Stanford, CA

James S. Powers, MD
Associate Professor of Medicine
Vanderbilt University Medical Center
Nashville, TN

Karen M. Prestwood, MD
Associate Professor of Medicine
UConn Center on Aging
University of Connecticut Health Center
Farmington, CT

Peter V. Rabins, MD
Professor of Psychiatry, Medicine, Mental Health and
    Health Policy and Management
Johns Hopkins Medical Institution
Baltimore, MD

John W. Rachow, PhD, MD
Assistant Clinical Professor
Department of Medicine
University of Iowa College of Medicine
Iowa City, IA

Paula A. Rochon, MD, MPH
Associate Professor
Department of Medicine and Health Policy
    Management and Evaluation
University of Toronto
Senior Scientist and Assistant Director
Kunin-Lunenfeld Applied Research Unit
Baycrest Centre for Geriatric Care
Scientist, Institute for Clinical Evaluative Sciences
Toronto, ON

David Sarraf, MD
Assistant Clinical Professor of Ophthalmology
Jules Stein Eye Institute, UCLA School of Medicine
    and the Greater Los Angeles
VA Healthcare Center
Assistant Professor of Ophthalmology
Martin L. King Medical Center/Charles R. Drew
    University of Medicine
Los Angeles, CA

Todd P. Semla, PharmD, MS
Clinical Pharmacy Specialist
Department of Veterans Affairs
Pharmacy Benefits Management & Strategic Health
    Group
Hines, IL
Associate Professor
Department of Psychiatry and Behavioral Sciences
The Feinberg School of Medicine
Northwestern University
Chicago, IL

Kenneth Shay, DDS, MS
Director of Geriatric Programs
Office of Geriatrics and Extended Care
VA Central Office, Washington, DC
Adjunct Professor of Dentistry
University of Michigan School of Dentistry
Ann Arbor, MI

Javaid I. Sheikh, MD
Professor
Department of Psychiatry and Behavioral Sciences
Stanford University School of Medicine
Stanford, CA
Chief of Staff
VA Palo Alto Health Care System
Palo Alto, CA

Gary W. Small, MD
Parlow-Solomon Professor of Psychiatry and
    Biobehavioral Sciences
Director, UCLA Center on Aging
University of California, Los Angeles
Los Angeles, CA

Stephanie A. Studenski, MD, MPH
Professor, Department of Medicine (Geriatrics)
Staff Physician
Veterans Affairs Pittsburgh Geriatric Research,
    Education and Clinical Center
Pittsburgh, PA

Mark A. Supiano, MD
Professor and Chief, Division of Geriatric Medicine
University of Utah Health Science Center
Director, Veterans Affairs Salt Lake City
Geriatric Research, Education and Clinical Center
Executive Director, University of Utah Center on
    Aging
Salt Lake City, UT

George Triadafilopoulos, MD
Clinical Professor of Medicine
Division of Gastroenterology and Hepatology
Stanford University School of Medicine
Stanford, CA

Bruce R. Troen, MD
Associate Professor of Medicine
Miller School of Medicine
University of Miami
Geriatric Research, Education and Clinical Center
Miami Veterans Affairs Medical Center
Miami, FL

Andrew C. Warren, MB, BS, DPhil
Attending Physician, Sheppard Pratt Hospital
Associate Professor of Psychiatry
The Johns Hopkins University School of Medicine
Baltimore, MD

Debra K. Weiner, MD
Associate Professor of Medicine, Psychiatry and
    Anesthesiology
University of Pittsburgh School of Medicine
Pittsburgh, PA

Kristine Yaffe, MD
Associate Professor
Departments of Psychiatry, Neurology, Biostatistics
    and Epidemiology
University of California, San Francisco
Chief, Geriatric Psychiatry
San Francisco Veterans Administration Medical Center
San Francisco, CA

GRS6 QUESTION AND CRITIQUE AUTHORS

Reva N. Adler, MD, MPH
Medical Director, STAT Centre and At-home
    Supports
Vancouver Hospital and Vancouver Community
    Health Services
Clinical Associate Professor
Division of Geriatric Medicine
University of British Columbia
Vancouver, BC

Kathryn A. Atchison, DDS, MPH
Professor and Associate Dean for Research
School of Dentistry
University of California, Los Angeles
Los Angeles, CA

Sidney T. Bogardus, Jr., MD
Associate Professor of Medicine
Yale University School of Medicine
New Haven, CT

Kenneth Brummel-Smith, MD
Charlotte Edwards Maguire Professor of Geriatrics
Chair, Department of Geriatrics
Florida State University College of Medicine
Tallahassee, FL

Susan Charette, MD
Assistant Clinical Professor
Division of Geriatrics
Department of Medicine
University of California, Los Angeles
Los Angeles, CA

Pejman Cohan, MD
Assistant Professor of Medicine
Co-Director, Pituitary Program
School of Medicine
University of California, Los Angeles
Los Angeles, CA

Leo M. Cooney, Jr., MD
Humana Foundation Professor of Geriatric Medicine
Chief, Section of Geriatric Medicine
Yale University School of Medicine
New Haven, CT

Robert S. Crausman, MD, MMS
Chief Administrative Officer
Rhode Island Board of Medical Licensure and
  Discipline
Providence, RI

James Cummins, MD
Staff Psychiatrist
OhioHealth Behavioral Health
Columbus, OH

Margaret A. Drickamer, MD
Associate Professor
Yale University School of Medicine
New Haven, CT

Edmund H. Duthie, Jr, MD
Professor of Medicine (Geriatrics/Gerontology)
Chief, Division of Geriatrics and Gerontology
Medical College of Wisconsin
Lead Physician, Geriatrics Section, Consultant Care
  Division
VA Medical Center, Milwaukee
Milwaukee, WI

Carmel Bitondo Dyer, MD
Associate Professor of Medicine
Baylor College of Medicine
Director, Geriatrics Program
Harris County Hospital District
Houston, TX

Michelle S. Eslami, MD
Associate Professor of Medicine
Division of Geriatrics
David Geffen School of Medicine
University of California, Los Angeles
Los Angeles, CA

Mark H. Fleisher, MD
Associate Professor of Psychiatry
Medical Director, Adult Community Psychiatry Clinics
Director, Neurodevelopmental Psychiatry
University of Nebraska College of Medicine
Omaha, NE

Alastair J. Flint, MB
Professor of Psychiatry
University of Toronto
Head, Geriatric Psychiatry Program
University Health Network
Toronto, ON

David G. Folks, MD
Professor of Psychiatry
University of Nebraska College of Medicine
Omaha, NE

Christine Himes Fordyce, MD
Medicare Medical Director
Group Health Cooperative
Seattle, WA

Andrea R. Fox, MD, MPH
Associate Director
Clinical Care GRECC
VA Pittsburgh Healthcare System
Associate Professor of Medicine
University of Pittsburgh
Pittsburgh, PA

Angela Gentili, MD
Associate Professor of Internal Medicine
Director, Geriatrics Fellowship Program
VA Medical Center/Virginia Commonwealth
  University
Richmond, VA

Mary Kane Goldstein, MD, MS
Associate Director for Clinical Services
Geriatrics Research Education and Clinical Center
VA Palo Alto Health Care Systems
Professor of Medicine
Center for Primary Care and Outcomes Research
Stanford University
Palo Alto, CA

Shelly L. Gray, PharmD, MS, BCPS
Director, Geriatric Pharmacy Program
Associate Professor, School of Pharmacy
Seattle, WA

Nathan Herrmann, MD
Professor, Department of Psychiatry
University of Toronto
Head, Division of Geriatric Psychiatry
Sunnybrook & Women's College Health Science
    Centre
Toronto, ON

Kevin Paul High, MD, MSc
Associate Professor of Medicine
Sections on Infectious Diseases and
    Hematology/Oncology
Wake Forest University School of Medicine
Winston Salem, NC

Michele Iannuzzi-Sucich, MD
Family Practice and Geriatrics
Modena Family Practice
Modena, NY

Gail Ishiyama, MD
Assistant Professor
Department of Neurology
Division of Neurotology
University of California, Los Angeles
Los Angeles, CA

Thomas Vincent Jones, MD, MPH
Associate Editor
The Merck Manuals
Merck & Co, Inc.
Blue Bell, PA

Fran E. Kaiser, MD
Chief Executive Officer
Kaiser and Associates Consulting
Clinical Professor of Medicine
University of Texas Southwestern Medical School
Dallas, TX
Adjunct Professor of Medicine
St. Louis University School of Medicine
St. Louis, MO

Anne Kenny, MD
Associate Professor of Medicine
UConn Center on Aging
University of Connecticut Health Center
Farmington, CT

Mary B. King, MD
Assistant Professor of Medicine
University of Connecticut School of Medicine
Geriatrician, Hartford Hospital
Division of Geriatric Medicine and Gerontology
Hartford, CT

George A. Kuchel, MD
Director, University Connecticut Center on Aging
Chief, Division of Geriatric Medicine
University of Connecticut Health Center
Farmington, CT

Robert K. Lee, DPM
Assistant Clinical Professor
David Geffen School of Medicine
University of California, Los Angeles
Los Angeles, CA

Michael C. Lindberg, MD
Director of Clinical Inpatient Services
Department of Medicine
Hartford Hospital
Clinical Associate Professor
University of Connecticut School of Medicine
Hartford, CT

Shari M. Ling, MD
Clinical Research Branch
National Institute on Aging
Intramural Research Program
Baltimore, MD

Constantine G. Lyketsos, MD, MHS
Professor of Psychiatry and Behavioral Sciences
Co-Director, Division of Geriatric Psychiatry and
    Neuropsychiatry
The Johns Hopkins University and Hospital
Baltimore, MD

Mathew S. Maurer, MD
The Advanced Cardiac Care Center
Columbia University
Irving Assistant Professor of Medicine
Director, Clinical Cardiovascular Research Laboratory
    for the Elderly
Columbia University College of Physicians and
    Surgeons
New York, NY

Ellen McMahon, MD
Assistant Professor
University of Massachusetts Medical School
Oak Bluffs, MA

Lynn McNicoll, MD
Assistant Professor of Medicine
Geriatrician
Division of Geriatrics
Rhode Island Hospital
Providence, RI

Daniel Ari Mendelson, MS, MD
Assistant Professor of Medicine
Division of Geriatrics
University of Rochester School of Medicine and
    Dentistry
Medical Director
Acute Care for Elders Unit, Highland Hospital
Medical Director
Visiting Nurse Service of Rochester and Monroe
    County
Rochester, NY

Laura Mosqueda, MD
Director of Geriatrics
Professor of Family Medicine
Ronald W. Reagan Endowed Chair in Geriatric
    Medicine
University of California, Irvine School of Medicine
Orange, CA

Benoit H. Mulsant, MD
Professor of Psychiatry
Center for Addiction and Mental Health
University of Toronto
Toronto, ON

Arash Naeim, MD, PhD
Assistant Professor of Medicine
University of California, Los Angeles
Los Angeles, CA

Joseph G. Ouslander, MD
Professor of Medicine and Nursing
Director, Division of Geriatric Medicine and
    Gerontology
Chief Medical Officer
Wesley Woods Center of Emory University
Director, Emory Center for Health in Aging
Research Scientist
Birmingham/Atlanta VA Geriatric Research, Education
    and Clinical Center
Atlanta, GA

Ronald Frederick Pfeiffer, MD
Professor and Vice Chair
Department of Neurology
University of Tennessee Health Science Center
Memphis, TN

James T. Pacala, MD, MS
Associate Professor
Distinguished University Teaching Professor
Department of Family Medicine and Community
    Health
University of Minnesota Medical School
Minneapolis, MN

Joe W. Ramsdell, MD
Professor and Head
Division of General Internal Medicine/Geriatrics
University of California, San Diego
UCSD Medical Center
San Diego, CA

Anthony E. Ranno, PharmD
Clinical Education Consultant
Pfizer Inc.
Sherwood, OR

Michael W. Rich, MD
Associate Professor of Medicine
Washington University School of Medicine
Director, Cardiac Rapid Evaluation Unit
Barnes-Jewish Hospital
St. Louis, MO

Debra Saliba, MD, MPH
Research Associate
VA Health Services Research and Development
Center for the Study of Healthcare Provider Behavior
Sepulveda, CA

Gary Schiller, MD
Department of Medicine
Division of Hematology/Oncology
School of Medicine
University of California, Los Angeles
Los Angeles, CA

Nancy Shafer Clark, MD
Assistant Professor, Medicine and Geriatrics
University of Rochester
Rochester, NY

Alan M. Singer, DPM
Department of Medicine
Division of Podiatry
University of California, Los Angeles
Los Angeles, CA

Upinder Singh, MD
Clinical Associate Professor
School of Medicine, UNR
Chief of Geriatrics
Southwest Medical Associates
Sierra Health Services
Las Vegas, NV

Monica Stallworth Kolimas, MD
Faculty, Harvard Division on Aging
Shattuck House, Harvard University
Boston, MA

David H. Stern, MD
Specialized Ambulatory Geriatric Evaluation Clinic
  (S+AGE)
Sherman Oaks, CA

Gwen K. Sterns, MD
Chief, Department of Ophthalmology
Rochester General Hospital
Clinical Professor of Ophthalmology
University of Rochester Eye Institute
Rochester, NY

Dennis H. Sullivan, MD
Director, Geriatric Research Education and Clinical
  Center
Central Arkansas Veteran's Healthcare System
Vice Chairman and Professor
Donald W. Reynolds Department of Geriatrics
University of Arkansas for Medical Sciences
Little Rock, AR

Mark Supiano, MD
Professor and Chief, Division of Geriatric Medicine
University of Utah Health Science Center
Director, VA Salt Lake City Geriatric Research,
  Education and Clinical Center
Executive Director, University of Utah Center on
  Aging
Salt Lake City, UT

Robert A. Sweet, MD
Associate Professor of Psychiatry
Vice-Chair, Institutional Review Board
University of Pittsburgh
Pittsburgh, PA

David C. Thomas, MD, MS
Associate Professor of Medicine and Rehabilitation
Department of Medicine, Division of General Internal
  Medicine
Medical Director, Ambulatory Care/Outpatient
  Services
Mount Sinai School of Medicine
New York, NY

Corina M. Velehorschi, MD
Adjunct Professor of Psychiatry
University of Western Ontario
Windsor Regional Hospital
Windsor, ON

Katherine Ward, MD
Assistant Clinical Professor
Division of Geriatric Medicine
University of California, Los Angeles
Los Angeles, CA

Michael R. Wasserman, MD
Senior Care of Colorado
Assistant Clinical Professor
University of Colorado Health Science Center
Denver, CO

Barbara E. Weinstein, PhD
Executive Officer, Clinical Doctoral Programs
The Graduate Center, CUNY
Professor, Lehman College, CUNY
Bronx, NY

Steven P. Wengel, MD
Chair, Department of Psychiatry
University of Nebraska Medical Center
Omaha, NE

Index

DISCLOSURE OF FINANCIAL INTERESTS

As an accredited provider of Continuing Medical Education, the American Geriatrics Society continuously strives to ensure that the education activities planned and conducted by our faculty meet generally accepted ethical standards as codified by the ACCME, the Food and Drug Administration, and the American Medical Association's Guide for Gifts to Physicians. To this end, we have implemented a process wherein everyone who is in a position to control the content of an education activity has disclosed to us all relevant financial relationships with any commercial interests as related to the content of their presentations and under which we work to resolve any real or apparent conflicts of interest. Faculty conflicts of interest in this particular CME activity have been resolved by having the content independently peer reviewed before publication by the Editorial Board and Question Review Committee.

The following faculty (and/or their spouses/partners) have reported real or apparent conflicts of interest that have been resolved through a peer review content validation process.

Harold Adams, MD
Dr. Adams has received speaking honorarium from Bayer (aspirin) and has received research grants from Bristol-Meyers-Squibb (clopidogrel).

Marc E. Agronin, MD
Dr. Agronin is a member of the Speaker's Bureau for Janssen (risperidone) and for Forest Laboratories (escitalopram oxalate).

William J. Burke, MD
Dr. Burke serves as a paid consultant and is a member of the Speakers Bureau for Forest Pharmaceuticals (psychopharmacology) and for Cyberonics (depression). He receives grants from Cyberonics (depression) and Merck (Alzheimer disease).

Anne L. Coleman, MD, PhD
Dr. Coleman receives grant support from Pfizer.

Catherine E. DuBeau, MD
Dr. DuBeau serves as a paid consultant and is a symposium speaker for Astellas (solifenacin), Indevus (trospium chloride), Novartis (darifenacin), and is a symposium speaker for Watson (oxybutynin).

William B. Ershler, MD
Dr. Ershler receives grant support and is a member of the Speaker's Bureau for Amgen.

Anne R. Fabiny, MD
Dr. Fabiny discloses that her spouse/partner serves as a paid consultant to Abgenix (bone and mineral metabolism).

Lisa J. Granville, MD
Dr. Granville serves as a paid consultant for Novartis and Pfizer in the area of incontinence.

Nathan Herrmann, MD
Dr. Herrmann serves as a paid consultant and is a member of the Speaker's Bureau for Janssen (risperidone).

Fran E. Kaiser, MD
Dr. Kaiser was CEO of Kaiser and Associates Consulting when she began work on the GRS-6 and is currently an employee of Merck & Co., Inc.

Gary J. Kennedy, MD
Dr. Kennedy discloses that he receives grant support and is a member of the Speaker's Bureau for Forest Laboratories (escitalopram), and is a member of the Speaker's Bureau for Pfizer (sertraline).

Melinda S. Lantz, MD
Dr. Lantz receives grant support from Bristol-Myers Squibb (aripiprazole) and from Forest Laboratories (memantine).

Courtney H. Lyder, ND, GNP
Mr. Lyder is a member of the Speaker's Bureau for ConvaTec (wound dressings), and for Hil-Rom (mattress replacements).

Constantine G. Lyketsos, MD, MHS
Dr. Lyketsos receives grant support and speaking honorarium from Forest, serves as a paid consultant and is a member of the Speaker's Bureau for Novartis, receives grant support and speaking honorarium from Pfizer, and receives speaking honorarium from GlaxoSmithKline.

Alison A. Moore, MD, MPH
Dr. Moore owns shares of Merck stock.

Thomas Mulligan, MD
Dr. Mulligan owns significant shares of Pfizer stock, and receives grant support from Ascend (dihydrotestosterone) and Solvay (testosterone).

Benoit H. Mulsant, MD
Dr. Mulsant is a member of the Speaker's Bureau for Pfizer (sertraline), and is a paid consultant and a member of the Speaker's Bureau for Forest Labortatories (citalopram, escitalopram).

Joseph G. Ouslander, MD
Dr. Ouslander serves as a paid consultant, receives grant support and is a member of the Speaker's Bureau for Pfizer (tolterodine).

Peter V. Rabins, MD
Dr. Rabins is a member of the Speaker's Bureau for Pfizer, AstraZeneca, Janssen, Eli Lilly, and Forest Laboratories.

Anthony E. Ranno, PharmD
Dr. Ranno is an employee of Pfizer (sertraline).

Michael W. Rich, MD
Dr. Rich is a member of the Speaker's Bureau for Merck & Co. (simvastatin, losartan) and receives grant support from Bristol-Myers Squibb (irbesartan).

Todd P. Semla, PharmD, MS
Dr. Semla serves as a paid consultant for Omnicare and Ovations (a part of United Healthcare) Pharmacy and Therapeutics Committees, and his spouse is employed by and holds shares of Abbott Laboratories.

Javaid I. Sheikh, MD
Dr. Sheikh is a member of the Speaker's Bureau for Pfizer, Forest, and Janssen Pharmaceutica.

Gary W. Small, MD
Dr. Small is a member of the Speaker's Bureau for Pfizer (donepezil) and Novartis (rivastigmine). He is a significant shareholder in MFI (educational information), and holds a license with Siemens for FDDNP-PET.

Stephanie Studenski, MD, MPH
Dr. Studenski serves as a paid consultant for Wyeth and receives grants from Eli Lilly and Co. and Ortho-Biotech for studies of measurement of physical function.

Dennis H. Sullivan, MD
Dr. Sullivan receives grant support from Bristol-Myers Squibb (megase).

George Triadafilopoulos, MD
Dr. Triadafilopoulos serves as a paid consultant, receives grant support, and is a member of the Speakers Bureau for Astra-Zeneca (omeprazole), Pfizer (celecoxib), TAP (lansoprazole). He is also a paid consultant and member of the Speaker's Bureau for Santarus (omeprazole).

Kristine Yaffe, MD
Dr. Yaffe serves as a paid consultant for Novartis.

The following faculty have returned disclosure forms indicating that they (and/or their spouses/partners) have no affiliation with, or financial interest in, any commercial interest that may have direct interest in the subject matter of their presentation(s):

Sumaira Aasi, MD

Itamar B. Abrass, MD

Reva N. Adler, MD, MPH

Cathy A. Alessi, MD

Neil B. Alexander, MD

Wilbert S. Aronow, MD

Kathryn A. Atchison, DDS, MPH

Priscilla F. Bade, MD, MS

Cynthia Barton, RN, MSN

Marc R. Blackman, MD

Caroline Blaum, MD

Harrison G. Bloom, MD

Sidney T. Bogardus, Jr., MD

Chad Boult, MD, MPH, MBA

Cynthia J. Brown, MD

Kenneth Brummel-Smith, MD

David M. Buchner, MD, MPH

Lynda C. Burton, ScD

David Bush, MD

Erin L. Cassidy, PhD

Susan Charette, MD

Gurkamal S. Chatta, MD

Colleen Christmas, MD

Pejman Cohan, MD

Leo M. Cooney, Jr., MD

Steven R. Counsell, MD

Robert S. Crausman, MD, MMS

James Cummins, MD

G. Willy Davila, MD

Margaret A. Drickamer, MD

Pamela W. Duncan, PhD

Edmund H. Duthie, Jr., MD

Carmel Bitondo Dyer, MD

G. Paul Eleazer, MD

E. Wesley Ely, MD, MPH

Michelle S. Eslami, MD

Mark H. Fleisher, MD

Alastair J. Flint, MB

David G. Folks, MD

Christine Himes Fordyce, MD

Andrea R. Fox, MD, MPH

Terry T. Fulmer, RN, PhD

Angela Gentili, MD

Thomas M. Gill, MD

Mary K. Goldstein, MD, MS

Shelly L. Gray, PharmD, MS

David A. Gruenewald, MD

Arthur E. Helfand, DPM

Kenneth W. Hepburn, PhD

Kevin P. High, MD, MSc

Chris Himes, MD

Michelle Iannuzzi-Sucich, MD

Gail Ishiyama, MD

Gordon L. Jensen, MD, PhD

Thomas V. Jones, MD, MPH

Donald A. Jurivich, DO

Jennifer M. Kapo, MD

Jurgis Karuza, PhD

Judith Kasper, PhD

Paul R. Katz, MD

Catherine Lee Kelleher, MD

Anne Kenny, MD

Douglas P. Kiel, MD, MPH

Mary B. King, MD

Kurt Kroenke, MD

George A. Kuchel, MD

C. Seth Landefeld, MD

Robert K. Lee, MD

Michael C. Lindberg, MD

Robert D. Lindeman, MD

Shari M. Ling, MD

David A. Lipschitz, MD, PhD

Dan L. Longo, MD

William L. Lyons, MD

Edward R. Marcantonio, MD, SM

Coleman O. Martin, MD

Alvin M. Matsumoto, MD

Matthew S. Maurer, MD

Robert M. McCann, MD

Ellen McMahon, MD

Lynn McNicholl, MD

Daniel A. Mendelson, MD

Barbara E. Moquin, PhD, MSN, APRN, BC-P

R. Sean Morrison, MD

Laura Mosqueda, MD

John B. Murphy, MD

Arash Naeim, MD, PhD

David W. Oslin, MD

James T. Pacala, MD, MS

Ronald F. Pfeiffer, MD

Stacie T. Pinderhughes, MD

Peter Pompei, MD

Jane F. Potter, MD

James S. Powers, MD

Karen M. Prestwood, MD

John W. Rachow, MD, PhD

Joe W. Ramsdell, MD

Paula A. Rochon, MD, MPH

Debra Saliba, MD, MPH

David Sarraf, MD

Gary Schiller, MD

Susan K. Schultz, MD

Nancy Shafer-Clark, MD

Kenneth Shay, DDS, MS

Alan M. Singer, DPM

Upinder Singh, MD

Monica Stallworth-Kolimas, MD

David H. Stern, MD

Gwen K. Sterns, MD

Gail M. Sullivan, MD, MPH

Mark A. Supiano, MD

Robert A. Sweet, MD

David C. Thomas, MD

Bruce R. Troen, MD

Corina M. Velehorschi, MD

Katherine Ward, MD

Andrew C. Warren, MB, BS, DPhil

Michael R. Wasserman, MD

Debra K. Weiner, MD

Barbara E. Weinstein, PhD

Steven P. Wengel, MD